MW00846555

Veterinary Image-Guided Interventions

Veterinary Image-Guided Interventions

Edited by

Chick Weisse
The Animal Medical Center
New York, NY, USA

and

Allyson Berent
The Animal Medical Center
New York, NY, USA

Section Editors

Matthew W. Beal
Michigan State University
East Lansing, MI, USA

Brian A. Scansen
Ohio State University
Columbus, OH, USA

William T.N. Culp
University of California – Davis
Davis, CA, USA

WILEY Blackwell

Editorial Offices
1606 Golden Aspen Drive, Suites 103 and 104, Ames, Iowa 50010, USA
The Atrium, Southern Gate, Chichester, West Sussex, PO19 8SQ, UK
9600 Garsington Road, Oxford, OX4 2DQ, UK

For details of our global editorial offices, for customer services and for information about how to apply for permission to reuse the copyright material in this book please see our website at www.wiley.com/wiley-blackwell.

Library of Congress Cataloging-in-Publication Data

Veterinary image-guided interventions / edited by Chick Weisse and Allyson Berent.
p. ; cm.
Includes bibliographical references and index.
ISBN 978-1-118-37828-1 (cloth)
1. Veterinary endoscopy. 2. Veterinary diagnostic imaging. 3. Veterinary medicine–Diagnosis. I. Weisse, Chick, editor. II. Berent, Allyson, editor.
[DNLM: 1. Radiography, Interventional–methods. 2. Radiography, Interventional–veterinary. 3. Diagnostic Techniques, Surgical–veterinary. 4. Surgery, Computer-Assisted–veterinary. SF 757.8]
SF772.55.V485 2015
636.089′607545–dc23

2014039226

A catalogue record for this book is available from the British Library.

Wiley also publishes its books in a variety of electronic formats. Some content that appears in print may not be available in electronic books.

Cover design by Meaden Creative

Set in 10/12.5pt Palatino LT Std by SPi Global, Pondicherry, India
Printed and bound in Singapore by Markono Print Media Pte Ltd

2 2016

CONTENTS

SECTION 3 GASTROINTESTINAL SYSTEM 109
Edited by Allyson Berent

SECTION 4 HEPATOBILIARY SYSTEM 199
Edited by Chick Weisse

List of Contributors

Larry G. Adams, DVM, PhD
Diplomate, ACVIM (SAIM)
Professor, Small Animal Internal Medicine
Department of Veterinary Clinical Sciences
Purdue University
West Lafayette, IN

Matthew W. Beal, DVM, DACVECC
Associate Professor, Emergency and
Critical Care Medicine
Director of Interventional Radiology Services
Chief of Staff, Small Animal Veterinary Teaching Hospital
College of Veterinary Medicine
Michigan State University
East Lansing, MI

Allyson Berent, DVM, DACVIM
Interventional Endoscopy/Interventional
Radiology Service
Director of Interventional Endoscopy
The Animal Medical Center
New York, NY

Sarah Boston, DVM, DVSc, DACVS
ACVS Founding Fellow of Surgical Oncology
Associate Professor of Surgical Oncology
Small Animal Clinical Sciences
University of Florida
Gainesville, FL

Stacy Kathleen Burdick, BS, DVM
Resident, Internal Medicine
The Animal Medical Center
New York, NY

Julie K. Byron, DVM, MS, DACVIM
Associate Professor – Clinical
Department of Veterinary Clinical Sciences
The Ohio State University
Columbus, OH

Dean J. Cerf, DVM
Director Laser Surgery
Ridgewood Veterinary Hospital
Ridgewood, NJ

Craig A. Clifford, DVM, MS, DACVIM (Oncology)
Director of Clinical Studies
Hope Veterinary Specialists
Malvern, PA

Steven G. Cole, DVM, DACVECC, DACVIM (Cardiology)
Los Angeles, CA

William T.N. Culp, VMD, DACVS
Assistant Professor
Department of Surgical and
Radiological Sciences
School of Veterinary Medicine
University of California – Davis
Davis, CA

Marilyn E. Dunn, DMV, MVSc, ACVIM (Internal Medicine) (Small Animal)
Professor of Small Animal Internal Medicine
Department of Clinical Sciences
Faculty of Veterinary Medicine
University of Montreal
Quebec, Canada

Amara H. Estrada, DVM, DACVIM (Cardiology)
Associate Chair and Associate Professor
Small Animal Clinical Sciences
Service Chief for Section of Cardiology
College of Veterinary Medicine
University of Florida
Gainesville, FL

Sonya G. Gordon, DVM, DVSc, DACVIM (Cardiology)
Associate Professor Cardiology
Department of Small Animal Clinical Science
College of Veterinary Medicine and Biomedical Sciences
Texas A&M University
College Station, TX

Amy M. Habing, DVM, DACVR
Assistant Professor – Clinical
Diagnostic Imaging and Radiation Oncology
Department of Veterinary Clinical Sciences
The Ohio State University
Columbus, OH

Elaine Holmes
Veterinary Specialty Hospital of the Carolinas
Cary, NC

Bruce W. Keene, DVM, MSc, DACVIM (Cardiology)
Professor of Cardiology
Department of Clinical Sciences
North Carolina State University
College of Veterinary Medicine
Raleigh, NC

Mandi E. Kleman DVM, DACVIM (Cardiology)
Cardiology Associate
Pacific Veterinary Specialists and Emergency Service
Capitola, CA

George A. Kramer, DVM, DACVIM (Cardiology)
Chief-of-Staff
Atlantic Coast Veterinary Specialists
Bohemia, NY

Rafael Latorre, DVM, PhD
Professor of Veterinary Anatomy
Department of Anatomy and Comparative Pathological Anatomy
University of Murcia
Murcia, Spain

Eric C. Lindquist, DMV, DABVP
Director of Operations, New Jersey Mobile Associates
Founder/CEO, SonoPath.com
Sparta, NJ

Andrea L. Looney, DVM, DACVAA, DACVSMR, CCRP
Anesthesia, Pain Management & Rehabilitation Services
InTown Veterinary Group (IVG) Hospitals
Woburn, MA

Christine Mullin, VMD
Resident in Medical Oncology
The Oncology Service, LLC
Washington, DC

Sean Murphy, DVM, DACVS
Staff Surgeon
Westvet Emergency and Specialty Center
Garden City, ID

E. Christopher Orton, DVM, PhD, DACVS
Professor
Department of Clinical Sciences
College of Veterinary Medicine and Biomedical Sciences
Colorado State University
Fort Collins, CO

Douglas A. Palma, DVM, DACVIM (Small Animal Medicine)
Staff Internist
Internal Medicine Department
The Animal Medical Center
New York, NY

Manuela Perego, DVM
Unità Operativa di Cardiologia
Clinica Veterinaria Malpensa
Samarate Varese, Italy

Roberto A. Santilli, DVM, PhD, DECVIM – CA (Cardiology)
Unità Operativa di Cardiologia
Clinica Veterinaria Malpensa
Samarate Varese, Italy

Ashley B. Saunders, DVM, DACVIM (Cardiology)
Associate Professor of Cardiology
Department of Small Animal Clinical Sciences
College of Veterinary Medicine and Biomedical Sciences
Texas A&M University
College Station, TX

Brian A. Scansen, DVM, MS, DACVIM (Cardiology)
Assistant Professor of Cardiology and Interventional Medicine
Director, Cardiac Catheterization and Interventional Medicine Laboratory
Department of Veterinary Clinical Sciences
The Ohio State University
Columbus, OH

Michael David Schlicksup, DVM, DACVS – SA
Staff Surgeon
Veterinary Specialty Care
Mount Pleasant, SC

Ameet Singh, DVM, DVSc, DACVS
Assistant Professor, Small Animal Surgery
Department of Clinical Studies
Ontario Veterinary College
University of Guelph
Guelph, Ontario, Canada

Christopher D. Stauthammer, DVM, DACVIM (Cardiology)
Assistant Clinical Instructor
Veterinary Medical Center
College of Veterinary Medicine
University of Minnesota
Saint Paul, MN

Fei Sun, MD
Coordinator
Endoluminal Therapy and Diagnosis Department
Jesús Usón Minimally Invasive Surgery Centre
Caceres, Spain

Sandra P. Tou, DVM, DACVIM (Cardiology and Internal Medicine)
Clinical Assistant Professor of Cardiology
Department of Clinical Sciences
North Carolina State University
College of Veterinary Medicine
Raleigh, NC

Chick Weisse, VMD, DACVS
Director of Interventional Radiology Services
The Animal Medical Center
New York, NY

Aaron C. Wey, DVM, DACVIM (Cardiology)
Upstate Veterinary Specialties, PLLC
Latham, NY

Allison Zwingenberger, DVM, DACVR, DECVDI, MAS
Associate Professor, Diagnostic Imaging
Department of Surgical and Radiological Sciences
School of Veterinary Medicine
University of California – Davis
Davis, CA

Acknowledgments

I would like to thank my entire extended family for their never-ending support, patience, and guidance; and for instilling in me the importance of always asking "**Why?**"

I would like to acknowledge my mentors, in particular Dr. Demetrius Bagley (Thomas Jefferson University), and Dr. Jeffrey Solomon, Dr. Constantin Cope, and the entire staff of the Hospital of the University of Pennsylvania Interventional Radiology Department. These talented and innovative individuals inspired me to always ask "**Why not?**"

I would like to dedicate this book to the countless clients who placed their trust in us to try new, unproven treatments in the hopes of benefiting their beloved pets and hopefully improving future care for the entire veterinary community.

Finally, I wish to thank my wife Allyson for providing me with the two most precious daughters in the world. She is the most dedicated, compassionate, and knowledgeable veterinarian I have ever met, and whose contributions to this profession are already vast and will only continue to expand. There is nobody of whom I am more proud or admiring.

Chick Weisse

I would like to dedicate this book to those people in my life that inspire me every day to push beyond the boundaries… to never take "no" for an answer… to search for solutions when poor options exist… to question myself and others… and to believe that anything and everything is possible: my tireless and amazingly motivated parents Shelley and Mark, my brilliant husband Chick, and our two little angels, Kai and Quincy.

Additionally, I would especially like to dedicate this book to two people who helped to make my career possible: Dr. Demetrius Bagley and Dr. Chick Weisse. They inspired me to prove the "imaginable" and refute the "impossible." Because of their encouragement and perseverance we have interventional options that have changed the way we practice veterinary medicine. They are the true definition of PROGRESS.

Allyson Berent

We would like to thank the individual authors without whom this book could never have become a reality. In addition, a very special thank you to each section editor whose knowledge, expertise, and time helped refine and enhance this textbook in numerous ways. Your contributions to this textbook, and veterinary image-guided interventions as a whole, are gratefully appreciated.

Chick Weisse and Allyson Berent

About the Companion Website

This book is accompanied by a companion website:

www.wiley.com/go/weisse/vet-image-guided-interventions

The website includes:

- Powerpoints of all figures from the book for downloading
- Video clips of interventional procedures

SECTION ONE

INTRODUCTION

Edited by Chick Weisse

CHAPTER ONE

Tools of the Trade – Interventional Radiology

Fei Sun
Endoluminal Therapy and Diagnosis Department,
Jesús Usón Minimally Invasive Surgery Centre, Caceres, Spain

Interventional radiology refers to image-guided interventions characterized by minimal invasiveness. Technically, these interventions employ various tools introduced via percutaneous access or through natural orifices, navigating to the target organ, and finally deploying specific devices or delivering drugs for therapeutic purpose. Image-guided interventions rely heavily on instrumentation. Ensuring the proper selection of a particular instrument and making rational combinations of the tools and devices available is key to improving technical success, shortening procedure times, and avoiding potential complications. Knowledge of basic instrumentation is of great importance to the clinical practice of interventional radiology. Some of the more commonly used devices will be introduced in this chapter.

Digital Fluoroscopy and Digital Subtraction Angiography

Digital fluoroscopy, also called digital radiography, is a computer-based digital image-processing technique by which real time radiographic images are projected on an image-intensifying fluorescent screen, and in turn converted or digitized for storage or reproduction through an image processor. Compared with conventional fluoroscopy, digital fluoroscopy has several advantages including: post processing that may greatly enhance contrast resolution, high speed image acquisition up to 30 frames/second, and digital image distribution and archiving.

In veterinary hospitals, the standard C-arm digital fluoroscopy system (Figure 1.1) is commonly located in an angiography suite or surgical operating room. It is a mobile and self-contained unit requiring no connections to other equipment. The image intensifier of the C-arm unit normally comes in 23 or 30 cm (9 inch or 12 inch) sizes and can provide a sufficient field of view for interventional procedures in small animals. Advanced hardware and software upgrades may allow the traditional C-arm unit to meet the requirements for more contemporary clinical applications, including cardiovascular, neurovascular, and urological interventions. More advanced digital flat-panel detectors attached to the ceilings or floors are becoming more popular among larger referral veterinary centers.

Currently, digital subtraction angiography (DSA) has become an indispensable tool in angiography and endovascular interventions. DSA refers specifically to techniques by which an initial no-contrast mask image is electronically subtracted from subsequent serial images following injection of contrast medium into the target vessels. After subtraction, the static anatomic structure common to both images is removed; the remaining blood vessels containing contrast medium are opacified. DSA (Figure 1.2) substantially improves the contrast resolution of angiography; however, any slight motion of the structures inside the field of view during the image acquisition may induce remarkable artifacts greatly compromising the image quality. Accordingly, temporarily controlled apnea by suspension of mechanical ventilation is often recommended for abdominal angiography when performing DSA.

Roadmapping (also called trace subtract fluoroscopy) is the fluoroscopic equivalent of DSA. It is widely used to guide and facilitate endovascular manipulation of the catheter and guide wire. During the procedure, a desired background angiogram, with or without subtraction, is obtained. With the patient remaining perfectly still, the background angiogram is used as a mask to perform subtraction fluoroscopy (roadmapping) in the same field of view. In contrast to DSA, the contrast-filled vessel in roadmapping will appear

Veterinary Image-Guided Interventions, First Edition. Edited by Chick Weisse and Allyson Berent.

Companion website: www.wiley.com/go/weisse/vet-image-guided-interventions

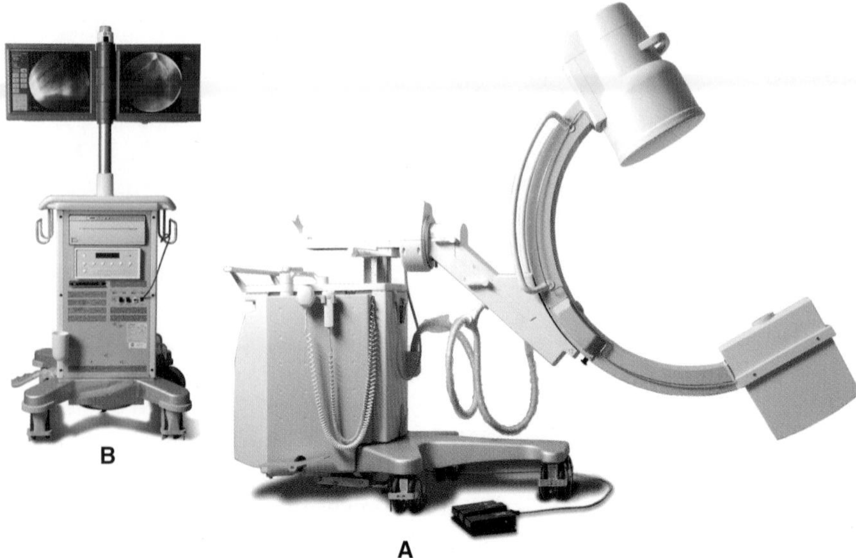

Figure 1.1 Mobile C-arm fluoroscopy system (BV Pulsera, Philips Medical Systems). (A) C-arm stand and imaging system; (B) mobile view station. Used with permission from Usón J, Sun F, Crisóstomo V, et al. (2010) Manual de técnicas endoluminales y radiología intervencionista en veterinaria. Jesús Usón Minimally Invasive Surgery Centre, Caceres, Spain.

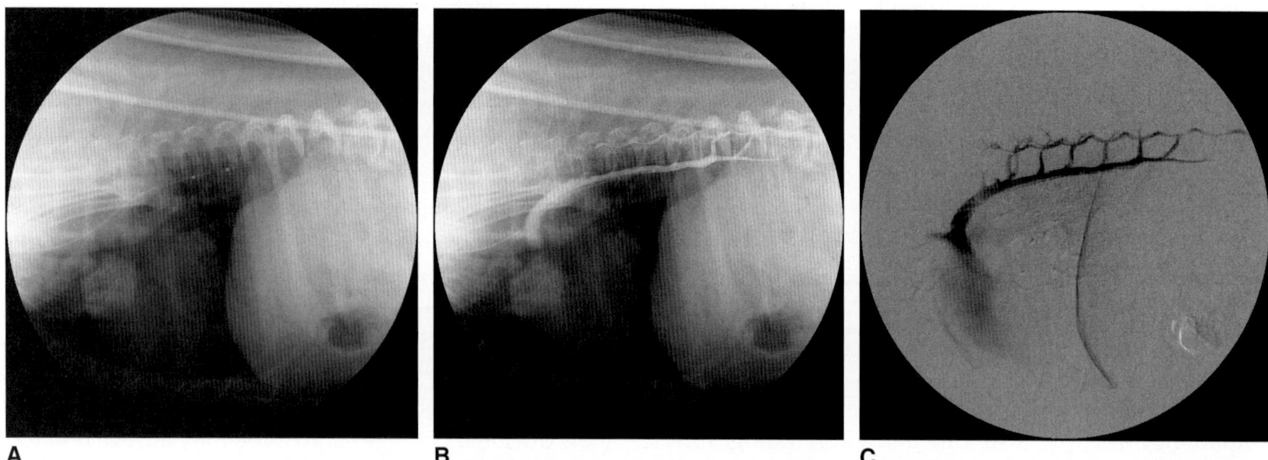

Figure 1.2 Selective digital subtraction angiography of the azygos vein (Lateral view). (A) mask image showing the background structures before injection of contrast medium; (B) The live or contrast image including azygos vein and surrounding anatomic structure; (C) digital subtraction angiogram of the azygos vein with background subtracted.

white, as opposed to black; images of a catheter and guide wire and their motion are visualized superimposed on the background mask image (Figure 1.3). Roadmapping may improve safety during catheter and guide wire manipulations, reduce radiation exposure and procedure times, and minimize contrast use.

Interventional radiology procedures may involve significant radiation exposure and associated risks for both staff and patients. Radiation protection is one of the main concerns in interventional radiology. For the operators and assistants, wearing an appropriate lead apron, lead glasses and thyroid collar is essential; maintaining maximal distance from the radiation source whenever possible, is also important. Techniques to minimize radiation exposure include the use of low frame rate pulsed fluoroscopy, lower dose exposure (higher kV, lower mA) and the option of last-image-hold, use of the collimator when necessary, maximizing the source-to-patient distance, minimizing the air gap between the patient and the image intensifier/digital flat panel, and limiting the use of electronic magnifications.

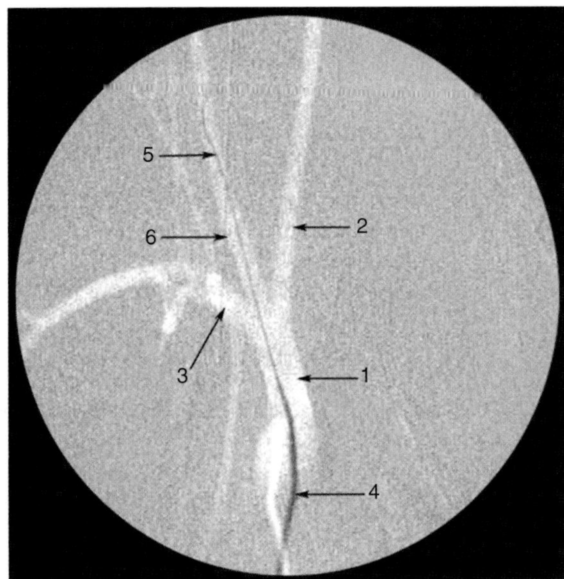

Figure 1.3 Roadmapping fluoroscopy as a guidance in manipulation of selective catheterization in the right common carotid artery. 1 – brachiocephalic trunk, 2 – left common carotid artery, 3 – right subclavian artery, 4 – angiographic catheter, 5 – guide wire, 6 – right common carotid artery. Used with permission from Usón J, Sun F, Crisóstomo V, et al. (2010) Manual de técnicas endoluminales y radiología intervencionista en veterinaria. Jesús Usón Minimally Invasive Surgery Centre, Caceres, Spain.

Access Needles

Percutaneous access needles are thin-walled with relative large lumens to allow passage of the guide wire. The gauge system is used for sizing the outer diameter of access needles; higher gauge means thinner needle. Commonly used vascular access needles range from 18 to 21 gauge (G). For non-vascular access, a fine needle of 21 G is frequently used in order to minimize the damage to target organs. The lumens of needles may vary in size even if they are of the same gauge in outer diameter. Generally a 18G needle allows for passage of a 0.038" and 0.035" guide wire; a 19G needle, however, accommodates 0.035" but not 0.038" guide wires. Before puncturing, it is important to ensure that the guide wire to be used can pass through the needle.

The traditional vascular access needle, also called a Seldinger needle, consists of two parts. The outer metallic cannula has a blunt tip into which a pointed inner stylet is placed (Figure 1.4). Standard Seldinger needles are 18G and 7 to 8cm long. The use of Seldinger needles involves the double-wall puncture technique to achieve vascular access. Both walls of the target vessel are punctured with the needle assembly. After removal of the inner stylet, the needle cannula is retracted slowly until its blunt tip is back within the lumen of the vessel identified by blood return. A guide wire is inserted through the needle into the target vessel and vascular access can be subsequently obtained. Currently, the Seldinger needle is used less frequently due to the complexity of its two-part design and the concern of potential complications from double-wall puncture such as bleeding and damage to more proximal vessels during access.

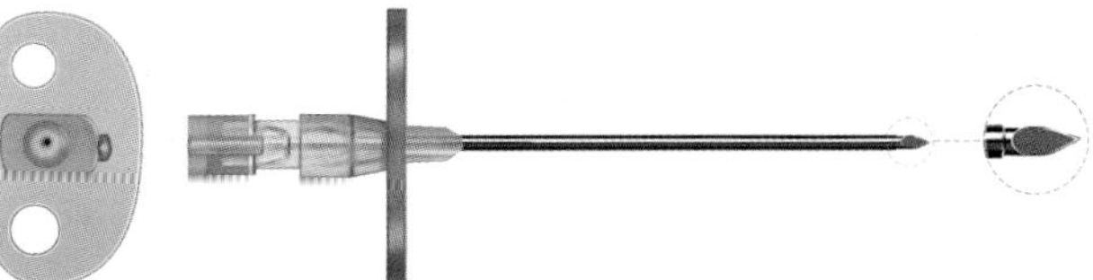

Figure 1.4 Seldinger needle (18G) consists of an outer cannula and a pointed inner stylet. Used with permission from Usón J, Sun F, Crisóstomo V, et al. (2010) Manual de técnicas endoluminales y radiología intervencionista en veterinaria. Jesús Usón Minimally Invasive Surgery Centre, Caceres, Spain.

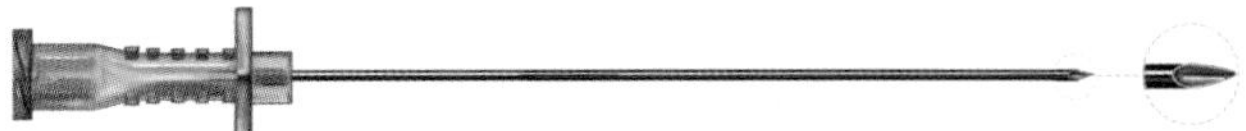

Figure 1.5 Single-wall puncture needle (19G) is also called a one-part needle. Used with permission from Usón J, Sun F, Crisóstomo V, et al. (2010) Manual de técnicas endoluminales y radiología intervencionista en veterinaria. Jesús Usón Minimally Invasive Surgery Centre, Caceres, Spain.

Instead, a single-wall puncture technique is more frequently used. The single-wall needle has only one part, a metallic cannula with a sharply beveled tip without an inner stylet (Figure 1.5). This needle is designed for puncturing the more superficial wall of the target vessel. When the sharp needle tip pierces the wall and enters the vessel lumen, the blood return is identified. When puncturing a small artery, however, it is more difficult to position the needle tip totally within the arterial lumen by using the single-wall technique. If the beveled needle tip is partially placed in the lumen, insertion of the guide wire into the lumen is difficult or impossible so that meticulous repositioning of the needle is required. Either a double-wall technique is used or preferably a micropuncture set.

In small animal practice, a micropuncture set is most commonly used when accessing smaller vessels. The micropuncture set combines the use of a fine puncture needle and a standard guide wire. It consists of a 21G puncture needle, an 0.018" guide wire, and a 4 or 5-Fr coaxial dilator assembly. The inner and outer coaxial

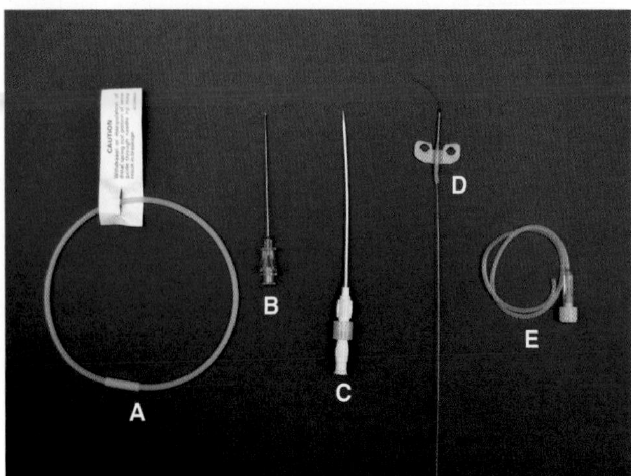

Figure 1.6 Vascular access by the use of butterfly infusion set (21 G). After the butterfly needle (D) punctures and enters the vessel, the silicon connection tube (E) is cut through which a 0.018" guide wire is inserted. The needle is removed and the microwire is replaced with a 0.035" wire using the coaxial dilators of a micropuncture set. A regular introducer sheath is inserted over the 0.035" wire. The micropuncture set includes 0.018" guide wire (A), 21G percutaneous needle (B), and coaxial dilators (C).

dilators accommodate an 0.018" and a 0.035" guide wire, respectively. During the procedure, the 0.018" guide wire is placed through the 21 G needle and the coaxial dilators are placed over the guide wire. After removal of the 0.018 " guidewire and the inner dilator leaving the outer dilator behind, a 0.035" guide wire can be placed though the outer dilator. In addition, the micropuncture set can be used in combination with the 22 G IV catheter or a 21 G butterfly infusion set (Figure 1.6). See Chapter 44 for more information on vascular access.

Guide Wires

A guide wire is a device used to facilitate the placement of catheters at a particular target site. It serves two objectives during manipulations: selecting a desired route and offering support for advancing catheters. Although appearing rather simple and universal, guide wires are highly specialized medical instruments that play a vital role during interventions.

The outer diameter of guide wires is expressed in inches. The standard guide wires are 0.035" in diameter and 145 cm in length. Guide wires of 0.038" are also commonly used and guide wires of 0.018" or less are called microwires. Guide wires should be selected to be twice as long as the catheters used in general. Exchange-length guide wires indicate those of 260 cm or longer and allow for removal and replacement of longer catheters without losing selective access. Other characteristics of guide wires include tip shape, taper, core stiffness, and coating.

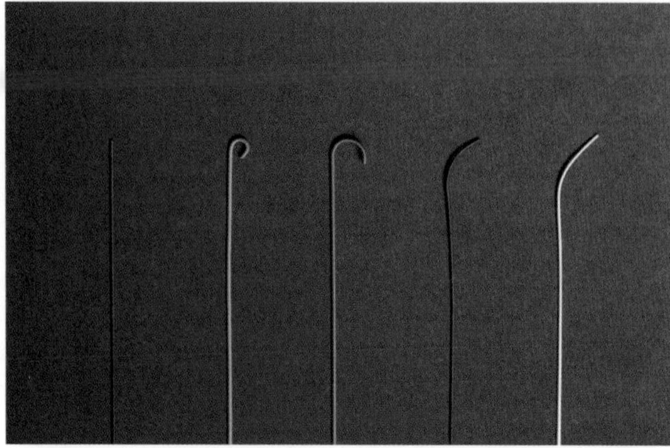

Figure 1.7 Guide wires (0.035") from the left to right: straight Glidewire, Rosen wire, Safe-T-J wire, curved Glidewire, and curved Roadrunner hydrophilic wire. Used with permission from Usón J, Sun F, Crisóstomo V, et al. (2010) Manual de técnicas endoluminales y radiología intervencionista en veterinaria. Jesús Usón Minimally Invasive Surgery Centre, Caceres, Spain.

The soft leading tips of guide wires are available in straight, angled, and "J" configurations (Figure 1.7). Angled-tip guide wires are steerable for selective catheterization. Some microwires have a shapeable floppy tip made from shape memory alloy that enables the floppy tip to be deformed by the operator prior to use and maintains the user-shaped tip during manipulations. Furthermore, the deformed shape can be reshaped if the initial modification of the tip configuration is not ideal. J-tipped guide wires are designed for safety considerations as the J-curve tip is less traumatic when passing through tortuous vessels. The curve of the J tip is described by its radius with a range up to 15 mm. The other advantage of the use of a J-tip guide wire is to avoid untoward entrance to branch vessels with diameters less than that of J-curve of the guide wire.

The length of taper is used to describe length of the distal flexible segment of the guide wire. It is constructed by a tapered mandrel core located within the central canal of guide wires, enabling a graduated transition from stiff to soft distal tip. The taper length of common guide wires ranges from 2 cm (e.g., Rosen wire) to 20 cm (e.g., Bentson wire). The size and stiffness of the mandrel determines the rigidity of guide wire shaft, which varies from regular or standard, stiff, extra stiff, super stiff to ultra stiff guide wires. Safe-T-J (Cook Medical) and Bentson (Cook Medical) wires have a standard stiffness of guide wire shaft. Terumo Glidewires and other hydrophilic wires have two subtypes: standard and stiff guide wires. Rosen guide wires are of intermediate stiffness, which are stiffer than the stiff type of Terumo Glidewires. Guide wires in the Amplatz family (Amplatz Stiff, Amplatz Extra Stiff, Amplatz Super Stiff, and Amplatz Ultra Stiff guide wires) are stiffer than Rosen guide wires but not as stiff as Lunderquist guide wires. Generally, a guide wire with a longer taper is easy to negotiate tortuous vessels or a branch vessel with a steeply angled origin, whereas a stiffer guide wire affords more controlled catheter manipulation and enough support for passage of catheters, balloons or stents. In addition, guide wires with longer tapers, such as Bentson or Newton guide wires, are usually used as a pusher to deliver thrombogenic coils for embolization because a short taper stiff guide wire may deform the tip of catheter and flip it out the target vessel leading to dislodgement of the coil elsewhere.

Guide wire surfaces have many different coatings that convey various advantages. Most guide wires are coated with polytetrafluoroethylene (PTFE, Teflon®) and heparin to reduce friction and thrombogenicity. PTFE-coated guide wires increase lubricity during manipulations but have proved more thrombogenic than stainless steel guide wires. Accordingly, some guide wires come with double coatings, such as the PTFE-Coated Stainless Steel with Heparin Coating guide wire (Bentson, Cook Medical). Hydrophilic polymer coatings have been a major breakthrough in guide wire technology, and more recently have been applied in the manufacturing of catheters and other devices. A hydrophilic-coated guide wire has an extremely low coefficient of friction when wet. It can be passed into small, tortuous vessels more easily. Before introducing a hydrophilic guide wire into the body or passing a catheter over the guide wire, it must be completely wet and the catheter flushed. Otherwise, there is increased friction generated between the wire and the catheter. In addition, hydrophilic-coated guide wires have been reported to be significantly less thrombogenic than the stainless steel spring guide wires. Unlike conventional stainless steel guide wires, hydrophilic-coated guide wires (e.g., Terumo Glidewires or Infiniti Medical Weasel Wires), consist of a nitinol alloy core with a polyurethane jacket and a hydrophilic polymer coating. Due to the super elastic property of nitinol alloy these wires are highly resistant to kinking. This property provides both their advantage and their failing. Once a hydrophilic wire is advanced into a tortuous vessel, it may have a tendency to recoil out of the target vessel. To prevent the wire recoiling, especially when advancing a catheter over the guide wire, a constant forward force is needed to apply to the guide wire by the use of a torque device. It is worth noting that the hydrophilic-coated guide wires should not be inserted or withdrawn through a beveled-tip needle or metal cannula because the hydrophilic coating may be sheared off leading to potential embolic debris.

Introducer Sheath

Once vascular access is achieved, an introducer sheath is typically placed. An introducer sheath (also called vascular sheath) is a thin-walled catheter placed percutaneously at the access site to facilitate insertion of catheters or other devices. An introducer sheath kit generally contains a dilator, sheath, and guide wire. The dilator is a thick-walled, stiff tube with a tapered leading end (Figure 1.8). Upon establishing percutaneous access, the coaxial dilator-sheath assembly is placed over the guide wire into the target vessel. Sheaths are labeled as French (Fr; 3 Fr = 1 mm) describing the inner diameters while dilators are named for the outer diameters. For example, a 5 Fr sheath can accommodate a catheter or dilator with maximal size of 5 Fr.

Vascular sheaths are most commonly used for two major purposes: protection of the vascular entry site and enabling exchanges of various catheters and other devices. Without the protection of the introducer sheath, the vascular wall at the entry site may be lacerated by repeated manipulations of catheters and other devices: e.g., twirling, advancing and withdrawing. A hemostasis valve and a side port are attached at the trailing end of the vascular sheath. The former enables

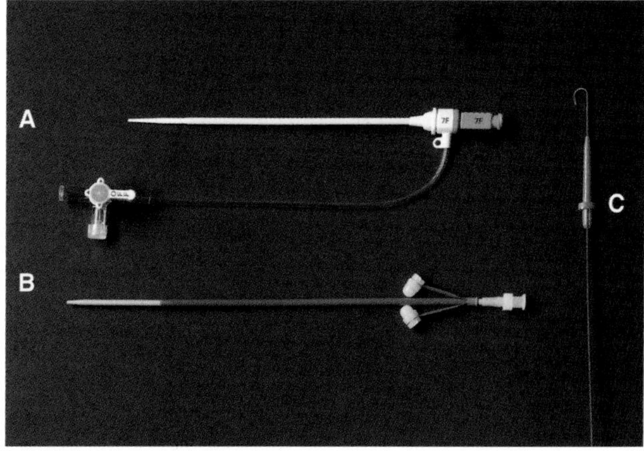

Figure 1.8 Check-flo introducer sheath (A), peel-away sheath (B), and guide wire (C). Used with permission from Usón J, Sun F, Crisóstomo V, et al. (2010) Manual de técnicas endoluminales y radiología intervencionista en veterinaria. Jesús Usón Minimally Invasive Surgery Centre, Caceres, Spain.

exchanges of catheters, guide wires, and other devices without blood loss or air aspiration, while the later allows pressure measurements, administration of heparinized saline, blood sampling, and injection of contrast medium.

Peel-away sheaths are another type of introducer sheath used in vascular or non-vascular procedures for implanting infusion or drainage catheters, pacemaker leads and other devices. The devices can be smoothly advanced into the desired location through the peel-away sheath. At completion of the procedure, the sheath is peeled off and removed, leaving the implanted devices in place.

Angiographic Catheters

An angiographic catheter is a flexible conduit that allows delivery of contrast medium for angiographic diagnosis and administration of therapeutic agents or passage of other devices for endoluminal therapy. The catheter is composed of three parts: the hub, shaft, and tip. Angiographic catheters are measured in French for the outer diameter of the shaft. Most commonly used catheters are 4 or 5 Fr, accepting 0.035″ or 0.038″ guide wires. The length of commonly used catheters is between 65 and 100 cm.

Angiographic catheters are constructed of polyurethane, polyethylene, Teflon, or nylon with radiopaque materials in the wall. Polyethylene is commonly used in angiographic catheters. Polyethylene has a flexibility property that allows for easy passage of catheters over the guide wire to the target vessel with less damage to the intima. However, polyethylene catheters tend to soften with time at body temperature, and lose their shape memory and torsional rigidity after repeated manipulation. To enhance shape memory and torqueability, a fine wire mesh (braid) is usually incorporated into the wall of polyethylene catheters.

Polyurethane catheters are similar to polyethylene catheters in respect to good trackability (advancement over the guide wire). Compared with polyethylene, polyurethane is softer, more flexible, but less slippery (increased friction).

Teflon is occasionally used for flush catheters because of its moderate stiffness. Other features of Teflon include good memory, kink resistance, and lower coefficient of friction when wet. Currently, Teflon is generally reserved for use in dilators and sheaths.

Nylon catheters have reasonable stiffness and high tensile strength, and withstand high pressure and high flow injections. In addition, some angiographic catheters are treated with a hydrophilic polymer coating on the outer surface and substantially improve the trackability and reduce the risk of direct injury to the vessel.

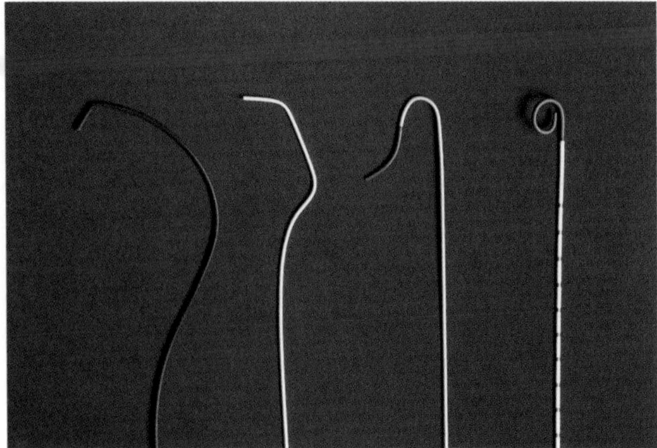

Figure 1.9 Angiographic catheters from the left to right: Cobra-II, Headhunter-I, Simmons-Sidewinder-I, and Pigtail catheters. Used with permission from Usón J, Sun F, Crisóstomo V, et al. (2010) Manual de técnicas endoluminales y radiología intervencionista en veterinaria. Jesús Usón Minimally Invasive Surgery Centre, Caceres, Spain.

Angiographic catheters are functionally divided into non-selective (flush) and selective categories (Figure 1.9). Flush catheters are commonly made of nylon or Teflon to allow for large-volume and high-pressure injections. They are straight or curled at the tip (pigtail catheter) with an end hole and typically 8 to 12 side holes. The pigtail tip keeps the end (hole) away from the vessel wall and multiple side holes along the distal shaft help evenly disperse contrast medium during injection without a single forceful jet effect that may cause unwinding of the looped tip or subintimal dissection. The side holes of flush catheters must be smaller than the end hole so that a guide wire accepted by the end hole cannot exit elsewhere.

All selective catheters share common criteria in design, including high torque control (torqueability), good radio-opacity, and adequate flexibility and trackability. The shape of the catheter tip varies greatly and is designed for specific functions. To selectively catheterize a target vessel, the catheter tip must be curved or angled. Some selective catheters can be used for many blood vessels; a particular blood vessel also can be cannulated by maneuvering various catheters with quite different shapes. Occasionally however, a slight change in the catheter tip configuration can make a big difference in the success or failure of a procedure. The shape of selective catheters can be simple or complex, depending on the number and fashion of curves at the leading end. The primary curve is defined as the one closest to the catheter tip. It is designed for seeking and engaging the origin of branch vessels. Additional curves (secondary or tertiary) beyond the primary curve enable stabilization of the engaged catheter tip in the branch vessels and help to force the catheter tip deeper in position. Berenstein and Vertebral catheters are typical simple curve catheters. Cobra catheter is a double curve catheter, in which the primary and secondary curves are in the same direction. Recurvant catheters (reverse curve catheters) indicate that the primary and secondary curves are in opposite orientation. Examples of recurvant catheters are Simmons and Sos-selective catheters.

When recurvant catheters are introduced over a guide wire into the aorta they must be re-formed to their original packaged configuration prior to manipulation for selective catheterization. Generally, recurvant catheters will resume their original shape spontaneously provided there is sufficient space in the vessel lumen and shape-memory capability of the catheter. Otherwise, the Waltman loop technique and other strategies can be used to re-form the catheter shape. Once the tip of a recurvant catheter engages the orifice of target vessel, manipulations in moving catheter tip have the opposite maneuvering effects; inserting the trailing end of the catheter withdraws the leading tip from the vessel and pulling on it advances it further into the vessel. In addition, removal of a recurvant catheter from deeply selective position requires careful disengagement under fluoroscopic guidance. The curves of the recurvant catheter should be straightened with a guide wire prior to removal from the patient.

Most selective catheters only have an end hole, which snugly fits the accepted guide wire size. Some selective catheters, such as the Cobra catheter, have two small side holes immediately adjacent to the catheter tip. The design of side holes is to diminish risky high-velocity jet effects during injection of contrast with a power injector. However, side hole catheters should not be used for embolization. When delivering coils, side holes may entangle the coil at the catheter tip. Gelfoam and PVA particles also tend to occlude the catheter tip because of decrements in pressure distal to the side holes. Cautions should be exercised when using side hole selective catheters because thrombi can more easily form between the side hole and catheter tip. Catheters with suspected tip occlusion should be immediately removed.

Balloon Catheters

Standard balloon catheters are wire-guided double lumen catheters that incorporate a balloon at the leading end. When a balloon catheter is inserted over a guide wire to a target site, the balloon can be inflated for therapeutic or diagnostic purposes. Two basic types of balloons are used in veterinary interventions: dilation and occlusion balloons. The dilation balloon is a high-pressure and non-elastic balloon used to apply force to dilate a local stricture, such as valvuloplasty in pulmonic stenosis (see Chapter 59) and esophageal dilation for benign esophageal strictures (see Chapter 13). The occlusion balloon is a low-pressure, elastomeric balloon and typically made of latex or silicone. Unlike dilation balloons, occlusion balloon inflation is guided by volume rather than pressure. In clinical practice, occlusion balloons are used for temporary occlusion of blood vessel to measure occlusive pressures or perform retrograde angiography.

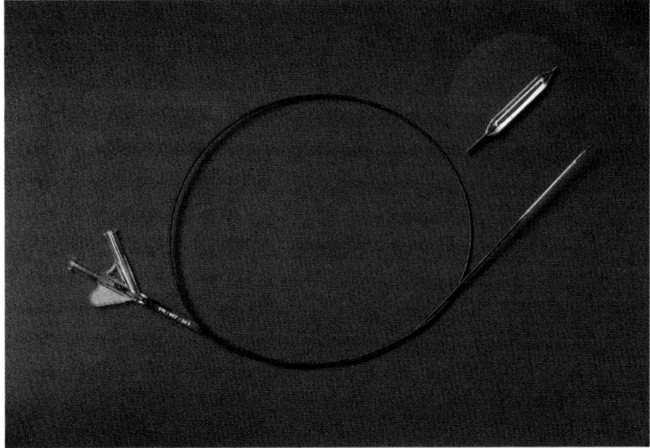

Figure 1.10 Angioplasty balloon catheter (5 Fr, 8 mm × 40 mm) before and after inflation. Used with permission from Usón J, Sun F, Crisóstomo V, et al. (2010) Manual de técnicas endoluminales y radiología intervencionista en veterinaria. Jesús Usón Minimally Invasive Surgery Centre, Caceres, Spain.

Typical dilation balloons are composed of four parts: the tip, balloon, shaft, and hub (Figure 1.10). The balloon catheter tip should taper well to fit the guide wire and aid in crossing tight stenoses. The commonly accepted guide wires are 0.035 and 0.038 inch but lower profile balloons are available for use with smaller diameter wires (0.014″ and 0.018″ for example). The hub has two ports; the main central port is used for insertion of the guide wire and the side port is for inflation and deflation of the balloon. The shaft is described in Fr for its outer diameter and in centimeters for its length. A standard balloon consists of a cylindrical body, two conical tapers, and two necks (proximal and distal). The balloon is measured by millimeters in diameter and length. Balloon diameter refers to nominal inflated balloon diameter measured at a specified pressure; balloon length refers to the working length or the length of the cylindrical body, typically indicated by a pair of radiopaque markers located underneath the balloon. Other technical details regarding inflation of the balloon include balloon nominal pressure (value at which the balloon reaches its labeled diameter), balloon rated burst pressure (value at which the probability of balloon rupture is < 0.1%), and balloon average burst pressure (value at which the probability of balloon rupture reaches 50%).

Compliance is another important characteristic of a balloon catheter that describes the extent to which a balloon will stretch beyond a predetermined diameter when a certain force is applied. A low-compliance dilation balloon might expand only 5–10% when inflated to the rated pressure, whereas a high-compliance dilation balloon might stretch 18–30%. If the material is compliant, the balloon will deform in the region of a stenosis, in a dog-bone fashion. This prevents the dilating force from being concentrated in the narrowed lesion and tends to over-distend the adjacent normal vessel. Therefore, noncompliant balloons are desirable when dilating rigid stenotic lesions. Balloon compliance is determined by the material from which it is constructed. Nylon, polyester (PET), and polyurethane are the most common materials used in dilation balloon production. PET balloons offer high tensile strength and low compliance while polyurethane is softer and of medium to high compliance. Compliance of nylon balloons is medium between PET and polyurethane.

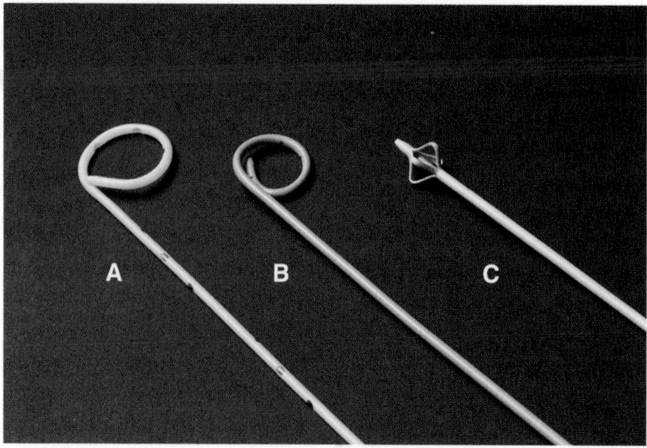

Figure 1.11 Common drainage catheters: biliary drainage catheter (A), nephrostomy drainage catheter (B), and Malcot nephrostomy catheter (C). Used with permission from Usón J, Sun F, Crisóstomo V, et al. (2010) Manual de técnicas endoluminales y radiología intervencionista en veterinaria. Jesus Uson Minimally Invasive Surgery Centre, Caceres, Spain.

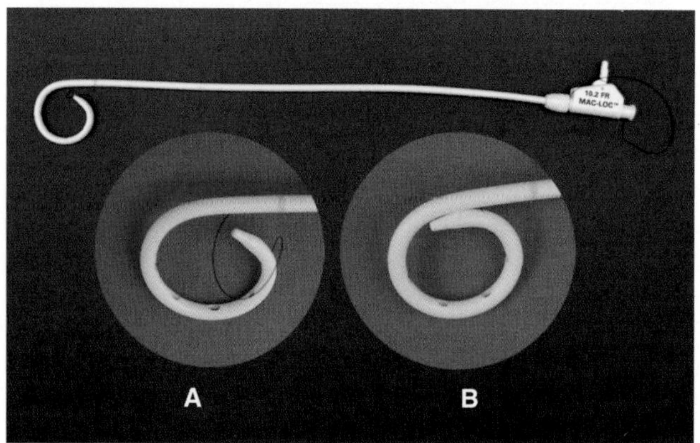

Figure 1.12 Mac-Loc® multipurpose drainage catheter (10.2 Fr, Cook Medical) with the distal loop before (A) and after locking (B).

Drainage Catheters

Percutaneous drainage catheters are commonly used for the management of various fluid collections: e.g., pleural and peritoneal drainage and lavage, nephrostomy and cystostomy drainage, and biliary drainage. Unlike angiographic catheters, drainage catheters are generally large bore (6–12 Fr), typically with a single large lumen allowing for a higher flow rate of viscous fluid. The tip of drainage catheters is designed with special configurations (pigtail or mushroom shape) to help prevent migration of the catheter (Figure 1.11). To enhance self-retention at the target site, a suture-locking-loop system is commonly used. The catheter has a suture passed through its proximal end and lumen. The distal end of suture is attached to the tip of the catheter. When the proximal end of suture is retracted, the distal pigtail is created. This configuration is maintained by a locking device at the hub of catheter. The locked pigtail protects again accidental dislodgement of the drainage catheter (Figure 1.12).

Typical drainage catheters (also called external drainage catheter) have multiple large side holes that are on the inside surface of the pigtail loop to maintain patency as the drained space surrounding the catheter collapses. Furthermore, the location of side holes at the inner aspect of the pigtail contains drainage to the target and decreases the likelihood of leakage back along the track, which potentially leads to infection and other complications. Some biliary drainage catheters are specially designed for purpose of internal/external drainage, with side holes extending several centimeters up to the catheter shaft so that they can be located above and below the obstruction of lesion. This enable bile to pass from obstructed ducts above a stricture through the catheter to the duodenum (Figure 1.11).

Drainage catheters may be introduced percutaneously either by a direct puncture utilizing a trocar needle or by Seldinger technique. In general, superficial collections are drained by the trocar method, using the trocar stylet for direct insertion; in deeper collections with complex anatomy the Seldinger technique is preferable in the placement of a drainage catheter. Drainage catheters require periodic exchange. If access of the drainage site is to be maintained when exchanging catheters, a straight guidewire is used to past the distal tip of the pigtail with less likelihood to exit a side hole because location of sideholes is on the inner curvature of the loop.

Stents

Stents are tubular devices made of metal, plastic, or bioabsorbable materials that are implanted into blood vessels or other structures to restore or preserve luminal patency. Most stents are metal and commonly used for both vascular and nonvascular lesions, whereas plastic stents are only employed in some nonvascular organs such as the ureter, biliary duct, and trachea. Stents can be placed percutaneously or deployed through natural orifices with or without endoscopic assistance, such as in ureteral or tracheal stenting. Currently available metal stents are mostly made of nitinol or stain-less steel alloy by modern manufacturing technologies, including laser cutting, laser welding, and mechanical braiding. Differences in design and materials for stent fabrication directly influence the physical properties of the stent which can ultimately determine the technical success or failure of a procedure. Metal stents have two major categories including balloon-expandable and self-expanding stents. Based on coverings and coatings of metal stents they are further divided into bare stent (uncovered stent), stent-graft (covered stent), and drug-eluting stent (Figure 1.13).

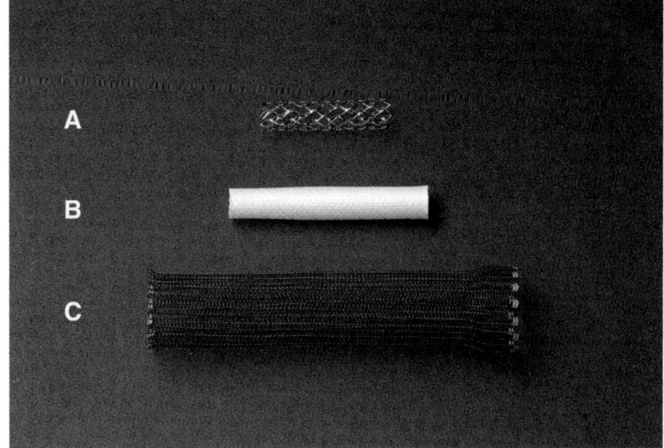

Figure 1.13 Metal stents from the top to bottom: balloon-expandable stent, covered self-expanding stent, and uncovered self-expanding stent. Used with permission from Usón J, Sun F, Crisóstomo V, et al. (2010) Manual de técnicas endoluminales y radiología intervencionista en veterinaria. Jesús Usón Minimally Invasive Surgery Centre, Caceres, Spain.

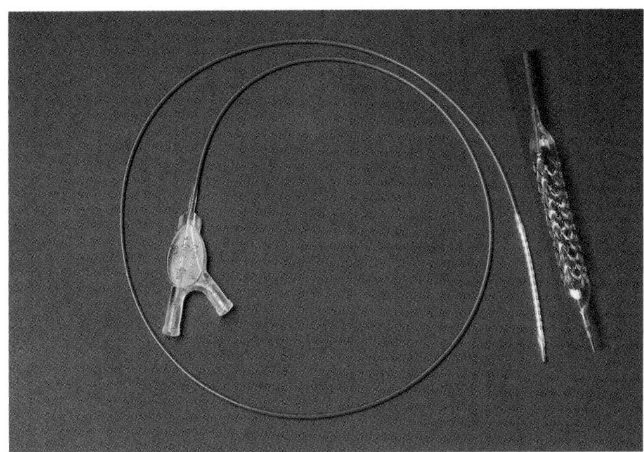

Figure 1.14 Balloon-expandable stent before and after balloon inflation.

A balloon-expandable stent (Figure 1.14) is a device used to perform dilation of a narrowed lumen and simultaneous implantation of a stent to support the wall, preserving long-term patency. The Palmaz stent was the first balloon-expandable stent and has undergone several modifications. Current balloon-expandable stents are constructed from a thin-walled stainless steel tube with parallel rows of staggered laser-cut slots. The stents are mounted onto a balloon catheter and placed across the target lesion. When the balloon is inflated, the rectangular slots open up to form diamond-shaped cells while the small tube is expanding into a cylindrical stent. After deflation and removal of the balloon catheter, the stent remains in place. Balloon-expandable stents have high radial force and hoop strength that resist deformation under a compressive load. They are most commonly used in stenting arterial ostial stenosis in humans. Other advantages of balloon-expandable stents include ease of implantation at a precise location and a precise stent diameter controlled by final inflation of the balloon at an indicated pressure. However, if an outer compressive force (beyond the stent's yield point) is applied to an implanted balloon expandable stent, it will be crushed with irreversible deformation (plastic deformation). Thus, balloon-expandable stents should not be used in locations where they may be compressed by external forces due to repetitive motion such as in the neck or over joints. Relative lack of flexibility and short length is another drawback of balloon-expandable stents, so that they cannot be readily deployed across bifurcations or in tortuous vessels. During the stenting procedure, a guiding catheter or guiding sheath is always recommended when advancing the stent-balloon device to the target site in order to avoid dislodgement of the un-deployed stent. Balloon-expandable stents are most commonly used in veterinary medicine for nasopharyngeal stenosis (see Chapter 6).

Self-expending stents are compressed within a delivery system and generally divided into mesh/woven types or laser-cut types. They are implanted by retracting the outer sheath while holding the stent delivery system in place. The exposed part of the stent, due to its spring-like tendency, immediately expands to reach its nominal diameter. To ensure secure fixation, most stents require oversizing 1–2 mm (or more) greater than the target lumen. The Wallstent (mesh stent) is a special self-expending stent that is composed of 18 to 24 Elgiloy stainless steel filaments, each 100 μm in diameter, woven in a crisscross pattern to form a tubular braid configuration. The filament crossing points are not fixed but are free to slide or pivot over each other. The special design allows the stent to be flexible, compressible and have a good radio-opacity. Another common example of a mesh stent is the Infiniti Medical nitinol Vet Stent-Trachea. One feature of most mesh stents is the reconstrainable nature of the delivery system. If the stent is partially released but at an undesirable position, the stent may be reconstrained at a variable percentage of its total length (up to 87% in the Wallstent) until its limit marker band ("point of no return") and repositioned or removed. However, caution should be exercised concerning the foreshortening of mesh stents. Stent foreshortening refers to the shortening of the stent that occurs as its diameter increases upon deployment. Foreshortening of mesh stents is substantial and can vary between 20% and 50% according to the final expansion during deployment. These mesh stents are most commonly used in veterinary medicine for tracheal stenting (see Chapter 7), GI stenting (see Chapter 17), and vascular stenting (see Chapters 21 and 49).

Currently, the most commonly used self-expanding stents in humans are laser-cut nitinol stents. Nitinol (an acronym for Nickel Titanium Naval Ordinance Laboratories) is an alloy composed of approximately 55% nickel and 45% titanium (wt.%), which has been found to have unique properties of shape memory and super-elasticity. Nitinol stents are magnetic resonance imaging (MRI) compatible and produce fewer artifacts than stainless steel stents. More importantly, laser-cut nitinol stents exhibit minimal foreshortening during deployment compared to mesh stents, and have a more predictable length and location after deployment. Common veterinary examples of laser-cut nitinol stents are the Infiniti Medical Vet Stent-Urethra or Vet Stent-Cava. It should be noted that some (Symphony stent) nitinol stents may exhibit significant foreshortening. Unlike stents made from laser-cut nitinol tubes, the Symphony stent is constructed from nitinol wire welded to form a closed-cell structure. Reported foreshortening of the Symphony stent may be up to 11.7%. Laser-cut stents are not typically reconstrainable making removal extremely difficult and not recommended, especially during deployment. Laser-cut stents are most commonly used in veterinary medicine for urethral tumors (see Chapter 34) and in the vasculature (see Chapters 21 and 49).

Fabric-covered stents or stent-grafts and drug-eluting stents are also available in balloon-expandable and self-expending types. In human medicine, vascular covered stents are used for exclusion of aneurysms or management of arterial rupture; non-vascular covered stents are used for malignant strictures. Drug-eluting stents have been developed to minimizing post-procedural vascular restenosis by local delivery of drugs that block cell proliferation. Covered stents are uncommonly used in veterinary practice but have been used in the urinary tract (see Chapter 31), nasopharynx (see Chapter 6), gastrointestinal tract (see Chapter 17), and vasculature (see Chapter 21).

A typical plastic stent used in veterinary practice is the ureteral stent composed of synthetic polymeric compounds including polyurethane, silicone and other proprietary polymeric materials. Functionally, it works as an internal drainage catheter designed with multiple sideholes and two pigtail-loop ends (also called double-pigtail stent) (Figure 1.15). To minimize the possibility of migration one loop is deployed within the renal pelvis and the other within the urinary bladder. Endoscopic implantation of the stent is the standard technique in dogs, whereas surgical stent placement is needed in patients without endoscopic access and cats typically (see Chapter 30). Some stents have a hydrophilic coating in order to decrease friction and reduce or eliminate biofilm formation and encrustation. The Vet Stent-Ureter (Infiniti Medical) stents are dedicated for veterinary use and come in a variety of sizes (2.5–6.0 Fr) and lengths (12–23 cm); the inner lumens of the stents accommodate various sized guide wires (0.018–0.035 inch).

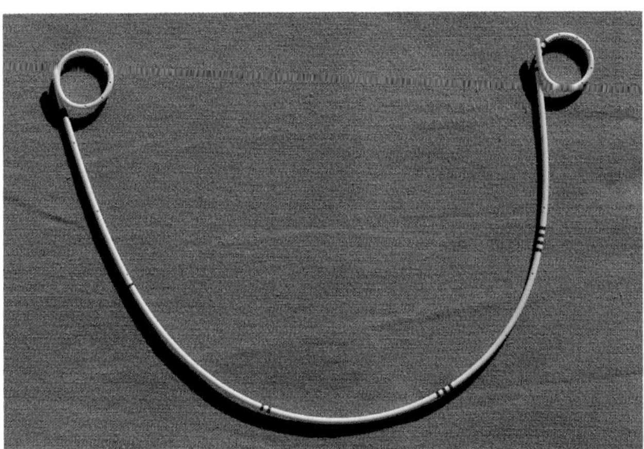

Figure 1.15 Universa™ double pigtail stent (4.7 Fr, Cook Medical).

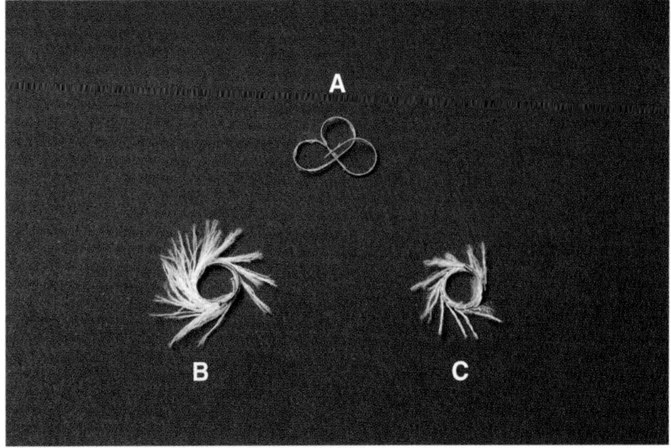

Figure 1.16 Coils with different size and shape with synthetic fibers: (A) complex helical fibered platinum coil-18 (Boston Scientific); (B) MReye-35 coils (Cook Medical); (C) fibered platinum coil-35 (Boston Scientific). Used with permission from Usón J, Sun F, Crisóstomo V, et al. (2010) Manual de técnicas endoluminales y radiología intervencionista en veterinaria. Jesús Usón Minimally Invasive Surgery Centre, Caceres, Spain.

Coils

Metallic coils are most frequently used for occlusion of abnormal vascular communications including portosystemic shunts (see Chapter 21) and patent ductus arteriosus (PDA) (see Chapter 58). The first-generation coil, Gianturco Coil, was initially developed by Drs. Gianturco and Wallace in 1975, which was comprised of a short stainless steel wire with diameter ranging from 0.025" to 0.038" packaged in a straight conformation within an introducer. When the coil is delivered into the target vessel, it assumes a spiral or other configuration with specified diameter and length. In theory, the deployed coils do not occlude the vessel lumen completely but rather induce thrombosis. To enhance thrombogenicity, the coil was subsequently modified by attaching wool strands or synthetic fibers (Figure 1.16). Newly developed MReye Embolization Coils (Cook Medical) are constructed of Inconel super alloy, which has similar physical characteristics to stainless steel, but has no ferro-magnetic properties. The coils are easily detected radiographically and are considered to be MRI compatible, with the potential for minor artifacts to be observed in the immediate vicinity of the device. Selection of proper coil size is extremely critical during coil embolization. Generally, the diameter of the deployed coil should be approximately 2 mm larger than that of target vessel. When the coil is too small, it may migrate distally, even into the pulmonary circulation through arteriovenous shunting if present. Conversely, if the coil is too large, it cannot retain its normal form, so that the proximal elongated portion protrudes out of the target vessel. Since the 1990s, smaller coils made of platinum have been available. The small platinum coils come in 0.010 to 0.018 inch in diameter and can be delivered through microcatheters to embolize tiny vessels. To control precise coil implantation and minimize the risk of coil migration, detachable coils (e.g., MReye Flipper coils by Cook Medical), have been widely used in occlusion of PDAs.

Amplatz Canine Duct Occluder

The Amplatz Canine Duct Occluder (ACDO, Infiniti Medical) is a self-expanding nitinol mesh device intended for endovascular closure of canine PDAs. The ACDO is specifically designed to fit the size and shape of the canine PDA. It has a short central waist that connects a flat distal disk and a cupped proximal disk (Figure 1.17). After implantation, the distal disk covers the pulmonary artery side of the ductal ostium, the waist spans the pulmonic ostium of the ductus, the dense nitinol mesh occludes the communication, and the proximal cupped disk expands and conforms to the shape of the ductal ampulla. The ACDO device is available in a wide range of waist sizes (3 mm–14 mm) that can meet the needs for closure of any size PDA. However, application of the ACDO is limited by the size of patient. In dogs under 2.5 kg of body weight the femoral artery is too small to accommodate the appropriate catheter size. Additionally, if the length of ductus is too short (e.g., the window type PDA), the ACDO is contraindicated because of the risk of interference with the aortic flow. The ACDO is recapturable (reconstrainable) before release and repositionable to

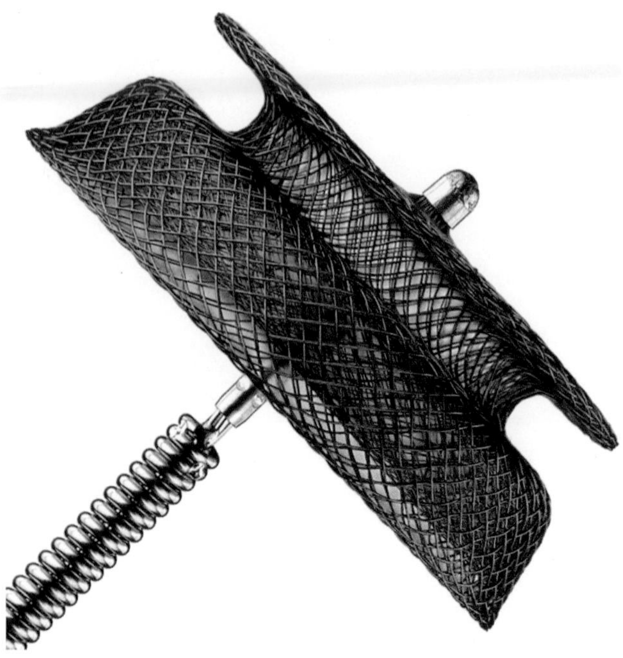

Figure 1.17 Amplatz Canine Ductal Occluder connecting to a delivery cable. (Copyright Infiniti Medical, LLC, Menlo Park, CA, USA.)

obtain a final stable and desired position improving technical success and safety. Furthermore, the transarterial approach used for ACDO placement makes selective placement of the device through the ductus much easier and avoids right heart catheterization and its associated complications such as arrhythmia and kinking of the device sheath. Since the development of the ACDO, this device has gained widespread popularity and become the treatment of choice for the majority of PDA occlusions. See Chapter 58 for more information on PDA occlusion.

Summary

Interventional procedures are indeed a process of maneuvering, threading, passing, and delivering a variety of special tools or medications to target organs for diagnostic and therapeutic purposes. Familiarity and proper selection of the optimal devices, as well as awareness of potential complications associated with their use are essential for any veterinarian performing these procedures.

Suggested Reading

Berent AC, Weisse C, Beal MW, Brown DC, Todd K, and Bagley D (2011) Use of indwelling, double-pigtail stents for treatment of malignant ureteral obstruction in dogs: 12 cases (2006–2009). *J Am Vet Med Assoc* 238(8), 1017–25.

Berent AC, Weisse C, Todd K, Rondeau MP, Reiter AM (2008) Use of a balloon-expandable metallic stent for treatment of nasopharyngeal stenosis in dogs and cats: six cases (2005–2007). *J Am Vet Med Assoc* 233(9), 1432–40.

Estrada A, Moïse NS, Renaud-Farrell S (2005) When, how and why to perform a double ballooning technique for dogs with valvular pulmonic stenosis. *J Vet Cardiol.* 7(1), 41–51.

Gonzalo-Orden JM, Altónaga JR, Costilla S, et al (2000) Transvenous coil embolization of an intrahepatic portosystemic shunt in a dog. *Vet Radiol Ultrasound* 41, 516–518.

Gordon SG and Miller MW (2000) Transarterial coil embolization for canine patent ductus arteriosus occlusion. *Clin Tech Small Anim Pract* 20(3), 196–202.

Leach KR, Kurisu Y, Carlson JE, et al (1990) Thrombogenicity of hydrophilically coated guide wires and catheters. *Radiology* 175(3), 675–7.

Nakagawa N, Yashiro N, Nakajima Y, Barnhart WH, and Wakabayashi M. (0000) Hydrogel-coated glide catheter: experimental studies and initial clinical experience. *AJR Am J Roentgenol* 163(5), 1227–9.

Reddy SC, Kamath P, Talwar KK, Saxena A, and Wasir HS (1997) Guide wire outer coat shearing and embolisation: an unusual complication of pericardiocentesis. *Int J Cardiol* 60(1), 15–8.

Rösch J, Keller FS, and Kaufman JA (2003) The birth, early years, and future of interventional radiology. *J Vasc Interv Radiol* 14(7), 841–53.

Singh MK, Kittleson MD, Kass PH, and Griffiths LG (2012) Occlusion devices and approaches in canine patent ductus arteriosus: comparison of outcomes. *J Vet Intern Med* 26(1), 85–92.

Spinosa DJ, Angle JF, Hagspiel KD, Pyle DA, and Matsumoto AH (1998) Iliac artery stenting: A review of devices and technical considerations. *Appl Radiol* 27(7), 10–24.

Sun F, Usón J, Ezquerra J, Crisóstomo V, Luis L, and Maynar M (2008) Endotracheal stenting therapy in dogs with tracheal collapse. *Vet J* 175(2), 186–93.

Tanaka R, Hoshi K, Nagashima Y, Fujii Y, and Yamane Y (2001) Detachable coils for occlusion of patent ductus arteriosus in 2 dogs. *Vet Surg* 30(6), 580–584.

Weisse C, Berent A, Todd K, Clifford C, and Solomon J (2006) Evaluation of palliative stenting for management of malignant urethral obstructions in dogs. *J Am Vet Med Assoc* 229(2), 226–34.

Weisse C, Berent AC, Todd KL, and Solomon JA (2008) Potential applications of interventional radiology in veterinary medicine. *J Am Vet Med Assoc* 233(10), 1564–74.

Weisse C, Schwartz K, Stronger R, et al (2002) Transjugular coil embolization of an intrahepatic portosystemic shunt in a cat. *J Am Vet Med Assoc* 221, 1287–91.

CHAPTER TWO

Tools of the Trade – Interventional Endoscopy

Allyson Berent
The Animal Medical Center, New York, NY

Introduction

Interventional endoscopy (IE) involves the use of endoscopic equipment with other contemporary imaging modalities, such as fluoroscopy and/or ultrasonography, to perform diagnostic and therapeutic procedures in virtually any part of the body amenable to endoscopic access (gastrointestinal, biliary, respiratory, urinary tract, etc.).

Currently, there is expanding investigation of the use of these novel techniques in veterinary medicine. The combination of endoscopy and fluoroscopy allows for one to visualize and gain access to small orifices that would otherwise require more invasive surgical techniques. A good example of this is the placement of a biliary stent into the common bile duct via the major duodenal papilla with endoscopic and fluoroscopic guidance. Many of these interventional procedures are considered the standard-of-care in human medicine, and are currently being routinely performed or investigated in veterinary medicine.

The invasiveness and morbidity associated with some traditional surgical techniques (i.e., ureterotomy for ureteral obstructions or strictures, biliary re-routing surgery, nasopharyngeal surgery for nasopharyngeal stenosis, etc.) makes the use of minimally invasive alternatives through IE techniques appealing. The advantages are not limited only to their minimally invasive nature but also to the lower morbidity, shorter hospital stays, and most importantly, the lack of alternative options in some patients. These procedures are technically challenging and require specialized equipment and training.

This chapter provides a brief overview of some of the equipment needed for the IE procedures that will be described in further detail throughout this textbook. It is important for the reader to note that the equipment footnoted below are commonly used in the author's practice, however there are dozens of other companies currently providing similar devices for veterinary use.

Equipment

Imaging Devices

A C-arm fluoroscopy unit is ideal for most IE procedures. This unit has the advantage of image mobility, permitting various tangential views without moving the patient and allowing patient positioning to facilitate endoscopic access (i.e. at the end of the table for rigid cystoscopy) (Figure 2.1). A portable ultrasound machine (Figure 2.2) is useful for percutaneous needle access into varies structures (gall bladder, renal pelvis, etc.).

Endoscopes are used to visualize an orifice for access within the body (i.e., common bile duct, ureteral orifice, etc.). Various flexible and rigid endoscopes are used for interventional endoscopic techniques. A light and camera box are needed to visualize the images on a monitor with appropriate illumination. The monitors should be strategically set up in the procedure room so that the operator is always looking straight ahead at the endoscopic image (Figure 2.3). Video flexible endoscopes provide a much higher quality image than the fiberoptic flexible scopes. Flexible gastroduodenoscopes (6 mm and 8 mm)[1] bronchoscopes,[2] and ureteroscopes (7.5–8.1 French)[3] (Figure 2.4) are classically used for various body system interventions. An adult (11.3 mm)[4] or pediatric (9 mm)[5] side-view duodensocope (Figure 2.5) is necessary for endoscopic retrograde cholangiopancreatography (ERCP) and biliary stenting (see Chapter 24). When performing an intervention through a flexible endoscope it is

Veterinary Image-Guided Interventions, First Edition. Edited by Chick Weisse and Allyson Berent.

Companion website: www.wiley.com/go/weisse/vet-image-guided-interventions

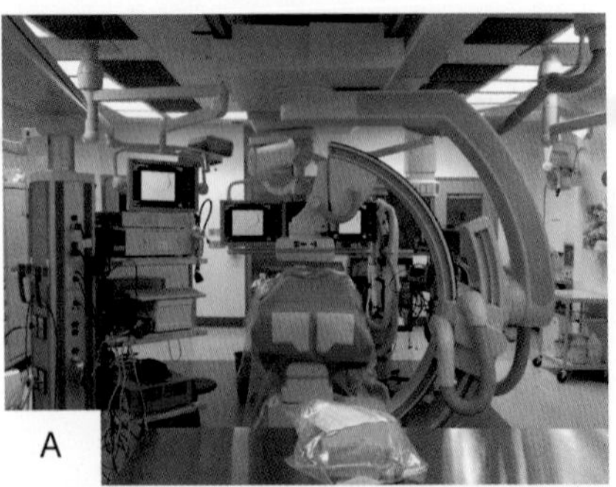

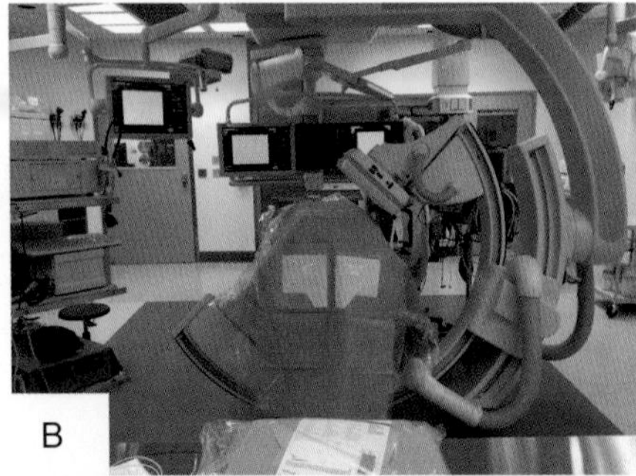

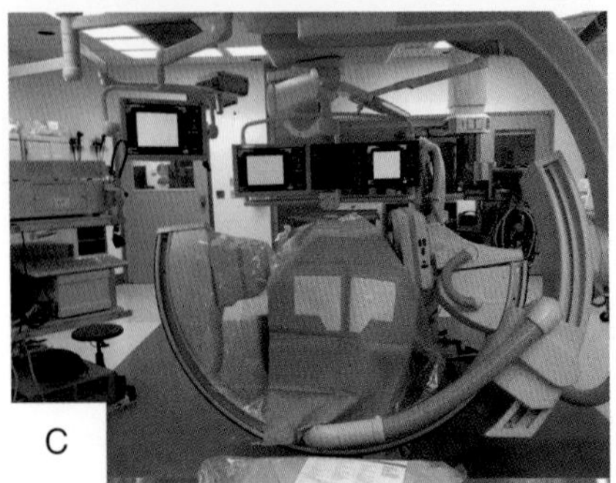

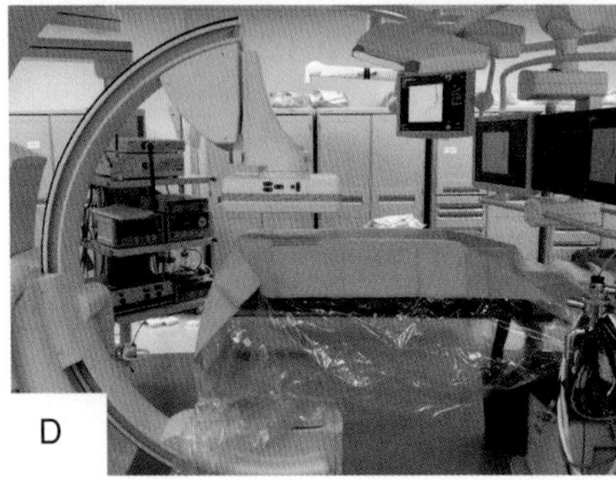

Figure 2.1 Integrated fluoroscopic and endoscopic operating room. (A) Standard set up for female cystoscopy. It is important to have visibility of the monitors during the procedure. (B) Notice the C-arm is at a 45 degree angle permitting an oblique view of the patient. (C) Notice the C-arm is at a 90 degree angle permitting a lateral view of the patient that is in dorsal recumbency. (D) Standard position of the C-arm during a surgically-assisted procedure, allowing the surgeons to stand on opposite sides of the table.

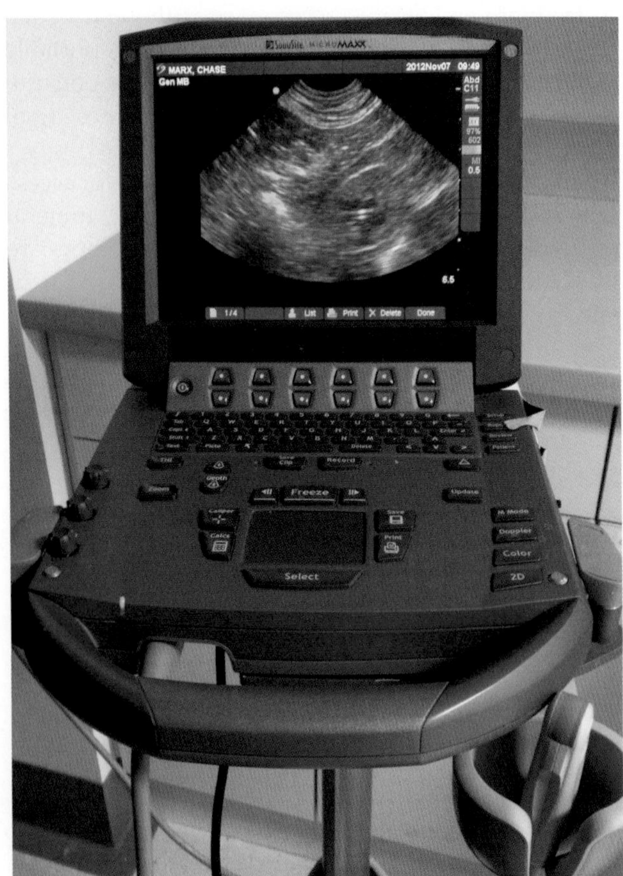

Figure 2.2 Portable ultrasonography machine used in the operating room.

important to use a guide wire that is at least double the length of the scope so that a guide wire exchange can be performed to pass the stent. This is called "exchange-length wire", and is typically 150–400 cm long (260–400 cm for flexible endoscopes). Other specialized catheters and guide wires are needed for each particular procedure, which will be expanded upon in each chapter.

Rigid cystoscopes (1.9–4.0 mm)[6–9] (Figure 2.6) are useful for cystoscopy and rhinoscopy and a 30-degree angle is recommended for improved 360-degree field-of-view when rotated. Rigid scopes utilize glass rod/lens technology that provides an image nearly as good as video technology. All cystoscopes should have a working channel either permanently attached (integrated sheath) or added separately (non-integrated sheath). The sheath has two fluid ports, one for ingress and one for egress.

Lithotripsy and Intracorporeal Ablation Devices

Lithotripsy ("the breaking of stones") is performed for stone removal (Figure 2.7). This procedure is typically performed for urinary tract stones. Extracorporeal shockwave lithotripsy (ESWL) utilizes a fluoroscopy unit that is attached to a lithotripter, where the shockwaves are guided through a water medium onto a

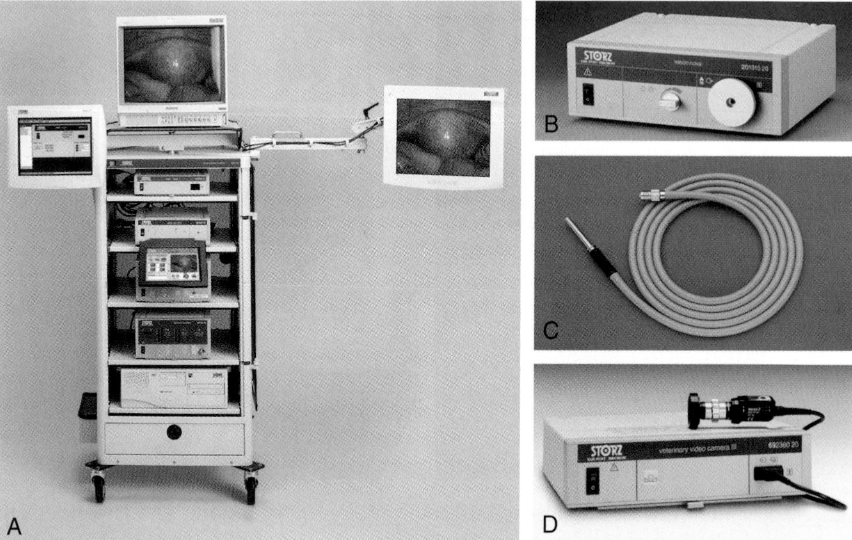

Figure 2.3 Equipment needed for endoscopy. (A) A mobile tower to hold the various camera boxes and light sources with multiple monitors attached. (B) Light source box. (C) Light guide cable. (D) Camera box. (Pictures courtesy of Karl Storz Endoscopy.)

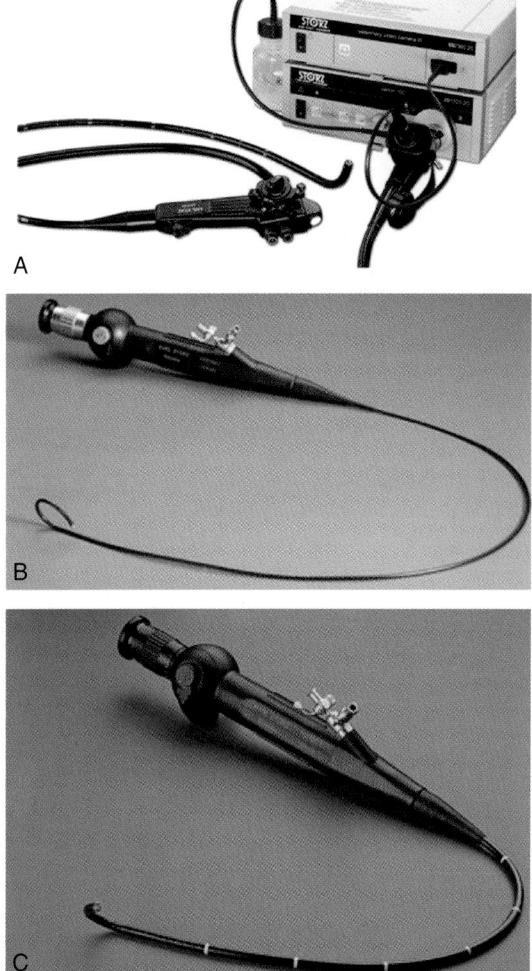

Figure 2.4 Flexible endoscopes. (A) Gastrointestinal video endoscope. (B) Flexible 8Fr fiberoptic ureteroscope. (C) Flexible bronchoscope. (Pictures courtesy of Karl Storz Endoscopy.)

stone(s) for fragmentation (typically 1–1.5 mm pieces). Each fragment is left to be voided over time (see chapters 27 and 30) For larger stone burdens intracorporeal lithotripsy is recommended (kidney, ureter, bladder, urethra). This can be done using laser (Holmium:YAG [yttrium, aluminum, garnet])[10], electrohydraulic, ultrasonic[11], pneumatic, and/or intracorporeal shockwave lithotripsy (Chapters 27 and 33), Each fragment is then fragmented in contact mode and manually removed during the procedure.

Lasers can be used for tissue ablations as well. All operators should be trained in laser safety and appropriate laser goggles should be worn by all OR personnel during any laser ablation procedure. A diode laser[12] and a Holmium:YAG (yttrium, aluminum, garnet) laser[10] are commonly used for the ablation of ectopic ureters (Chapter 32), inflammatory polyps of the urinary tract (Chapter 35), laser ablation of bladder/urethral tumors (Chapter 37), and cauterization of hemorrhagic lesions. The diode laser provides continuous firing at 980 nm providing both coagulation and cutting, with essentially no hemorrhage. The laser fiber is larger for the diode (600 or 1000 μm) making it harder to manipulate during flexible cystoscopy. The Hol:YAG laser works at a wavelength of 2100 nm but has a pulsed activity that results in more of an intermittent surge of pulsing energy resulting in a jumping action during the ablation, reducing precise control. This laser also results in a mild amount of hemorrhage and some tissue edema that can obscure the endoscopic image. This is typically of no clinical consequence for the patient post-operatively. To avoid excessive bleeding with the Hol:YAG laser, the contact mode should be

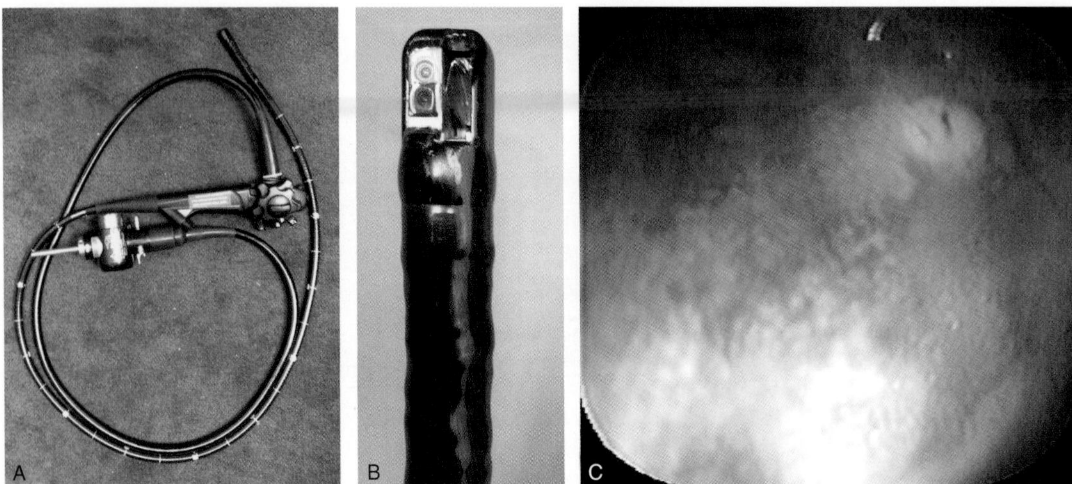

Figure 2.5 Side-view duodenoscope used for biliary interventions. (A) The video endoscope is 150 cm long. (B) Note the side location of the lens and working channel. (C) The major duodenal papilla in a dog visualized with the side-view lens permitting direct visualization for cannulation.

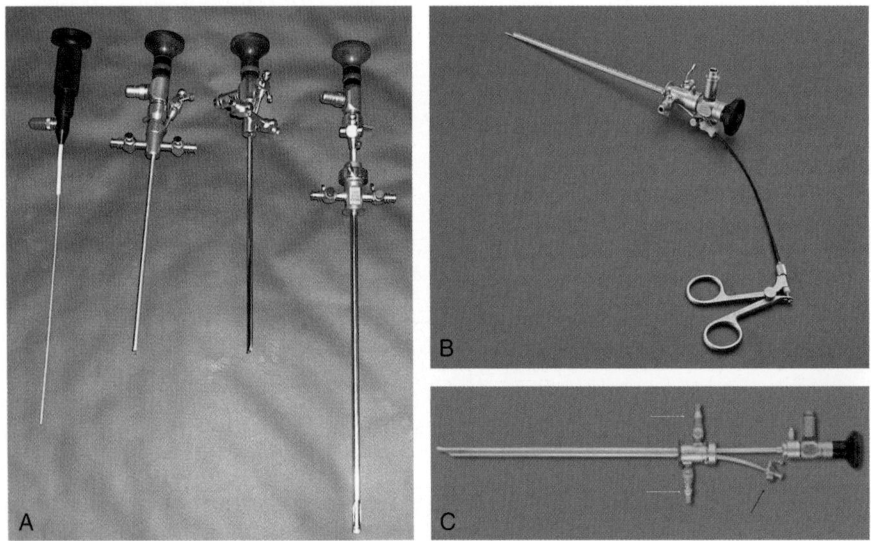

Figure 2.6 Rigid endoscopes used for cystoscopy and rhinoscopy. (A) Various sized scopes (left to right) including a 1-mm semi-rigid male cat cystoscope, a 1.9-mm rigid female cat or small female dog cystoscope, 2.7-mm rigid female dog cystoscope, and a 4.0-mm rigid female dog cystoscope. (B) An instrument placed through the working channel of the endoscope. (C) Notice the 30-degree angle at the end of the endoscope that allows for 360-degree visibility in a lumen through rotation. Also notice the ingress and egress valves (white arrows) and the working channel (black arrow).

avoided and the laser fiber should be situated 0.1 to 0.5 mm from the desired tissue to be ablated allowing the power to coagulate, rather than cut the tissue directly. For stone therapy the Hol:YAG laser should be used only in contact mode. The laser fibers available for the Hol:YAG are 200, 400, 600, and 1000 μm. Since the advent of laser lithotripsy, more veterinarians have a Hol:YAG laser available than a diode, making this a reasonable alternative for tissue ablations as it is more versatile (see Chapter 33).

Endoscopic cautery with a bugbee electrode[13,14] can also be used to cauterize and ablate tissue. This electrode fiber is typically between 100 and 300 μm in diameter and allows great flexibility in small endoscopes (see Chapter 28). This electrode is attached to a regular electrocautery unit and requires a foot pedal and adaptor for the electrode (Figure 2.8). This is more commonly used for laser ablation of small bleeding lesions, and should not be used in lumens with high oxygen content (airway).

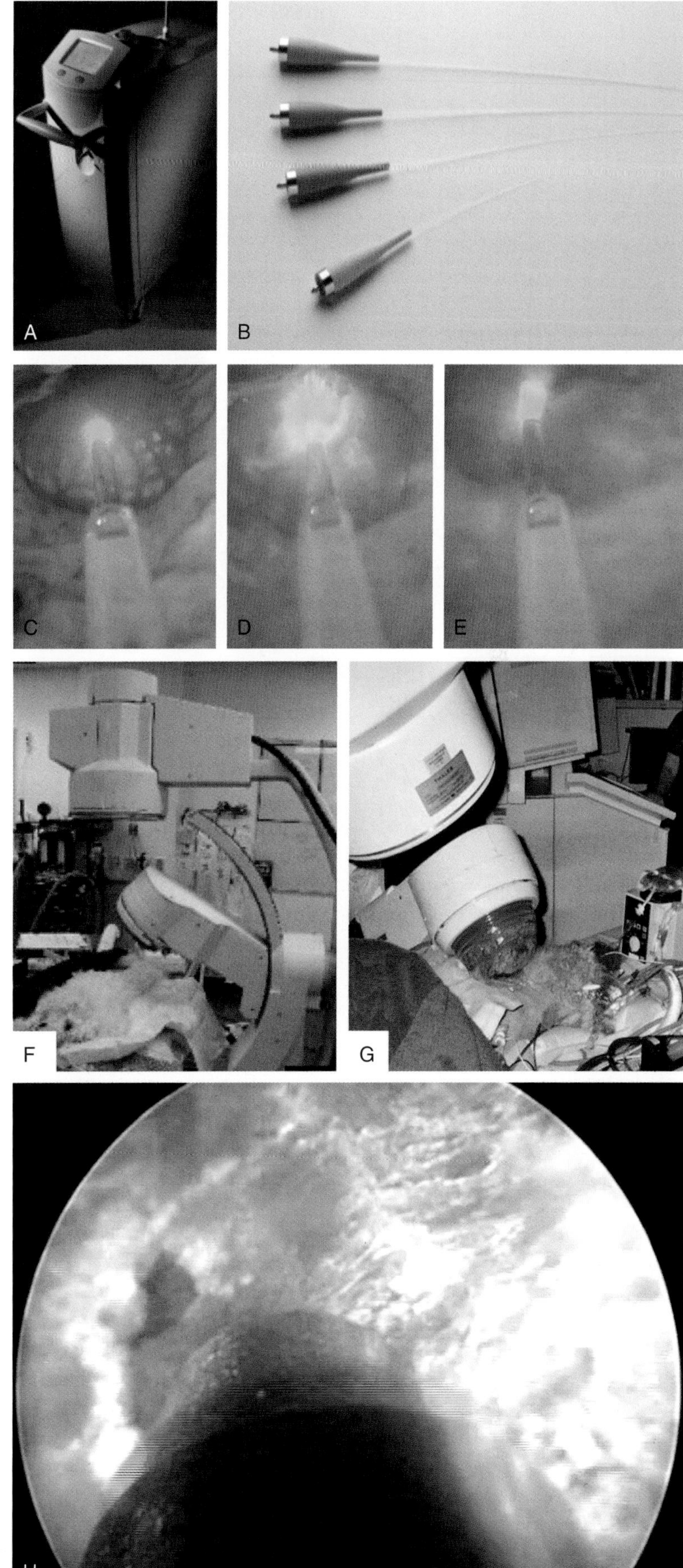

Figure 2.7 Lithotripsy equipment. (A) A Holmium:YAG laser machine. (B) Laser fibers available in different sizes for the intracorporeal lithotripter. (C–E) the Hol:YAG laser fiber in direct contact with a bladder stone in a dog during cystoscopy. Notice the stone breaking until it is cracked in half (E) and the green laser beam. (F) Dry extracorporeal shockwave lithotripsy (ESWL) machine. (G) The water bag placed onto the skin of a dog during ESWL of a nephrolith. (H) Intracorporeal lithotripsy during percutaneous nephrolithotomy in a dog. Notice the ultrasonic probe through the working channel of the nephroscope.

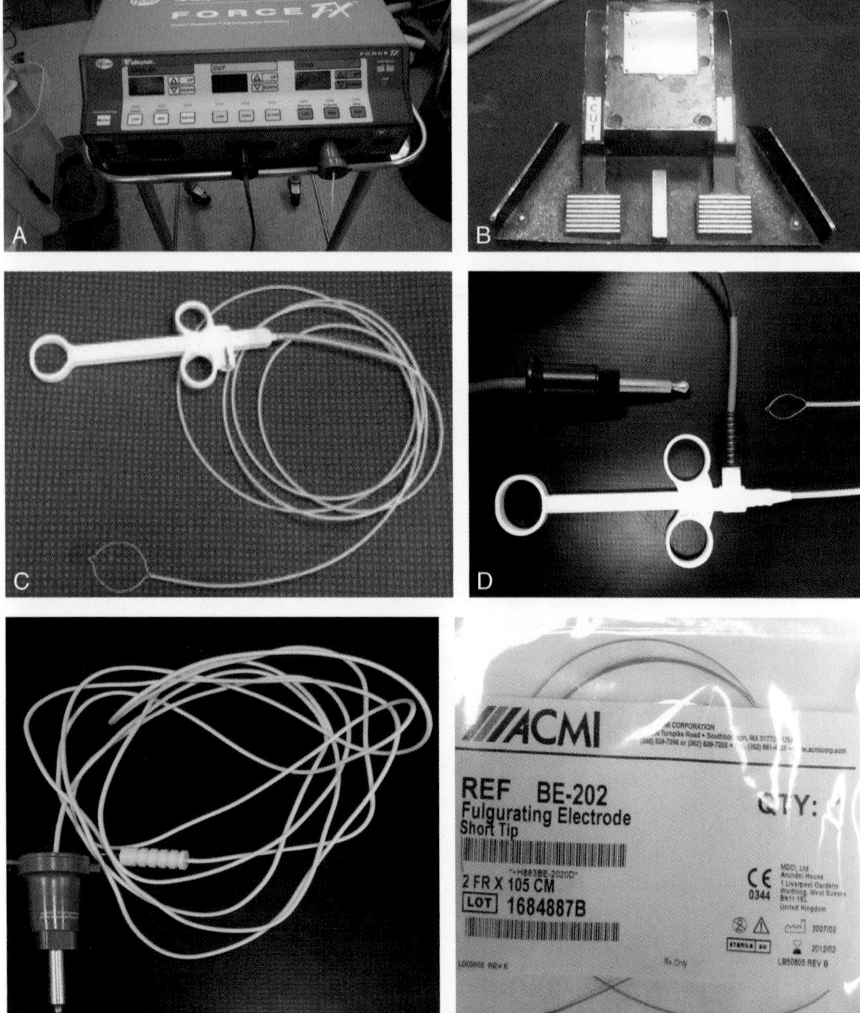

Figure 2.8 Electrocautery unit with various accessories. (A) The electrocautery device attached to a red and blue/yellow adaptor. (B) The foot pedal needed to activate the devices. (C) A polypectomy snare device that is then attached (D) to the red adaptor that connects to the electrocautery unit. (E) The adaptor for the Bugbee cautery probe (F).

Supplies/Disposables

Guide wires of various sizes (0.014″, 0.018″, 0.025″, 0.035″), shapes (angled or straight), length (80, 150, 180, 260, 300, 460 cm), and stiffness (soft, stiffened, super stiff, etc), as well as catheters (straight, angled, reverse-curved, etc.) and stents of various materials (metal, plastic, silicone, etc.), shapes, and sizes are needed for each procedure. These devices were expanded upon in Chapter 1.

Stents

The stents most commonly used in IE cases are either metallic (balloon expandable metallic stents [BEMS] or self-expanding metallic stents [SEMS]) (Figure 2.9, Figure 2.10. Figure 2.11, Figure 2.12, and Figure 2.13) or polyurethane (double pigtail ureteral stents or biliary stents) (Figure 2.14 and Figure 2.15). Each chapter will emphasize the preferred type of stent, wire, and catheter for the specific condition considered. The polyurethane stents are typically retrievable, whereas the metallic stents (unless they are completely covered as with esophageal or colonic stents) are not typically considered retrievable.

A BEMS[15–17] (Figure 2.9) is classically placed for nasopharyngeal stenosis (NPS). These stents are preloaded on a percutaneous transluminal angioplasty (PTA) balloon and once this balloon is inflated the stent is deployed. If this stent were to get compressed, it would remain compressed and would need to be re-ballooned to be re-expanded. The advantage of these stents is the ability to place them precisely across a short stenosis. A SEMS[18–27] is a stent that is classically used for tracheal, urethral, esophageal, and colonic stenting. There are 2 main types of SEMS, a laser-cut SEMS (Figure 2.10) (urethral) and a mesh SEMS (Figure 2.11) (tracheal, esophageal, colonic stents). The laser-cut SEMS[18,25] is cut from a tube of metal (typically NiTiNOL = nickel and

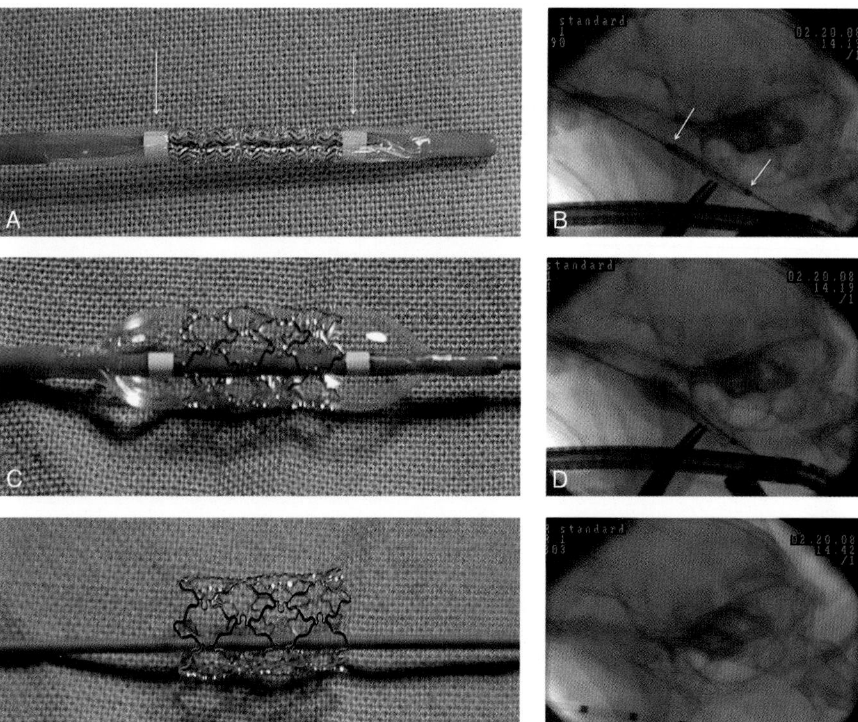

Figure 2.9 Deployment of a balloon expandable metallic stent (BEMS). Images B, D, and F are fluoroscopic images in a cat with nasopharyngeal stenosis during stent placement. The nares are to the left of these images. (A) Percutaneous transluminal angioplasty balloon (PTA) with a metallic stent compressed on top of the balloon. Two radiopaque marks (white arrows) identify each end of the stent. (B) Un-deployed stent in the nasopharynx of a cat. (C,D) Inflating the balloon with 50/50 contrast and saline. (E,F) The stent is deployed after the balloon is deflated and removed.

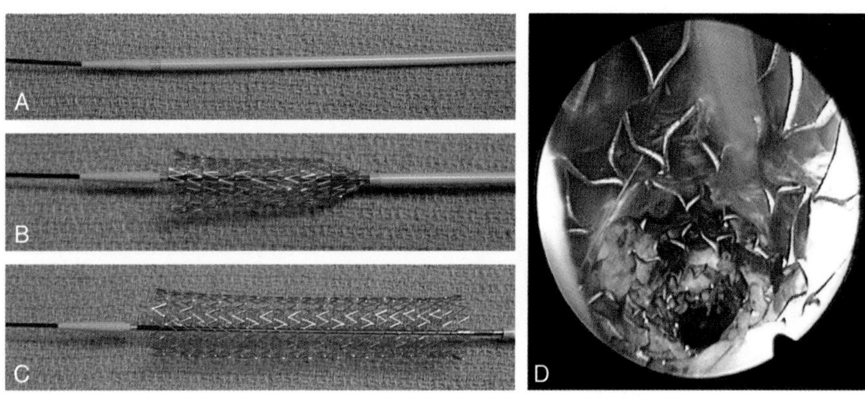

Figure 2.10 A laser-cut self-expanding metallic stent (SEMS) during and after deployment. (A) The stent is compressed onto the delivery system and covered with a sheath. The delivery system is placed over a black guide wire. (B) The stent is opening as the sheath is withdrawn. (C) The stent is fully deployed. (D) The deployed stent within the urethra of a dog with obstructive transitional cell carcinoma.

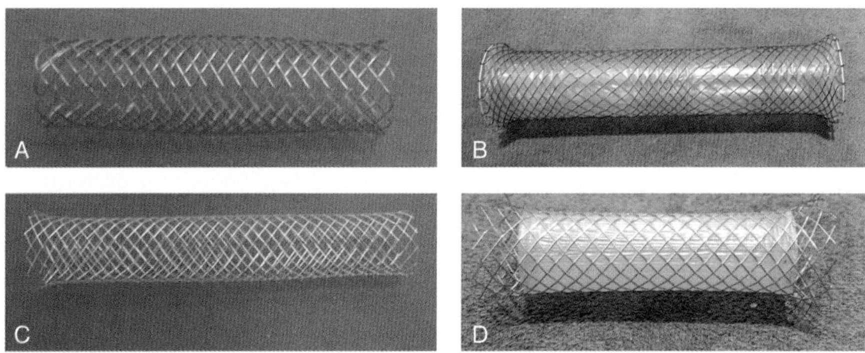

Figure 2.11 Various types of mesh self-expanding metallic stents (SEMS). (A) Tracheal stent with soft rounded edges. (B) Mesh stent with sharp edges. (C) A fully covered retrievable esophageal stent. Notice the flared ends to help to prevent migration. (D) A partially covered stent. The partial covered incorporates into the mucosa to prevent migration.

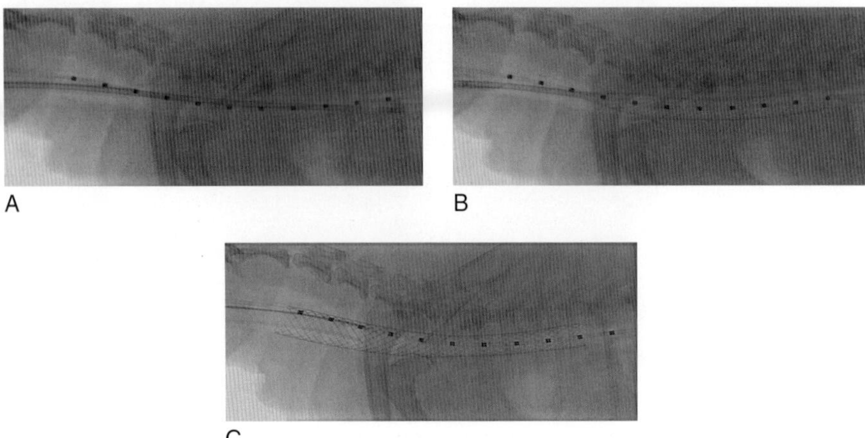

Figure 2.12 Fluoroscopic images of a mesh SEMS showing the length of the stent before and after deployment to demonstrate foreshortening. Fluoroscopic images are of a dog in lateral recumbency with tracheal collapse during stent placement. The head is to the left in each image. There is a marker catheter in the esophagus. (A) The stent is on the delivery system and measures to be over 115 mm long. (B) The stent is visualized mid-deployment and now the stent is measuring about 110 mm long. (C) Once the stent is deployed it is measuring approximately 95 cm long.

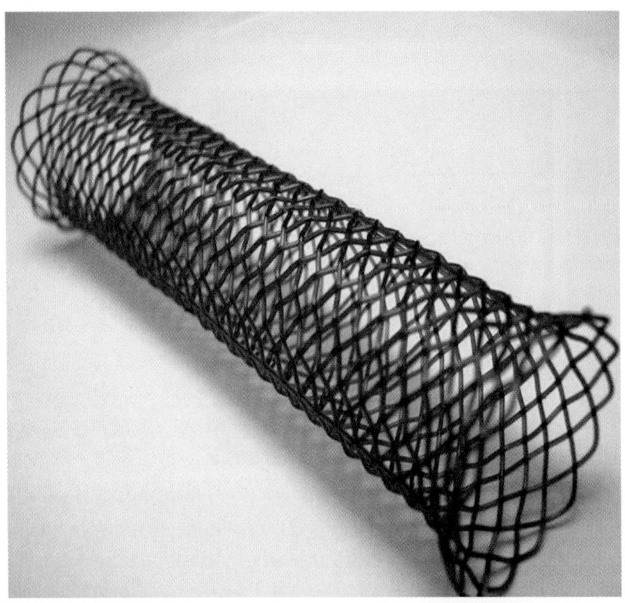

Figure 2.13 Bioabsorbable esophageal stent. This is a self-expanding stent. Notice the flared ends to prevent migration.

titanium alloy developed at the Naval Ordinal Laboratory), that is expanded and set to retain a predetermined length and diameter. The laser creates the mesh-like design making it very flexible. The stent is super-cooled and compressed onto a delivery system (typically 6–10 Fr) that allows the relatively large stent to be delivered through a small hole or orifice. Once the stent reaches body temperature it resumes its pre-determined size. When the sheath is removed the stent will expand and does not foreshorten substantially, regardless of the ultimate diameter achieved (Figure 2.10).

The mesh SEMS[19–27] is either a single wire, or many wires, woven together. It is very flexible and resistant to fatigue as the wires move across one another during motion. It is compressed onto a delivery system like the laser cut stent, but during compression the design of the stent results in lengthening; During the deployment the stent will foreshorten to its original length (Figure 2.12) (see Chapter 1 and Chapter 7). This characteristic facilitates reconstraint of many of these stents but also creates unpredictability during deployment as to the ultimate length achieved. It also means that with time, if the stent continues to expand, it will foreshorten further. Esophageal and colonic SEMS often have a dog-bone shape to help prevent stent migration (Figure 2.11 and Figure 2.13). These come either bare (uncovered) or covered (stent grafts) with various materials[21,22,26,27] and are typically metal, plastic, or biodegradable (e.g. polydioxanone)[27]. These stents often have a retrieval string on the ends so that they can be repositioned or removed if necessary (Figure 2.11B).

A double pigtail ureteral stent[28–30] is available in various sizes (2.5–8 Fr) and lengths (12–32 cm). These stents have one loop to coil inside the renal pelvis, one loop to coil inside the urinary bladder, and a multi-fenestrated shaft to travel within the lumen of the entire ureter (Figure 2.14). There is a ureteral cancer stent for dogs with an unfenestrated distal 1/3 of the stent to prevent tumor ingrowth as is traverses the trigonal tumor and exits at the ureterovesicular junction (UVJ). Aside from bypassing the ureteral obstruction, another main benefit to this stent is the passive ureteral dilation that occurs over 2 days–2 weeks, increasing ureteral flow of urine. Ureteral stents are typically placed

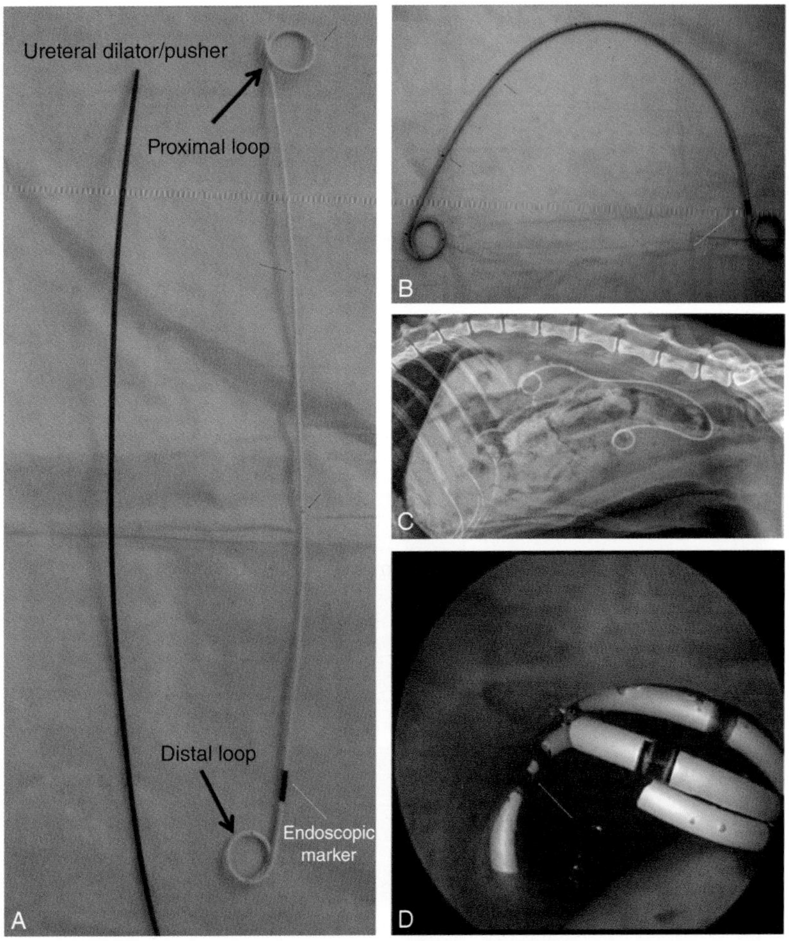

Figure 2.14 Double pigtail ureteral stents. (A) Feline 2.5 Fr ureteral stent with tapered dilation catheter (0.034″). Notice the loops on each end of the stent to prevent migration. The stent is multi-fenestrated (red arrows) for better drainage. The distal end of the shaft has a black mark that is used to mark the end of the stent during endoscopic placement. (B) Ureteral stent used in cases with trigonal neoplasia. The distal shaft of the stent does not have any fenestrations to prevent tumor ingrowth. (C) Lateral radiograph of a cat after ureteral stent placement. Notice the proximal loop is within the renal pelvis and the distal loop is in the urinary bladder. (D) Endoscopic image of a dog with a ureteral stent in the urinary bladder. Notice the endoscopic marks (white arrow) on the stent as it exits the ureterovesicular junction.

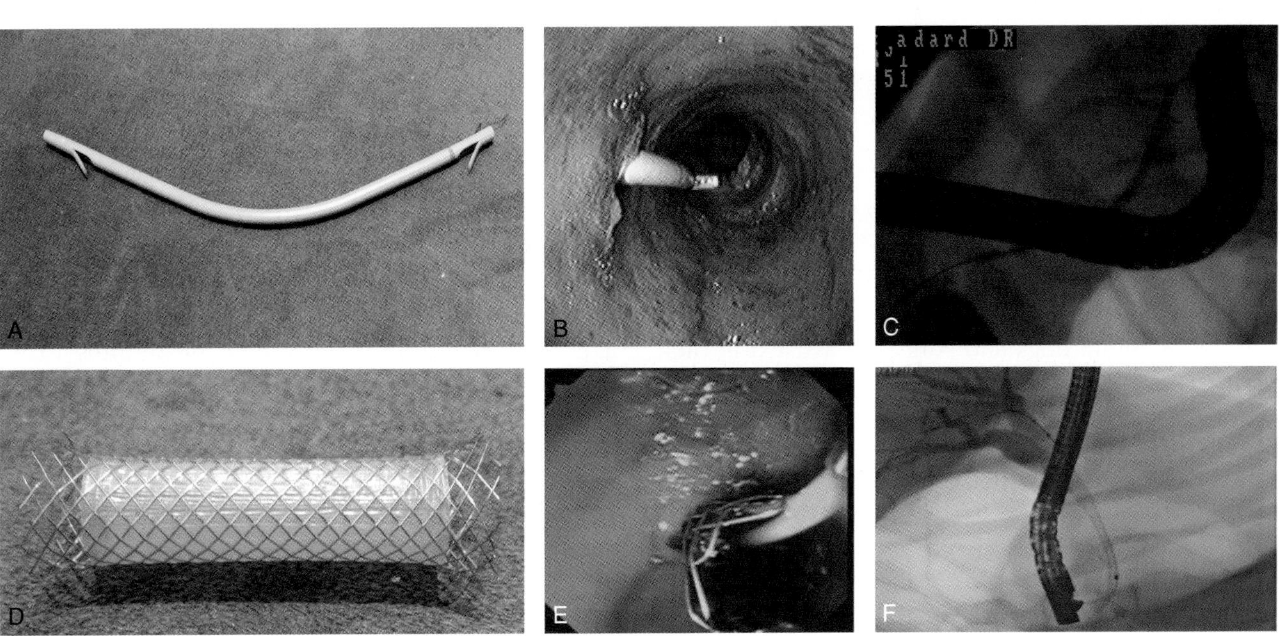

Figure 2.15 Various types of biliary stents. (A) Polyurethane biliary and pancreatic stent that come in different sizes. The flanges help to prevent stent migration. (B) Endoscopic image of a dog with a biliary stent exiting the common bile duct (CBD) at the major duodenal papilla (MDP). (C) Fluoroscopic image of the stent within the CBD approaching the level of the gall bladder. (D) Biliary SEMS that is partially covered. These are most commonly used for common bile duct strictures or tumors. (E) SEMS as it exits the CBD at the MDP and bile coming out of the stent. (F) Fluoroscopic image of the SEMS within the CBD.

TABLE 2.1
Ureteral stenting equipment chart

Ureteral stent size (French)	Guidewire size	Open-ended ureteral catheter size	Rigid cystoscope lens size (working channel diameter)	Over the needle catheter size (gauge) for antegrade placement
2.5-feline	0.018″	3 Fr or 0.032–0.034″ ureteral dilator	1.9 mm (3 Fr)	21 or 22
3.7-small dog	0.025″	4 Fr	2.7 mm (5 Fr)	20
4.7-medium/large dog	0.035″	5 Fr	2.7 mm (5 Fr)	18
6.0-large dog/cancer stent	0.035″	5–6 Fr	4 mm (6 Fr)	18

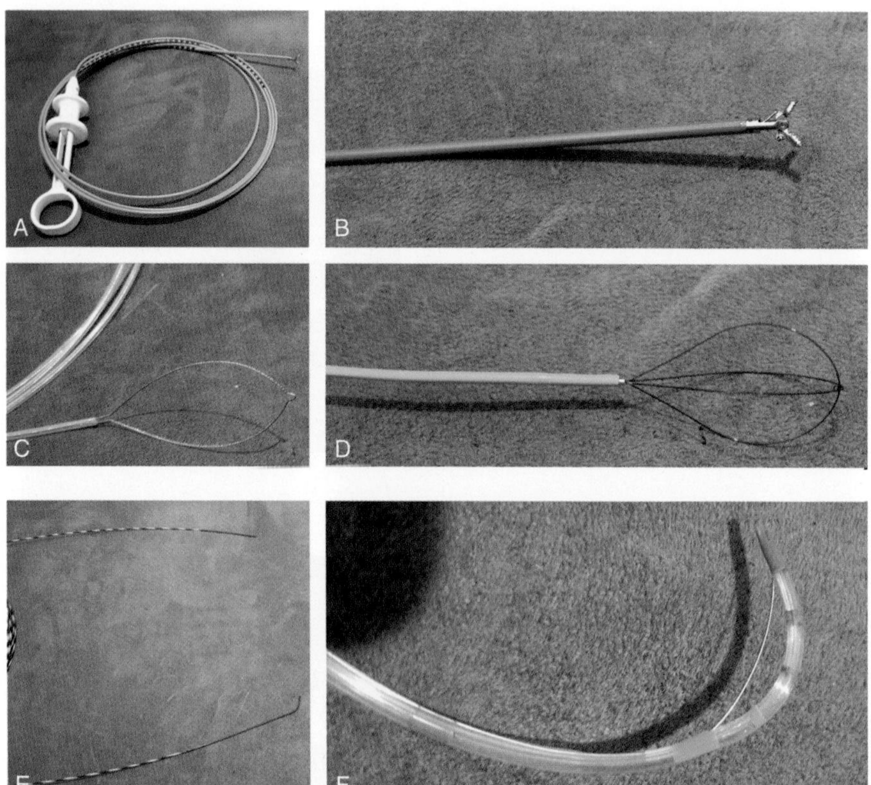

Figure 2.16 Various accessories that can be used through the working channel of an endoscope. (A and B) various types of biopsy instruments. (C) Endoscopic polypectomy snare. (D) Endoscopic basket. (E) Guide wire used for gastrointestinal and/or biliary access. (F) Sphinctertome used for common bile duct access through a side view duodenoscope.

endoscopically in dogs and surgically-assisted in cats (see chapters 30 and 31) making appropriately sized wires, catheters and endoscope working channels very important (see Table 2.1).

The polyurethrane biliary stent[31] has a flange on each end to prevent migration up the common bile duct or down into the duodenum (Figure 2.15). Metallic stents can also be used for permanent placement, most commonly for malignant obstructions.

Snares / Baskets / Needles

Using an endoscopic snare polypectomy device,[32] also attached to the electrocautery unit as above, with a slightly different adaptor (Figure 2.8) allows various endoscopic polypectomy procedures to be performed. This is most commonly done in the stomach, colon, trachea and urinary bladder (see Chapters 10, 15, 33, 35, and 37). It is important this device is used either in air at 21% oxygen (trachea), within an evacuated colon (to prevent accumulation of gases), or using D5W instead of 0.9% saline during bladder irrigation.

Baskets and stone retrieval devices are very useful for stone removal during cystoscopy, nephroscopy and urethroscopy. After lithotripsy is performed these baskets are needed to retrieve the fragments, or if the stones are small enough they can be removed with basketing alone without the need for lithotripsy[33–35] (Figure 2.16). Baskets for removal of foreign

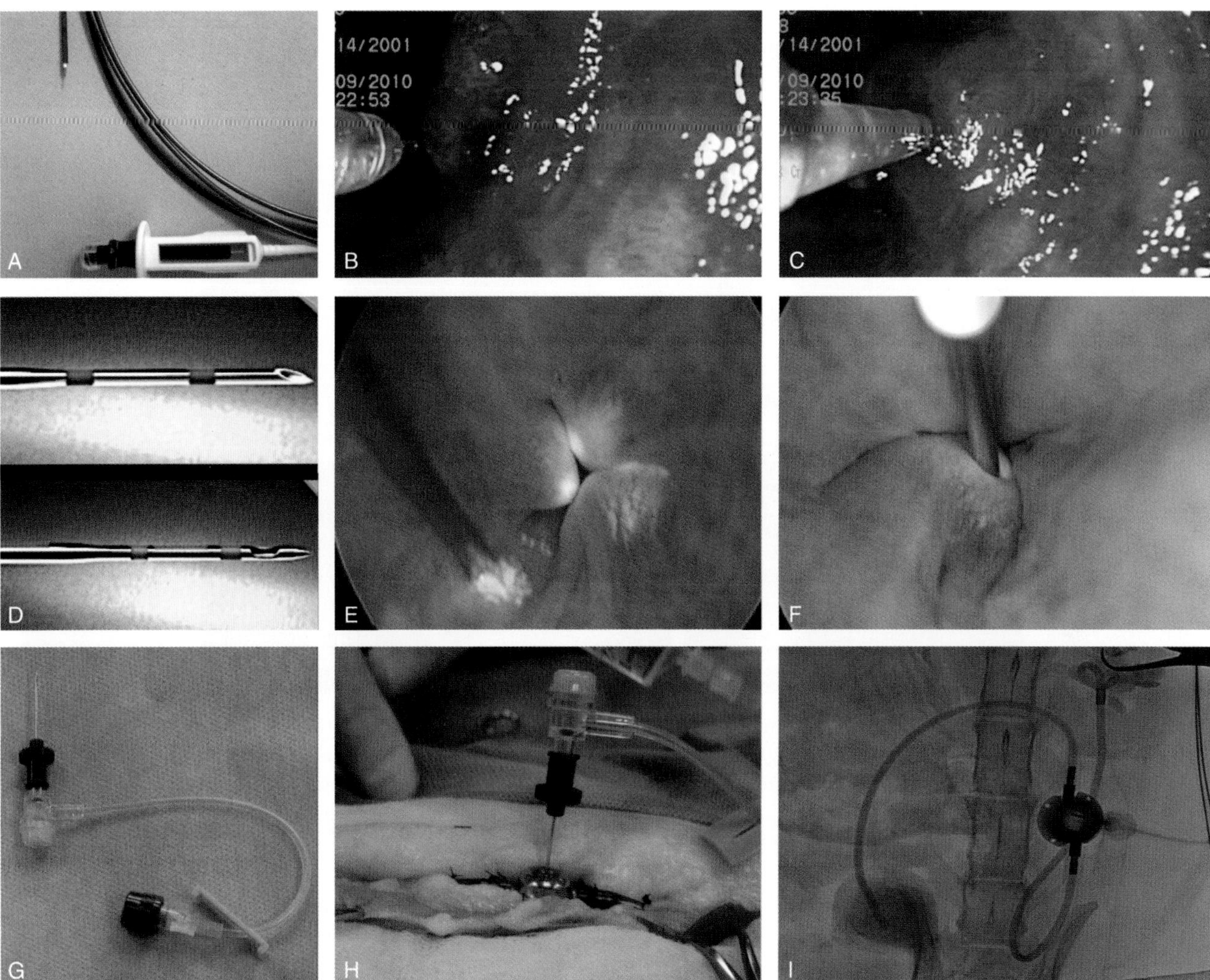

Figure 2.17 Various types of injection needles. (A) Endoscopic injection needle. (B) Needle from (A) being placed through the endoscope working channel into the lumen of the colon. (C) Needle inserted under the mucosal tissue to inject saline prior to polyp resection. (D) Bulking agent injection needles. Marks provide reference of depth during endoscopic transurethral injection. (E) Needle through working channel of the endoscope prior to penetration into the urethral tissue. (F) Needle after penetration into the urethral tissue during bulking-agent injection. (G) Non-coring Huber needle attached to a T-port. (H) Insertion of the Huber needle into an access port during a subcutaneous ureteral bypass (SUB) placement in a cat. (I) Fluoroscopic image taken during injection of contrast through the Huber needle and SUB device.

bodies (tracheal, nasopharyngeal, and intestinal) are also very helpful. The operator should be aware that the basket should be appropriately sized for the endoscope in use (diameter and length), and the object to be removed. The basket should be sterile if being used in the urinary tract. These are typically meant for one time use only, however they can often be re-sterilized and reused if not damaged. Baskets are also commonly used to remove a ureteral stent from the urinary bladder cystoscopically, when needed.

Injection needles[33–35] (Figure 2.17) are used for various reasons. Submucosal triamcinolone injections of strictures of the urethra, esophagus, nasopharynx and colon, or for endoscopic mucosal resections (EMR) of sessile gastric or colonic polyps using saline. The needles are typically 25 gauge diameter and 4 mm long (Figure 2.17A) attached to the tip of a 2 mm catheter/sheath system that can fit through all GI scopes, a bronchoscope, and a 2.7 mm or 4 mm cystoscope. Bulking agent urethral injections are typically infused through a larger 21 gauge Huber needle (Figure 2.17B).[34] A Huber needle[35] is non-coring and prevents making a large hole in the urethral tissue; Instead it is meant to pierce the tissue and spread it apart to inject the bulking material

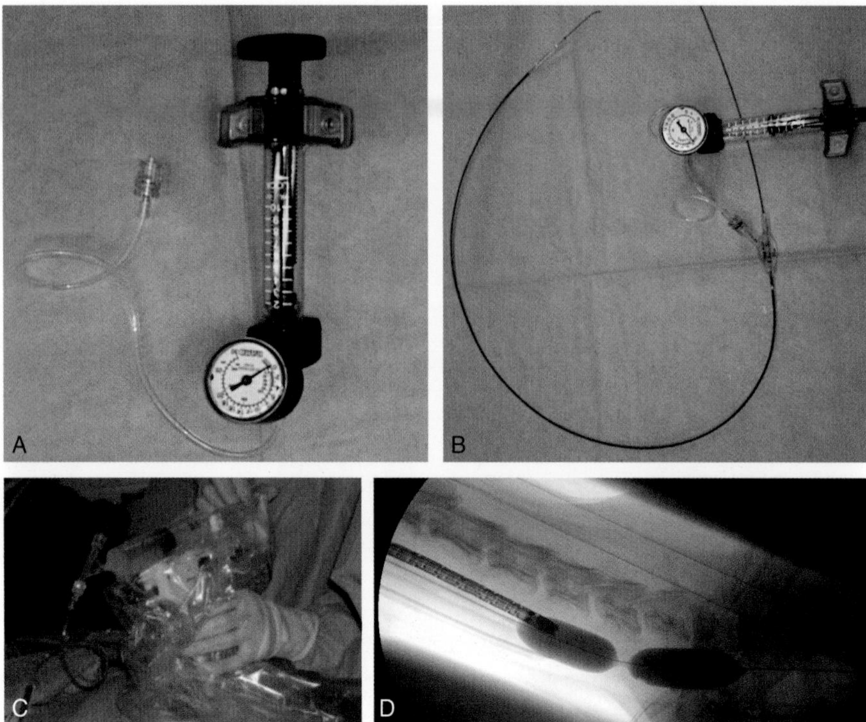

Figure 2.18 Balloon dilation catheter equipment. (A) Insufflation device for balloon dilation catheter. (B) Balloon dilation catheter with two ports on the end. One for guide wire access and the other for balloon inflation/deflation. (C) Inflating a balloon inside a patient. (D) Fluoroscopic image of the balloon inflating an esophageal stricture. The balloon is inflated with a 50% contrast solution.

into the lumen. This is also the needle used to flush a subcutaneous ureteral bypass device (SUB)[35] (Figure 2.17C).

Balloons

Balloon dilation catheters[36–42] are used to dilate strictures throughout the body (nasopharynx, esophagus, colon, urethra, ureter) using endoscopic and/or fluoroscopic-guidance. Balloon diameter, length, catheter diameter, and rated burst pressures are very important to know prior to choosing a balloon. Balloons should be inflated using a commercially available inflation device[42] (Figure 2.18) as the manual pressure exerted by hand inflation is typically insufficient to reach the pressure required to efface a stricture (e.g. 8–22 atm). The inflation device should be filled with a 1:1 mixture of contrast and saline so that the balloon can be seen during fluoroscopy and the stricture can be monitored while breaking; air is too compressive for stricture dilation. The author recommends monitoring with both endoscopy and fluoroscopy to confirm the entire stricture has been broken rather than just mucosal tearing (Figure 2.18).

Miscellaneous Devices

A subcutaneous ureteral bypass device (SUB)[43] is currently placed with surgical-assistance under fluoroscopic guidance (see Chapter 29). This device is a combination nephrostomy and cystostomy tube that is hooked up subcutaneously to a shunting access port (Figure 2.19) that can be flushed intermittently with a Huber needle to prevent accumulation of debris.

Special Recommendations

Setting up an IE suite appropriately requires meticulous organization. When setting up for an IE procedure it is important that the operator has all the equipment necessary, the procedure is well thought out, and the room is appropriately organized. Easy viewing of both fluoroscopy and endoscopy simultaneously on monitor(s) is very important, and if possible, two monitors for endoscopy should be placed in the room to allow better visibility. The operator should have more than one wire, catheter, needle, balloon, laser fiber, basket, etc., available in the event one breaks, gets contaminated, or becomes

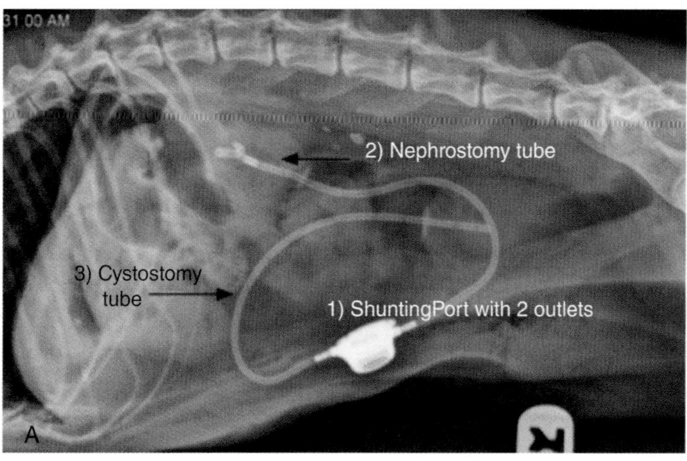

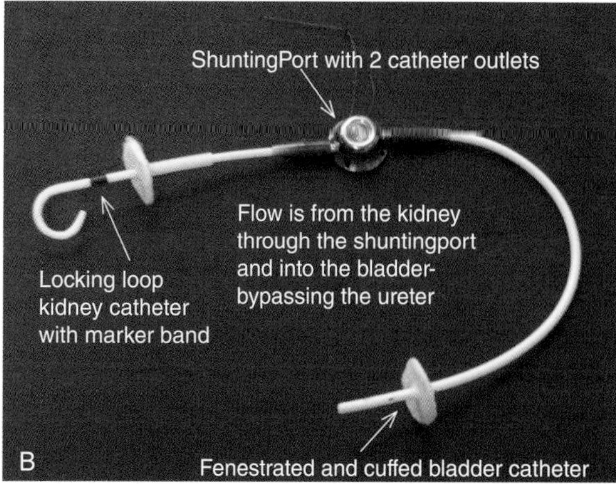

Figure 2.19 Subcutaneous ureteral bypass device (SUB). (A) Lateral radiograph of the SUB device inside a cat that was obstructed with numerous ureteroliths. Notice the three pieces: Nephrostomy tube, shunting port and cystostomy tube. (B) The same device showing all of its parts.

difficult to use over time (wires and baskets, especially). Ideally this should be a sterile operating room so that if surgical conversion is necessary, this is easily performed.

Notes

Note the equipment on this list are only examples of what is used in the author's practice and various alternatives would be considered appropriate.

1. GIF-XP180, GIF-160 5.9 and 8.6 mm, Video flexible gastroduodenoscope, Olympus, Southborough, MA.
2. BF-Q180 Flexible 5.5 mm bronchoscope, Olympus, Southborough MA.
3. Flex X^2 Flexible ureteroscope, Karl Storz Endoscopy, Culver City, CA.
4. Side-view duodenoscope, TF-160VF, 11.3 mm, Olympus, Southborough, MA.
5. Side-view duodenoscope, pediatric, PJF-160, 7.5 mm, Olympus, Southborough, MA.
6. Rigid endoscope, 1.9-mm 30° lens, Karl Storz Endoscopy, Culver City, CA.
7. Rigid endoscope, 2.7-mm integraded sheath 30° lens, Richard Wolf, Vernon Hills, IL.
8. Rigid endoscope, 2.7-mm 30° lens, Karl Storz Endoscopy, Culver City, IL.
9. Rigid endoscope, 4-mm 30° lens, Karl Storz Endoscopy, Culver City, IL.
10. 200 or 400-μm Holmium:YAG laser fiber and 30-W Hol:YAG Lithotrite, Odyssey, Convergent Inc, Alameda, CA.
11. bbCyberwand Dual Ultrasonic Lithotriptor, Olympus, Gyrus/ACMI, Southborough, MA.
12. z600-μm diode laser fiber and 100-W diode Lithotrite, Vectra, Convergent Inc, Alameda, CA.
13. Cautery machine Valley Lab Force FX, Electrosurgical Generator, Covideien, Boulder, CO.
14. Fulgurating electrode Bugbee cautery, 2 Fr, short tip, ACMI-Olympus, Southborough, MA.
15. Balloon Expandable Metallic Stents, Infiniti Medical, LLC, Menlo Park, CA.
16. Palamaz Genesis Transhepatic Biliary Stent, Cordis Corp, Miami, FL.
17. iCast Covered stent, Atrium Medical, Hudson, NH.
18. VetStent Urethra, Infiniti Medical LLC, Menlo Park, CA.
19. SEMS Tracheal stent, Infiniti Medical LLC, Menlo Park, CA.
20. WallStent, Boston Scientific, Natick, MA.
21. Wallflex Covered and Uncovered Esophageal Stent, Boston Scientific, Natick, MA.
22. VetStent Covered esophageal stent, Infiniti Medical LLC, Menlo Park, CA.
23. Vet Stent Colon, Infiniti Medical LLC, Menlo Park, CA.
24. WallFlex Colonic Stent (covered or uncovered), Boston Scientific, Natick, MA.
25. Fluency Covered stent graft, Bard Medical, Covington, GA.
26. PolyFlex Esophageal Stent, Boston Scientific, Natick, MA.
27. PDS Esophageal stent, Infiniti Medical LLC, Menlo Park, CA.
28. Vet Stent ureter 2.5-4.7 Fr double pigtail ureteral stent, Infiniti Medical LLC, Menlo Park, CA.
29. Bard In-Lay ureteral stent (4.7-8.0 Fr), Bard Medical, Covington, GA
30. Vet Stent Ureter-Cancer stent 6 Fr, Infiniti Medical LLC, Menlo Park, CA. MA
31. Cotton-Huibregtse Biliary Stent Set, 7 Fr., Cook Medical, Bloomington IL.
32. SnareMaster Polypectomy snare, Olympus, Southborough MA.
33. Endoscopy injection needle, 25 ga. × 4 mm, US Endoscopy, Mentor, OH.
34. Coaptite needle for injection, 21 ga. Boston Scientific, Natick, MA.

35. 22 gauge Huber needle, Norfolk Vet, Skokie, IL.
36. Dimenstion® Basket, 2.4 Fr, Bard Medical, Covington, GA.
37. N-Compass™ stone retrieval basket, Cook Medical, Bloomington, IN.
38. Sur-Catch® NT, No Tip Nitinol Basket, Olympus/Gyrus ACMI, Southborough MA.
39. Balloon dilation catheters, Infiniti Medical, LLC, Menlo Park CA
40. Balloon dilation catheters, Conquest, Bard Medical, Covington, GA.
41. Esophageal balloon dilation catheters CRE, Boston Scientific, Natick, MA.
42. Balloon inflation device, Bard Medical, Covington, GA.
43. Subcutaneous ureteral bypass device (SUB), Norfolk Vet, Skokie, IL.

CHAPTER THREE

Oncology for the Interventionalist

Christine Mullin[1] and Craig A. Clifford[2]
[1]*The Oncology Service LLC, Washington, DC*
[2]*Hope Veterinary Specialists, Malvern, PA*

Introduction

Interventional oncology (IO) is a rapidly evolving, dynamic specialty in which clinicians are trained to perform a myriad of image-guided, minimally invasive techniques and procedures to assist in the diagnosis and management of cancer patients. The need for such a specialty comes as a result of the unique challenges faced by the veterinary oncologist – the administration of less than maximally tolerated dosages of chemotherapy with a greater focus on the improvement in quality of life and not necessarily true eradication of the cancer. This more palliative approach to chemotherapy administration often results in reduced tumor response rates, primary tumor recurrence, and the subsequent development of metastatic lesions; scenarios which often have few viable long-term therapeutic options. As previously described by Weisse et al., these limitations in veterinary oncology have inspired various innovative, image-guided regional tumor therapies that can now be offered to veterinary patients (Weisse et al, 2008).

Although IR in veterinary oncology is still in its relative infancy and a paucity of information exists in the veterinary literature, significant progress has been made in the use of regional techniques that include, but are not limited to, the following:

- Percutaneous tumor ablation (radiofrequency, microwave, laser thermal, cryoablation, and percutaneous ethanol injection)
- Intra-arterial chemotherapy
- Transcatheter arterial embolization/chemoembolization
- Palliative stenting for malignant vascular, urinary, respiratory, and gastrointestinal obstructions
- Catheter-directed thrombolysis for arterial and venous thromboembolic disease
- Port placement for effusion drainage (thoracic, peritoneal, retroperitoneal, other) and access for intracavitary chemotherapy administration
- Subcutaneous vascular access port placement for repeated chemotherapy administration or frequently anesthetized radiation therapy patients
- Feeding tube placement.

As with its human counterpart, veterinary IO is increasingly being utilized in both academic and referral institutions to help palliate cancer patients in which traditional therapies have failed or demonstrated minimal benefit. The goal with these techniques is to maximize local therapy and minimize systemic toxicity while improving quality of life. In many cases, even though still considered "palliative techniques", improved survival times, disease-free intervals, and recurrence rates have been documented.

The goal of this chapter is to provide the IO clinician with the basics of veterinary oncology in regards to the current tumor staging systems for relevant tumors, an understanding of the chemotherapy basics including commonly used drugs, proper administration, disposal, toxicities and their associated grading schemes, basics of radiation therapy, an introduction to tyrosine kinase inhibitors and their expanding use in veterinary medicine, and standard criteria for defining responses in an effort to further standardize studies that evaluate cancer therapies. Useful charts and handouts for chemotherapy are provided to be modified by the IO clinician as needed.

Tumor Staging

Staging describes the severity of a patient's cancer based on the size and/or extent/dimensions of the tumor and whether metastasis is present. Staging is

Veterinary Image-Guided Interventions, First Edition. Edited by Chick Weisse and Allyson Berent.

Companion website: www.wiley.com/go/weisse/vet-image-guided-interventions

BOX 3.1

Staging criteria for tumors commonly treated with IR

WHO TNM Staging System for Canine Urogenital Cancer (Knapp and McMillan, 2013)

T – Primary Tumor

Tis	Carcinoma in situ
T0	No evidence of primary tumor
T1	Superficial papillary tumor
T2	Tumor invading the bladder wall, with induration
T3	Tumor invading neighboring organs including prostate, uterus, vagina, pelvic canal

N – Regional Lymph Node (Internal and External iliac)

N0	No regional lymph node involvement
N1	Regional lymph node involvement
N2	Regional lymph node involvement and juxtaregional lymph node involved

M – Distant Metastases

M0	No evidence of metastasis
M1	Distant metastasis present

WHO TNM Staging System for Canine Nasosinal Tumors (Turek and Lana, 2013)

T – Primary Tumor

T0	No evidence of primary tumor
T1	Tumor ipsilateral, minimal or no bone destruction
T2	Tumor bilateral and/or moderate bone destruction
T3	Tumor invading neighboring tissue

N – Regional Lymph Node

N1	No evidence of lymph node involvement
N2	Movable ipsilateral nodes
N3	Fixed nodes

M – Distant Metastasis

M1	No evidence of distant metastasis
M2	Distant metastasis detected (including nodes)

Modified Adams Staging System for Canine Nasosinal Tumors (Turek and Lana, 2013)

Stage 1 Confined to one nasal passage, paranasal sinus, or frontal sinus, with no bone involvement beyond turbinates

Stage 2 Any bone involvement (beyond turbinates) but no evidence of orbit/subcutaneous/submucosal mass

Stage 3 Orbit involved or nasopharyngeal or subcutaneous or submucosal mass

Stage 4 Tumor causing lysis or the cribriform plate

important to help the clinician develop an appropriate treatment plan (local vs. systemic therapy), determine the patient's prognosis, identify appropriate patients for a clinical trial, and enable investigators to use common terminology for study comparison of patient populations.

The most common staging system is the World Health Organization (WHO) TNM staging system (Box 3.1). Specifically this is based on the size and/or extent of the primary tumor (T), presence or absence of lymph node involvement (N), and whether metastasis (M), has occurred.

Chemotherapy

Chemotherapy is an important adjunctive therapy to IR and as such, it is important for the IR clinician to have at least a broad understanding regarding the usage and indications, safety precautions, the most commonly used agents, common side effects, and associated toxicities. Clearly the information provided is not intended to be a substitute for the training and expertise of a medical or radiation oncologist, but rather to provide a basic background regarding chemotherapy along with useful handouts for clinical application (Table 3.1, Table 3.2, and Table 3.3).

Chemotherapy Usage/Indications

- *Adjuvant*: The administration of chemotherapy after surgery, radiotherapy, or IR procedures. Aimed at eliminating residual disease at the primary tumor site and delaying the onset of metastatic disease. May entail single or multi-agent protocols.
- *Neoadjuvant*: The administration of chemotherapy prior to treatment with other modalities including surgery, radiation, or IR procedures. Aimed at reducing the tumor volume before definitive therapy. May entail single or multi-agent protocols.
- *Metronomic (low dose chemotherapy)*: The continuous administration of low doses of chemotherapy (generally oral) over a prolonged period of time (generally daily). Mechanisms of action include a direct cytotoxic effect on the vascular endothelial cells, an indirect effect via inhibition of angiogenic growth factors thus preventing further vessel expansion, suppression of the recruitment of bone marrow-derived endothelial progenitor cells, and reduction in the number of regulatory T cells that are involved in tumor-induced immune tolerance. Efficacy has been documented in dogs with a variety

TABLE 3.1
Commonly used chemotherapy agents

Agent	Class/MOA [1]	Dose	Neutrophil Nadir	Screening/ contraindications	Side effects	Concomitant medications	Follow-up
Doxorubicin	Anthracycline antitumor antibiotic	>15 kg: 30 mg/m^2 <15 kg: 1 mg/kg q 1–3 weeks	7–10 days	• CBC • Renal/hepatic profile before first dose • Echocardiogram recommended if suspected or known pre-existing cardiac disease or at-risk breed	*Acute*: • Infusion-rate dependent hypersensitivity[2] • Extravasation *Delayed*: • Anorexia/vomiting/ diarrhea • Myelosuppression • Cumulative cardiotoxicity (dogs)[3] • Cumulative renal tubular damage (cats)[4]	• Maropitant injection (1 mg/ kg SQ or IV) as pre-medication & (2 mg/kg PO on days 2-5) • Ondansetron/ metronidazole PRN *Optional*: • Diphenhydramine as pre-medication • TMS[5] (15–30 mg/ kg PO q12 × 7 days)	CBC/7 days
Carboplatin	Platinum	> 15 kg: 300 mg/ m2; <15 kg: 10 mg/kg q 3 weeks	10–14 days	• CBC • BUN/Creat/USG[6] • Cats: May calculate dose based on GFR[7]	• Myelosuppression • Anorexia/vomiting (less than Cisplatin)	Ondansetron/ metronidazole PRN	CBC/10 days
Cisplatin	Platinum	50–70 mg/ m^2 q 3 weeks	Bimodal: 7–10, 15–21 days	• CBC • BUN/Creat/USG	*Acute*: • Emesis during infusion *Delayed*: • Myelosuppression • Nephrotoxicity • Fatal pulmonary edema (Cats: DO NOT USE)	• Butorphanol (0.4 mg/kg IV) and Cerenia injections as pre-medication • Diuresis before/ during/after administration • Ondansetron/ metronidazole PRN	CBC/7–10 & 21 days
Mitoxantrone	Synthetic anthracycline derivative	5–6.5 mg/m^2 q 2–3 weeks	7–10 days	CBC	• Myelosuppression • Anorexia/vomiting/ diarrhea	Ondansetron/ metronidazole PRN	CBC/7–10 days
Cyclophoshamide	Nitrogen mustard alkylating agent	IV or PO: 200–250 mg/m2 q 7 days *Metronomic*: 12.5–15 mg/m^2 daily to EOD	7 days	CBC, UA	• Myelosuppression • Anorexia/vomiting • Sterile hemorrhagic Cystitis (dogs) • Alopecia (at-risk breeds)	Furosemide 2 mg/kg IV or PO when given IV or PO	• IV: CBC/ 7 days • Metronomic: Monthly UA/ sediment analysis; CBC every other month

[1] Mechanism of action.
[2] If signs of anaphylaxis develop, stop the infusion, administer dexamethasone (1 mg/kg IV) and diphenhydramine (2 mg/kg SQ or IM).
[3] Dose range considered to be safe in dogs: 180–240 mg/m^2.
[4] Re-assess renal values prior to the 3rd administration.
[5] Trimethoprim Sulfa (Chretin et al. *JVIM* 2007).
[6] Urine specific gravity.
[7] Glomerular filtration rate (Bailey et al. *AJVR* 2009).

TABLE 3.2
Chemotherapy flow sheet

Hope Veterinary Specialists
___Dr. ____________ ___Dr. ____________ Dr. ______________

CANINE CARBOPLATIN & DOXORUBICIN PROTOCOL Stage:
Patient Name: ID #:

DUE DATE	WK	WGT	CHEMO/PROCEDURE	DOSE	TX DATE	WBC	NEU/GRA	HCT %	PLT
	1		Carboplatin 300 mg/m² IV						
Notes Box:									
	2		CBC 1 week post						
	3								
	4		Doxorubicin 30 mg/m² IV						
	5		CBC						
	6		Carboplatin 300 mg/m² IV						
	7		CBC 1 week post						
	8								
	9		Doxorubicin 30 mg/m² IV						
	10		CBC						
	11		Carboplatin 300 mg/m² IV						
	12		CBC 1 week post						
	13								
	14		Doxorubicin 30 mg/m² IV						
	15		OFF or CBC						

- BUN and CREA must be performed prior to Carboplatin treatments.
- In case of azotemia, examine urine specific gravity (USG). If USG is normal, then ok to give chemo. If USG is abnormal, then ask doctor prior to chemo.

of neoplasms in the microscopic and macroscopic disease setting.

- *Radiosensitization*: The administration of chemotherapy during a radiotherapy protocol so that an additive or synergistic cytotoxic effect is achieved. Involved mechanisms include the promotion of cell cycling and thus enhanced sensitivity to both methods of cell-killing as well as increased tumor oxygenation and thus susceptibility to radiation-induced cell death.
- *Intra-arterial chemotherapy*: The fluoroscopically guided, super-selective catheterization of the arteries feeding the tumor region, thus allowing for intra-arterial administration of chemotherapeutic

TABLE 3.3
Body surface area chart

kg	m²	kg	m²	kg	m²
2	0.159	8.6	0.42	36	1.101
2.2	0.169	8.8	0.426	37	1.121
2.4	0.179	9	0.433	38	1.142
2.6	0.189	9.2	0.439	39	1.162
2.8	0.199	9.4	0.445	40	1.181
3	0.208	9.6	0.452	41	1.201
3.2	0.217	9.8	0.458	42	1.22
3.4	0.226	10	0.464	43	1.24
3.6	0.235	11	0.5	44	1.259
3.8	0.244	12	0.529	45	1.278
4	0.252	13	0.553	46	1.297
4.2	0.26	14	0.581	47	1.302
4.4	0.269	15	0.608	48	1.334
4.6	0.277	16	0.641	49	1.352
4.8	0.285	17	0.668	50	1.371
5	0.292	18	0.694	52	1.412
5.2	0.3	19	0.719	54	1.448
5.4	0.307	20	0.744	56	1.484
5.6	0.315	21	0.769	58	1.519
5.8	0.323	22	0.785	60	1.554
6	0.33	23	0.817	62	1.588
6.2	0.337	24	0.84	64	1.622
6.4	0.345	25	0.864	66	1.656
6.6	0.352	26	0.886	68	1.689
6.8	0.36	27	0.909	70	1.722
7	0.366	28	0.931	72	1.755
7.2	0.373	29	0.953	74	1.787
7.4	0.38	30	0.975	76	1.819
7.6	0.387	31	0.997	78	1.851
7.8	0.393	32	1.018	80	1.882
8	0.4	33	1.029		
8.2	0.407	34	1.06		
8.4	0.413	35	1.081		

drugs directly to the tumor. With this technique, greater concentrations of drug are delivered to the tumor (local dose escalation) without the adverse systemic effects that would be encountered had the necessary equivalent dosage been administered intravenously.

- *Chemoembolization*: The super-selective, intra-arterial delivery of chemotherapeutic drugs in conjunction with subsequent or simultaneous particle embolization. This results in an even greater increase in intratumoral drug concentrations compared with IA or IV administration. Particle embolization has a synergistic effect with the intra-arterial delivery of chemotherapeutic drugs because the subsequent ischemia inhibits tumor cell excretion of the chemotherapeutic drugs, resulting in higher retained drug concentrations within the cell. Chemoembolization is commonly utilized for non-resecTable hepatic neoplasia in human and, more recently, veterinary medicine.

Common Chemotherapy Related Definitions

- *Therapeutic index*: The ratio between the toxic dose and the therapeutic dose.
- *Maximum tolerated dose (MTD)*: The highest dose of a given drug that can be administered without causing unacceptable or irreversible side effects.
- *Biologically effective dose (BED)*: The measured response of a putative or surrogate target (e.g. a particular chemistry value, phosphorylated protein, etc.) that is related to the mechanism of action of the drug. Frequently used in response assessment for molecularly-targeted and anti-angiogenic therapies.
- *Dose intensity*: The measure of dose per unit of time.

Chemotherapy Handling and Safety

In physician-based oncology, there is minimal risk to hospital workers due to the adequate routine safety measures undertaken during chemotherapy handling (Wick et al., 2003). Similar measures outlined below are routinely practiced by veterinary oncologists and chemotherapy technicians.

- All chemotherapy drugs should be drawn into syringes, reconstituted, or prepared inside of the biological safety cabinet (BSC). If chemotherapeutic drugs are prepared in your practice then only trained staff members should attempt to mix, prepare, or administer the drugs. Of course, eating, drinking, smoking, chewing gum, applying cosmetics, and food storage are all prohibited in the preparation and administration areas. Use the list below as a guideline for safe preparation:
  - Protective equipment:
    - Protective chemotherapy gowns, eyewear and unpowdered chemotherapy gloves with the

glove over the cuff of the gown should be utilized. If chemotherapy gloves are unavailable, double glove with disposable latex gloves.
  - When transported, chemotherapy should be kept in a labeled zip-lock bag and the syringe with the patient's name, the date, and the appropriate syringe label.
  - Place all disposable supplies in an appropriate receptacle marked "Chemotherapy". Do not recap remaining needles – dispose of them directly in a sharps container.
- Chemotherapy spill kit: A chemotherapy spill kit should be assembled and maintained near the site where chemotherapy drugs are mixed or administered. Each spill kit should contain at least the following: two pairs of latex gloves, plastic-backed absorbent pad, and zip-lock bag for disposal. The addition of a gown, mask and eye protection is also recommended. If a spill occurs, absorb the spilled liquid with absorbent pads or kitty litter. Wearing gloves, use paper towels to clean up the remaining liquid. The contaminated materials should then be placed in an appropriate zip-locked receptacle marked "Chemo". The contaminated area can then be cleaned with water and detergent.
- Closed chemotherapy administration system: Using a closed-system drug transfer device is very important when administering chemotherapy as numerous studies have documented widespread, low-level contamination of the environment by chemotherapy drugs in areas where the drugs are handled. Studies have found traces of chemotherapy drugs in numerous locations throughout the treatment area including: workbenches, floors, gloves, gowns, shoes, office chair, syringes, carts, and trash cans. Contamination can be found dispersed in the environment anywhere hazardous drugs have been used. Once contamination has occurred, it is extremely difficult to eradicate.
  - One example is the PhaSeal® System which is currently considered the highest rated closed-system drug transfer device on the market. It represents a closed, double-membrane system for ensuring leak-free transfer of drugs, has been shown to reduce environmental and personnel exposure compared with existing processes for the preparation and administration of chemotherapy drugs. PhaSeal uses a dry-connection system for drug transfer, with each element sealed off with a membrane cover. The injecTable drug is transferred via a specially cut injection cannula. When the components of the PhaSeal system are separated after transfer, the membranes act as tight seals preventing leakage. The system is made up of several adaptors that easily fit onto a syringe and catheter used for chemotherapy administration. The benefits of such a closed system include:
  - Prevention of the transfer of environmental contaminants (such as bacteria) into the drug vial and the syringe; therefore, a sterile environment is maintained and helps prevent unnecessary infections in the patient.
  - Inhibition of the escape of hazardous chemotherapy aerosols or vapors into the environment, thereby protecting your pet and our staff from unnecessary chemotherapy exposure.

Of unique concern in veterinary oncology is the routine exposure to patient excrement in which chemotherapeutic residues have been documented (Knobloch et al, 2010). This risk is especially concerning for immunosuppressed or pregnant adults, and children in the homes of veterinary patients receiving chemotherapy. Many oncology centers provide owners with handouts pertaining to chemotherapy safety and hygiene in the home. Guidelines that may be included in such handouts are listed in Box 3.2.

BOX 3.2

At-home chemotherapy safety guidelines

If administrating oral chemotherapy at home:
- Keep the medication in the vial and do not store it in the kitchen.
- Ensure children and pets do not have access to the drugs.
- Do not eat, drink, or chew gum when giving the medication.
- Do not crush or break the pills.
- Wear unpowdered latex gloves when handling the medication (unless allergic to latex, then wear nitrile gloves). Dispose of the gloves promptly, and wash hands thoroughly after administration.
- Gloves and empty vials should be returned to the oncology facility.

Cleaning up after your pet:
- It is normal that a small amount of chemotherapy is excreted in the urine and feces for about 12–72 hours after chemotherapy administration.
- Wear gloves if handling feces or urine.
- Wash hands after cleaning up after your pet.
- Keep children away from excrement.
- Soiled bedding should be washed normally.

Accidental exposure:
- Wash skin thoroughly and if the skin becomes irritated, seek physician assistance.
- Use detergent to clean floors, carpets or countertops. Wear gloves when cleaning.

Patient safety is also of the utmost importance considering that the patient experiences the highest level of chemotherapy exposure. Extravasation and immediate hypersensitivity reactions are the most common risks to the patient during chemotherapy administration. The following guidelines should be followed for all chemotherapy treatments.

Chemotherapy administration guidelines

1. All patients should be properly restrained. If any question exists regarding the ability to properly restrain the animal for safe chemotherapy administration, then sedation should be used to ensure safety.
2. Clean "first-stick" catheter/needle placement is imperative when administering vesicants.
3. Each catheter is checked for patency with saline flushes prior and after drug administration. For severe vesicants, flush with a minimum of 6 ml of saline.
4. During administration of drugs, the catheters should be checked for patency by periodic aspiration.
5. The catheter site must be visually monitored for patency at all times.
6. If extravasation or hypersensitivity should occur, immediate action should be taken.

Extravasation of vesicant chemotherapeutic agents may cause local pain, discomfort, regional tissue damage, and even extensive tissue necrosis. Extravasations can occur as a result of multiple punctures of the same vein, inadequate restraint of patients predisposing to catheter dislodgement, and negligence of the person administering the drug. Doxorubicin is the most commonly used chemotherapeutic agent, is a severe vesicant, and therefore carries a high risk with extravasation.

Guidelines for doxorubicin extravasation

(The first three steps below are standard no matter what type of agent has been extravasated.)

1. Alert the attending clinician.
2. Do not remove the catheter. Draw back as much of the chemotherapy agent as possible.
3. Once as much drug is withdrawn as possible, remove IV catheter.
4. Apply cold compress for 20 minutes every 4–8 hours for 48 hours.
5. Place IV catheter in a different vein to administer dexrazoxane (Zinecard®) at 10 times the doxorubicin dose, at the following intervals (Venable et al., 2012):
   a. Immediately (within 3 hours of extravasation)
   b. 24 hours
   c. 48 hours (1/2 dose)
6. *Optional:* Topical DMSO application (Bertelli et al, 1995).
7. *Optional*: Intralesional hyaluronidase (Spugnini 2002).

Doxorubicin-induced tissue sloughing usually appears 7–10 days after extravasation and progressively will worsen over the next 2–3 months. Surgical consultation may be required if tissue sloughing occurs and debridement is indicated. A possible sequelae to Doxorubicin extravasation includes limb amputation if medical management and local tissue debridement is unsuccessful in addressing the pain and tissue damage.

Hypersensitivity reactions are uncommon but can result in an emergent situation. Most are generally immediate in nature and doxorubicin is a common agent associated with hypersensitivity reactions. Below are recommendations in case a hypersensitivity reaction occurs secondary to doxorubicin.

1. Discontinue doxorubicin infusion immediately.
2. Administer diphenhydramine (2 mg/kg) IM. Dose can be repeated to effect.
3. Administer Cerenia® (1 mg/kg IV) for acute emesis if not already given as pre-medication. Alternatively, Anzemet® (dolasetron, 0.2 mg/kg IV) may be given.
4. Steroids (0.25 mg/kg dexamethasone sodium phosphate) may be administered if patient is not already on steroids or if a lack of response to Benadryl is noted.
5. Provide emergency intervention (oxygen, endotracheal intubation, etc.) as indicated.
6. Infusion may be resumed at ½ the previous rate if clinical signs subside quickly.

Chemotherapy is designed to affect rapidly dividing cells; hence, the unique susceptibility of cancer cells versus normal tissue. Some tissues, including the gastrointestinal tract and the bone marrow, have normal cells with increased replication rates which are susceptible to the effects of chemotherapy leading to possible side effects. Since the dose intensity of chemotherapy administered in veterinary medicine is significantly less than that in human oncology, the side effect rate is generally 15–20%, with most side effects mild and self-limiting. Patient side effects may be related to the presence of concurrent illness, organ dysfunction, tumor burden, and/or specific breed sensitivities. Theoretically, regionally delivered chemotherapeutics should result in less gastrointestinal and bone marrow exposure and subsequently fewer systemic side effects. A published grading scheme for chemotherapy related side effects exists and should be referred to for consistency (Table 3.4).

TABLE 3.4

Veterinary Cooperative Oncology Group – common terminology criteria for adverse events (VCOG CTCAE 2012)

	Grade				
Adverse event	1	2	3	4	5
Packed cell volume (PCV)	Dog: 30%-LLN[1] Cat: 25%-LLN	Dog: 20–<30% Cat: 20–<25%	Dog: 15–<20% Cat: 15–<20%	Dog: <15% Cat: <15%	Death
Neutropenia	1500-LLN	1000–1499	500–999	<500	Death
Thrombocytopenia	100 000-LLN	50 000–99 999	25 000–49 999	<25 000	Death
Lethargy/Fatigue/General Performance	Mild lethargy over baseline; diminished activity from predisease level, but able to function as an acceptable pet	Moderate lethargy causing some difficulty with performing ADL[2]; ambulatory only to the point of eating, sleeping and consistently defecating and urinating in acceptable areas	Compromised, severely restricted in ADL; unable to confine urinations and defecation to acceptable areas; will consume food if offered in place	Disabled, must be force fed and helped to perform ADL	Death
Weight loss	<10% from baseline, intervention not indicated	10–15% from baseline, nutritional dietary modification indicated	>15% of baseline	–	Death
Anorexia	Coaxing or dietary change required to maintain appetite	Oral intake altered (≤3 days) without significant weight loss; oral nutritional supplements/appetite stimulants may be indicated	Of >3 days duration; associated with significant weight loss (≥10%) or malnutrition; IV fluids, tube feeding or force feeding indicated	Life-threatening consequences; TPN[3] indicated; >5 days duration	Death
Diarrhea	Increase of up to 2 stools per day over baseline; no increase in frequency, however, consistency decreased over baseline	Increase of 3–6 stools per day over baseline; medications indicated; parenteral (IV or SC) fluids indicated ≤48 h; not interfering with ADL	Increase of >6 stools per day over baseline; incontinence >48 h; IV fluids >48 h; hospitalization; interfering with ADL	Life-threatening (e.g. hemodynamic collapse)	Death
Vomiting	>3 episodes in 24 h, medical intervention not indicated	3–10 episodes in 24 h; <5 episodes/day for <48 h; parenteral fluids (IV or SQ) indicated <48 h, medications indicated	Multiple episodes >48 h and IV fluids or PPN[4]/TPN indicated > 48 h	Life-threatening (e.g. hemodynamic collapse)	Death
Cystitis (hematuria/pyuria included)	Asymptomatic; microscopic hematuria/pyuria, not requiring attributed drug discontinuation	Pollakiuria with dysuria; macroscopic hematuria, transient and not requiring attributed drug discontinuation	Transfusion indicated; pain or antispasmodic medication; bladder irrigation indicated; requiring attributed drug discontinuation	Catastrophic bleeding; non-elective intervention indicated	Death
ALT	Dog: >ULN[5] to 1.5× ULN Cat: >ULN to 1.25× ULN	Dog: >1.5–4.0× ULN, transient (<2 weeks) Cat: >1.25–1.5× ULN, transient (<2 weeks)	Dog: >4.0–10× ULN Cat: >1.5–2.0× ULN	Dog: >10× ULN Cat: >2× ULN	—
BUN	>1 – 1.5× baseline; >ULN to 1.5× ULN	>1.5 – 3× baseline; >1.5–2.0× ULN	>3× baseline; >2.0–3× ULN	>3× ULN	—
Creatinine	>1–1.5× baseline; >ULN to 1.5× ULN	>1.5–3× baseline; >1.5–2.0× ULN	>3× baseline; >2.0–3× ULN	>3× ULN	—

Modified with permission from John Wiley & Sons.

[1]Lower limit normal.

[2]Adequate daily life.

[3]Total parenteral nutrition.

[4]Partial parenteral nutrition.

[5]Upper limit normal.

Common Chemotherapy Toxicities

Gastrointestinal

Chemotherapy-induced gastrointestinal disturbances are often a result of the destruction of the rapidly diving cells present within the inner lining of the gastrointestinal tract. Agents may also directly or indirectly stimulate pathways to the chemoreceptor trigger zone and/or emetic center leading to nausea or vomiting. In the average patient, transient mild lethargy and inappetance, with or without an episode of nausea/vomiting and diarrhea, are to be expected and should be considered acceptable by the clinician and owner. In general, these are mild and self-limiting with the addition of supportive therapies. A 10–25% risk of moderate gastrointestinal signs including anorexia and/or >3 episodes of vomiting or diarrhea) does exist and can often require hospitalization and supportive therapy.

Prophylactic medications are commonly used to prevent and/or decrease the severity of adverse events related to chemotherapy administration. These are the commonly used prophylactic/symptomatic medications and recommended dosing:

- Cerenia® (maropitant): 1 mg/kg SQ or IV; 2 mg/kg PO q24 × 5 days, longer if needed
- Zofran® (ondansetron): 0.2–0.5 mg/kg PO q8–24
- Reglan® (metoclopramide): 0.2–0.5 mg/kg PO q8–24
- Flagyl® (metronidazole): 7.5–15 mg/kg PO q12
- Pepcid® (famotidine): 0.5–1 mg/kg PO q12–24
- Prilosec® (omeprazole): 1 mg/kg PO q24.

Bone marrow

Most systemically administered chemotherapeutic agents will cause some degree of neutropenia and thrombocytopenia at predictable time points after dosing, corresponding to the nadir(s) of the agent. Mild non-regenerative anemia is possible with longer chemotherapy protocols, but is usually not clinically significant. A 1–5% risk of life-threatening side effects associated with marked neutropenia resulting in an increased risk for sepsis secondary to gastrointestinal bacterial translocation exists.

These are general risks for all chemotherapeutic agents, with each having a slightly variable side effects profile (Table 3.1). An uncommon (<5% incidence) and reversible but significant side effect of cyclophosphamide use is sterile hemorrhagic cystitis (SHC). Other risks that can be encountered with chemotherapy include cardiac, renal, hepatic, and extravasation toxicities, specific to the agent administered.

Dose adjustments (treatment delay, dose reductions) are made as indicated by the severity of the adverse event. In general, a 20–25% dose reduction is indicated for moderate to severe gastrointestinal and bone marrow toxicities. As a general rule, a treatment delay is indicated if neutrophil count is less than 2000/µL or if platelet count is less than 100 000/µL (cut-off values may vary with clinician experience). Oral antibiotics are recommended for moderate neutropenia (<1000/µL) in the absence of fever or severe clinical signs requiring hospitalization, and in fact, avoidance of hospitalization is recommended if at all possible during an asymptomatic neutropenic episode. Intravenous antibiotics and aggressive in-hospital supportive measures are indicated in the case of febrile neutropenia.

Helpful hints

Establish an accepted routine for each time a patient is treated with chemotherapy. Maintaining good record keeping and utilizing a standard protocol is helpful. A checklist may be helpful for this purpose, as follows:

1. Refer to patient's chemotherapy flow sheet (Table 3.2)
   a. Check to make sure correct patient chart
   b. Check CBC for adequate cell counts (liver/kidney values may also be considered depending upon agent to be administered)
   c. Check for adverse events related to previous dosing of drug in question (i.e. GI or myelosuppression)
   d. Modify dose if indicated
   e. Ensure m^2 matches kilogram weight (Table 3.3)
   f. Ensure mg/m^2 dose for agent is appropriate
2. Technician or oncologist calculates dose for patient
3. Oncologist or technician (different that person who initially calculated dose) independently calculates dose (double check calculation)
4. Check concentration of agent on bottle to ensure appropriate volume of drug
5. Two staff members check volume of agent in syringe and verbally agree before administration
6. Ensure proper personal protective equipment (PPE) in place
7. Ensure adequate patient restraint
8. Ensure adequate placement and patency of IV catheter before administration

Tyrosine Kinase Inhibitors

Receptor tyrosine kinases (RTKs) are cell-surface receptors for extracellular growth factors that facilitate signaling to the cell interior, mediating functions such as growth, survival, invasion, and angiogenesis in normal cells. Upon binding of the appropriate ligand, dimerization occurs which induces a conformational change in the receptor that allows phosphorylation of tyrosine residues in the intracellular domain. This then triggers several different intracellular second messenger cascades leading to altered gene expression. Examples of surface RTKs include KIT, epidermal growth factor receptor (EGFR), vascular endothelial growth factor receptor (VEGFR), and platelet-derived growth factor receptor (PDGFR).

Dysregulation of these RTKs can lead to uncontrolled cell growth and survival and is one of many underlying causes of some cancers. Examples in veterinary medicine include mutations in the c-Kit gene in canine and feline mast cell tumors as well as gastrointestinal stromal tumors in dogs. Dysregulation of the angiogenic RTKs (VEGF and PDGF) are likely present in a variety of canine and feline cancers including injection site sarcomas (feline), osteosarcoma, anal sac/anal gland carcinoma, squamous cell carcinoma (canine and feline), thyroid carcinoma, and nasal carcinoma.

With this understanding, the dysregulation within RTKs has lead to the development of novel "target" therapy in the form of a new class of molecules called tyrosine kinase inhibitors. Currently, toceranib phosphate (Palladia®; Zoetis Animal Health) is fully licensed and Masitinib (Kinavet®, AB Science) is conditionally licensed by the FDA for treatment in canine mast cell tumors. Multiple TKIs are entering the pipeline and will soon be available within the veterinary market. The current discussion regarding these agents is where best to include them in treatment protocols, whether along with current chemotherapy protocols or as a maintenance therapy to minimize recurrence/metastasis in the setting of microscopic disease. Side effects are common with these agents and are related to the specific receptors being targeted that are often also present in normal tissue. Although they can be serious, most side effects are mild and self-limiting.

Radiation Therapy

Radiation therapy (RT) is a standard modality in the treatment of cancer and a general understanding of its nuances is important for the IO clinician. RT may be used in the adjuvant or neoadjuvant setting, as well as a single modality or concurrently to chemotherapy. The response of tumor and normal tissues between dose fractions throughout the course of radiation therapy is dictated by the "4 R's":

- *Repair* – of cellular DNA damage inflicted by radiation. Cells that are unable to repair radiation-induced DNA damage will die.
- *Redistribution* – cells that are in the relatively radiation-resistant late S-phase progress to other parts of the cell cycle, thus becoming more susceptible to radiation-induced death.
- *Reoxygenation* – when hypoxic tumor cells become aerobic and thus more sensitive to radiation.
- *Repopulation* – proliferation of tumor (and normal) cells in between radiation doses.
- Radiation types
  - *Definitive (Full course) RT*: Curative intent. 2.4–4 Gray per fraction, 3 to 5 times per week for a total dose of 42 to 57 Gray; used most commonly in the adjuvant setting.
  - *Palliative RT*: Coarsely fractionated (once to twice weekly for 4–6 doses) radiation given to a lower total dose (20–32 Gray); aimed at controlling the pain and swelling of a primary tumor but offers little direct anti-tumor benefit.
  - *IMRT*: Intensity-modulated radiation therapy. Uses inverse planning to optimize and contour a highly sculpted dose (similar fractionation schemes to definitive RT) to the tumor while sparing surrounding tissues; especially useful for tumors or tumor beds with complex geometry.
  - *SRT*: Stereotactic radiation therapy. Involves the use of high doses per fraction (usually 1–5 total fractions) that highly targets a specified tumor volume (using advanced planning equipment) with a dramatic dose drop-off, thus sparing the surrounding normal tissues.
- Common Indications for RT:
  - Oral tumors
  - Nasal tumors
  - Thyroid tumors
  - CNS tumors
  - Urogenital tumors
  - Soft tissue sarcomas
  - Osteosarcoma
  - Subcutaneous/Intramuscular hemangiosarcoma
- Side effects:
  - *Acute/Early* (3–4 weeks post-treatment initiation): oral mucositis, moist desquamation, gastrointestinal sloughing (with abdominal irradiation)
  - *Late* (months to years post-treatment): fibrosis/stricture, necrosis, loss of function, radiation-induced tumors

Tumor Response Assessment Criteria

It is important for the clinician to have a general understanding of the current systems created to assess responses to a given criteria. The two commonly used systems include the Response Evaluation Criteria in Solid Tumors (RECIST) and the WHO Tumor response Criteria (Table 3.5 and Table 3.6). The

TABLE 3.5

Response Evaluation Criteria in Solid tumors (RECIST guidelines 1.1)

Method: Unidimensional measurements (Sum of longest diameters/LDs)

Response	Criteria
Complete response (CR)	Disappearance of all target lesions for at least 4 weeks. Any pathological lymph nodes (whether target or non-target) must have reduction in short axis to <10 mm.
Partial response (PR)	≥30% decrease in the sum of diameters of target lesions compared to baseline or lowest sum diameter, for at least 4 weeks.
Progressive disease (PD)	≥20% increase in the sum of diameters of target lesions, taking as reference the smallest sum on study (this includes the baseline sum if that is the smallest on study). In addition to the relative increase of 20%, the sum must also demonstrate an absolute increase of at least 5 mm. (Note: the appearance of one or more new lesions is also considered progression).
Stable disease (SD)	Neither sufficient regression to qualify for PR nor sufficient increase to qualify for PD, taking as reference the smallest sum diameters while on study. Required duration determined by study protocol.

Modified from Eisenhauer EA, et al. 2009.

TABLE 3.6

Tumor response criteria, World Health Organization (WHO) (Miller et al., 1981)

Method: Bidimensional measurements (Sum of (Longest diameter × largest perpendicular diameter) + Sum of LD of unidimensionally measured lesions)

Response	Criteria
Complete response (CR)	Disappearance of all target lesions.
Partial response (PR)	≥50% decrease in tumor load compared to baseline or lowest measurement.
Progressive disease (PD)	≥25% increase in sum tumor load compared to baseline or lowest measurement; ≥25% increase in 1 lesion; appearance of any new lesion.
Stable disease (SD)	Neither sufficient regression to qualify for PR nor sufficient increase to qualify for PD, compared to baseline or lowest measurement.

TABLE 3.7

Outcomes with Chemotherapy and RT for most common tumors treated with IR techniques

Tumor type	Best response rate (PR + CR) with systemic chemotherapy (%)[1]	Best clinical benefit rate (PR + CR + SD) with systemic chemotherapy (%)	Best MST with chemotherapy (days)	Best response rate with radiotherapy	Best MST with radiotherapy (months)
Urogenital carcinoma	38 (Boria et al. 2005)	88	307	Subjective response rates reported only (Improvement in associated clinical signs)	21.8 (Nolan et al. 2012) – Many included chemotherapy, NSAIDs, and/or surgery
Hepatocellular carcinoma	N/A <25% in human patients	N/A	983 for all dogs (Elpiner et al. 2011) –Many included surgery 197 for non-resectable HCC (Elpiner et al. 2011)	N/A	N/A
Sinonasal tumors	75 (Langova, et al. 2004)	100 (*n*=8 dogs)	140 (Hahn et al. 1992)	Subjective response rates reported only (Improvement in associated clinical signs)	19.3 (Lana et al. 2004)

[1]Does not include data from cisplatin/piroxicam studies, as this combination is not recommended due to frequent renal toxicity.

use of a standardized system creates uniformity amongst trials allowing for the ability to compare results of a given technique or treatment. Although the literature is lacking regarding tumor responses in IO studies a review is listed in Table 3.7. Variations of RECIST (modified RECIST or mRECIST) have been introduced in human IO in response to criticism from HCC chemoembolization studies in which tumor length remains unchanged although PET and perfusion scans demonstrate complete tumor death. Similar conditions have been identified in dogs with HCC chemoembolization.

References

Bertelli, G., Gozza, A., Forno, G.B., et al. 1995. Topical dimethylsulfoxide for the prevention of soft tissue injury after extravasation of vesicant cytotoxic drugs: a prospective clinical study. *J Clin Oncol*, 13, 2851–2855.

Boria, P.A., Glickman, N.W., Schmidt, B.R., et al. 2005. Carboplatin and piroxicam in 31 dogs with transitional cell carcinoma of the urinary bladder. *Vet Comp Oncol*, 3, 73–78.

Eisenhauer, E.A., Therasse, P., Bogaerts, J., et al. 2009. New response evaluation criteria in solid tumours: Revised RECIST guideline (version 1.1). *Eur J Cancer*, 45, 228–247.

Elpiner, A.K., Brodsky, E.M., Hazzah, T.N., et al. 2011. Single-agent gemcitabine chemotherapy in dogs with hepatocellular carcinomas. *Vet Comp Oncol*, 9(4), 260–268.

Hahn, K.A., Knapp, D.W., Richardson, R.C., et al. 1992. Clinical response of nasal adenocarcinoma to cisplatin chemotherapy in 11 dogs. *J Am Vet Assoc*, 200(3), 355–357.

Knapp, D.W., McMillan, S.K. 2013. Tumors of the Urinary System. In *Withrow and MacEwen's Small Animal Clinical Oncology*, 5th edition, Eds Withrow SJ, Vail DM, Page RL. Elsevier Saunders, St. Louis, MO, 572–582.

Knobloch, A., Mohring, S.A., Eberle, N., et al. 2010. Cytotoxic drug residues in urine of dogs receiving anticancer chemotherapy. *J Vet Intern Med*, 24, 384–390.

Lana, S.E., Dernell, W.S., Lafferty, M.H., et al. 2004. Use of radiation and a slow-release cisplatin formulation for treatment of canine nasal tumors. *Vet Radiol Ultrasound*, 45, 1–5.

Langova, V., Mutsaers, A.J., Phillips, B., et al. 2004. Treatment of eight dogs with nasal tumours with alternating doses of doxorubicin and carboplatin in conjunction with oral piroxicam. *Aust Vet J*, 82(11), 676–680.

Miller, A.B., Hoogstraten, B., Staquet, M., et al. 1981. Reporting Results of Cancer Treatment. *Cancer*, 47, 207–14.

Nolan, M.W., Kogan, L., Griffin, L.R., et al. 2012. Intensity-modulated and image-guided radiation therapy for treatment of genitourinary carcinomas in dogs. *J Vet Intern Med*, 26, 987–995.

Spugnini, E.P. 2002. Use of hyaluronidase for the treatment of extravasation of chemotherapeutic agents in six dogs. *J Am Vet Med Assoc*, 221, 1419, 1420, 1437–1440.

Turek, M.M., Lana, S.E. 2013. Nasosinal tumors. In *Withrow and MacEwen's Small Animal Clinical Oncology*, 5th edition, Ed Withrow SJ, Vail DM, Page RL. Elsevier Saunders, St. Louis, MO, 435–451.

Venable, R.O., Saba, C.F., Endicott, M.M., et al. 2012. Dexrazoxane treatment of doxorubicin extravasation injury in four dogs. *J Am Vet Med Assoc*, 240, 304–307.

Veterinary Cooperative Oncology Group – common terminology criteria for adverse events (VCOG-CTCAE) following chemotherapy or biological antineoplastic therapy in dogs and cats v1.1. *Vet Comp Oncol* 2012. Epub ahead of print.

Weisse, C., Berent, A., Todd, K., et al. 2008. Potential applications of interventional radiology in veterinary medicine. *J Am Vet Med Assoc*, 233(10), 1564–74.

Wick, C., Slawson, M.H., Jorgenson, J.A., et al. 2003. Using a closed-system protective device to reduce personnel exposure to antineoplastic agents. *Am J Health-Sys Pharm*, 60(15), 2314–2320.

Supplementary Reading

Bailey, D.B., Rassnick, K.M., Prey, J.D., et al. 2009. Evaluation of serum iohexol clearance for use in predicting carboplatin clearance in cats. *Am J Vet Res*, 70, 1135–1140.

Chretin, J.D., Rassnick, K.M., Shaw, N.A., et al. 2007. Prophylactic trimethoprim-sulfadiazine during chemotherapy in dogs with lymphoma and ostoesarcoma: A double-blind, placebo-controlled study. *J Vet Intern Med*, 21, 141–148.

Rau, S.E., Barber, L.G., Burgess, K.E., et al. 2010. Efficacy of maropitant in the prevention of delayed vomiting associated with administration of doxorubicin to dogs. *J Vet Intern Med*, 24, 1452–1457.

Thamm, D.H., Vail, D.M. 2007. Aftershocks of cancer chemotherapy: managing adverse effects. *J Am Anim Hosp Assoc*, 43, 1–7.

Villalobos, A. 2006. Dealing with chemotherapy extravasations: a new technique. *J Am Anim Hosp Assoc*, 42, 321–325.

SECTION TWO

Respiratory System

Edited by Chick Weisse

CHAPTER FOUR

Epistaxis Embolization

Chick Weisse
The Animal Medical Center, New York, NY

Background/Indications

Epistaxis results from primary nasal diseases or systemic disease processes and is typically responsive to conservative treatment modalities including management of the underlying systemic condition, strict rest, cold packs, sedation or tranquilization, local vasoconstrictors, blood transfusions, and/or packing of the external nares and caudal nasopharynx with epinephrine-soaked gauze (Mahony, 2000). Nasal hemorrhage that is refractory to conservative treatment, defined as "intractable epistaxis", can be a life-threatening condition. Dogs have a well-developed vertebral basilar arterial system that permits ligation of the carotid artery without deleterious consequences. Surgical options have therefore been limited to ligation of the carotid artery that is performed to reduce the pressure-head behind the hemorrhage to allow hemostasis to occur. Experimental studies (Clendenin and Conrad, 1979a, b) reveal that extensive collateralization develops after unilateral and bilateral occlusion of the common carotid arteries. Collateral vessels connected to the caudal auricular and occipital artery develop from the ipsilateral cranial thyroid and vertebral artery and the contralateral vertebral artery after unilateral ligation (Clendenin and Conrad, 1979). Retrograde blood flow from the proximal portion of the caudal auricular artery is thought to supply the terminal branches of the external carotid artery. Anastomotic connections from the internal carotid artery to the maxillary artery and the internal carotid artery to the ascending pharyngeal artery develop bilaterally after bilateral ligation of the common carotid artery (Clendenin and Conrad, 1979). Therefore, the benefits of carotid artery ligation are only transient, and the procedure may not be able to be repeated. When epistaxis recurs after collateral vessels have developed, surgical treatment options are limited. This is an important feature of embolization with regard to the etiology of the epistaxis in veterinary patients. In most instances, whether epistaxis is caused by an intrinsic abnormality of the nasal passage, or by a systemic condition like a coagulopathy or vasculitis, the primary problem will often persist after either type of vascular intervention. Although carotid ligation and embolization may treat hemorrhage acutely, only embolization will be effective in the future if the underlying condition does not resolve and hemorrhage recurs. One of the most common causes of intractable epistaxis requiring embolization in the author's experience has been nasal cancer (pre- or post-radiation therapy) or thrombocytopathia (e.g. Scott Syndrome). Because there is no definitive treatment for these conditions there will always be a risk of life-threatening hemorrhage recurrence, and therefore transarterial embolization seems to be the most appropriate treatment, which can be repeated on an as needed basis when necessary.

Intractable epistaxis is also a therapeutic challenge in humans (Elahi et al., 1995). Reported failure rates of 9.5% to 15% and complication rates of 40% to 47% after ligation of the internal maxillary artery have spawned investigation into the efficacy of embolization to control hemorrhage (Schaitkin et al., 1987). A catheter and embolic agent can be used to selectively occlude a vascular distribution at a desired level. The level of occlusion can be much further distal than that achieved during an open surgical procedure. Super-selective, distal embolization reduces the development of substantial collateralization compared with proximal ligation. When bleeding recurs, repeated embolization can still be performed because larger, more proximal vessels remain patent. In humans, successful control of hemorrhage has been reported to be 87% to 91% with a single embolization of the internal maxillary artery and 96% to 97% with embolization of supplementary vessels (Vitek, 1991).

Veterinary Image-Guided Interventions, First Edition. Edited by Chick Weisse and Allyson Berent.

Companion website: www.wiley.com/go/weisse/vet-image-guided-interventions

Patient Preparation

Prior to performing nasal embolization, a complete work-up is required to rule-out the more common causes of epistaxis that might be controlled medically (hypertension, coagulopathy, hyperviscosity, neoplasia, fungal infection, chronic rhinitis, nasal parasites, etc.). Important pre-operative information includes the severity of the hemorrhage, whether it is always unilateral or bilateral, and whether the dog has melena (swallowing blood or not). Unilateral hemorrhage is commonly treated with unilateral embolization as the procedure is faster and likely associated with a lower risk of ischemic complications. Bilateral epistaxis will require bilateral embolization. If the dog is not swallowing blood, the bleed may be more rostral, suggesting a better chance of embolization stopping the hemorrhage. If large quantities of melena are being produced, the bleed is either very serious, more caudally located, or both. This is important as the embolization is performed rostral to the ophthalmic artery and therefore not likely to stop nasal bleeding originating caudal to the medial canthus (nasopharynx).

Cross-sectional imaging and rhinoscopy (angegrade and retrograde) is highly recommend prior to performing the embolization procedure in order to rule out neoplasia, foreign bodies, and erosion of the cribriform plate suggesting communication with the brain. Additionally, other medically treated conditions should be ruled out prior to considering embolization. If emergent treatment is necessary, the contrast load associated with contrast computerized tomography (CT) scans may prevent a therapeutic interventional study to be performed simultaneously. In those cases possible options include cross-sectional imaging with the procedure the following day or possible MRA (using gadolinium) rather than CT. Dual-phase CT scans provide information regarding the individuals' vascular anatomy and possible presence of arteriovenous fistulas or potential hamartomas to target. The scan may also reveal the possible location of the lesion and help determine whether embolization will be able to target the region of interest; for instance if the only abnormal region is in the nasopharynx, this region will not be supplied by the vessels typically targeted in nasal embolization. In those cases with cribriform erosion, the risk of stroke or complications following swelling extending into the calvarium is greatly increased. Should neoplasia be diagnosed, consultation with an oncologist is critical for developing a treatment plan and ensuring standard-of-care therapies have been discussed. Embolization can be performed with chemotherapy (see Chapter 10).

TABLE 4.1
Procedural and post-procedural medical management

- Antibiotics:
  - Intra-operative: Cefoxitin (30 mg/kg IV once, then 20 mg/kg IV q2 hr)
  - Postoperative: Clavamox (13.75 mg/kg PO BID × 14 days)
- Anti-inflammatories:
  - Intraoperative: Dexamethasone SP (0.01 mg/kg IV once at induction)
  - Postoperative: Prednisone if indicated (1 mg/kg/day PO × 3 days, then 0.5 mg/kg/day PO × 3 days, then 0.5 mg/kg/q2days PO × 3 days)
- Analgesics:
  - Perioperative: Opioid premedications
  - Postoperative: Tramadol (2–4 mg/kg PO q8–12 hr × 3–5 days

Premedications include broad-spectrum antibiotic coverage, anti-inflammatories (corticosteroids), and analgesics (Table 4.1).

Potential Risks/ Complications/ Expected Outcomes

Reported complications in humans such as pain are typically minor. More important and severe complications are uncommon and related to non-target embolization and tissue necrosis related to embolization that occurs too distally. Such procedures should therefore be attempted only by individuals with experience in embolization procedures and superselective catheterizations cranial to the aortic arch. As opposed to peripheral embolization procedures, complications specifically related to neuroembolization include stroke, blindness, and cranial nerve injury that can be devastating (Connors and Wojak, 1999). These injuries can result from non-target embolization, guide wire- and catheter-induced trauma, and pericatheter thrombosis.

An absolute contraindication to arteriography is a known severe allergy to contrast media. Relative contraindications might include coagulopathy, diminished renal function, and inability to tolerate general anesthesia. Contraindications to the embolization procedure itself include inability to selectively catheterize the bleeding vessel, visible communications to the internal carotid artery distribution or brain, and possibly bacteremia or sepsis. Additional care should be taken during catheter manipulations in previously radiated areas because local vessels are prone to rupture and dissection. In addition, because radiation results in microvascular angiopathy, there is a theoretically increased risk of embolization-induced ischemia. This risk can be minimized by less vigorous embolization (i.e., leaving more blood flow to the area), which is also performed when embolization is performed prior to radiation therapy. The owner should be made aware of the rare risk of neuroembolization which can result in post-procedural neurologic deficits, circling, ataxia, and potentially intractable seizures. This can be prevented by keeping the embolization as distal as possible and rostral to the ophthalmic artery. When a tumor is present, aberrant circulation from the mass to the brain could occur resulting in inadvertent embolization.

Clients should be informed that the embolized region (muzzle and mucous membranes depending upon target vessel) might be temporarily tender or painful to the touch for the first week. Non-steroidal anti-inflammatory drugs (NSAIDs) seem to provide sufficient analgesia (assuming no corticosteroids have been administered) but care should be taken during mucous membrane evaluation and perhaps soft foods should be recommended initially, particularly in those dogs receiving bilateral nasal embolization. In addition, while serious hemorrhage should stop immediately, there may be mild bloody mucus discharge for the first week due to discharge of previous blood clots and sloughing of superficial mucosa. These are typically dark blood clots and not bright red arterialized blood; it is important to explain the difference to the client. Warning clients that this may occur, as well as melena from swallowed and digested blood, will help reduce any potential alarm. The author has rarely appreciated very mild nasal planum tip necrosis when aggressive, bilateral embolization has been performed but this has not required any subsequent treatment.

The durability of embolization likely depends upon the disease process, target vessels, and degree of embolization performed. The author has seen dogs require repeat embolization procedures in as short as a few months to not needing them again ever or for many years (e.g., Scott syndrome). When follow-up cross-sectional imaging has been performed, there has been occasional substantial turbinate loss identified, presumably due to ischemic necrosis following embolization. In general, the procedure in dogs can be expected to generally be safe, well tolerated, and typically effective in dogs with rostral lesions (rostral to the medial canthus) when performed by people with experience performing neuroembolization procedures (Weisse, 2004).

Equipment

A list of recommended equipment can be found in Figure 4.1 and Figure 4.2. Transarterial embolization procedures require very little equipment but the fluoroscopy unit must provide adequate imaging detail to identify very small caliber vessels using digital subtraction angiography (DSA) and the ability to obtain orthogonal imaging when necessary. Failure to identify collateral vessels could lead to non-target embolization and severe consequences.

Fluoroscopic Procedure

Antimicrobials are administered perioperatively. The hair on the caudoventral portion of the abdomen, inguinal areas, and both medial thigh regions is clipped. The dog is positioned in dorsal recumbency with one hind limb extended, abducted, and secured in place to allow access to the inguinal area. The skin of the inguinal area is aseptically prepared and draped. Femoral artery access is described in detail in Chapter 44. A 4-F angled catheter[1] and 0.035-inch angled guide wire[2] combination are passed through the femoral artery sheath, into the aorta, and advanced to the common carotid artery and then the external carotid artery on the patient's affected side (Figure 4.3). A digital subtraction angiogram is performed to define the anatomic features; it is imperative that the patient's

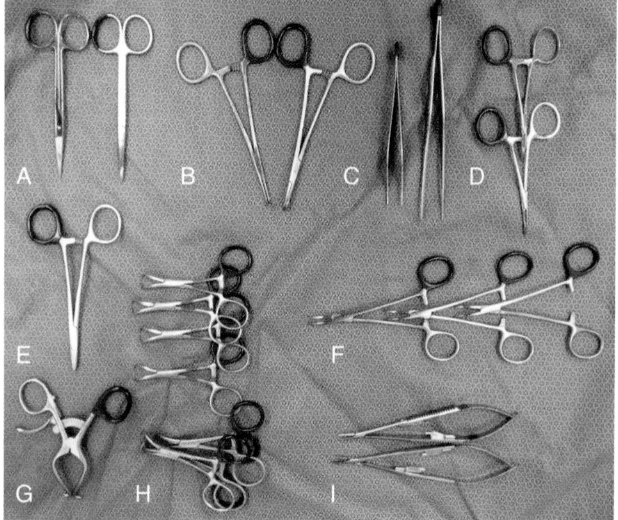

Figure 4.1 Sample surgical cut-down set. (A) Sharp-sharps and small Metzenbaum scissors. (B) Right-angled forceps. (C) Brown–Adson and Debakey forceps. (D) Mosquito hemostats. (E) Needle drivers. (F) Kelly hemostats. (G) Small Gelpi retractors. (H) Small Babcock towel clamps. (I) Castroviejo needle drivers for vessel repair.

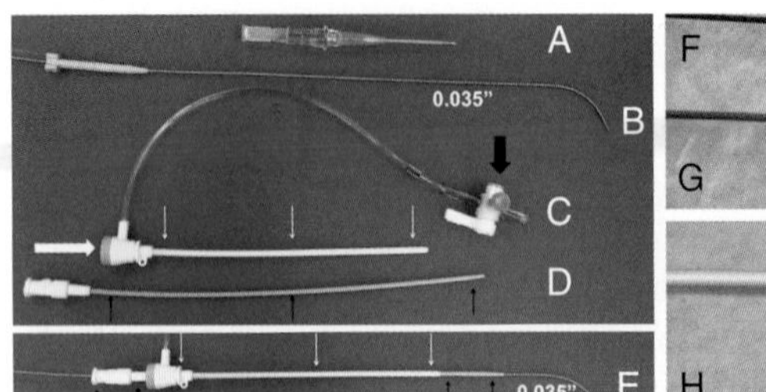

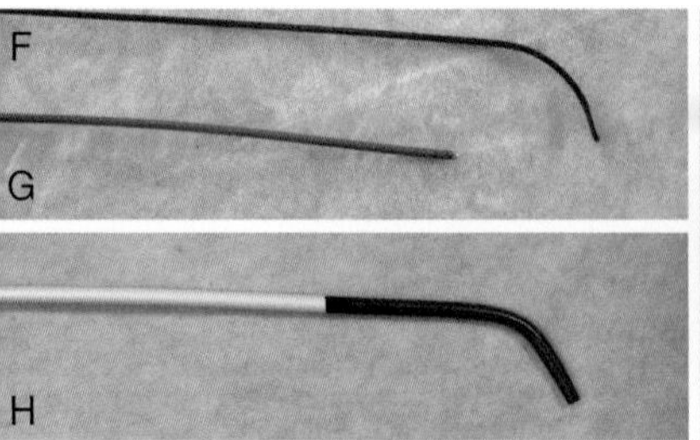

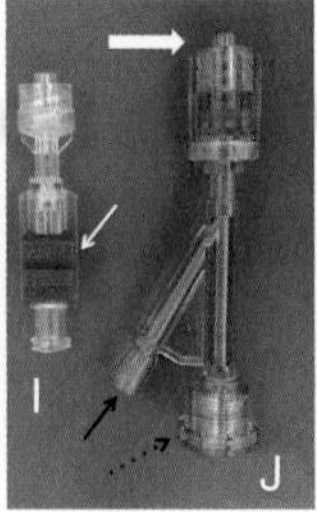

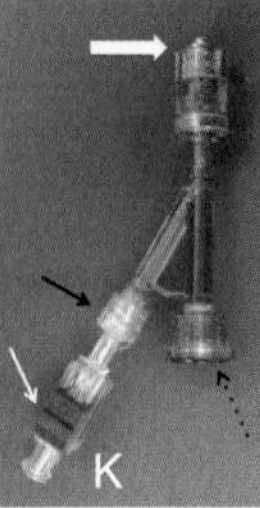

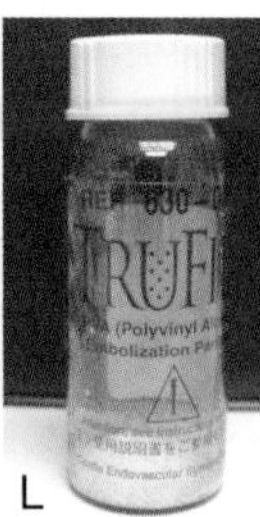

Figure 4.2 Equipment for standard neuroembolization (epistaxis) procedure. (A) 18-gauge over-the-needle catheter. (B) 0.035″ guide wire with gentle bend manual performed on shapeable tip. The bend permits operator to turn the wire during introduction if it does not pass easily. A straight wire will not change course. (C) 5Fr vascular introducer sheath made up of shaft (white arrows) with 5Fr inner diameter, hemostasis valve (white block arrow) to prevent bleeding, and three-way stopcock (black block arrow) to flush and/or aspirate. (D) 5Fr Dilator with 5Fr outer diameter shaft (black arrows). (E) Combination 5Fr vascular introducer sheath (white arrows) and dilator (black arrows) making smooth transition down to the 0.035″ guide wire. (F) 0.035″ angled, hydrophilic guide wire. (G) Standard 0.035″ Teflon guide wire. (H) 4Fr Berenstein (hockey stick) angiographic catheter. (I–K) Flo-switch (I) and Touhy-Borst adapter (J) which connect (K) to form a hemostasis valve (dotted black line) and side-port that can be switched on or off (white arrow) for flushing or aspirating. This device is attached to the hub of the 4Fr catheter (at white block arrow) and allows coaxial passage of a microcatheter/microwire through the 4Fr catheter. (L) Poly-vinyl alcohol particles (or PVA hydrogel microspheres can be used instead).

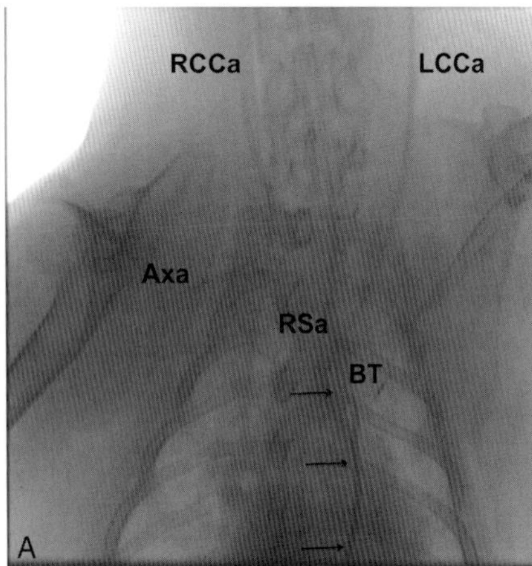

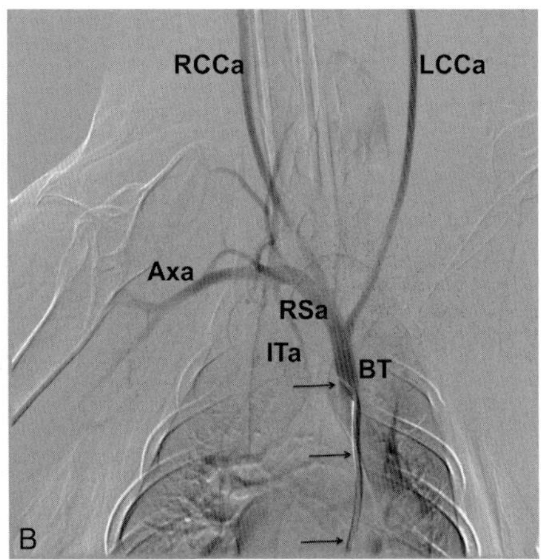

Figure 4.3 Ventrodorsal angiogram (A) and digital subtraction angiogram (B) of a dog with intractable epistaxis during embolization procedure. A 4Fr Berenstein catheter (black arrows) placed via the femoral artery has been positioned in the brachiocephalic trunk (BT). The subsequent angiograms demonstrate the right subclavian (RSa), axillary (Axa), and right (RCCa) and left (LCCa) common carotid arteries. The internal thoracic artery (ITa) is apparent on the DSA study (B).

head be positioned as evenly as possible and motionless prior to the DSA (Figure 4.4). A Touhy-Borst adapter[3] and Flo-switch[4] are attached to the 4Fr catheter. With the tip of the 4Fr catheter securely positioned in the external carotid artery, a microcatheter[5,6] and compatible angled microwire[7,8] are used to select the maxillary artery using the fluoroscopy roadmap setting.

At this point the head is rotated in a lateral position (or the c-arm rotated 90 degrees) and another angiogram is performed to define the anatomic features of the nasal cavity (Figure 4.5). The microcatheter/microwire combination is advanced beyond the origin of the external ophthalmic artery to a point just proximal to the origins of the minor palatine artery, the common trunk of the sphenopalatine and major palatine arteries, and the infraorbital artery (Figure 4.6). This location is chosen to ensure adequate embolization of the nasal cavity while sparing the external ophthalmic artery and its anastomotic ramus to the internal carotid artery. Reflux of embolization material into the external ophthalmic artery could result in blindness and stroke. More recently the author has been targeting just the sphenopalatine artery when possible as this vessel is responsible for the majority of the intranasal blood supply and therefore limits collateral non-target

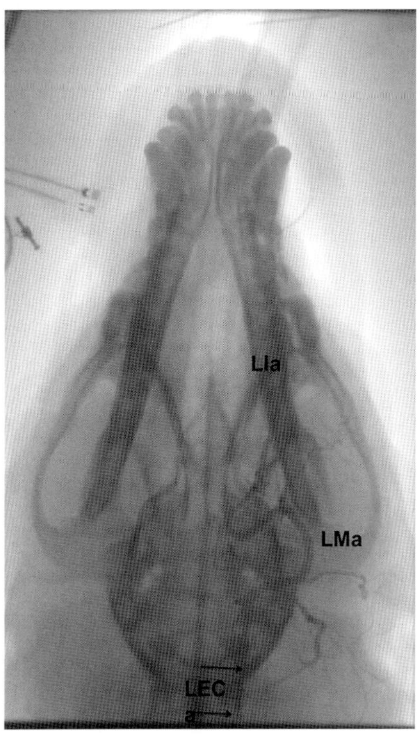

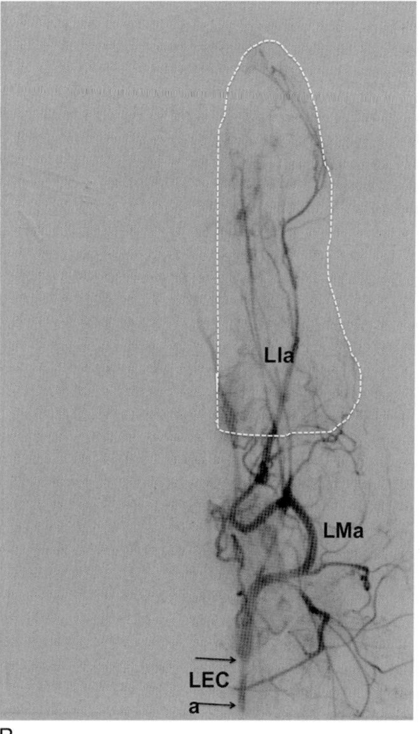

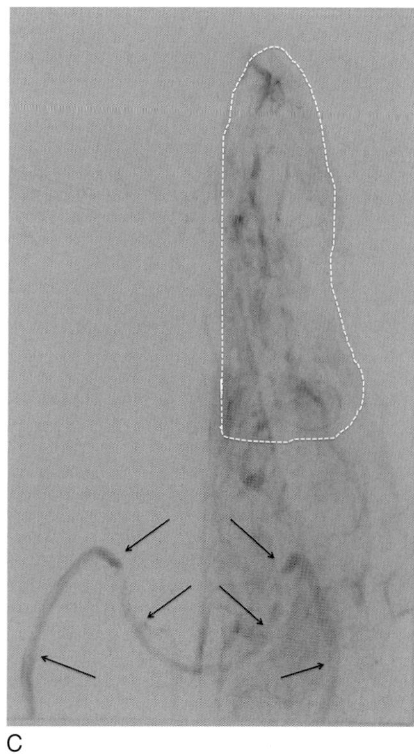

Figure 4.4 Ventrodorsal arteriogram (A), digital subtraction arteriogram (B), and digital subtraction venogram (C) of the head of a dog with intractable epistaxis. In the arteriograms (A/B), the tip of the catheter (black arrows) can be seen within the left external carotid artery (LECa). Also visible are the left maxillary (LMa) and left infraorbital (LIa) arteries. In the DSA study (B), the area supplied by the vessels to be embolized is surrounded by a white dotted line. C. This image shows the venous phase demonstrating the bilateral venous drainage (black arrows) of an angiogram performed unilaterally in the head.

embolization of the minor and major palatine arteries and the infraorbital artery. Care must be taken when selecting this vessel as it is often small and can spasm easily or the catheter can be occlusive preventing embolization. If spasm occurs, it may relax after 5 or 10 minutes. Alternatively, some have recommended infusion of lidocaine to minimize vessel spasm. If both strategies fail, one may have to treat the contralateral side first (if a bilateral case), wait longer, or return at a later date.

After proper location of the microcatheter is confirmed angiographically, embolization can be safely performed with an embolic and iohexol[9] slurry until flow through the vessels is substantially diminished angiographically (Figure 4.5 and Figure 4.6). When performing neuroembolization procedures, it is imperative to prevent air emboli due to the risk of stroke, blindness or cranial nerve damage. When removing the microwire, do so slowly and infuse saline into the hub during microwire removal to prevent the vacuum created from sucking air into to the catheter hub. Alternatively, place the hub of the catheter into a basin filled with sterile saline during microwire removal. The appropriate size of polyvinyl alcohol (PVA) or other embolization particles[11] (see Chapter 1) are chosen on the basis of vascular architecture. Use of undersized particles carries the risk of extreme distal vascular occlusion and increases the risk of necrosis and tissue sloughing. On the other hand, use of inappropriately large particles carries the risk of proximal vessel thrombosis, which may allow for development of collateral vessels that bypass the proximal occlusion and re-establish perfusion over time. In cases with spontaneous arteriovenous shunting, proximal occlusion may be preferred to mitigate the risk of embolization of particles to the lungs. In the nasal cavity, there is often rapid venous blushing from hyperemia; this must be differentiated from AV shunting. The author has used PVA-200 particles[8] (180–300 μm) or 300–500 μm PVA hydrogel microspheres[9] for nasal embolization. The chosen embolic is primed for delivery by preparing it as a slurry with iodinated contrast material. To do so using PVA, the embolic is loaded into a syringe, the plunger replaced, and all of the air evacuated to densely compact the material. This syringe is connected with a three-way stopcock to a second syringe filled with contrast material, and the

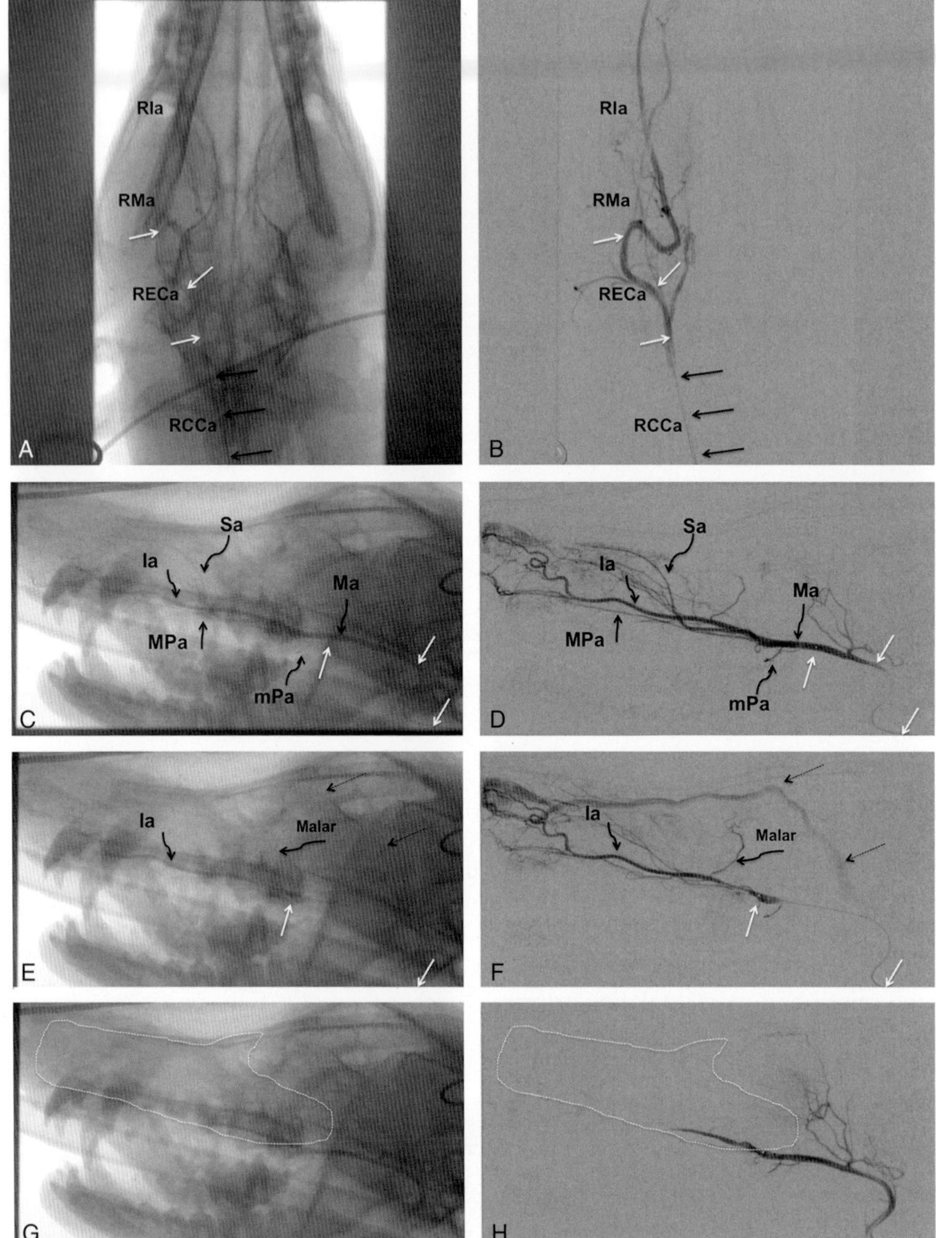

Figure 4.5 Serial fluoroscopic images of a dog with right-sided intractable epistaxis. (A/B) Right common carotid arteriogram (A) and DSA (B) with the tip of the 4Fr catheter (black arrows) in the right common carotid artery (RCCa) and the microcatheter (white arrows) passing through the right external carotid artery (RECa) up to the right maxillary artery (RMa). The right infraorbital artery (RIa) is more evident on the DSA study. (C/D) Lateral arteriogram (C) and DSA (D) through the microcatheter (white arrows) with the tip in the maxillary artery (Ma). Arterial perfusion to the muzzle is evident through the minor palatine (mPa), major palatine (MPa), infraorbital (Ia), and the sphenopalatine (Sa) arteries. (E/F) Lateral arteriogram (E) and DSA (F) through microcatheter during embolization demonstrating progressive diminished perfusion, identification of the malar artery (Malar), and venous drainage (black arrows). (G/H) Final lateral arteriogram (G) and DSA (H) demonstrating diminished perfusion to the nasal cavity (white dotted line) after embolization has been completed.

contents are vigorously mixed to form the slurry. The viscosity is adjusted by additional dilution of the PVA with sterile saline as necessary to match the caliber of the delivery catheter and the flow in the vessel to be embolized. Relatively dilute concentrations are required to prevent occlusion of microcatheters or clumping within the small caliber vessels and subsequent proximal embolization. Microspheres can just be gently mixed with a contrast/saline mixture to keep them evenly suspended.

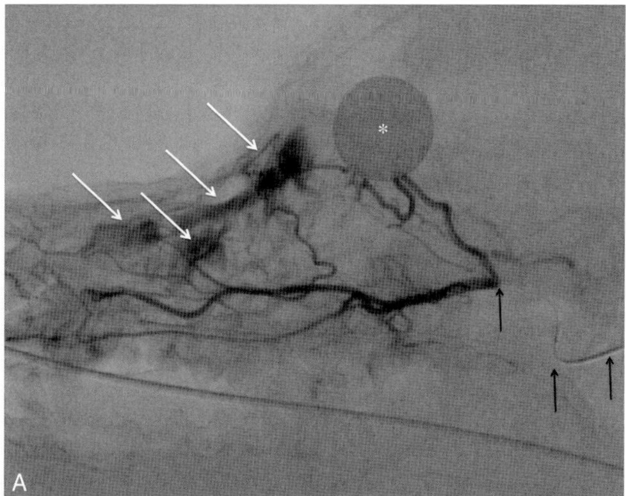

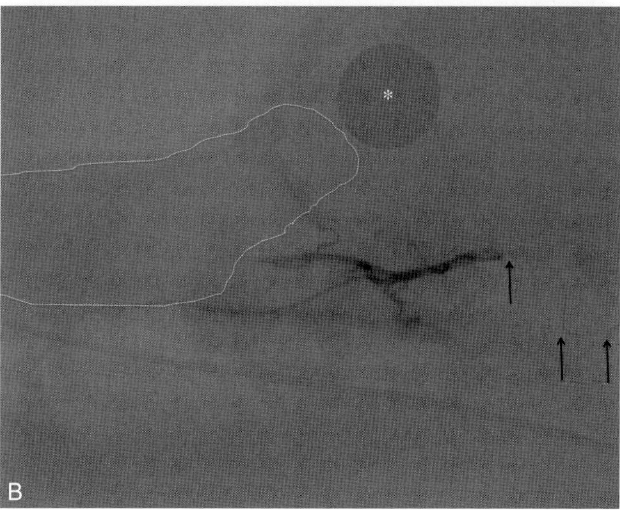

Figure 4.6 Lateral DSA studies through microcatheter (black arrows) in maxillary artery before (A) and after (B) nasal embolization. There are areas of vascular blushing/hyperemia (white arrows) before (A) embolization that no longer enhance (B) when the embolized area (white dotted line) is no longer perfused. A coin (*) was placed over the eye to locate the globe during embolization.

Embolization is performed by injecting the slurry via a 1 ml luer-lock polycarbonate syringe[12] through a selectively placed microcatheter under fluoroscopic visualization using digital roadmapping software. The slurry is radio-opaque due to the contrast mixture and can thus be seen perfusing the nasal cavity. Care is taken to prevent reflux of particles into non-target vessels. As embolization proceeds, flow decreases. Embolization is performed subjectively to near-stasis of blood flow; complete stasis is avoided to permit future embolization if hemorrhage recurs, reduce the risk of tissue necrosis, and reduce the risk of embolic material reflux and non-target embolization. Prior to complete bloodflow stasis (and periodically during the embolization procedure), the catheter is flushed of slurry by injecting saline solution gently. A gentle injection avoids flushing particles into non-target vessels. Selective arteriography is performed to evaluate the success of the procedure. If embolization is successful, little to no flow is seen in the target vessels. When performing bilateral nasal embolization, the author prefers to embolize until reduced flow is present rather than complete bloodflow stasis as bilateral embolization carries more risk of ischemic consequences. The microcatheter is withdrawn and repeat external carotid angiography is performed through the 4Fr catheter to identify persistent perfusion through other vessels or decreased perfusion elsewhere due to non-target embolization. This procedure can be repeated on the contralateral side by using the 4Fr catheter and guide wire combination to select the contralateral common carotid artery. The procedure is then repeated, as above.

Following embolization, the catheter and sheath are removed. Hemostasis of the femoral artery access site is typically achieved with femoral artery ligation. The dog is recovered in the intensive care unit for monitoring overnight. Treatment instructions include intravenous fluids at maintenance rates (unless contraindicated) or higher rates if excessive (>3 ml/kg) volumes of iodinated contrast were necessary. Analgesics are typically recommended but often not necessary; NSAIDs seem to provide sufficient palliation for any discomfort from the surgical cut-down site (unless corticosteroids have been administered prior).

Follow-Up

Patients are routinely discharged the following day. On occasion, some dogs demonstrate mild discomfort around the gums and/or muzzle on the embolized side for approximately 1 week. This is usually identified during physical examination while checking mucus membranes. Typically, NSAIDs provide sufficient analgesia. Antibiotics are prescribed for 10 days due to diminished bloodflow and possible ischemic consequences although these are uncommonly encountered. The owners are warned that passage of blood from the nose will occasionally continue for 1 week or so as blood clots are discharged and superficial mucosal sloughing occurs. Warning about possible melena due to swallowed blood will help reduce any potential alarm from the clients. Activity is limited for 2 weeks while the groin incision heals, until suture removal 10–14 days later.

Special Considerations/ Alternative Uses/ Complication Examples

The author has successfully performed nasal embolization prior to rhinotomy in one case in order to reduce intra- and post-operative hemorrhage. In some cases, surgical exploration of the nasal cavity may be necessary for diagnosis and/or treatment such as with chronic inflammatory rhinitis, foreign bodies, or neoplastic disease. Hemorrhage at the time of surgery can be minimized by temporary occlusion of the common carotid arteries (Hedlund et al., 1983) however this requires a second surgical approach and only provides temporary control of hemorrhage. Embolization was successful at reducing hemorrhage and improving visual evaluation at the time of surgery and does not require packing the nasal cavity with gauze.

If carotid ligation has been performed previously, the author has successfully accessed the ligated carotid via surgical cut-down and sheath placement rostral to the ligation weeks later. Interestingly, a pulse was present as might be expected due to the collateral blood supply, further supporting the theory that only temporary relief is provided through carotid ligation.

Notes

(Examples; Multiple vendors available)

1. Berenstein catheter, Infiniti Medical, Menlo Park, CA.
2. Weasel wire, Infiniti Medical, Menlo Park, CA.
3. Touhy–Borst adapter, Cook Medical, Bloomington, IN.
4. Flo-switch, Boston Scientific, Natick, MA.
5. Renegade or Tracker microcatheter, Boston Scientific, Natick, MA.
6. Microcatheter, Infiniti Medical, Menlo Park, CA.
7. 0.018 Transend or V-18 microwire, Boston Scientific, Natick, MA.
8. 0.014 Microwire or 0.018 Weasel wire, Infiniti Medical, Menlo Park, CA.
9. Omnipaque (iohexol) injection, Amersham Health Inc., Princeton, NJ.
10. PVA-200 particles, Cook Medical Inc., Bloomington, IN.
11. Beadblock 300–500 μm PVA hydrogel microspheres, Biocompatibles UK Limited, Farnham, UK.
12. 1 cm^3 polycarbonate syringes, Merit Medical, South Jordan, UT.

References

Clendenin, M.A., Conrad, M.C. (1979a) Collateral vessel development, following unilateral chronic carotid occlusion in the dog. *Ame J Vet Res* 40, 84–88.

Clendenin, M.A., Conrad, M.C. (1979b) Collateral vessel development after chronic bilateral common carotid artery occlusion in the dog. *Am J Vet Res* 40, 1244–1248.

Connors, J.J., Wojak, (1999) Epistaxis. In: Connors JJ, Wojak JC, eds. *Interventional Neuroradiology: Strategies and Practical Techniques*. Philadelphia: WB Saunders Co., 147–156.

Elahi, M.M., Parnes, L.S., Fox, A.J., et al. (1995) Therapeutic embolization in the treatment of intractable epistaxis. *Arch of Otolaryngol Head Neck Surg* 121, 65–69.

Hedlund, C.S., Tanger, C.H., Elkins, A.D., et al. (1983) Temporary bilateral carotid artery occlusion during surgical exploration of the nasal cavity of the dog. *Vet Surg* 12, 83–85.

Mahony, O. (2000) Bleeding disorders: epistaxis and hemoptysis. In: Ettinger SJ, Feldman EC, eds. *Textbook of Veterinary Internal Medicine.* 5th ed. Philadelphia: WB Saunders Co, 213–218.

Schaitkin, B., Strauss, M., Houck, J.K. (1987) Epistaxis: medical versus surgical therapy: a comparison of efficacy, complications, and economic considerations. *Laryngoscope* 97, 1392–1397.

Vitek, J. (1991) Idiopathic intractable epistaxis: endovascular therapy. *Radiology* 181, 113–116.

Weisse, C., Nicholson, M.E., Rollings, C., et al. (2004) Use of percutaneous arterial embolization for treatment of intractable epistaxis in three dogs. *J AmVet Med Assoc* 224[8]), 1307–11.

Suggested Reading

Brooks MB, Catafamo JL, Brown HA, et al (2002) A hereditary bleeding disorder of dogs caused by a lack of platelet procoagulant activity. *Blood* 99, 2434–41.

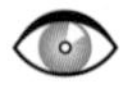 Video clips to accompany this chapter can be found in the online material at **www.wiley.com/go/weisse/vet-image-guided-interventions**

CHAPTER FIVE

Nasal/Sinus Tumors

William T.N. Culp
School of Veterinary Medicine, University of California – Davis, Davis, CA

Background/Indications

Neoplasia affecting the nasal cavity and paranasal sinuses is uncommon. Carcinomas are the most frequently diagnosed tumor of the nasal cavity, however other tumor types including chondrosarcoma, fibrosarcoma, osteosarcoma, squamous cell carcinoma and mast cell tumor have also been diagnosed (Henry et al., 1998, Kondo et al., 2008, Mellanby et al., 2002, Rassnick et al., 2006). Most dogs with nasal neoplasia are evaluated for clinical signs secondary to local disease including epistaxis, sneezing, and/or facial deformity. Metastatic disease is uncommon at the time of diagnosis (Rassnick et al., 2006). Euthanasia is often performed due to progression of local disease; the treatment of local disease is therefore the primary recommended course of action (Adams et al., 1987, Buchholz et al., 2009, Evans et al., 1989, Henry et al., 1998, LaDue et al., 1999, Lana et al., 2004, Rassnick et al., 2006, Theon et al., 1993).

Several treatment modalities have been proposed and reported in the veterinary literature including surgery, chemotherapy, immunotherapy and several versions of radiation therapy (Buchholz et al., 2009, Evans et al., 1989, Mellanby et al., 2002, Theon et al., 1993). While surgery as a single treatment option has been reported, radiation therapy is considered by most as the current treatment of choice (Buchholz et al., 2009, Evans et al., 1989, LaDue et al., 1999, MacEwen et al., 1977, Theon et al., 1993). Outcomes with radiation therapy are likely dependent on the tumor type, grade, and stage, as well as the timing and type of radiation therapy utilized. Reported median survival times range from 4.9 to 23.4 months (Adams et al., 2009, Buchholz et al., 2009, Hunley et al., 2010, LaDue et al., 1999, Mellanby et al., 2002, Northrup et al., 2001, Gieger et al., 2008). Due to poor long-term outcomes, it is necessary to investigate alternative treatment options that may improve the prognosis of dogs affected with nasal/sinus neoplasia.

Encouraging outcomes have been reported in two separate canine studies evaluating the use of slow release cisplatin in combination with radiation therapy for the treatment of nasal tumors suggesting an advantage of combination therapies (Lana et al., 1997, 2004). In the first study, a slow release delivery system containing cisplatin was placed intramuscularly, and the dogs received a median total radiation dose of 49.5 Gy (Lana et al., 1997). The median survival times in these dogs was 580 days which was significantly longer than the median survival time in a group of historical control dogs (325 days) (Lana et al., 1997). A follow-up study reported a median survival time of 474 days in the dogs receiving slow release cisplatin and radiation therapy. No other factors (including tumor type, disease stage and invasion into the cribriform plate) significantly affected survival (Lana et al., 2004).

Intra-arterial delivery of chemotherapy is a commonly utilized technique in human patients with head and neck cancers (Lee et al., 1989, Robbins et al., 2005, Samant et al., 1999). There are several advantages to delivering chemotherapy directly into the tumor bed. When intra-arterial chemotherapy is delivered directly to a tumor, the tumor receives markedly higher concentrations of chemotherapy as compared to intravenous administration (Eckman et al., 1974, Stephens, 1983, von Scheel and Golde, 1984). Additionally, the side effects associated with certain chemotherapy administration tend to occur less commonly when delivered intra-arterially (Eckman et al., 1974, Stephens, 1983, von Scheel and Golde, 1984).

The use of intra-arterial chemotherapy for the treatment of nasal/sinus tumors in veterinary patients has only been reported in one case in combination with the delivery of an embolic agent (chemoembolization). In this cat, chemoembolization was pursued as part of

Veterinary Image-Guided Interventions, First Edition. Edited by Chick Weisse and Allyson Berent.

Companion website: www.wiley.com/go/weisse/vet-image-guided-interventions

the treatment of a cystic nasal adenocarcinoma and the superficial temporal artery was embolized (Marioni-Henry et al., 2007). Embolization has been utilized in the treatment of dogs with idiopathic epistaxis (non-oncologic disease), and the technique utilized in that study is similar to what is described here for oncologic disease (Weisse et al., 2004).

Many human tumors in various locations are treated on a regular basis with thermal ablation techniques including radiofrequency ablation, cryoablation, microwave ablation, and laser ablation. Generally speaking, the thermal ablation treatment options work through the destruction of tumor cells that are within the limited treatment zone of the ablation probe (Simon et al., 2005). Chemical ablation with ethanol, hot saline and acetic acid is also performed in human patients (Moser et al., 2008); however, the current applications for veterinary patients have been limited to date (Murphy et al., 2011).

Patient Preparation

It is recommended for all patients that are undergoing anesthesia to undergo clinical laboratory testing such as a complete blood count, biochemistry profile, and urinalysis. As patients with nasal/sinus tumors often present for epistaxis, evaluation of coagulation profiles and platelet-function testing should also be considered to rule-out the presence of other diseases. While metastatic disease is not a common finding early in the treatment of nasal tumors, chest radiographs are recommended to evaluate for spread of cancer to the pulmonary parenchyma or for the presence of other intrathoracic disease. Additionally, as many cases of nasal neoplasia occur in older companion animals, abdominal ultrasonography can be performed to evaluate the patient for comorbidities.

Specific characterization of the nasal/sinus tumor and the associated vascularity is regularly performed with a computerized tomography (CT) scan, particularly multiple phase CT-angiography when available, to assess tumor vascularity. Cross sectional imaging provides improved detail compared to routine radiography and/or rhinoscopy, and reveals the presence of cribriform plate lysis and local lymphadenopathy. Several systems have been utilized in veterinary patients to stage nasal tumors and two recent examples are discussed below. The first is a modified World Health Organization (WHO) system described by Adams et al. (1998) for dogs, and this utilizes four stages. Dogs in this study with stage 1 or 2 had a longer relapse free interval and longer median survival times than dogs with stage 3 or 4 (Adams et al., 1998). The four stages identified included:

- Stage 1: Tumor is confined to one nasal passage, paranasal sinus or frontal sinus, with no bony involvement
- Stage 2: Any bony involvement, but with no evidence of orbit, subcutaneous, or submucosal mass
- Stage 3: Involvement of orbit, or a subcutaneous, or submucosal mass
- Stage 4: Tumor extension into nasopharynx or cribriform plate.

The CT-based tumor staging system (Kondo et al., 2008) evaluates six parameters evaluated on the CT images including: (1) tumor invasion to the bilateral nasal/paranasal sinus, (2) nasal bone destruction and tumor growth on the nasal planum or face, (3) involvement of the oral cavity with destruction of the hard palate, (4) orbital involvement with lateral compression of the orbit, (5) frontal sinus involvement, and (6) brain involvement with the destruction of the cranium or the cribriform plate. In this staging system, dogs with Stage 1 do not have any of the above six parameters noted on CT. Dogs with Stage 2 have one of the findings in (1–5) and dogs with Stage 3 have two or more of these findings. Dogs with parameter (6) are considered Stage 4. Similar to the above study, dogs with lower CT stages had improved median survival times as compared to dogs with higher CT stages.

As with all oncologic cases, it is important to develop a team-based approach when treating nasal and sinus tumors. The interventional techniques utilized for these tumors (see below) involve detailed discussions about potential chemotherapy agents that may be administered during the procedures as well as the potential for combination of intra-arterial chemotherapy and intravenous chemotherapy. Additionally, some of the interventional procedures may be considered in addition to procedures that are more regularly utilized such as radiation therapy. Active communication between members of the medical oncology, radiation oncology, surgical oncology and interventional oncology teams is crucial to maximize the success of the chosen treatment (see Chapter 3 for more information).

Potential Risks/Complications/Expected Outcomes

When an embolization procedure is being considered for tumors above (cranial to) the aortic arch, it is absolutely crucial that vascular selection is accurate and the delivery of embolic agents is executed precisely. Many

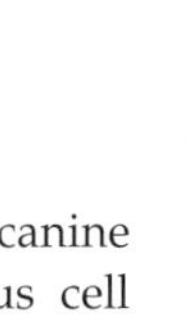

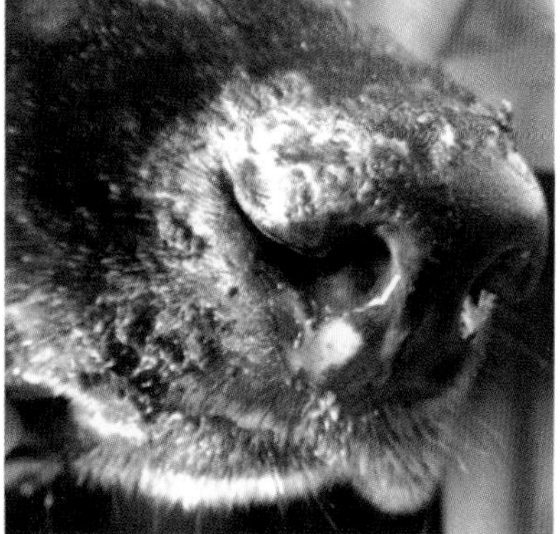

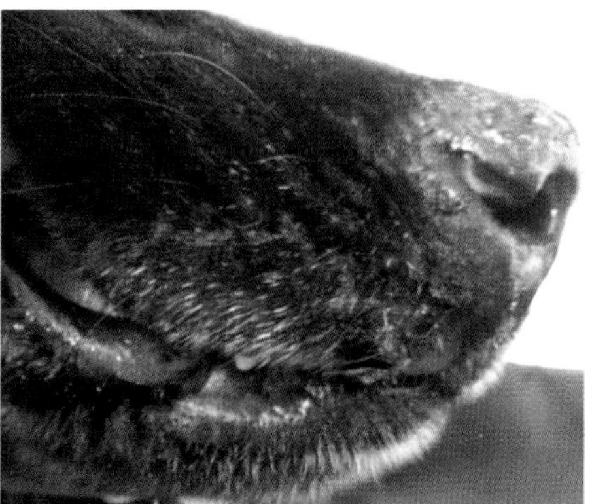

Figure 5.1 Muzzle of a canine patient with a nasal squamous cell carcinoma. (A) Note the depigmentation and scaling of the nostril. (B) The rostral lip margin has been partially devascularized and a section of skin has undergone necrosis.

of the vessels above the aortic arch communicate, and the potential end-organ for these procedures is the brain. As such, stroke is a major complication that can occur secondary to an embolization in this region if non-target injection of an embolic agent occurs; it is highly recommended that an excellent understanding of the anatomy in this region and experience with this procedure be obtained prior to pursuing embolizations above the aortic arch. Additionally, the injection of air should be avoided. Due to the close proximity of the eye and cranial nerves, blindness and cranial nerve injury is possible. Skin necrosis can occur (Figure 5.1) and while this injury often resolves with time, repair of the necrotic region may be required due to extensive tissue sloughing. Many dogs appear to have muzzle tenderness post-embolization and may occasionally paw at the nasal cavity or overlying skin temporarily following the procedure.

A clinician considering the use of an image-guided procedure in the treatment of nasal/sinus neoplasia should evaluate the CT images closely in regards to the vascular supply of the tumor and the surrounding structures. Patients that have penetration of the cribriform plate are generally not considered suitable candidates for intravascular therapies due to the risk associated with non-target embolization of the brain (with subsequent stroke/ischemia) or post-procedural swelling. Additionally, the owners of patients with tumor extension through the palate or bones of the maxilla should be forewarned that a positive response to therapy may result in an oronasal fistula or open exposure of the nasal cavity.

When chemotherapy is included in the treatment protocol, clients should be warned of the general side effects and complications that can be encountered. Some dogs may experience the typical chemotherapy side effects including neutropenia and/or the development of gastrointestinal side effects such as nausea, anorexia, vomiting, diarrhea and lethargy. While rare, clients should also be warned about the potential for immediate toxicity due to infusion hypersensitivity as well as sepsis and death secondary to chemotherapy administration.

Intravascular Therapies

Intra-arterial Chemotherapy and Embolization/Chemoembolization

Equipment

Some recommended equipment is shown in Figure 5.2, and the application of this equipment can be found in the section describing the procedure. The use of fluoroscopy, and if available, concurrent CT-angiography or magnetic resonance imaging-angiography is essential to perform intravascular therapies of nasal tumors. As a surgical approach is utilized, a basic surgical pack and sterile drapes are needed.

Relevant anatomy and fluoroscopic procedure

An intimate knowledge of the vascular anatomy and associated structures is mandatory prior to performing neurointerventional procedures (Figure 5.3). The external carotid artery branches off the common carotid artery bilaterally and provides the arterial blood to the ipsilateral half of the head. Several branches of the external carotid artery exist with the largest of the terminal branches being the maxillary artery (Evans, 1993). The maxillary artery has three major components: mandibular portion, pterygoid portion, and pterygopalatine portion (Evans, 1993). The pterygopalatine portion is the component that supplies the majority of the nasal cavity and sinuses. Several branches of the pterygopalatine portion of the maxillary artery should be avoided with superselective catheterization when pursuing embolization/chemoembolization of the nasal cavity or sinuses including the external ophthalmic artery (supplies

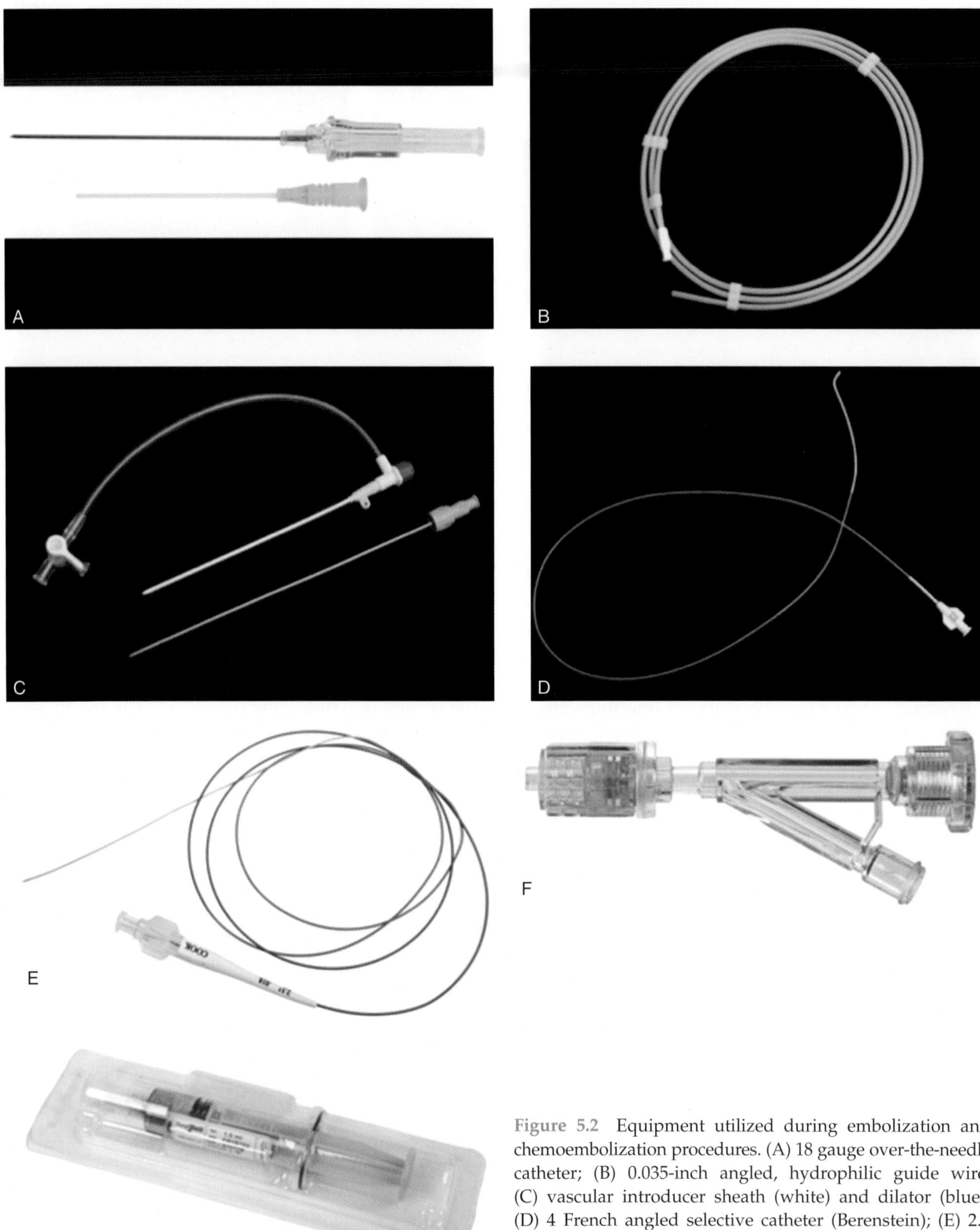

Figure 5.2 Equipment utilized during embolization and chemoembolization procedures. (A) 18 gauge over-the-needle catheter; (B) 0.035-inch angled, hydrophilic guide wire; (C) vascular introducer sheath (white) and dilator (blue); (D) 4 French angled selective catheter (Berenstein); (E) 2.5 French microcatheter; (F) Touhy–Borst adapter; (G) Polyvinyl alcohol particles (Bead Block).

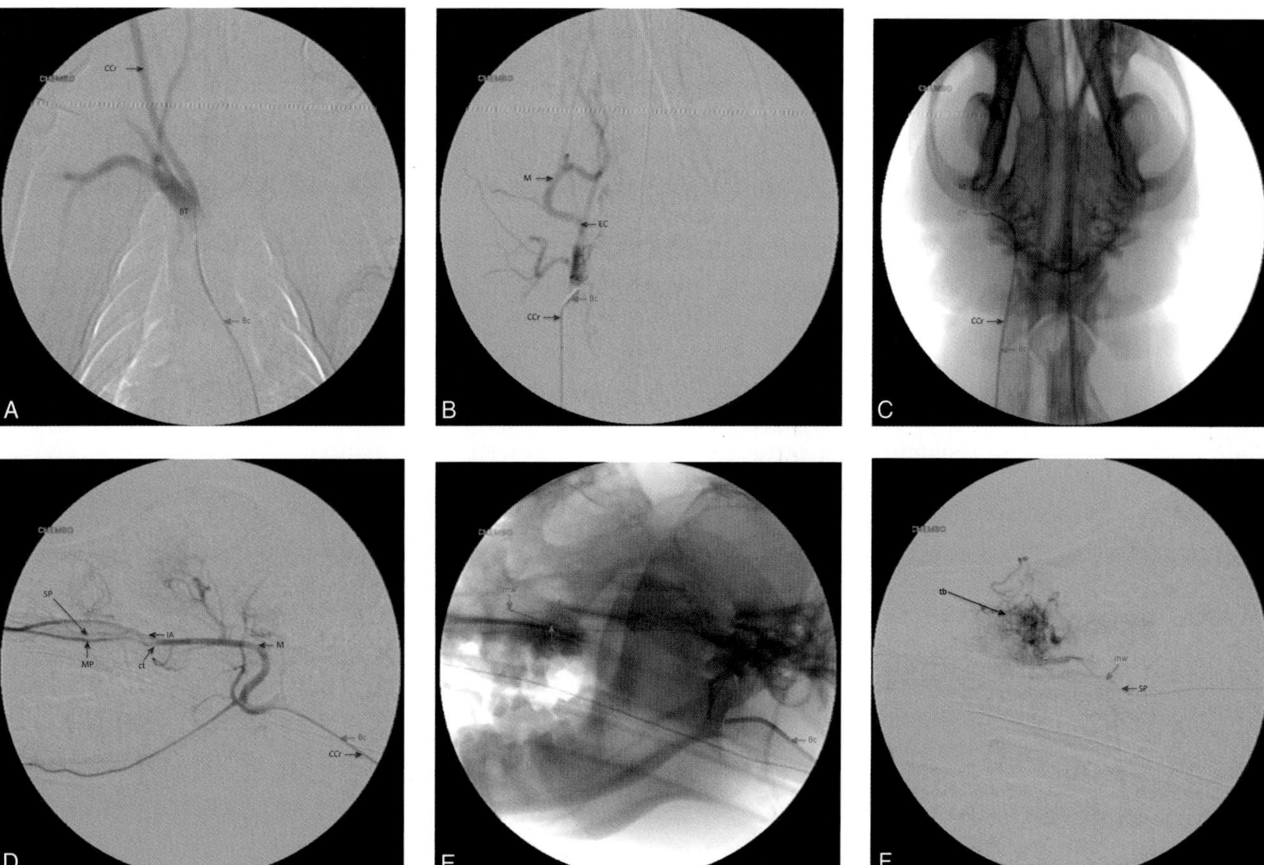

Figure 5.3 (A) Dorsoventral projection of the cranial chest and caudal cervical region. Femoral arterial access has been established in this dog who is undergoing chemoembolization of a nasal squamous cell carcinoma. A Berenstein catheter (Bc) has been passed to the level of the brachiocephalic trunk (BT) at the point of branching of the right common carotid artery (CCr), and an angiogram (subtracted) has been performed. (B) Dorsoventral projection of the cranial neck and caudal skull region. In Image B, a Berenstein catheter (Bc) has been advanced into the right common carotid artery (CCr) and a subtracted angiogram has been performed. The external carotid artery (EC) branch is continuing rostrally, and the maxillary artery (M) is branching directly off this vessel. (C) Dorsoventral projection of the cranial neck and caudal skull region. Image C is an unsubtracted image showing much of the same anatomy as Image B. In this image, the Berenstein catheter (Bc) has been advanced from the right common carotid artery (CCr) into the external carotid artery (EC) and a guide wire (gw) has been used to select the maxillary artery (M). (D) Lateral projection of the head. After selection of the maxillary artery with the Berenstein catheter, the patient is positioned in lateral recumbency. Image D shows the position of the Berenestein catheter (Bc) extending from the right common carotid artery (CCr) into the maxillary artery (M). An angiogram has been performed through the Berenstein catheter and the branches of the maxillary artery can be seen: infraorbital (IA) and the common trunk (ct) of the major palatine (MP) and the sphenopalatine (SP). (E) Lateral projection of the head. Image E is an unsubtracted image demonstrating the position of the Berenstein catheter (Bc) and the microcatheter (mc) and associated microwire (mw) that have been passed through the Berenstein catheter into the infraoribital artery (IA). (F) Lateral projection of the head. In this subtracted image, a microwire (mw) has been advanced into the sphenopalatine artery (SP) and an angiogram has been performed. The tumor blush (tb) can be clearly identified in this region, and chemoembolization can be pursued in this vessel as no non-target vessels are opacifying.

orbit and anastomoses with skull vessels), rostral deep temporal artery (supplies temporal muscle), buccal artery (supplies medial pterygoid muscle, masseter muscle, temporal muscle, buccinator muscles, and zygomatic gland) and minor palatine (supplies hard and soft palate and palatine glands) (Evans, 1993). The maxillary artery terminates in three major arteries that are the focus of a nasal embolization/chemoembolization procedure; these arteries include the sphenopalatine and major palatine arteries that share a common trunk and the infraorbital artery (Evans, 1993). The major palatine artery supplies the mucosa of the oral surface of the hard palate, the periosteum and the alveolar bone, and anastomoses exist with the sphenopalatine artery and lateral nasal artery (Evans, 1993). The major palatine artery also gives off the rostral septal branches that supply the nasal septum (Evans, 1993). The sphenopalatine artery supplies the mucoperiosteum of the side and floor of the nasal fossa, the nasal septum, nasal conchae and nasolacrimal duct (Evans, 1993). The branches of the infraorbital artery (malar, rostral dorsal alveolar, middle dorsal alveolar, caudal dorsal alveolar, lateral nasal, and dorsal nasal) supply the alveolar canals of the teeth as well as the muzzle (Evans, 1993).

With many intra-arterial chemotherapy and embolization/chemoembolization procedures, complete ventilatory control by the anesthetic team is necessary (e.g., liver embolization/chemoembolization) to allow for angiography to be performed without image disruption. This is generally not necessary in nasal/sinus tumor cases once access of the external carotid artery has been achieved. Neuromuscular-blocking agents such as succinylcholine and the aminosteroids are also generally not necessary in these cases. Opioid medications should be considered as part of the premedication and post-procedure drug protocols of these patients to assist with pain control.

The arterial supply of the nasal and sinus cavities can be accessed through the carotid or femoral artery. The author prefers femoral arterial access as both carotid arteries can be selected during the procedure to allow for bilateral treatment. Patients are placed in dorsal recumbency at the initiation of the procedure, and both inguinal regions are clipped and prepared with aseptic technique. The patient is draped, and the fluoroscopy unit is placed over the abdomen to allow for monitoring of guide wire passage from the femoral artery into the aorta.

When performing embolization of a nasal or sinus tumor, the treating clinician will need to decide if the goal is to cause vascular stasis of the blood supply to the tumor. When an embolization is performed, vascular recanalization may or may not occur. If this occurs, further treatment of the tumor through the previously embolized blood vessel is possible; if the vessel remains embolized, further treatment of that tumor is no longer possible. However, many clients may not have the opportunity to perform multiple locoregional procedures and an attempt to alter the tumor vascularity as much as possible (via complete stasis) may be elected in those cases.

The method for arterial vascular access can be found in Chapter 51. The largest catheter utilized during nasal/sinus intra-arterial chemotherapy or embolization is generally 4–5 French in diameter; therefore, a 5 French vascular access sheath[1] in the femoral artery is recommended. Once the vascular access sheath is in place, vascular selection can commence with fluoroscopic-guidance.

A guide wire (hydrophilic 0.035-inch angled)[2] is passed through the vascular access sheath into the femoral artery and further into the aorta. The fluoroscopy unit generally needs to be repositioned over the chest to allow for visualization of the aortic arch and the bifurcation into the brachiocephalic trunk and the left subclavian artery. A catheter with an angled-tip (a 4–5 French Berenstein catheter)[3] is passed over the guide wire to the point of the bifurcation. The brachiocephalic trunk is selected with the guide wire and catheter combination, and further selection of either the left or right common carotid artery is performed, depending on the side that is going to be treated. If selection of the blood vessels is difficult or vascular localization is not possible, a contrast arteriogram can be performed by removing the guide wire from the catheter and injecting a contrast[4]/saline mixture (generally 50%/50%) to obtain a vascular map. Extreme care must be exercised during neurointerventional procedures as air or clot emboli can have severe consequences in this region.

Once the appropriate common carotid artery has been selected, the catheter and guide wire combination is passed into the external carotid artery and further into the maxillary artery. The 4 or 5 French catheter remains in the relatively larger external carotid artery and a coaxially placed microcatheter[5] is used for all further vessel selections. An alternative technique to consider is placement of the catheter in the common carotid artery and utilization of the microcatheter to select the external carotid artery and subsequently the maxillary artery. Once the maxillary artery has been selected, the vascular anatomy is more easily evaluated with a lateral projection, and the patient's head is turned from dorsal recumbency into lateral recumbency, or the C-arm is repositioned (Figure 5.3). A Touhy–Borst adapter[6] with attached flow switch[7] is attached to the hub of the Berenstein catheter. A microwire (0.010-inch or 0.014-inch)[8] is passed into the microcatheter (1.9 French to 2.7 French), and the combination is passed through the Touhy-Borst adapter and into the Berenstein catheter after removal of the 0.035-inch guide wire. The microwire and microcatheter combination are passed from the maxillary artery to the point of trifurcation of the maxillary artery into the major palatine, sphenopalatine and infraorbital arteries. The microcatheter should be secured in position with the Touhy–Borst adapter, and an arteriogram obtained at this point to assess the local vascular anatomy and tumor location. While this positioning is generally used for intractable epistaxis when the location of the lesion is unknown, a more specific super selective location may need to be chosen for nasal/sinus tumors.

When administering intra-arterial chemotherapy, the operator should decide if the dose will be divided between the left and right side of the patient. If administering only intra-arterial chemotherapy, the blood supply to the tumor should be selected with the microcatheter. The chemotherapeutic agent is mixed with contrast to allow for visual monitoring of the delivery of chemotherapy; chemotherapy delivery should be performed slowly with the intention of delivering maximum chemotherapy dose directly to the tumor, minimizing reflux.

In preparation for the delivery of chemotherapy, several precautions should be taken. Any personnel within the catheterization laboratory should be wearing hand and eye protection as well as a protective gown. The surgical site should be isolated with gowns or towels designed for chemotherapy safety. A separate region of the sterile instrument table should be established to prevent contamination of all equipment with chemotherapy. Syringes designed for chemotherapy should be utilized.

If an embolic agent is to be administered in combination with the chemotherapy (chemoembolization), selection of the appropriate vessel is critical. Once the blood vessel or vessels supplying the tumor are selected, the microcatheter is locked in place by gently securing the microcatheter with the Touhy–Borst adapter.

The chemotherapy should be mixed with an agent for contrast enhancement, which may include either an iodinated contrast material or ethiodized oil (see Chapter 23). Very little ethiodized oil is necessary; excessive amounts will lead to premature embolization. These materials can be combined by utilizing syringes of each that have been attached to a three-way stopcock. When this combination has been obtained, a separate syringe containing embolic particles (generally polyvinyl alcohol particles or microspheres)[9] can then be attached to the three-way stopcock; the author generally utilizes 100–300 µm or 300–500 µm polyvinyl alcohol particles for nasal/sinus embolization. A combined slurry of the embolic agent, chemotherapy and contrast agent is then created and individual treatments can be suctioned into 1 mL polycarbonate chemotherapy-safe syringes[10] for delivery. When delivering the slurry, it is crucial to inject slowly and closely monitor the flow of the injection to prevent non-target embolization or reflux of the injected material.

After the procedure, pain control is recommended. Patients may experience discomfort in the nasal/sinus region. The author generally administers opioid pain medication for approximately 24 hours post-procedure, as well as non-steroidal anti-inflammatories (NSAIDs), if no contraindications exist. Patients are often sent home with tramadol and/or an NSAID for continued pain relief. Alternatively, steroids may be utilized instead of NSAIDs in some cases. In cases where chemotherapy has been administered, the clinician should also consider prescribing anti-emetics and anti-diarrhea medications.

Ablation Therapies

Equipment

Several radiofrequency and cryoablation units are available; examples include the Covidien Cool-tip™ RF Ablation System[11] and Galil Medical Cryoablation System[12] (Figure 5.4 and Figure 5.5). For radiofrequency ablation procedures a generator is required as well as grounding pads and probes for delivering the radiofrequency waves. For cryoablation procedures, the argon and helium gases are both required in sufficient tank volumes; generally two tanks should be available per procedure.

Image-Guided Procedure

Discussion will be focused on the use of radiofrequency ablation and cryoablation, as these have been the most frequently explored options in veterinary medicine. Ablation procedures are performed with the patient under general anesthesia. When performing these procedures for the treatment of nasal or sinus tumors, ultrasound or CT guidance should be utilized. These imaging modalities allow the clinician performing the treatment to specifically place probes within the tumor tissue, and often probes are able to be placed transnasally. For both therapies, the goal is to cause destruction of tumor tissue and increase the zone affected by the thermal ablation beyond the visible tumor as detected by either ultrasonography or CT. When systems allow, several probes can be placed to cause an overlapping of the treated fields.

When utilizing radiofrequency ablation, a radiofrequency generator produces a current that is delivered through an electrode (Moser et al., 2008). The current generates heat, which results in subsequent cell necrosis

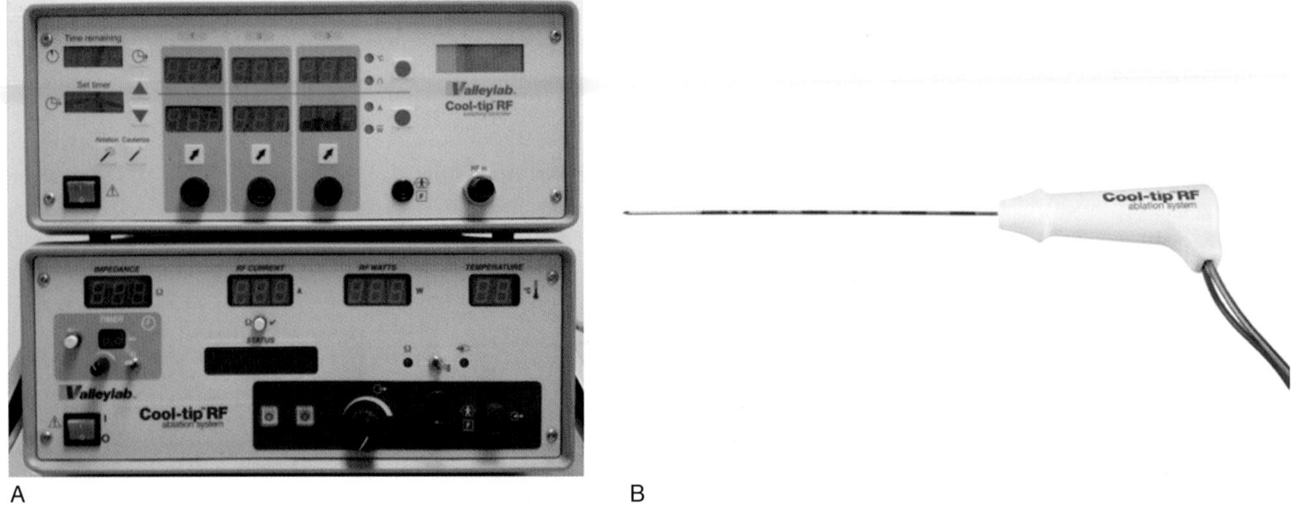

Figure 5.4 Cool-tip RF™ Ablation System, Covidien, Mansfield, MA. (A) Generator; (B) electrode.

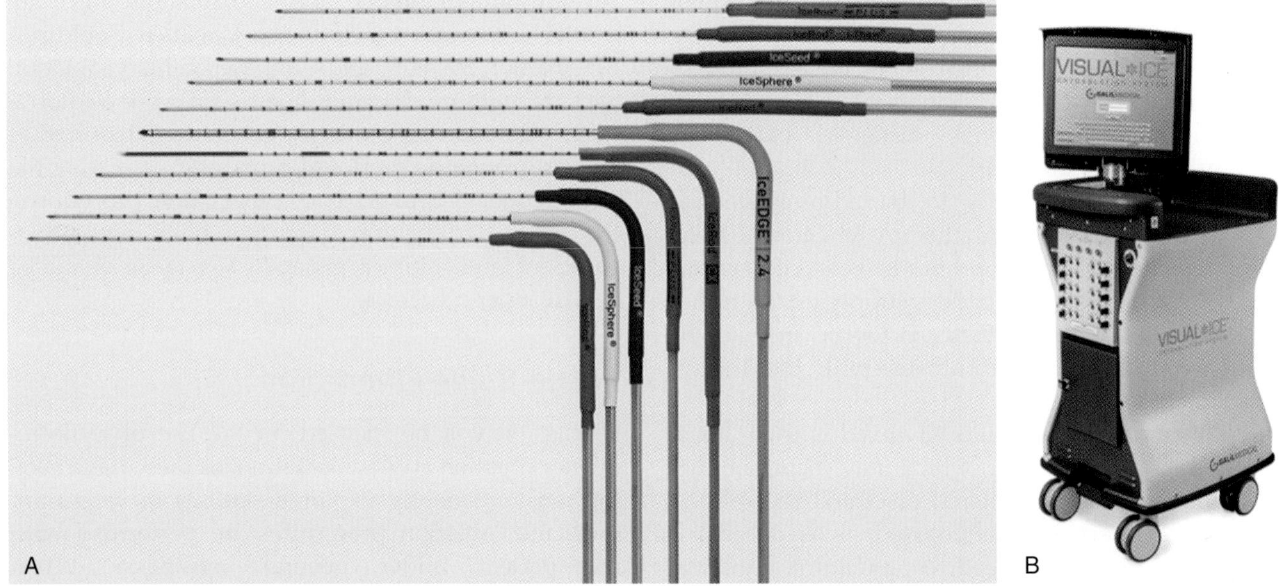

Figure 5.5 SeedNet™ Cryoablation System, Galil Medical Inc., Arden Hills, MN. (A) Electrodes; (B) generator.

(D'Ippolito and Goldberg, 2002, Mahnken et al., 2009). When a monopolar system is utilized a single probe is inserted into the tumor; bipolar systems are also available (D'Ippolito and Goldberg, 2002).

Current techniques of cryoablation require the use of two gases: argon and helium. With the use of ultrasonography or CT, the probe or probes are positioned within the tumor tissue. A single large probe generally results in the formation of an ice ball that is approximately 3.5 cm diameter, but varying sizes and shapes of ice balls can be generating using a variety of available probes (Callstrom and Kurup, 2009, Moser et al., 2008). The argon is administered through the cryoprobe to cause a rapid freeze. After a period of freezing, the helium is then administered through the probe to result in active thawing (Padma et al., 2009). Most recommendations for freeze–thaw cycles include a period of 10 minutes of freezing followed by 5 minutes of thawing; however, the freeze time can be altered as the size of the ice ball is monitored by the chosen imaging modality (ultrasonography or CT) (Callstrom and Kurup, 2009). After the thawing period, freezing of the lesion should again be performed (10 minutes) (Callstrom and Kurup, 2009, Moser et al.,

2008). The operator should allow the probe to warm prior to removal (Callstrom and Kurup, 2009, Moser et al., 2008).

A case report of the use of cryoablation to treat canine nasal tumors exists (Murphy et al., 2011). In this study, a dog was treated with transnasal cryoablation and the response was monitored by CT. The ice ball region appeared to respond as eventual resolution of the primary tumor volume was noted. Long-term clinical signs were limited to mild chronic nasal discharge, and the dog was eventually euthanatized for separate disease (Murphy et al., 2011). Studies evaluating the use of chemical ablation in the treatment of companion animals with nasal/sinus neoplasia are lacking.

Follow-Up

Patients with nasal or sinus tumors that have been treated with an image-guided therapy can be monitored via several techniques. As many of these patients are originally evaluated for clinical signs, the improvement of signs such as epistaxis, epiphora, nasal discharge, and sneezing should be noted. However, signs such as nasal discharge and sneezing may persist secondary to the impact of the image-guided treatment on the tumor.

Advanced imaging is likely the best method for assessing tumor response and tumor volume. A post-treatment CT scan is generally performed in the author's practice at a time period of 4–12 weeks post-treatment. The post-treatment CT scan is utilized to assess the response to the treatment as well as to determine if further therapies can be considered.

As chemotherapy may have some impact on nasal/sinus tumors (Lana et al., 1997, 2004), the administration of intra-venous chemotherapy in-between image-guided therapies can be considered. Appropriate timing of chemotherapy is still essential to prevent excessive side effects or diminished quality of life. As stated above, communication with other members of the oncologic treatment team is essential with these cases.

Special Considerations/ Alternative Uses/ Complication Examples

When an image-guided option is going to be pursued in the treatment of a nasal or sinus tumor, the treating clinician must consider which of the above options is most appropriate. One of the first choices is whether chemotherapy should be administered to a particular patient. Owners should be aware of the potential complications that can occur with chemotherapy administration, and the use of these agents may not be appropriate in all cases. In patients with epistaxis secondary to the tumor, embolization offers the added benefit of cessation of bleeding in addition to tumor devascularization. Ablation procedures require specialized equipment; while specific instrumentation is utilized for intra-arterial chemotherapy and embolization/chemoembolization cases, this equipment is generally significantly less expensive. The use of intra-arterial chemotherapy or embolization/chemoembolization is contraindicated in cases with cribriform plate destruction; however, the use of ablation also carries the risk of significant swelling post-treatment that can result in a negative outcome in cases of cribriform plate erosion as well.

In some cases, increased efficacy of the procedure can lead to new complications. While the infraorbital artery often provides some of the blood supply to a tumor, this vessel also supplies the skin of the muzzle. When this artery is embolized, devascularization of the muzzle skin can also occur leading to necrosis and skin sloughing (Figure 5.1 and Figure 5.6). When ablation procedures are utilized, massive tumor and/or skin necrosis can occur (Figure 5.7).

Several studies in human patients have evaluated the combined use of intra-arterial chemotherapy and radiation therapy. Delivering a radiosensitizing chemotherapy agent such as cisplatin directly to a tumor that is being irradiated may improve the efficacy of radiation therapy thus allowing for improved tumor response with simultaneous organ preservation (Robbins et al., 2005, Samant et al., 1999).

Intra-arterial chemotherapy has been combined with radiation therapy and reported in a few veterinary studies. In a study evaluating the combination of intra-arterial chemotherapy (cisplatin) with radiation therapy for treatment of bladder cancer, two dogs demonstrated an objective reduction in tumor size (McCaw, 1988). Additionally, three studies have combined intra-arterial chemotherapy with radiation therapy in the treatment of canine osteosarcoma (Heidner et al., 1991, Powers et al., 1991, Withrow et al., 1993). Studies specifically evaluating the use of intra-arterial chemotherapy combined with radiation therapy in the treatment of nasal and sinus neoplasia have not been performed in veterinary patients, but the concept warrants further investigation.

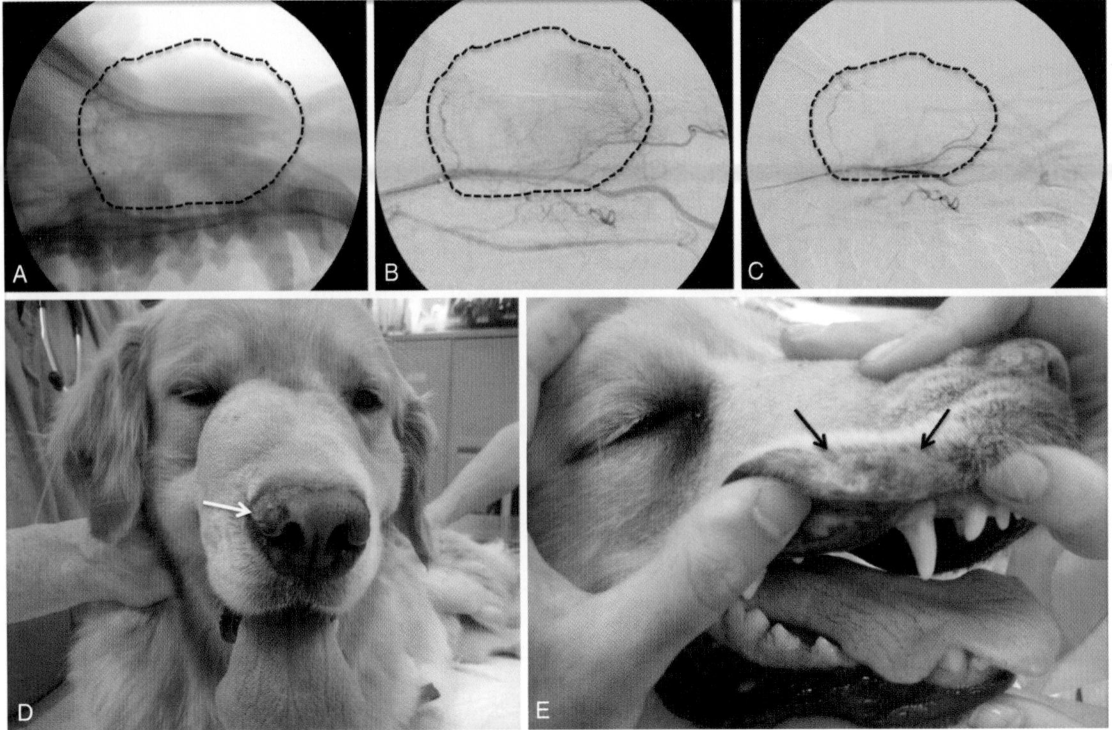

Figure 5.6 Embolization of a maxillary fibrosarcoma. Lateral nasal fluoroscopic (A) and digital subtraction angiography (B,C) images of a dog with nose to the right of the images. (A) Image demonstrates microcatheter in maxillary artery with mass (black dotted line) evident. (B) Pre-embolization digital subtraction angiogram (DSA) demonstrating tumor blush (black dotted line). (C) Post-embolization DSA demonstrating lack of perfusion to tumor compared to pre-embolization image. (D/E) Recheck examination one week later demonstrating very mild nasal planum erosion (white arrow) and lip margin ulceration (black arrows) due to distal embolization and ischemia. Both healed uneventfully without treatment.

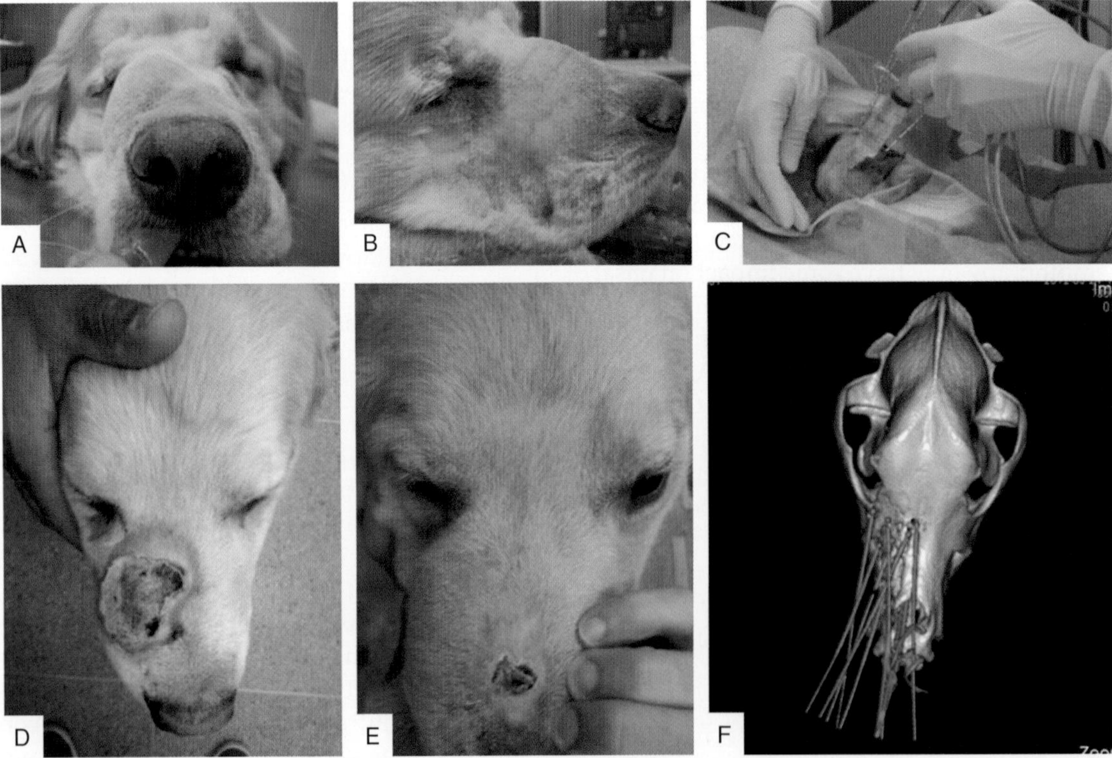

Figure 5.7 Cryoablation of a maxillary fibrosarcoma. (A/B) Pre-operative images demonstrating a large right maxillary mass. (C) Hydro-dissection (injection of saline under the skin) is being performed to raise the skin off the tumor to reduce the risk of skin necrosis for such a superficial tumor. (D) Approximately one week later demonstrating patch of skin necrosis and then a few weeks later (E) demonstrating progressive healing of the superficial wound with tumor regression. (F) 3-D CT reconstruction of subsequent cryoablation performed in same patient with additional probes in overlapping positions.

NOTES

(Examples; Multiple vendors available)

1. Vascular introducer sheath, Infiniti Medical, Menlo Park, CA.
2. Weasel wire, Infiniti Medical, Menlo Park, CA
3. Berenstein catheter, Infiniti Medical, Menlo Park, CA.
4. Omnipaque (iohexol) injection, Amersham Health Inc., Princeton, NJ.
5. Microcatheter, Infiniti Medical, Menlo Park, CA.
6. Touhy–Borst adapter, Cook Medical, Bloomington, IN.
7. Flo-switch™, Boston Scientific, Natick, MA.
8. Microwire, Infiniti Medical, Menlo Park, CA.
9. Bead Block® PVA hydrogel microspheres, Biocompatibles UK Limited, Surrey, England.
10. 1 ml polycarbonate syringes, Merit Medical, South Jordan, UT.
11. Cool-tip RF™ Ablation System, Covidien, Mansfield, MA
12. SeedNet™ Cryoablation System, Galil Medical Inc., Arden Hills, MN.

References

Adams WM, Kleiter MM, Thrall D, et al (2009) Prognostic significance of tumor histology and computed tomographic staging for radiation treatment response of canine nasal tumors. *Vet Radiol Ultrasound* 50, 330–5.

Adams WM, Miller PE, Vail DM, Forrest LJ, and Macewen EG (1998) An accelerated technique for irradiation of malignant canine nasal and paranasal sinus tumors. *Vet Radiol Ultrasound* 39, 475–81.

Adams WM, Withrow SJ, Walshaw R, et al (1987) Radiotherapy of malignant nasal tumors in 67 dogs. *J Am Vet Med Assoc* 191, 311–5.

Buchholz J, Hagen R, Leo C, Ebling A, Roos M, Kaser-Hotz B, and Bley CR (2009) 3D conformal radiation therapy for palliative treatment of canine nasal tumors. *Vet Radiol Ultrasound* 50, 679–83.

Callstrom MR and Kurup AN (2009) Percutaneous ablation for bone and soft tissue metastases--why cryoablation? *Skeletal Radiol* 38, 835–9.

D'ippolito G and Goldberg SN (2002) Radiofrequency ablation of hepatic tumors. *Tech Vasc Interv Radiol* 5, 141–55.

Eckman WW, Patlak CS, and Fenstermacher JD (1974) A critical evaluation of the principles governing the advantages of intra-arterial infusions. *J Pharmacokinet Biopharm* 2, 257–85.

Evans HE (1993) The heart and arteries. In: *Miller's Anatomy of the Dog*, 3rd edn (Evans HE, ed.). W.B. Saunders Company, Philadelphia, PA.

Evans SM, Goldschmidt M, Mckee LJ, and Harvey CE (1989) Prognostic factors and survival after radiotherapy for intranasal neoplasms in dogs: 70 cases (1974–1985). *J Am Vet Med Assoc* 194, 1460–3.

Gieger T, Rassnick K, Siegel S, et al (2008) Palliation of clinical signs in 48 dogs with nasal carcinomas treated with coarse-fraction radiation therapy. *J Am Anim Hosp Assoc* 44, 116–23.

Heidner GL, Page RL, Mcentee MC, Dodge RK, and Thrall DE (1991) Treatment of canine appendicular osteosarcoma using cobalt 60 radiation and intraarterial cisplatin. *J Vet Intern Med* 5, 313–6.

Henry CJ, Brewer WG, Jr, Tyler JW, et al (1998) Survival in dogs with nasal adenocarcinoma: 64 cases (1981–1995). *J Vet Intern Med* 12, 436–9.

Hunley DW, Mauldin GN, Shiomitsu K, and Mauldin GE (2010) Clinical outcome in dogs with nasal tumors treated with intensity-modulated radiation therapy. *Can Vet J* 51, 293–300.

Kondo Y, Matsunaga S, Mochizuki M, et al (2008) Prognosis of canine patients with nasal tumors according to modified clinical stages based on computed tomography: a retrospective study. *J Vet Med Sci* 70, 207–12.

Ladue TA, Dodge R, Page RL, Price GS, Hauck ML, and Thrall DE (1999) Factors influencing survival after radiotherapy of nasal tumors in 130 dogs. *Vet Radiol Ultrasound* 40, 312–7.

Lana SE, Dernell WS, Larue SM, et al (1997) Slow release cisplatin combined with radiation for the treatment of canine nasal tumors. *Vet Radiol Ultrasound* 38, 474–8.

Lana SE, Dernell WS, Lafferty MH, Withrow SJ, and Larue SM (2004) Use of radiation and a slow-release cisplatin formulation for treatment of canine nasal tumors. *Vet Radiol Ultrasound* 45, 577–81.

Lee YY, Dimery IW, Van Tassel P, De Pena C, Blacklock JB, and Goepfert H (1989) Superselective intra-arterial chemotherapy of advanced paranasal sinus tumors. *Arch Otolaryngol Head Neck Surg* 115, 503–11.

MacEwen EG, Withrow SJ, and Patnaik AK (1977) Nasal tumors in the dog: retrospective evaluation of diagnosis, prognosis, and treatment. *J Am Vet Med Assoc* 170, 45–8.

Mahnken AH, Bruners P, and Gunther RW (2009) Local ablative therapies in HCC: percutaneous ethanol injection and radiofrequency ablation. *Dig Dis* 27, 148–56.

Marioni-Henry K, Schwarz T, Weisse C, and Muravnick KB (2007) Cystic nasal adenocarcinoma in a cat treated with piroxicam and chemoembolization. *J Am Anim Hosp Assoc* 43, 347–51.

McCaw DL (1988) Radiation and cisplatin for treatment of canine urinary bladder carcinoma. *Vet Radiol* 29, 264–8.

Mellanby RJ, Stevenson RK, Herrtage ME, White RA, and Dobson JM (2002) Long-term outcome of 56 dogs with nasal tumours treated with four doses of radiation at intervals of seven days. *Vet Rec*, 151, 253–7.

Moser T, Buy X, Goyault G, Tok C, Irani F and Gangi A (2008). Image-guided ablation of bone tumors: review of current techniques. *J Radiol* 89, 461–71.

Murphy SM, Lawrence JA, Schmiedt CW, et al (2011) Image-guided transnasal cryoablation of a recurrent nasal adenocarcinoma in a dog. *J Small Anim Pract* 52, 329–33.

Northrup NC, Etue SM, Ruslander DM, et al (2001) Retrospective study of orthovoltage radiation therapy for nasal tumors in 42 dogs. *J Vet Intern Med* 15, 183–9.

Padma S, Martinie JB, and Iannitti DA (2009) Liver tumor ablation: percutaneous and open approaches. *J Surg Oncol* 100, 619–34.

Powers BE, Withrow SJ, Thrall DE, et al (1991) Percent tumor necrosis as a predictor of treatment response in canine osteosarcoma. *Cancer* 67, 126–34.

Rassnick KM, Goldkamp CE, Erb HN, et al (2006) Evaluation of factors associated with survival in dogs with untreated nasal carcinomas: 139 cases (1993–2003). *J Am Vet Med Assoc* 229, 401–6.

Robbins KT, Kumar P, Harris J, et al (2005) Supradose intra-arterial cisplatin and concurrent radiation therapy for the treatment of stage IV head and neck squamous cell carcinoma is feasible and efficacious in a multi-institutional setting: results of Radiation Therapy Oncology Group Trial 9615. *J Clin Oncol* 23, 1447–54.

Samant S, Kumar P, Wan J, et al (1999) Concomitant radiation therapy and targeted cisplatin chemotherapy for the treatment of advanced pyriform sinus carcinoma: disease control and preservation of organ function. *Head Neck*, 21, 595–601.

Simon CJ, Dupuy DE, and Mayo-Smith WW (2005) Microwave ablation: principles and applications. *Radiographics* 25 Suppl 1, S69–83.

Stephens FO (1983) Pharmacokinetics of intra-arterial chemotherapy. *Recent Results Cancer Res*, 86, 1–12.

Theon AP, Madewell BR, Harb MF, and Dungworth DL (1993) Megavoltage irradiation of neoplasms of the nasal and paranasal cavities in 77 dogs. *J Am Vet Med Assoc* 202, 1469–75.

Von Scheel J and Golde G (1984) Pharmacokinetics of intra-arterial tumour therapy. An experimental study. *Arch Otorhinolaryngol* 239, 153–61.

Weisse C, Nicholson ME, Rollings C, Hammer K, Hurst R, and Solomon JA (2004) Use of percutaneous arterial embolization for treatment of intractable epistaxis in three dogs. *J Am Vet Med Assoc*, 224, 1307–11.

Withrow SJ, Thrall DE, Straw RC, et al (1993) Intra-arterial cisplatin with or without radiation in limb-sparing for canine osteosarcoma. *Cancer*, 71, 2484–90.

CHAPTER SIX

Interventional Treatment of Nasopharyngeal Stenosis

Allyson Berent
The Animal Medical Center, New York, NY

Background/Indications

Nasopharyngeal stenosis (NPS) is a pathologic narrowing within the nasopharynx caudal to the choanae resulting in inspiratory and/or expiratory stertor. This can occur as a congenital anomaly similar to choanal atresia or, more commonly, secondary to an inflammatory condition (chronic inflammatory rhinitis/aspiration rhinitis), surgery, trauma, or a space-occupying lesion. One of the most common causes in dogs is secondary to aspiration rhinitis following general anesthesia. Within a few days the patient displays difficulty passing air through the nose; these patients can exhibit obligate open-mouth breathing when the obstruction is complete. Nasopharyngeal stenosis has only been described in a small number of cases in the veterinary literature but the condition is likely more common than described. Minimally invasive interventions are recommended due to the common recurrence of stenosis after attempted surgical repair. The most common intervention advocated for this condition is balloon dilatation or metallic stent placement. Both have been shown to be effective.

Patient Preparation

All patients should have a thorough physical examination. Respiratory signs are often consistent with that of a fixed obstruction (inspiratory and expiratory in nature) and should resolve during open-mouthed breathing. Blood work should be evaluated prior to anesthesia. A computerized tomography (CT) scan is recommended. This should be performed with 1 mm slices to get an exact measurement of stenosis length and nasopharyngeal diameter, both rostral and caudal to the stenosis (Figure 6.1). Some lesions are very short and can be missed if larger CT slices are taken. Imaging should be done from the tip of the nares to the larynx, including the entire nose and nasopharynx. Many patients have a large amount of mucus accumulation within the sinuses and bullae. Contrast CT is often helpful in differentiating mucus accumulation around the stenosis with the fibrous tissue associated with the lesion; this can make a substantial difference when choosing stent length. These lesions can also be secondary to chronic inflammatory rhinitis so biopsies of the turbinates should be obtained if deemed appropriate.

A thorough oral examination should be completed to ensure there are no palatal defects. These can be seen in cases of congenital malformations, trauma, tumors, or those that had previous surgery in the area.

Potential Risks/Complications/Expected Outcomes

Nasopharyngeal stenosis (NPS) can be rostral or caudal within the nasopharynx but is most often located at the level of the junction of the hard and soft palate. For lesions that are very thin (<5 mm length) balloon dilation alone is initially recommended. This has been successful in 30–50% of cases with a very thin membrane but may require two to three separate dilation procedures. For lesions that are more caudally located and have less than 1 cm of soft palate between the stricture and oropharynx, balloon dilation alone should be attempted prior to considering the placement of a nasopharyngeal stent. This is because a stent that is in the caudal nasopharynx can result in excessive gagging and oropharyngeal irritation due to the position of the stent and subsequent reflux of oral contents into the nasopharynx during feeding.

Complications seen with nasopharyngeal balloon dilation or stents include restenosis (through the

Veterinary Image-Guided Interventions, First Edition. Edited by Chick Weisse and Allyson Berent.

Companion website: www.wiley.com/go/weisse/vet-image-guided-interventions

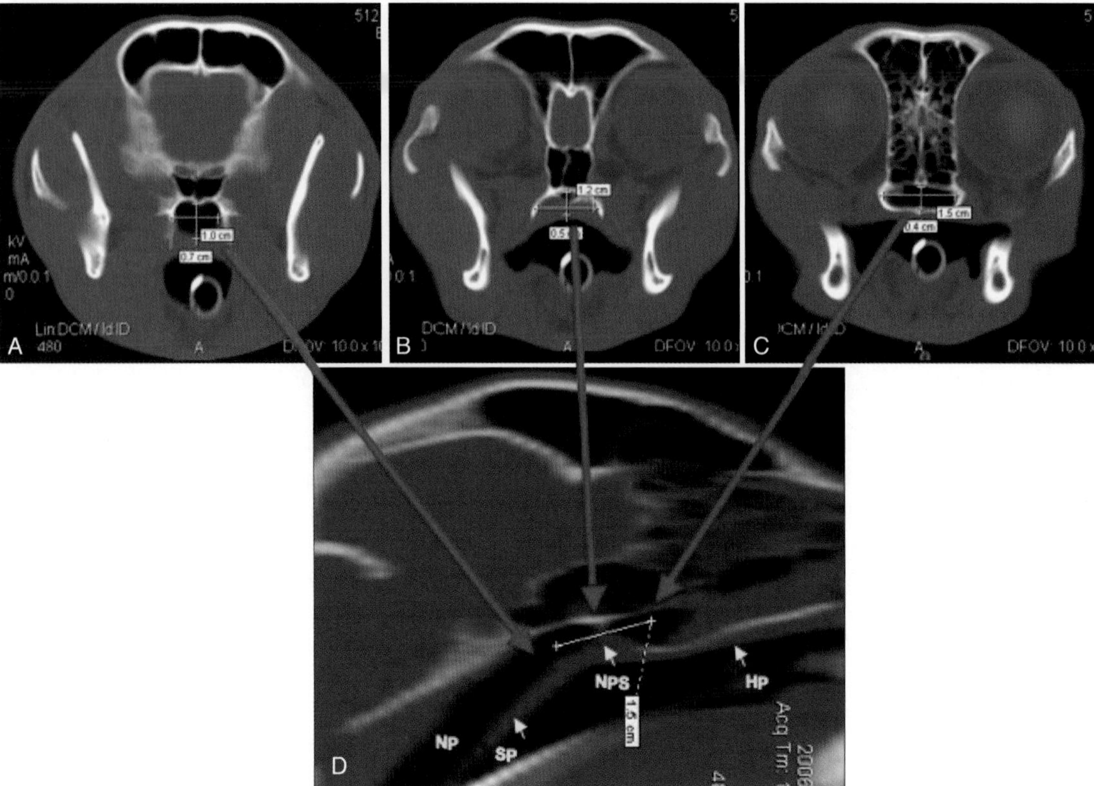

Figure 6.1 Computed tomography of a feline patient with NPS. (A) Transverse image of the patient showing the normal nasopharynx caudal to the stenosis. This area (the hamular processes of the pterygoid bones) is used to obtain measurements of the normal nasopharynx for stent sizing. (B) Transverse image of the patient at the level of the NPS. Notice the narrow opening with soft tissue opacity occluding over 90% of the nasopharynx. (C) Transverse image of the patient just rostral to the NPS. Notice this is the area of the nasopharynx just rostral to the junction of the hard and soft palate. This is a common location for NPS. (D) Sagittal image of the same patient. This image assists in measuring the length of the nasopharyngeal stenosis (NPS). Notice the hard palate (HP), soft palate (SP) and open nasopharynx (NP) caudal to the stricture (NPS). This view also shows the NPS sitting just caudal to the junction of the hard and soft palate.

uncovered stent or after balloon dilation alone), stent compression and/or migration, pharyngeal irritation, stent reaction/irritation, nasopharyngeal reflux, chronic infections, soft palate tear, stent fracture, and the development of an oronasal fistula. There are far fewer complications with balloon dilation alone than with balloon expandable stent placement, but these complications are relatively uncommon, and balloon dilation alone has a higher failure rate in the author's experience.

The stent used is typically a balloon expandable metallic stent (BEMS) although self-expanding stents have also been described, and are becoming more commonly used in the author's practice. Stents are typically bare (uncovered). If a covered stent is chosen the author recommends the covered material be made of silicone, rather than Dacron or Teflon. The silicone-covered stents are usually mesh self-expanding metallic stents (SEMS) so are more difficult to place in a short stenotic segment and deploy differently than the BEMS (see Chapters 1 and 2). Covered nasopharyngeal stents are not typically recommended unless absolutely necessary due to the risk of migration and recurrent infections. Because these stents do not get incorporated into the nasopharyngeal mucosa like the uncovered stents, nasal debris accumulates and chronic infections can occur. They can also migrate and the operator may consider suturing them in-place through the soft palate. Uncovered stents are very well tolerated and should be placed for NPS when balloon dilatation fails or the operator has one chance to address the stenosis (typically due to financial constraints). The cost of multiple serial balloon dilation procedures (×2) versus single NPS stenting is similar; many owners therefore elect for a stent be placed early in the course of treatment.

In patients with congenital NPS and under 6 months of age the nasopharynx can grow and the stent may ultimately be undersized at the time of placement. This was seen in two cats, both of which resulted in stent movement. The edges did not incorporate within the mucosa of the nasopharynx and this movement presumptively resulted in palatal irritation and subsequent oronasal fistula formation. In similar cases, performing balloon dilation until the pet is fully grown is now encouraged.

In patients with a completely closed membrane (no patency through the lumen of the nasopharynx) balloon dilation or uncovered stents do not provide durable results in the author's experience. This is most commonly seen in animals that develop the NPS after aspiration rhinitis. These are very aggressive strictures often with no opening, or a very small opening. The stenosis will routinely grow through an uncovered stent, so a covered stent can be considered.

In the author's practice, approximately 1/4 of the cases had completely closed stenoses and 3/4 had patent (open) strictures. In cats, the stent size chosen is typically 8–10 mm diameter × 15–30 mm length and in dogs 7–14 mm diameter × 18–40 mm length. In cases recently evaluated, covered stents were used in 8/12 closed membranes; Three of the four that did not have a covered stent placed developed tissue ingrowth. One cat that did not grow through had a very thin membrane. Other complications in approximately 46 cases include stent migration ($n = 1$), BEMS deformation ($n = 5$), oronasal fistula development ($n = 7$), exaggerated swallowing ($n = 2$) and hairball entrapment ($n = 1$). One cat also developed global brain ischemia (GBI) (post-stent blindness, dullness, and behavior changes) after anesthesia, presumed to be secondary to receiving ketamine at induction in the presence of theoretical chronic hypoxia. GBI has been associated with ketamine pre-anesthetic hypoxia. This did resolve over 3 months. We have seen tissue ingrowth through the uncovered BEMS in approximately 35% of patent NPS cases as well, though this usually requires re-ballooning or restenting with permanent resolution in most cases; Owners should be prepared for potential repeat procedures.

Clinical outcome in approximately 46 cases performed to date is typically excellent in the short-term with 76% of owners in a recent case series reporting immediate resolution of clinical stertor and reduced nasal discharge. Owners describe the personality, activity, and appetite all improved immediately. Considering the larger number of patients now treated in our practice, there have been two dogs that were ultimately euthanized; one due to chronic nasal discharge in which an oronasal fistula developed, and the other due to tissue ingrowth through an uncovered stent; this owner declined covered stent placement.

Equipment

Endoscopy is typically performed with a flexible bronchoscope[1] (5.5 mm) with concurrent fluoroscopy. A traditional fluoroscopic C-arm is sufficient for visualization. Fluoroscopy entails the risk of radiation exposure so care must be taken to reduce exposure through beam collimation, reducing dose, and wearing standard radiation protection gear. A 0.035″ hydrophilic angle-tipped guide wire[2] and a 5 Fr marker catheter[3] are needed. If the membrane is not patent then a 4–7 Fr vascular access sheath[4] is needed, along with a 15–25 cm 18 gauge renal access trocar needle[5] for transnasal puncture of the NPS.

If balloon dilation alone is being performed than an appropriately sized (typically 8–14 mm × 2–4 cm) high-pressure percutaneous transluminal angioplasty (PTA) balloon (e.g. 8–15 atm)[6] is used to break the stenosis. The balloon size needed is based on the CT scan (Figure 6.1) or a nasopharyngeogram. If a stent is not placed the author recommends instilling 2.5–5.0 ml of 0.1% topical mitomycin C[7], or endoscopically injecting triamcinolone (0.2 mg/kg) under the mucosal tissue using a 25 gauge endoscopic injection needle.[8] (See Table 6.1)

TABLE 6.1
Medications commonly used for NPS

Medication	Dosage	Indication
Mitomycin C	0.1% solution dwelled for 5 minutes: 2.5 ml in a cat and 5.0 ml in a dog	Antifibrosis when a BEMS is not being placed
Triamcinolone	0.2 mg/kg divided into 4 quadrants as submucosal injections	Antifibrosis
Bupivicaine	0.3 mg/kg diluate in 3 ml of saline topically	Local analgesia into the nares and nasopharynx
Buprenoriphine	0.008–0.01 mg/kg IV or sublinqual q 8 hours	Analgesia as needed
Amoxicillin-clavulanic acid	13–18 mg/kg BID PO	Antibiotic
Prednisone (prednisolone-cats)	0.5 mg/kg BID for 5 days, then taper over 2–4 weeks	Anti-inflammatory

A balloon expandable metallic stent (BEMS)[9,10] typically comes pre-loaded on the PTA balloon (see Chapters 1 and 2). The BEMS is positioned across the stenosis using fluoroscopic and endoscopic guidance. For animals requiring a covered stent, a self-expanding silicone covered metallic stent (SEMS)[11] is currently recommended.

Procedure

The patient is placed in lateral recumbency, and a mouth gag is placed on the dependent canine teeth. The anesthetist should be sure the endotracheal tube cuff is appropriately inflated as contrast studies and rigorous flushing will occur. Packing the back of the pharynx is not possible during this procedure when the scope is also in place. In some cases neuromuscular blockade is helpful to prevent excessive gagging during endoscope placement and other manipulations in this sensitive area. This is usually unnecessary once the endoscope is in place.

The flexible bronchoscope should be placed in a retroflexed manner transorally and positioned over the soft palate into the nasopharynx so the NPS is clearly visualized (Figure 6.2). Under fluoroscopic guidance a 0.035-inch hydrophilic angle-tipped guide wire is advanced through the naris into the ventral nasal meatus and directed caudally to the stenosis (Figure 6.3). For animals with patent NPS the guide wire is directed through the small opening and down the esophagus (Figure 6.3 and Figure 6.4).

For patients in which no orifice is visible a 4–7 French access sheath is advanced through the one naris, over the guide wire to the stenosis (Figure 6.5 and Figure 6.6). To create an opening the NPS is viewed via retroflexed rhinoscopy and the scope is advanced rostrally to the stenosis to visualize the caudal aspect of the membrane. A guide wire can be used through the endoscope to mark the caudal aspect of the stenosis fluoroscopically (Figure 6.5b and Figure 6.6a). An 18 gauge renal access trocar needle is advanced through the access sheath to pierce the membrane, visualizing it simultaneously with rhinoscopy (Figure 6.5) and fluoroscopy (Figure 6.6). The needle is directed in a dorsomedial direction to avoid piercing the soft palate, and aiming to stay on midline. Once through the membrane the stylette is removed and the guide wire is advanced through the trocar needle and down the

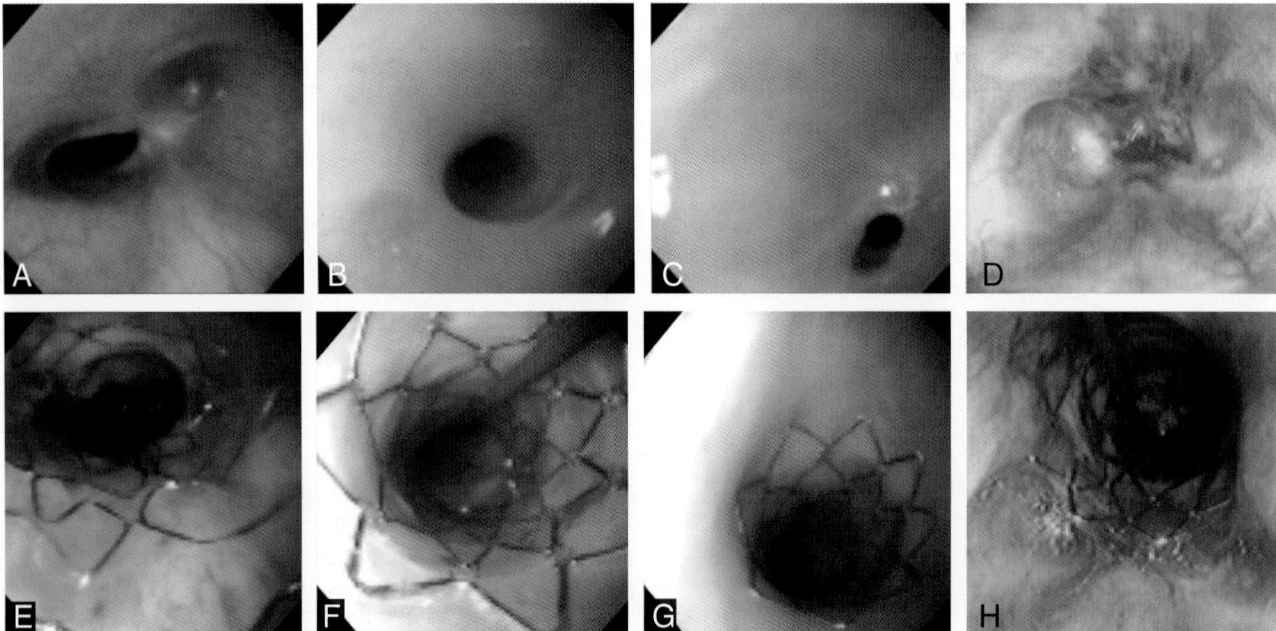

Figure 6.2 Retroflex view of various types of NPS. (A–D) are images of the NPS prior to treatment; and images (E–H) are the respective cases after nasopharyngeal stent placement in each patient. (A) A dog that developed an NPS after soft palate surgery for a benign tumor. (B) Feline patient with a 6-year history of chronic lymphoplasmacytic rhinitis that developed severe inspiratory stertor at age 8. (C) Feline patient that was born with severe inspiratory stertor that would result in intermittent periods of open-mouth breathing. (D) A dog that was an obligate open-mouth breather that developed 3 days after ovariohysterectomy surgery. This is a non-patent NPS.

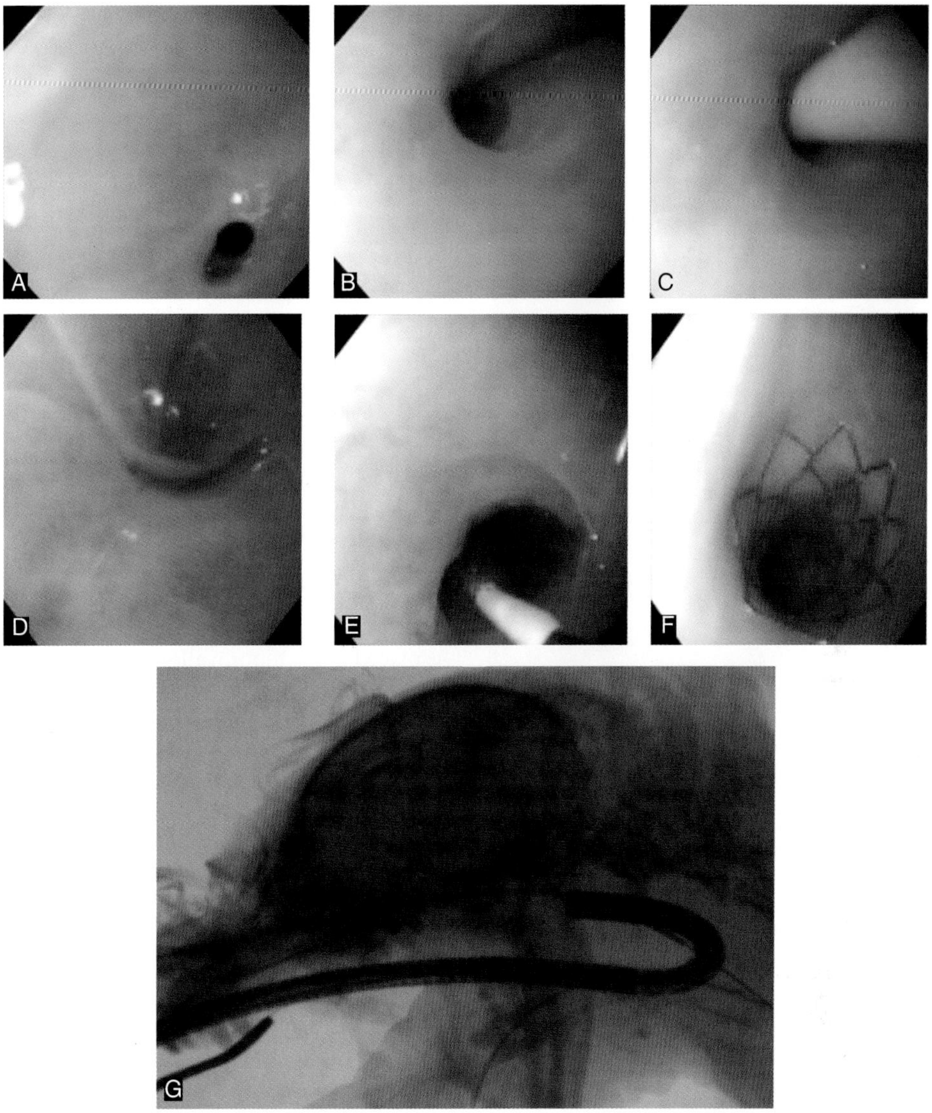

Figure 6.3 Endoscopic and fluoroscopic images of a cat with NPS during balloon dilation and BEMS placement. The patient is in lateral recumbency. (A) Retroflex rhinoscopic view of the NPS prior to intervention. (B) Guide wire passed from the ventral nasal meatus of the naris, through the NPS and down the nasopharynx. (C) Measuring catheter placed over the guidewire through the NPS. (D) Rhinoscopic image of the inflated balloon dilation catheter placed over the guide wire to dilate the NPS. (E) Dilation of the NPS after the balloon is withdrawn showing the tear in the nasopharyngeal mucosa. (F) Image of the NPS after a BEMS had been placed. (G) Fluoroscopic image that is simultaneously being taken during the procedure described above.

esophagus. The needle and sheath are removed, and an 8 French vascular dilator[12] is passed over the wire to expand the orifice large enough to accept a balloon dilation catheter.

Next, the distal end of the stenosis is appreciated rhinoscopically and its location confirmed fluoroscopically using anatomical landmarks (i.e., bullae or other landmarks) (Figure 6.4G,H). An appropriately sized PTA balloon is advanced over the guide wire, through the stenosis, and visualized endoscopically and fluoroscopically. The balloon is inflated with 50% iohexol and 50% saline (0.9% NaCl) solution via fluoroscopic guidance using an appropriate insufflation device. This should not be done with hand-pressure as it is typically not strong enough to efface the stricture. The waist of the stenosis is viewed to expand the stricture and the balloon is deflated and removed over the wire. If no stent is being placed than this balloon should be 1 mm larger than the pre-determined diameter of the nasopharynx in this area. If a stent is to be placed than the balloon diameter should be 50–60% of the nasopharyngeal diameter or the BEMS can just be placed primarily. It is important to remember that the animals with a totally closed stenosis should not be ballooned

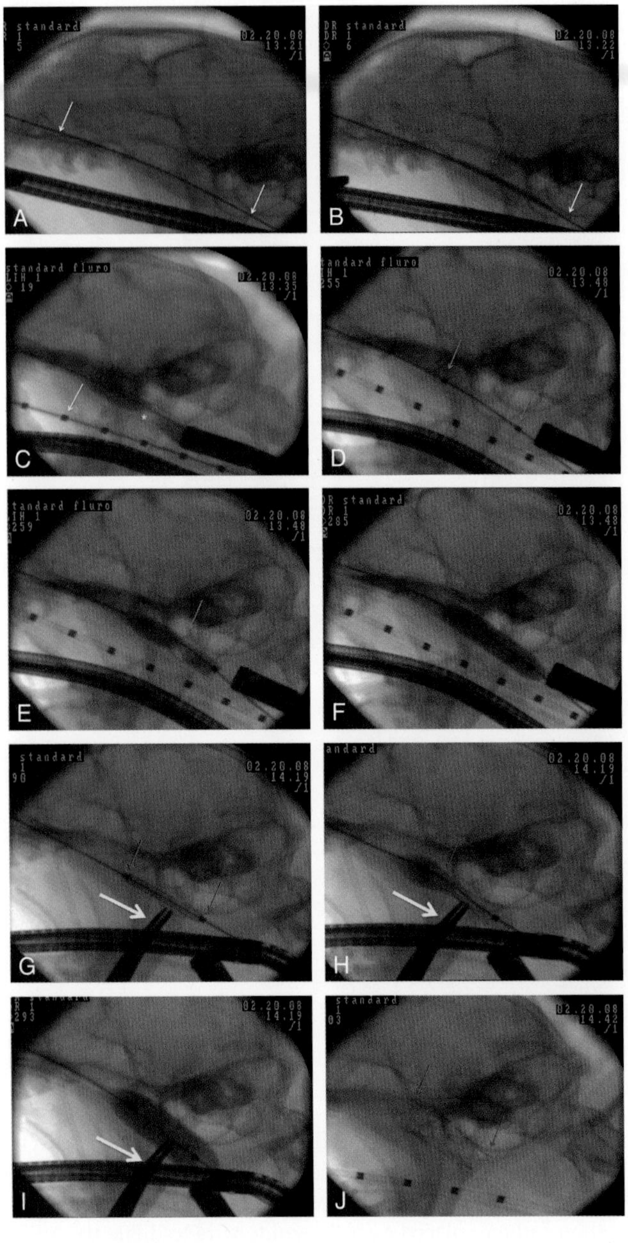

Figure 6.4 Fluoroscopic images of a cat with a patent NPS during BEMS placement. (This is the same patient as described above in Figure 6.3.) The patient is placed in lateral recumbency. The nares are to the left of the image. (A) A guidewire (white arrows) is being passed from the nares, down the ventral nasal meatus, and through the NPS into the esophagus. (B) Over the guide wire (white arrow) a catheter (red arrow) is placed through the stenosis. (C) This is a contrast nasopharyngeogram. A marker catheter (yellow arrow) is placed in the mouth, allowing measurement of the stenosis and adjustment for magnification. This measurement is typically not needed unless a CT is not available. Contrast is injected rostral to the stenosis through the catheter placed in image B and through the working channel of the endoscope. This allows fluoroscopic visibility of the NPS (yellow asterisk). (D) A balloon dilation catheter (blue arrows) is advanced over the guide wire, and crosses the NPS. The radiopaque marks are seen on each end of the balloon. (E) Inflation of the balloon catheter (blue arrow) at the NPS using a 50% mixture of contrast to visualize the stenosis breaking as seen in Figure F. (G) The BEMS (red arrows) is placed over the guide wire. Landmarks can be marked to ensure proper placement of the stent across the stenosis. In this image a hemostat (yellow arrow) is clamped to the fur at the stenosis. You can also use the exact location on the bullae. (H) BEMS (red arrow) being deployed as the balloon is inflated. (I) BEMS fully open. (J) The BEMS (red arrows) is in place after the balloon and guidewire are withdrawn.

alone as a sole procedure as this has a very high chance of recurrence (>90%).

Balloon Dilation Alone

If no stent is placed than when the NPS is broken satisfactorily (Figure 6.7) topically 0.1% MMC can be instilled in the region of the stenosis. For cats 2.5 ml is used and for dogs 5 ml is used. After 5 minutes this region should be flushed vigorously with saline. The operator and anesthetist should wear chemotherapy safety gloves during and after the infusion. If MMC is unavailable then mucosal/submucosal injections using 0.2 mg/kg of triamcinolone, divided into four quadrants, can be injected through the working channel of the bronchoscope into the effaced fibrous tissues. Some advocate injecting the triamcinolone prior to effacing the stenosis.

NPS Metallic Stenting

After the NPS is pre-balloon dilated (50–60% of diameter), the pre-mounted stent is advanced over the wire, centered across the stenosis, and deployed using both endoscopic and fluoroscopic guidance (Figure 6.3, Figure 6.4, Figure 6.5, and Figure 6.6). For the BEMS, the balloon is inflated with a 50% contrast/50% saline mixture until the stenosis is effaced under fluoroscopic

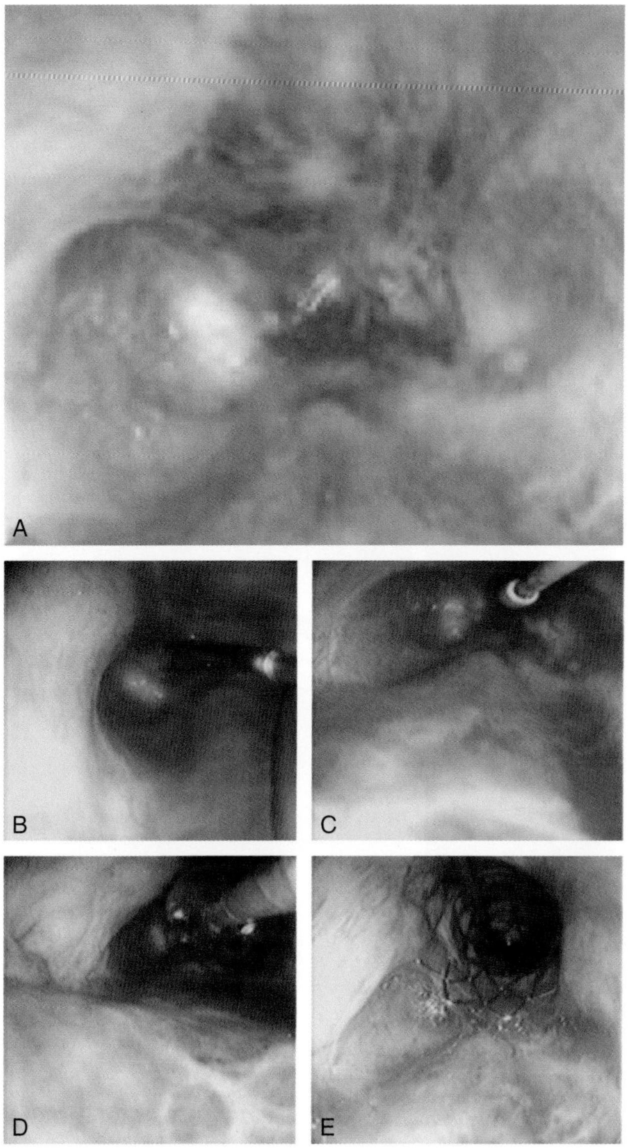

Figure 6.5 Endoscopic images of piercing a non-patent NPS during BEMS placement. This patient is in lateral recumbency. The trocar needle is passed through an access sheath from the upper nare, and using endoscopic and fluoroscopic guidance, remains on midline and pierces the stenosis. (A) Retroflexed endoscopic image of a non-patent NPS. (B) Trocar needle as it pierces the NPS visualized from a retroflexed rhinoscopic view. (C) Guidewire passed through the trocar after the stylette is removed. (D) Balloon dilation catheter passed over the guide wire as the NPS is pre-dilated prior to stent placement. (E) NPS after the BEMS is placed. Notice the choanae positioned rostral to the stenosis.

guidance. If the stenosis is more caudally positioned within the nasopharynx then it is important the operator leaves at least 1 cm of unstented soft palate caudal to the stent. Similarly, if the stenosis is very rostral, just behind the choanae, care should be taken to know exactly where the nasal septum ends so the proximal end of the stent is not placed down one nasal passage. This will result in excessive mucous accumulation in the covered nasal passage because drainage will be compromised. Sometimes this cannot be achieved and the stent is placed on one side, however this is not ideal and should be avoided whenever possible. One way to help prevent this from occurring is to pass a red rubber catheter down each nasal passage so that you can endoscopically visualize through the pre-dilated stenosis where the septum lies (where both catheters are seen to meet). This area is marked on the fluoroscopic image (using molars/hard palate location), and the stent is then deployed caudal to this region.

Following stent deployment the balloon (in the BEMS) is deflated and removed over the wire, leaving the expanded stent in place across the now expanded lesion (Figure 6.4J and Figure 6.6I). A catheter is placed over the wire, the wire is removed, and vigorous nasal flushing is performed with sterile saline solution to try and clear the nasal passages and sinuses of mucous and debris that has previously accumulated. The endoscope is maintained in place to suction out all the material and care should be taken to ensure this is not flushed down into the trachea around the endotracheal tube cuff. Finally, prior to removing the catheter a local anesthetic (bupivicaine, 1 mg/kg [0.45 mg/lb], dog; 0.2 mg/kg [0.9 mg/lb], cat) is injected at the level of the stenosis.

Postprocedural and Follow-Up Care

For the first 12 hours, buprenorphine (0.008–0.01 mg/kg [0.004–0.005 mg/lb] IV) is given as needed. Patients are discharged with an antimicrobial (amoxicillin-clavulanic acid, 13–18 mg/kg [5.9–8.2 mg/lb], PO, q 12 h, for 7–14 days) and a 4–6 week tapering dose of corticosteroids (prednisone, 0.5 mg/kg [0.23 mg/lb], PO q 12 h, initially). At 1 and 3 months a VD and lateral radiograph should be obtained to ensure the stent is in place and not compressed.

If a BEMS is used they can get deformed if exposed to excessive compressive pressures (Figure 6.8A). Because of this moist food is recommended and the animals should not be encouraged to play with hard treats or toys. Various complications can occur from weeks to years after BEMS placement and patients should be monitored based on clinical sign recurrence (Figure 6.8).

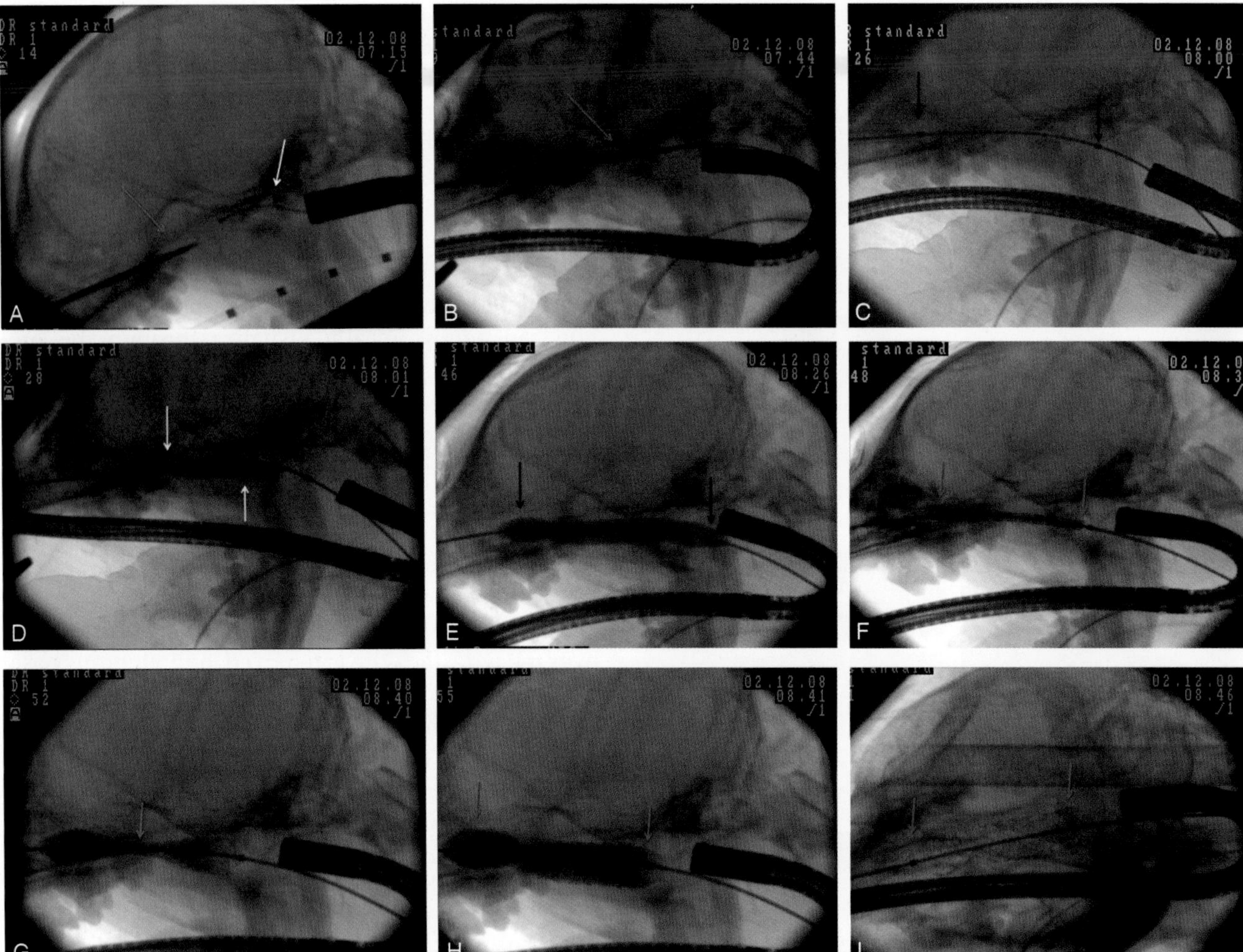

Figure 6.6 Fluoroscopic images of piercing a non-patent NPS during BEMS placement. This is the same patient described endoscopically in Figure 6.4. The patient is in lateral recumbency with the nares to the left of the image. (A) Trocar needle (red arrow) is advanced through an access sheath in the ventral nasal meatus to the level of the rostral aspect of the stenosis. A guide wire (white arrow) is advanced through the working channel of the endoscopic during retroflex rhinoscope marking the caudal aspect of the stenosis. (B) The trocar needle (red arrow) is advanced on midline toward the endoscope, and through the stenosis. The stylette is removed and a guide wire is advanced through the trocar needle. (C) Over the guide wire a balloon dilation catheter (black arrows) is advanced across the stenosis to pre-dilate the tract prior to stent placement. (D) The balloon is inflated with contrast and the rostral and caudal ends of the stenosis are visualized (yellow arrows). (E) The balloon catheter (black arrows) effaces the NPS. (F) The BEMS (blue arrows) is advanced over the wire, through the nares and lined up to cover the entire stenosis. (G) The BEMS (blue arrow) is deployed by balloon inflation. Notice the ends deploy before the center. This helps to keep the stent in place during deployment. (H) The BEMS (blue arrows) after maximal balloon inflation. Notice the narrowing at the junction of the hard and soft palate. This is very common due to the oblong shape of the rostral nasopharynx. (I) BEMS (blue arrows) in place after the balloon is deflated.

Prognosis

The prognosis for dogs and cats with NPS should be considered good. The owner should be aware that complications, as described above, are possible but they are usually manageable. If an owner has financial constraints, if the stenosis is longer than 5–10mm, or if there is not a patent membrane, then a stent is recommended instead of balloon dilation alone. If there is no patency, a covered stent is likely needed but owners should be aware that these can result in chronic nasal discharge and chronic infections so the author prefers to use a bare (uncovered) stent initially when possible (such that another procedure can be performed in the future if necessary).

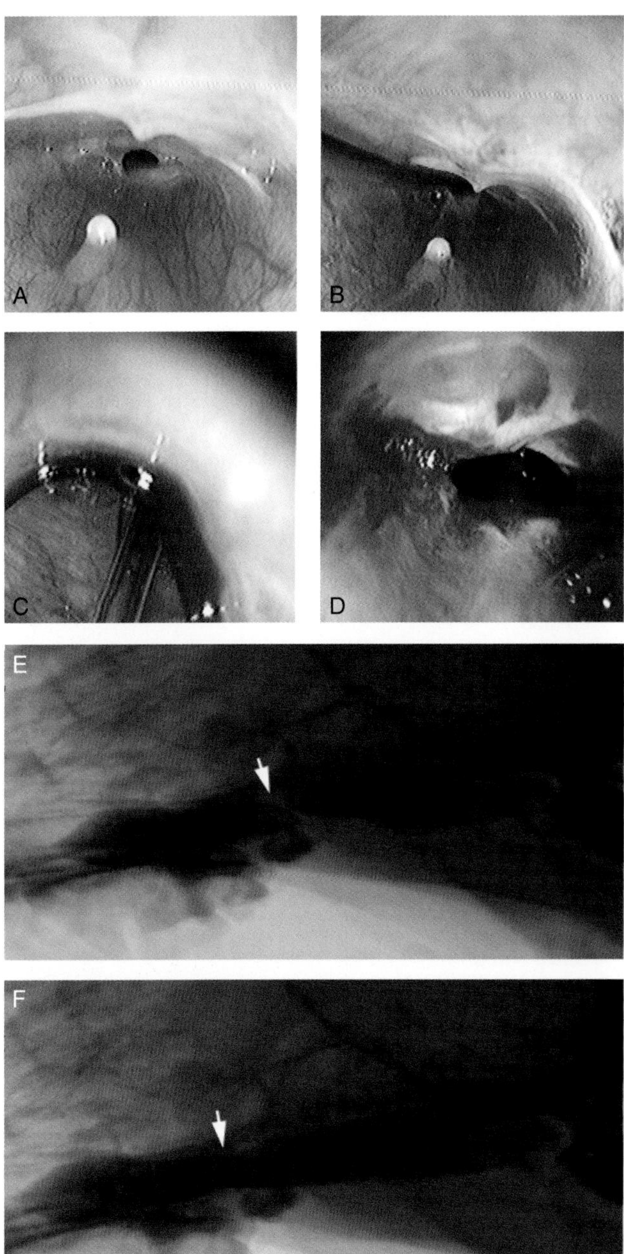

Figure 6.7 Endoscopic and fluoroscopic images of a patient during balloon dilation of a NPS. No stent was placed in this patient. The patient is placed in lateral recumbency and in the fluoroscopic images the nares are to the left of the image. (A) Retroflex endoscopic image of the NPS in the proximal nasopharynx. (B) Guide wire passed from the nares and through the opening of the NPS. (C) Balloon inflated over the guide wire, across the NPS. (D) Open NPS after balloon dilation. Notice the choanae rostral to the NPS. There is still a slight narrowing of the NPS. (E) Fluoroscopic image of the NPS during balloon dilation prior to effacing the stenosis. (F) Same image as (E) after effacement of the NPS.

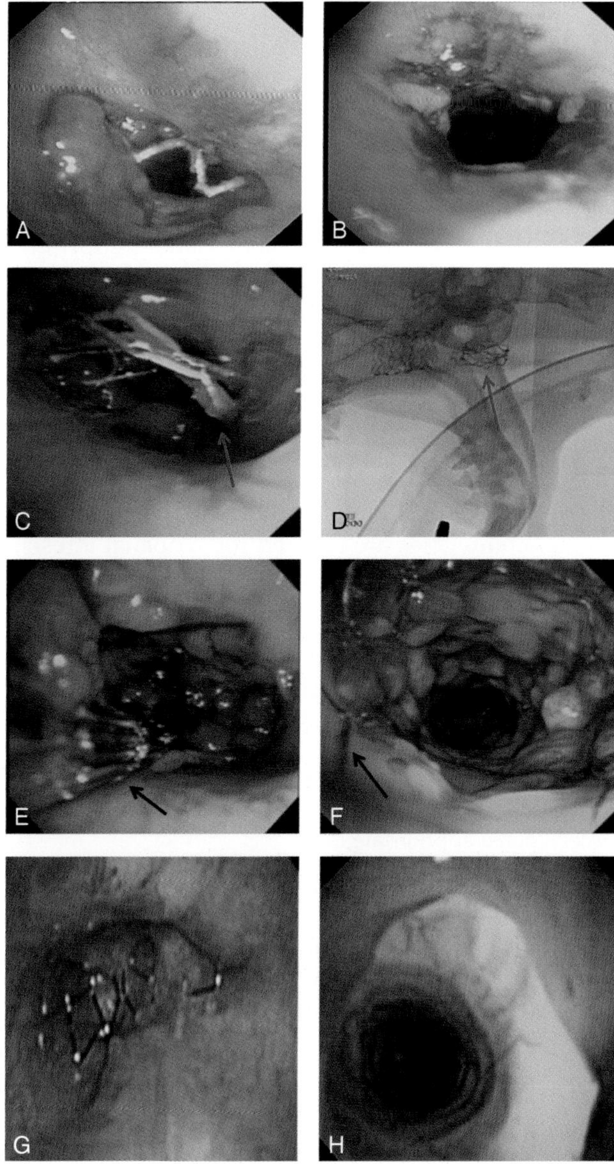

Figure 6.8 Complications seen with NPS stenting. (A and B) Retroflex endoscopic image of a cat 1 year after NPS placement. (A) Notice the deformity to the caudal end of the stent. (B) After re-balloon dilation of the stent. The deformity is corrected. (C and D) Endoscopic (C) and fluoroscopic (D) images of a cat with NPS 2 years after stent placement with fracture of the distal end of the stent and proliferative tissue ingrowth around the fragment (red arrows). (E and F) Endoscopic images of a cat with a proliferative reaction within the stent found 1.5 years after placement, likely associated with chronic infections. (E) A new BEMS (black arrows) prior to deployment placed through the proliferative tissue within the lumen of the first BEMS. (F) The nasopharynx after the new BEMS is deployed (black arrow) showing patency. This cat has not reobstructed in 2.5 more years. (G and H) Endoscopic images of a dog with a closed membrane NPS. (G) 6 weeks after a bare BEMS was placed the stricture grew through the stent aggressively. (H) A covered BEMS placed through the first bare stent.

Special Considerations

Choanal atresia with or without interventional management has been rarely reported in dogs and cats. Most reported cases were treated surgically and NPS developed subsequently. For this condition the authors would recommend piercing each nasal passage with a needle, as described above and performing balloon dilation on each side until both nasal passages are open. In humans these can be laser ablated or stented. If a stent is used, temporary stenting using a red rubber catheter or endotracheal tubes sutured to the nares for 6 weeks can be attempted. If this does not maintain patency than double-barreled stents (one placed in each nasal passage) can be considered. The operator should be confortable interpreting the CT scan as many cases are referred for "choanal atresia" and they are actually NPS. These two conditions would be treated very differently.

Notes

Note the equipment on this list are only examples of what is used in the author's practice and various alternatives would be considered appropriate.

1. BF-Q180 Flexible 5.5 mm bronchoscope, Olympus, Southborough MA.
2. Weasel wire 0.035", Infiniti Medical, Menlo Park, CA.
3. Marker Catheter, Infiniti Medical, Menlo Park, CA.
4. 4–7 French vascular access sheath, Infiniti Medical, Menlo Park, CA.
5. Disposable Trocar Needle, 18 g x 15 cm, Cook Medical, Bloomington, IN.
6. Valvuloplasty balloon, Medi-Tech Boston Scientific, Natick, MA.
7. Mitomycin C, Bristol-Myers Squibb, New York, NY.
8. Endoscopy injection needle, 25 ga. X 4 mm, US Endoscopy, Mentor, OH.
9. Balloon Expandable Metallic Stents, Infiniti Medical, LLC, Menlo Park, CA.
10. Palamaz Genesis Transhepatic Biliary Stent, Cordis Corp, Miami, FL.
11. Covered SEMS (silicone), Infiniti Medical, Menlo Park, CA.
12. 8 French vascular dilator, Infiniti Medical, Menlo Park, CA.

Suggested Reading

Berent A, Kinns J, and Weisse C (2006) Balloon dilatation of nasopharyngeal stenosis in a dog. *J Am Vet Assoc* 229, 385–388.

Berent A, Weisse C, Rondeau M, et al (2008) Metallic stenting for benign nasopharyngeal stenosis in 3 dogs and 3 cats. *J Am Vet Assoc* 233(9),1432–1440.

Coolman BR, Marretta SM, McKiernan, et al (1998) Choanal atresia and secondary nasopharyngeal stenosis in a dog. *J Am Anim Hosp Assoc* 34, 497–501.

Glaus TM, Gerber M, Tomsa K, et al (2005) Reproducible and long-lasting success of balloon dilation of nasopharyngeal stenosis in cats. *Vet Rec* 157, 257–259.

Mitten RW (1988) Nasopharyngeal stenosis in four cats. *J Small Anim Pract* 29, 341–345.

Prasad M, Ward RF, April MM, et al (2002) Topical mitomycin as an adjunct to choanal atresia repair. *Arch Otolaryngol Head Neck Surg* 128, 398–400.

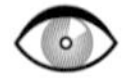 Video clips to accompany this chapter can be found in the online material at **www.wiley.com/go/weisse/vet-image-guided-interventions**

CHAPTER SEVEN

Intraluminal Tracheal Stenting

Chick Weisse
The Animal Medical Center, New York, NY

Background/Indications

Intraluminal stenting is a palliative, minimally invasive therapy used for restoration of an obstructed or narrowed tracheal lumen. While the most common indication is for treatment of intractable dyspnea, honking/raspy breathing, and/or possible coughing associated with the tracheal collapse syndrome (Figure 7.1 and Figure 7.2), stenting can also be performed in animals with obstructions secondary to strictures or tumors in both dogs and cats. As with other interventional procedures, case selection and management of owner expectations are important aspects that will help ensure the best possible outcome, as will a basic understanding of the equipment and placement techniques involved. Please use the suggested references for additional information regarding the diagnostic work-up and medical management of each individual disease process.

Patient Preparation

Prior to performing tracheal stenting for tracheal collapse, a full diagnostic work-up is recommended to appropriately evaluate each individual patient for related comorbidities that may require initial or concurrent medical or surgical therapies. The majority of patients identified with tracheal collapse often have either mild or no clinical signs. Basic conservative management options such as weight loss, improving environmental air quality through smoke reduction and ambient dehumidification, the use of harnesses instead of neck leads, etc. can dramatically improve clinical signs and avoid, at least temporarily, more invasive procedures. In addition, the toy and small breed dogs often treated for tracheal collapse are also susceptible to various other common conditions that can produce similar respiratory signs such as cardiac disease or lower airway disease. The clinical signs associated with these conditions can often improve dramatically with appropriate medical therapy prescribed prior to tracheal stent placement. Medical management for tracheal collapse often includes a combination of a variety of medications such as corticosteroids, anti-tussives, antibiotics, bronchodilators, tranquilizers/sedatives/anxiolytics, and/or anti-histamines among others (Box 7.1). Approximately 70% of appropriately medicated dogs can remain asymptomatic for over 12 months. Those patients that have had appropriate therapy for identified comorbidities and have failed aggressive medical management can be considered candidates for tracheal stent placement.

Potential Risks/Complications/Expected Outcomes

The most substantial acute risk of tracheal stenting is the anesthetic procedure itself. The anesthetist should be familiar with the stenting procedure and constant communication between the anesthetist and stent operator is critical. A variety of endotracheal tube sizes should be available and emergency drug doses should be calculated and available. Both early and late complications are most often due to inexperienced operator error in terms of stent sizing and/or stent misplacement within the carina or cricoid. As with any procedure, the risk of complications is reduced with experience. Long-term complications reportedly include continued collapse beyond the

Veterinary Image-Guided Interventions, First Edition. Edited by Chick Weisse and Allyson Berent.

Companion website: www.wiley.com/go/weisse/vet-image-guided-interventions

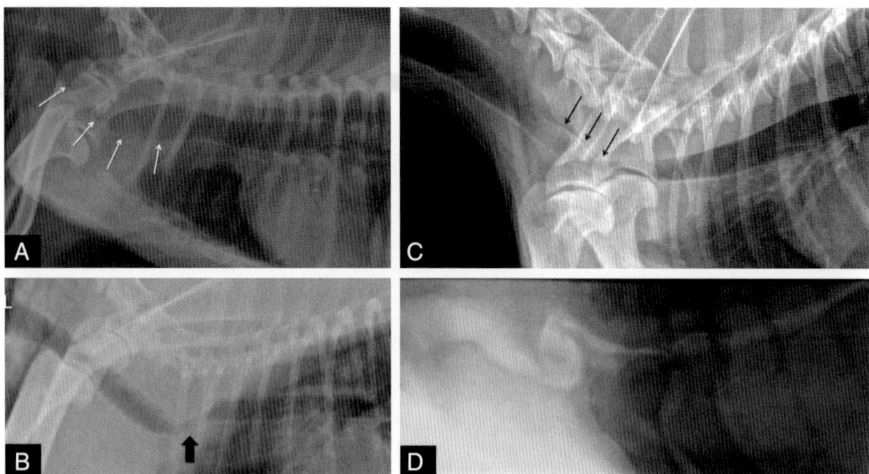

Figure 7.1 Radiographic variations of tracheal collapse syndrome. (A) Cervical chondromalacia (white arrows) with enlarged trachea. (B) Segmental tracheal narrowing (black arrow). (C) Segmental tracheal malformation with dorsal luminal narrowing (black arrows). (D) Diffuse chondromalacia with tracheal folding due to loss of integrity.

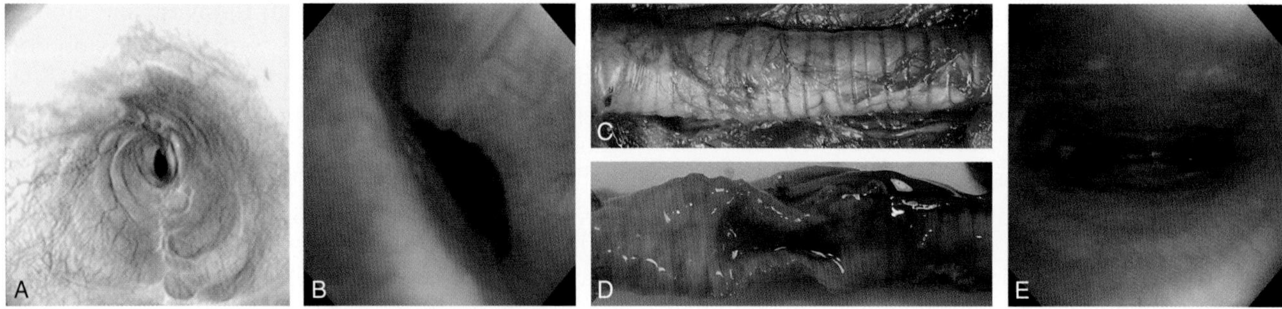

Figure 7.2 Endoscopic and gross variations of tracheal collapse/narrowing. (A) Endoscopic view of congenital tracheal stricture/stenosis. (B) Endoscopic view of tracheal malformation with lateral compression of tracheal rings. (C) Normal post mortem specimen of ventral aspect of canine trachea. (D) Gross mortem specimen of ventral aspect of canine tracheal malformation with "W"-shaped tracheal cartilages. (E) Endoscopic view of "W"-shaped cartilage in canine tracheal malformation demonstrating narrowed lumen. Note the "W" rather than "C" shaped cartilage rings.

BOX 7.1
Medical management

- Antitussives:
  - Hydrocodone (0.25–1.0 mg/kg PO q4–8 hr until sedation)
  - Dextromethorphan (1 ml/kg of 2 mg/ml solution PO q8–12 hr)
  - Butorphanol (0.5–1.0 mg/kg PO q4–6 hr)
- Anti-inflammatories:
  - Prednisone (1–2 mg/kg/day PO)
  - Inhaled fluticasone 220 μg (1–2 puffs q12 hr using pediatric spacer)
- Bronchodilators:
  - Theophylline – extended release (5–20 mg/kg PO q12 hr – dogs)
- Anxiolytics/sedatives:
  - Trazodone 2–4 mg/kg PO q12 hr
  - Acepromazine 0.005–0.02 mg/kg SQ or IV prn

stent, stent shortening (up to 83% of cases), stent migration (typically only when undersized), pneumonia, bacterial tracheitis (up to 58%), inflammatory and/or granulation tissue development (up to 16–28%), stent fracture (up to 42% with some stents), and death. The higher ends of these reported incidences seem excessive and are uncommon in the author's experience. Stenting has largely replaced extraluminal prostheses in some veterinary hospitals as clinical improvement rates of 75–90% are similar for both techniques, with fewer perioperative complications associated with stenting including lower (0–8%) perioperative mortality rates. Long-term complications are still largely unknown due to limited small retrospective studies currently available using different stent types, however stent fractures are reported in 10–42% of cases and likely occur somewhere in-between depending upon stent type and material, technical considerations such as sizing and placement, period of follow-up, and severity of disease (such as lower airway involvement/collapse). In the author's experience of over 200 cases currently stented, periprocedural morbidity (<10%) and mortality (~6%) is extremely rare, but long-term complications, as discussed earlier, are not uncommon. Fortunately, many of the complications associated with stenting are technical errors associated with stent selection and placement; these mistakes can often be prevented with experience and training. Other complications, such as stent fracture, may be avoided or minimized with aggressive and routine re-evaluations, aggressive antitussive therapy, and re-stenting when necessary. Intraluminal stents have been in place for over 10 years in some patients. Patients with dynamic airway obstructions and honking/raspy breathing seem to respond best to tracheal stenting. Patients with coughing as the most profound presenting clinical sign can improve with stenting, but these are the patients in whom predicting outcomes is most difficult. Continued coughing should be anticipated in patients with concurrent symptomatic bronchial collapse. Owners should be warned of a possible worse prognosis when bronchial collapse is present, however many of these dogs respond well to tracheal stenting when the clinical signs are associated with the tracheal rather than bronchial component of the collapse. Regular post-stent monitoring and owner compliance with medical management instructions likely will improve outcomes and identify complications sooner before catastrophic problems arise.

Equipment

A list of recommended equipment can be found in Figure 7.3. Mesh, self-expanding metallic stents are most commonly used for tracheal stenting procedures, as balloon-expandable and laser-cut stents have been associated with unacceptable risks of migration and fracture, respectively. Tracheal stenting can be performed using fluoroscopy, endoscopy, or digital radiography. Fluoroscopy is the author's preferred method as it can be performed patiently and under controlled circumstances, as the patient remains intubated providing constant oxygen and anesthetic delivery. In addition, the entire stent, cricoid, and carina remain visible at all times limiting the chance for accidental stent dislodgement or misplacement during the procedure. Fluoroscopy and digital radiography entails risk of substantial radiation exposure, so care must be taken to reduce operator exposure through beam collimation, reducing dose, and wearing standard radiation protection gear.

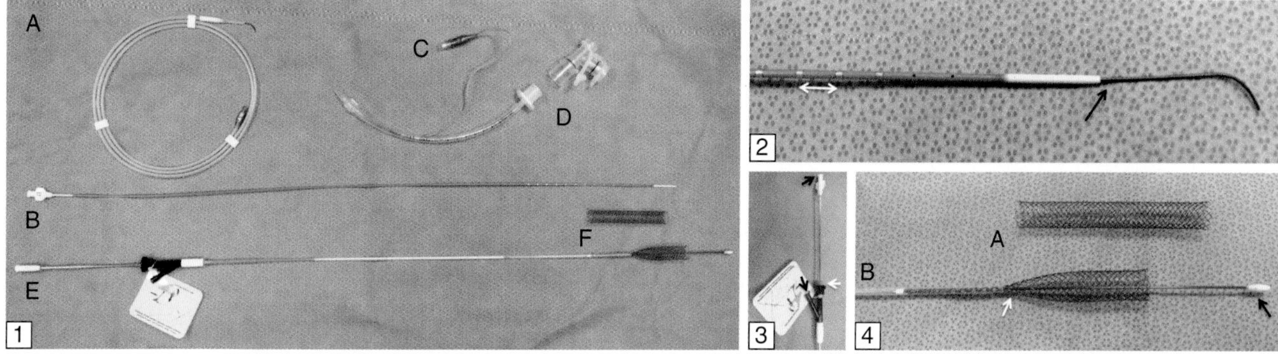

Figure 7.3 Equipment needed for tracheal stenting procedure. 1A. Hydrophilic 0.035" angled guide wire. 1B. 5Fr Marker catheter. 1C. Radio-opaque endotracheal tube of at least 4mm internal diameter. 1D. Bronchoscope adapter. 1E. Tracheal stent on delivery system with partial stent deployment. 1F. Deployed tracheal stent (not necessary; for demonstration only). 2. Close-up view of marker catheter with guide wire (black arrow) extending 3–5cm out the tip prior to advancement down the esophagus. Note the distance from the beginning of one mark to the beginning of the next (white arrow) is 10mm. 3. Close-up view of the tracheal stent delivery system. Prior to use sterile saline is injected in the proximal port and side port (black arrows) to remove air and moisten stent. The diaphragm is then unlocked by twisting the dial on the Y-piece (white arrow). 4A. Close-up view of deployed tracheal stent. 4B. Partially constrained tracheal stent. Prior to placement within the patient the stent is only slightly deployed to make certain everything is working. Note the partially constrained stent and partially deployed stent (white arrow). As the stent is deployed, it retracts away from the nose cone (black arrow).

Tracheoscopy

Although not required, the author recommends and standardly performs an oral and laryngeal exam and tracheoscopy prior to intubation using a flexible bronchoscope. Endoscopy helps provide information on the type of collapse present (such as weakened dorsal tracheal membrane, tracheal malformation, etc.) and variability between tracheal width and height. Tracheoscopy is repeated following stent placement to ensure the cricoid and carina are not engaged by the stent and there is appropriate apposition between the stent and tracheal wall. An endotracheal lavage is also performed to obtain samples for cytology and microbial culture and sensitivity testing.

Fluoroscopic Procedure

Refer to Chapter 1 for further information regarding each piece of recommended equipment. A radio-opaque endotracheal (ET) tube with an inner diameter (ID) of at least 4 mm (4.5 mm or larger preferred when possible) is recommended. The patient is placed in lateral recumbency with the neck flexed in order to straighten the trachea as much as possible. A combination 5Fr marker catheter[1] with a 0.035″ angled hydrophilic guide wire[2] extending approximately 5 cm out the catheter tip is placed in the mouth and advanced down the esophagus until the radio-opaque markers span the length of the trachea. The endotracheal (ET) tube cuff is deflated and under fluoroscopic guidance the ET tube is withdrawn until the cuff is at the level of the cricoid where it is reinflated. The patient is hyperventilated to reduce breathing during radiograph exposure. The positive/negative pressure device (Figure 7.4) is attached to the ET tube and two subsequent images are obtained; one during positive pressure ventilation at 20 cmH_2O and a second at −10 to −15 cmH_2O (Figure 7.5). Make certain there is no air leak during acquisition of these images. The negative pressure ventilation image will help define the extent of the tracheal and bronchial collapse that is often underestimated using static radiographs or (non-dynamic) tracheobronchoscopy.

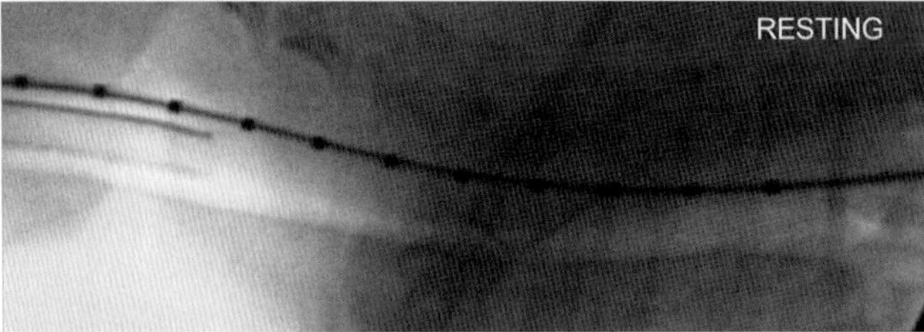

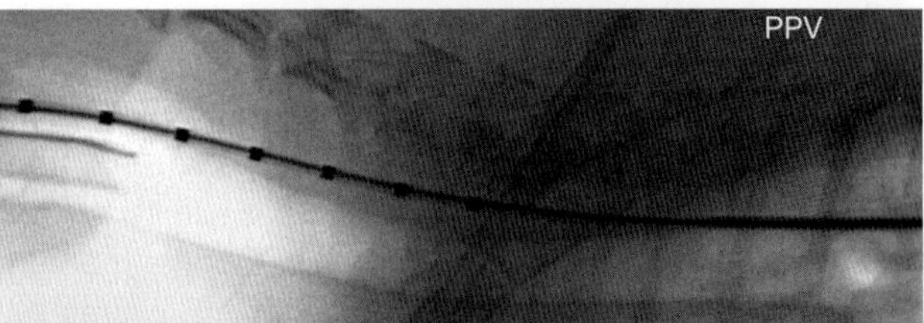

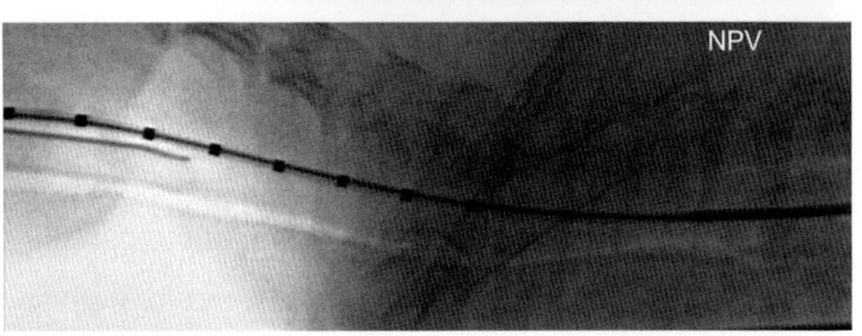

Figure 7.4 Serial lateral radiographs in a dog demonstrating variability under static versus dynamic ventilatory pressures. RESTING: Static radiograph demonstrating minimal degree of collapse. PPV: 20 cmH_2O positive pressure ventilation demonstrating maximal tracheal diameter. NPV: −10 to −15 cmH_2O demonstrating diffuse tracheal and carinal collapse.

Tracheal Stent Diameter

On the positive pressure ventilation radiograph, use the esophageal marker catheter to determine the maximal tracheal diameter of the area you wish to span with your stent (typically the cervical and intrathoracic portions) and the degree of radiographic magnification (Figure 7.6). As tracheal stent sizes are typically available in 2 mm diameter increments, the author tends to choose a tracheal stent diameter 2–3 mm larger than the maximal tracheal diameter measured. The largest diameter is typically found in the cervical tracheal region. The measurement tools available on the radiography or fluoroscopy machine should not be used to obtain dimensions without the calibration of the marker catheter within the esophagus.

Tracheal Stent Length

On the same radiograph identify the carina and cricoid. Leaving approximately 10 mm of safety distance from each of these locations, measure the distance between them using the marker catheter. This will be the MAXIMUM length of trachea to stent, NOT the tracheal stent length. Using the stent shortening chart provided by most mesh, self-expanding metallic stent manufacturers, one can determine the estimated length of stent necessary to cover this area and ultimately the necessary stent length. Oversizing the stent diameter will hold the stent in place and also prevent complete stent expansion; if the stent does not expand to its

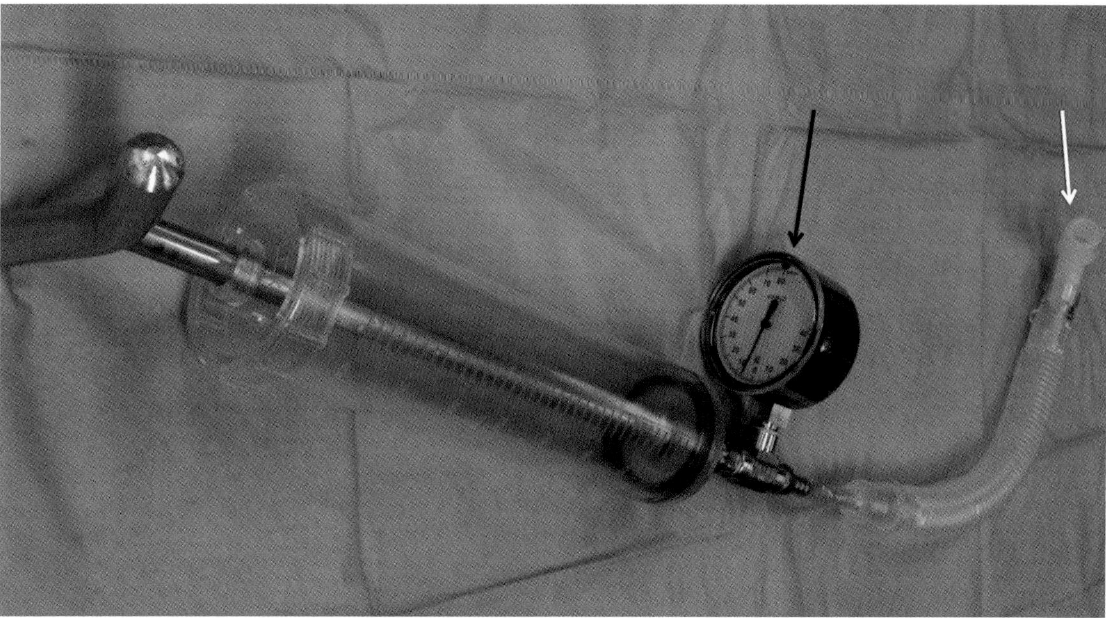

Figure 7.5 Positive (PPV) and negative pressure ventilation (NPV) device. Positive pressure can be achieved with the anesthesia machine but this device is necessary to perform NPV. A dosing syringe is attached to a sphygmomanometer (black arrow) and anesthesia tubing with an adapter (white arrow) to attach to the ET tube. PPV at 20 cmH_2O and NPV at −10 to −15 cmH_2O are performed.

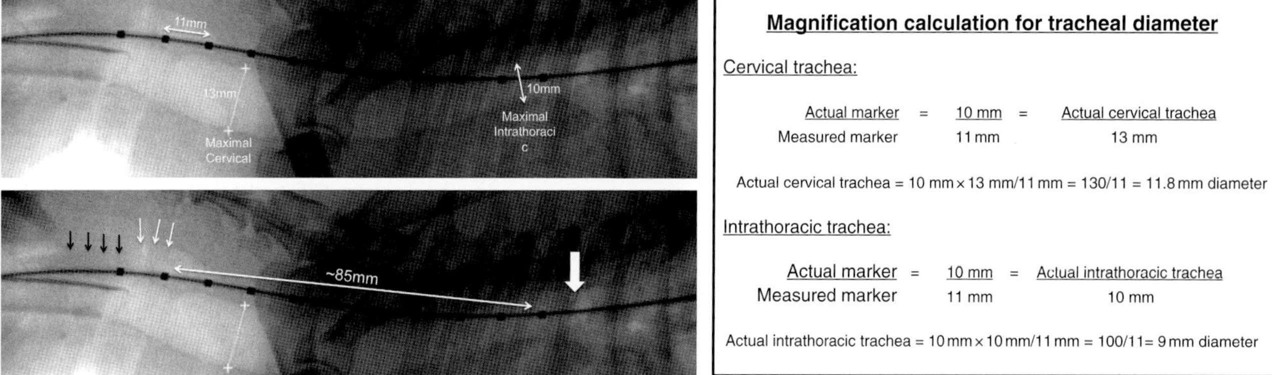

Figure 7.6 Lateral 20 cmH_2O positive-pressure radiographs with esophageal marker catheter in place performed for determining maximal tracheal diameter and length of stent necessary. Top: Measurement from the beginning of one marker to the next is 11 mm. Maximal cervical and intrathoracic tracheal diameters are 13 mm and 10 mm, respectively, prior to accounting for radiographic magnification. Bottom: Cricoid cartilage (black arrows) identified rostral to air in the esophagus (white arrows) and the carina (white block arrow) mark the extent of the trachea. Using a 10 mm safety margin from each of these landmarks, a maximum of 85 mm of trachea will be stented. Right: Radiographic magnification is calculated and used to determine the actual maximum cervical and intrathoracic tracheal diameters of 11.8 mm and 9 mm, respectively.

full diameter, it will not shorten completely. Therefore, using the maximal cervical and intrathoracic tracheal diameters, one can anticipate the degree of stent diameter expansion that will occur. Using the stent shortening chart (Figure 7.7), one will then be able to anticipate the ultimate length a particular stent will achieve following placement, assuming it opens slightly larger than the maximal measurements in each area obtained (via the outward radial force of the stent as well as the generally larger width of the oval trachea compared to the height that is measured on the lateral radiograph). Remember that each manufacturer will have different sizing/shortening charts and they should be not interchanged.

Shortening chart of vet stent - trachea 14 mm diameter nominal dimensions of the stent		Dimensions of the stent during expansion	
Nominal (Relaxed) outer diameter	Nominal (Relaxed) Length [mm]	Expanded diameter [mm]	Length at expanded diameter [mm]
14	30	On delivery system	54
		7	50
		10	44
		12	39
14	40	On delivery system	75
		7	69
		10	61
		12	53
14	58	On delivery system	105
		7	97
		10	85
		12	74
14	72	On delivery system	131
		7	121
		10	106
		12	92
14	85	On delivery system	157
		7	144
		10	127
		12	110
14	100	On delivery system	183
		7	168
		10	148
		12	128

Figure 7.7 Stent shortening chart for 14 mm tracheal stents (www.infinitimedical.com). For the trachea in Figure 7.4, a 14 mm diameter stent will be used in order to be 2–3 mm greater diameter than maximum measured. The chart above demonstrates the various lengths different 14 mm diameter stents will achieve when expanded to different diameters. A 14 × 58 mm stent expanding between 9 mm and 11.7 mm will ultimately expand to approximately 85 mm.

Stent Placement

Please refer to individual manufacturer guidelines regarding preparation, deployment, and specific characteristics (reconstrainability, degree of foreshortening, etc.) of individual stents prior to use. In general, the stent delivery systems[3] are handled with sterile gloves. Flush the delivery system hub and sheath with sterile saline to expel air and wet the stent. Loosen the Y-piece on the stent delivery system to facilitate stent deployment; this does not need to be completely unscrewed, just loosened. For reconstrainable stents, deploy approximately 10 mm of the stent and reconstrain it to make certain the delivery system is working properly prior to placement. Attach the bronchoscope adapter to the endotracheal tube, hyperventilate the patient, and consider an injectable anesthetic bolus when indicated to prevent patient movement and coughing during stent placement. Confirm appropriate patient and fluoroscopic positioning such that the trachea is straight, the ET tube is at the level of the cricoid, and the cricoid and carina are both identified in the field of view. Remember, a radiopaque endotracheal tube should be used to visualize the end of the tube at all times during stent deployment. Deflate the ET tube cuff and untie the endotracheal tube from around the neck or muzzle. Under direct fluoroscopic visualization, advance the stent delivery system through the bronchoscope adapter, down the trachea, and proceed with deployment. To proceed with stent deployment, the sheath is gently withdrawn as the stent is slowly advanced into the trachea (Figure 7.8). This results in the nose cone being advanced down the trachea and the leading (caudal) edge of the stent remaining in the same position (Figure 7.9). After approximately 1/3 to 1/2 of stent length deployment, gently push and pull the delivery system to confirm the partially deployed

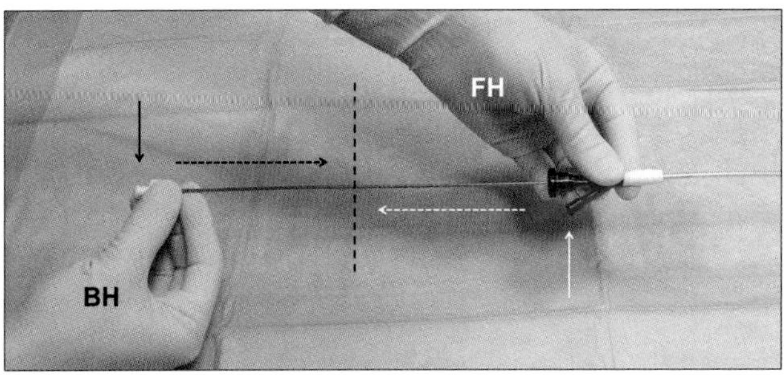

Figure 7.8 Stent deployment. The stent delivery system is held with two hands, the front hand (FH) holds the Y-piece connector of the delivery system (white arrow) and the back hand (BH) holds the hub (black arrow). During deployment, the two hands move together to meet in the middle (the dotted black line). As the FH moves back, the stent is exposed. As the BH pushes forward, the stent is advanced down the trachea. If done correctly, the leading edge of the stent is motionless as the stent is deployed. The nose cone of the delivery system will advance down the trachea and the stent will shorten from the cranial edge. During deployment, remember that the BH determines the location of the stent and the FH deploys it.

stent is engaging the trachea and not sliding back and forth; If the stent is moving within the trachea it is undersized and should be reconstrained and removed before complete deployment and a larger size should be chosen. If the trachea moves back and forth with gentle movement of the delivery system while the stent is engaged, continue deployment. During every few centimeters of stent deployment, push the delivery system inward softly to gently force the stent to expand; it is important NOT to have excessive back tension on the delivery system that will result in stretching and narrowing of the stent. Pay close attention to the ET tube so that it is withdrawn during stent deployment, preventing entrapment of the stent inside the tube; it is occasionally necessary to extubate the dog during stent deployment and then reintubate by advancing the ET tube over the delivery system under fluoroscopic guidance after the stent is fully deployed. If at any time the stent diameter or length appears inadequate prior to complete deployment, gently reconstrain the stent and remove the entire delivery system. Different stents have different characteristics but in general (to be safe) one should not deploy more than approximately 80% of the stent length with hopes of reconstrainment. Remove the delivery system under fluoroscopic guidance to avoid engaging the stent with the delivery system nose cone. Once the stent is fully deployed take a still image in both lateral and VD dimensions so that final stent location is documented for future comparisons and to ensure the stent is not placed into the mainstem

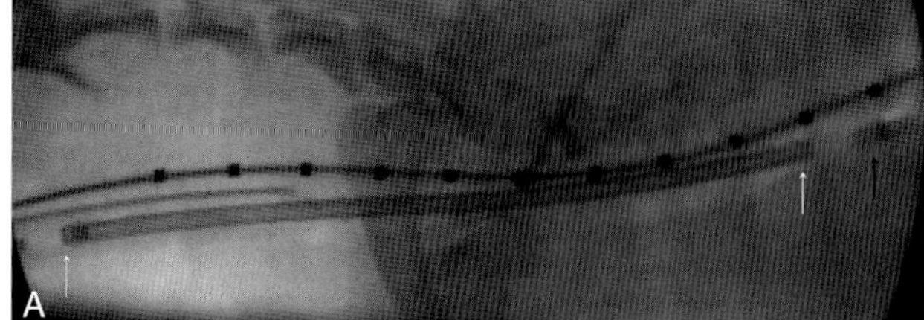

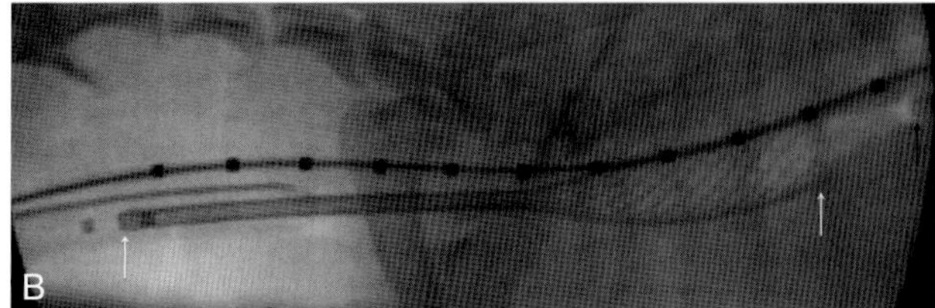

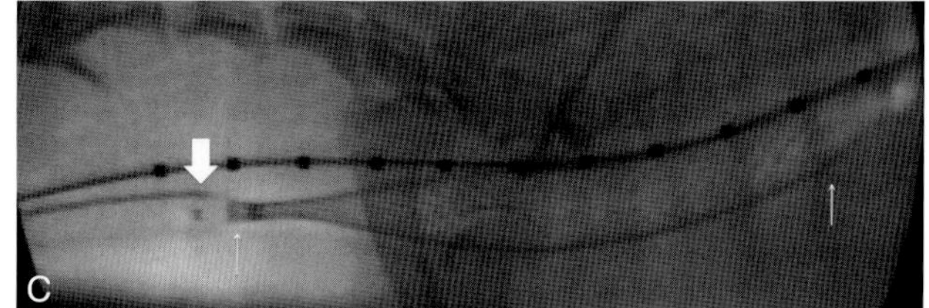

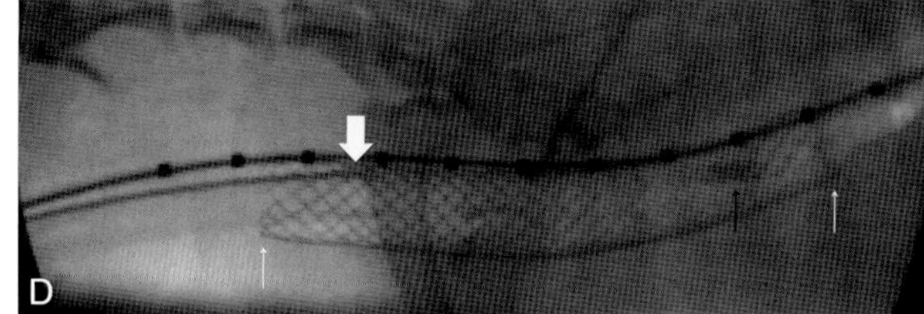

Figure 7.9 Serial images taken during stent deployment. (A) Constrained stent (white arrows) in place prior to deployment. Note the location of the nose cone (black arrow). (B) As deployment proceeds, the stent (white arrows) expands from the leading edge and the nose cone advances down the trachea (black arrow) as the stent shortens from the cranial edge. At this time gentle back and forth movement of the delivery systems confirms friction and an appropriate stent diameter. (C) Just before final deployment retract ET tube (white block arrow). (D) After deployment the ET tube (white block arrow) is advanced over the delivery system and the nose cone (black arrow) is gently retracted with the delivery system. Note the stent (white arrows) is substantially shorter than it was in the delivery system prior to deployment (A).

bronchus or larynx. As mentioned above, repeat tracheoscopy is recommend following stent deployment.

Follow-Up

The patient is recovered in the intensive care unit and medical therapy including antitussives (hydrocodone 0.25–1.0 mg/kg PO q6 hr), corticosteroids (prednisone 0.5–1.0 mg/kg PO q12 hr to taper after 2 weeks of therapy), and antibiotics (10–14 days of broad-spectrum antibiotics) are continued. Trazodone

(2–4 mg/kg PO q12 hr) is administered to patients in whom anxiety or excitement historically exacerbate clinical signs. Patients with bronchial collapse and/or an observed "expiratory push" during exhalation may benefit from bronchodilator therapy. Patients have three-view thoracic radiographs the following day prior to discharge. Owners are instructed to call with updates weekly until the first recheck examination in one month. Three-view thoracic radiographs are always recommended in these patients with the forelimbs pulled forward in one lateral and pulled caudally in the other to make certain the entire trachea is visualized. A mild, dry cough should be anticipated for the first 3–4 weeks as the stent becomes incorporated into the tracheal mucosa. While some dogs respond immediately, for others the first month post-stenting can be difficult for owners necessitating frequent phone calls and medication adjustments. As long as they have been warned this does not come as a surprise. Dogs with bronchial collapse should be expected to have continued coughing and will likely need to be maintained on antitussive therapy for life. The majority of dogs with tracheal stents will require some form of lifelong medication; the owners should be aware of this prior to stent placement. Recheck examinations are scheduled every 3 months for the first year or sooner if there are problems; examinations are then scheduled every 3–6 months. Owners are also instructed to rate coughing, honking/raspy breathing, and dyspnea levels routinely and call if there are acute changes in any of these parameters as this may be indicative of a problem requiring further intervention.

Special Considerations/ Complication Examples

In general, it appears that clinical signs associated with honking/raspy breathing and dyspnea/airway obstruction respond very favorably to tracheal stenting. Coughing can be due to tracheal collapse, bronchial collapse, lower airway disease, cardiac disease, pneumonia, and other comorbidities. Resolution or improvement of coughing following tracheal stenting is less predictable and, in rare occasions, can actually worsen in cases of lower airway collapse with expiratory push/effort. The variety of disorders included in the "tracheal collapse syndrome" including chondromalacia, weakened/redundant dorsal tracheal membranes, and tracheal ring malformations ("W"-shaped cartilage rings, lateral compressions, etc.) makes prognosis difficult, however some complications are shared amongst them. Common stent placement problem and complications are demonstrated in Figure 7.10 for reference. The most severe problems include stent fracture or inflammatory/granulation tissue proliferation, both of which can lead to progressive airway obstruction. Restenting of these conditions (a second stent placed within the first) can substantial alleviate clinical signs in these patients in the short term (months to years); however, the durability of these treatments is still unclear in the long term (many years). When re-stenting is performed it is recommended that the second stent be placed directly inside the first stent. This procedure should be done over a soft guide wire being careful to prevent lung

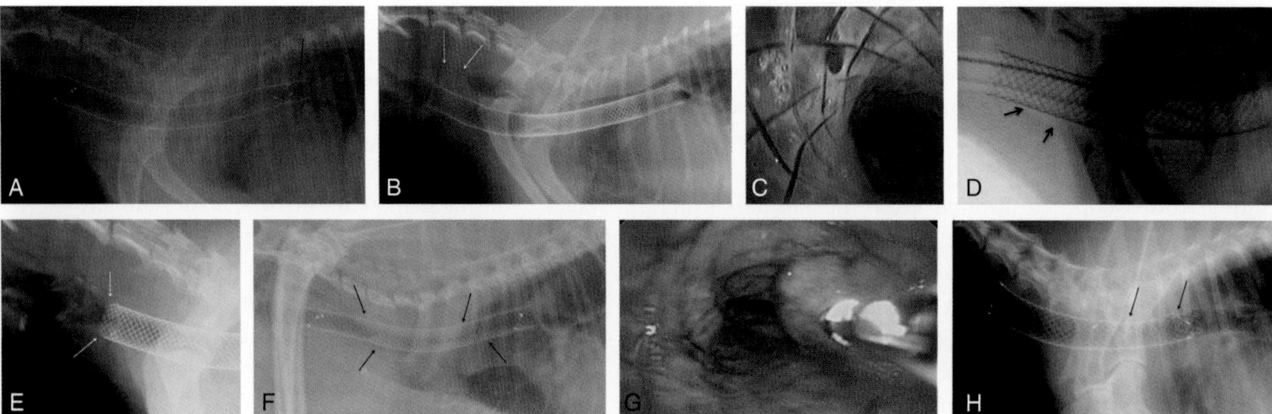

Figure 7.10 Various tracheal stent complications. (A) Stent placed into mainstem bronchus. Note stent tapering at level of carina (black arrow). (B) Stent placed within cricoid. Note stent tapering (black arrow) ventral to the cricopharyngeus muscle (white arrows). (C) Undersized stent with incomplete tracheal contact and mucus accumulation. (D) Stent undersizing with gap (black arrows) between stent and tracheal wall on radiographs. (E) Inflammatory tissue development at cranial aspect of stent (white arrows) resulting in luminal narrowing. (F) Tissue ingrowth at thoracic inlet (between black arrows). (G) Inflammatory/granulation tissue (asterisk) identified and biopsied during tracheoscopy. (H) Early stent fracture (black arrows) along dorsal, intrathoracic portion of the stent.

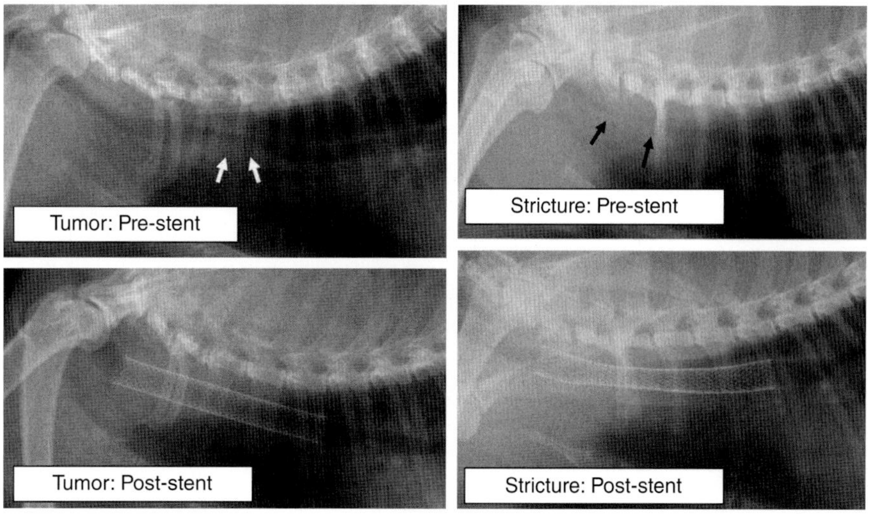

Figure 7.11 Lateral thoracic radiographs in two cats with tracheal obstructions. Left: Cat with tracheal tumor and subsequent airway obstruction prior to (above) and following (below) self-expanding, mesh metallic stent placement. Right: Cat with benign tracheal stricture prior to (above) and following (below) laser-cut, self-expanding stent placement.

parenchymal perforation and to ensure that the wire is through the lumen of the first stent and not lateral to it. The new constrained stent should be evaluated prior to deployment in two views (lateral and DV/VD) to ensure it is within the lumen of the first stent. Alternatively the guide wire can be placed through the bronchoscope first placed through the lumen of the prior fractured stent. The first stent should be covered at least 50% by the second stent, and if re-stenting is for a fracture, the entire stent should be covered as this patient is likely at increased risk for future fracture. When stenting for tracheal malformations, incomplete tracheal wall apposition by the stent is one of the most common complications encountered. This can result in "gutters" to exist at the ventrolateral aspects of the trachea along the malformation and permit mucus accumulation and subsequent infections and tissue ingrowth. Tracheoscopy performed prior to and following stent placement can help identify these cases and ensure there is good wall apposition; if not, the endotracheal tube cuff (or angioplasty balloon) can be used to gently expand the stent to improve wall apposition.

Tracheal Tumors and Strictures

Intraluminal stenting has also been used for tracheal tumors and strictures in both dogs and cats (Figure 7.11). The procedure is similar to that described above but there are a few differences. As these lesions tend to be more focal, shorter stents can typically be used. The lesions are spanned by at least 10mm on each side and care should be taken when using very short stents as they may have a tendency to "watermelon seed" or slide cranially or caudally when eccentrically placed across a narrowing. In addition, while laser-cut stents are not recommended for tracheal collapse cases due to considerable fracture rates with currently available stents, laser-cut stents have been successfully used for tracheal tumors and strictures. The author believes this is likely due to the fact that the tracheal cartilage integrity is fairly preserved in the latter cases (unlike the tracheal collapse cases) providing support and rigidity for the stents. Patients with tumors and strictures subjectively appear to tolerate tracheal stents very well, often with considerably fewer clinical signs than tracheal collapse patients. One recent report of using a tracheal stent in 3 cats for a stricture (2) and neoplasia (1) resulted in excellent short- and long-term outcomes (>3 years for stricture cases).

Notes

(Examples; Multiple vendors available)

1. Measuring catheter, Infiniti Medical, Menlo Park, CA.
2. Weasel wire, Infiniti Medical, Menlo Park, CA.
3. Vet Stent-Trachea, Infiniti Medical, Menlo Park, CA.

Suggested Reading

Buback JL, Boothe HW, Hobson HP, et al (1996) Surgical treatment of tracheal collapse in dogs: 90 cases (1983–1993) *J Am Vet Assoc* 208(3), 380–4.

Culp WT, Weisse C, Cole S, et al (2007) Intraluminal tracheal stenting for treatment of tracheal narrowing in three cats. *Vet Surg* 36, 107–13.

Johnson LR and Fales WH (2001) Clinical and microbiologic finding in dogs with bronchoscopically diagnosed tracheal collapse: 37 cases (1990–1995). *J Am Vet Assoc* 219, 1247–50.

Mittleman E, Weisse C, Mehler SJ, et al (2004) Fracture of an endoluminal nitinol stent used in the treatment of tracheal collapse in a dog. *J Am Vet Med Assoc* 225(8), 1217–1221.

Moritz A, Schneider M, and Bauer N (2004) Management of advanced tracheal collapse in dogs using intraluminal self-expanding biliary wallstents. *J Vet Intern Med* 18, 31–42.

Nelson AW (2002) Diseases of the trachea and bronchi. In: *Textbook of Small Animal Surgery*, 3rd edn (Slatter D, ed). WB Saunders Co, Philadelphia, p. 858.

Sun F, Uson J, Ezquerra J, et al (2008) Endotracheal stenting therapy in dogs with tracheal collapse. *Vet J* 175, 186–93.

Sura PA and Krahwinkel DJ (2008) Self-expanding nitinol stents for the treatment of tracheal collapse in dogs: 12 cases (2001–2004). *J Am Vet Med Assoc* 232(2), 228–36.

Weisse C and Berent A (2010) Tracheal stenting in collapsed trachea. *Textbook of Veterinary Internal Medicine*, 7th edn (Feldman, ed.) pp. 1088–1096.

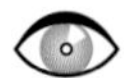
Video clips to accompany this chapter can be found in the online material at **www.wiley.com/go/weisse/vet-image-guided-interventions**

CHAPTER EIGHT

Bronchial Collapse and Stenting

George A. Kramer
Atlantic Coast Veterinary Specialists, Bohemia, NY

Background/Indications

Bronchial collapse in dogs is associated with a number of causes including chronic bronchitis, neoplasia, heart disease, chondromalacia, and strictures. Collapse can occur focally, diffusely, or may be an extension of tracheal collapse. Symptoms of bronchial collapse include coughing, dyspnea, tachypnea, expiratory push, wheezing, syncope, and cyanosis. Treatment for most cases of bronchial collapse consists of a combination of medical therapies including cough suppressants, antibiotics, bronchodilators, anti-inflammatory medications (e.g., corticosteroids), and sedatives (Box 8.1). Patients with bronchial collapse/compression associated with cardiomegaly should also be treated with a negative chronotropic drug (e.g., digoxin or diltiazem) to decrease the heart rate and cyclic compression of the affected bronchus. In certain cases, intraluminal stenting may be an option if medical therapy has failed. When treating these cases, either medically or via intraluminal stenting, it is important to manage the owner's expectations. The causal conditions leading to bronchial collapse are typically chronic conditions and as a general rule of thumb, treatments (including stenting) are palliative rather than curative.

The indication for bronchial stenting is the inability of medical therapy to adequately control clinical signs and provide a reasonable quality of life. Careful case selection is very important to ensure a positive outcome. The best candidates for stenting should have discrete collapse in one or two bronchi with normal appearing airways throughout the rest of the bronchial tree. Patients with chronic bronchitis and multifocal collapse or diffuse chondromalacia are not good candidates for this procedure.

The author has previously shown an association between cardiomegaly in small breed dogs due to chronic valvular heart disease and bronchial collapse. The patient population in that study consisted of dogs with severe chronic valvular disease (CVD), cardiomegaly, and a chronic cough, but were not in congestive heart failure. Individuals in this cohort of patients may be suitable candidates for stenting and should be further assessed. Although this chapter focuses on patients with heart disease and bronchial collapse/compression, patients with other causes of discrete collapse of a principle or lobar bronchus (i.e., chronic airway disease, neoplasia, or a stricture) could also be potential candidates for stenting. Some dogs with tracheal collapse may also present with bronchial collapse; the vast majority of these dogs do not require bronchial stenting. If the bronchial collapse is discrete and persistently clinical after tracheal stenting has been performed, the author believes the patient may benefit from bronchial stenting as well (see Figure 8.1). At the time of writing this article, the author has placed bronchial stents in 28 dogs. Twenty-four of them were dogs with severe discrete collapse of LB2 and LB1 in association with cardiomegaly. The remaining four dogs presented with tracheal collapse and had tracheal stents placed either at the time of bronchial stent placement or several months prior to bronchial stent placement.

Patient Preparation

While fluoroscopy and chest radiography are helpful, the extent of bronchial collapse is best made via bronchoscopy. In addition, samples can be obtained for cytology, culture, and biopsy when indicated. The initial workup should include chest radiographs, echocardiogram, complete blood count, chemistry profile, heartworm and lungworm testing. Cross-sectional imaging (e.g., computerized tomography (CT) scan, magnetic resonance imaging (MRI), etc.)

Veterinary Image-Guided Interventions, First Edition. Edited by Chick Weisse and Allyson Berent.

Companion website: www.wiley.com/go/weisse/vet-image-guided-interventions

BOX 8.1
Commonly used drugs for the medical management of bronchial collapse

- *Antitussives*
  - Butorphanol (0.5–1.0 mg/kg PO q4–12 hr)
  - Hydrocodone (0.25–1.0 mg/kg PO q4–8 hr)
  - Dextromethorphan 2 mg/ml (1 ml/kg q8–12 hr)
- *Anti-inflammatory*
  - Inhaled fluticasone 220 μg (1–2 puffs q12 hr)
  - Prednisone (0.5–1.0 mg/kg q12 hr); avoid use if the patient has significant underlying heart disease
- *Antibiotics*
  - Broad-spectrum antibiotic, or one based on culture and sensitivity
- *Bronchodilators*
  - Theophylline, extended release (5–20 mg/kg PO q12 hr); avoid use in dogs with underlying cardiac disease if it induces sinus tachycardia.
- *SEDATIVES*
  - Acepromazine (0.005–0.02 mg/kg SC or IV q 4–12 hr)

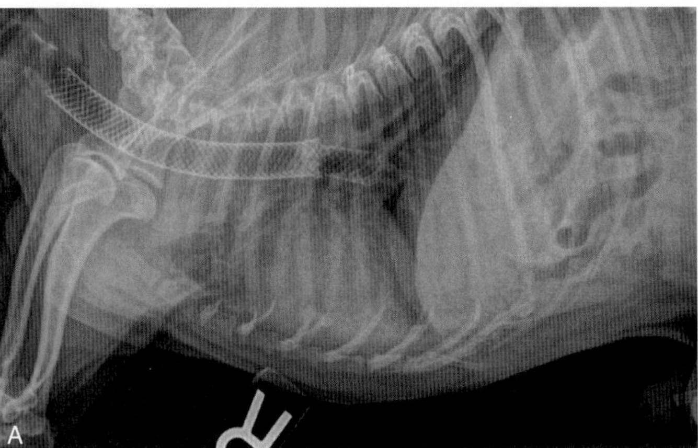

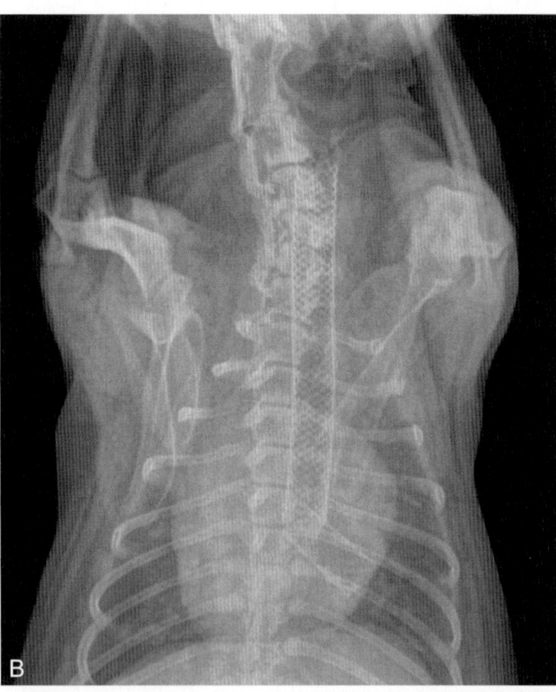

Figure 8.1 Chest radiograph of a patient that had a bronchial stent placed in LPB 8 months after placement of the tracheal stent.

may be helpful after the initial workup; however the author has not utilized these modalities in the cases described to date.

Understanding bronchial anatomy is a prerequisite. There are species variations in bronchial anatomy that are important and should be reviewed. Figure 8.2 diagrams the canine bronchial tree. The left principal bronchus (LPB) and right principal bronchus (RPB) are often referred to as mainstem bronchi. The lobar bronchi branch off of the principal bronchi. The LPB splits into the left cranial lobar bronchus (LB1) and the left caudal lobar bronchus (LB2). The RPB splits into the right cranial lobar bronchus (RB1), middle lobar bronchus (RB2), accessory lobar bronchus (RB3) and caudal lobar bronchus (RB4). In the author's opinion, tertiary bronchi distal to the lobar bronchi are not candidates to stent due to their smaller size and tight branching pattern and due to the fact then when there is collapse of tertiary bronchi, typically multiple bronchi are affected. However, further investigation in the future may prove that collapsed tertiary bronchi could be candidates for stenting.

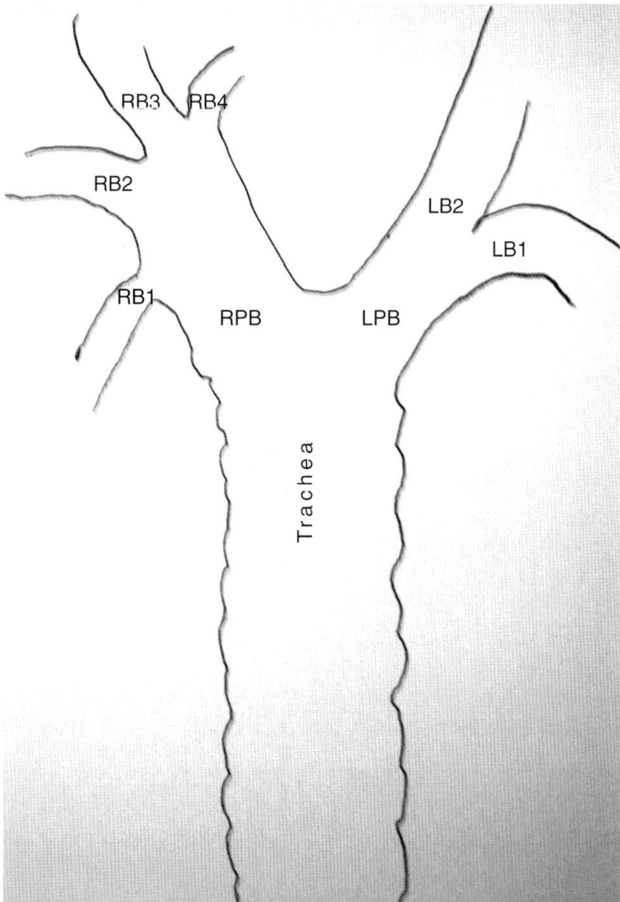

Figure 8.2 Canine bronchial tree showing the left principal bronchus (LPB), left cranial lobar bronchus (LB1), and the left caudal lobar bronchus (LB2), right principal bronchus (RPB), right cranial lobar bronchus (RB1), right middle lobar bronchus (RB2), right caudal lobar bronchus (RB3), right accessory lobar bronchus (RB4). Modified from Amis and McKiernan, Am J Vet Res 1986, 47:2649–2657.

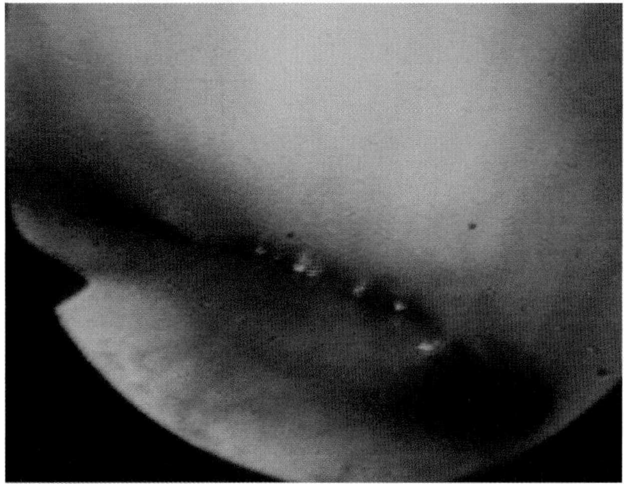

Figure 8.3 Bronchoscopic image showing grade 4 collapse of LB2 and LB1.

The author uses a system to grade bronchial collapse similar to that described for tracheal collapse; Grade 1 is 25% collapsed, grade 2 is 50% collapsed, grade 3 is 75% collapsed and grade 4 is 100% collapsed. In the chronic valvular disease cohort described above, LB2 is usually most severely collapsed (usually grade 4), followed by LB1 (usually grade 3 or 4). The principal bronchi and the right lobar bronchi are usually normal or minimally collapsed (assuming chronic bronchitis is not a comorbidity). Stenting is only recommended for grade 3 or 4 collapse (see Figure 8.3).

Potential Risks/Complications/Expected Outcomes

The most serious risks associated with the procedure are those resulting from anesthesia, especially considering most of the patients also have severe cardiac disease. A dedicated individual needs to monitor anesthesia, cardiac rhythm, blood pressure and most critically, make sure the patient is getting adequately ventilated, maintaining an appropriate SpO_2.

Potential complications associated with bronchial stenting are similar to those encountered with tracheal stenting, including stent migration, infection, stent fracture and excessive granulation or inflammatory tissue formation. Proper sizing of the stent can reduce the risk of migration. Antibiotic therapy may limit the risk of infection. Although bronchospasm and pneumothorax are complications that have been reported in humans with tracheobronchial stenting, they have not yet been reported in dogs with bronchial stents. Overall complication rates are low. To date the author has performed 28 bronchial stenting procedures. Migration has occurred in two cases, infection in one case and excessive granulation tissue formation in one case.

In addition to patient selection, managing client expectations is vital. Clients need to understand that the underlying condition(s) are chronic and treatment is palliative. Most of the patients will require ongoing medical therapy after stenting. With proper case selection, clinical signs can be significantly reduced. Owners, when questioned two weeks after the bronchial stenting procedure, have reported 60–90% reduction in coughing, decreased tachypnea, and improved quality of life. The most dramatic improvements seem to be in patients that have minimal airway disease except for the stented bronchus.

Equipment

A list of equipment needed for this procedure is listed in Figure 8.4. A flexible bronchoscope is required. Fluoroscopy and/or digital radiography may be helpful in sizing the stent, but it is not recommended to place bronchial stents solely with fluoroscopic or radiographic guidance. There have been a variety of stent types used to treat bronchial collapse in humans including polymer stents and a variety of metal stents (Gianturco, Palmaz, Wallstent, and Ultraflex stents). There have been frequent complications reported in humans and dogs with laser-cut stents and balloon expandable stents in the bronchi and trachea. The best type of stent for bronchial stenting in the author's opinion is an

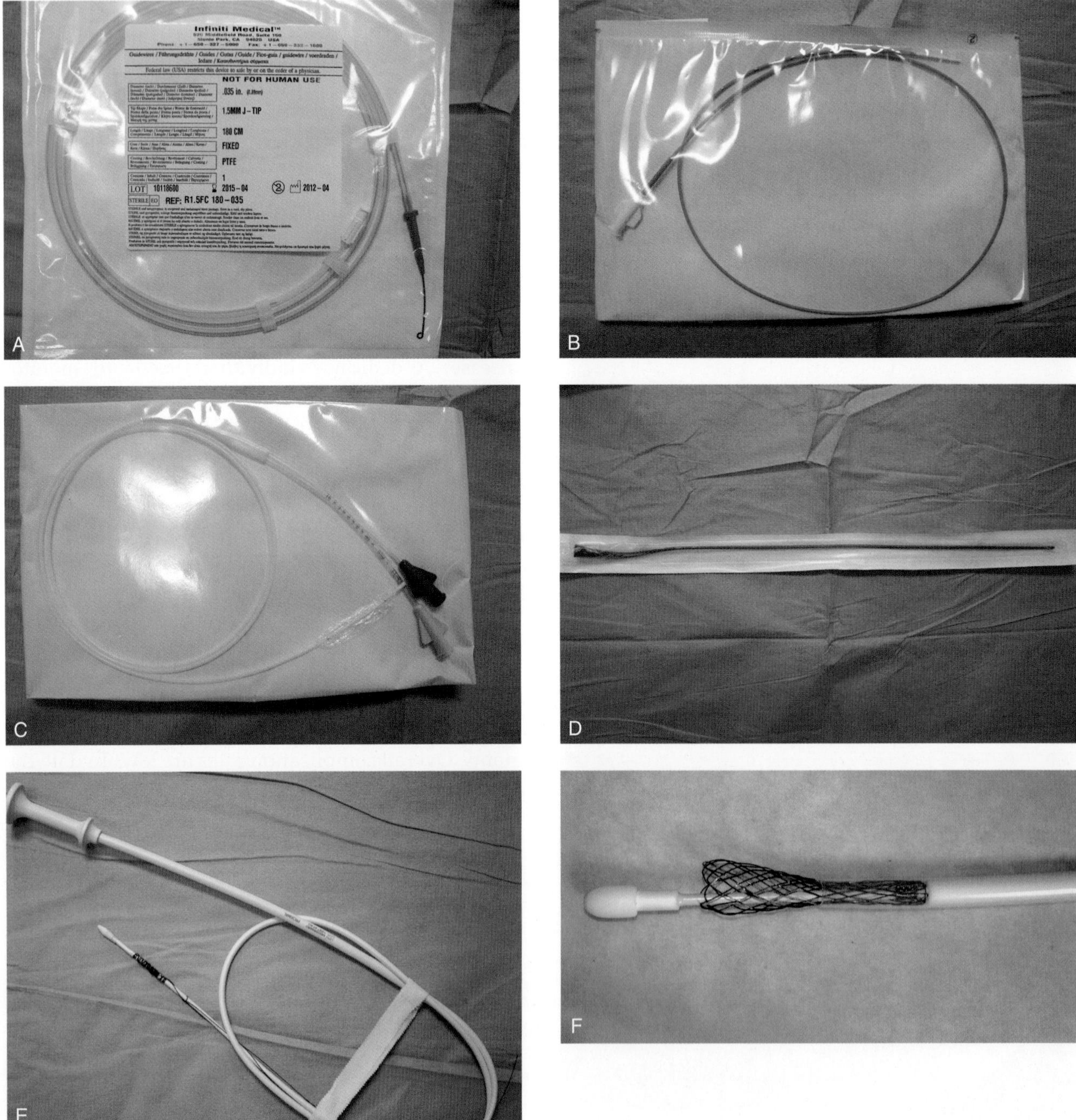

Figure 8.4 Equipment used for bronchial stenting; (A) 0.035″ j-tip guide wire. (B) 5Fr Sizing catheter. (C) Sizing balloon. (D) Red rubber catheter. (E) Ultraflex proximal release stent. (F) Partially deployed custom sized (8 × 20 mm) tracheal stent (for demonstration).

uncovered mesh self-expanding nitinol stent. Uncovered stents are preferred over covered stents to help maintain mucociliary function. The stents can be either proximally or distally released. With the current stent designs that are commercially available, the proximally releasing Ultraflex stents seem to work best. An alternative to the Ultraflex stent is a custom-sized, self-expanding, nitinol tracheal stent. The author currently has a bifurcating stent in development that will stent both LB1 and LB2. Additional equipment needed include a guide wire, measuring catheter, and balloon catheter.

Procedure

The majority of candidates for bronchial stenting have significant underlying valvular heart disease. Care must be taken to ensure that the heart disease is well regulated and the patient is not in congestive heart failure at the time of the procedure. The patient should be premedicated with hydromorphone and induced with either propofol or a ketamine/ diazepam combination. The plane of anesthesia should be kept very light, just enough to pass the bronchoscope without inducing coughing. Because these patients have significant heart disease every effort should be made to keep the procedure time within 30 minutes.

Once anesthetized, a measuring catheter is placed within the esophagus. The bronchoscope can be passed through an adaptor on the endotracheal tube, size permitting. Alternatively, a red rubber catheter can be used for oxygen delivery and the bronchoscope can be passed directly into the trachea without an endotracheal tube (the author's preferred method). Examination of the trachea, principal, lobar, and tertiary bronchi bilaterally is performed. LB2 is the bronchus that is usually most severely collapsed (grade 4) in these cases. Frequently LB1 will also have grade 3 or 4 collapse. If it is cost prohibitive to stent both bronchi, choose to stent the more severely collapsed bronchus. Once that stent is deployed, local tissue traction may slightly reduce the degree of collapse of the adjacent bronchus.

Once it is determined the patient is a candidate for stenting (i.e., there is focal collapse), cytology and culture samples are taken from the bronchus via a sterile brush catheter. The guide wire is then passed through the biopsy channel and advanced through the collapsed bronchus. It should be passed several centimeters down into distal branches to be secured in place. Special care is taken to avoid puncturing through the lung distally.

Sizing the Stent

The length of the stent required can be determined by placing the tip of the bronchoscope at the opening of the collapsed bronchus and using the centimeter markings on the scope. Measure how far the scope needs to be advanced to traverse the collapse. The stent should be slightly longer than the area of collapse. Typically, in most dogs, a 20 mm length stent is chosen. The guide wire is then held fixed in space while the bronchoscope is removed. The measuring balloon catheter is advanced over the guidewire into the trachea. The bronchoscope is repositioned into the carina and the bronchus is visualized to confirm the guide wire is still in position. The measuring balloon is then advanced into the bronchus and inflated with air or contrast agent until the bronchus fully opens. Care should be taken not to over-inflate the balloon. Using the measuring catheter scale, measurements of the balloon diameter are determined on the fluoroscopic or digital radiographic image (Figure 8.5). The stent should be 1.2–1.5 times the diameter of the balloon. In most small breed dogs, that is usually an 8 or 10 mm diameter stent. A less accurate and less time consuming alternative method to determine the stent diameter is utilizing the known diameter of the scope tip. Place the tip at the opening of the bronchus and estimate the width of the collapsed bronchus by direct visualization. A cytology brush of known size can also be used as a scale for comparison. Alternatively, the width of a grade 4 collapsed bronchus approximates half of the circumference of the bronchus. Using the equation $D = C/\pi$ to solve for diameter, multiply the

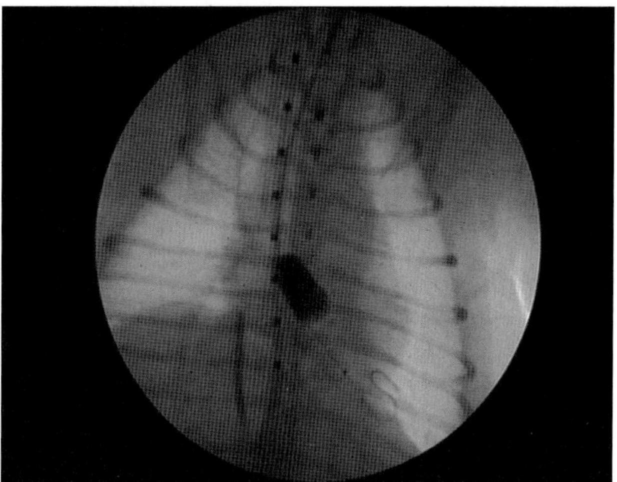

Figure 8.5 Fluoroscopic image of a Tyshak balloon distending LB2 to its normal diameter. A measuring catheter is in place in the esophagus to provide a centimeter scale to measure the balloon diameter.

width estimate by two (Width of grade 4 collapsed bronchus × 2 ~ Circumference) and divide by π (3.14) to determine the estimated diameter of the bronchus.

Deployment

The balloon is removed leaving the guide wire in place. The stent delivery system is passed over the guide wire and advanced into the lumen of the collapsed bronchus and the stent is deployed (see Figure 8.6 and Video 8.1). The delivery system should be positioned so that when the stent is deployed, it extends a few millimeters proximal to the opening of the bronchus. Once the stent is deployed, the delivery system and guide wire are carefully removed. Chest radiographs should be taken to document the stent position and serve as a standard for future comparison. The patient remains on supplemental oxygen during recovery. If the vital signs are stable the patient can be placed on room air within an hour after stent placement. Cough suppressant therapy is continued and the patient is monitored in ICU and discharged the following day.

Follow-Up

The patient is discharged on a broad-spectrum antibiotic for two weeks. Cough suppressant therapy (butorphanol 0.5–1.0 mg/kg TID) and the cardiac medications are continued. Bronchodilator therapy is not necessary unless significant small airway disease was noted during the pre-operative bronchoscopy. Inhaled fluticasone (220 μg puff BID) is used in patients with concurrent lower airway disease. Oral corticosteroids should be avoided if possible in the cohort of dogs with severe underlying CVD due to the risk developing decompensated CHF. The patient should be rechecked in 2 weeks with chest radiographs to confirm there has been no stent migration. Routine

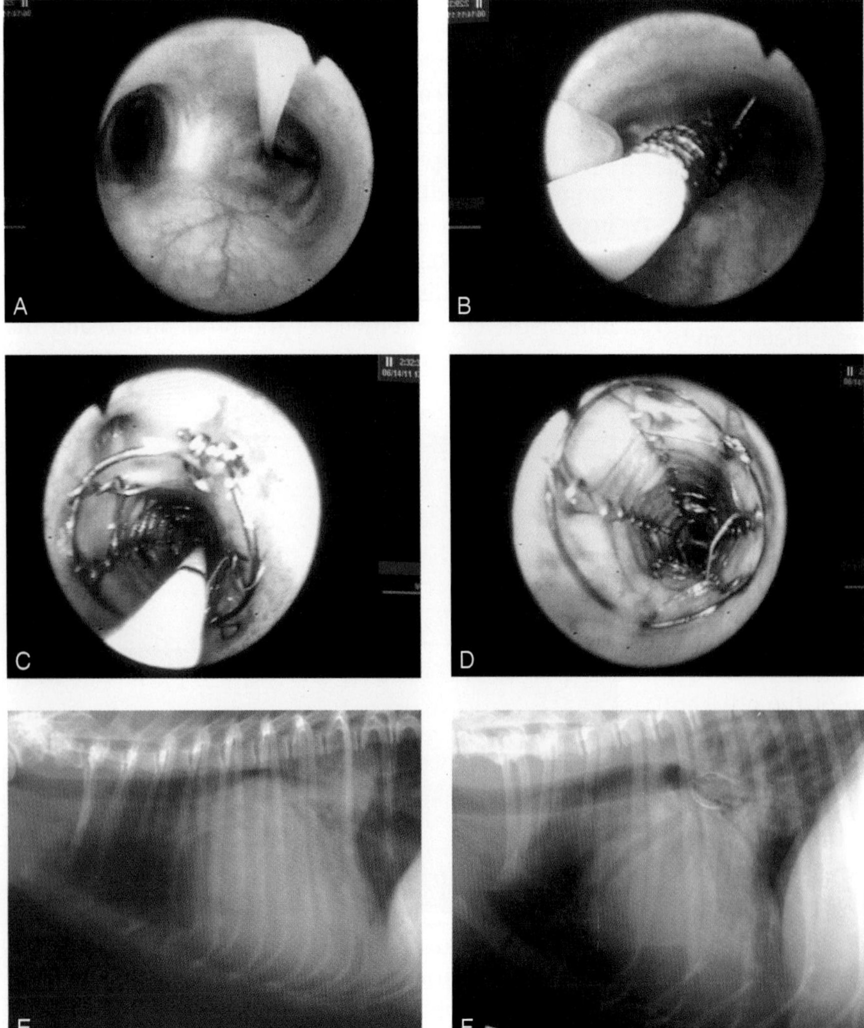

Figure 8.6 Procedural steps for bronchial stenting; (A) Guide wire being advanced through LB2. (B) 5Fr Stent delivery system being passed over the guide wire into LB2. (C) Partial deployment of stent. (D) Complete deployment of stent after removal of the delivery system and guide wire. (E) Pre-procedure lateral chest radiograph. (F) Post-procedure lateral chest radiograph showing the deployed stent.

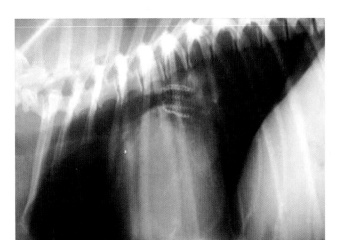

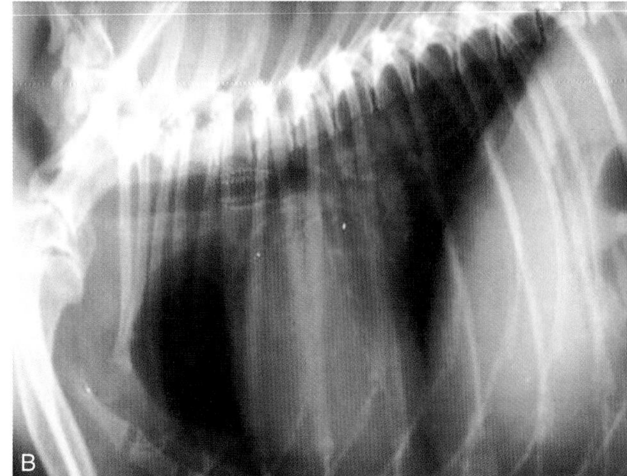

Figure 8.7 (A) Post-procedure chest radiograph documenting bronchial stent position in LB2. (B) Chest radiograph taken the day after the procedure demonstrating migration of the stent into the trachea.

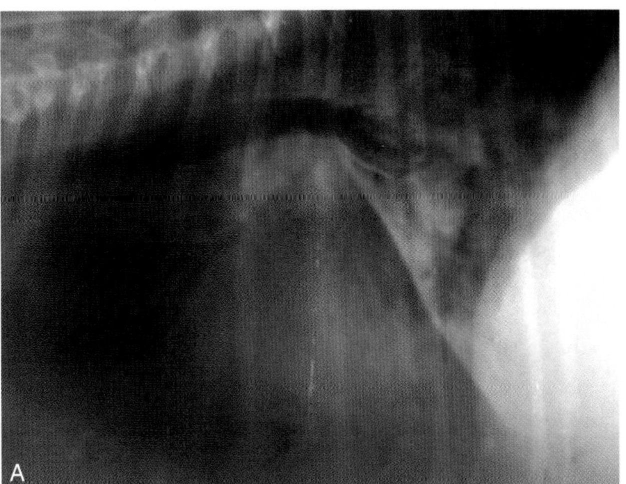

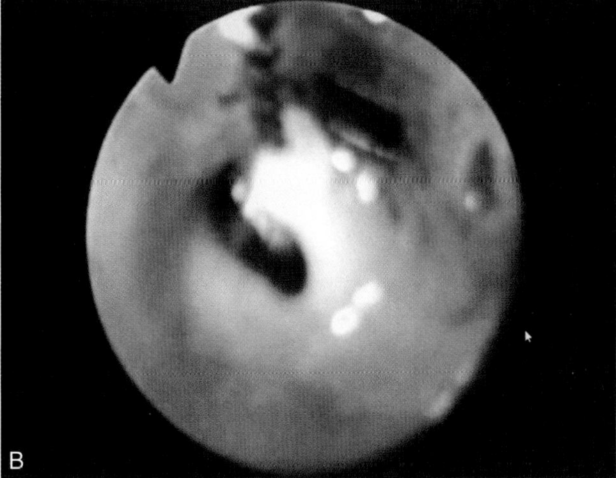

Figure 8.8 (A) Chest radiograph taken three months after bronchial stent placement indicating a lobar pneumonia. (B) Bronchoscopic image from the same patient showing sample collection from the infected stent for cytology and culture.

rechecks should initially be performed every three months in conjunction with the management of any concurrent underlying heart disease and/or airway disease.

Special Considerations/ Complication Examples

Although the complication rates are low, care must still be taken to identify them early to minimize negative outcomes. Chest radiographs should be taken during the routine follow-up exams to check for evidence of infection or stent migration. If migration has occurred (Figure 8.7) the stent should be removed and replaced with a larger stent. If there is evidence of infection, bronchoscopy should be performed to inspect the stent and obtain samples with a cytology brush for cytology, culture, and sensitivity (Figure 8.8). Appropriate antibiotic therapy should be instituted. The patient in the example shown had a *Pasteurella* sp. infection and made a full recovery with antibiotic therapy.

Suggested Reading

Kramer G, McKiernan B, and Burk R (2008) Evaluation of bronchial collapse in dogs with chronic heart disease. [Abstract] *J Vet Intern Med* 22: 687–824.

Johnson LR and Pollard RE (2010) Tracheal collapse and bronchomalacia in dogs: 58 cases (7/2001–1/2008). *J Vet Intern Med* 24: 298–305.

Nelson AW (2002) Diseases of the trachea and bronchi. In: *Textbook of Small Animal Surgery*. 3rd edn. W Saunders Co, Philadelphia.

Radlinsky MG, Fossum TW, Walker MA, et.al (1997) Evaluation of the Palmaz stent in the trachea and mainstem bronchi of normal dogs. *Vet Surg* 26: 99–107.

Weisse C and Berent A (2010) Tracheal stenting in collapsed trachea. In: *Textbook of Veterinary Internal Medicine*. 7th edn (Feldman and Nelson eds). Elsevier, New York, pp. 1088–96.

Woods DE (2004) Tracheal and bronchial stenting. In: *Surgery of the Trachea and Bronchi* (HC Grillo ed.). BC Decker Inc, Hamilton, Ontario, pp. 763–790.

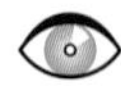

Video 8.1 This video shows the bronchoscopic examination of the trachea, the principle, lobar and tertiary bronchi. There is grade 4 collapse of LB2 and grade 3 collapse of LB1. Note the addition dynamic compression that occurs as a result of cardiac motion. The distal tertiary bronchi appear unaffected. As the procedure progresses, the guidewire is passed through LB2 into the tertiary bronchi. The stent delivery system is then passed over the guidewire into the lumen of LB2. The constraining thread is removed and the stent is deployed. The delivery system and then the guided wire are removed. Post-deployment inspection of the bronchus shows normal luminal patency. This video can be found in the online material at **www.wiley.com/go/weisse/vet-image-guided-interventions**

CHAPTER NINE

Pleural Space Disease – Thoracic Drainage and Port Placement

William T.N. Culp

School of Veterinary Medicine, University of California – Davis, Davis, CA

Background/Indications

Pneumothorax and pleural effusions are common causes of respiratory distress in companion animals. Many different diseases can result in pneumothorax or pleural effusion, and primary treatment of the underlying cause should be pursued when possible. Persistent air or fluid accumulation in the pleural space requires that drainage options be considered to stabilize these patients and improve quality of life.

In most cases, the goal of placing a thoracic drainage catheter is palliation of the associated adverse clinical signs; however, intrathoracic drains can be utilized to administer intracavitary chemotherapy or local anesthetics as well. The catheter may be placed temporarily or can be attached to an indwelling port for long-term drainage. The suspected or known underlying disease process should be considered when determining the length of time that a thoracic drain will remain in place.

Patient Preparation

When respiratory distress is detected, initial diagnostics in the stable patient should include bloodwork (complete blood count, biochemistry panel), urine evaluation, thoracic radiographs, and fecal evaluation. If effusion is present, fluid should be obtained by thoracocentesis, and cytological and biochemical analysis of the fluid performed, as well as culture in some circumstances. Other diagnostics that may be considered include echocardiography, abdominal ultrasonography, and thoracic computerized tomography scan.

Initial treatments for pneumothorax and pleural effusion generally include thoracocentesis and pleural cavity drainage. When a primary treatment option can be pursued (e.g., chylothorax), this should be offered to improve the opportunity for a successful outcome. In cases where primary treatment has been unsuccessful or not pursued, drainage can be attempted on a temporary or permanent basis.

Potential Risks/Complications/Expected Outcomes

A few veterinary studies have recently evaluated the use of thoracic drains (Brooks and Hardie, 2011, Cahalane and Flanders, 2012, Valtolina and Adamantos, 2009). Temporary thoracic cavity drainage was achieved with a small-bore chest tube placed utilizing a modified Seldinger technique in one study (Valtolina and Adamantos, 2009). In that study, 29 drains were placed with the most common indication being pyothorax. Placement of the drains was quick and complications were uncommon (Valtolina and Adamantos, 2009). For long-term drainage, the attachment of a thoracic drain to a subcutaneous port has been reported in two studies (Brooks and Hardie, 2011, Cahalane and Flanders, 2012). In one case series of six dogs and four cats, a thoracic drain designed for veterinary patients (PleuralPort device™, Norfolk Vet Products, Skokie, IL) was utilized with good success (Brooks and Hardie, 2011). The drains in that study were placed either percutaneously or during thoracotomy. Results of that study were promising, however a few complications were encountered including pneumothorax in one cat resulting in death and port obstruction in three cases. In the remaining six cases, the port functionality varied

Veterinary Image-Guided Interventions, First Edition. Edited by Chick Weisse and Allyson Berent.

Companion website: www.wiley.com/go/weisse/vet-image-guided-interventions

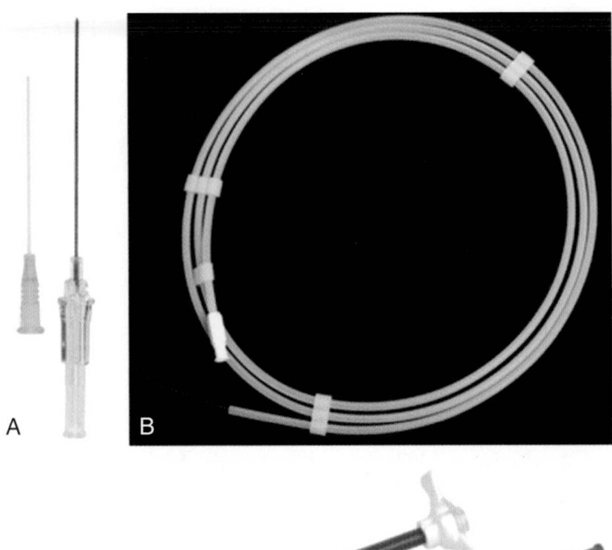

Figure 9.1 Equipment utilized to gain entrance into intrathoracic cavity. (A) 18 gauge over-the-needle catheter; (B) 0.035-inch hydrophilic guide wire; (C) peel-away sheath (1) and dilator (2).

from 6 to 391 days (Brooks and Hardie, 2011). Port migration, irritation, or infection were not noted (Brooks and Hardie, 2011). Pleural access ports were also successfully utilized in two dogs with recurrent pneumothorax although the ports were only utilized for 14 and 17 days (Cahalane and Flanders, 2012).

Equipment

A list of recommended equipment for both temporary and permanent pleural drainage can be found in Figure 9.1, Figure 9.2, Figure 9.3, and Figure 9.4. The use of fluoroscopy is recommended for placement of the pleural drainage catheter when not performed through an open procedure. A surgical approach is used for placement of the port associated with permanent pleural drainage and a basic surgical pack and sterile drapes are needed.

To place a temporary pleural drainage catheter, a locking-loop pigtail catheter[1] is needed. The chosen catheters are generally 5–14 French depending on the size of the animal and the pleural disease being drained (i.e., smaller catheters can be used for air drainage while larger catheters are recommended for fluid drainage).

To place a permanent pleural drainage catheter, several specific pieces of equipment are needed:

- 18 gauge over-the-needle catheter[2]
- 0.035-inch hydrophilic angled guide wire[3]

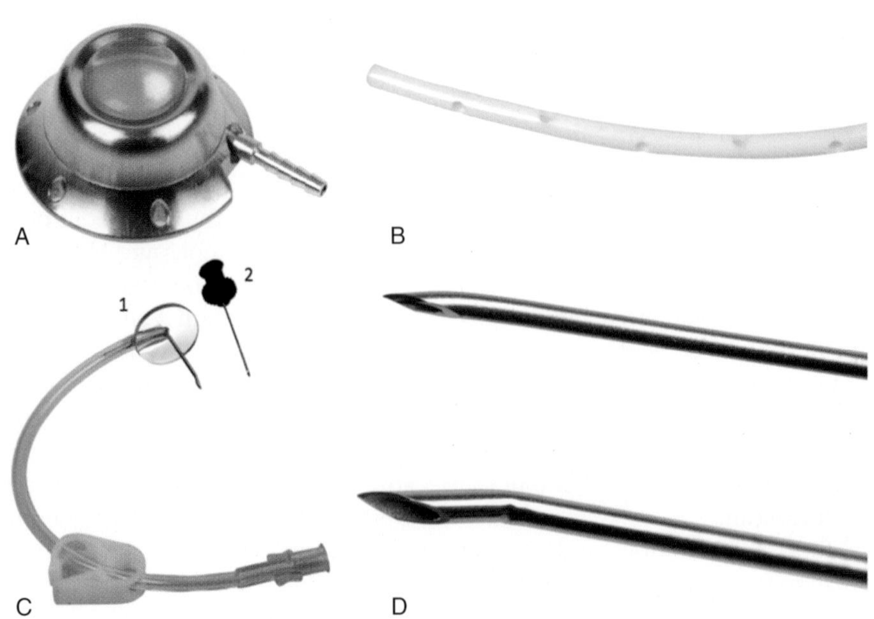

Figure 9.2 Equipment utilized during permanent thoracic drain placement. (A) Subcutaneous port. (B) Multi-fenestrated thoracic drainage catheter. (C) Two versions of Huber needles – 1. Huber needle with attached tubing, 2. Huber needle alone. (D) Close-up images of two Huber needle points.

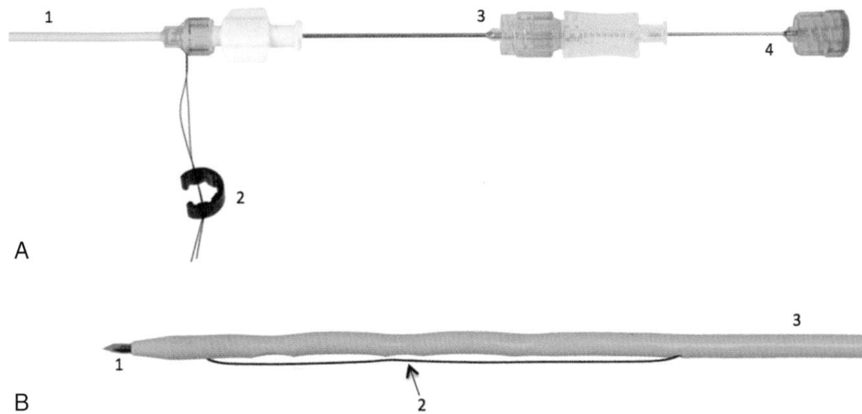

Figure 9.3 Locking-loop pigtail catheter and associated equipment. (A) 1. Proximal end of locking-loop pigtail catheter, 2. Clasp utilized to fasten the suture, 3. Cannula, 4. Stylet. (B) 1. The stylet has been advanced and locked into the cannula to expose the distal pointed/sharp tip, 2. Exposed suture that can be pulled to lock the pigtail loop in place when the stylet and cannula have been removed, 3. Locking-loop pigtail catheter.

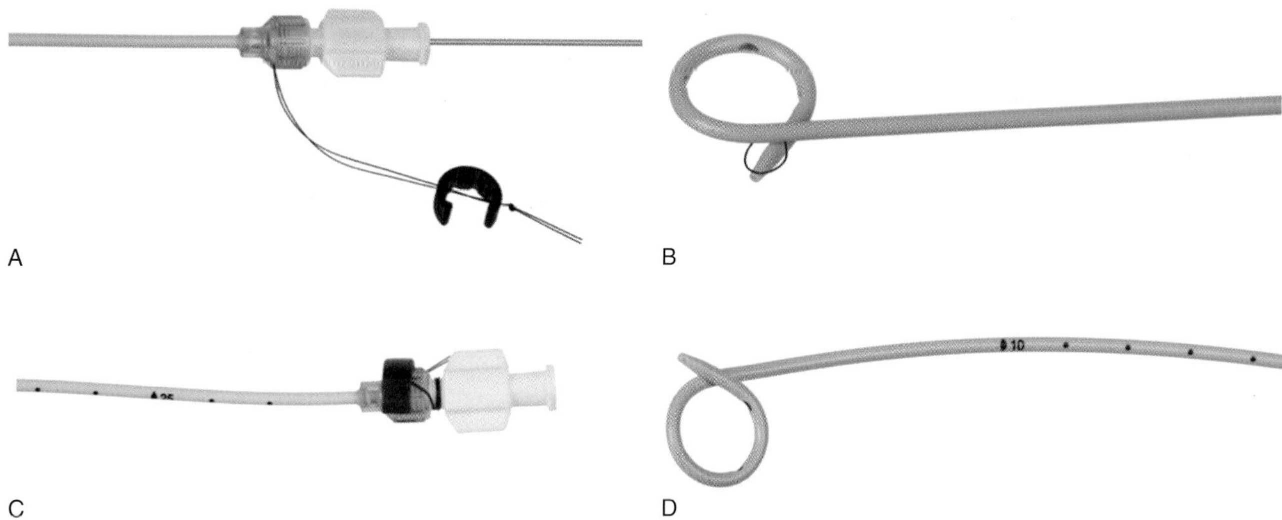

Figure 9.4 (A) Locking-loop pigtail catheter with clasp unlocked. (B) When the pigtail catheter is unlocked and the cannula and stylet have been removed, the pigtail loop is still formed; however, the suture responsible for locking the loop is loose and the loop can be easily undone. (C) Locking-loop pigtail catheter with clasp locked. (D) When the pigtail catheter is locked, the suture responsible for locking the loop cannot be visualized as it is tightened. The loop is not easily undone in this position.

- 9 French peel-away sheath (dogs) and dilator/7 French peel-away sheath (cats) and dilator[4]
- 9 French fenestrated thoracic drain (dogs)/7 French fenestrated thoracic drain (cats) and drainage port[5]
- Huber point needle[6].

Temporary Pleural Drainage Procedure

Temporary drainage of the thoracic cavity can be easily achieved through the placement of an intra-thoracic catheter (Figure 9.5 and Figure 9.6). These temporary catheters are placed in patients with the hope that the air or fluid accumulating intrathoracically is transient, as these patients will need to be monitored closely in a hospital environment.

Pigtail catheters (Figure 9.3 and Figure 9.4) are often utilized for temporary drainage due to ease of placement and usage. These catheters can be placed with sedation and allow for short-term drainage of pleural effusions. These catheters often contain a locking mechanism that improves the security of the catheter and decreases the likelihood of inadvertent catheter removal (see Chapter 2).

The placement of temporary drainage catheters can be performed with either sedation or general anesthesia.

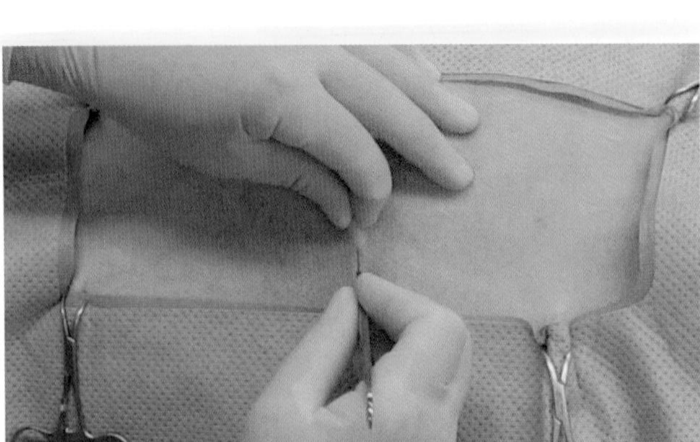

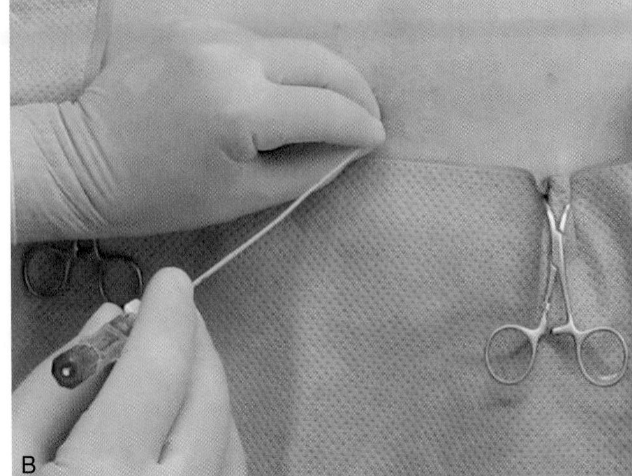

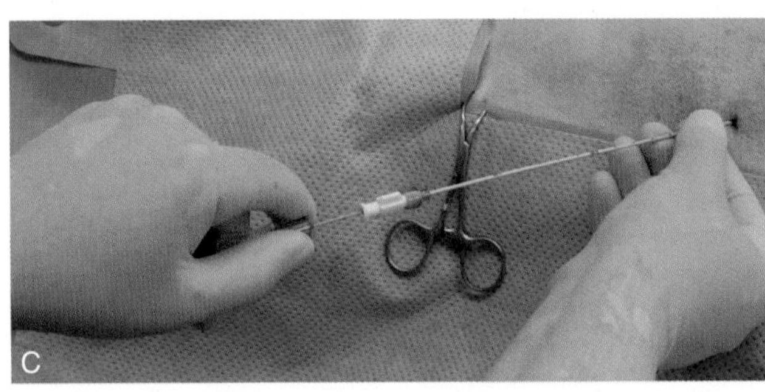

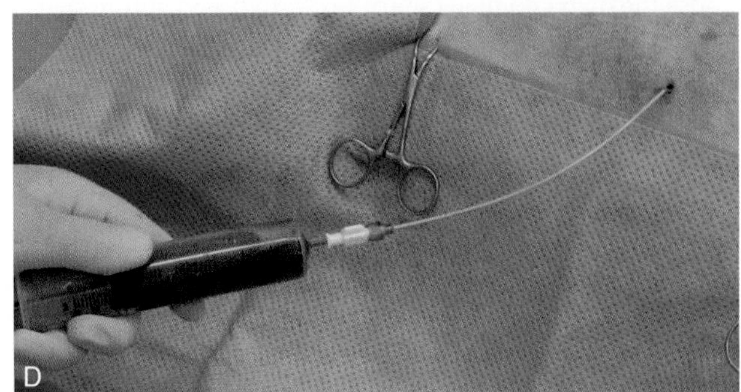

Figure 9.5 Placement of a locking-loop pigtail catheter for temporary drainage into the pleural space without a guide wire. A stab incision (A) can be made to facilitate entrance of the locking-loop catheter into the pleural space, or the locking-loop pigtail catheter and associated stylet and needle can be advanced directly into the pleural space (B). Once the locking-loop pigtail catheter has been introduced into the pleural space, the catheter can be passed over the stylet into the pleural space (C). When positioned correctly, a syringe can be attached to the catheter to allow for fluid or air aspiration (D).

The caudolateral thoracic cavity should be clipped and prepared with aseptic technique. Patients can be placed in lateral, ventral, or dorsal recumbency. The author recommends the use of locking-loop pigtail catheters for temporary drainage, and catheter size should reflect what is to be drained; air will require a relatively small catheter whereas fluid may require a larger bore catheter depending upon the viscosity of the fluid to be drained. Pigtail catheters can be placed using either of two common techniques:

Pigtail Catheter Without Guide Wire

Most pigtail catheters are equipped with a cannula and a sharp stylet for placement (Figure 9.3). The cannula is utilized to provide stiffness to the catheter, and the stylet is advanced so that the sharp tip is visualized. When all three components are attached together, the entire unit can be advanced through the skin, subcutaneous tissue and muscles and then further through the pleura into the thoracic cavity. Depending on the size of the catheter, a very small skin incision may be necessary. The positioning of the catheter is dependent on the disease being treated; in cases of pleural effusion, the catheter is generally placed in the ventral third of the thoracic cavity in intercostal space 7–10. When the entire unit (including the catheter) has just entered the thoracic cavity, the needle can be removed leaving the cannula in place; the cannula provides rigidity but does not extend beyond the catheter minimizing iatrogenic trauma to intrathoracic structures. After removal of the stylet, the catheter-cannula combination can be advanced further into the thoracic cavity, and the cannula can be removed to allow the pigtail aspect of the catheter to take shape. It is crucial that all holes of the pigtail catheter are within the pleural space. When the pigtail catheter is positioned, the locking mechanism can be engaged (the suture attached to the locking mechanism is wrapped around the hub of the catheter, the clasp is fastened to the hub,

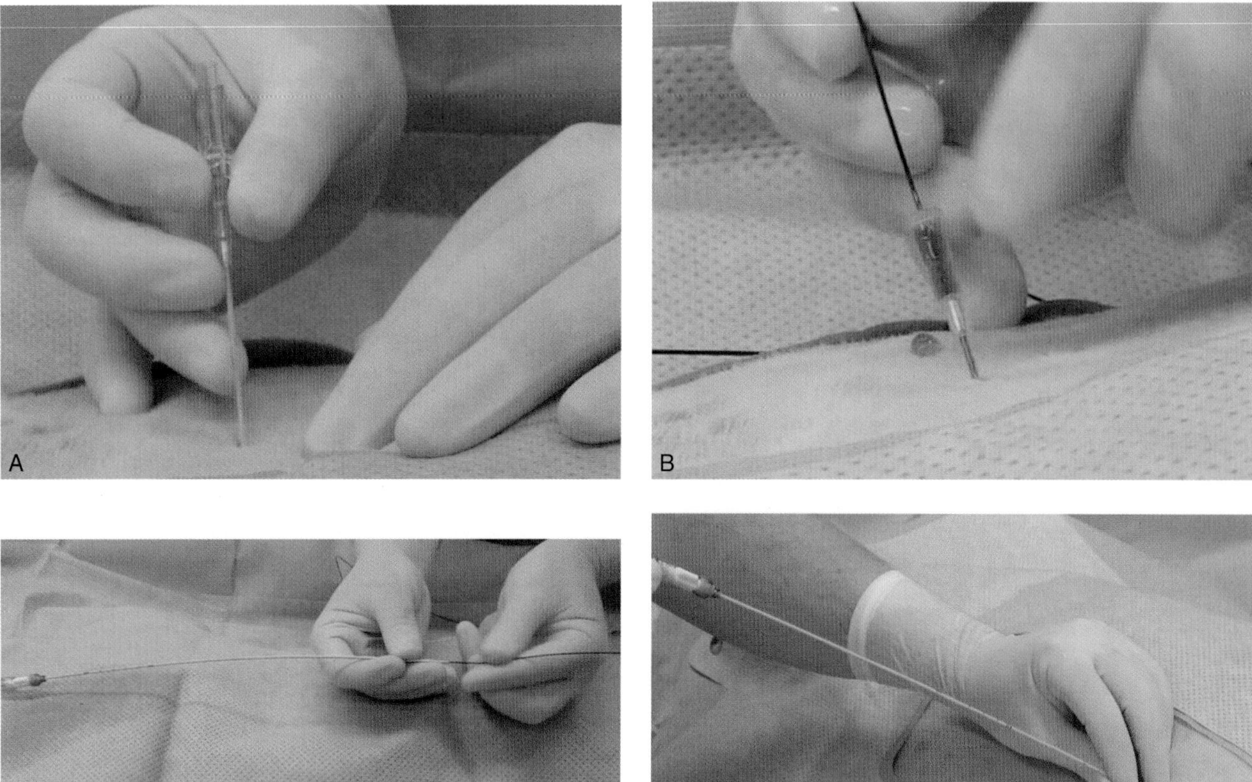

Figure 9.6 Placement of a locking-loop pigtail catheter for temporary drainage into the pleural space with a guide wire. An 18 gauge over-the-needle catheter is introduced into the pleural space (A). When fluid is obtained, the needle is removed and a 0.035-inch hydrophilic guide wire is introduced through the catheter into the pleural space with fluoroscopic-guidance (B). The locking-loop pigtail catheter is flushed with saline, as the catheter will be passed over the hydrophilic guide wire (C). The catheter is passed over the guide wire to the body wall (D) and then eventually into the pleural space. Once the holes of the catheter have been completely introduced into the pleural space, the guide wire can be removed.

and the hub is screwed down to the catheter), and the thoracic cavity can be drained of air or fluid. Different companies have different locking loop catheter configurations and locking mechanisms; make certain to review these prior to use. When the thoracic cavity is sufficiently emptied, the hub of the catheter is capped. The catheter should be secured to the skin to prevent the tube from being inadvertently removed. An Elizabethan collar and thoracic bandage can also be placed to prevent the patient from traumatizing the catheter.

Pigtail Catheter With Guide Wire

Some clinicians may choose to place a pigtail catheter with the use of a guide wire to allow for alteration of the position of a catheter or for an increased level of safety. To perform this technique, an 18 gauge over-the-needle catheter is introduced into an intercostal space as described above. The needle is removed, and the catheter is monitored for drainage of air or fluid (depending on the disease process). When air or fluid is obtained, a 0.035-inch hydrophilic guide wire is passed through the over-the-needle catheter and into the pleural space. The position of this guide wire can be changed via fluoroscopic-guidance to allow the clinician to place the catheter into a specific region of the thoracic cavity or have it extend through the mediastinum. When the guide wire has been properly positioned, the drainage catheter can be passed over the guide wire and into position; the catheter can be passed with the cannula in place to improve pushability or it can be passed without the use of the stiffening cannula. The guide wire can then be removed which allows the pigtail aspect of the catheter to take shape. The locking mechanism is engaged as described above and the catheter is secured in position.

Permanent Pleural Drainage Procedure

Permanent pleural drainage can be accomplished by the placement of an intra-thoracic drain that is attached to a subcutaneous port (Figure 9.2). Several different devices have been developed to be utilized as drains, and the author most commonly uses a multi-fenestrated drain designed for this purpose (Figure 9.2). A Jackson–Pratt drain can be attached to a catheter and employed as well.

Port placement (Figure 9.7) is always performed with the patient under general anesthesia and controlled ventilation. A 5 cm skin incision is made in the dorsal 3rd of the lateral thorax in the region of the 10th intercostal space. A stab incision is made in the 8th or 9th intercostal space in the middle third of the lateral thorax. A hemostat is passed subcutaneously from the dorsal incision to the stab incision, and the thoracic drain is passed between the two incisions. The anesthetist pauses respiration under direction of the operator as an 18 gauge over-the-needle catheter is inserted into the stab incision and into the pleural space. The needle is removed leaving the catheter in the pleural space, and the 0.035-inch guide wire is passed into the thoracic cavity. Controlled respiration can again resume. Fluoroscopic-guidance can be utilized to pass the guide wire into the proper location. The peel-away sheath and dilator combination are passed over the

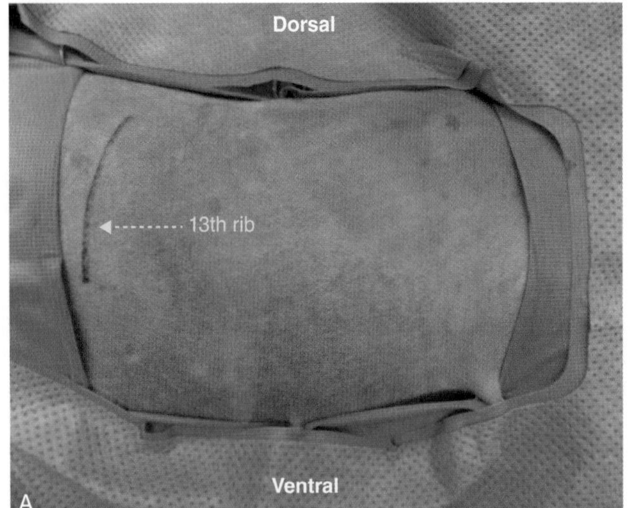

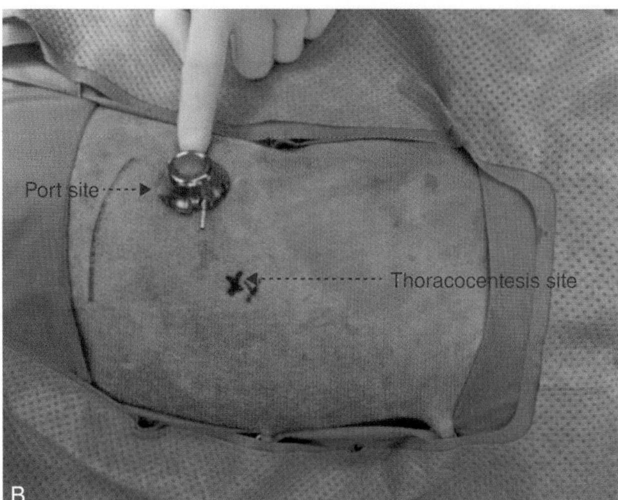

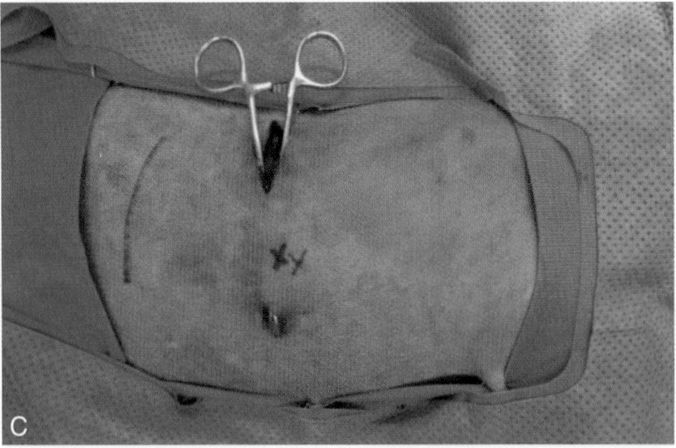

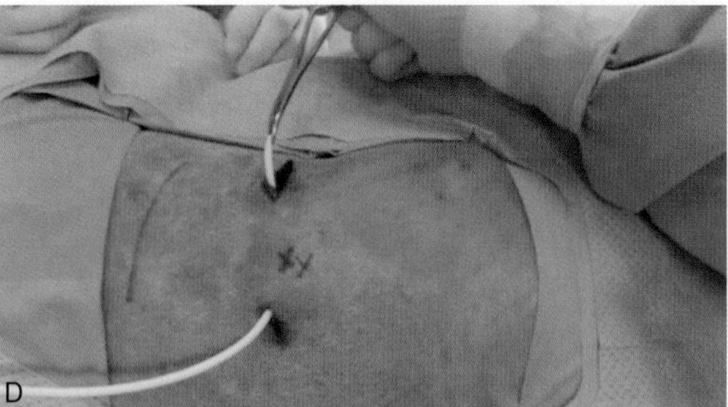

Figure 9.7 Placement of a thoracic drainage catheter and subcutaneous port for permanent pleural space drainage. The lateral thorax is clipped, prepared with aseptic technique and draped (A). The location of the port (10th intercostal space) and thoracocentesis site (8th–9th intercostal space) are determined (B). A hemostat is passed (C) subcutaneously from the dorsal incision to the stab incision (at the thoracocentesis site). The thoracic drainage catheter is passed between the incisions (D). After thoracocentesis, the 0.035-inch hydrophilic guide wire (gw) is passed into the pleural space through the 18 gauge over-the-needle catheter with fluoroscopic-guidance (see Figure 9.6). A peel-away sheath (ps) is placed over the guide wire into the pleural space after removal of the catheter. The thoracic drainage catheter can then be passed through the peel-away sheath.

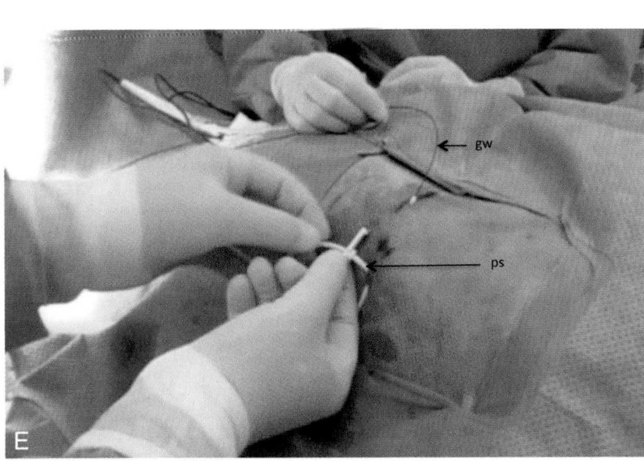

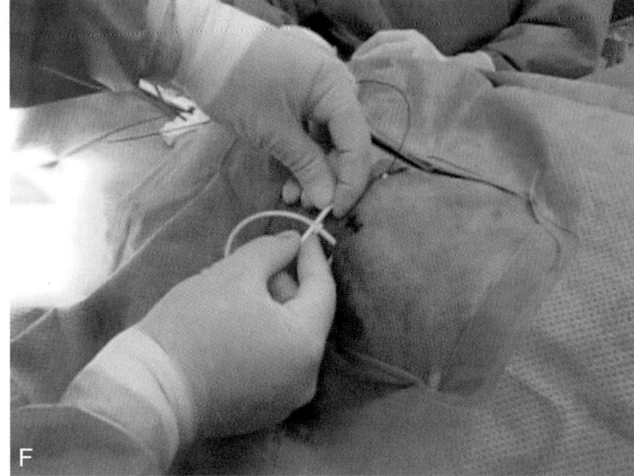

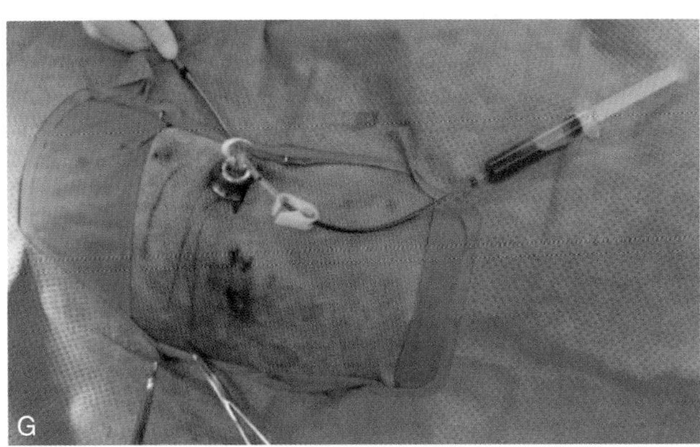

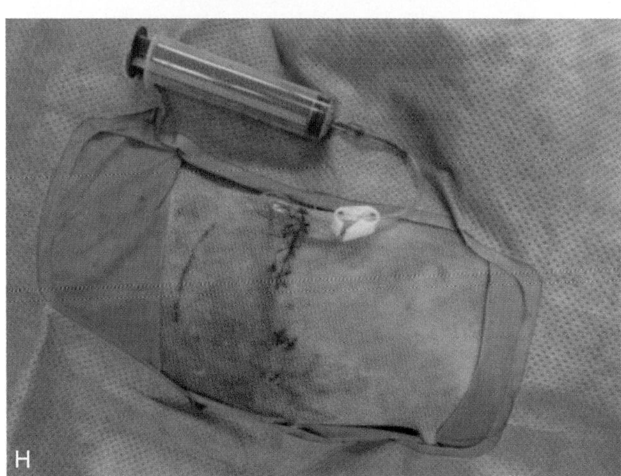

Figure 9.7 (*Continued*) (E). When the thoracic drainage catheter has been placed sufficiently into the pleural space (fluoroscopy is utilized to determine that all holes are located intra-thoracically), the peel-away sheath can be peeled down leaving the catheter in place (F). After the fenestrated end of the thoracic drainage catheter has been placed into the pleural space, the external end is attached to the port, and the port is placed into the subcutaneous pocket (G). A Huber needle should be inserted into the port to test for the removal of fluid and air; this can be done both prior to and after closure of the port (dorsal) incision (G and H).

guide wire and into the thoracic cavity. When the dilator is removed, the chest cavity is effectively open to the atmosphere; the anesthetist should be warned prior to dilator removal. Once the dilator is removed, the thoracic drain is placed over the guide wire through the peel-away sheath and into the thoracic cavity. Once the thoracic drain has been properly positioned in the thoracic cavity (fluoroscopic-guidance is again recommended), the guide wire can be removed, and the peel-away sheath can be peeled down until removal is possible. The external end of the thoracic drain can then be attached to the subcutaneous port. The port is secured subcutaneously with non-absorbable suture in a position that allows for easy percutaneous access. The skin incision is closed routinely.

Follow-Up

All cases should be monitored for accumulation of air or fluid via clinical signs, physical examination, thoracic radiographs (Figure 9.8) or thoracic ultrasonography. If respiratory compromise is noted or quality of life has diminished, the pleural space should be drained via the thoracic drainage catheter. For cases with a permanent thoracic drainage catheter, the port should be used for drainage. It is essential that a Huber needle be utilized to access the port as this needle has a specific non-coring point which allows the material within the port (silicone) to be deflected (Figure 9.2); use of a traditional needle will core a piece of the silicone, leaving a hole and subsequently predisposing to leakage.

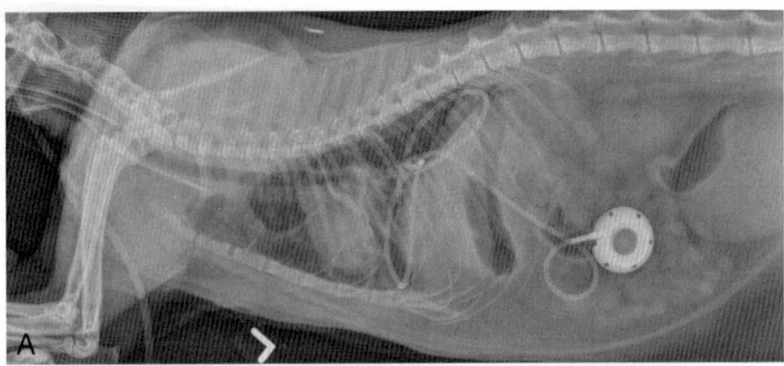

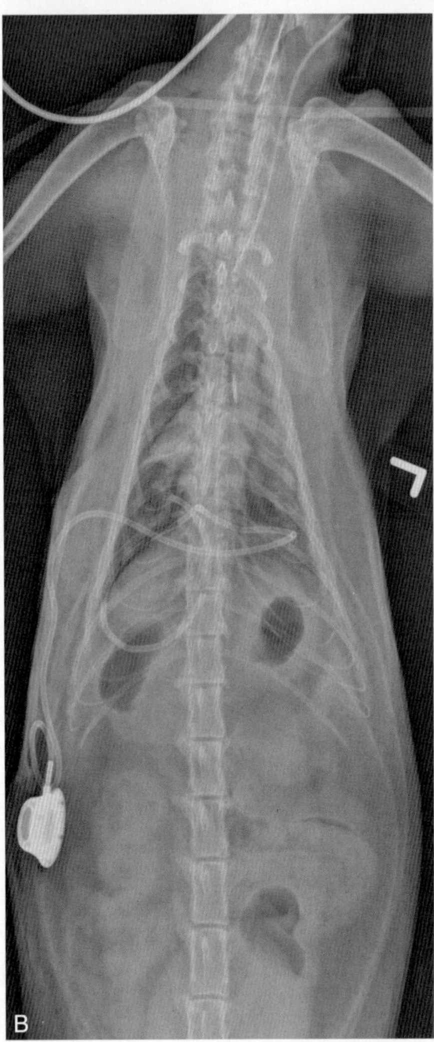

Figure 9.8 Ventrodorsal and lateral radiographic projections of a cat with a thoracic drainage catheter and subcutaneous port. The drainage catheter was placed to remove air in this cat who was developing pneumothorax secondary to a congenital pulmonary parenchyma abnormality.

To access the port, an area of fur over the port site is clipped and the site is prepared with sterile technique. Sterile gloves are worn, and the port is grasped with the non-dominant hand and stabilized. A Huber needle attached to a collection system is inserted into the port until the metal base plate can be felt at the tip of the needle. When the Huber needle is properly positioned, suction can commence. When the pleural space has been drained, the catheter is injected with a locking solution. The author generally uses a mixture of saline and heparin (100 units per ml) as a locking solution, although, others also infuse the catheters with antibiotics such as gentamicin. After infusion of the locking solution, the port is again stabilized and the needle is removed.

Special Considerations/ Alternative Uses/ Complication Examples

Several studies have evaluated the use of pigtail catheters in human patients (Klein et al., 1995, Liang et al., 2009, Parulekar et al., 2001). The outcome appears to be similar in human patients that have undergone placement of a small-bore catheter (such as pigtail catheters) when compared to large-bore chest tubes (Clementsen et al., 1998, Parulekar et al., 2001). Additionally, comfort levels also appear to be improved in patients requiring thoracic drainage when small-bore tubes are utilized (Clementsen et al., 1998).

A few veterinary studies have documented successful short- and long-term drainage utilizing drains placed intrathoracically (Brooks and Hardie, 2011, Cahalane and Flanders, 2012, Valtolina and Adamantos, 2009). In some cases, pneumothorax has resolved and the accumulation of pleural effusion has diminished over time allowing for removal of the drains (Brooks and Hardie, 2011, Cahalane and Flanders, 2012, Valtolina and Adamantos, 2009). These devices have the benefit of being able to be placed with low morbidity, and in some instances, with minimal sedation. In certain cases, clients can be taught how to utilize the subcutaneous ports which may allow for decreased patient distress and improved quality of life.

As stated above, thoracic drainage catheters can also be used for infusion. There is limited data evaluating intrathoracic chemotherapy treatments in veterinary patients but this therapy has been considered when treating neoplasia such as mesothelioma that can be present diffusely throughout the pleural cavity. Alternatively, cases of pyothorax, in which medical management is being pursued, may require thoracic lavage and drainage. The temporary thoracic drainage catheters can be used for this purpose; however, ports should not be used as they may become occluded or infected after suction.

Notes

(Examples; Multiple vendors available)

1. Locking-loop pigtail catheter, Infiniti Medical, Menlo Park, CA.
2. Insyte™ IV catheter, BD Medical, Franklin Lakes, NJ.
3. Weasel wire, Infiniti Medical, Menlo Park, CA.
4. Peel-away sheath®, Cook Medical Inc., Bloomington, IN.
5. PleuralPort™, Norfolk Vet Products, Skokie, IL.
6. Huber point needle, Norfolk Vet Products, Skokie, IL.

References

Brooks AC and Hardie RJ (2011) Use of the PleuralPort device for management of pleural effusion in six dogs and four cats. *Vet Surg* 40, 935–41.

Cahalane AK and Flanders JA (2012) Use of pleural access ports for treatment of recurrent pneumothorax in two dogs. *J Am Vet Med Assoc* 241, 467–71.

Clementsen P, Evald T, Grode G, Hansen M, Krag Jacobsen G, and Faurschou P (1998) Treatment of malignant pleural effusion: pleurodesis using a small percutaneous catheter. A prospective randomized study. *Respir Med* 92, 593–6.

Klein JS, Schultz S, and Heffner JE (1995) Interventional radiology of the chest: image-guided percutaneous drainage of pleural effusions, lung abscess, and pneumothorax. *AJR Am J Roentgenol* 164, 581–8.

Liang SJ, Tu CY, Chen HJ, et al (2009) Application of ultrasound-guided pigtail catheter for drainage of pleural effusions in the ICU. *Intensive Care Med* 35, 350–4.

Parulekar W, Di Primio G, Matzinger F, Dennie C, and Bociek G (2001) Use of small-bore vs large-bore chest tubes for treatment of malignant pleural effusions. *Chest* 120, 192–5.

Valtolina C and Adamantos S (2009) Evaluation of small-bore wire-guided chest drains for management of pleural space disease. *J Small Anim Pract* 50, 290–7.

CHAPTER TEN

Interventional Treatment of Large Airway Obstructions: Ablations, Balloon Dilation, and Foreign Body Retrieval

Allyson Berent
The Animal Medical Center, New York, NY

Background/Indications

Tracheal and bronchial obstructions can occur secondary to a benign or malignant process and lead to substantial respiratory distress or even death. Safe curative resection or removal may not always be possible, making palliative options appealing. Causes of obstruction, aside from tracheal and bronchial collapse, include strictures, tumors (benign and malignant), and foreign body inhalation. There is very little reported in the veterinary literature on the treatment options for these types of conditions. In humans, primary tumors are most commonly associated with benign lesions (lipomas, leiomyomas, hamartomas, and inflammatory polyps) and strictures are most commonly associated with endotracheal tube trauma following anesthesia, congenital malformations, or post-surgical damage. Obstructive lesions can be associated with static stridor, wheezing, hemoptysis, coughing, chronic pneumonia, and varying degrees of dyspnea. In recent years endoscopic treatments have become increasingly more available in human and veterinary medicine.

Therapeutic endoscopy utilizing resection by electrocautery, argon plasma coagulation (APC), laser ablation, brachytherapy, cryosurgery, and balloon dilation, is routinely performed in human medicine. These techniques are highly effective, safe, and minimally invasive, offering an outpatient procedure for an otherwise highly morbid surgery. Of these options, laser resection and electrocautery are the only two options that produce rapid tissue destruction in a single procedure, providing immediate improvement in life-threatening clinical signs while awaiting a diagnosis. The goal of this chapter is to focus on interventional endoscopic and radiologic techniques for the resection of large airway tumors and strictures, as well as foreign body retrieval, which are currently available for veterinary patients.

Patient Preparation

Once the patient is stabilized a thorough history should be obtained including change in bark, coughing, hemoptysis, difficulty eating or drinking, inspiratory and/or expiratory noise, presence of cyanosis or syncope, known foreign body inhalation, travel history, other concurrent conditions, duration of signs, and acute or chronic progression. All patients should have an airway secured if severe dyspnea is apparent. Care should be taken during intubation to avoid accidentally tearing a stricture or pushing a foreign body farther into a bronchus. A small endotracheal tube to provide oxygen should be the first consideration and preparation for a tracheostomy should be made if indicated.

Three-view thoracic radiographs should be obtained if the patient can tolerate the procedure. It is important that the larynx, cervical and intrathoracic trachea are all visualized on the radiographs. The forelimbs should

Veterinary Image-Guided Interventions, First Edition. Edited by Chick Weisse and Allyson Berent.

Companion website: www.wiley.com/go/weisse/vet-image-guided-interventions

be moved forward and backward in two different views to visualize the thoracic inlet clearly. A blood gas analysis should be obtained to ensure hypercapnia is controlled. If a lesion is not seen on radiographs, and the patient is stable, than a computerized tomography (CT) scan can be considered. It is important to remember to pull the endotracheal tube back to the level of the larynx so that the entire trachea can be clearly visualized during the thoracic radiographs and/or CT scan. It is also important to identify those patients that may not be stable enough to undergo these various diagnostic tests without a secured airway. Upon patient triage, owner consent for intubation and emergency tracheotomy should be obtained.

Potential Risks/Complications/Expected Outcomes

Ideally, a highly experienced endoscopist and anesthetist should perform this procedure. The most substantial risk is severe hypoxia from airway occlusion, airway perforation, fistula formation, bleeding, and ignition/explosion due to flammable material in the airway during laser ablation or electrocautery use. The close proximity of the endotracheal tube, high oxygen content of the inspired air, and high ignition source of a laser or electrocautery unit can result in hazardous explosions and fires. It is very important that the patient be maintained at no greater than 21% FiO_2 to prevent this from occurring and to avoid contact of the endotracheal tube with any of the thermal ablation devices.

Equipment

Endoscopy is typically performed with a flexible or rigid bronchoscope.[1,2] Ideally the scope should be placed through an endotracheal tube, but this requires a 5.0–7.0mm inner diameter endotracheal tube or larger. Most flexible bronchoscopes are between 5 and 6mm in diameter. If the scope is to be placed through the endotracheal tube than a bronchoscope adaptor (see Chapter 7) is recommended to maintain the patient on the anesthesia circuit. The working channel is typically no larger than 2.0mm so all devices guided through the working channel should be appropriately sized. A traditional fluoroscopy unit may be needed.

Devices (Figure 10.1) that may be necessary include polypectomy snares of various sizes,[3,4] retrieval baskets (ranging in basket diameter of 1–4cm),[6,7] compliant and non-compliant balloons,[7] a Bugbee cautery probe[8] with adaptor, a diode laser,[9] laser safety goggles, an electrosurgical knife,[10] and various sized self-expanding metallic stents[11,12] (see Chapter 7 and Chapter 2). A soft hydrophilic angle-tipped guide wire[13] placed down the trachea, beyond the mass or foreign body, is also useful to maintain distal access beyond the lesion should it get displaced during manipulations.

Procedures

Preparation

At the time of intubation the pharyngeal and laryngeal region should be carefully visualized. If signs are consistent, a dynamic laryngeal exam should be performed to confirm normal arytenoid function. Additionally, the epiglottis should be evaluated during inspiration to ensure there is no evidence of epiglottic retroversion. If no mass or web lesions are seen then the patient should be intubated carefully with a relatively small endotracheal (ET) tube unless the endoscope is to be placed through the ET tube. If the patient is a cat or small breed dog, direct bronchoscope intubation should be performed after respiratory stabilization is achieved. Oxygen can be delivered through the working channel of the endoscope or via jet ventilation. Jet ventilation utilizes a small catheter passed into the airway, adjacent to or through the bronchoscope. A small tidal volume is delivered through the catheter at a high rate to maintain lung expansion, alveolar ventilation, and oxygenation. The entire tracheal, major bronchial, and laryngeal lumens should be carefully visualized for a lesion. If no lesion is visualized then retroflex nasopharyngoscopy should be performed to ensure there is not a nasopharyngeal stenosis (NPS) or mass (see Chapter 6).

Tissue Resection

Resection should be considered for polypoid-type masses (Figure 10.2) that have a narrow base. For more sessile masses that are non-resectable (Figure 10.3) a self-expanding metallic stent can be placed. The most common large airway masses reported are tracheal and laryngeal polyps, polypoid extramedullary plasmacytomas, tracheal and laryngeal lymphoma, and pyogranulomatous masses (sterile and infectious). Tissue resection can be used for both diagnostic and therapeutic purposes by obtaining a histopathology sample and restoring a patent airway. Once the large airways have been thoroughly evaluated endoscopically and a lesion is identified that will require resection, the endoscope

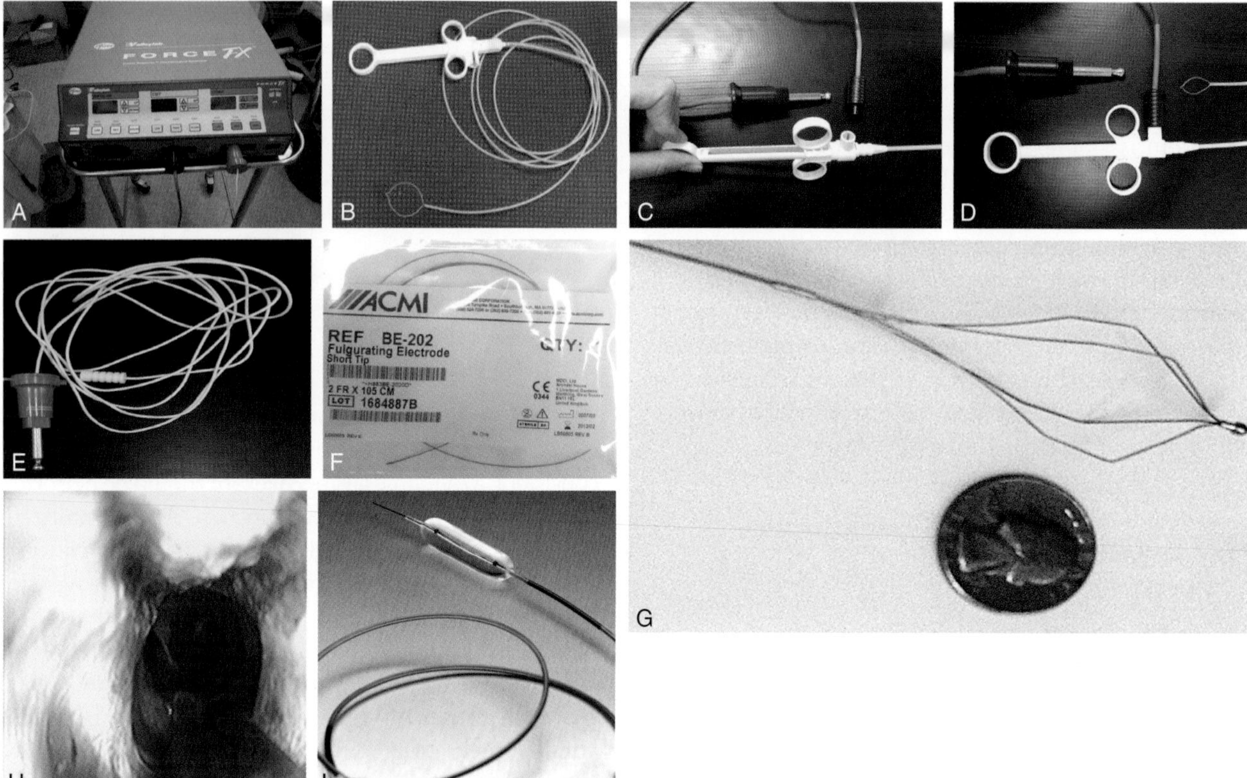

Figure 10.1 Equipment used for various large airway interventions. (A) Electrocautery unit that has both monopolar, bilpolar and blend settings. Notice the two adaptors (red for attachment to the polypectomy snare, and blue/yellow for the Bugbee cautery probe). (B) This is a snare polypectomy device. (C) The snare with the adaptor on the handpiece, which is attached to the electrocautery unit (red adaptor). (D) Once the adaptor is connected it will allow activation of the snare that is controlled by a foot pedal. (E) Adaptor for the Bugbee cautery probe. (F) Bugbee cautery probe. (G) Foreign body retrieval basket. (H) Hot-knife electrocautery probe through the working channel of the bronchoscope. It is creating defects in a tracheal stricture in a dog prior to balloon dilation. (I) Balloon dilation catheter with a soft tip to aid in dilation of tracheal strictures.

is removed and the patient is re-intubated (if it is too small for concurrent intubation). The oxygen should be discontinued and the patient maintained on injectable anesthesia and ventilated with room air. This can be accomplished with a bag valve mask, or "Ambu-Bag". After 3–5 minutes the FiO_2 should be approximately 0.21, making electrocautery or laser ablation safe.

An electrocautery snare device (Figure 10.1B) is effective and safe for polypectomy when there is a polypoid mass that has a relatively narrow base (Figure 10.2). The grounding pad needs to be placed on the patient as with routine surgical electrocautery procedures. The snare is enclosed within a plastic sheath and is loaded into the working channel of the endoscope. Once it is seen to exit the scope within the tracheal lumen it is minimally deployed so the tip is in contact with the mass (Figure 10.2b). Starting at 15 watts in the blend mode (allowing for some coagulation and some cutting capacity) the power is advanced up (maximal 30 W) as one area of the tissue is gently ablated to identify the ideal power setting. This is done using the monopolar foot pedal (see Chapter 2, Figure 2.8). Ablation is typically effective between 18 and 22 W. This part of the procedure is not performed to completely ablate the mass; rather it is performed to identify the proper setting prior to snare cauterization removal of the mass. Next the snare is opened and placed around the base of the mass and gently closed once the loop is around the base (Figure 10.2D, E). The mass is pulled cranially to ensure the front of the snare is not touching the normal tracheal wall caudal to the mass. Once this is ensured, with very gentle traction, the mass is pulled cranially as the electrocautery is activated. If there is sufficient space within the trachea adjacent to the scope, a grasping instrument can be placed as well so that the polyp can be held during the cauterization

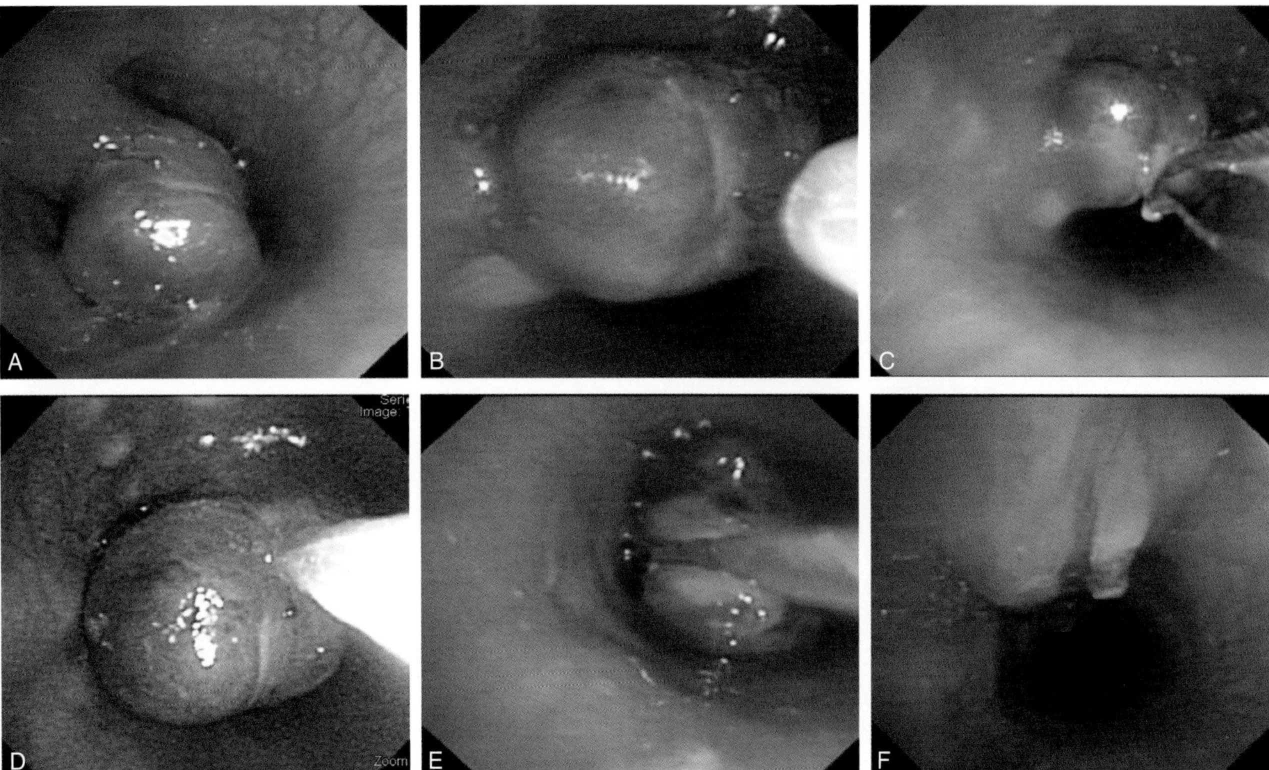

Figure 10.2 Endoscopic images of a dog with a polypoid lesion arising from the dorsal tracheal membrane occluding the tracheal lumen. (A) Thick stalk of the mass visualized. (B) Polypectomy device being used to test the power settings using the tip on the mass. (C) The snare being placed around the mass. (D) The snare entrapping the base of the polypoid mass as it is pulled cranially toward the scope to prevent electrocautery caudally. (E) Removal of the polypoid mass once it fell from the base of the stalk. (F) The resultant base of the mass after polypectomy.

process to prevent it from falling into the bronchial lumen once it is resected. The mobile mass is removed through the mouth with the grasping instrument, a retrieval basket, or the snare device, and submitted for histopathological analysis. The scope should then be replaced into the tracheal lumen to ensure there are no areas of bleeding or tracheal tears. If there is bleeding identified, the tip of the snare can be used to cauterize (in coagulation mode) the bed of tissue and stop any persistent hemorrhage.

If the mass is more broad based and resection is desired over tracheal stenting while awaiting biopsy results, then either diode or ND:YAG (neodymium-doped yttrium aluminum garnet) laser ablation can be performed. As described above, once 21% inspired oxygen is achieved the laser fiber can be directed through the working channel of the endoscope and used to ablate the tissue to open the airway lumen. The biopsy should be obtained prior to laser ablation as it will make the tissue very difficult to evaluate histopathologically due to the ablation and charring artifact.

Tissue Ablation

For benign and malignant tracheal lesions, argon plasma coagulation (APC) therapy and cryotherapy can be considered. Neither of these modalities have been used in the author's practice. These techniques are described in humans for the treatment of tracheal-esophageal fistulas, malignant tracheal/bronchial obstructions, and endotracheal tube induced stenosis. APC provides rapid coagulation with minimal mechanical trauma to the target tissue by the use of a jet of ionized argon gas (plasma) directed through an endoscopic probe. With a high frequency electrical current conducted through the gas, coagulation occurs without any contact of the probe to the tissue, making it safe for surrounding tissues. Cryotherapy is a newer type of thermal energy platform that maintains the integrity of the extracellular matrix providing the structural framework for appropriate wound repair, resulting in less long-term scarring than other modalities when used for benign airway strictures or tumors.

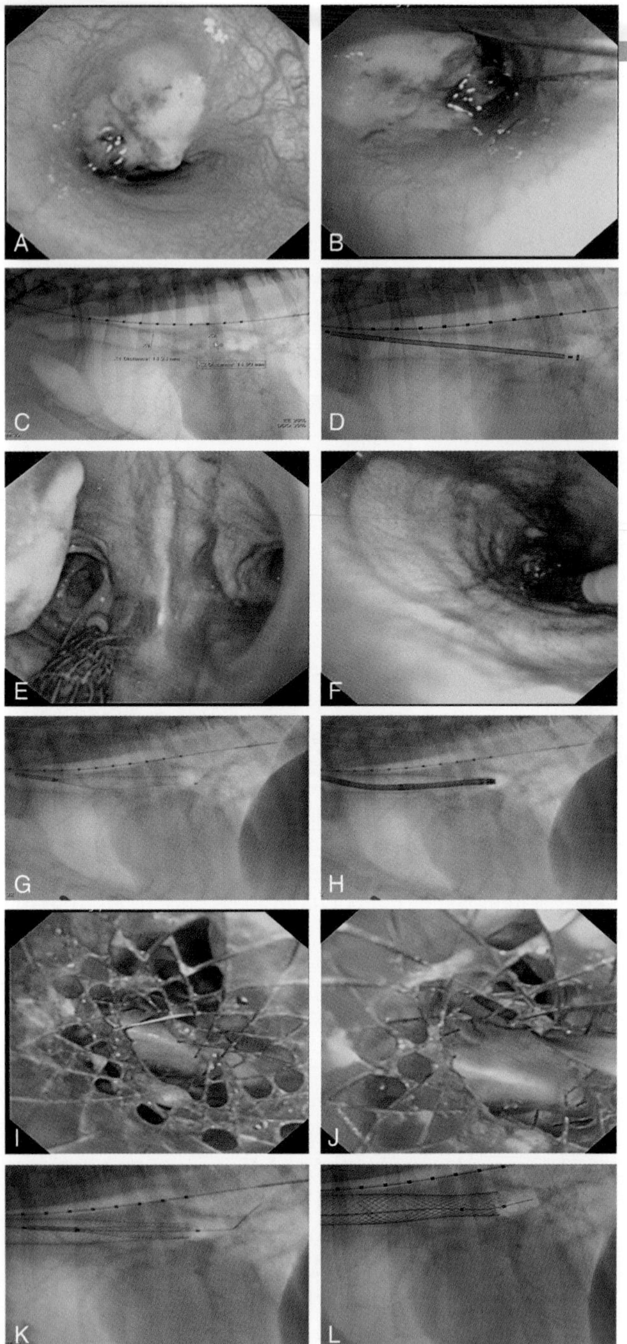

Figure 10.3 Endoscopic and fluoroscopic images of a dog with a broad-based, non-resectable, granuloma of the trachea sitting at the carina. (A) Tracheoscopic image of the mass occluding 90% of the lumen. (B) Unsuccessful attempt at polypectomy/electrocautery of this mass to open the airway. (C) Fluoroscopic image during positive pressure ventilation (20 cmH_20) with a marker catheter in the esophagus. This allowed for measurements of the tracheal lumen for stent placement. (D) Placement of the stent within the tracheal lumen under fluoroscopic guidance. (E) Endoscope placed next to the delivery system of the stent during initial deployment because the mass extends to the carina. Care is taken not to place the stent down one of the mainstem bronchi. (F) Once the caudal aspect of the stent was determined to be in an appropriate position the endoscope was withdrawn to the cranial aspect of the stent prior to deployment. (G) The stent being deployed under fluoroscopic guidance. (H–I) The endoscope visualizing the caudal end of the stent using both endoscopic and fluoroscopic guidance. (J) Due to the caudal end of the stent remaining compressed just cranial to the carina a guide wire is placed through the lumen of the stent using both endoscopic and fluoroscopic guidance to allow a second stent to be placed to reinforce the first (K) and balloon dilate the distal end (L).

Laryngeal webbing is a rare condition that is most commonly associated with previous laryngeal surgery. In humans this is typically treated with CO_2, diode or ND:YAG laser ablation and has been met with good to excellent results.

Balloon Dilation

Tracheal stenosis is most commonly due to congenital or acquired strictures. Acquired strictures can occur following endotracheal tube damage, caustic inhalation, surgical manipulation, and trauma. The various treatment options include electrocautery (hot knife ablation), balloon dilation, APC, cryotherapy, and palliative stenting. Most interventional pulmonologists do not recommend balloon dilation alone, as the risk of creating a propagating tracheal tear is high. Instead, an electrosurgical knife[14] is used to cut the tissue in three or four areas (Figure 10.4) to weaken the stricture evenly. This is performed using an electrocautery adaptor, similar to that used for a snare device. After this tissue is cut balloon dilation will allow the strictured mucosal tissue to tear evenly at the created areas of weakness, avoiding a full thickness tracheal perforation. In humans this

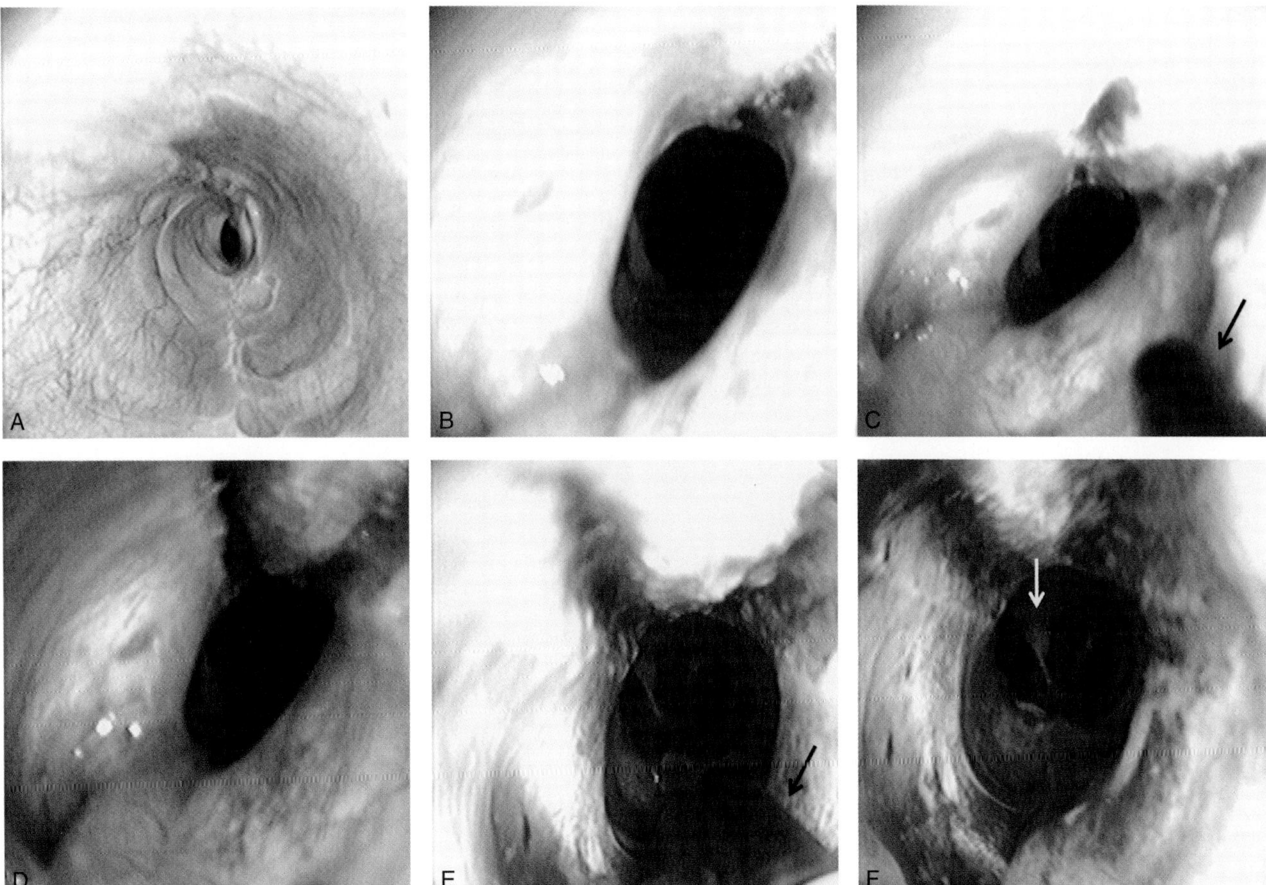

Figure 10.4 A 3-month-old dog with an intrathoracic tracheal stricture, likely secondary to trauma. Due to the small size and expected growth of the patient a stent was not used and instead the lesion was cut with an electrosurgical knife and balloon dilated. (A) Endoscopic image of the stricture in the distal intrathoracic tracheal lumen. (B–E) Cutting the strictured tissue with the electrosurgical knife (black arrows) using endoscopic guidance in three areas. (F) The tracheal lumen after balloon dilation. The carina (yellow arrow) can now be seen through the stricture (images courtesy of Dr. Chick Weisse).

procedure often needs to be repeated two to four times and tracheal metallic stenting is usually avoided for strictures due to the excessive granulation tissue ingrowth at the stenosis site. When balloon dilation is performed, a marker catheter[10,15] should be used to determine the appropriate tracheal luminal diameter measurement under positive pressure ventilation (20 cmH_2O) on fluoroscopy (Figure 10.3). Once the luminal diameter is determined an appropriate size balloon is chosen. The balloon should not be oversized so as to avoid tracheal perforation. Inflation should be performed using a commercially available inflation device.[15]

Tracheal or Bronchial Stenting

This procedure is described in more detail in Chapters 7 and 8. If laser ablation or electrocautery/balloon dilation procedures fail for amenable cases then a tracheal stent can be well tolerated, especially for nonresectable tumors that are non-surgical (Figure 10.3).

Foreign Body Retrieval

This procedure can be easily performed in veterinary patients using either endoscopic or fluoroscopic assistance. If a patient is small and intubation with tracheoscopy is difficult then endoscopic foreign body retrieval may be risky. Under these circumstances, if the foreign body can be visualized with fluoroscopy, than fluoroscopic-assisted removal is recommended. Fluoroscopic-assisted removal (Figure 10.5) is best done after a patient is intubated. An angle-tipped hydrophilic guide wire should be placed through the tube and monitored under fluoroscopic guidance to make sure it is easily passed beyond the foreign body without pushing it farther into a bronchus. A retrieval basket can then be used to entrap the foreign body and remove it through (or with) the endotracheal tube. Once it is successfully removed the guide wire is removed. If the foreign body is not easily seen fluoroscopically then endoscopic assistance is required. A grasping instrument (alligator forceps, basket, snare, or bag) can be used through the

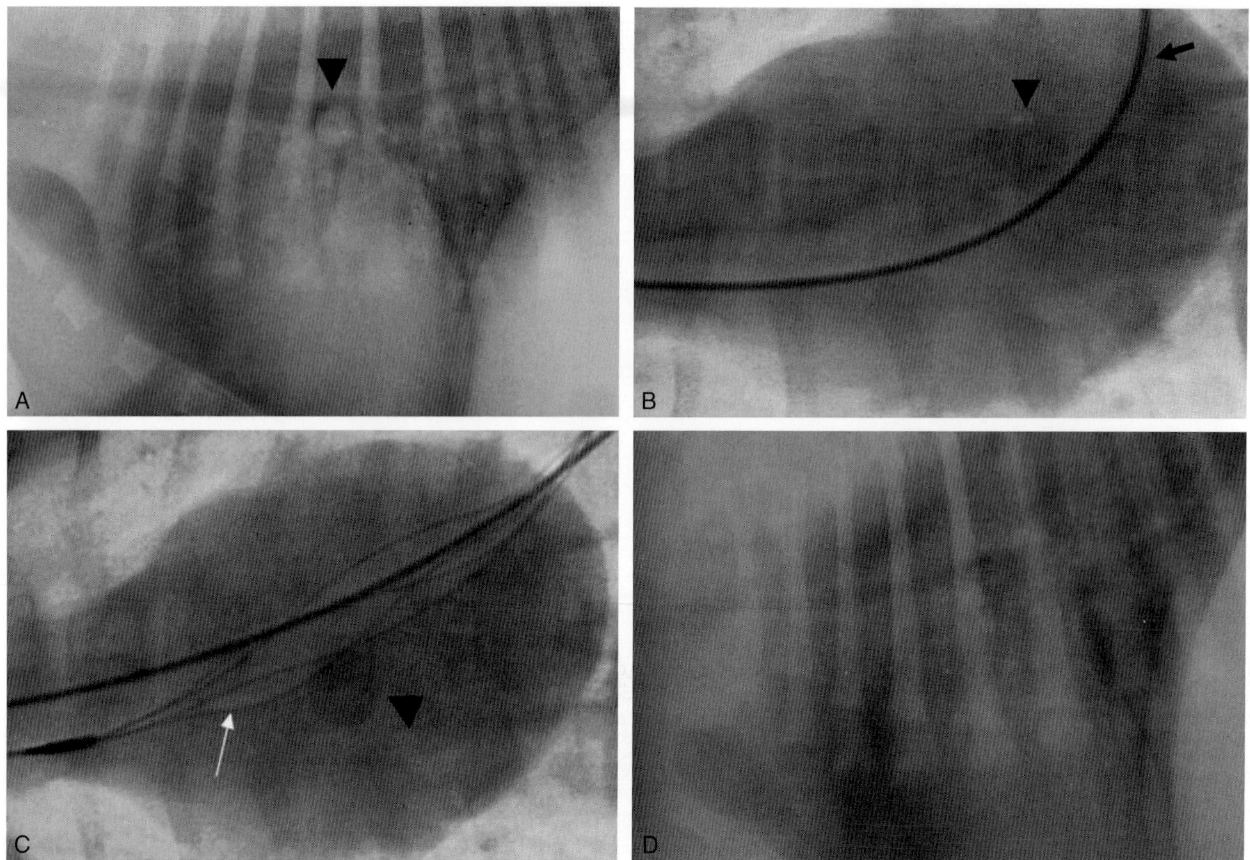

Figure 10.5 Radiographic and fluoroscopic images of an 8-week-old Pug with a foreign body (FB) at the carina. (A) Lateral radiograph of a round object (black arrowhead) sitting at the carina. (B) V/D fluoroscopic image of the dog after a guide wire (black arrow) is placed through the endotracheal tube, down the trachea, and into the right bronchus beyond the FB. (C) A FB retrieval basket (white arrow) placed next to the wire to entrap the FB (black arrowhead). (D) Lateral radiograph of patient after FB removed (images courtesy of Dr. Chick Weisse).

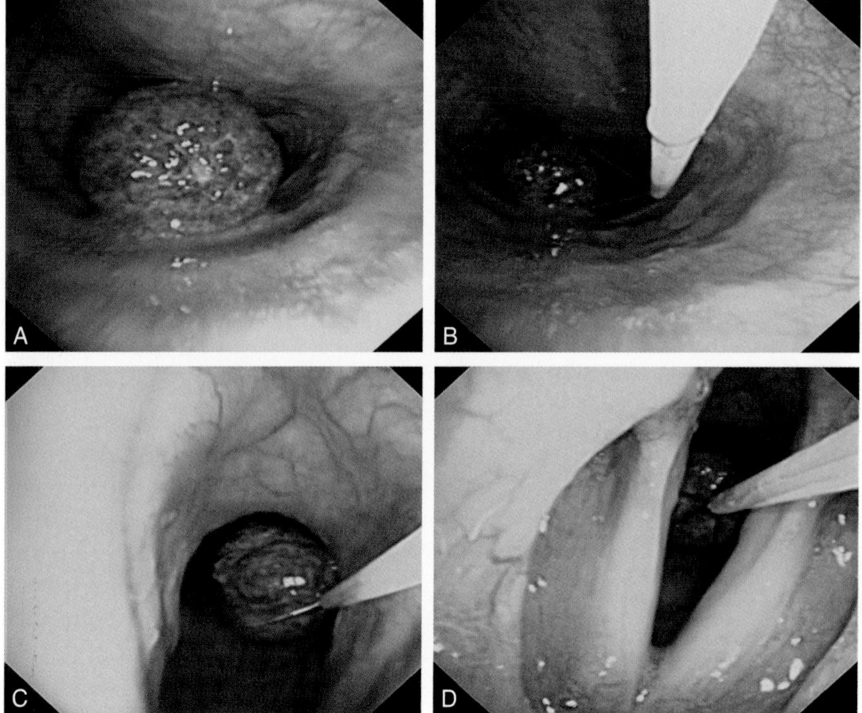

Figure 10.6 Endoscopic images of a Labrador Retriever with a 1-week history of chronic cough. Tracheal opacity seen on radiographs. (A) Tracheal foreign body (FB) seen endoscopically. (B) FB retrieval basket used through the working channel of the endoscope to entrap the object. (C) The FB is being removed through the tracheal lumen. (D) The FB seen before it exits the larynx.

working channel of the endoscope to remove the object carefully and quickly. (Figure 10.6)

Postprocedural and Follow-Up Care

Patients should be recovered with oxygen support and monitored carefully until they are extubated and breathing well. A 5–10-day course of broad-spectrum antibiotics is typically recommended after stenting or ablation. For tracheal strictures, re-scoping of the lesion and subsequent balloon dilation may be necessary, though this is based on recurrence of clinical signs. If the patient has a tumor that was successfully ablated follow-up with appropriate chemotherapy or radiation therapy should be considered.

Prognosis

There are no long-term or large studies in veterinary patients looking at any of these techniques for the treatment of either benign or malignant conditions. In people interventional endoscopic therapy for tracheal stenosis and tumors is typically associated with a good outcome, but repeated treatments may be necessary.

Notes

Note, the equipment on this list are only examples of what is used in the author's practice and various alternatives would be considered appropriate.

1. BF Q180 Flexible 5.5 mm bronchoscope, Olympus, Southborough, MA.
2. Rigid bronchoscope, Karl Storz, Culver City, CA.
3. SnareMaster Polypectomy snare, Olympus, Southborough, MA.
4. Lariat snare, 1.8 mm sheath, 4.0 cm × 3.0 cm, US Endoscopy, Mentor, OH.
5. Flacon rotatable retrieval basket, US Endoscopy, Mentor, OH.
6. Sur-Catch® NT, No Tip Nitinol Basket, Olympus/Gyrus ACMI, Southborough, MA.
7. CRE™ Pulmonary Balloon Dilator, Boston Scientific, Natick, MA.
8. Fulgurating electrode Bugbee cautery, 2 Fr, short tip, ACMI-Olympus, Southborough, MA.
9. 600-μm diode laser fiber and 100-W diode Lithotrite, Vectra, Convergent Inc, Alameda, CA.
10. Huibregtse® Single Lumen Needle Knife, Cook Medical, Bloomington, IN.
11. Vet Stent Trachea, Infiniti Medical, LLC, Menlo Park, CA.
12. WallStent, Boston Scientific, Natick, MA.
13. Weasel Wire 0.035-inch hydrophilic angle-tipped guidewire, Infiniti Medical LLC, Menlo Park, Calif.
14. 5 Fr Marker catheter, Infiniti medical, LLC, Menlo Park, CA
15. Balloon inflation device, Bard, Covington, GA

Suggested Reading

Dekeratry D, Downie G, Finley D, et al. (2011) Feasibility of spray cryotherapy and balloon dilation for non-malignant strictures of the airway. *Eur J Cardio-Thorac Surg*, 40, 1177–1180.

Riffat F, Palme CE, et al. (2012) Endoscopic treatment of glottis stenosis: a report on the safety and efficacy of CO_2 laser. *J Laryngol Otol*, 126(5), 503–505.

Rodrigues A, Coelho D, Azevedo Dias Junior S, et al. (2011) Minimally invasive bronchoscopic resection of benign tumors of the bronchi. *J Brasil Pneumol*, 37(6), 796–800.

SECTION THREE

Gastrointestinal System

Edited by Allyson Berent

CHAPTER ELEVEN

Oral Tumors

William T.N. Culp
School of Veterinary Medicine, University of California – Davis, Davis, CA

Background / Indications

While oral tumors only account for 6% of canine and 3% of feline tumors (Hoyt and Withrow, 1984), the impact that these tumors can have on quality of life is profound. The most common tumors encountered in the canine oral cavity include malignant melanoma, squamous cell carcinoma, and fibrosarcoma. Cats are most likely to be diagnosed with oral squamous cell carcinoma and fibrosarcoma. Tumors of the oral cavity can be identified as affecting the maxilla, mandible/s, tongue, or tonsils. While surgery and/or radiation therapy may be employed in an attempt to cure certain types of oral neoplasia, this is not always possible and other treatment options may need to be considered.

Maxillectomy and mandibulectomy techniques are well-described in veterinary medicine. Dogs tolerate these procedures well and are often able to account for changes in jaw and tongue position as well as loss of bone with little adjustment on their part. Cats, likely due to the smaller size of the maxilla and mandibles, are less tolerant of major maxillary and mandibular surgeries; however, some surgical options may exist. Several studies have discussed surgical techniques for tongue resection (Beck et al., 1986, Syrcle et al., 2008).

Radiation therapy is generally reserved for cases of oral tumors that are deemed non-resectable or in cases when an incomplete margin is obtained or anticipated during surgical resection. Several different radiation therapy modalities have been utilized and can be effective for local control of certain oral tumors (Brooks et al., 1988, Freeman et al., 2003, Proulx et al., 2003, Theon et al., 1997a, b). Acute side effects associated with radiation therapy of oral tumors are common with late effects being diagnosed less regularly.

Treatment of oral tumors can be difficult due to the limited anatomical space to perform large surgical procedures and the close association of many important structures. In some circumstances, surgery is deemed an unacceptable option for certain tumors and radiation therapy may have limited benefit with tumors that are very large. In these cases, alternative options should be considered; these options, while still uncommonly performed in veterinary medicine, may include locoregional therapy via intravascular techniques or directly-applied ablation.

The use of intravascular therapies in the treatment of human oral tumors has been performed. Oral tumors can be treated with intra-arterial chemotherapy alone, embolization/chemoembolization, or a combination of intra-arterial chemotherapy and radiation therapy (Bonet-Coloma et al., 2011, Ikushima et al., 2008, Kobayashi et al., 2010, Korogi et al., 1995, Ohba et al., 2012, Suzuki et al., 2011, Wu et al., 2010). These techniques have been rarely performed in veterinary patients for the treatment of oral tumors and studies are lacking. One report of a dog with a maxillary fibrosarcoma treated with combined therapy of transarterial embolization, systemic cyclophosphamide, and cryoablation exists (Weisse et al., 2011); in that study, a femoral artery approach was utilized to gain access to the sphenopalatine artery, which was subsequently embolized.

The potential for incorporating ablation therapies in the treatment of oral tumors is promising. The use of thermal ablation techniques such as radiofrequency ablation (RFA) and cryoablation have been described for oral lesions (Bozkaya et al., 2006, Leboulanger et al., 2008, Schirmang et al., 2007), although the volume of literature dedicated to this topic is minimal. As stated above, a case of a dog with a maxillary fibrosarcoma that had cryoablation as part of the treatment regimen has been reported (Weisse et al., 2011). Reports of the clinical use of RFA to treat malignant neoplasia in companion animals are lacking.

Veterinary Image-Guided Interventions, First Edition. Edited by Chick Weisse and Allyson Berent.

Companion website: www.wiley.com/go/weisse/vet-image-guided-interventions

Patient Preparation

Diagnostic tests including complete blood count, biochemistry profile, urine evaluation, chest radiography, and abdominal ultrasonography are often employed as staging tools for companion animals with oral neoplasia. Additionally, fine-needle aspiration of local lymph nodes should be performed when possible to determine the extent of neoplastic spread. While fine-needle aspiration of oral tumors can be performed, a pre-treatment biopsy is typically recommended to properly plan definitive therapy.

When considering definitive treatments such as surgery, radiation, or the image-guided therapies discussed below, advanced imaging is recommended. Computerized tomographic (CT)-angiography provides an excellent depiction of bone and soft tissue involvement as well as vascular supply of the oral tumor. As some oral tumors are highly malignant, a CT scan can include thoracic evaluation to determine if metastasis has occurred to the pulmonary parenchyma.

Potential Risks/ Complications/ Expected Outcomes

Intra-Arterial Chemotherapy and Embolization/Chemoembolization

Equipment

Some recommended equipment can be found in Figure 11.1, and the application of this equipment can be found in the section describing the procedure. The use of fluoroscopy, and if available, concurrent CT-angiography or magnetic resonance imaging-angiography is essential to perform intravascular therapies of oral tumors. As a surgical approach is utilized, a basic surgical pack and sterile drapes are needed.

Relevant anatomy and fluoroscopic procedure

The arterial blood supply of the head originates from the brachiocephalic trunk branches. Prior to giving off the axillary branch to the forelimbs both the right and left subclavian arteries provide a vertebral artery branch; the right and left vertebral arteries are important to identify, as it is not uncommon to accidentally select these branches during an attempt to select the common carotid arteries. As the vertebral artery courses cranially, several branches are produced. As the vertebral artery perforates the dura and the arachnoid to subarachnoid space, both cranial and caudal branches are formed; the cranial branches form the basilar artery which is the largest source of blood to the brain (Evans and de Lahunta, 2013).

The left and right common carotid arteries originate from the brachiocephalic trunk and course cranially within the cervical region and then bifurcate into the external and internal carotid arteries. The external carotid artery provides the arterial blood to the ipsilateral half of the head whereas the internal carotid artery continues into the skull. Several branches of the external carotid artery exist, including the occipital, cranial laryngeal, ascending pharyngeal, lingual, facial, caudal auricular, parotid, superficial temporal, and maxillary arteries. Collectively, these branches supply the ear, larynx, pharynx, hard and soft palate, tongue, lips, cheeks, nasal cavity components, nose, eye, orbit, nerves of the face, salivary glands, lymph nodes, teeth, and alveoli (Evans and de Lahunta, 2013).

Particular branches of the external carotid artery that may require targeting during the treatment of oral tumors include:

- Occipital artery: supplies mucosa of the roof of the pharynx
- Lingual artery: supplies tongue, and a branch of the lingual artery, the tonsillar artery, supplies the tonsil
- Superficial temporal artery: supplies the upper and lower eyelids
- Maxillary artery: supplies the mandible via the mandibular alveolar artery, the soft palate via the buccal artery, the hard and soft palate via the major palatine artery, and the muzzle and upper lip via the infraorbital artery.

The arterial supply of the head can be accessed through the carotid or femoral artery. The femoral artery is preferred by the author as both carotid arteries can be selected during the procedure to allow for bilateral treatment. Patients are placed in dorsal recumbency at the initiation of the procedure, and both inguinal regions are clipped and prepared with aseptic technique. The patient is draped and the fluoroscopy unit is placed over the abdomen to allow for monitoring of guide wire passage from the femoral artery into the aorta.

The method for arterial vascular access can be found in Chapter 44. The largest catheter utilized during vascular therapies is generally 5 French in diameter; therefore, a vascular access sheath[1] in the femoral artery of at least 5 French is recommended. Once vascular access into the femoral artery has been achieved and the vascular access sheath is in place, vascular selection can commence with fluoroscopic-guidance.

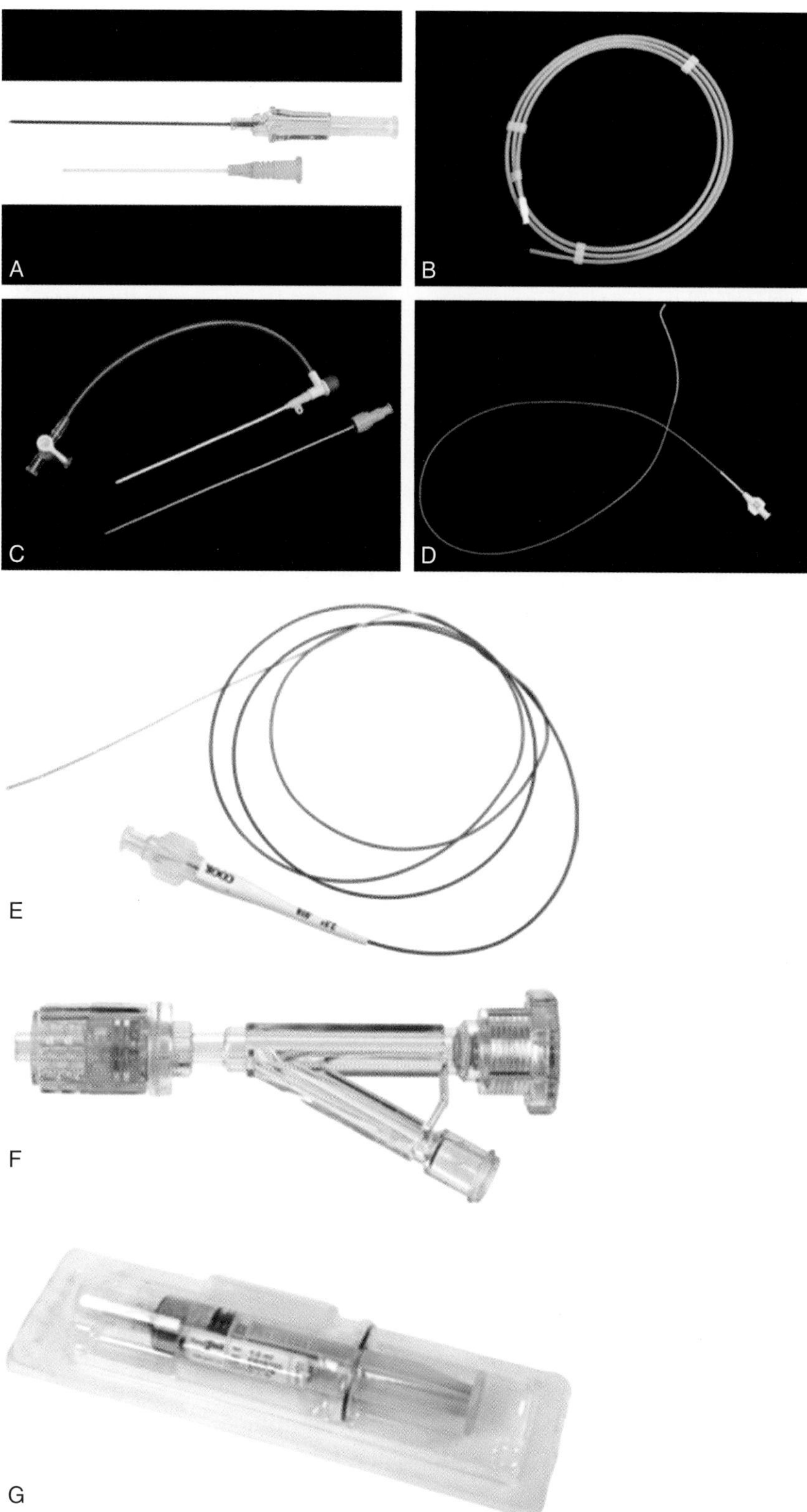

Figure 11.1 Equipment utilized during embolization and chemoembolization procedures. (A) 18 gauge over-the-needle catheter. (B) 0.035-inch angled, hydrophilic guide wire. (C) Vascular introducer sheath (white) and dilator (blue). (D) 4 French angled selective catheter (Berenstein). (E) 2.5 French microcatheter. (F) Touhy–Borst adapter. (G) Polyvinyl alcohol particles (Bead Block).

A guide wire (hydrophilic 0.035-inch angled)[2] is passed through the vascular access sheath into the femoral artery and further into the aorta. The fluoroscopy unit generally needs to be repositioned over the chest to allow for visualization of the aortic arch, the brachiocephalic trunk, and the left subclavian artery. A catheter with an angled-tip (a 4–5 French Berenstein catheter)[3] is passed over the guide wire and the brachiocephalic trunk is selected with the guide wire and catheter combination, and further selection of either the left or right common carotid artery is performed, depending on the side that is going to be treated. If selection of the blood vessels is difficult or vascular localization is not possible, a contrast arteriogram can be performed by removing the guide wire from the catheter and injecting a contrast[4]/saline mixture (generally 50%/50%) to obtain a vascular map.

When the appropriate carotid artery has been selected, the catheter and guide wire combination is passed into the external carotid artery and further into the particular artery that needs to be targeted for treatment. The patient's head may need to be repositioned into a lateral position to allow for better visualization of certain tumor vascular beds. To administer intra-arterial chemotherapy or perform embolization/chemoembolization, a microcatheter[5] is generally utilized. A Touhy–Borst adapter[6] with attached flow switch[7] is attached to the hub of the Berenstein catheter, and a microwire (0.010-inch or 0.014-inch)[8]/microcatheter (2.0 French to 2.7 French) combination is passed through the Touhy-Borst adapter and into the Berenstein catheter after removal of the 0.035-inch guide wire. The microwire and microcatheter combination are passed into the vessel that is to be treated.

When administering intra-arterial chemotherapy, the treating clinician should decide if the dose will be divided between the left and right side of the patient. If administering only intra-arterial chemotherapy, the blood supply to the tumor should be selected with the microcatheter. The chemotherapeutic agent is mixed with contrast to allow for monitoring of the delivery of chemotherapy; chemotherapy delivery should be performed slowly with the intention of delivering maximum chemotherapy dose directly to the tumor.

In preparation for the delivery of chemotherapy, several precautions should be taken. Any personnel within the catheterization laboratory should be wearing hand and eye protection as well as a protective gown. The surgical site should be isolated with gowns or towels designed for chemotherapy safety. A separate region of the sterile instrument table should be established to prevent contamination of all equipment with chemotherapy. Syringes designed for chemotherapy should be utilized.

If an embolic agent is to be administered in combination with the chemotherapy (chemoembolization), selection of the appropriate vessel is critical. Once the blood vessel or vessels supplying the tumor are selected, the microcatheter is locked in place by securing the microcatheter with the Touhy–Borst adapter.

During chemoembolization, the chemotherapy should be mixed with an agent for contrast enhancement which may include either an iodinated contrast material or ethiodized oil (see Chapter 31). These materials can be combined by using syringes of each that have been attached to a 3-way stopcock. When this combination has been obtained, a separate syringe containing embolic particles (generally polyvinyl alcohol particles or microspheres)[9] can then be attached to the three-way stopcock. A combined slurry of the embolic agent, chemotherapy and contrast agent is then created, and individual treatments can be suctioned into 1 ml chemotherapy-safe syringes[10] for delivery. When delivering the slurry, it is crucial to inject slowly and closely monitor the flow of the injection to prevent non-target embolization or reflux of the injected material.

Ablation Therapies

Equipment

Several RFA and cryoablation units are available; examples include the Covidien Cool-tip™ RF Ablation System[11] and Galil Medical Cryoablation System[12] (see Chapter 5). For RFA procedures, a generator is required as well as grounding pads and probes for delivering the radiofrequency waves. For cryoablation procedures, the argon and helium gases are both required in sufficient tank volumes; generally two tanks should be available per procedure.

Image-guided procedure

Several basic principles are shared between RFA and cryoablation. For both techniques, probes are placed into the tumor tissue to allow for the application of a thermal energy (Figure 11.2) (Abbas et al., 2009, Callstrom and Kurup, 2009, El Dib et al., 2012). The goal of both procedures is to cause cell destruction, and this is performed while treating the tumor tissue plus a margin of normal tissue. Both RFA probes and cryoprobes are placed with image-guidance, generally ultrasonography, fluoroscopy, CT or magnetic resonance imaging (Figure 11.2). Additionally, the extent of treatment and response to treatment are monitored with these imaging modalities.

These two techniques differ in how the actual tumor ablation is performed. RFA involves the application of current that is produced from a generator and passed through a probe. The subsequent tissue destruction occurs from heating the cell and coagulative necrosis (D'Ippolito and Goldberg, 2002). With cryoablation, an ice ball is created through the use of alternating freeze–thaw cycles; these cycles result in cell death through

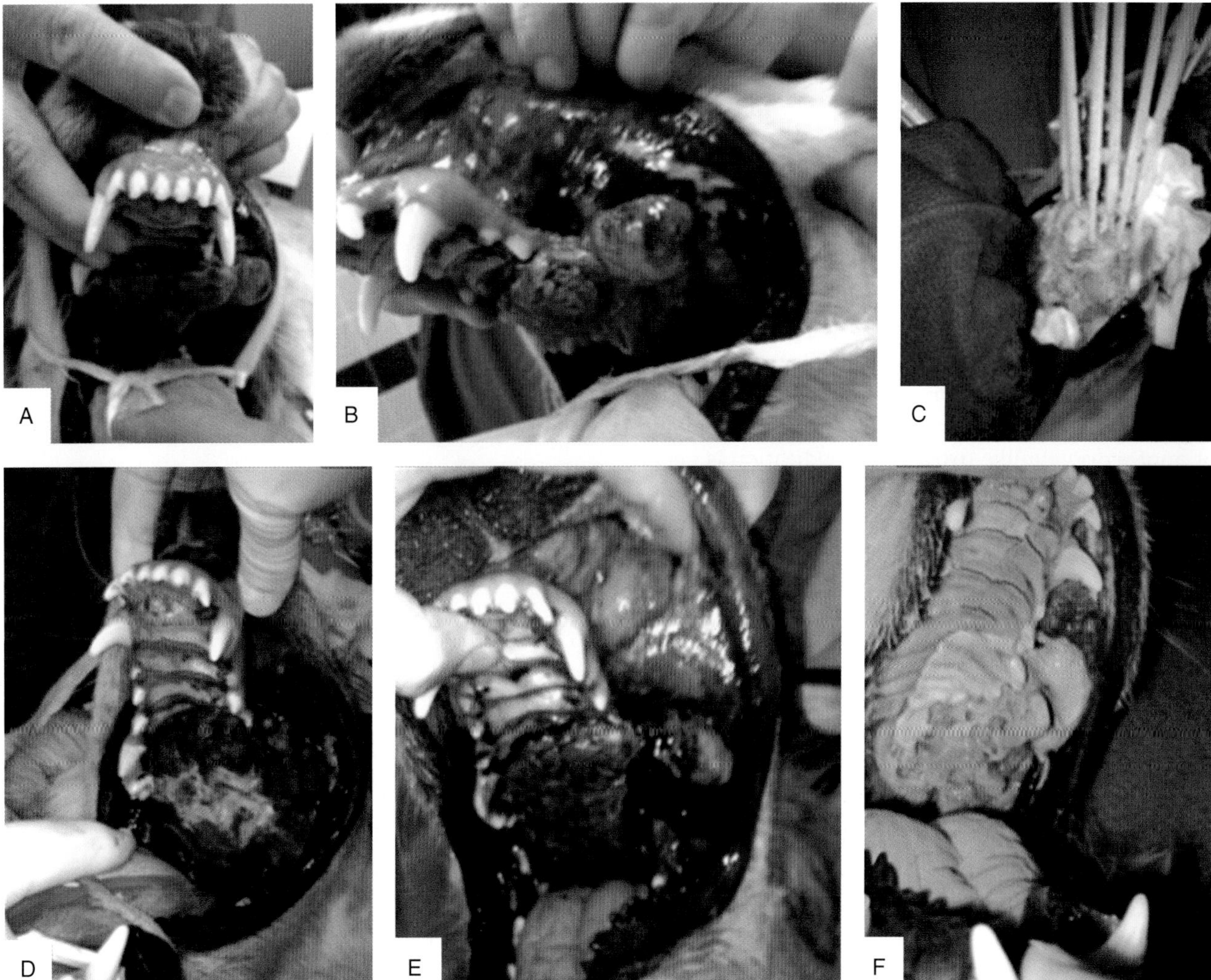

Figure 11.2 Hard palate melanoma: Serial images in a dog with an extensive hard palate malignant melanoma with partial nasal cavity occlusion and dysphagia. (A/B) Preoperative images demonstrating extent of mass on oral hard palate, crossing midline, and extending laterally. (C) Cryoablation performed with CT-guidance with multiple probes demonstrating frozen tumor and probes. (D) Immediately post-cryoablation demonstrating severely hyperemic tumor. (E) One day post-cryoablation demonstrating darkening and necrosis of tumor. (F) A few weeks post-cryoablation demonstrating sloughed tumor and ulcerated hard palate with tissue necrosis and clear margin of cryoablation zone. The dog was eating and did not appear overtly sensitive to this area likely due to the diffuse necrosis. (Pictures courtesy C. Weisse.)

several mechanisms including cellular crenation and lysis and intracellular ice formation resulting in cell damage (Vestal, 2005).

These ablation modalities hold tremendous potential in the treatment of oral tumors in companion animals, as there are several potential advantages. First, the extent of ablation can be controlled through close monitoring of probe position and the zone of tissue that is being treated. As the oral cavity contains many important structures, preventing trauma to adjacent organs is critical. Second, certain bone tumor cases may be encountered where other treatment options such as surgery or radiation therapy are not offered or elected due to the potential morbidity. Both cryoablation and RFA have been shown to be effective in the treatment of bony lesions (Ahrar and Stafford, 2011, Callstrom and Kurup, 2009, Castaneda Rodriguez and Callstrom, 2011, Lane et al., 2011, Mavrogenis et al., 2012, Nazario et al., 2011, Piccioli et al., 2011). Finally, the location of many oral tumors allows for accurate positioning of probes with minimal morbidity or limited or no surgical approach. As an example, probes placed for tumors of the maxilla, mandible, tongue or tonsils can likely be placed under direct visualization; however, subsequent administration of either RFA or cryoablation should be monitored closely with available imaging.

Follow-Up

After the utilization of an image-guided procedure, the patient should be monitored closely in hospital for side effects. While these procedures are minimally invasive, extended hospitalization may still be required to monitor patients for complications that can develop. During the early post-treatment period, side effects such as postembolization syndrome, bleeding from the vascular access site or treatment site, reactions to chemotherapy, and pain can be encountered.

Pain management may include the use of a non-steroidal anti-inflammatory medication (if not contra-indicated due to a comorbidity), gabapentin, tramadol or another opiate-like drug. Pain medication is generally administered for 4–7 days post-treatment unless a complication results in further morbidity and pain.

Patients should be monitored after treatment with comprehensive oral examinations (i.e., open-mouth investigation, palpation of intraoral and extraoral structures) and imaging. Skull radiographs can be useful to evaluate the patient for bone changes that have occurred secondary to the procedure or recurrence or progression of bony disease. CT is considered the imaging modality of choice to monitor both response to the treatment and progression of disease; however, the placement of some patients under anesthesia may not be recommended.

If intra-arterial chemotherapy is utilized as part of the image-guided procedure, the treating clinician may consider the use of intravenous chemotherapy at future visits. When chemotherapy is administered, proper preparation of clients should include a discussion of the potential complications (e.g., neutropenia, sepsis, nausea, vomiting, diarrhea, lethargy, anorexia) and the handling of waste products. Some tumors affecting the oral cavity have metastatic potential (e.g., osteosarcoma and malignant melanoma) and systemic chemotherapy may be recommended as treatment for metastasis.

Special Considerations/ Alternative Uses/ Complication Examples

Complications seen with treatment of oral tumors can include the development of fistulas through the skin or hard palate. Oronasal fistulas can occur when tumor extends through the hard or soft palate and response to therapy is robust. When oronasal fistulas develop, treatment is generally recommended, and the use of flaps may need to be considered; if a flap is utilized, it is highly recommended that a region not undergoing treatment be utilized. In addition to fistulas, erosion of the skin and mucosa can also occur due to devascularization (Figure 11.2).

Post-embolization syndrome can occur when an embolization technique has been pursued and may include signs such as fever, nausea, vomiting, lethargy and pain. Alterations in white blood cell count can also occur. In general, post-embolization syndrome, while being poorly described in veterinary patients, has been shown to be self-limiting in humans, although extended hospital stays may be required.

Notes

1. Vascular introducer sheath, Infiniti Medical, Menlo Park, CA.
2. Weasel wire, Infiniti Medical, Menlo Park, CA.
3. Berenstein catheter, Infiniti Medical, Menlo Park, CA.
4. Omnipaque (iohexol) injection, Amersham Health Inc., Princeton, NJ.
5. Microcatheter, Infiniti Medical, Menlo Park, CA.
6. Touhy–Borst adapter, Cook Medical, Bloomington, IN.
7. Flo-switch™, Boston Scientific, Natick, MA.
8. Microwire, Infiniti Medical, Menlo Park, CA.
9. Bead Block® PVA hydrogel microspheres, Biocompatibles UK Limited, Surrey, England.
10. 1 ml polycarbonate syringes, Merit Medical, South Jordan, UT.
11. Cool-tip RF™ Ablation System, Covidien, Mansfield, MA
12. SeedNet™ Cryoablation System, Galil Medical Inc., Arden Hills, MN.

References

Abbas G, Pennathur A, Landreneau R J, and Luketich JD (2009) Radiofrequency and microwave ablation of lung tumors. *J Surg Oncol* 100, 645–50.

Ahrar K and Stafford RJ (2011) Magnetic resonance imaging-guided laser ablation of bone tumors. *Tech Vasc Interv Radiol* 14, 177–82.

Beck ER, Withrow SJ, McChesney AE. et al (1986) Canine tongue tumors: a retrospective review of 57 cases. *J Am Anim Hosp Assoc* 22, 525–532.

Bonet-Coloma C, Minguez-Martinez I, Palma-Carrio C, Galan-Gil S, Penarrocha-Diago M, and Minguez-Sanz JM (2011) Clinical characteristics, treatment and outcome of 28 oral haemangiomas in pediatric patients. *Med Oral Patol Oral Cir Bucal* 16, e19–22.

Bozkaya S, Ugar D, Karaca I, Ceylan A, Uslu S, Baris E, and Tokman B (2006) The treatment of lymphangioma in the buccal mucosa by radiofrequency ablation: a case report. *Oral Surg Oral Med Oral Pathol Oral Radiol Endod* 102, e28–31.

Brooks MB, Matus RE, Leifer CE, Alfieri AA, and Patnaik AK (1988) Chemotherapy versus chemotherapy plus radiotherapy in the treatment of tonsillar squamous cell carcinoma in the dog. *J Vet Intern Med* 2, 206–11.

Callstrom MR and Kurup AN (2009) Percutaneous ablation for bone and soft tissue metastases--why cryoablation? *Skeletal Radiol* 38, 835–9.

Castaneda Rodriguez WR and Callstrom MR (2011) Effective pain palliation and prevention of fracture for axial-loading skeletal metastases using combined cryoablation and cementoplasty. *Tech Vasc Interv Radiol* 14, 160–9.

D'ippolito G and Goldberg SN (2002) Radiofrequency ablation of hepatic tumors. *Tech Vasc Interv Radiol* 5, 141–55.

El Dib R, Touma NJ, and Kapoor A (2012) Cryoablation vs radiofrequency ablation for the treatment of renal cell carcinoma: a meta-analysis of case series studies. *BJU Int* 110, 510–6.

Evans HE and De Lahunta A (2013) The heart and arteries. *Miller's Anatomy of the Dog*. 4th edn. Elsevier Saunders, St. Louis.

Freeman KP, Hahn KA, Harris FD, and King GK (2003) Treatment of dogs with oral melanoma by hypofractionated radiation therapy and platinum-based chemotherapy (1987 1997). *J Vet Intern Med* 17, 96–101.

Hoyt RF and Withrow SJ (1984) Oral malignancy in the dog. *J Am Anim Hosp Assoc* 20, 83.

Ikushima I, Korogi Y, Ishii A, et al (2008) Superselective intra-arterial infusion chemotherapy for stage III/IV squamous cell carcinomas of the oral cavity: midterm results. *Eur J Radiol* 66, 7–12.

Kobayashi W, Teh BG, Sakaki H, et al. (2010) Superselective intra-arterial chemoradiotherapy with docetaxel-nedaplatin for advanced oral cancer. *Oral Oncol* 46, 860–3.

Korogi Y, Hirai T, Nishimura R, et al. (1995) Superselective intraarterial infusion of cisplatin for squamous cell carcinoma of the mouth: preliminary clinical experience. *AJR Am J Roentgenol* 165, 1269–72.

Lane MD, Le HB, Lee S, et al (2011) Combination radiofrequency ablation and cementoplasty for palliative treatment of painful neoplastic bone metastasis: experience with 53 treated lesions in 36 patients. *Skeletal Radiol* 40, 25–32.

Leboulanger N, Roger G, Caze A, Enjolras O, Denoyelle F, and Garabedian E N (2008) Utility of radiofrequency ablation for haemorrhagic lingual lymphangioma. *Int J Pediatr Otorhinolaryngol* 72, 953–8.

Mavrogenis AF, Rossi G, Palmerini E, et al (2012) Palliative treatments for advanced osteosarcoma. *J BUON* 17, 436–45.

Nazario J, Hernandez J, and Tam AL (2011) Thermal ablation of painful bone metastases. *Tech Vasc Interv Radiol* 14, 150–9.

Ohba S, Yokoyama J, Fujimaki M, et al (2012) Significant improvement in superselective intra-arterial chemotherapy for oral cancer by using indocyanine green fluorescence. *Oral Oncol* 48, 1101–5.

Piccioli A, Ventura A, Maccauro G, Spinelli MS, Del Bravo V, and Rosa MA (2011) Local adjuvants in surgical management of bone metastases. *Int J Immunopathol Pharmacol* 24, 129–32.

Proulx DR, Ruslander DM, Dodge RK, et al (2003) A retrospective analysis of 140 dogs with oral melanoma treated with external beam radiation. *Vet Radiol Ultrasound* 44, 352–9.

Schirmang TC, Davis LM, Nigri PT, and Dupuy DE (2007) Solitary fibrous tumor of the buccal space: treatment with percutaneous cryoablation. *AJNR Am J Neuroradiol* 28, 1728–30.

Suzuki G, Ogo E, Tanoue R, et al (2011) Primary gingival angiosarcoma successfully treated by radiotherapy with concurrent intra-arterial chemotherapy. *Int J Clin Oncol* 16, 439–43.

Syrcle JA, Bonczynski JJ, Monette S, and Bergman PJ (2008) Retrospective evaluation of lingual tumors in 42 dogs: 1999–2005. *J Am Anim Hosp Assoc* 44, 308–19.

Theon AP, Rodriguez C, Griffey S, and Madewell BR (1997a) Analysis of prognostic factors and patterns of failure in dogs with periodontal tumors treated with megavoltage irradiation. *J Am Vet Med Assoc* 210, 785–8.

Theon AP, Rodriguez C, and Madewell BR (1997b) Analysis of prognostic factors and patterns of failure in dogs with malignant oral tumors treated with megavoltage irradiation. *J Am Vet Med Assoc* 210, 778–84.

Vestal JC (2005) Critical review of the efficacy and safety of cryotherapy of the prostate. *Curr Urol Rep* 6, 190–3.

Weisse C, Berent A, and Solomon S (2011) Combined transarterial embolization, systemic cyclophosphamide, and cryotherapy ablation for "Hi-Lo" maxillary fibrosarcoma in a dog. *Proceedings 8th Annual Meeting Veterinary Endoscopy Society*, 22.

Wu CF, Huang CJ, Chang KP, and Chen CM (2010) Continuous intra-arterial infusion chemotherapy as a palliative treatment for oral squamous cell carcinoma in octogenarian or older patients. *Oral Oncol* 46, 559–63.

CHAPTER TWELVE

Esophageal Foreign Body Retrieval

Douglas A. Palma
The Animal Medical Center, New York, NY

Background/Indications

Esophageal obstruction is a common emergency seen in veterinary medicine, most commonly associated with a foreign body. Other causes include esophageal neoplasia, polyps, strictures, gastroesophageal achalasia, granulomas, and extraluminal obstructions (i.e., mediastinal disease, vascular anomalies) (Figure 12.1). These conditions are similar in their clinical presentation but may vary in clinical progression. Additionally, these conditions can overlap with concurrent non-obstructive esophageal diseases (i.e., esophagitis, gastroesophageal reflux, hiatal hernias, diverticuli) and dysmotility issues. While they can occur in any patient, it should be noted that esophageal foreign body obstruction is more likely to occur in small dogs and may have a slight predisposition towards Terrier breeds (Juvet, 2010).

The diagnosis of an esophageal foreign body is critical for timely treatment. Differentiating vomiting from regurgitation can often be done with thorough questioning of the owner. Radiographic evaluation can diagnose the majority of foreign body obstructions since there is a tendency of these obstructions to be radiodense (bones) and highlighted by regional air-filled structures (i.e., lungs, gas-filled esophageal dilations) (Figure 12.2). Occasionally, regional anatomy may make diagnosis difficult due to various overlapping structures (at the thoracic inlet, caudal cervical region). In these cases, utilization of contrast radiography with traditional liquid barium or paste can be helpful. Barium paste has a more reliable ability to coat intraluminal foreign objects. Contrast evaluations may also help to identify local perforations, determine whether the obstruction is extraluminal, and define esophageal motility. Care must be taken when considering a contrast esophagram, as most contrast agents are highly irritating to the tissues surrounding the esophagus, and if a perforation is present, or aspiration occurs, this could result in a severe mediastinitis or pneumonitis. In addition, if barium is present in the esophagus during esophagoscopy the endoscope can be severely damaged. The gold standard for the diagnosis of esophageal disease is esophagoscopy. This can aid in simultaneous diagnosis and treatment.

Potential Risks/Complications/Expected Outcomes

The major risk associated with esophageal foreign body retrieval is esophageal perforation. This complication is uncommon but can be exacerbated by devitalized esophageal tissue, delayed intervention (chronic foreign bodies), bone foreign bodies, use of rigid instrumentation, pushing of foreign objects aborally, and excessive insufflation of the esophagus. Endoscopic features associated with increased risk of perforation include discolored mucosa (black, purple, burgundy), presence of deep ulcerations, and observed defects in the wall (Figure 12.3). Perforation may be clearly visualized or never observed if small. Other complications include esophagitis, esophageal ulceration, esophageal stricture formation and the development of aspiration pneumonia. Esophagitis is common (Figure 12.4), though rarely results in subsequent stricture formation. If a stricture were to occur it typically starts 7–10 days after the procedure. Some strictures may result in a noticeable narrowing on esophagoscopy but no clinical signs. Circumferential ulceration or deep ulceration may have higher rates of stricture formation (see Chapter 13).

The majority of esophageal foreign bodies can be successfully removed or displaced aborally (for removal from the stomach via gastrotomy or digestion). Owners should be aware of all potential risks prior to removal of the foreign body.

Veterinary Image-Guided Interventions, First Edition. Edited by Chick Weisse and Allyson Berent.

Companion website: www.wiley.com/go/weisse/vet-image-guided-interventions

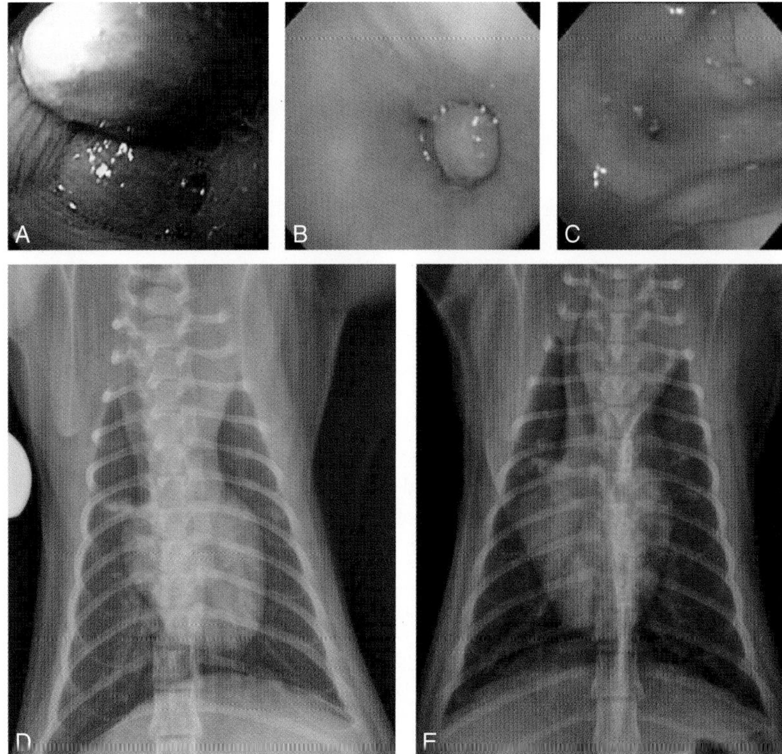

Figure 12.1 Endoscopic images of various esophageal obstructions. (A) Esophageal tumor with food proximal. (B) Esophageal polyp, (C) esophageal stricture, (D,E) radiographs of a dog with an esophageal mass showing the contrast of air outlining the lesion.

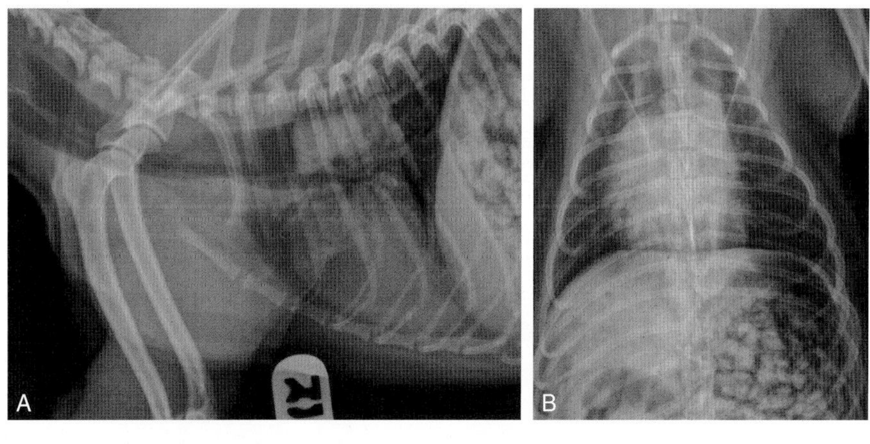

Figure 12.2 Lateral and VD radiographs of a dog with a bone esophageal foreign body.

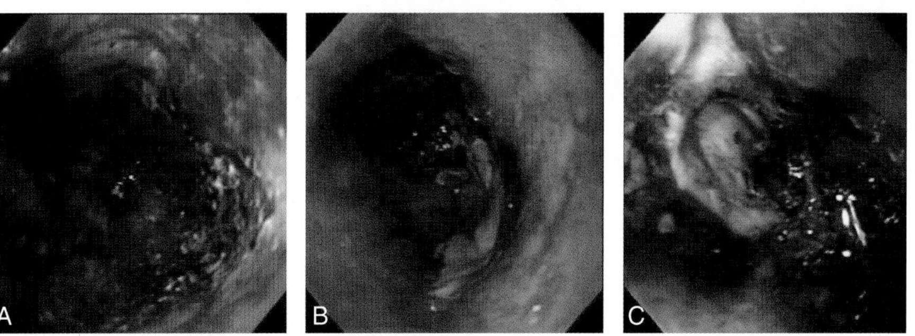

Figure 12.3 Endoscopic images of various esophageal lesions after foreign body removal with a high risk of perforation. (A) The black, bluish mucosal color is indicative of severe mucosal injury, however this lesion is superficial. (B) Esophageal lesion that has a blue-blackish discoloration, moderate depth of injury, and the white superficial, necrotic mucosal layer. (C) Esophageal lesion with hemorrhagic discoloration and moderate-severe depth of injury.

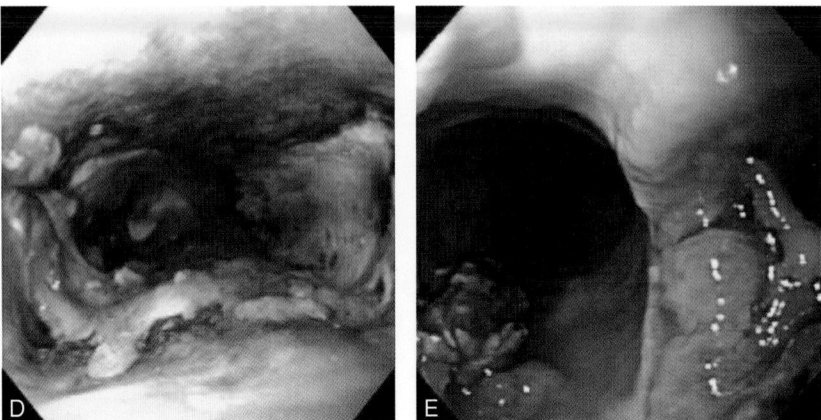

Figure 12.3 (*Continued*) (D) Esophageal lesion that is necrotic and pale. This has a high risk of perforation. The true depth of the injury cannot be assessed in this case until the superficial necrotic layer is debrided. (E) While this lesion is not overtly discolored, the depth of injury puts this patient at great risk of perforation. Note that it is not possible to determine whether small perforation exists in this patient. Radiography and antibiotic therapy is recommended.

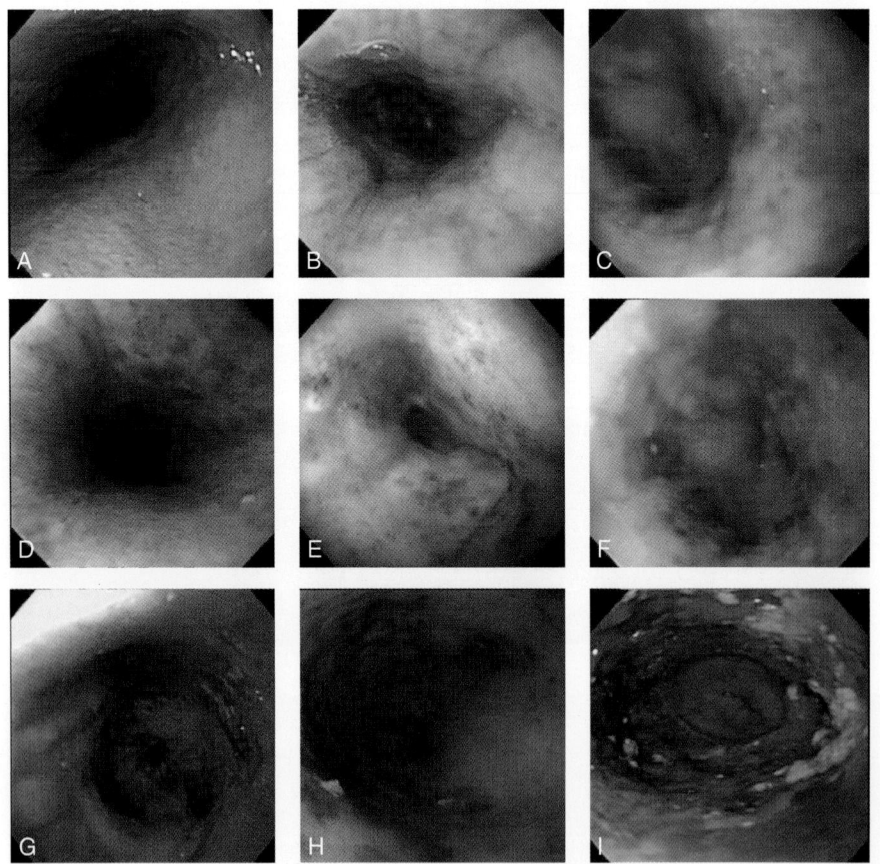

Figure 12.4 Endoscopic images of various esophageal lesions after foreign body removal at low risk of perforation. Note varying degrees of esophagitis with some patients having focal, multifocal or concentric diffuse changes. Additionally, patients have variable degrees of mucosal defects ranging from superficial erosions to deep ulcers. Variations in mucosal color can be observed; as dictated by the degree of mucosal compromise and duration of foreign body contact.

Equipment

Many tools exist for potential extraction of the foreign body (Table 12.1) including: (1) endoscopic equipment, (2) laparoscopic equipment, and (3) balloon dilators. Each instrument will better assist in foreign body retrieval in a given case, therefore, it is crucial to have access to a wide variety of options. The instrument that provides the most purchase of the foreign object is likely to be the most successful.

TABLE 12.1
Commonly Used Endoscopic Equipment (see Figure 12.5)

Endoscopic equipment
- Retrieval forceps (eg. rat tooth,[1,2] alligator type,[3,4] shark tooth,[5] rubber tip.[6])
- Baskets (eg. 3 wire,[7] 4 wire,[8] 6 wire,[9,10], 4 wire rotatable.[11])
- Endoscopic snares: non-rotating[12], rotating[13]
- Nets (eg. Roth net,[14] Nakao Spider-Net.[15])
- Endoscopic graspers (eg. 2 prong,[16] 3 prong,[17] 4 prong,[18] 5 prong.[19])
- Biliary stent remover (eg. Soehendra stent retriever.[20])
- Endoscopic balloons (eg. Multi-diameter,[21] or single diameter balloons.[22])

Laparoscopic equipment
- Forceps[23]
- Scissors[24,25]

Endoscopic attachments
- Overtubes[26,27]
- Endoscopic hood[28]

Non-traditional equipment
- Suture/guide wire
- Plastic bags

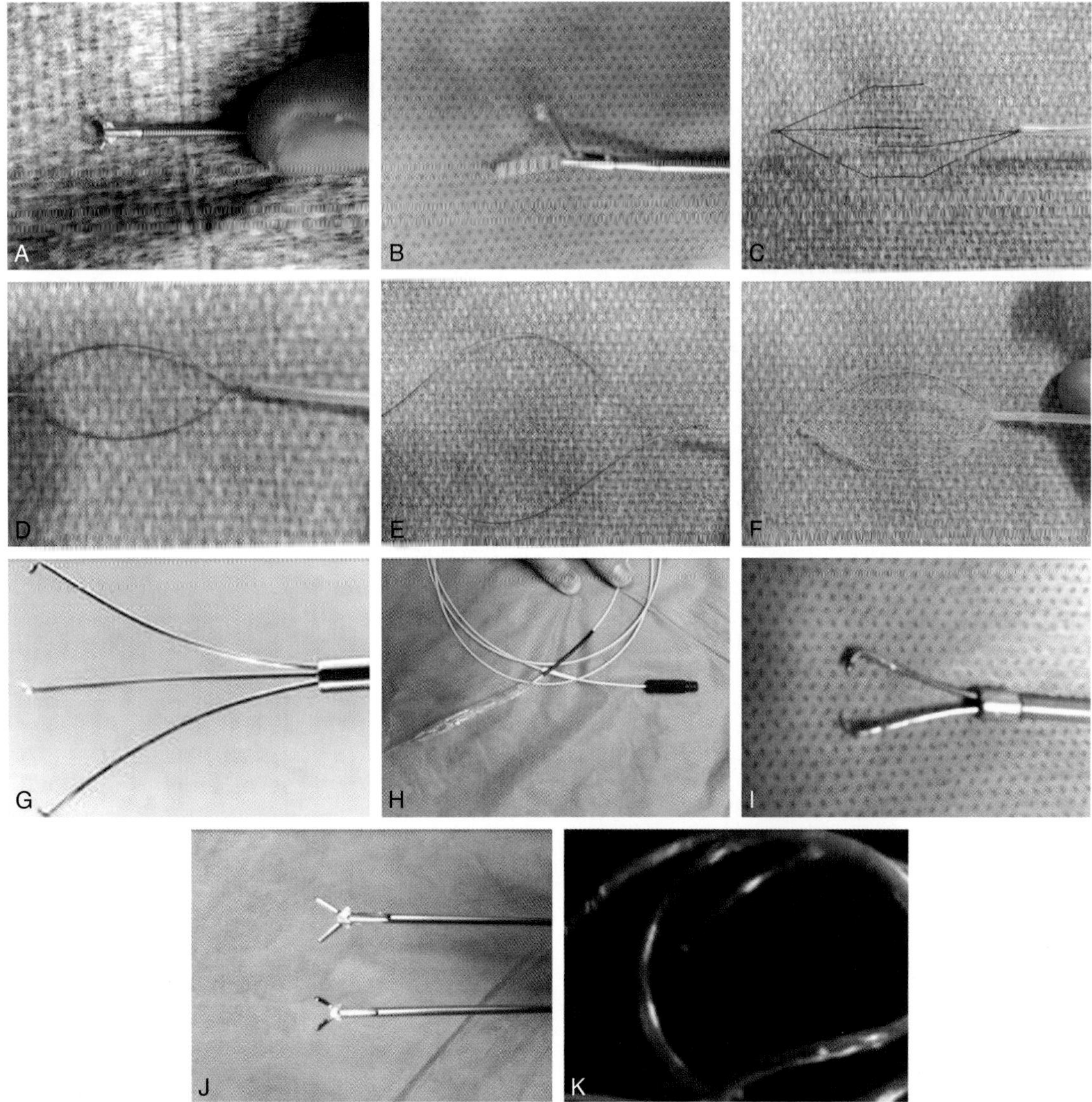

Figure 12.5 Various equipment used for foreign body retrieval. (A) rat tooth retrieval forceps; (B) longer rat tooth retrieval forceps; (C) 4 wire basket; (D) small non-rotating endoscopic snare; (E) large non-rotating endoscopic snare; (F) roth net; (G) 3 prong grasper; (H) multidiameter endoscopic balloon; (I) rigid rat tooth gasper; (J) laparoscopic forceps; (K) orogastric tube ("overtube").

Patient Preparation

Given the emergent nature of this procedure, minimal preoperative preparation is possible. A radiograph should be taken prior to any intervention, because if a pneumomediatinum, indicating an esophageal perforation, the approach will be different. Esophageal perforation is a risk from the presence of the foreign object, and from the manipulation of the esophagus during retrieval. Documentation of its presence prior to any intervention is always ideal. A pneumomediastinum can progress to a pneumothorax, and during anesthesia this should be carefully monitored for. In addition, one might find the presence of a pneumothorax, pleural effusion, pyothorax, and/or other comorbidities like concurrent gastrointestinal foreign bodies and aspiration pneumonia (Figure 12.6).

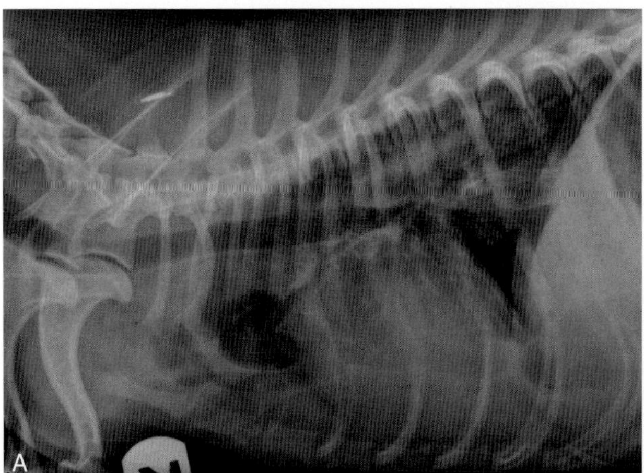

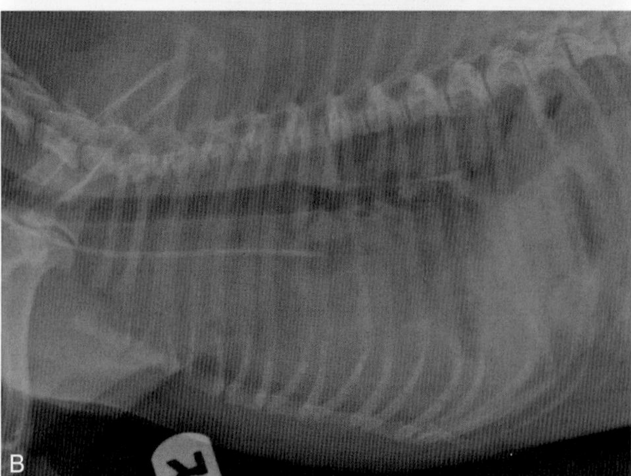

Figure 12.6 Radiographs of two dogs with esophageal perforations from foreign bodies resulting in pyothorax. When large effusions are present, foreign objects may be difficult to identify. These patients are at great risk of developing a pneumothorax during the retrieval procedure.

The patient is placed under general anesthesia using a fully inflated endotracheal tube. The patient is then placed in left lateral recumbency for routine esophagoscopy. If aspiration pneumonia is a concern than an endotracheal wash should be considered prior to anesthetic recovery.

Procedure

The upper esophageal sphincter is intubated gently with a well-lubricated endoscope. Careful attention during continued visualization of the lumen is necessary to ensure that proximal foreign bodies are not encountered or disrupted without determination of the ideal approach for retrieval.

When the foreign body is encountered, a complete examination of the surrounding mucosa is made to look for areas of weakness and increased risk of perforation with manipulation. If the endoscope can safely pass around the irregular shaped foreign body then this is done to determine the length, anatomy, and areas of weakness caudally.

After the foreign body is encountered the proper instrument is chosen. The instrument is ideally passed through the working channel of the endoscope, and the scope is withdrawn partially to allow the instrument to be visualized as it exists the endoscope, for controlled placement during retrieval. When the endoscope and retrieval device are too close to the foreign object, precise manipulation of the instrument is difficult. Additionally, bending of the instrument can occur, causing damage and preventing repeated usage (Figure 12.7).

After the instrument has exited from the scope it is opened and attempts are made to advance the instrument around the object to entrap it (with a snare, basket, bag, or net), or to grasp the object on an edge with a forcep or grasper (Figure 12.8). This should be attempted at an area where a predicted area of "purchase" can be achieved; this may be dorsal, ventral or lateral depending on the object. Creativity is often necessary during retrieval, and in some circumstances non-traditional equipment is used (bags, condoms, lubrication, etc.).

If this technique is unsuccessful, then the instrument (i.e., snare, basket, bag, or net) is inserted between the foreign object and the esophageal wall in an unopened fashion. Care is taken to ensure perforation does not occur. The instrument is gradually opened and manipulated so that the wires can engage around the object. When the instrument is opened to its maximal diameter it is gradually retracted until it is seen to purchase the object (Figure 12.9). When this is visualized, the endoscope is positioned with the directional controls

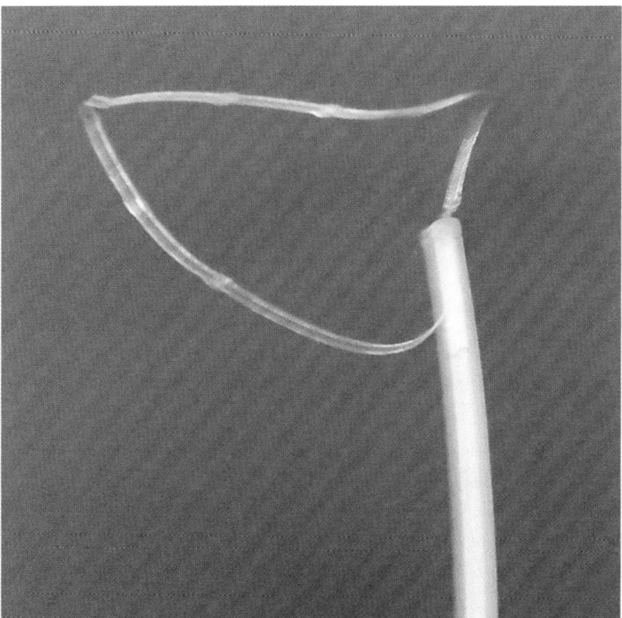

Figure 12.7 Deformed endoscopic loop, which can occur with inappropriate use. The equipment should be carefully manipulated over/around foreign material and not opened directly onto the foreign body, as it will become deformed.

in the opposite direction of the instrument/wall to facilitate pulling the instrument over the object to entrap it. This technique is often effective but requires patience.

Proximal esophageal foreign bodies can be amendable to removal with rigid instrumentation in select cases, though this holds greater risk, as the instruments are not directed through the working channel of the endoscope (Figure 12.10). Placement of rigid instrumentation under endoscopic visualization across the upper esophageal sphincter (UES) is dependent on the size of the patient. As the instrument is passed, careful attention is placed on maneuvering the instrument without placing excessive pressure on the esophageal mucosa. Given the limited size of the UES and concurrent scope passage across this region, a combination of cervical manipulation, and angling of the instrument carefully in line with the endoscope will facilitate passage without injury. Occasionally, open-ended stomach tubes, large vascular access sheaths, or large gauge red rubber catheters can be used as an overtube or sheath for the passage of an instrument across the UES.

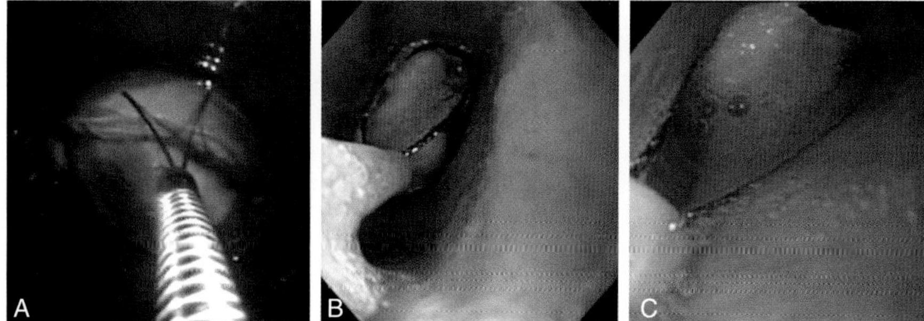

Figure 12.8 Endoscopic images of three dogs during foreign body retrieval. (A) A 3-pronged grasper is directed into the foreign body for purchase; (B) an endoscopic basket is placed over the object for engagement; (C) a loop is manipulated around the edge of the foreign object. Firm purchase of a small piece of the foreign object may help with extraction.

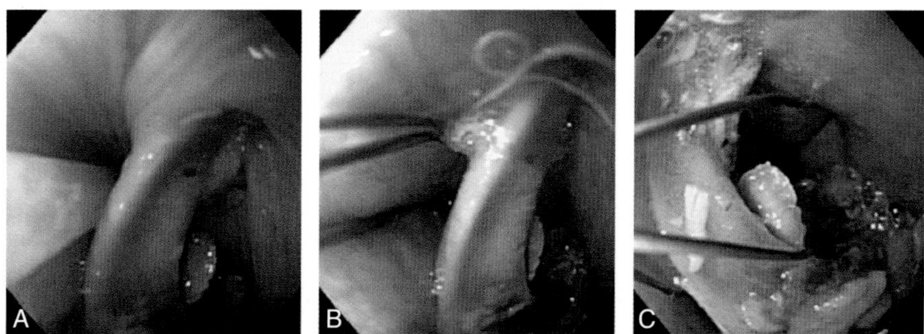

Figure 12.9 Endoscopic images of a dog with an esophageal foreign body during basket retrieval. (A) The instrument is passed beyond the foreign body in a closed position. (B) The instrument is opened and then pulled forward to line-up around the foreign body. (C) The basket is moved back and forth encouraging the wires to engage the foreign object.

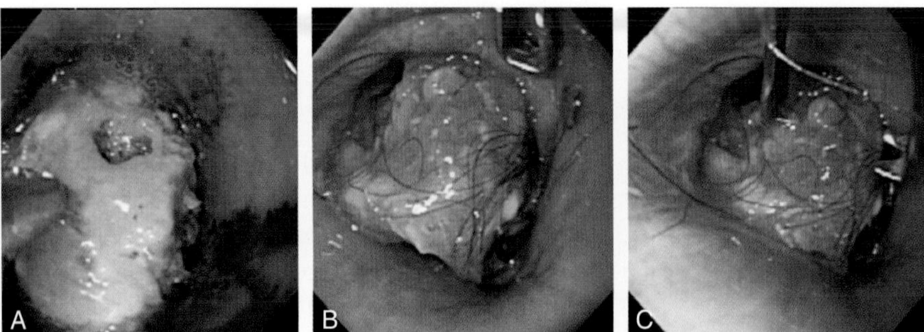

Figure 12.10 Endoscopic images of foreign body retrieval using a rigid instrument. Note that this these instruments engage the foreign objects carefully and under direct endoscopic visualization. Passage of these rigid instruments may require manipulation of the cervical region to "straighten out" the esophagus and reduce iatrogenic mucosal trauma.

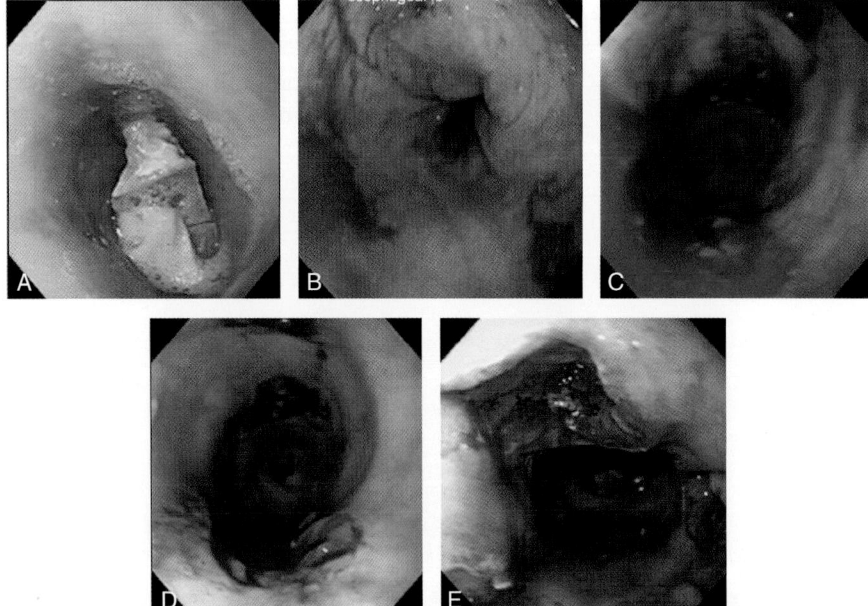

Figure 12.11 Endoscopic images with various points of engagement in the esophageal wall. (A) The foreign body is fixed in place within the esophagus. It is tough to appreciate the depth of mucosal engagement that is present. (B–F) Various depths of foreign body engagement prior to endoscopic removal. These points represent areas of weakness; the endoscopist should be aware that putting excessive pressure on these areas may cause esophageal perforation.

Regardless of the technique used appropriate esophageal distension with air will aid in successful removal or dislodgement of a foreign object. This may require external cervical compression to maintain air distension. When foreign bodies are very tight and difficult to manipulate, passing a red rubber catheter down the esophagus to the level of the foreign body and infusing around the object 60 mL of a sterile lubrication/warm water mixture can make the edges of the object lubricious so that dislodgement is facilitated.

Occasionally, foreign objects cannot be removed from the esophagus orally and may need to be pushed into the stomach for digestion (i.e., bones) or for surgical gastrotomy. Pushing foreign bodies into the stomach requires careful attention to detail to prevent injury to the insertion tube and to not result in unnecessary pressure on the areas of weakness within the esophagus (usually areas of object contact or point of engagement with the mucosa) (Figure 12.11). Soft foreign bodies or food may be manipulated with the endoscope alone. However, an overtube can be very helpful to protect the scope during this procedure (Figure 12.12) and is generally recommended for hard/sharp objects (ASGE Technology Committee et al, 2009). A standard stomach tube can also be used as a make-shift over tube if necessary. The scope/overtube combination are advanced lateral to the foreign object, and between the esophageal wall and the material. The insertion tube/

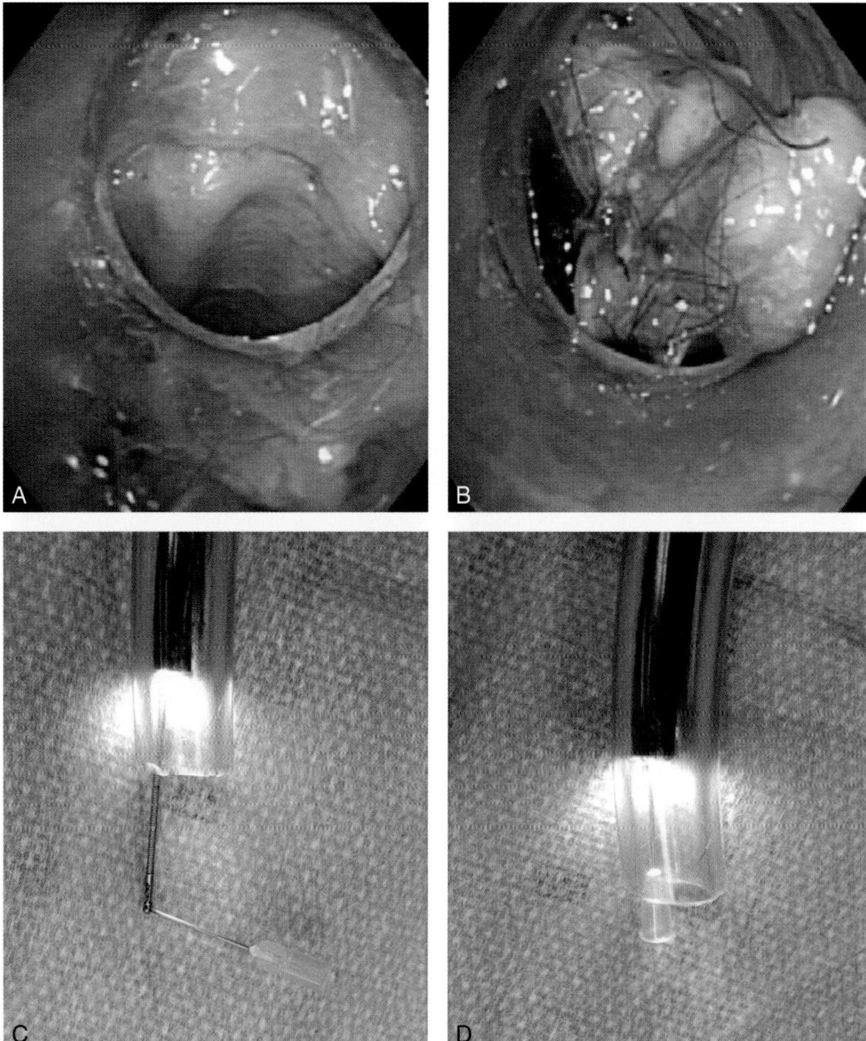

Figure 12.12 Overtube usage. (A) Use of an overtube to help with dislodgement of a fixed esophageal foreign body. The overtube is placed around the endoscope and directed between the foreign object and the wall. This pushes the wall laterally to disengage points of fixation and protects the scope. (B) The overtube is contacting the foreign object on the side, not directly. Occasionally, the overtube can dilate the esophagus wide enough to allow for retraction of the foreign object into its lumen for removal. (C,D) A model showing the use of an overtube to retract a sharp foreign body for protection of the esophageal lumen during retraction.

overtube are advanced distally while simultaneously insufflating. As the wall is pushed laterally, the foreign body's point of engagement in the mucosa will be dislodged. Small movements with firm steady pressure are made and this is repeated circumferentially until the foreign body is rotated or seamlessly moves distally. This "push technique" is designed to remove the points of fixation of the foreign body from the esophageal wall, as these points are the sites or mucosal weakness, and are typically deeper due to regional edema and central ulceration. If you attempt to push a foreign body directly, you increase the risk of perforation within these areas of weakness (Figure 12.13).

Percutaneous Endoscopic Gastrotomy Tube Placement

The author does not typically place a percutaneous endoscopic gastrotomy (PEG) tube unless perforation or near perforation has occurred. The esophagus can heal quickly in the majority of cases. The presence of esophageal discoloration, ulceration, bleeding, or length of esophagitis do not reliably predict the healing process of the esophagus. PEG tubes are utilized in cases where perforation has occurred and mediastinal or pleural contamination needs to be limited. A PEG tube is not believed to limit the formation of strictures,

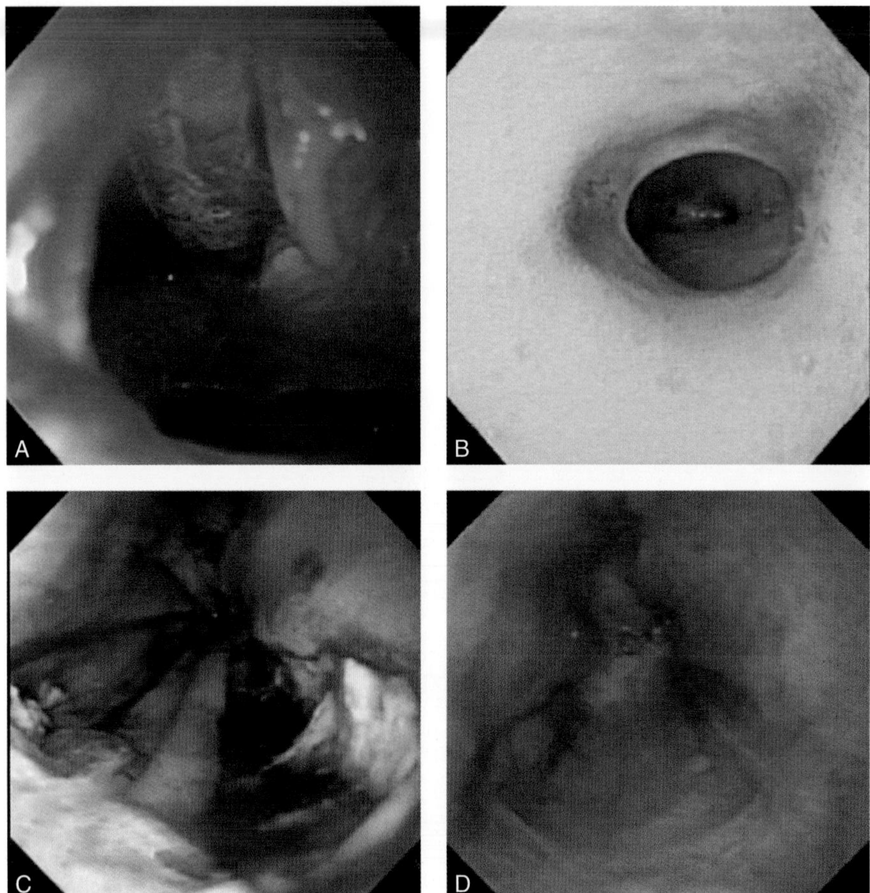

Figure 12.13 Endoscopic images of patients with esophageal perforations. (A) Mediastinal defect in the esophagus and the separate defect in the mediastinum, entering the pleural space. This patient required a thoracic tube. Note the potential for insufflation causing severe respiratory compromise from pneumothorax. (B) The same patient as image A evaluated 1 month following the procedure with complete healing and a slight stricture at the perforation site. (C) A perforation that was not overtly obvious on observation; this patient had a pyothorax managed with thoracic tubes. (D) Rapid healing is observed. This image is 10 days after image C was taken.

and feeding may prevent esophageal collapse, which may ultimately prevent stricture formation.

Dealing with a Perforation

If a perforation is observed, and the foreign body was not successfully removed, then surgical intervention is indicated. If perforation is observed, the endoscopist must be cognizant of air insufflation, as small perforations can result in a one way valve leading to accumulation of air in the mediastinum and pleural space. The esophagus and mediastinum should be immediately deflated, and if the foreign body was removed a PEG tube should be placed. Following the procedure, the stomach air is evacuated and the scope is withdrawn carefully. Interrogation of the esophageal perforation is done carefully with minimal insufflation. Information regarding the location and size of perforation should be recorded. The patient is recovered and broad spectrum antibiotics are initiated. Post-operatively, the patient is placed on aggressive acid suppression (i.e., omeprazole 1 mg/kg q 12), nothing per os and potentially gastroesophageal sphincter tonicity manipulation (i.e., cisapride 0.5 mg/kg q 8). Alternatively, metoclopramide could be given, but is considered less effective. Placement of a nasogastric feeding tube could be considered in cases where PEG tubes are not available, though this could result in reflux due to the tube crossing the LES. These should ideally be placed via a guide wire through the endoscope to prevent inadvertent placement through the esophageal defect. A radiograph should be taken prior to recovery to ensure and

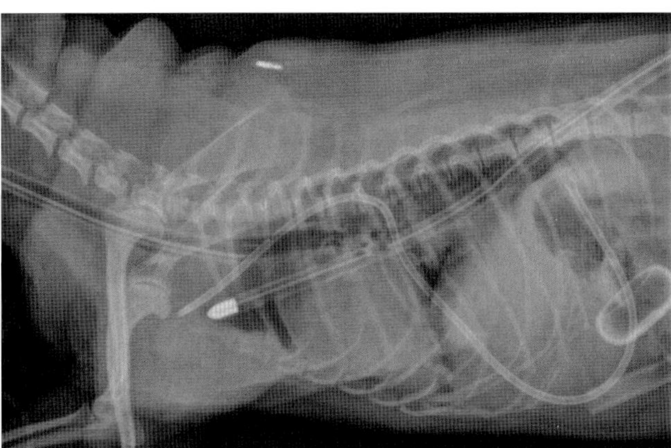

Figure 12.14 An intraoperative radiograph demonstrating bilateral thoracic tubes placed for pneumothorax after an esophageal perforation. Note the PEG tube placed to bypass the esophageal defect esophageal.

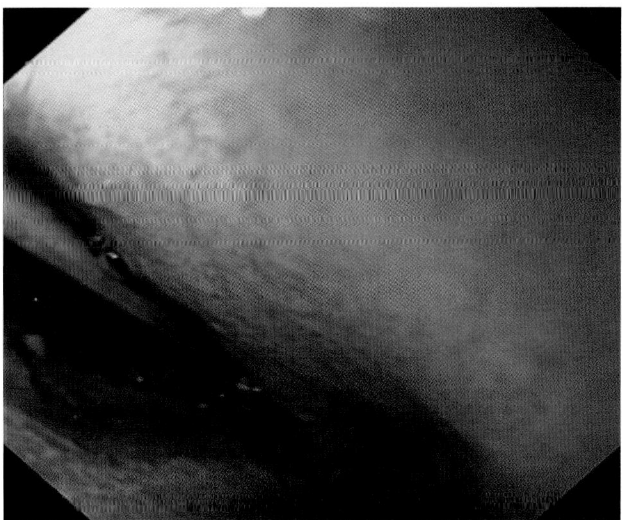

Figure 12.15 Nasomediastinal tube placement following mediastinal penetration. These tubes can be used to evacuate air during perforation or for post-operative drainage

document the presence and degree of pneumomediastinum and/or pneumothorax.

The decision to place a thoracic tube for a pneumothorax is based on the size of the perforation, the presence pneumothorax, and the degree of respiratory impairment. In cases with rapid respiratory decompensation, time can be essential and decompression should be immediate with thoracocentesis (Figure 12.14). Rare utilization of nasomediastinal tubes to provide drainage of fluid, purulent material, air accumulation or to decontaminate particulate matter could be employed (Figure 12.15). These tubes can be placed over a guide wire under endoscopic or fluoroscopic assistance and placed antegrade, through the nares using a red rubber catheter.

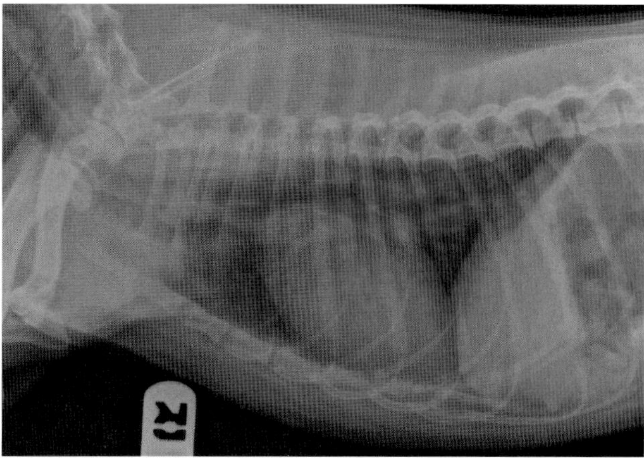

Figure 12.16 Lateral radiograph of a dog with a pneumomediastinum associated with an esophageal perforation. This was not observed during esophagoscopy.

Repeat endoscopic procedures are essential prior to oral feeding to ensure that the esophageal defect is clearly healed. Caution should be taken to avoid overdistension with air. It should be noted that even large esophageal defects can heal without surgical intervention quickly. In one human study, 100% of the esophageal perforations treated non-surgically were healed by time of discharge regardless of size. Patients with spontaneous perforation however, had a longer hospitalization than those with iatrogenic perforations (Vogel, 2005).

Some perforations are not observed endoscopically, but the devitalized tissue permits air to track into the mediastinum. In any patient with significant esophageal devitalization, thoracic radiographs should be acquired prior to anesthetic recovery to evaluate for a pneumomediastinum and/or pneumothorax (Figure 12.16). These patients could be managed as above with feeding tubes but may be managed more conservatively with NPO and parenteral nutrition. Serial contrast radiography can be used to evaluate for continued leakage before oral feeding, but the risk of mediastinitis and pleuritis must be considered. A seal may be obtained in 24–48 hours in many patients. Contrast esophagography with iodinated contrast is generally preferred for this technique due to reduced likelihood of inflammatory reaction in cases of perforation, however, in cases where a small perforation is strongly suspected barium may be more sensitive (Bueker et al, 1997) (Figure 12.17).

Post-Procedural and Follow-Up Care

Following the procedure, the author recommends treatment of esophagitis with acid suppression for 5–7 days. Carafate is added to patients with

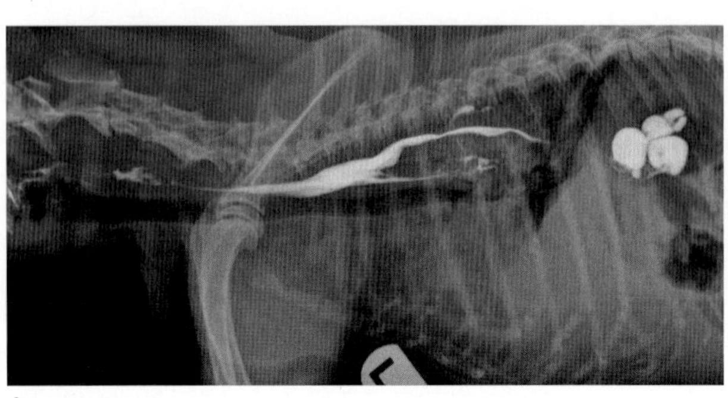

A

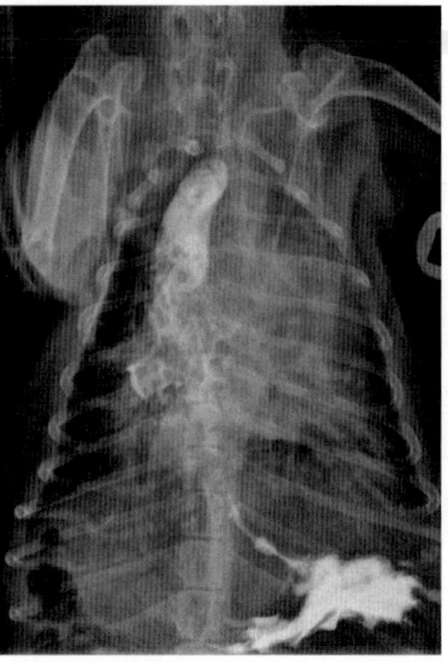

B

Figure 12.17 Barium esophagrams done preoperatively. The radiograph shows the esophageal foreign body and a perforation is observed dorsal to the esophagus detected radiographically.

moderate to severe esophagitis. The author tends to utilize antibiotic therapy for patients with deep, ulcerative or suspected devitalized esophageal tissue for 5–7 days. A concern involves the utilization of acid suppression with residual gastric bones that have been pushed into the stomach. The author consistently uses acid suppressive medications in these cases and does not believe that this delays gastric digestion of the bone. In the author's experience, it generally takes 3–5 days for the stomach to dissolve a bone; however, this is dependent on the size, density and surface area. Additionally, the author recommends feeding a soft diet for the first 24–48 hours following the procedure if significant esophagitis is observed.

Following removal or dislodgement of the esophageal foreign body we commonly are faced with residual esophageal disease. Esophagitis is common and can range from focal erythema, erosions/ulcerations, mucosal discolorization (i.e., black, purple, white) to more generalized/circumferential changes and ultimately strictures. Owners need to be aware of these risks (Rousseau et al, 2008).

Animals with esophageal perforations should have a PEG tube placed to prevent contamination of the site with food. In the author's experience, the majority of perforations will be healed in 7–10 days with only partial thickness residual defects. However, serial assessments of the esophageal integrity with esophagoscopy are recommended to assess for healing, prior to feeding orally. If the gross lesions suggest potential residual perforation, then avoidance of oral feeding is recommended for an additional 7–10 days before repeat assessment. Patients should remain on antibiotic therapy during this time. The PEG tube can be removed after oral feedings are well tolerated.

Prognosis

The prognosis following the removal of an esophageal foreign body is excellent. Complications following the procedure are uncommon and complete resolution of signs due to associated esophagitis are expected.

Notes

1. Maxum® Reusable Forceps Cook Medical, Winston-Salem, NC.
2. Rat tooth retrieval forceps, Olympus America, Center Valley, PA.
3. Alligator jaw retrieval forceps, Olympus America, enter Valley, PA.
4. Rat tooth alligator jaw retrieval forceps, Olympus America, Center Valley, PA.
5. Shark tooth retrieval forceps, Olympus America, Center Valley, PA
6. Rubber tip retrieval forceps, Olympus America, Center Valley, PA
7. 3 wire, Helical Retrieval Baskets: Reusable, Hobbs Medical. Stafford Springs, CT.
8. 4-Wire Basket w/3-Ring Handle, Olympus America, Center Valley, PA.
9. 4-wire foreign body basket, Medi-Globe,Tempe, AZ.
10. 6-wire foreign body basket, Medi-Globe, Tempe, AZ.

11. Falcon rotatable retrieval basket, US Endoscopy, Mentor, OH.
12. AcuSnare® One Piece Disposable Snare Cook Medical, Winston-Salem, NC.
13. RotaSnare® Rotating and with Multifilament Loop, Medi-Globe, Tempe, AZ.
14. Roth Net Platinum retriever - universal, US Endoscopy, Mentor, OH.
15. Nakao Spider-Net, ConMed, Billerica, MA.
16. Foreign Body Retriever – Grasper with Forked Jaws, Medi-Globe, Tempe, AZ.
17. Caesar® Grasping Forceps Cook Medical, Winston-Salem, NC.
18. Reusable Retrieval Forceps, 4 prong, Hobbs Medical, Stafford Springs, CT.
19. Pentapod grasping forceps, Olympus America, Center Valley, PA.
20. Soehendra stent retriever, Cook Medical, Winston-Salem, NC.
21. CRE Single-Use Fixed wire Esophageal Balloon Dilators, Boston Scientific, Natick, MA.
22. Maxforce TTS Single Use Balloon Dilators, Boston Scientific, Natick, MA.
23. Kelly Forceps, AEM Laparascopic Instruments, Encision, Boulder CO.
24. Hook scissors AEM Laparascopic Instruments, Encision, Boulder CO.
25. Straight scissors AEM Laparascopic Instruments, Encision, Boulder CO.
26. Guardus overtube – esophageal, US Endoscopy, Mentor, Ohio.
27. ConMed Endoscopic Overtube, ConMed, Utica, NY.
28. Foreign body hood protector, Kimberly-Clark, Roswell, GA.

References

ASGE Technology Committee, Tierney WM, Adler DG, et al (2009) Overtube use in gastrointestinal endoscopy. *Gastrointest Endosc* 70 (5), 8288–34.

Bueker A, Wein BB, Neuerburg JM, et al (1997) Esophageal perforation: comparison of use of aqueous and barium containing contrast media. *Radiology* 202(3), 6836–86.

Diehl DL, Adler DG, Conway JD, et al (2009) Endoscopic retrieval devices ASGE Technology Committee, *Gastroinest Endosc* 69(6), 9971–3.

Juvet F, Pinna M, Shiel RE, et al (2010) Oesophageal foreign bodies in dogs: factors affecting success of endoscopic retrieval. *Irish Vet J* 63(3), 163–8.

Rousseau A, Prittie J, Broussard JD, et al (2008) Incidence and characterization of esophagitis following esophageal foreign body removal in dogs: 60 cases (1999–2003). *J Vet Emerg Crit Care* 17, 159–63.

Vogel SB, Rout WR, Martin TD, et al (2005) Esophageal perforation in adults: aggressive, conservative treatment lowers morbidity and mortality. *Ann Surg* 241(6), 1016–21.

Suggested Reading

Bexfield NH, Watson PJ, and Herrtage ME (2006) Esophageal dysmotility in young dogs. *J Vet Intern Med* 20, 1314–18.

Houlton JEF, Herrtage ME, Taylor, et al (1985) Thoracic oesophageal foreign bodies in the dog: a review of 90 cases. *J Small Anim Pract* 26, 521–36.

Leib MS and Sartor LL (2008) Esophageal foreign body obstruction caused by a dental chew treat in 31 dogs (2000–2006). *J Am Vet Med Assoc* 232, 1021–5

Narra S and Al-Kawas FH (2010) The importance of preparation and innovation in the endoscopic management of esophageal foreign bodies. *Gastroenterol Hepatol* 6(12), 795–7.

Sale CS and Williams JM (2006) Results of transthoracic esophagotomy retrieval of esophageal foreign body obstructions in dogs: 14 cases (2000–2004). *J Am Anim Hosp Assoc*. 42, 450–6.

Spielman BL, Shaker EH, and Garvey MS (1992) Esophageal foreign body in dogs: a retrospective study of 23 cases. *J Am Anim Hosp Assoc* 28, 570–4.

CHAPTER THIRTEEN

Esophageal Obstruction: Strictures/Tumors – Balloon, Bougie, Injections, Stent

Douglas A. Palma and Allyson Berent
The Animal Medical Center, New York, NY

Background/Indications

Esophageal obstructions can be a result of extraluminal or intraluminal occlusion. While foreign bodies are the most common cause of obstructive esophageal disease, esophageal strictures are the next most common cause, followed by esophageal neoplasia, granuloma, or intussusception. Strictures occur secondary to local esophageal injury often associated with gastroesophageal reflux (GERD) or direct damage (esophageal trauma, caustic irritation, post surgical inflammation). The esophageal mucosal lining is made of non-keratinized, stratified squamous epithelium and is not equipped to deal with the acidity and enzymes present within the gastric fluids. This injury causes esophageal erythema, erosions, ulcerations and fibrosis. The fibrosis occasionally leads to a circumferential narrowing of the lumen, which is the classic benign stricture.

Anesthetic agents result in relaxation of the lower esophageal sphincter (LES), predisposing the esophagus to the reflux of gastric contents. Other factors that may play a role include the duration of anesthesia, patient positioning, and the manipulation of abdominal organs, which can all increase the duration of gastric acid contact time with the esophageal mucosa.

Treatment for benign esophageal strictures includes medical management, bougienage, balloon dilation, resection and anastomosis, and salvage esophageal stenting. Medical management is aimed at controlling esophageal reflux and subsequent mucosal damage, however resolution of strictures with medical management alone is unlikely. A subjectively "good" outcome has been reported following balloon dilation or bougienage (70–88%) for benign esophageal strictures in dogs and cats, though only 14–25% ever regain the ability to eat dry food without regurgitation. A subset of strictures are termed refractory benign esophageal strictures (RBES) and recur despite multiple attempts at dilation. These are, by definition, strictures that fail despite greater than three dilation sessions .

Both balloon dilation and bougienage have been used in animals for the management of benign esophageal strictures. Bougienage was the primary method of stricture management until the late 1980s when balloon dilation was described in veterinary medicine and adopted as a "safer" and "superior" technique. Safety concerns with bougienage on the esophageal integrity have been proposed, with the frequent citation of the progressive proximal to distal application of longitudinal and radial forces compared to controlled radial forces of balloon dilation. Despite the absence of randomized studies in humans or animals documenting superiority, it rapidly became the primary method of dealing with esophageal strictures in veterinary and human medicine.

The majority of veterinary literature highlights balloon dilation, with bougienage being only rarely discussed. Recently, a retrospective study demonstrated safety and efficacy of bougienage in both cats and dogs. The results of this study, and human data, suggests that both procedures can be used successfully.

In humans, indwelling esophageal stents have been used for the palliation of dysphagia from RBES. Gentle dilation through gradual expansion of the stent may cause less trauma to the stricture and the continual

Veterinary Image-Guided Interventions, First Edition. Edited by Chick Weisse and Allyson Berent.

Companion website: www.wiley.com/go/weisse/vet-image-guided-interventions

presence may reduce the risk of restenosis. Although long-term clinical resolution of strictures with stents only occurs in 50% of patients with RBES, this can offer patients improved palliation when balloon dilation or bougienage repeatedly fails.

The use of esophageal stents has been described in separate reports encompassing 9 dogs, two cats, and a ferret with benign esophageal strictures, and in a dog with a malignant esophageal obstruction. In a recent report of nine dogs, various types of stents were used including biodegradable stents, self-expanding metallic stents (SEMS), self-expanding plastic stents (SEPS), as well as uncovered and covered stents. Stents were found to immediately improve the dysphagia score, but were met with some complications, most commonly discomfort from the presence of the stent or chronic esophageal distension. This resulted in excessive gagging, nausea and ptyalism. Stent migration occurred in 3/9 patients and recurrence of the stricture occurred in 6/9 cases after the stent either absorbed (biodegradable) or migrated. Due to the unpredictability of stent tolerance in dogs with RBES, this procedure should be reserved for those that have failed dilation of the stricture multiple times or the owners financially cannot afford to perform serial balloon dilations, as stenting is considered a salvage procedure. If a stent is placed dogs should be monitored carefully for stent migration, recurrence after dissolution of absorbable stents, and discomfort. The stents seem to be well tolerated for malignant lesions and are not seemingly associated with discomfort, gagging, nausea or migration.

General Appearance

Strictures can be associated with non-malignant and malignant pathology. In general benign strictures are relatively smooth in appearance with no mass effect. The residual lumen is generally central within the esophagus. The mucosa is usually pale pink to white. If a mass is present, or the meatus is eccentrically located, irregular, or discolored (Figure 13.1).

Potential Risks/ Complications/ Expected Outcomes

The main complications of benign esophageal stricture dilation procedures include perforation, mucosal bleeding, and poor functional outcomes. Esophageal perforation may or may not be visualized on endoscopy depending on the size of the perforation. If perforation is suspected, intra-operative radiography may help to identify the presence of air within the mediastinum or pleural cavity. This complication can be minimized with appropriate selection of balloon sizes and careful visualization of the procedure. Additionally, use of wire-guided balloons and concurrent fluoroscopy may reduce iatrogenic mucosal injury.

The median number of dilation sessions required is variable between patients but is, in general, two to five, regardless of technique used. The risk of esophageal perforation is uncommon and estimated to be between 2–9% per case or 0.8–3% per session.

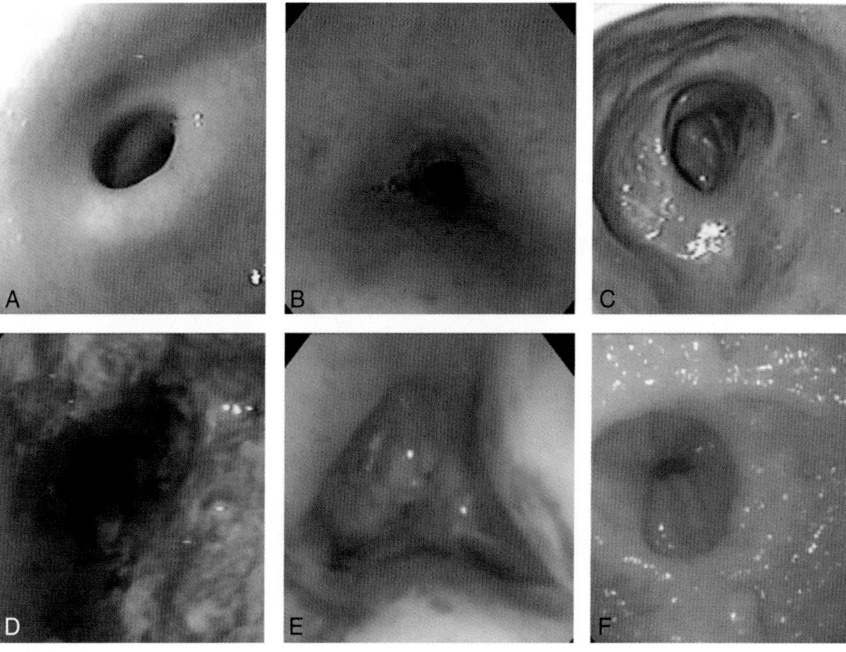

Figure 13.1 Endoscopic images of esophageal strictures. (A–C) Characteristic benign esophageal strictures. Note the smooth mucosal margin. Note that the diameter may be more subtly narrowed (C). (D) Note the irregular, discolored mucosa associated with local esophageal disease due to neoplasia. (E) Completely closed esophageal stricture with no lumen present. (F) Eosinophilic esophagitis.

In the authors' practice esophageal stents have been placed for both malignant and benign obstructions in a small number veterinary patients. The main complications are stent intolerance, with signs like excessive gagging, ptyalism. and nausea. Humans complain of a feeling of a constant "lump in the throat" after esophageal stenting. This is not seen as common when stents are placed for malignant obstructions. The cause of this difference is not clear, but it may be due to the lack of nerves in a tumor. This is why a covered, retrievable stent or a biodegradable stent (BDS) is typically recommended to provide temporary relief while the stenosis heals, with the goal of a short-term palliation and ultimate removal or absorption after 6–12 weeks. For malignant obstructions an uncovered SEMS is recommended, and typically well tolerated. As with intestinal stents (see Chapter 17), migration is an issue more commonly with covered stents, so the author typically sutures these stents in place, as described below.

Equipment (Figure 13.2, Table 13.1)

A standard flexible gastrointestinal endoscope is needed for any of these procedures. The author prefers the video gastroduodenoscope.[1] A traditional fluoroscopic C-arm is sufficient for visualization deep to the mucosal surface. Some operators prefer the combination of fluoroscopy and endoscopy for balloon

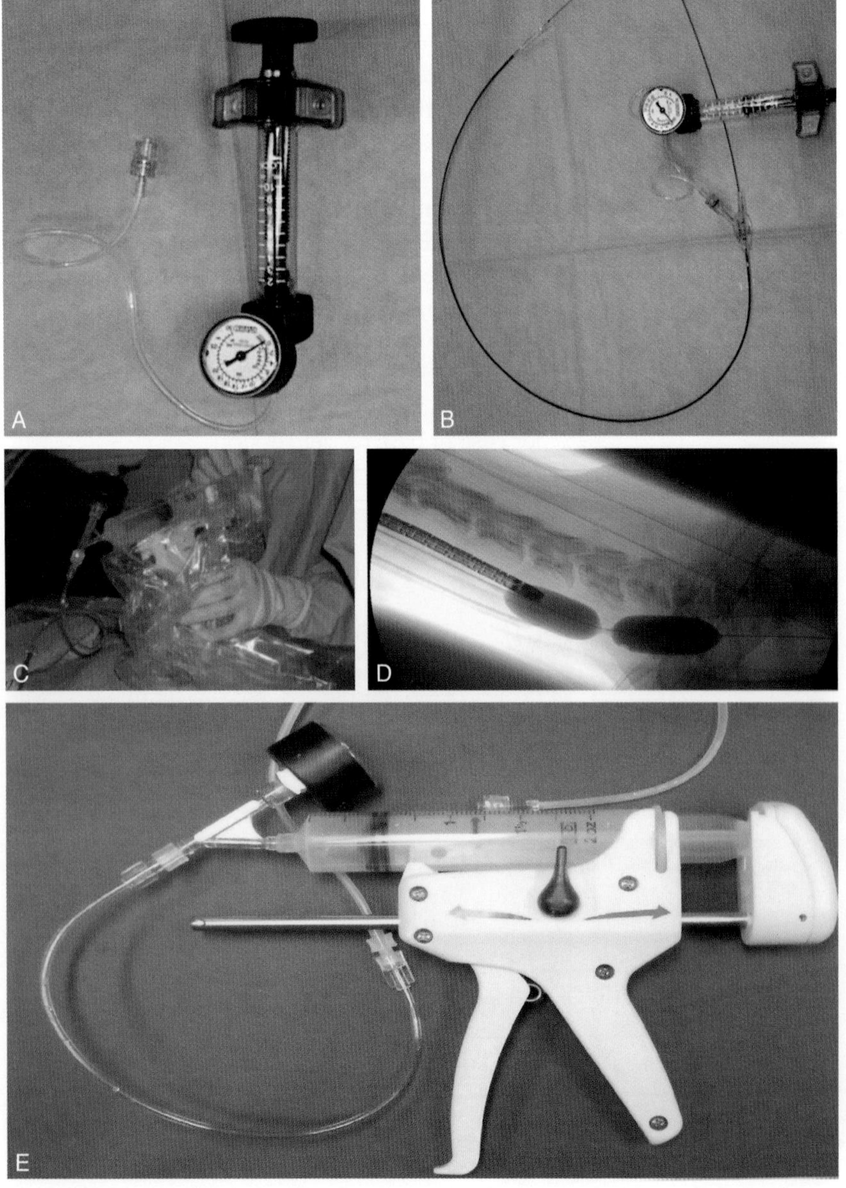

Figure 13.2 Equipment. (A) Screw insufflation device for balloon dilation catheter. (B) Balloon dilation catheter with two ports on the end. One for a guide wire and the other for a balloon dilation device. (C) Inflating a balloon inside a patient. (D) Fluoroscopic image of the balloon inflating an esophageal stricture. The balloon is inflated with a 50% contrast solution to make it visible during fluoroscopy. (E) Gun-type inflation device.

TABLE 13.1
Equipment or medications often used in the management of esophageal strictures

Triamcinolone[2]	Dose of 3 mg/kg (total 6 mg) injected in 4 quadrants at 0.5 ml per quadrant
Injection catheters[3]	Used to inject triamcinolone into stricture prior to balloon dilation
Mitomycin C[4]	0.1% solution (2.5 ml per cat and 5.0 ml per dog) dwell for 5 minutes per stricture
Guidewire[5]	0.035″ angle-tipped hydrophilic wire. Used to pass balloons across stricture meatus. Only utilized with balloon dilators that have an internal guidewire channel.
Marker catheter[6]	A catheter used to measure the esophageal diameter and stricture length for appropriate balloon selection or stent sizing.
Balloon[7]	Balloons that are distended to provide a controlled radial force across a stricture. Balloons come in a multitude of diameters and lengths. Additionally, each balloon system will have its own working pressure and burst pressure. It is critical that these are recorded, as they can vary greatly. Some balloons have an internal channel for contrast studies and/or passage of a guide wire, while others do not. Additionally, some balloons can provide a variable diameter based on pressure.
Balloon inflation device[8]	Device that is used to distend balloons with saline in a controlled fashion.These devices can measure the relative radial force that the balloon is encountering with the stricture during distension.These pressures are recorded on attached pressure gauges.These pressures are used to determine diameter of balloon distention and when potential that balloon rupture may occur. These dilators can maintain constant pressure by maintaining a closed system.Two common types are encountered in practice including the "gun-type"systems and the "screw-type" system.

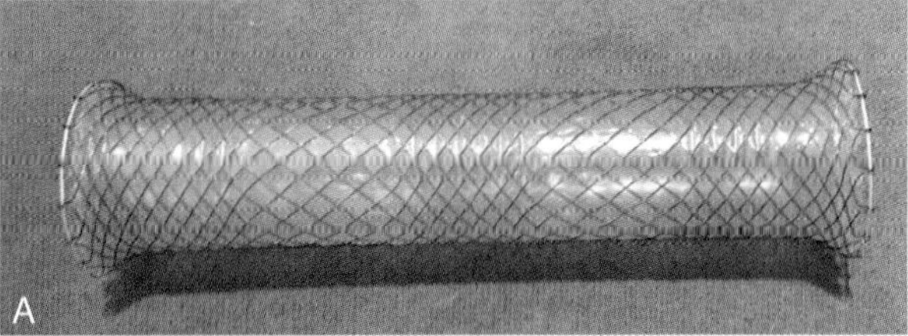

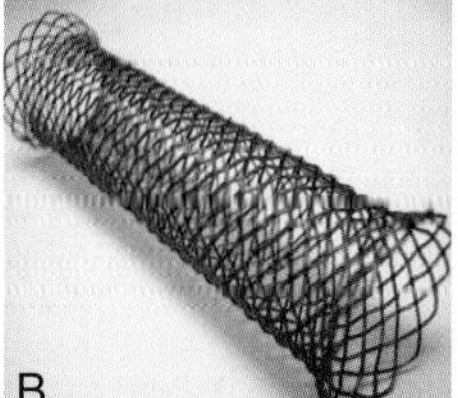

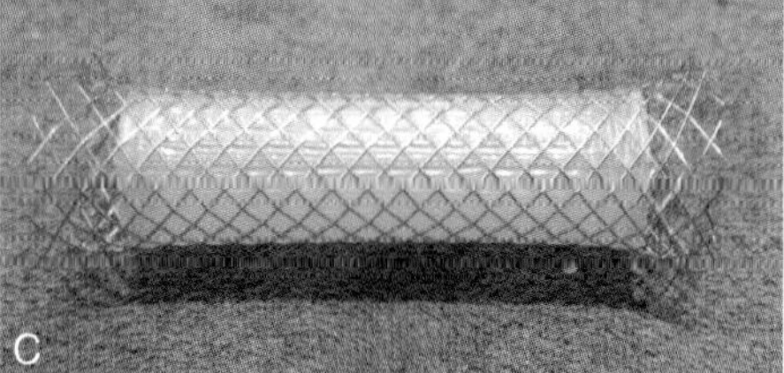

Figure 13.3 Various esophageal stents. (A) A covered metallic self-expanding stent. Notice the string at the ends for retrieval. Notice the dumbbell shape on the ends of the stents in (B) A biodegradable self-expanding stent. (C) Partially covered metallic self-expanding stent. The flanged ends are to help prevent stent migration.

dilation, bougienage, and esophageal stent placement. This allows the operator to see when the entire stricture is effaced, within the muscular wall of the esophagus. The endoscope only confirms the mucosal surface is effaced (Figure 13.2D).

The balloon dilation catheters require an insufflation device to get the proper pressure (Figure 13.2). For esophageal balloon dilation, a wide variety of balloon types are available. Both variable[13,14,21,22] or fixed external diameters[15,19,20,23] are available. Additionally, wire-guided[14,20,22,23] and non-wire-guided options are available.[13,19,21] Balloon dilation devices are available as "screw-type"[16,17] or "gun-type" systems.[18] A wide variety of balloon sizes should be available to the clinician. The author recommends sizes ranging from 4 mm to 25 mm, as this will facilitate balloon dilation of small strictures and complete serial dilations in both dogs and cats. If the balloon diameter sizes you have are not large enough you could double balloon so that you can get a larger diameter (12 mm and 12 mm next to one another). This is best done under fluoroscopic guidance and care should be taken to avoid overdilation.

For esophageal stricture bougienage procedures, placement of a wire guide[24] prior to placement of a bougie[25] is recommended. The author only recommends Savary–Gilliard wire guides and bougies at this time. Variable bougie sizes are necessary to facilitate successful dilation; it is recommended that bougies be stocked from 5–15 mm. A 7 piece[26] or 16 piece[27] dilator set can be purchased with variable dilator sizes; 5–15 mm and 5–20 mm, respectively.

For esophageal stent placement[9–12] a 0.035″ hydrophilic angle-tipped guide wire[5] and marker catheter[6] is used to estimate esophageal diameter and obstruction length. This aids in sizing. Various balloons are needed for pre-dilation.[7]

Esophageal stents are either biodegradable (BDS) made of polydioxonone suture material,[9] metallic (SEMS),[10,11] or plastic (SEPS).[12] They are either uncovered, partially covered, or fully-covered. The advantages of a covered stent is a lower rate of re-obstruction, especially with strictures, but a higher rate of migration, due to the failure of tissue in-growth. Esophageal stents have a dumb-bell shape at each end, to aid in preventing migration (Figure 13.3), and the covered stents,

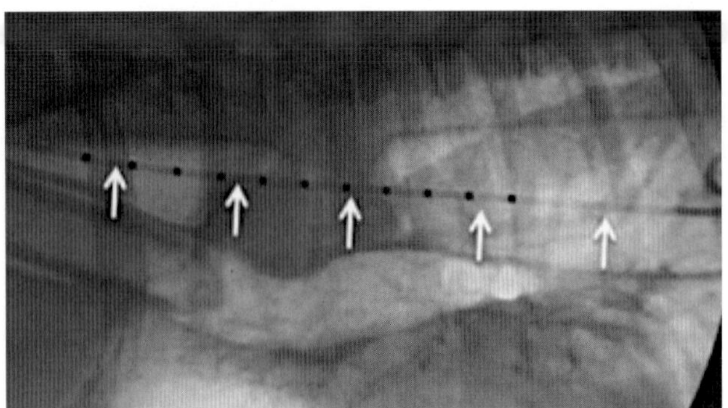

Figure 13.4 Fluoroscopic image of a dog in lateral recumbency with an esophageal tumor. Air is infused into the esophagus through the endoscope or catheter demarcating the borders of the esophageal wall (black arrows). A marker catheter (white arrows) is advanced through the tumor allowing for measurements of the esophageal diameter and stenosis length.

since they are intended for short-term use, have a string around each end so that they can be removed endoscopically with a grasping instrument.

Patient Preparation

Patients are fasted prior to balloon dilation procedures for a minimum of 12 hours to reduce likelihood of aspiration and residual esophageal contents. Endoscopic evaluation requires a minimum of 12 hours between barium contrast procedures to reduce scope damage. The author routinely incorporates opoids (hydromorphone, oxymorphone, methadone) in the anesthetic protocol for intraoperative analgesia prior to induction.

Procedure

Balloon Selection

The approximate diameter of the meatus is estimated based on the known external diameter of the endoscope. The length of the stricture is estimated when possible by direct visualization of the most proximal and distal aspect of the narrowing. However, accurate determination of stricture length is best determined with a contrast study (air or iodinated contrast agents) under radiographic or fluoroscopic guidance, using a marker catheter to adjust for magnification (Figure 13.4). Contrast studies are performed using diluted (50:50 mixture) iodinated contrast material with saline. A standard esophageal balloon dilation catheter or marker catheter can be used to measure. The balloon dilation catheter should have radiopaque marks of a predetermined length on each end to allow one to adjust for magnification and measure the stricture length and normal esophageal luminal diameter. If a marker catheter is used than the catheter is strategically placed across the stricture so that some fenestrations are placed on each side of the stricture and then contrast is infused both cranial and caudal to the stricture simultaneously. This allows measurement of both esophageal diameter and stricture length. The balloon or marker catheter should have an open lumen so that they can be advanced over a guide wire, through the meatus of the stricture. This helps to prevent iatrogenic esophageal perforation and/or false passage into the fibrous tissue.

Once the stricture length is determined an appropriately sized balloon is selected. The main principle for balloon selection is to use a balloon that is a minimum of 1 cm longer than both the oral and aboral aspect of the stricture. The initial balloon size is selected to be approximately 2–3 mm greater than the estimated meatus diameter, and sized up in 2–4 mm increments until the diameter of the normal esophagus is achieved. Prior to balloon dilation, concentric injections of local steroids (triamcinolone) can utilized to reduce stricture re-formation.

Triamcinolone Injections

A 23–25-gauge, 4–5-mm length endoscopic sclerotherapy injection needle[3] is preloaded with the appropriate dose of triamcinolone (6–8 mg/patient in 0.5 ml aliquots per quadrant). In human medicine higher doses are commonly used with a 40 mg/ml solution. The author commonly uses higher doses, trying to remain within a total dose of 3 mg/kg. The potency is 1.25 times that of prednisone.

The needle is passed through the working channel, extracted from the sheath and gently directed into the mucosa proximal to the stricture. The needle should be nearly parallel to the esophageal wall so it can penetrate superficially. The esophageal wall is very thin and injecting through the entire wall of the esophagus is possible. Once the tip is engaged, directional controls on the endoscope provide radial pressure on the wall. While maintaining this pressure the injection catheter is advanced slightly to further engage the tip. Ideally, the bevel of the catheter should be directed towards the lumen to reduce leakage of the solution. Once the steroids are injected a bleb of fluid should be seen under the mucosal tissue (Figure 13.5).

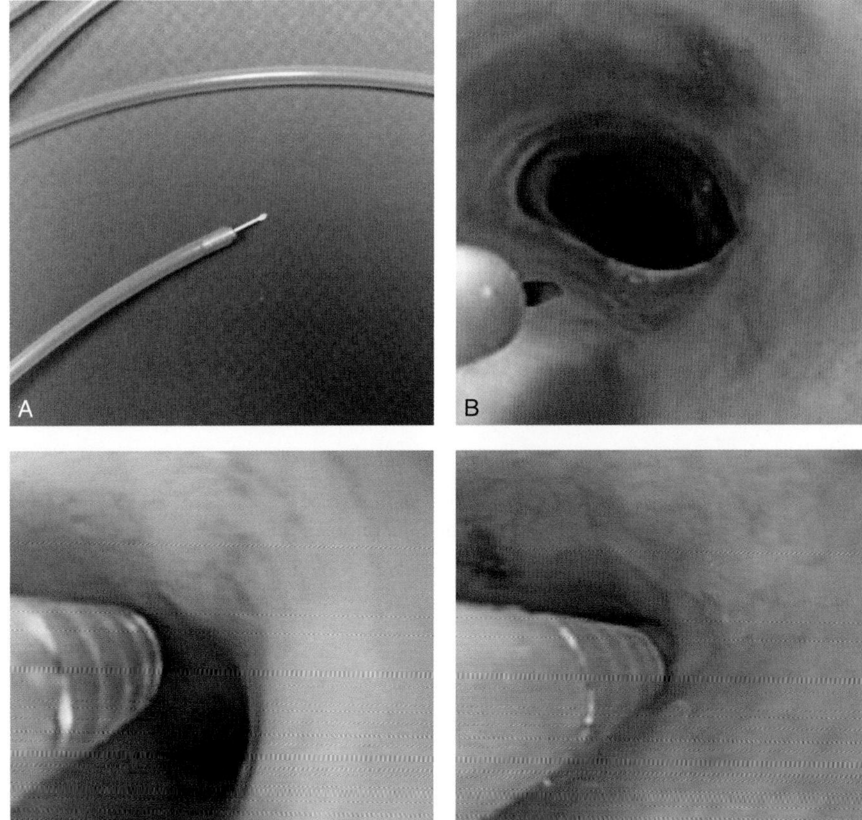

Figure 13.5 (A) Standard 23 gauge endoscopic, 5-mm long sclerotherapy injection needle. (B) Endoscopic image during triamcinolone injections in a dog with an esophageal stricture. Note that the needle is directed with the bevel towards the lumen and advanced towards the proximal aspect of the stricture. (C, D) The needle is introduced into the wall carefully and then maintained slightly parallel to the wall during injection.

This procedure is repeated with 4 separate injections being made at equidistant sites (i.e., 12, 3, 6 and 9 o'clock positions). It is recommended to inject at the proximal aspect of the stricture prior to balloon dilation. For long strictures (>2 cm), injection within the stricture is also recommended following dilation.

Balloon Dilations

Some balloons come with a central lumen for guide wires and others do not. In general, those that do not have channels for guide wires tend to be more durable and may last longer, but may also be more risky and allow for a false passage through a tight stricture resulting in iatrogenic perforation. The endoscope is advanced to the level of the stricture and the meatus is visualized. A lubricated guide wire can be placed alongside, or through the working channel and manipulated through the meatus of the stricture. The guide wire is then advanced into the gastric lumen. The balloon catheter is lubricated and the central lumen flushed with saline. The balloon catheter is advanced over the guidewire, through the stenosis, under direct observation (Figure 13.6).

Once the balloon is across the stenosis, with at least 1 cm of the balloon extending beyond the cranial and caudal borders, a balloon inflation device is used to distend the balloon. If this is done using fluoroscopic guidance is used, than a 50% mixture of contrast and saline is used, if this is done with endoscopy alone than just saline can be used. It is important that the operator uses an inflation device as this will appropriately inflate the balloon to the ideal recommended pressure, which is typically greater than a human can do manually (Figure 13.2A). It is important to watch the placement of the balloon during the inflation as there is a tendency to migrate orally or aborally, this may require tension or traction to help remain in position. The rated burst pressure and recommended dilation pressure is typically available on the package of each balloon and should be recorded and followed. Manual inflation with a syringe and hand is not strong enough to reach the rated inflation pressure and will likely not appropriately break the stricture. An inflation device should always be used.

Once the stricture is engaged, the balloon can be left in place for 1–2 minutes before deflation. No current consensus exists in human medicine on whether the

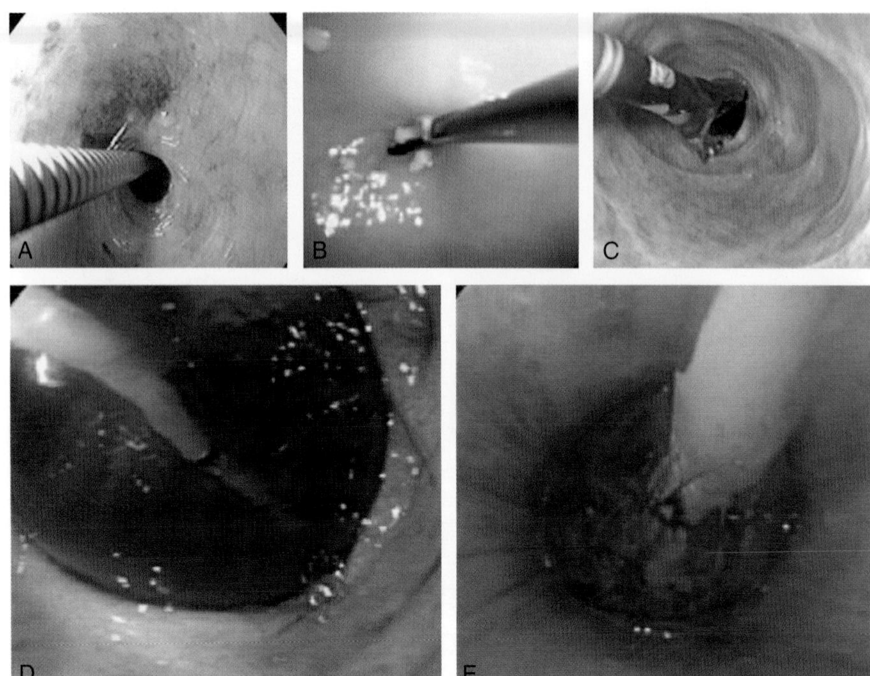

Figure 13.6 Endoscopic images during balloon dilation of an esophageal stricture in a dog. (A, B) Note the passage of various guide wires to aid in balloon passage through the stricture. (C) The balloon is passed through the stricture in a deflated state until "coverage" is observed across the stenosis both proximal and distal to the stricture. This balloon is being reused. (D, E) Note that as the balloon is inflated adequate engagement of stricture is maintained and the balloon does not slide/disengage.

balloon needs to remain inflated once the stricture is broken. Occasionally, for highly resistant strictures, longer durations of dilation can be performed and friction by moving the balloon back and forth can be done. The procedure is repeated with sequentially larger balloons at 2 mm increments, with a goal of reaching the target diameter determined from the initial measurements of the esophagus and visibility of the stricture being effaced under fluoroscopic and/or endoscopic guidance. Small incremental increases in diameter are commonly employed in human and veterinary medicine but no standardization exists. The target diameters will vary with the patient size, therefore, generalizations cannot be made reliably. Smaller patients commonly have a smaller target diameter than larger patients. However, it should be noted that some smaller patients, may be able to tolerate balloon sizes up to 18 mm. Most adult feline patients require balloons that are 6–12 mm in diameter, however dogs are quite variable depending on the breed (10–30 mm in diameter).

In addition to estimated target diameters, the decision to stop dilation sessions is also based on the degree of mucosal tearing/injury and the refractoriness of a stricture. Some degree of mucosal tearing and bleeding should be expected. What constitutes excessive injury and reasonable injury is very subjective. In general, mucosal tearing that extends linearly beyond the stricture, deep/submucosal tearing, or excessive bleeding are appropriate times to stop the session (Figure 13.7 and Figure 13.8). Some clinicians feel that some degree of tearing is necessary to break the fibrotic tissue and reduce recurrence. However, others feel that a more gentle approach will limit stricture recurrence to avoid excessive inflammation of fibrin development. The author feels that a great degree of variability exists between strictures, with some recurring with the more gentle approach and some recurring with the more aggressive approach. This is also likely influenced by the interval between balloon dilations. The author *generally* prefers a controlled amount of mucosal tearing at each session, however, this may differ with other strictures (see refractory strictures below).

The authors have found that it is often helpful to monitor the balloon dilation of the stricture with fluoroscopic and endoscopic guidance simultaneously (Figure 13.7). For the recurrent strictures, there is often a muscular component to the fibrosis and by monitoring only the mucosal/submucosal tearing, there may still be a ring in the muscle that would only be visualized using fluoroscopy.

Tremendous variation exists on the recommended interval between balloon dilations. The veterinary community has not standardized this interval and opinions vary greatly. In human medicine, weekly dilation sessions are commonly employed for patients with tight strictures or for patients with a high risk for recurrence ("non-peptic" causes of stricture, fibrous strictures, and a maximum dilator size less than 14 mm). The author prefers to repeat balloon dilation at 5–7 day intervals with the theory that the more immature tissue is more easily torn. Longer intervals may

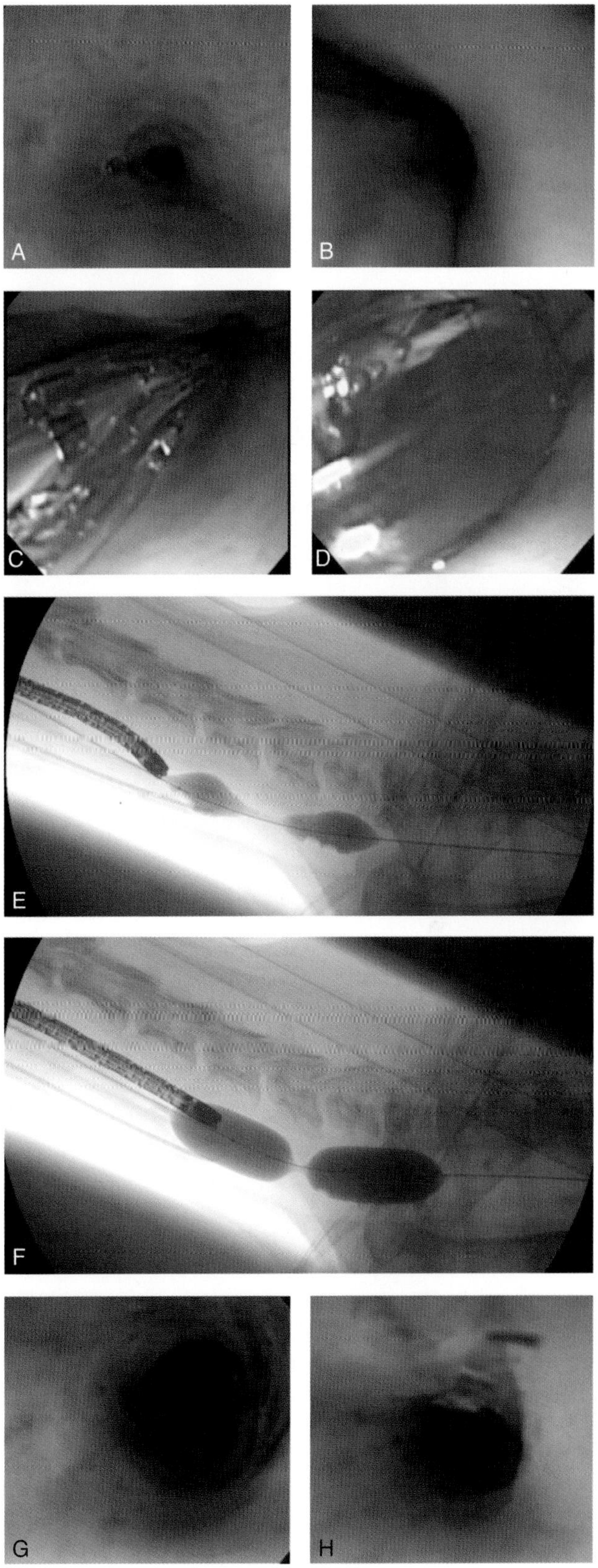

Figure 13.7 Endoscopic and fluoroscopic images during balloon dilation of an esophageal stricture in a dog. (A) Endoscopic image of a stricture in the esophageal lumen. (B) Guide wire passed through the stenosis. (C) Deflated balloon passed over the guide wire, through the stenosis. (D) Inflation of the balloon within the stricture. (E) Fluoroscopic image of the dog in lateral recumbency during balloon dilation of the stricture. Notice the narrowing in the center of the balloon and the endoscope sitting in front of the balloon. (F) Fluoroscopic image of the stricture during balloon dilation showing the severe narrowing of the esophagus, which is a muscular stenosis that is very difficult to break. (G) Endoscopic image of the dog after balloon inflation when a waist was still present during fluoroscopy supporting that endoscopic visualization alone may underestimate the degree of stricture defacement. H) Endoscopic image after the stricture was effaced on fluoroscopic imaging showing the desired longitudinal mucosal tear.

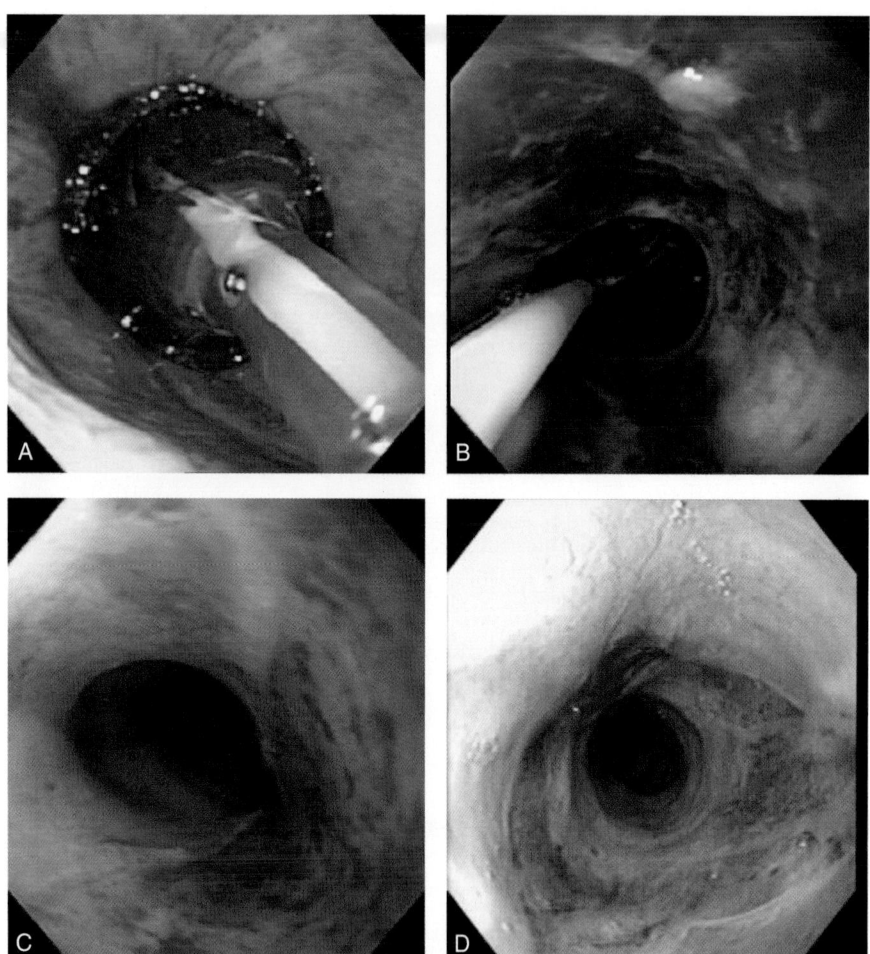

Figure 13.8 Endoscopic images during and after balloon dilation in different dogs. (A) Note the small amount of bleeding during insufflation suggesting mucosal injury/stretching. (B) Superficial mucosal tearing following balloon dilation. (C) Mucosal trauma/tear following balloon dilation. (D) Note the already healing esophageal tearing 5 days post balloon dilation.

result in complete stricture recurrence, though repeated anesthesia events may increase the risk of reflux.

Pinhole-Meatus

When the meatus is excessively small (Figure 13.6B) a guide wire should be used. It is passed through the working channel of the endoscope and guided into the hole. This is best done using fluoroscopic assistance as well so the caudal aspect of the stricture can be monitored with contrast to ensure there is no false passage of the wire. Additionally, the use of small endoscope may allow direct intubation of a small meatus in some cases (bronchoscope, flexible cystoscope/ureteroscope). Once the meatus is cannulated than a multi-fenestrated marker catheter can be advanced over the wire and a contrast study (with air or iodinated contrast material) can be performed using fluoroscopic guidance to ensure the catheter is within the esophageal lumen and measurements of stricture length and esophageal diameter can be made (Figure 13.4). Then, balloon dilation can be performed, as discussed above.

Complete Stenosis/Imperforate Membrane

When a complete stenosis is encountered (Figure 13.1E) an endoscopic procedure could be considered, but only in select cases. If the length of the stricture is known based on advanced imaging, or due to illumination of the scope across the stricture, and is thought to be short, this technique can be considered. Care should be taken to avoid penetrating the large vessels in the mediastinum and cervical region with an access needle. If this is to be attempted than an access sheath is introduced adjacent the scope, through a protective access sheath. This will contact the stenosis, providing some rigidity. An access needle, which has a hollow trocar and sharp stylette, is then introduced through the sheath, using both endoscopic and fluoroscopic guidance. The needle must have a large enough lumen to accept an appropriately sized guide wire (0.035″ typically) once the imperforate membrane is penetrated. Fluoroscopic assistance will help to ensure that the positioning is appropriate. Once the needle is across the membrane than the guidewire is passed through the hollow trocar into the stomach to ensure you are in the lumen. If there is any concern than air or contrast can be infused. Once the hollow trocar and sharp stylet of the access needle are through the membrane with the guide wire advanced into the stomach, the access needle is removed over the wire. Next, a dilation catheter, through the access sheath, can be advanced over the wire to dilate a tract that will accommodate the first balloon. This will also allow for a contrast study to confirm location without losing wire access. Once this is dilated the balloon can be used to fully dilate the stricture. In these cases new balloons should be used as they are narrower than used balloons. These strictures are often very tight and pressure will be needed to obtain the first dilation. Contrast should be used to ensure the endoscopist is in the lumen prior to balloon dilation. Once the lumen is established, standard balloon dilation can be performed.

Refractory Benign Esophageal Strictures (RBES)

In general, refractory strictures need more dilation procedures over a short duration in order to facilitate efficacy. Repeat procedures at 5–7 day intervals with a special focus on limiting mucosal tearing may reduce the likelihood for recurrence. Significant mucosal tearing can result in healing between the walls when the esophagus is collapsed and recurrent structuring. There is also argument that these recur due to the muscular nature of these strictures, and by not using fluoroscopy to guide the balloon dilations, the strictures continue to recur because the operator is only tearing the mucosal and submucosal components (Figure 13.7).

Occasionally, strictures fail to dilate effectively despite appropriate technique, requiring over 5–15 dilation procedures. This can occur from dense fibrotic tissue, focal fibrous bands, or a concurrent muscular component (Figure 13.9). When this occurs consideration should be made to: (1) attempt controlled cutting of the fibrous ring/band using electrocautery; (2) bougeinage procedures; (3) triamcinolone injections; (4) topical mitomycin C infusions; or (5) salvage esophageal stenting. In addition, the authors have found that placing an esophagostomy tube through a stricture to keep the tissue apart and prevent collapse of the esophageal lumen may decrease the rate of re-stricture. This is completely anecdotal.

Fibrous rings/bands can be cut by several methods. Cervical fibrotic bands may be carefully cut with laparoscopic or endoscopic scissors that are introduced

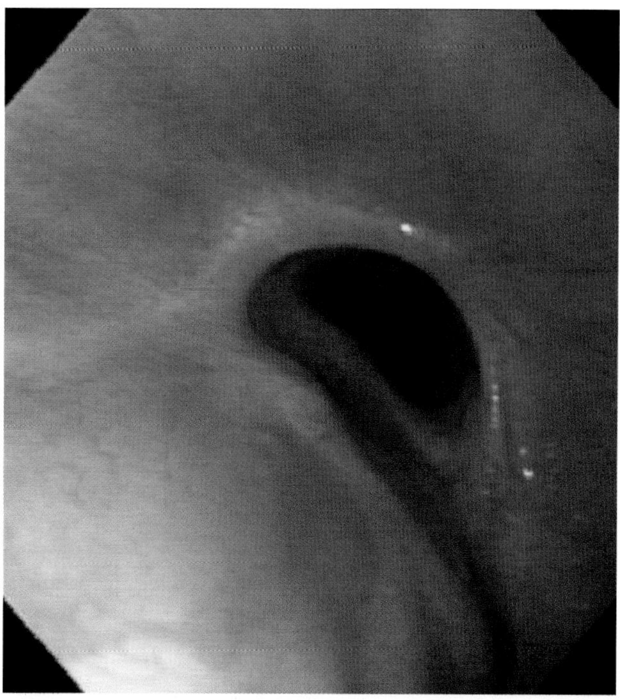

Figure 13.9 Endoscopic image of a dog with an esophageal stricture. This characteristic fibrous ring may not be responsive to standard balloon dilation and may require cutting with laparoscopic equipment or electrocautery.

alongside the scope, or through the working channel. By cutting the band of tissue that fails to dilate, an area of weakness is created which permits stretching or tearing with subsequent balloon dilations. It is critical that the instrument be introduced carefully and only under direct visualization, to limit excessive pressure on the wall and limit the risk of perforation. If the stricture fails to dilate, a standard polypectomy snare can be introduced through the endoscopic working channel, and placed across through the stricture. When introduced through the stricture, the snare is gradually opened until the surface of the mucosa is just encountered. This will create two points of contact between the snare and the stricture. While this is held in place, electrocautery is connected to the instrument, as described in Chapter 15. Coagulation cautery is used and a small current is introduced starting at 15 W and gradually increasing to a maximum of 25 W, or until small defects are made in the mucosa. It is critical that excessive current not be utilized and that the surface of the stricture be minimally contacted with the snare. This will reduce thermal injury to the esophageal wall and limit depth of the electrocautery penetration. It is critical that the snare be a safe distance from the distal end of the insertion tube to prevent injury to the endoscope. This procedure can also be performed with "hot" needle knife[28], or less optimally a "hot" biopsy instrument[29, 30], at controlled sites equidistant from one another (i.e., 12, 3, 6 and 9 o'clock). Recently, the use of a cutting balloon has been used aid in opening of a fibrotic ring.[31]

Bougienage Procedure (Figure 13.10)

Bougie size is selected based on estimations of the stricture diameter using comparison to external scope diameter, biopsy forceps, and bougie sizes available. The initial bougie selected is generally estimated to be 1–2 mm greater then the diameter of the stricture. Each subsequent dilation utilizes a bougie 1–3 mm greater than the previous dilation.

With endoscopic or fluoroscopic visualization, a guide wire is introduced across the stricture and a well lubricated bougie is passed over the guide wire to engage centrally. When the bougie is centered into the meatus, firm steady pressure is applied until the bougie pops into the more distal esophageal segment. It is critical that pressure be applied along the long access of the stricture and not directed into the wall; this can lead to perforation.

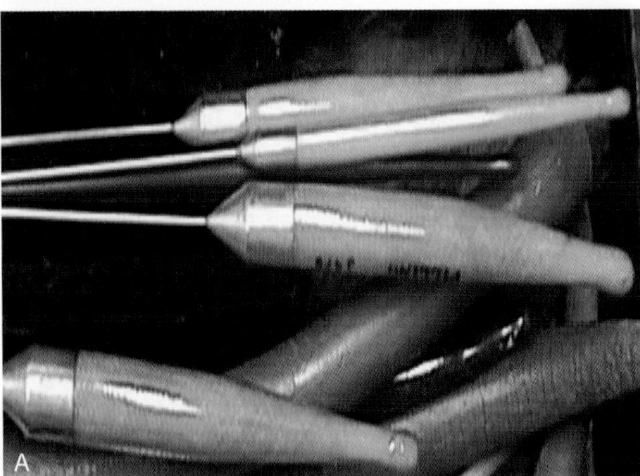

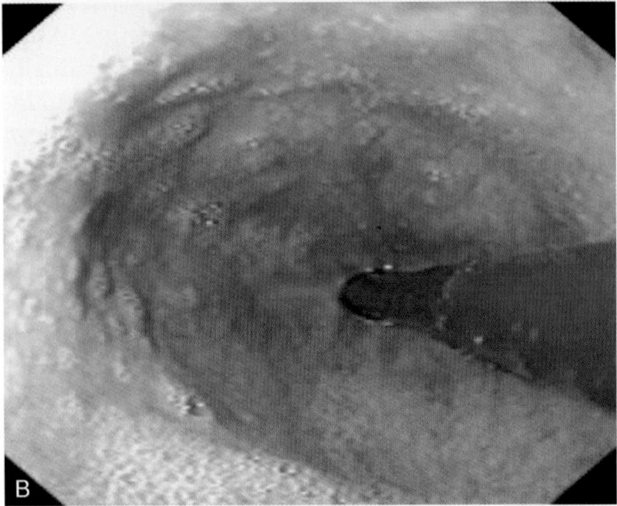

Figure 13.10 Bougienage. (A) Standard bougienage set; note the variable sizes. (B) The bougie is passed similarly to standard balloons through the center of the stricture.

Topical Mitomycin C Infusion

Mitomycin C (MMC) is an antibiotic that is produced by *Streptomyces caespitosus*. This drug is carcinostatic containing a ring of azauridine, a quinone group, and an octane group. Besides being an antibiotic, it is antineoplastic, causing single-band breakage and cross-linking of DNA at the adenosine and guanine molecules. It inhibits RNA and protein synthesis. It selectively inhibits the expression of inducible genes. As an antiproliferative agent, MMC inhibits fibroblast proliferation and decreases scar tissue formation. The antiproliferative properties on fibroblasts have been shown in vivo and vitro. MMC can be considered as another potential preventative treatment for recurrent esophageal stricture formation and has been shown in children to hold benefit in preventing stricture recurrence. In veterinary medicine we typically use 2.5–5 ml of a 0.1% MMC solution soaked on a gauze sponge and placed endoscopically over the stricture topically. This is left on the stricture for 5 minutes and then the stricture is flushed with sterile saline after the sponge is removed.

Esophageal Stenting

Dogs are placed under general anesthesia and positioned on a fluoroscopic table in dorsal or lateral recumbency. The ventral cervical region is clipped and aseptically prepared if tacking sutures are to be placed. A mouth gag is placed on the dependent canine teeth, and a flexible gastrointestinal endoscope is inserted into the esophagus to identify the location and length of the stricture(s). If the patient is going to have the stent sutured into the esophageal wall through the cervical region, than the patient remains in dorsal recumbency while the fluoroscopic C-arm is rotated to get a lateral projection of the patient. This aids in visualization of the esophagus for measurements and during stent placement.

Using fluoroscopic guidance a marker catheter is passed over an angle-tipped hydrophilic guidewire into the esophagus, next to then endoscope, to aid in radiographic measurement of the diameter of the normal esophagus and the length of the stricture while accounting for radiographic magnification (Figure 13.4). The wire can also be placed through the working channel of the endoscope if the opening is very small and the wire needs to be guided. The stricture is typically pre-ballooned partially (not to the full esophageal diameter) to permit safe passage of the endoscope through the lumen to help visualize the caudal aspect of the abnormal tissue, aiding in stent placement (Figure 13.7). Stent sizes are approximated to the normal esophageal diameter caudal to the stent when possible (although routinely the diameters are undersized compared to the dilated oral esophagus). Stent length is chosen to extend at least 1–2 cm cranial and caudal to the stricture, and even farther cranially to the level of the thoracic inlet if sutures is to be placed to prevent stent migration. Sutures can also be placed using a double lumen endoscope and this would prevent the need for such a long stent.

Under fluoroscopic and endoscopic guidance, the constrained stent is advanced over the guidewire, alongside the endoscope, through the stricture, and into the distal esophagus. The stent is deployed with 60% of its length being placed cranial to the stricture when possible. This is to minimize aboral stent migration. Further dilation of the stricture with a balloon can be performed but is not usually necessary. Stent patency and position is confirmed using endoscopy and fluoroscopy (Figure 13.11 and Figure 13.12).

If tacking sutures are placed, a 4–5 cm midline approach to the cervical esophagus prior to stent deployment, while the endoscope is within the esophagus. Blunt dissection is used to locate the cervical esophagus where the endoscope could be palpated. Once the area of the esophagus is isolated where the cranial aspect of the stent will land, the stent is deployed using fluoroscopic and endoscopic guidance. The endoscope is used to monitor that placement of two or three synthetic monofilament polypropylene sutures, which are used to secure the stent in the cervical esophagus (Figure 13.11 and Figure 13.12). The incision is routinely closed using a synthetic monofilament absorbable suture. Alternatively, an endoluminal suture-anchoring device can be used, or the stent can be anchored to an

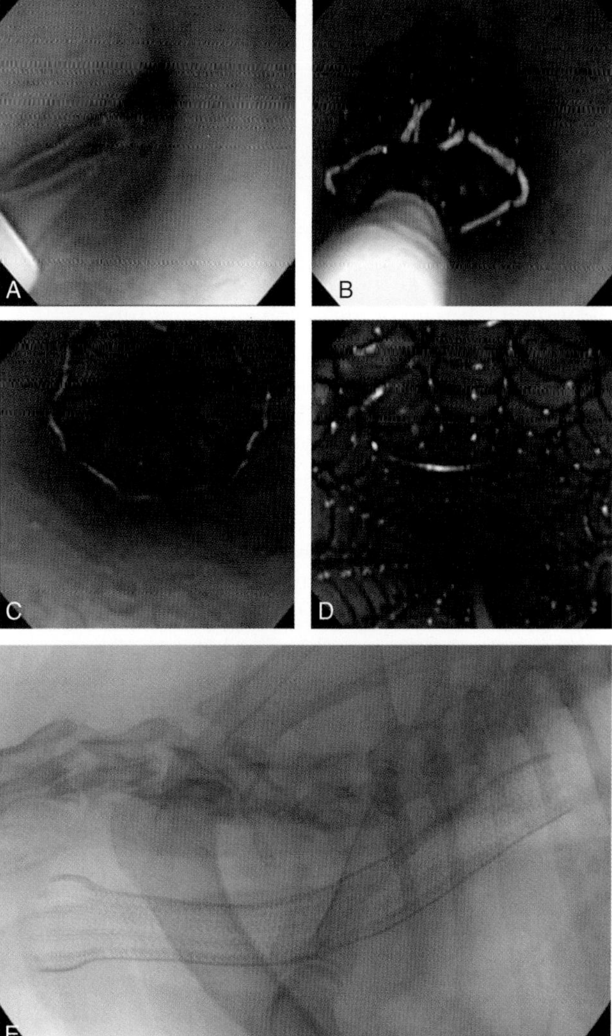

Figure 13.11 Endoscopic and fluoroscopic images of a dog with an esophageal stent placed after 15 balloon dilation procedures failed. (A) Endoscopic image of a balloon catheter across the stenosis during pre-dilation of the stricture so that the delivery system can be easily passed through the diseased tissue and the caudal aspect of the stricture can be clearly identified endoscopically. (B) Deployment of the stent being monitored endoscopically. (C) The cranial aspect of the stent seen endoscopically prior to suture placement. Notice the string at the cranial aspect of the stent, which is preset for stent retrieval if needed. (D) Two sutures are placed through the esophageal wall, engaging the stent, to prevent stent migration. (E) Lateral fluoroscopic projection of the esophageal stent after deployment, showing appropriate deployment. Notice the dumb-bell shape, which is meant to help prevent migration.

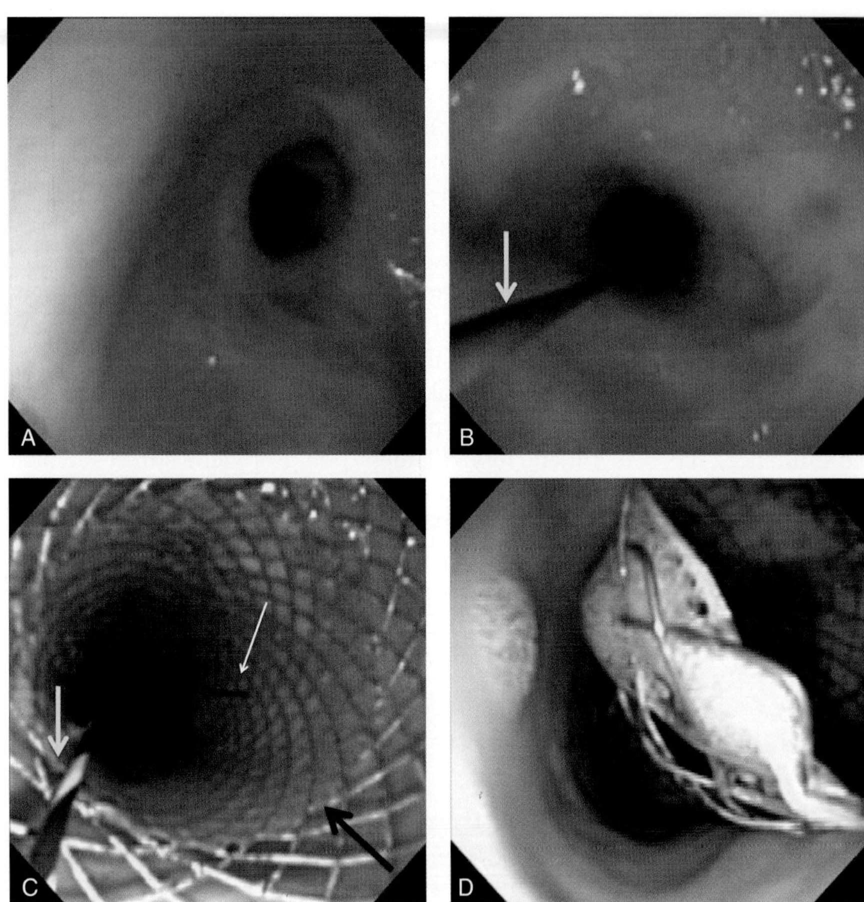

Figure 13.12 Refractory esophageal stricture in a dog before and after covered metallic stent placement. (A) intrathoracic stricture. (B) Guide wire (yellow arrow) through the lumen of the stricture. (C) Partially covered metallic esophageal stent over deployed within the esophagus. Notice the guide wire (yellow arrow) is still through the lumen of the stent. Also notice the suture (white arrow) through the wall of the esophagus and mesh of the stent. Notice the junction of the covered and uncovered aspect of the stent (black arrow). (D) Endoscopic image of the cranial aspect of the esophageal stent. Notice the dumb bell shape of the stent and the space between the stent and the wall. These stents are typically undersized.

esophagostomy tube using a long non-absorbable suture tied around the cranial aspect of the stent and through the lumen of the esophagostomy tube.

As mentioned above, the authors recommend covered stents that are sutured in place so they can be remove if they are poorly tolerated (Figure 13.12).

Esophageal stenting for malignant obstructions

Numerous studies have documented the safety and efficacy of palliative stenting for malignant esophageal obstructions in people. This has only been reported in one dog (Hansen, 2012). The technique for this procedure is the same as described above, although an uncovered stent is typically used and no suturing is necessary, as these stents have a low migration rate in people. Additionally, tumors rarely grow through the stents, so a covered stent is likely unnecessary.

Post-Procedural and Follow-Up Care

Patients are discharged the same day of the procedure. Patients are fed a soft food in small frequent meals. Patients are discharged with proton pump inhibitors (Omeprazole 1 mg/kg q 12) for 7 days. Consideration to a dispensing a sucralfate suspension (0.25–1 g PO q 8) is made for patients with severe mucosal tearing. Lower esophageal sphincter tonicity manipulation (cisapride: 0.5 mg/kg PO q 8) is considered in patients with distal esophageal strictures, refractory strictures or patients with chronic regurgitation (i.e., brachycephalic breeds, hiatal hernias).

Prognosis

Outcomes of balloon dilation have a reported success rate of 77–88%. It is important to note that definitions of efficacy vary between study with some reporting moderate success as regurgitation <50% of original and others defining success as tolerance of *any* dietary consistency. This included patients that could only tolerate gruel consistency. Additionally, animals that were euthanized or died were removed from statistical analysis in some studies, making assessment of true success rate difficult.

A recent retrospective study of bougienage by Bisset et al (2009) demonstrated a "good" outcome, defined as tolerance of solid food and regurgitation <1x per week, in 70% of dogs and 75% of cats.

Special Considerations

Esophageal stents should only be considered for patients that have failed traditional balloon dilation or bouigienage procedures. Owners should be aware that an esophageal stent is not meant for long-term use, unless it is placed for a malignant obstruction, and using a covered stent that can be removed after 6–12 weeks should be considered if the stent is not well tolerated. If it is tolerated long-term than it can remain in place. To remove the stent the retrieval string can be engaged with an endoscopic grasper and this will ultimately pull out the stent. If the stent is uncovered than damage to the esophageal mucosa will occur when the stent is removed because this metal will have incorporated into the esophageal tissue. If the stent is sutured than either endoscopic scissors, a laser, or elecrocautery probe can be used to cut the suture prior to removal.

Additionally, there is some thought that the placement of an esophagostomy feeding tube, of a relatively large diameter (18–20 Fr), across the stricture will prevent the stricture edges from meeting and reforming. This has not been proven to be effective but the authors have had some success.

Notes

These are only a few of the possible options for this procedure.

1. 6 mm gastroduodenoscope, Olympus, Melville, NY.
2. Triamcinolone, 2 mg/ml *Vetalog® Parenteral* (BIVI).
3. Endoscopy injection needle, 23–25 ga. × 4–5 mm, US Endoscopy, Mentor, OH.
4. Mitomycin C.
5. Weasel wire 0.035″ 260 cm, Infiniti Medical, Menlo Park, CA.
6. Marker Catheter, Merit Medical UHF, South Jordan, UT.
7. Esophageal balloon dilation catheters CRE, Boston Scientific, Natick, MA.
8. Balloon inflation device, Bard Medical, Covington, GA.
9. PDS Esophageal stent, Infiniti Medical LLC, Menlo Park, CA.
10. Wallflex Covered and Uncovered Esophageal Stent, Boston Scientific, Natick, MA.
11. VetStent Covered esophageal stent, Infiniti Medical LLC, Menlo Park, CA.
12. PolyFlex Esophageal Stent, Boston Scientific, Natick, MA.
13. CRE Single-use fixed wire esophageal balloon dilators, Boston Scientific, Natick, MA.
14. CRESingle-use wireguided esophageal/pyloric/biliary balloon dilators, Boston Scientific, Natick, MA.
15. Maxforce TTS Single-use Balloon Dilators, Boston Scientific, Natick, MA.
16. Sphere Inflation Device, Cook Endoscopy, Winston Salem, NC.
17. Quantum Inflation Device, Cook Endoscopy, Winston Salem, NC.
18. Alliance II Inflation System, Boston Scientific, Natick, MA.
19. Quantum TTC® Balloon Dilators, Cook Endoscopy, Winston Salem, NC.
20. Eclipse TTC™ Wire Guided Balloon Dilator, Cook Endoscopy, Winston Salem, NC.
21. Hercules® 3 Stage Balloon, Cook Endoscopy, Winston Salem, NC.
22. Hercules® 3 Stage Wire Guided Balloon, Cook Endoscopy, Winston Salem, NC.
23. Vet Balloons, Infiniti Medical, Menlo Park, CA.
24. Savary-Gilliard wire guide, Cook Endoscopy, Winston Salem, NC.
25. Savary-Gilliard Dilators, Cook Endoscopy, Winston Salem, NC.
26. Savary-Gilliard Dilator set (Standard Set of 7) , Cook Endoscopy, Winston Salem, NC.
27. Savary-Gilliard Dilator set (Standard Set of 16) , Cook Endoscopy, Winston Salem, NC.
28. Huibregtse® Single Lumen Needle Knife, Cook Endoscopy, Winston Salem, NC.
29. Radial Jaw™ 3 Hot Biopsy Forceps, , Boston Scientific, Natick, MA.
30. EndoJaw Disposable Biopsy Forceps, Olympus, Melville, NY.
31. Cutting balloon, Boston Scientific, Natick, MA.

References

Bissett SA, Davis J, Subler K, et al. (2009) Risk factors and outcome of bougienage for treatment of benign esophageal strictures in dogs and cats: 28 cases (1995–2004). *J Am Vet Med Assoc* 235, 844–50.

Hansen KS, Weisse C, Berent AC, et al. (2012) Use of a self-expanding metallic stent to palliate esophageal neoplastic obstruction in a dog. *J Am Vet Med Assoc* 240, 1202–7.

Suggested Reading

Adamama-Moraitou KK, Rallis TS, Prassinos NN, et al (2002) Benign esophageal stricture in the dog and cat: a retrospective study of 20 cases. *Can Jo Vet Res* 66, 55–9.

Battersby I and Doyle R (2010) Use of a biodegradable self-expanding stent in the management of a benign oesophageal stricture in a cat. *J Small Anim Pract* 51, 49–52.

Burk RL, Zawie DA, and Garvey MS (1999) Balloon catheter dilation of intramural esophageal strictures in the dog and cat: a description of the procedure and a report of six cases. *Semin Vet Med Surg (Small Anim)* 2, 241–7.

Dua, KS (2011) Expandable stents for benign esophageal disease. *Gastrointestinal Endosc Clin N Am* 21, 359–76.

Gallagher AE and Specht AJ (2013) The use of a cutting balloon for dilation of a fibrous esophageal stricture in a cat. *Case Rep Vet Med* Article ID 467806.

Glanemann B, Hildebrandt N, Schneider MA, et al (2008) Recurrent single oesophageal stricture treated with a self-expanding stent in a cat. *J Feline Med Surg* 10, 505–9.

Glazer A and Walters P (2008) Esophagitis and esophageal strictures. *Compendium Continuing Education* 30, 281–292.

Harai BH, Johnson SE, and Sherding RG (1995) Endoscopically guided balloon dilatation of benign esophageal strictures in 6 cats and 7 dogs. *J Vet Intern Med* 9, 332–5.

Kochhar R and Poornachandra KS (2010) Intralesional steroid injection therapy in the management of resistant gastrointestinal strictures. *World J Gastrointest Endosc* 2(2), 61–8.

Kochman ML, McClave SA, and Boyce HW (2005) The refractory and the recurrent esophageal stricture: a definition. *Gastrointest Endosc* 62, 474–5.

Siersema PD (2009) Stenting for benign esophageal strictures. *Endoscopy* 41, 363–73.

de Wijkerslooth LRH, Vleggaar FP and Siersema PD (2011) Endoscopic management of difficult or recurrent esophageal strictures *Am J Gastroenterol* 106, 2080–91.

Lam N, Weisse C, Berent AC, et al (2013) Preliminary evaluation of esophageal stenting for treatment of refractory benign esophageal strictures in dogs: 9 cases. *J Vet Intern Med* 27(5), 1064–70.

Leib MS, Dinnel H, Ward DL, et al (2001) Endoscopic balloon dilation of benign esophageal strictures in dogs and cats. *J Vet Intern Med* 15, 547–52.

Melendez LD, Twedt DC, Weyrauch EA, et al (1998) Conservative therapy using balloon dilation for intramural, inflammatory esophageal strictures in dogs and cats: a retrospective study of 23 cases (1987–1997). *Eur J Comp Gastroenterol* 3, 31–6.

Pereira-Lima JC, Ramires RP, Zamin I Jr, et al (1999) Endoscopic dilation of benign esophageal strictures: report on 1043 procedures. *Am J Gastroenterol* 94, 1497–501.

Ramage JI Jr, Rumalla A, Baron TH, et al (2005) A prospective, randomized, double-blind, placebo-controlled trial of endoscopic steroid injection therapy for recalcitrant esophageal peptic strictures. *Am J Gastroenterol* 100, 2419–25.

Riley SA and Attwood SEA (2004) Guidelines on the use of oesophageal dilatation in clinical practice. *Gut* 53(I), i1–i6.

Said A, Brust DJ, Gaumnitz EA, et al (2003) Predictors of early recurrence of benign esophageal strictures. *Am J Gastroenterol* 98, 1252–6.

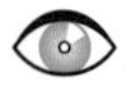
Video clips to accompany this chapter can be found in the online material at **www.wiley.com/go/weisse/vet-image-guided-interventions**

CHAPTER FOURTEEN

Gastrointestinal System – Gastric Foreign Body Retrieval

Douglas A. Palma
The Animal Medical Center, New York, NY

Background

Gastric foreign bodies are a common emergency in veterinary medicine and require appropriate case management for the most successful outcomes. Some foreign material may pass through the gastrointestinal tract without incident, while others may become obstructed within the stomach or more distally. Most patients present with acute or chronic, intermittent or excessive, vomiting. Other common presenting complaints include hematemesis, lethargy, restlessness, retching/gagging, abdominal pain, anorexia, or abdominal distension. Many patients may be asymptomatic based on incidental radiography or owner observation of inappropriate ingestion. The most commonly reported gastric foreign bodies in dogs include plastic, sharp objects, wood, toys, balls, stones, and bones (Gianella, 2009). In the author's experience cloth, coins and plastic toys/material are the most common in the canine, while hair ties, rubber bands, linear pieces of leather, small pieces of soft rubber (i.e.., ear plugs, etc.) are the most common in cats

The most definitive way to obtain a diagnosis of a gastric foreign body is via gastroscopy. This requires general anesthesia and is expensive, so having a diagnosis with other imaging modalities and historical information is often very helpful. Traditional radiography can be helpful to identify gastric foreign bodies and often times provides solid evidence of foreign material, particularly when the foreign material is radiopaque. Ultrasound can be used to detect foreign material as well, but associated with the intrinsic difficulty of imaging the stomach and its associated gas. Contrast radiography can help in cases where intraluminal foreign bodies are not highlighted. In many cases, gastroscopy is necessary to provide a definitive diagnosis. This is more common in the feline patient given the tendency to not swallow radiopaque objects. Conversely, demonstration of soft tissue opacities within the stomach does not always definitively mean that foreign material is present or that intervention is necessary. The clinician should consider the clinical history and strength of imaging findings before recommending intervention.

Knowledge of the most recent meal may aid in determining whether there is residual gastric contents and delayed gastric emptying. Normal gastric emptyting is influenced by the consistency, volume, and fat content of food. Smaller volume, low-fat, and liquid diets are most quickly emptied. In normal dogs solid diets may take up to 10 hours to empty completely (Miyabayashi, 2005). The author considers gastric foreign material when residual content is observed >18 hours. A compatible clinical history of vomiting and/or a known predisposition for eating foreign material can be helpful in substantiating intervention. It should be noted that some patients with gastric foreign bodies may show intermittent clinical signs or no clinical signs at all. It should also be noted that delayed gastric emptying and the persistent presence of material in the stomach, despite vomiting, can provide evidence to a suspicion of a gastric foreign body. Owners must be aware that a negative gastroscopy for foreign material is always possible. Patients with gastrointestinal disease, certain metabolic conditions, and regional inflammation can have alterations in gastric emptying. These conditions could result in unnecessary gastroscopy.

Additionally, acid–base evaluation may provide clues in some cases that an obstructive process is present. A hypochloremic metabolic alkalosis can indicate a proximal gastrointestinal obstruction. Imaging that supports a pyloric obstruction (i.e., gastric fluid distension, gastric foreign material), and absence of a recent meal ingestion encourages endoscopic evaluation.

Veterinary Image-Guided Interventions, First Edition. Edited by Chick Weisse and Allyson Berent.

Companion website: www.wiley.com/go/weisse/vet-image-guided-interventions

Additionally, some foreign bodies may approach the upper limits of endoscopic success. Knowledge about the size and type of foreign body can help to determine if gastrotomy would be more appropriate. Occasionally, a large volume of foreign material is present in the stomach that can be successfully removed but could take excessive amounts of time, making endoscopy inappropriate (Figure 14.1). Unfortunately, it is not always possible to predict, but an experienced endoscopist can quickly determine whether or not they can be successful. If attempts are made to remove foreign material that is difficult, a time limit should be considered to avoid excessive anesthesia times.

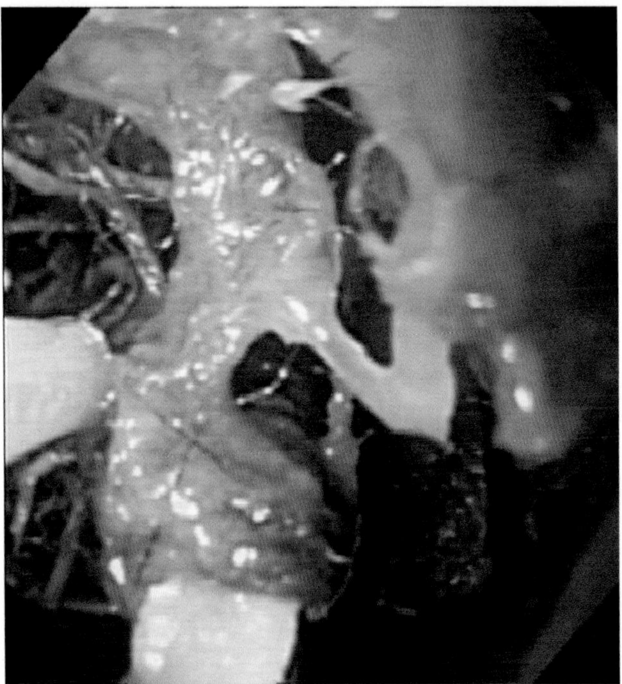

Figure 14.1 Endoscopic image of a volume of material in the stomach that could take hours to remove.

Potential Risks/Complications/Expected Outcomes

Gastric foreign body retrieval is generally a low-risk procedure with minimal risk for perforation or iatrogenic injury to the mucosa. If the appropriate case is selected, the expected outcome is typically excellent.

Equipment

A standard gastroduodenoscope is utilized to visualize the foreign body. A wide variety of instruments including baskets, nets, graspers, snares and forceps can be utilized for retrieval (Figure 14.2 and Table 14.1). Each foreign body is individualized to the type, location and size of the pet.

Some of the author's biases for the retrieval of foreign bodies are shown in Figure 14.3 and Table 14.2. *Please note that each clinician's preferences may differ.*

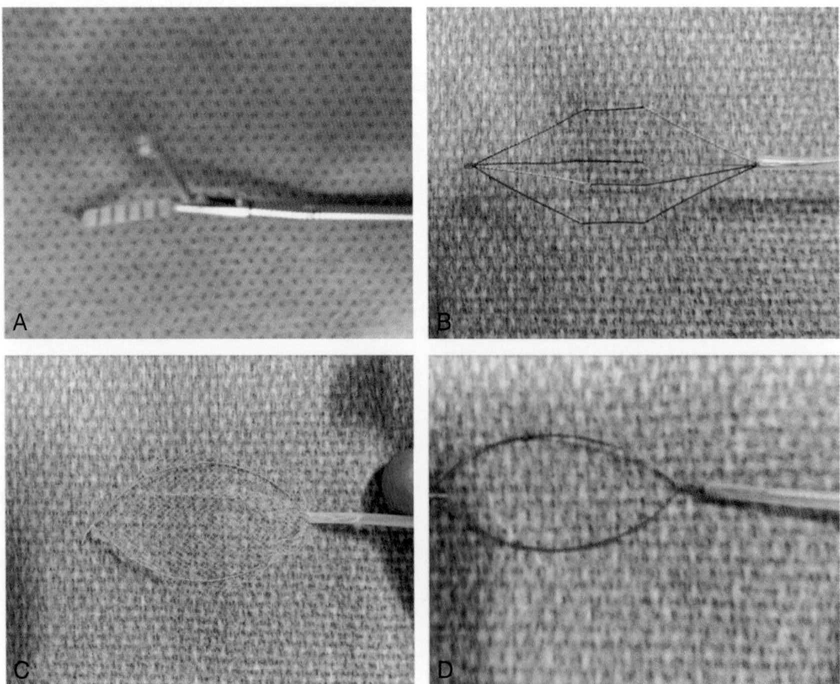

Figure 14.2 Various instruments that can be used for endoscopic foreign body retrieval. (A) rat tooth retrieval forceps; (B) 4 wire basket; (C) Roth net; (D) endoscopic loop.

TABLE 14.1
Commonly used equipment in imaging of foreign bodies

Endoscopic equipment
- Retrieval forceps (e.g., rat tooth,[1,2] alligator type,[3,4] shark tooth,[5] rubber tip.[6])
- Baskets (e.g., 3 wire,[7] 4 wire,[8] 6 wire,[9,10] 4 wire rotatable.[11])
- Endoscopic snares: non-rotating,[12] rotating[13]
- Nets (e.g., Roth net,[14] Nakao Spider-Net.[15])
- Endoscopic graspers (e.g., 2 prong,[16] 3 prong,[17] 4 prong,[18] 5 prong.[19])
- Biliary stent remover (e.g., Soehendra stent retriever.[20])
- Endoscopic balloons (e.g., Multi-diameter, [21] or single diameter balloons.[22])

Laparoscopic equipment
- Forceps[23]
- Scissors[24,25]

Endoscopic attachments
- Overtubes[26,27]
- Endoscopic hood[28]

Non-traditional equipment
- Suture/guide wire
- Plastic bags
- Condoms
- Lubrication

TABLE 14.2
Instruments for the retrieval of foreign bodies

Cloth material	Instruments with teeth: graspers, pronged grabbers (2-pronged, 3-pronged)
Coins Flat, firm thin objects	Graspers, net basket, rubber retrieval forceps, condom held by a grasping forcep
Bones	Loops>baskets
Balls	Baskets (when size permitting), Net
Hair	Loops, baskets, nets
Large volume debris	
Non-obstructive, small, large volume debris	May consider gastric lavage to reduce time of retrieval

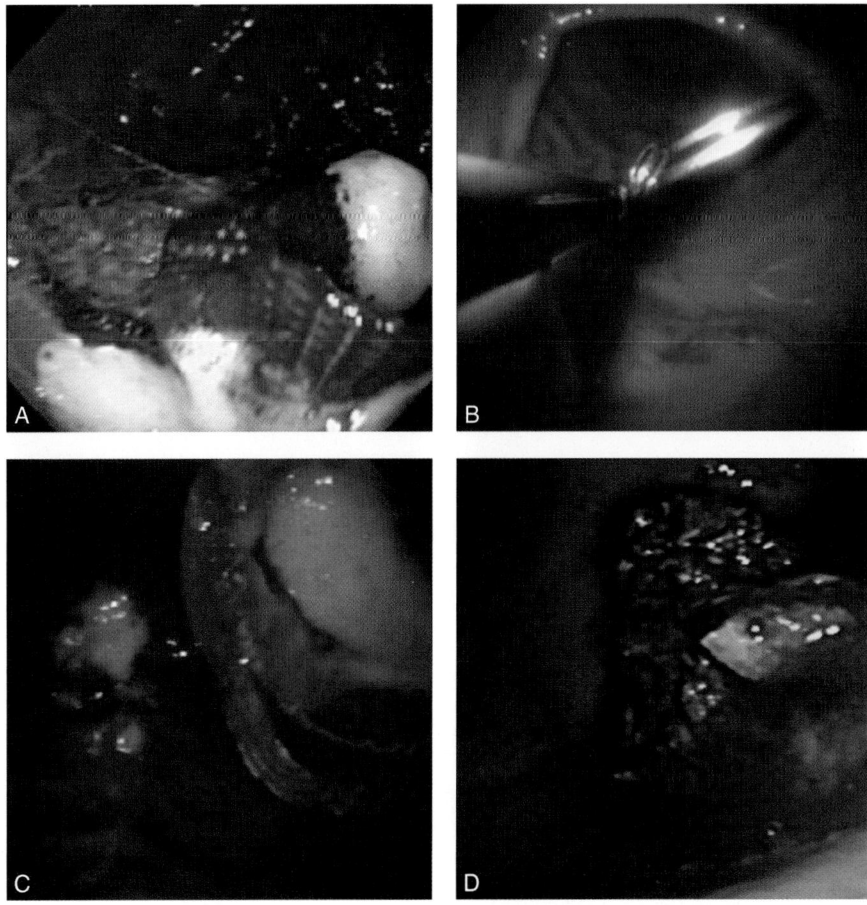

Figure 14.3 Endoscopic images in the stomach. (A) Cloth foreign body in the stomach. This was grasped with an endoscopic grasper and gently retracted through the LES. (B) A penny. (C) A piece of a rubber ball. (D) A bone.

Procedure

Basic Technique

No one technique or tool will be effective for retrieval of all gastric foreign bodies. Unlike an esophageal foreign body, the endoscopist has a greater ability to maneuver the endoscope due to the size of the foreign body relative to the internal diameter of the stomach. Additionally, gastric foreign bodies can be manually manipulated by repositioning the patient, collapsing an inflated stomach, or by pushing/pulling/rolling the object to achieve a better angle of approach.

The endoscopist should try and approach each foreign object perpendicularly, which allows an ideal position to entrap it in any device. Controlled manipulation of the scope using both gentle torque/rotation of the insertion tube with fine movements of the directional controls, aid in getting the retrieval device around the object.

The endoscope should be far enough away from the foreign object to be able to see the retrieval device and maintain visibility on the screen during manipulation. Working too close will have a tendency to deform the instruments, while working too far away will reduce the ability to engage the object securely.

The endoscopist should evaluate the foreign body at all angles to find a point of engagement that matches the particular instrument being used, providing a firm grip so that when it is removed through the lower esophageal stricture (LES), and into the esophagus is it not dislodged. Long foreign bodies (i.e., marrow bones,) should be manipulated on each end, so the most narrow aspect of the object is pulled through the LES first (Figure 14.4). When the foreign body is engaged, it is pulled against the insertion tube of the endoscope, and held firmly with the working instrument. The endoscope and instrument are then withdrawn together. Firm, consistent tension is needed at the LES to allow for some objects to be moved into the caudal esophagus. If the object is getting stuck at the LES than the endoscopist can entrap it at a different angle, or consider using lubrications (60 ml of sterile lubrication and warm water mixed in a syringe and injected through a catheter placed transorally, down the esophagus, next to the endoscope at the LES). Instrument selection is the key to being successful. Each clinician will develop preferences for instrumentation, however, having a wide variety of instruments will improve efficacy. Regardless of instrument selection, appropriate use of instrumentation will help to maximize efficiency (Figure 14.5).

Tips in the Stomach

The large stomach allows the positioning of a foreign body into an area that gives the endoscopist the most maneuverability. This can be accomplished by grasping an object and dragging it but also can be accomplished by pushing the object with the endoscope or manipulating the patient (e.g., externally pushing on the stomach, switching body position). Additionally, altering the degree of gastric distension will allow for movement towards or away from the instrument making engagement easier.

Finding an object, like a small coin or nail/needle, can be difficult. Always thoroughly evaluated the entire gastric lumen, paying closest attention to the point of dependency. If the patient is in left lateral recumbency, than the most dependant portion of the stomach, where a heavy object will be found, would be around the cardia/very lateral aspect of the fundus/greater curvature. This means that the endoscopist must look carefully in a retroflexed manner at the cardia (Figure 14.6).

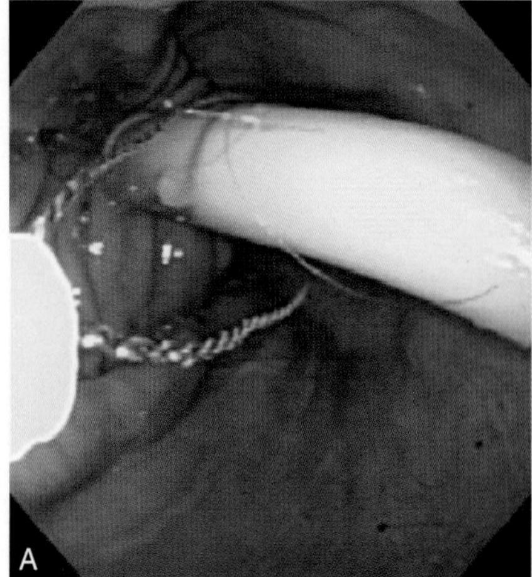

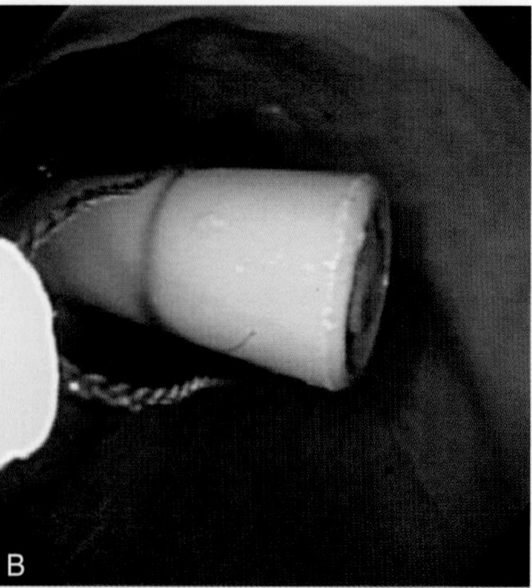

Figure 14.4 Pen cap foreign body in the stomach. (A) Object with grabbed in the center making it hard to pull through the GES. (B) The object that the instrument is grabbed with the loop at the end of the pen cap to facilitate passage through the lower esophageal sphincter.

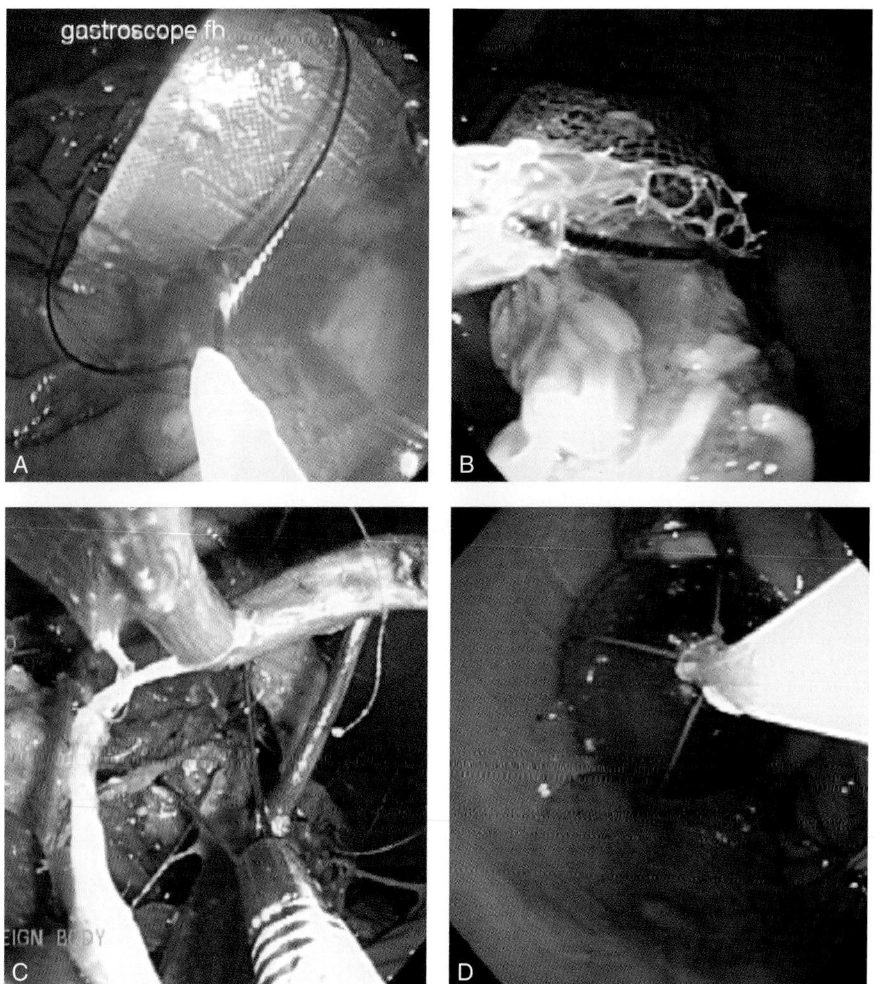

Figure 14.5 Various objects being removed with various pieces of equipment. (A) The endoscopic loop as it is opened and gently manipulated over the foreign object without deforming the instrument. (B) The Roth net is laid onto the object before it is pulled onto the object as it is closed. (C) The three prong graspers are opened and directed into the center of a mass of objects or is directly placed around a specific object. (D) A basket is opened and gently laid onto the object. As this occurs, the wires spread open and large objects become solidly engaged.

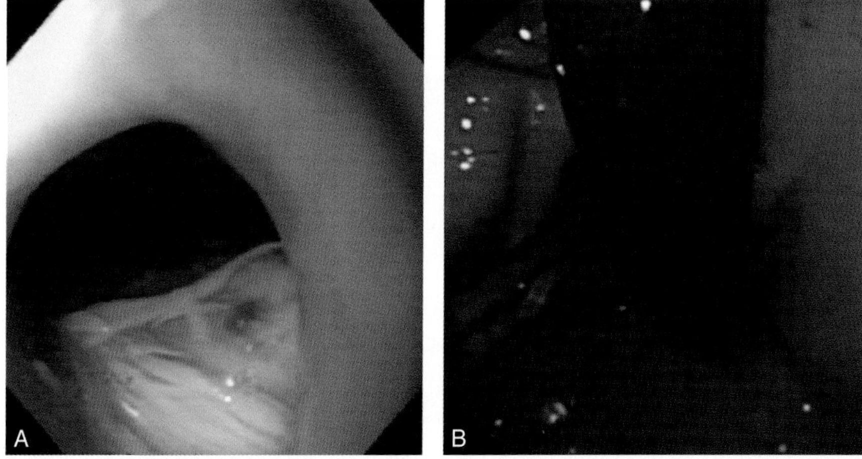

Figure 14.6 Foreign bodies at the lower esophageal sphincter. (A) Note that that the foreign body is located just aboral to the LES making visualization difficult. Manipulation of the instrument across the sphincter is difficult; retroflexion may provide the optimal visualization in this case. (B) The object at the cardia is easily visualized at the cardia with retroflexion. This object was not seen on passage of the scope in an antegrade fashion.

No Assistant vs. Assistant

The author believes that the majority of foreign objects can be removed successfully without the help of an assistant, even when available. It is the author's opinion that an experienced endoscopist will be able to control the small manipulations better individually. Often, these fine movements of the instrument cannot be verbalized well to an assistant. Occasionally, having an extra set of hands is of great value, but that is not always the case. Therefore, knowing when to utilize an assistant, having an experienced assistant, and knowing when to perform retrieval on your own is important. In addition, it is often helpful to have the assistant hold the endoscope in place while you work the retrieval device and torque the insertion tube gently as needed. This is where appropriate finesse is required.

Through the Pylorus

Every endoscopic foreign body retrieval should include a duodenoscopy, as there could be an additional foreign body in the duodenum. Occasionally, a foreign body is lodged in the pylorus (Figure 14.7, Figure 14.8,

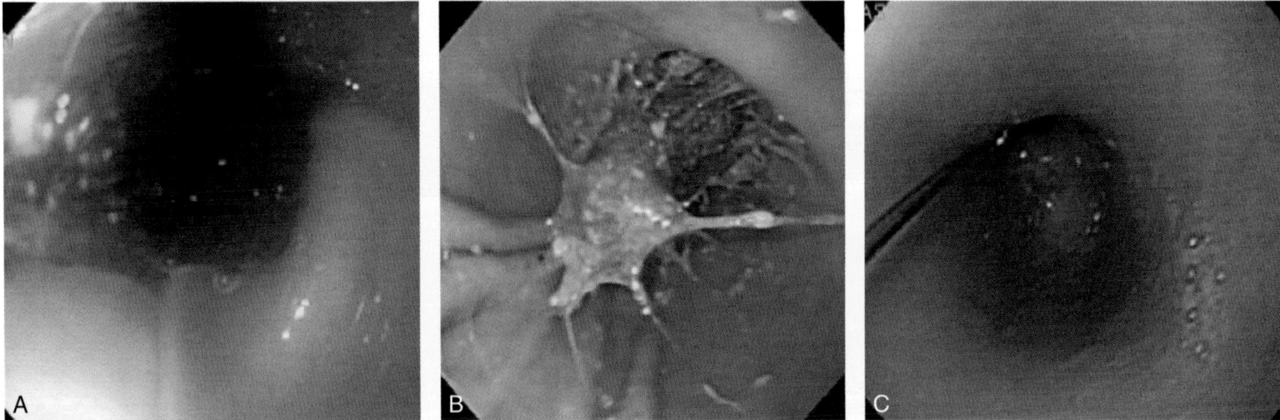

Figure 14.7 Endoscopic images of foreign bodies across the pylorus. The distal extent of the FB cannot often be assessed from endoscopy. Abdominal imaging can sometimes be helpful to determine pulling is appropriate or likely realistic.

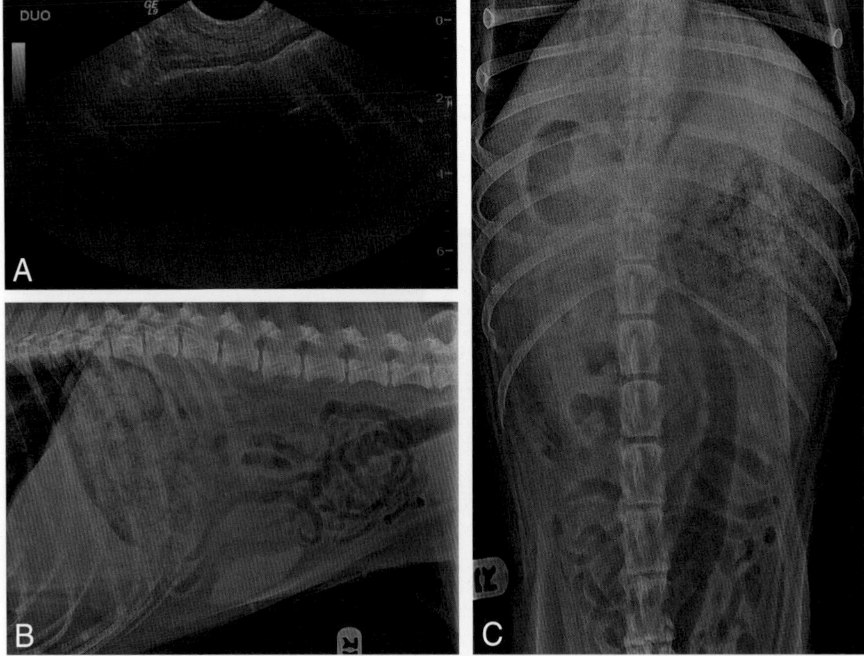

Figure 14.8 Imaging can be helpful to determine the distance that a foreign object may extend and evaluate for evidence of peritonitis. (A) ultrasound image showing a shadowing object without plication or regional peritonitis. The object can be traced to normal bowel, providing the clinician information regarding how far the foreign body extends. (B, C) Radiographs showing the extent of a pyloric foreign body into the descending duodenum and does not reveal evidence of pneumoperitoneum, loss of peritoneal detail, or intestinal plication.

and Figure 14.9). While successful manipulation of the FB is possible in many cases, knowledge of this is ideal prior to endoscopy. Occasionally, the proximal duodenum may have evidence of regional peritonitis, which can not be observed endoscopically, or a linear foreign body can be present aboral, necessitating a surgical approach. Appropriate knowledge of the leading edge of foreign body via imaging may help decide when surgery could be necessary (i.e., presence of plication, peritonitis, suspected perforation) (Figure 14.8). Generally speaking, string foreign bodies should not be pulled. However, cloth objects can be removed when gentle tension allows easy retrieval. Care should be taken, however, to not insufflate extensively, as this can dilate the small intestinal lumen and encourage the object to migrate aborally. Dilation is minimized until the object is engaged. In rare cases, the pylorus is too small to pull the foreign body orally and attempts at balloon dilation of the pylorus could be performed. The author has used up to 12 mm balloons in dogs and 10 mm balloons in cats.

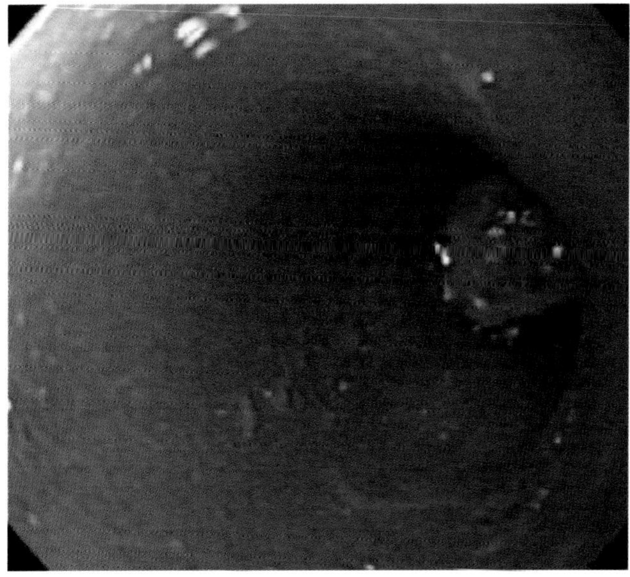

Figure 14.9 Duodenal foreign body. Note that with excessive dilatation of the small intestinal wall, duodenal foreign bodies may migrate beyond reach.

The Stubborn LES

The most frustrating aspect of gastric foreign body retrieval involves resistance that is encountered at the LES that continually dislodges the foreign body from engagement (Figure 14.10). This can be minimized by selecting and instrument that complements the foreign body and provides the most rigid, firm grasp possible, minimizing slipping. In addition, the use of lubrication can be incredibly helpful, as mentioned above.

Insufflation of the stomach can increase intragastric pressure on the LES and may increase its diameter. Additionally, utilization of an assistant pushing on an insufflated stomach in a caudal to cranial, subcostal direction, while the endoscopist simultaneously pulls can help to negotiate the foreign body into the esophagus. The author has occasionally passed a bougie across the LES prior to engaging the foreign body. Following engagement, retraction of the bougie simultaneously with the endoscope/instrument will allow the pylorus to stretch. Rarely, balloon dilation of the LES is needed to stretch the sphincter for passage. This may predispose to gastroesophageal reflux by reducing LES tonicity (Figure 14.11). Utilization of anesthetic protocols that may promote relaxation

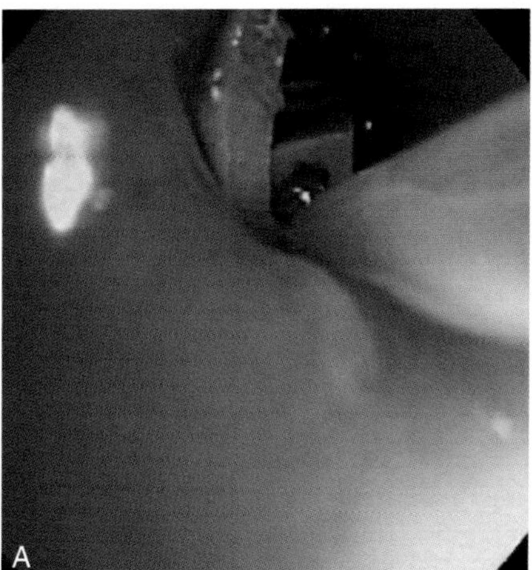

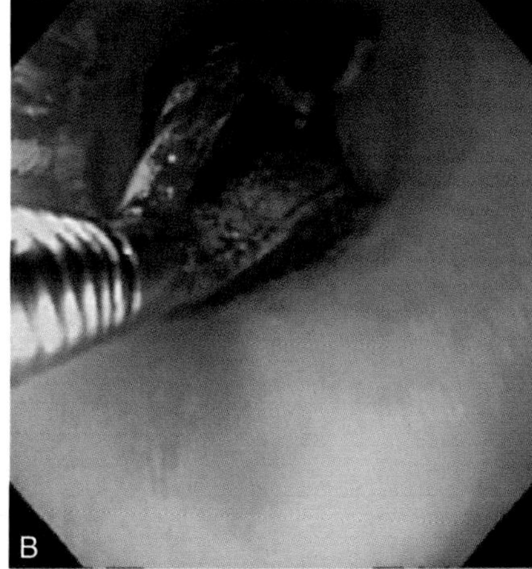

Figure 14.10 Endoscopic images of foreign bodies wedged in the LES. Note the resistance that is met at the lower esophageal sphincter during extraction of gastric foreign bodies.

could be helpful: gas anesthesia, benzodiazepines and/or opioids). Finally, utilization of regional injection of local anesthetics (i.e., lidocaine, bupivacaine) into the sphincter may provide relaxation. Finally, utilization of an overtube may help to dilate the LES and allow for objects to be partially pulled into the lumen for removal (Figure 14.12). Cutting the distal end of the over tube for 2–3 cm perpendicular to its long axis may allow for larger objects to be retracted partially into the lumen. The tapered effect of the tube may facilitate removal of the object (Figure 14.13). When this is done the tube is compressed around the object as it is pulled across the LES.

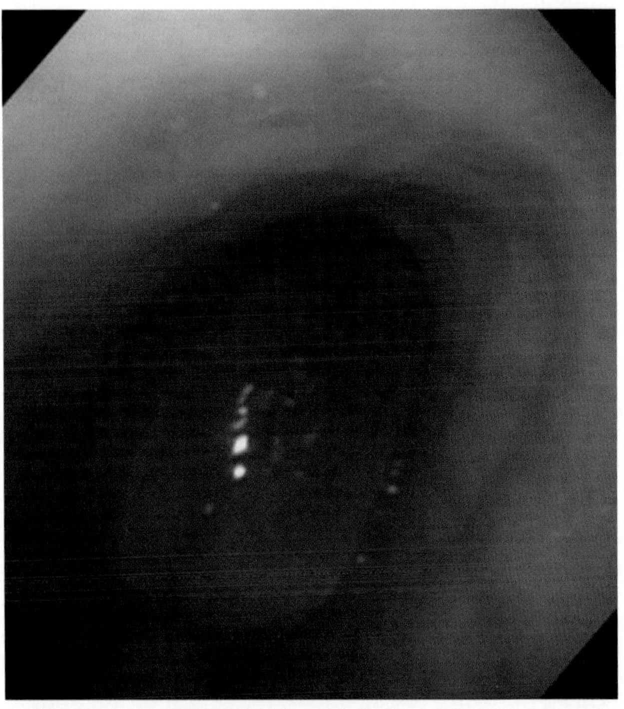

Figure 14.11 Balloon used at the LES to help remove a foreign body.

Post-Procedural and Follow-Up Care

Following the procedure, the patient is discharged the same day. Patients with ulcerative gastritis are treated with proton pump inhibitors (omeprazole 1 mg/kg q 12) and Carafate (0.25–1 g/kg q 8) for 3–5 days. No additional therapy is needed in non-ulcerative cases.

No further follow up is necessary in most cases.

Prognosis

The prognosis following successful removal of a gastric foreign body is excellent when all pieces are removed. All animals should have a concurrent duodenoscopy to ensure there are no additional objects lodged in the intestinal tract, and all owners should be warned that if there is an intestinal foreign body that you cannot see with the endoscope, this patient may require additional interventions.

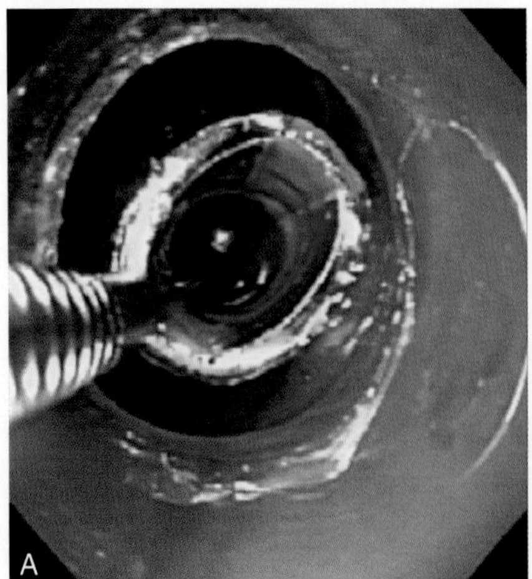

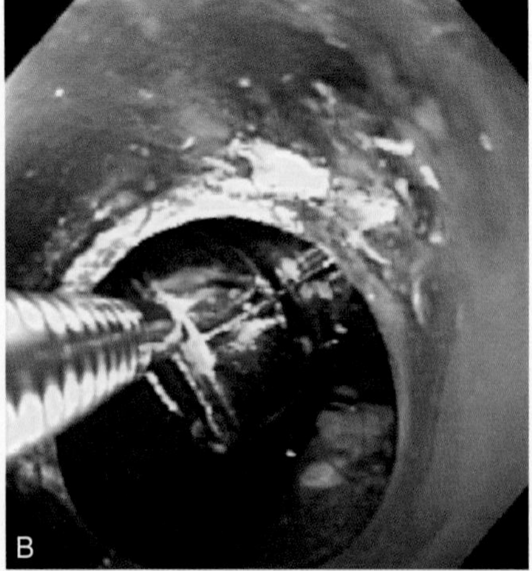

Figure 14.12 Using an overtube to remove a large object form the stomach. A large Christmas ornament is retracted into the lumen of an overtube for retraction across the LES. The tube maintains patency of the LES while it is retracted from the stomach. The resistance at the LES previously had resulted in repetitive disengagement of the instrument with the foreign object before this technique was employed.

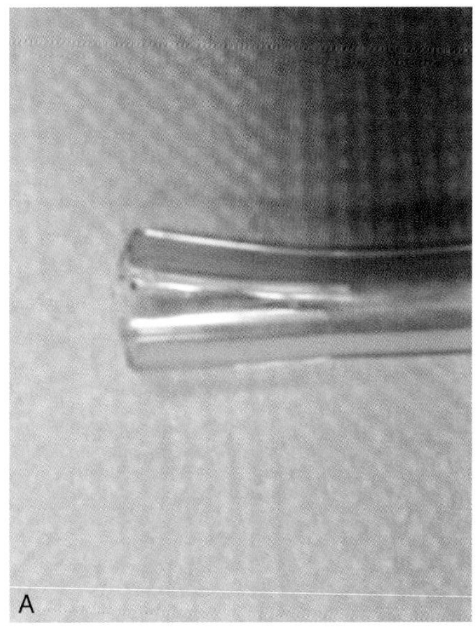
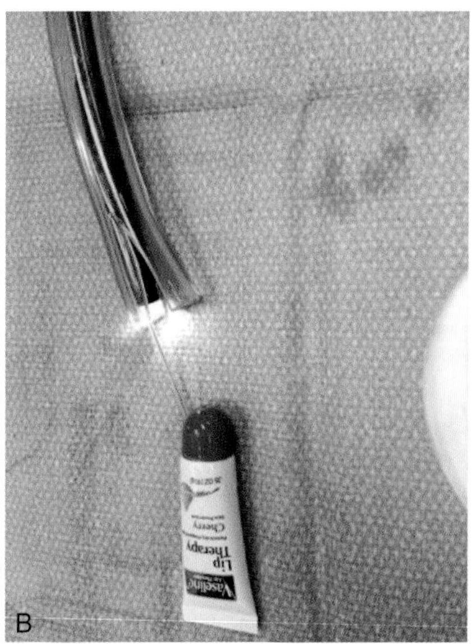
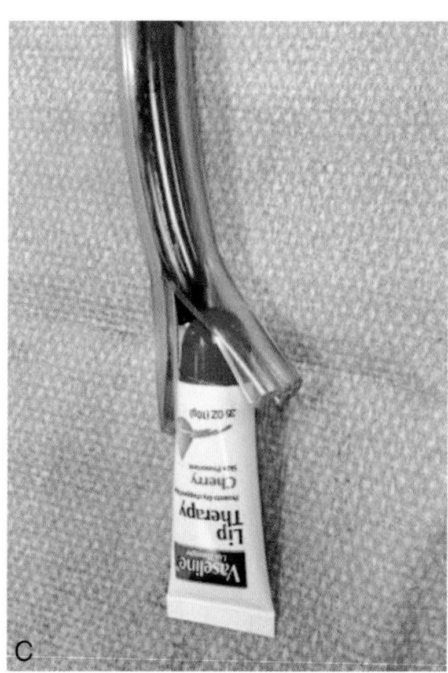

Figure 14.13 Use of the overtube. (A) A gastric tube is cut at the end to allow for larger objects to be pulled into the lumen for retrieval across the LES. (B, C) An object is grasped and pulled into the flared end of the tube for retraction across the LES.

Notes

1. Maxum® Reusable Forceps Cook Medical (Winston-Salem, NC).
2. Rat tooth retrieval forceps, Olympus America (Center Valley, PA).
3. Alligator jaw retrieval forceps, Olympus America (Center Valley, PA).
4. Rat tooth alligator jaw retrieval forceps, Olympus America (Center Valley, PA).
5. Shark tooth retrieval forceps, Olympus America (Center Valley, PA).
6. Rubber tip retrieval forceps, Olympus America (Center Valley, PA).
7. 3 wire, Helical Retrieval Baskets: Reusable, Hobbs Medical (Stafford Springs, CN).
8. 4-Wire Basket w/3-Ring Handle, Olympus America (Center Valley, PA).
9. 4-wire foreign body basket, Medi-Globe (Tempe, AZ).
10. 6-wire foreign body basket, Medi-Globe (Tempe, AZ).
11. Falcon rotatable retrieval basket, US Endoscopy (Mentor, OH).
12. AcuSnare® One Piece Disposable Snare Cook Medical (Winston-Salem, NC).
13. RotaSnare® Rotating and with Multifilament Loop, Medi-Globe (Tempe, AZ).
14. Roth Net Platinum retriever - universal, US Endoscopy (Mentor, Ohio).
15. Nakao Spider-Net, ConMed (Billerica, Mass).
16. Foreign Body Retriever – Grasper with Forked Jaws, Medi-Globe (Tempe, AZ).
17. Caesar® Grasping Forceps Cook Medical (Winston-Salem, NC).
18. Reusable Retrieval Forceps, 4 prong, Hobbs Medical (Stafford Springs, CN).
19. Pentapod grasping forceps, Olympus America (Center Valley, PA).
20. Soehendra stent retriever, Cook Medical (Winston-Salem, NC).
21. CRE Single-Use Fixed wire Esophageal Balloon Dilators, Boston Scientific (Natick, MA).
22. Maxforce TTS Single Use Balloon Dilators, Boston Scientific (Natick, MA).
23. Kelly Forceps, AEM Laparascopic Instruments, Encision, Boulder CO.
24. Hook scissors AEM Laparascopic Instruments, Encision, Boulder CO.
25. Straight scissors AEM Laparascopic Instruments, Encision, Boulder CO.
26. Guardus overtube – esophageal, US Endoscopy (Mentor, OH).
27. ConMed Endoscopic Overtube, ConMed, Utica, NY.
28. Foreign body hood protector, Kimberly-Clark (Roswell, GA).

References

Gianella P, Pfammatter NS, and Burgener IA (2009) Oesophageal and gastric endoscopic foreign body removal: complications and follow-up of 102 dogs. *J Small Anim Pract* 50(12), 649–54.

Miyabayashi T and Morgan JP (2005). Gastric emptying in the normal dog: a contrast radiographic technique. *Vet Radiol* 25(4), 187–91.

Suggested Reading

Hall JA, Magne ML, and Twedt DC (1987) Effect of acepromazine, diazepam, fentanyl-droperidol, and oxymorphone on gastroesophageal sphincter pressure in healthy dogs. *Am J Vet Res* 48(4), 556–7.

Leevy CM (1980) Effect of diazepam on the lower esophageal sphincter. A double-blind controlled study. *Rushnak Am J Gastroenterol* 73(2), 127–30.

CHAPTER FIFTEEN

GASTROINTESTINAL POLYPECTOMY

Douglas A. Palma and Allyson Berent
The Animal Medical Center, New York, NY

BACKGROUND/INDICATIONS

Gastric and colonic polyps are rare findings in veterinary medicine, with limited data reported. Malignant transformation of polyps is a major concern in human medicine, and is thought to be more common for colonic polyps (Miller et al, 2010). For gastric polyps, exposure to proton pump inhibitors, age, genetics, and *Helicobacter* gastritis has not been documented as risk factors in veterinary patients, as it has in human medicine (Ally et al, 2009; Gencosmanoglu et al, 2003).

In dogs, colorectal neoplasia is uncommon, and these lesions are typically adenocarcinoma (~60%), adenomatous polyps (~20%), or carcinoma *in situ* (~15%). Colorectal polyps are considered to be the most common benign colorectal tumor in dogs with an increased prevalence suggested in Poodles, Airedale terriers, German Shepherd dogs, and Collies. Colorectal polyps can undergo a malignant transformation (~18% when diffuse of multiple and 7% when solitary), like that seen in humans, making resection desired. If a lesion is sessile or pedunculated in nature, single, and a biopsy is suggestive of a benign inflammatory polyp, then endoscopic polypectomy with mucosal resection can be recommended. If the lesion is progressing, atypical (i.e., poorly demarcated or "napkin-ring" in nature), or histopathologically malignant, then surgical resection should be recommended, whenever possible (transanal rectal pull-through, colorectal resection and anastomosis, excision by mucosal eversion, etc.).

Most polyps are histologically considered either hyperplastic or adenomatous, and the epithelial changes do not cross the mucosal basement membrane to the lamina propria. While polyps (adenoma or hyperplasia) have an unknown cause, it is thought that they are typically associated with local irritation, which may occur from inflammation, parietal gland hyperplasia, gastrinomas, infectious etiologies, or chronic diarrhea.

Gastroscopy and colonoscopy are the mainstay for diagnosis and therapy when evaluating and treating gastrointestinal polyps in human medicine. Polypectomy is the mainstay of treatment in human gastroenterology and has been shown to reduce the risk of cancer progression. This progression is most commonly seen with carcinoma *in situ*. Because of this risk, the associated clinical signs seen, and the need for accurate histopathologic evaluation, their removal is indicated.

The term polypectomy is used when referring to removal of lesions measuring less than 2 cm with an electrosurgical snare alone, and the term endoscopic mucosal resection (EMR) is used when the polypectomy is done after fluid (saline, sterile water, epinephrine, or methylene blue solution) is infused in the submucosal tissue under the base of the mass separating the mucosa from the muscular layers, to assist in a clean and safe resection. This is typically done for larger more sessile lesions, allowing a safer resection, wile protecting the deeper tissue from both thermal injury and perforation during electrocautery.

POTENTIAL RISKS/COMPLICATIONS/EXPECTED OUTCOMES

Gastrointestinal polypectomy is met with few major complications. The most common concerns include gastrointestinal (GI) perforation, hemorrhage, recurrence, failure to remove the entire lesion, barotrauma from enemas, or a condition known as post-polypectomy syndrome. Post-polypectomy syndrome is more common following removal of a sessile polyp using electrocautery, resulting in a transmural burn and localized perforation. With an experienced operator taking proper prophylactic measures (EMR, epinephrine injections, band ligation, clipping, etc.), the incidence of these complications is

Veterinary Image-Guided Interventions, First Edition. Edited by Chick Weisse and Allyson Berent.

Companion website: www.wiley.com/go/weisse/vet-image-guided-interventions

reduced. If endoscopic removal is elected then the instruments that should be available include the polypectomy snare device, endoscopic injection needles, grasping/biopsy forceps, endoscopic clips, and baskets.

If the complete excision of a benign mass is accomplished, the prognosis for full recovery and elimination of clinical signs are generally good to excellent. If the benign mass is incompletely excised, recurrence and malignant transformation are possible and should be monitored for.

General Appearance

Similar to other regions of the body, gastrointestinal polyps generally appear as superficial pedunculated lesions of the mucosa without gross suggestion of deeper invasion. Most pedunculated polyps and have a relatively narrow stalk (Figure 15.1). The sessile, flat, broad-based polyps, are rarely seen in the stomach, but are commonly seen in the colon (Figure 15.2). The surface of a gastric polyp is generally homogeneous

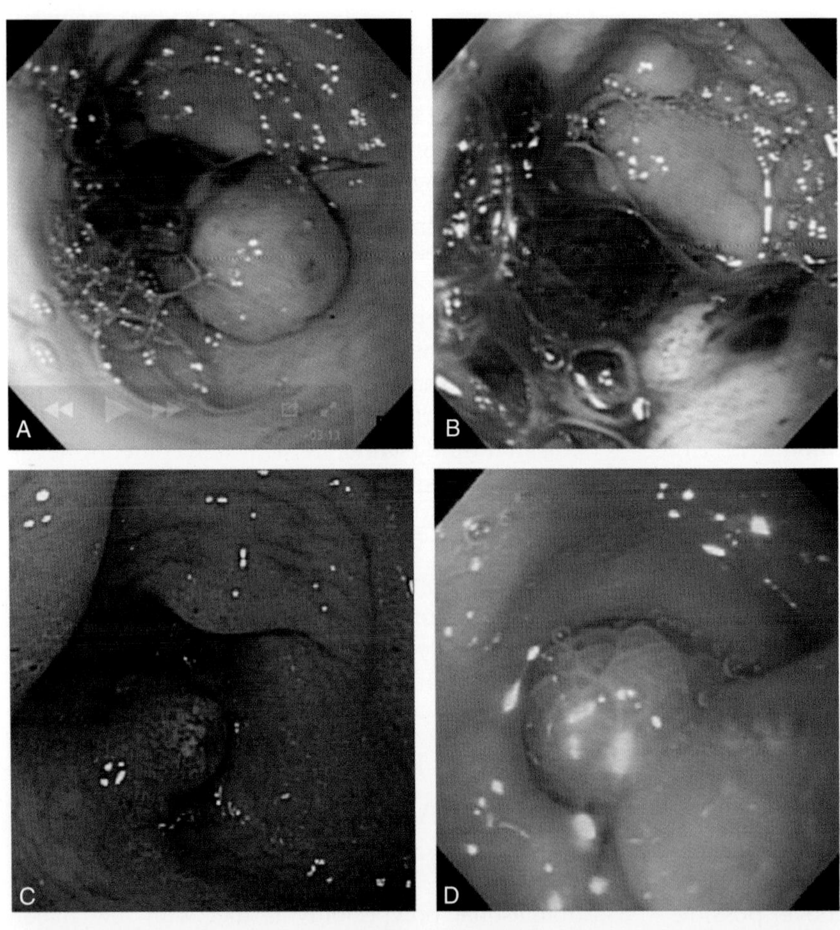

Figure 15.1 Endoscopic images of gastric polyps. (A, B) Bleeding gastric polyp in the antrum of the stomach of a dog. (C) A gastric polyp in the antrum of the stomach of a cat. (D) A gastric polyp obstructing the pylorus in a cat.

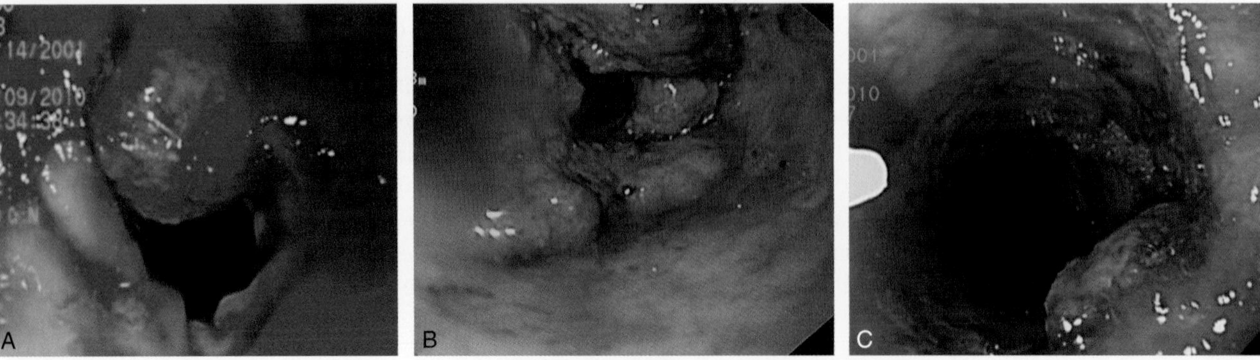

Figure 15.2 Colorectal polyps in three dogs. (A) broad based polyp prior to EMR. (B) Napkin ring polyp. (C) Flat sessile polyp at the colorectal junction.

throughout and can range from smooth to slightly textured. Gastric lesions are usually the same color as the remaining gastric mucosa and are rarely ulcerated or grossly well vascularized.

Colonic polyps typically are found in the distal colon of dogs and cats at the colorectal junction. They may also be found more proximally. When polyps are found in this region, they are characterized based upon their gross appearance and adherence to the colon wall. Most appear dark red or pink and are often soft, friable, and hemorrhagic. The three most commonly described varieties of colonic polyps are sessile, pedunculated, and flat (Figure 15.2). Napkin ring or apple core polyps are rare and typically have a more aggressive behavior (Figure 15.2B).

Interventional Decisions

Many patients with gastric polyps are asymptomatic and generally, the reason for endoscopic investigation is unrelated. Therefore, polypectomy should be considered carefully to prevent unnecessary complications. The most common location for gastric lesions is in the pyloric antral region, along the lesser curvature of the stomach and the incisura angularis. In cats these masses can be large, resulting in a pyloric outflow obstruction (Figure 15.1C, D).

Equipment

A standard flexible endoscope is needed for this procedure. The author prefers the video gastroduodenoscope.[1,2] Electrocautery (snare polypectomy) requires infusion with air, and a cautery pad needs to be placed on a patient for grounding. A snare polypectomy device is available in various shapes and sizes[5,6] (Figure 15.3 and Figure 15.4), and one should be chosen that is large enough to get around the polypoid mass while small enough to fit through the working channel of the endoscope (typically the 2 mm snare catheter fits through the 6–8 mm GI scope and the 2.4 mm catheter through the larger 8–10 mm GI scope). Retrieval baskets, ranging in basket diameter can be used to remove the mass once it is ablated.

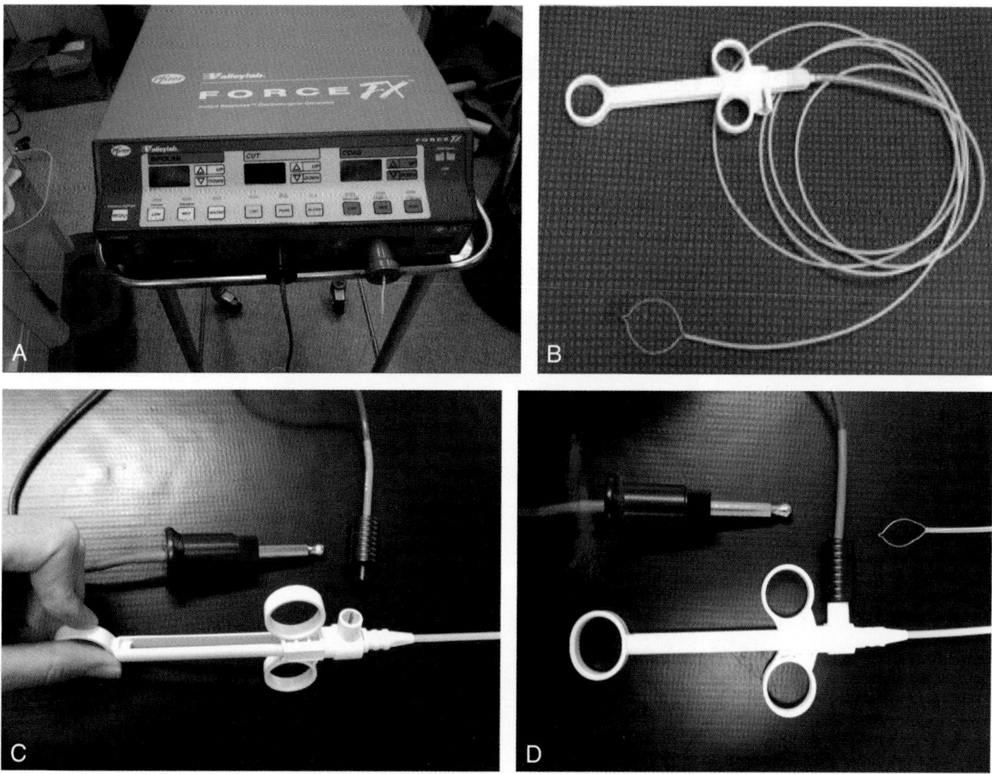

Figure 15.3 Equipment used for electrocautery polypectomy. (A) The electrocautery machine attached to a red and blue/yellow adaptor. (B) A polypectomy snare device. (C) Location on the polypectomy device where the electrocautery adaptor attaches. (D) The adaptor attached.

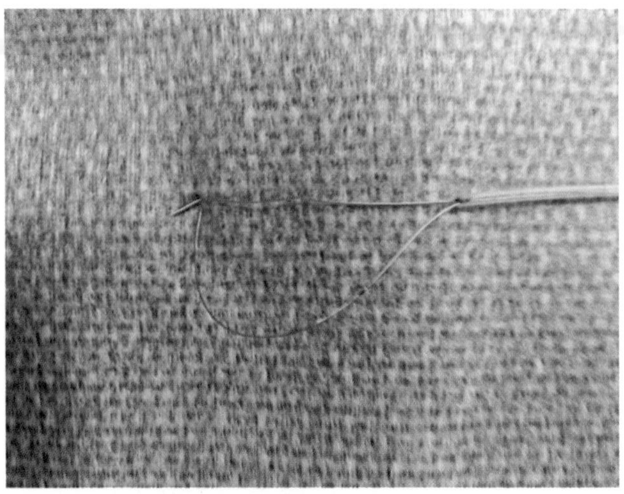

Figure 15.4 Crescent shaped polypectomy snare.

If endoscopic mucosal resection is to be performed than an injection needle is needed[6] that is able to fit through the working channel of the endoscope (see Chapter 2) (Figure 15.5).

Some clinicians prefer the use of EMR caps to facilitate removal of polyps. These caps act as extensions of the endoscope, allowing for the application of suction to the lesion. Application of caps may facilitate resection of flatter more sessile lesions more easily. The different angulations and consistencies available allow for appropriate positioning over the lesion despite the positioning of the lesion on the wall.[7] Standard snares can be loaded into EMR caps, however, the author prefers a crescent shaped snare polypectomy device, designed to be preloaded into these caps[8] (Figure 15.4).

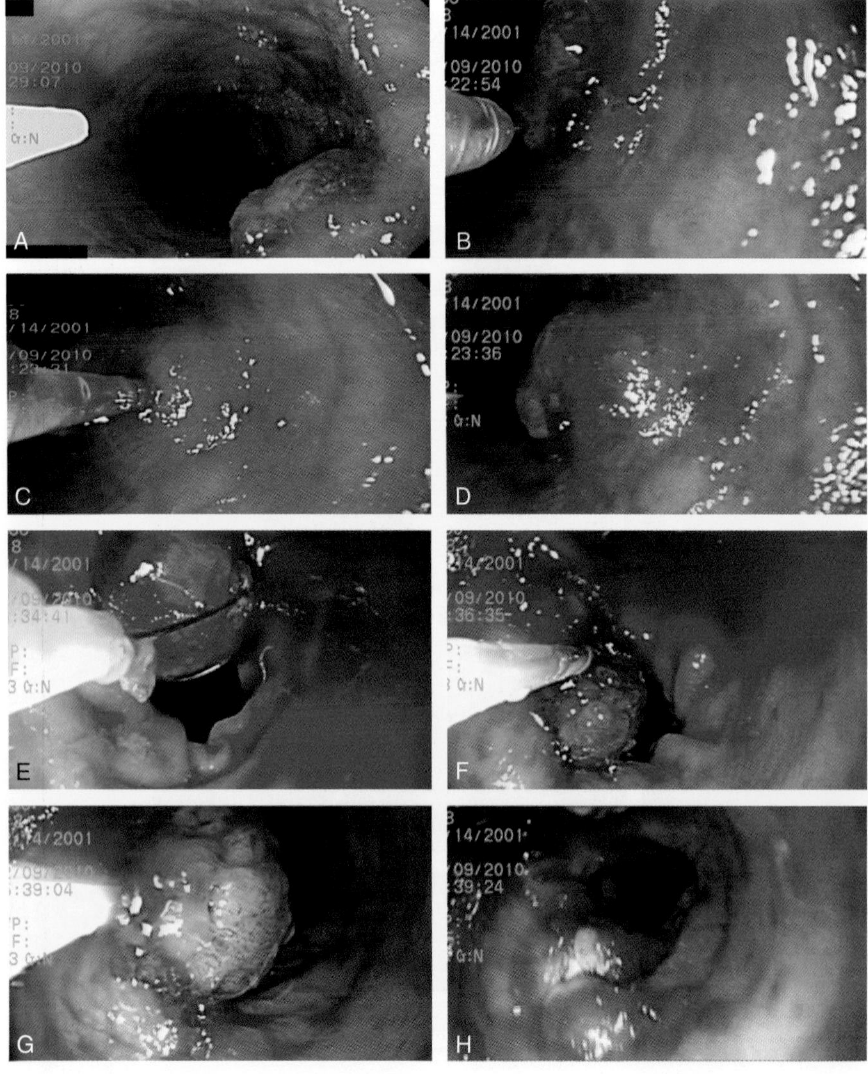

Figure 15.5 Colorectal polypectomy using endoscopic mucosal resection (EMR) in a dog with a colorectal sessile polyp. (A) Colonoscopic image of the flat sessile polyp. (B) Endoscopic needle through the working channel of the endoscope at it approaches the base of the polyp. (C) The needle inserted under the base of the polyp in the submucosal tissue as saline is injected between the tissue planes. (D) A lift is performed creating a more pedunculated mass. (E) Endoscopic polypecotmy snare being placed around the polyp. (F) The snare is engaging the base of the polyp at the lift site. (G) Electrocautery is activated at the base. (H) A clean base after polypectomy showing a mucosal defect with minimal hemorrhage.

Patient Preparation

For routine endoscopy the patient should be appropriately fasted and colonic cleansing performed. The patient should be pre-treated with broad-spectrum antibiotics, covering for intestinal microflora (anaerobes, Gram-negative bacteria). The author uses cefoxitin (30 mg/kg IV first dose, than 20 mg/kg IV q 4–6 hours) or metronidazole (10 mg/kg BID PO or IV) and enrofloxacin (10 mg/kg IV or PO q 24 hours in dogs and 5 mg/kg IV or PO q 24 hours in cats) for colonic polypectomy.

Prior to considering polypectomy a thorough endoscopy should be performed (gastroscopy or colonoscopy). If a sessile, ulcerated, poorly demarcated mass or a "napkin-ring" lesion (colon) is present than it may not be amenable to EMR and more aggressive treatment may need to be considered. In human medicine, flat sessile masses are often lifted with endoscopic submucosal saline injections (EMR). If a lift is achieved it is considered a superficial lesion that has not crossed the basement membrane and polypectomy will be performed via EMR. If there is no lift seen during the injection than they will send the patient for surgical removal.

Procedure

The technique for polypectomy of gastrointestinal lesions is similar to polypectomy in other sites (see Chapters 10 and 35). First, it is important to select appropriate cases. If the mass is sessile or broad-based than you must use a saline lift to elevate the lesion. Once the lesion is removed it may be necessary to clean up the margins, and this should be done carefully as this could result in perforation. Elevation of the lesion is done with a submucosal bleb of "fluid". The type of fluid used is not standardized amongst clinicians and can be either saline, D5W, or a mixture of D5W and epinephrine and/or methylene blue. The author commonly uses a 1:9 solution of epinephrine (1:10 000):D5W and then adds 1–2 drops of methylene blue to make a slightly blue color. (Munakata and Uno, 1994) The blue color usually is not taken up by the polypoid lesion, but only the submucosal tissue, making a clear demarcation of normal and abnormal tissue, ensuring mucosal resection. This helps to guide the depth of resection and improve the safety of getting the entire mucosal lesion (see later).

For colonic polypectomy (Figure 15.5) a 8–10 mm gastroduodenoscope is used to perform a colonoscopy. The entire colon should be evaluated endoscopically and biopsied. Using an endoscopic polypectomy device, of an appropriate loop size and shape, the mass is manipulated to assess the base. If it is broad-based with a sessile stalk, than a 25 gauge endoscopic injection needle is inserted through the working channel of the endoscope to aid in a saline lift for EMR (Figure 15.5). As mentioned above this can be done with either 0.9% bacteriostatic sterile saline solution, D5W, or a mixture with methylene blue. The needle device is primed to remove all the air in the syringe. The needle is inserted under the base of the polyp into the submucosal tissue and the fluid is injected creating a large enough pocket to separate the mucosa from the other layers of the colon and visualize a "lifting" bleb. This confirms the superficial nature of the mass as well as allowing the mass to become more pedunculated so that it could be resected carefully at the base without perforation. Then the needle is removed, and the snare device is placed around the base of the mass, including the bleb. This assists in an appropriate depth of resection while protecting the deeper tissues from thermal burn and perforation. The snare device is attached to the electrocautery unit (Figure 15.3). Using the electrocautery footpedal, a power of 15–20 W of monopolar coagulation cautery is used to remove the mass. Caudal traction is placed on the mass with the snare device to prevent it from touching the wall of the colon orad to the mass, which is not easily visualized during the polypectomy. Snare cautery quickly removes the polyp from its base, and the polyp is retrieved from the colonic lumen using the same snare device or an endoscopic basket. Once the mass is removed, it should be submitted for histopathology to confirm margins were obtained. Endoscopic evaluation of the site should then be performed with insufflation to confirm the integrity of the colonic wall. Using a 50% mixture of contrast and saline under fluoroscopic guidance, a colonogram can confirm there is no extravasation or perforation. Endoscopic clips can be used to close any questionable regions if necessary.

As mentioned above, this can be performed successfully in the stomach for gastric polyploid lesions, using the same technique (Figure 15.6). Given the frequent nature of the lesions in the pyloric antrum, occasionally, the lesion will migrate through the pylorus making clear delineation of the polyp base difficult. In these cases, passing the endoscope distal to the lesion and slowly retracting it will help to "pull"

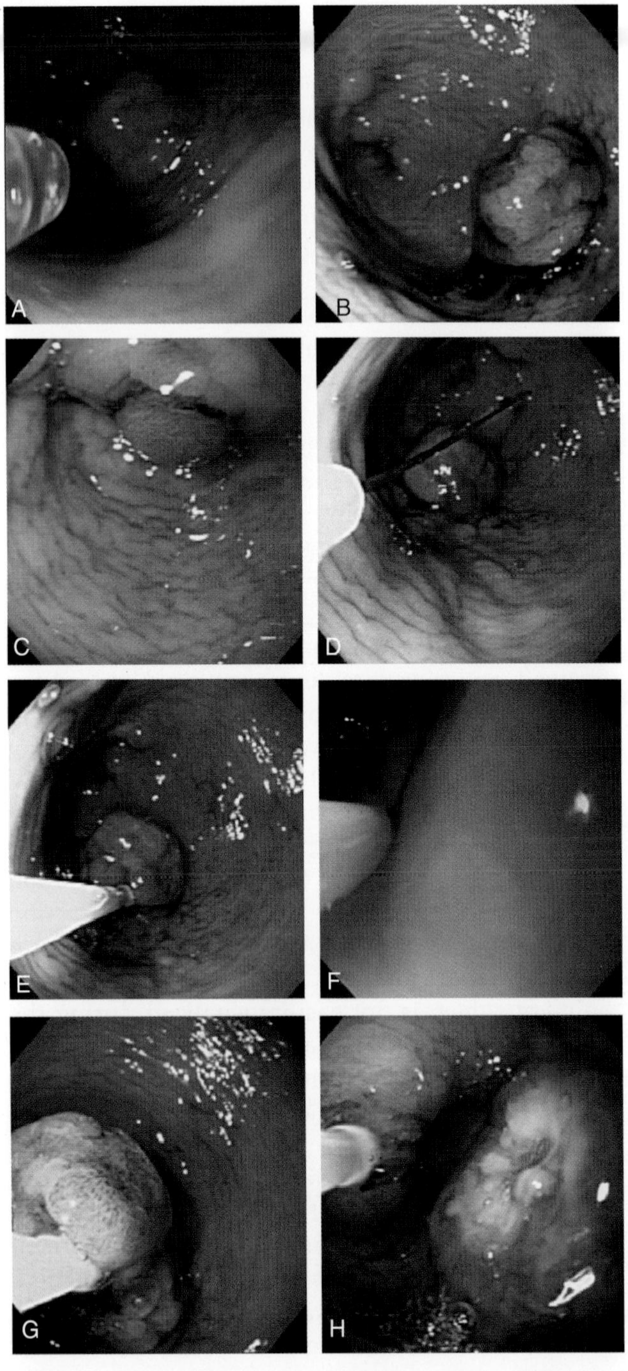

Figure 15.6 Gastric polypectomy using EMR and methylene blue injection. (A) Polypoid mass in the stomach of a cat. (B) Saline and methylene blue is injected at the base of the mass. (C) Lift of the lesion. (D, E) The snare encircles the lesion and is closed down at the base. (F) Perpendicular positioning of the snare helps to encompass the base of the lesion. (G) Cautery is applied and discoloration of the polyp can be observed before removal. (H) removal of the polyp from the surface of the stomach with the lesion free within the gastric lumen.

the polyp through the pylorus and into the stomach (Figure 15.7). The gastric site is inspected for excessive depth of resection. This is thought to be less of a concern in the stomach, due to gastric wall thickness relative to the colon (Figure 15.8).

EMRC (endoscopic mucosal resection with transparent plastic cap-fitted) can be utilized for polypectomy of sessile lesions. After visualization of the lesion, an appropriate cap is attached to the distal end of the endoscope. The appropriate cap is based on the endoscopist's ability to cover the lesion effectively and is largely determined on lesion positioning within the wall and the ability to angle the endoscope perpendicular to the lesion. A sclerotherapy needle is introduced through the working channel and a routine submucosal injection is performed. With the lesion elevated, the cap is centered on the lesion and a crescent shaped snare is inserted through working channel. The snare is opened within the internal diameter of the cap and the cap is pushed up against the surrounding healthy tissue. A brief suction is applied to the lesion, pulling the lesion into the center of the cap, and allowing the snare to loop circumferentially along the rim of the base. Additional suction is applied to the lesion and the snare is closed tightly at the base of the lesion. Suction is then terminated and the target site is observed. If placement is deemed appropriate, the electrosurgical snare device is activated and the lesion is resected (as described above) (Figure 15.9).

Post-Procedural and Follow-Up Care

After gastric polypectomy, the patients are discharged the same day with a proton pump inhibitor (omeprazole) and canned food for the next 3–5 days. Given the low sensitivity of non-invasive imaging and low likelihood of recurrence, no surveillance is indicated unless clinical signs are appreciated. Repeat gastroscopy would be indicated in these cases.

Patients after colorectal polypectomy are sent home the same day with metronidazole and a high fiber diet. There is some thought to use long-term non-steroidal anti-inflammatory therapy in the event there is malignant transformation of the polypoid mass, but this is no longer routinely done in humans. For colonic polyps that were diagnosed on digital palpation monthly rectal examinations should be performed for 3–6 months to confirm the mass does not recur. In humans repeat colonoscopy is recommended in 6–12-month intervals.

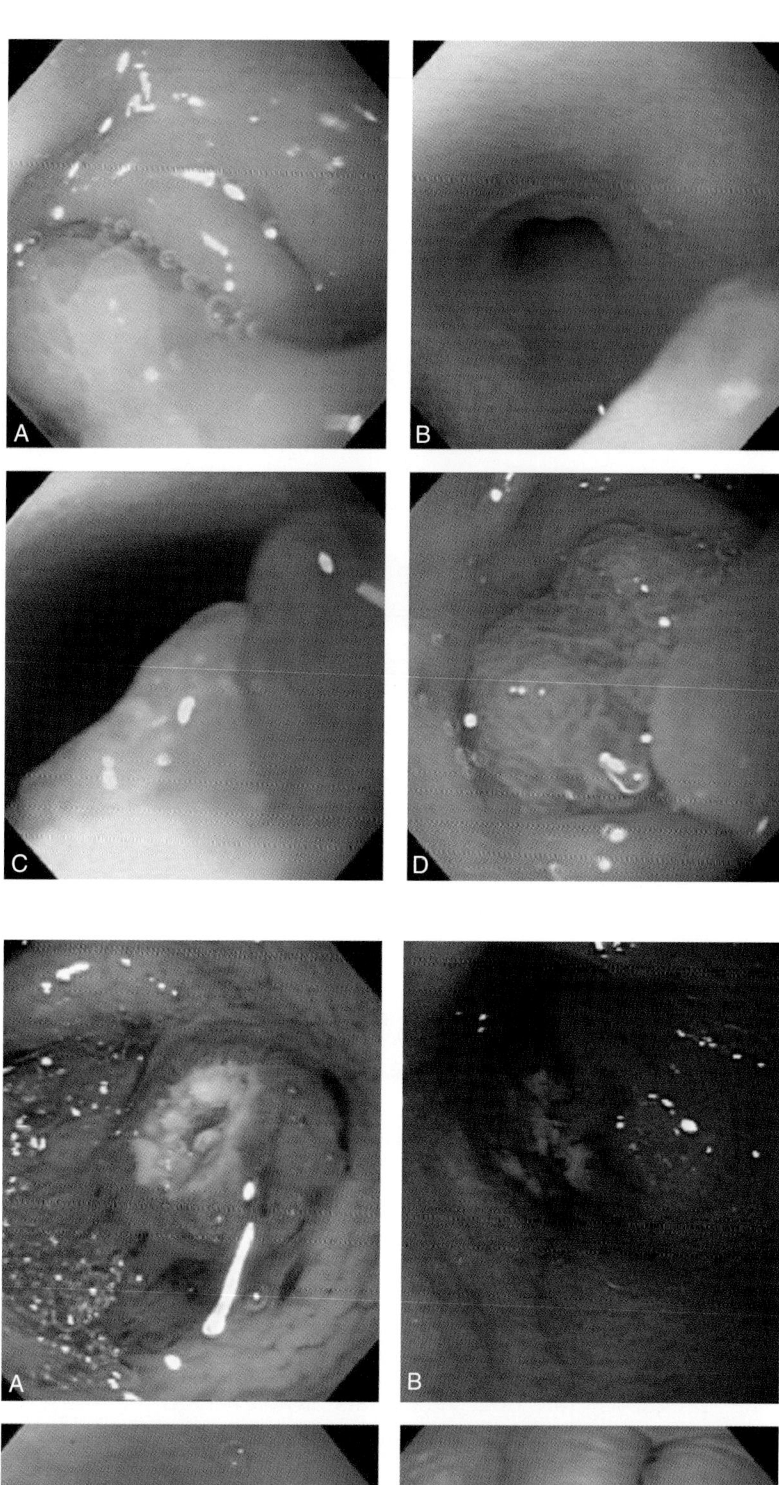

Figure 15.7 Endoscopic images of a gastric polyp in a cat at the pylorus. (A) Note the gastric polyp across the pylorus creating a partial obstruction. (B, C) The endoscope is distal to the polyp into the duodenum. It is slowly retracted and the polyp is pulled into the stomach; note the polyp on the lower right. (D) As the endoscope is retracted the true extent of the polyp can be observed and the based on the polyp more easily accessed.

Figure 15.8 Post gastric polypectomy in 4 different patients. (A) A bleeding polyp that resolved after removal. (B, C) Base after polypectomy. (D) The gastric polyp removed en bloc.

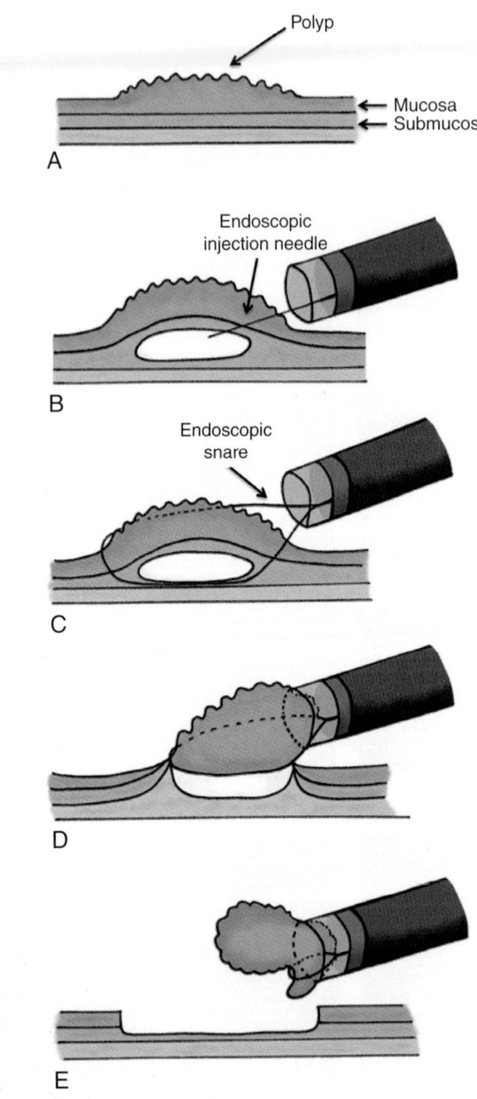

Figure 15.9 Endoscopic mucosal resection with a plastic cap (EMRC). Courtesy of Alice Defarges.

Prognosis

The prognosis for dogs and cats with benign gastrointestinal polyps is excellent after appropriate polypectomy is performed. Those with colonic polyps should be followed more carefully for malignant transformation, as the suggested rate is 7–18%.

Notes

1. 6 mm gastroduodenoscope, XP160, Olympus, Southborough, MA.
2. 9.9 mm gastroduodenoscope, Q160, Olympus, Southborough, MA.
3. Polypectomy snare US endoscopy, Mentor, OH.
4. Polypectomy snare, Olympus, Southborough MA.
5. Cautery machine Valley Lab Force FX, Electrosurgical Generator, Covideien, Boulder, CO.
6. 25 gauge endoscopic injection needle, Olympus, Southborough, MA.
7. EMR transparent plastic-fitted cap (hard straight, soft oblique, and hard oblique), Olympus, Southborough MA.
8. Electrosurgical snares, SnareMaster, Olympus, Southborough, MA.

References

Ally MR, Veerappan GR, Maydonovitch CL, et al (2009) Chronic proton pump inhibitor therapy associated with increased development of fundic gland polyps. *Dig Dis Sci* 54, 2617.

Miller J, Mehta N, Feldman M, et al (2010) Findings on serial surveillance colonoscopy in patients with low-risk polyps on initial colonoscopy. *J Clin Gastroenterol* 44(3), 46–50.

Munakata A and Uno Y (1994). Colonoscopic polypectomy with local injection of methylene blue. *Tohoku J Exp Med* 173, 377–82.

Suggested Reading

Church EM, Mehlhaff CJ, and Patnaik AK (1987) Colorectal adenocarcinoma in dogs: 78 cases (1973–1984). *J Am Vet Med Assoc* 191, 727–30.

Fyock CJ and Draganov PV. (2010) Colonoscopic polypectomy and associated techniques. *World J Gastroenterol* 16(29), 3630–7.

Gencosmanoglu R, Sen-Oran E, Kurtkaya-Yapicier O, et al (2003) Gastric polypoid lesions: analysis of 150 endoscopic polypectomy specimens from 91 patients. *World J Gastroenterol* 9 (10), 2236–9.

Ginsberg GG, Al-Kawas FH, Fleischer DE, et al (1996) Gastric polyps: relationship of size and histology to cancer risk. *Am J Gastroenterol* 91(4), 714.

Goddard AF,Badreldin R, Pritchard DM, et al. (2010) The management of gastric polyps. *Gut*. 59,1270.

Morais DJ, Yamanaka A, Zeitune JM, et al (2007) Gastric polyps: a retrospective analysis of 26,000 digestive endoscopies. *Arq Gastroenterol* 44(1),14

Park DY, et al. (2008) Gastric polyps: Classification and management. *Arch Pathol Lab Med*132, 633.

Valerius KD, Powers BE, McPherron MA, et al (1997) Adenomatous polyps and carcinoma in situ of the canine colon and rectum: 34 cases (1982–1994). *J Am Anim Hosp Assoc* 33, 156–60.

Waye JD and Lauwers GY (1997) New methods of polypectomy. *Gastrointest Endosc Clin N Am* 7, 413–22.

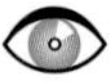 Video clips to accompany this chapter can be found in the online material at **www.wiley.com/go/weisse/vet-image-guided-interventions**

CHAPTER SIXTEEN

PEG Tube Placement

Douglas A. Palma
The Animal Medical Center, New York, NY

Background/Indications

Gastrostomy tubes are indicated for patients with disease of the esophagus, oropharyngeal cavity, or patients with chronic disease that require long-term feeding supplementation. These tubes can be placed percutaneously, surgically, or endoscopically. Percutaneous endoscopic gastrostomy tubes (PEG) are often the preferred method of gastric tube placement because visibility is ideal and the procedure is fast, effective, and safe. The benefit of a gastrostomy tube is that it is a larger diameter tube than esophagostomy, nasoesophageal/nasogastric, and jejunostomy tubes, increasing the versatility in dietary selection for patients. Additionally, they offer the ability to perform gastric suctioning in patients with delayed gastric emptying and/or high aspiration risk, and provide access to the stomach for the placement of a gastrojejunostomy tube when necessary. Surgically placed gastrotomy tubes are generally elected when wound healing is in question or if a laparotomy is required. These tubes offer the benefit of creating an adhesion between the stomach and body wall, ensuring stoma formation and minimizing complication risk. Non-endoscopic methods of placement have been described using an eld, or percutaneous gastrostomy tube placing, device. This method involves non-visualized placement of a gastrostomy tube and offers a viable alternative when diagnostic endoscopy is not needed; however, complication rates may be higher when anatomy is not visualized during placement. This procedure is beyond the scope of this chapter. See Chapter 18 for more details of other methods of interventional nutrition management.

Potential Risks/Complications/Expected Outcomes

While uncommon, clinicians should be aware of the potential complications associated with PEG tube placement and maintenance. The most common complications in our practice include PEG tube insertion site infection, peristomal pain, peristomal leakage, chewing of tube by the patient, inadvertent dislodgement, and tube occlusion. Other less common complications include injury to bystander organs during insertion of the catheter/sytlet (e.g., spleen, colon, small intestine and hepatic), bleeding (e.g., intraperitoneal, gastrointestinal, hepatic, abdominal wall), buried bumper syndrome, and gastric outflow obstruction.

A common problem with PEG tubes is cracking or ripping of the feeding tube or feeding adaptor, which commonly occurs over time. Generally, replacement adapters can be used otherwise exchange for a low-profile tube can be done (Figure 16.1).

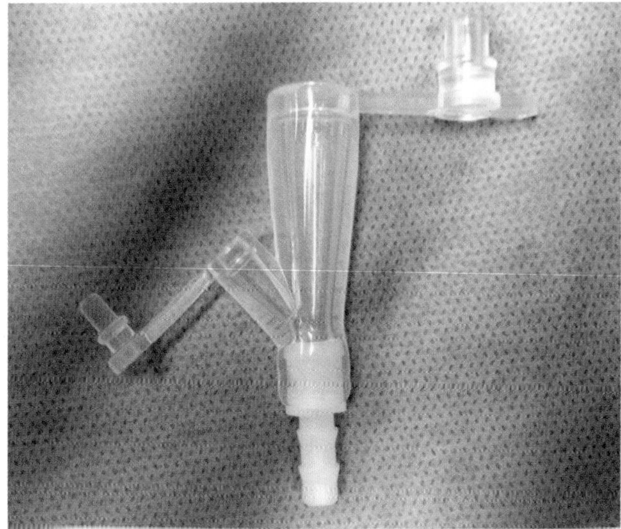

Figure 16.1 Replacement injection adaptor for the PEG tube.

Equipment

A standard gastroduodenoscope is utilized to facilitate placement of the feeding tube. PEG tubes are made by multiple manufacturers. These manufacturers make

Veterinary Image-Guided Interventions, First Edition. Edited by Chick Weisse and Allyson Berent.

Companion website: www.wiley.com/go/weisse/vet-image-guided-interventions

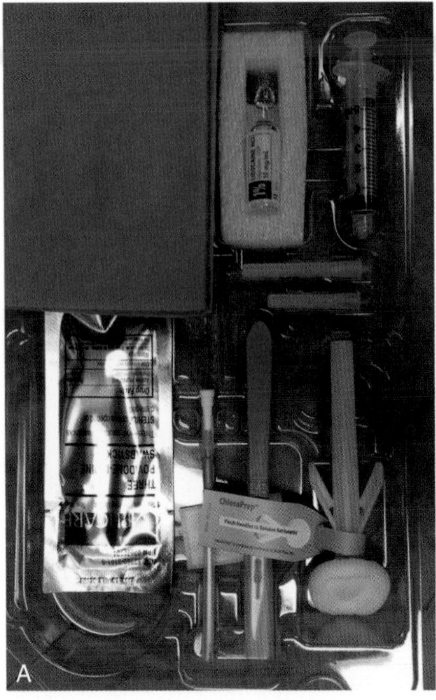

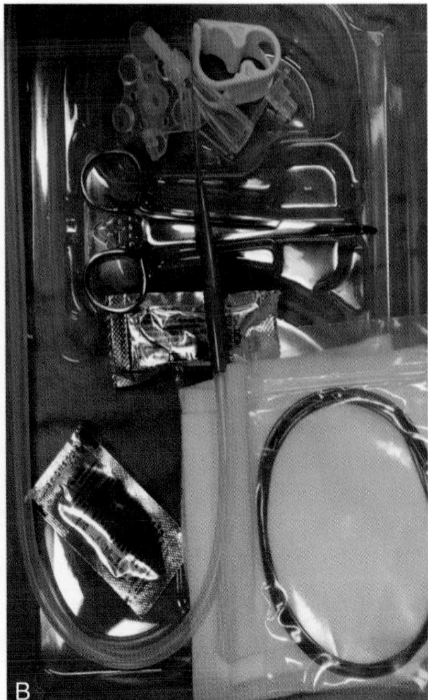

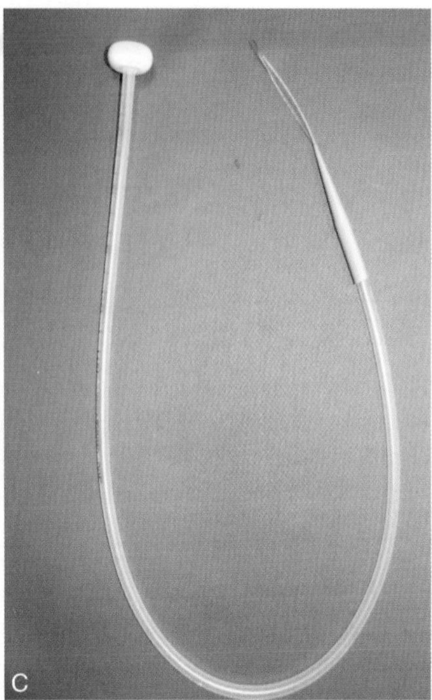

Figure 16.2 (A, B) Commercially available PEG tube kit containing all the necessary equipment needed for placement. (C) Standard PEG tube; note the tapered end with a snare and the mushroom style feeding tube.

"PEG tube kits"[1,2,3,4] that include everything one would need for placement of the feeding tube (Figure 16.2). These kits include the following basic pieces of equipment: gastrostomy tube, over the needle catheter, snare/wire, lubrication, materials for aseptic preparation, sterile drapes for aseptic technique, and local anesthetics for multi-modal analgesia. While these kits are not necessary, they are extremely convenient. The tubes are usually 16–24 French diameter.

For placement of a low-profile feeding tube (Figure 16.3) through an existing stoma a measuring device is needed to know the appropriate tube length in order to maintain the appropriate fit (Figure 16.4). Various commercially available low-profile feeding tubes are available from multiple manufacturers[5,6,7,8] (Figure 16.3). The low-profile tube diameter is selected based on the initial PEG tube diameter, with selection of an equal or lesser external diameter. For initial placement of a low profile feeding tube, only one manufacturer makes a tube that can be placed without an intact stoma [9] (Figure 16.3D).

Patient Preparation

Patients should be fasted for a minimum of 12 hours prior to the procedure to facilitate gastric emptying and visualization. The patient is generally positioned in right lateral recumbency. Traditional upper endoscopic techniques and complete evaluation of the pylorus, pyloric antrum, and duodenum are not easily performed in this position. It should be noted that body positioning can influence the difficulty of this procedure, which is most notable in large, deep-chested patients. Occasionally, placing the patient on a slight incline (reverse Trendelenberg), and/or placing a sandbag under the thorax, will move the stomach caudally, away from the ribs.

Procedure

The patient is placed in right lateral recumbency and the left lateral caudal thoracic/cranial abdomen region is clipped. The clipping should extend from the dorsal foramina to the sternum, including the entire abdominal wall between. The region is aseptically prepared and draped. Prophylactic antibiotic therapy (cefazolin 22 mg/kg or cefoxitin 30 mg/kg) is given within 30 minutes of the procedure.

The patient is placed into right lateral recumbency for PEG tube placement and the area mentioned above is clipped, asceptically prepared and draped (Figure 16.5). The stomach is distended with air via endoscopic insufflation until the rugal folds are flattened and the wall is percutaneously palpable. This may

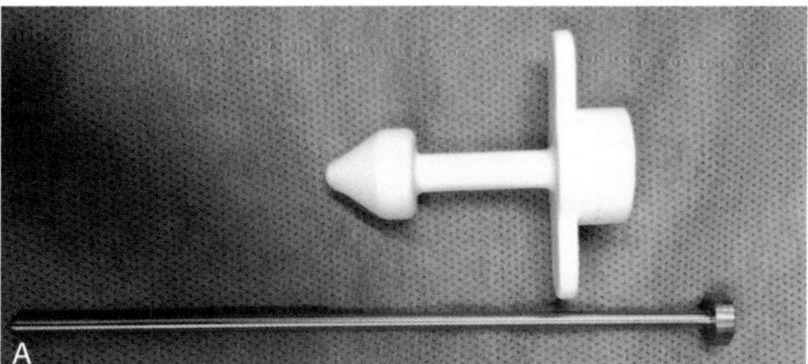

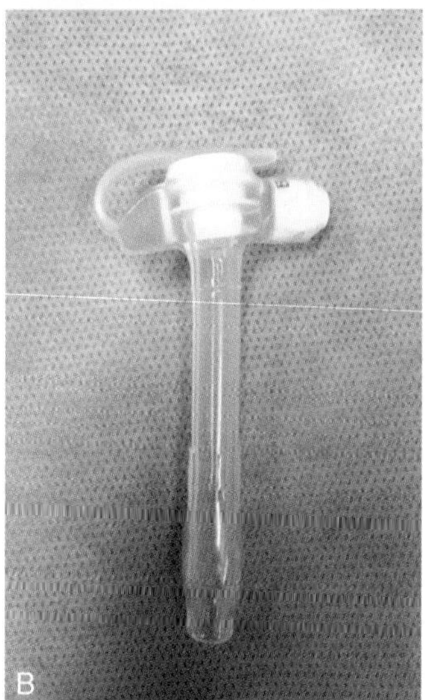

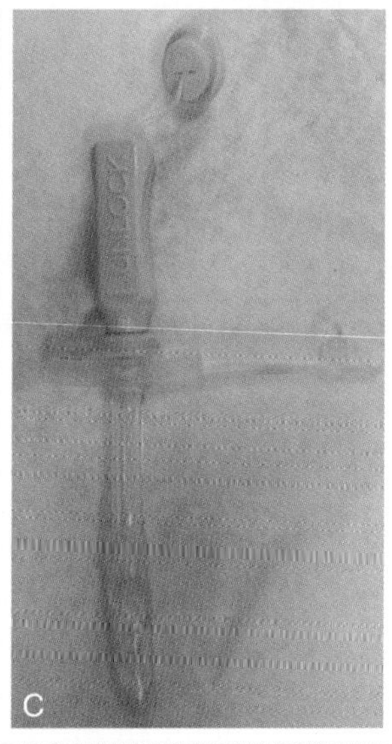

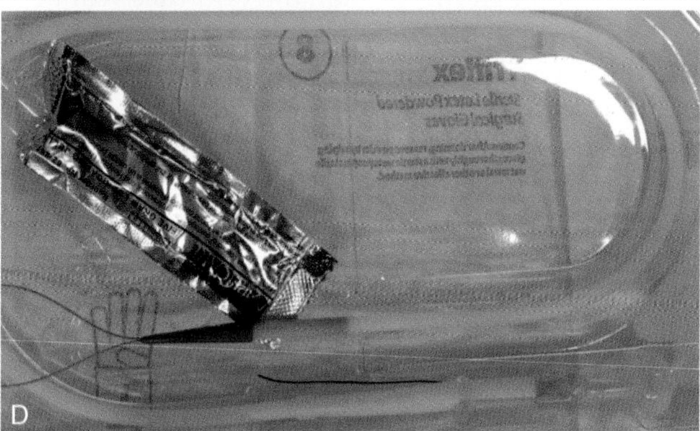

Figure 16.3 Commercially available low profile (LP) feeding tubes. (A) styleted LP feeding tube. (B) Non-styleted, balloon inflatable LP feeding tube. (C) Non-styleted, non-balloon inflatable, capsule type LP feeding tube. (D) One step button; note that this is looks like a traditional PEG tube prior to deployment.

require digital cervical compression to maintain distension in some patients. With the stomach distended, the assistant will sterilely palpate the fundus digitally with the endoscopist guiding the optimal region for catheter assess (Figure 16.6). This is typically caudal to the last rib by about 2–5 cm and halfway between the xiphoid and transverse process of the vertebrae, aiming at an approximate 45 degree angle cranially. When this location is noted, a small stab incision in made in the skin. The light of the endoscope should be seen illuminating through the body wall, and this helps ensure that the spleen is not sitting between the stomach and the body wall. Conversely, the stomach can be illuminated through the body wall without a superficial incision (Figure 16.5). Then, the assistant takes the over-the-needle introducer catheter (14 g), and places it through the abdominal wall at the desired site of insertion. This is typically done with a rapid thrust to penetrate the gastric wall. If the needle is not inserted with force, the stomach wall will push away from the needle and it may not pierce the mucosa. If the catheter does not penetrate the lumen the catheter should be re-directed perpendicular to the gastric lumen while the stomach remains insufflated. Occasionally, rotating the catheter with the sharp needle/stylet will help to remove residual tissue (Figure 16.6). Special positioning techniques, like raising the head and thorax above the abdomen (reverse Trendelenberg) can be employed to facilitate gastric penetration in larger patients.

Once the stomach wall is penetrated, the stylet is removed and the catheter covered digitally to prevent air from escaping, aiding to keep the stomach distended. Continued pressure should be applied to the catheter to prevent backing out/loss of the catheter. The assistant quickly places the snare end of the guide wire, which comes with the PEG tube set, through the catheter and into the gastric lumen (Figure 16.6 and Figure 16.7). The assistant should pass enough wire into the gastric lumen to aid grasping while simultaneously preventing the catheter from backing out. The endoscopic instrumentation (grasper, loop) are used to grasp the end of the snare. The instrument is gently retracted until it reaches the tip of the endoscope and is stabilized as the scope/wire/grasping instrument are slowly retracted retrograde out of the mouth. Slack should remain on the wire as it is pulled through the catheter and out the mouth. This provides through-and-through wire access. After the wire is released the snare is secured to the tapered end of the gastrotomy tube (Figure 16.7) Most commercially available tubes have one end with a "mushroom" tip and the other end with a tapered adaptor with a snare loop swaged onto it. This will facilitate securing the wire snare to the tube snare. If a snare or wire is not present on the distal end of the PEG tube than the through-and-through wire can be passed through the end of the tube using a large gauge needle (Figure 16.8). When secure, sterile lubrication is applied to the entire tube and tapered end/wire, and the assistant provides traction on the wire from the

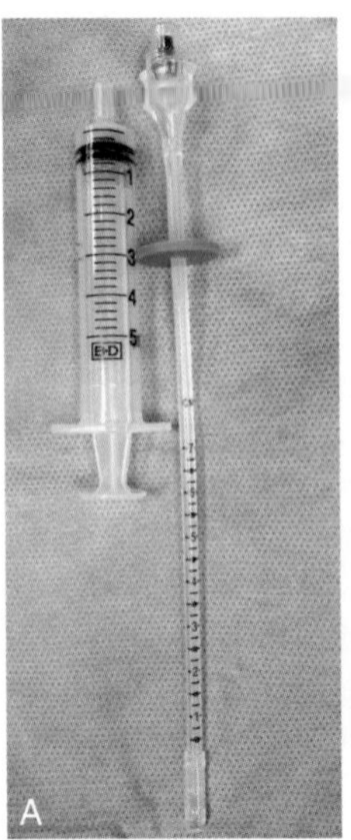
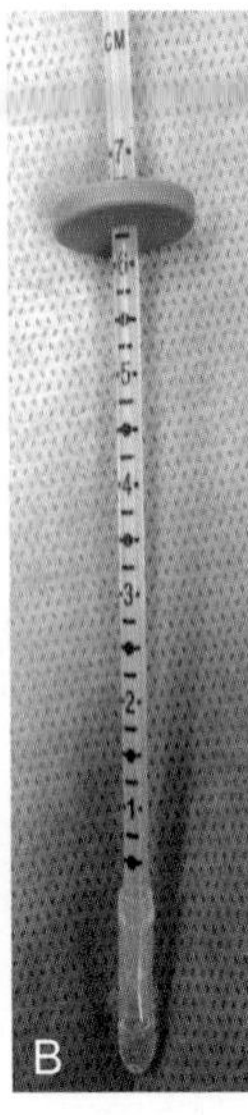
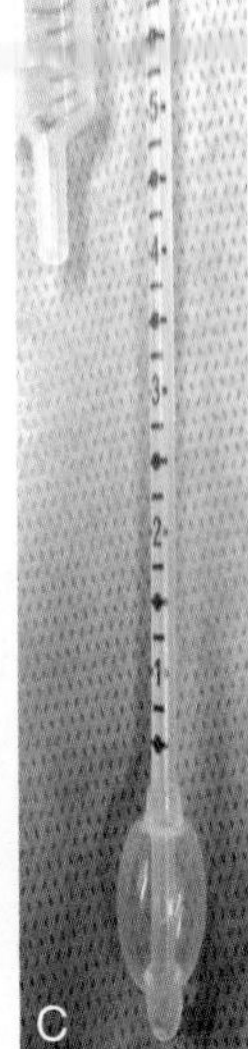
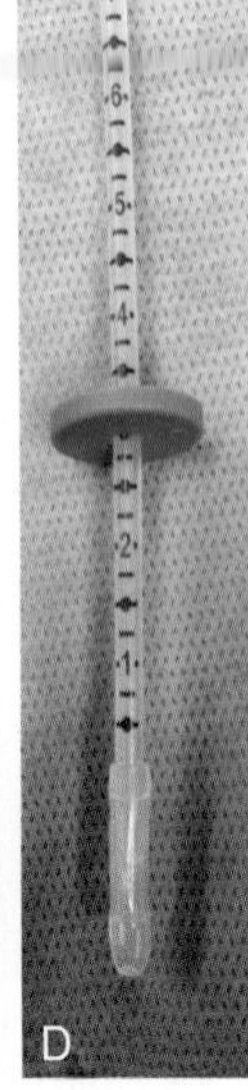
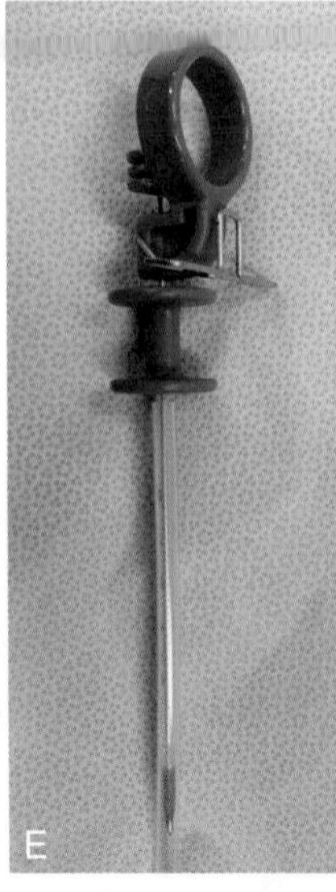

Figure 16.4 Stoma measuring device. (A, B) The balloon is distended within the stomach and pulled to the body wall. (C, D) The external marker is slid down to the body wall, marking the appropriate LP tube length. (E. One-step percutaneous stoma measuring device (PSMD).

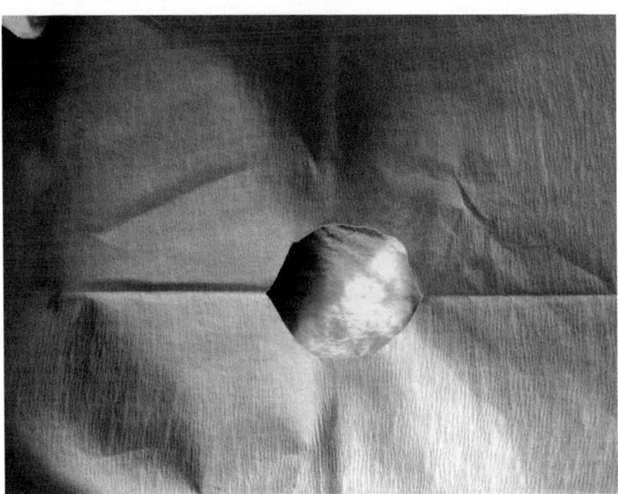

Figure 16.5 Illuminated stomach wall; the illumination is more pronounced when the external lights are turned down.

body wall as the distal end of the tube is pulled. The endoscopist ensures that the mouth is opened wide and that the tube does not encircle the endotracheal tube, anesthetic "ties", or monitoring equipment during passage (Figure 16.9). As the PEG tube moves aborally, resistance is often met at the sphincters (i.e., cricopharyngeal and gastroesophageal), and again at the insertion site through the body wall. With continued tension, the tapered end of the tube will appear at the surface of the skin and can then be pulled through the body wall gently. If necessary, the stab incision initially made may need to be extended to assist in pulling the tube through the body wall and skin. The tube is gently retracted until the mushroom/button is flush with the gastric wall. This should be assessed with the endoscope to ensure that the tube is not too tight to result in pressure necrosis, but tight enough that a gastropexy can form (Figure 16.10 and Figure 16.11). External markings on the tube help ensure that the tube is pulled to the body wall and not meeting resistance at the lower esophageal sphincter (Figure 16.10).

To maintain air insufflation the PEG tube will need to be clamped at the end otherwise air will escape and the endoscopist will not get a great visualization of the tube length. Once the length of the PEG tube is considered ideal the distal end of the tube outside of the body wall is cut, leaving about 5–8 cm of length, so that it fits into the appropriate adaptor (Figure 16.12). Each tube has a different method to secure to the body wall. One way is with a rubber stopper, which is placed over the tube and contacts the skin. An alternative is to use a hand-made flange from the excessive tube material (Figure 16.12). Hemostats can be used to open the hole in the rubber stopper or flange, and facilitate sliding it down the tube. The rubber stopper is slid to the body wall and generally should be slightly snug but not tight, which is generally about 0.5 cm from the body wall (Figure 16.13). The tube should be able to rotate comfortably with some in-and-out freedom to prevent pressure necrosis. Tissue swelling and external contact of the stopper with the body wall can result in tissue devitalization of the skin, muscle and gastric wall; this is limited by reducing tension. The open-ended tube is then closed with the provided injector cap (Figure 16.1). Routinely, in our hospital, we reinforce the junction between the injection port and the tube using a cable tie, as this can occasionally become dislodged at home.

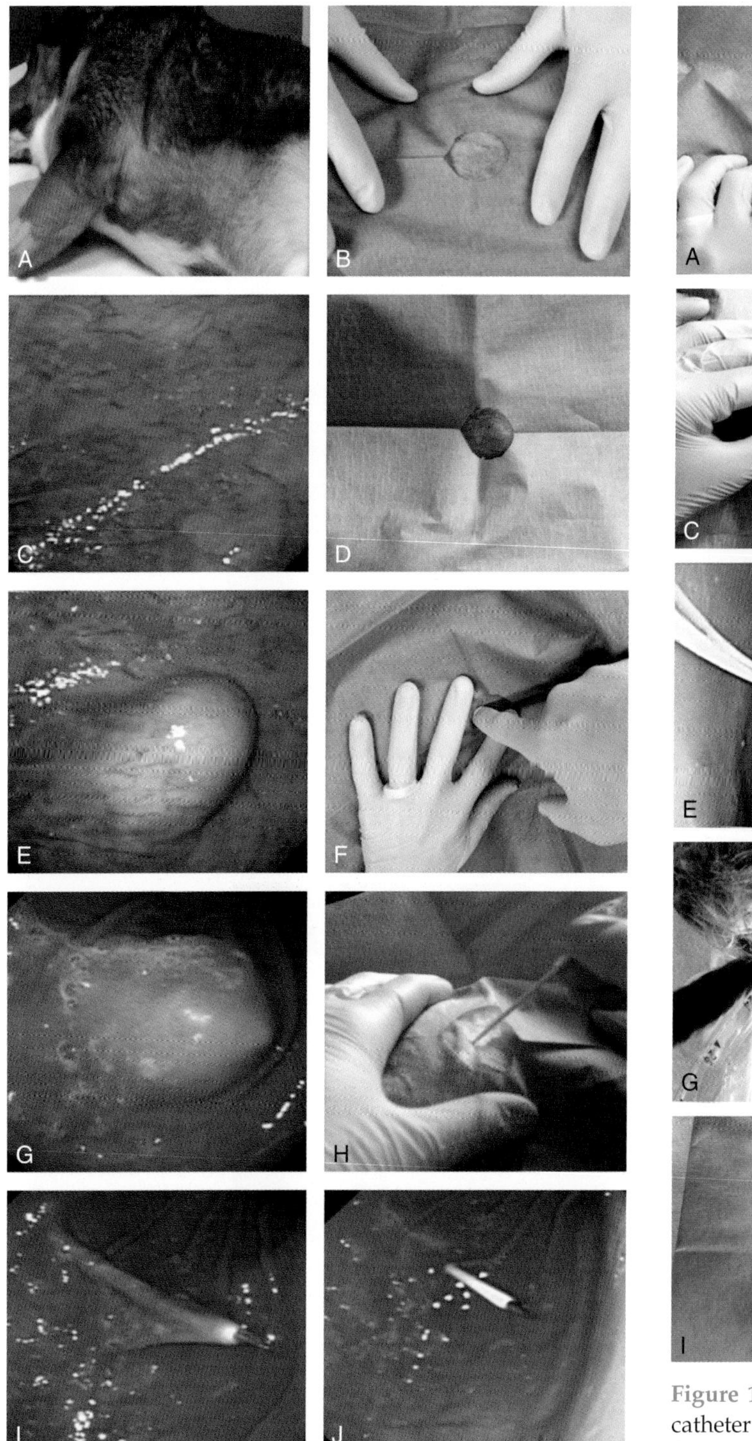

Figure 16.6 Placement of a PEG tube in a dog. (A) the patient is placed in right lateral recumbency. (B) The dog is draped just caudal to the last rib. (C) Endoscopic image of the gastric fundus when it is distended. (D–F) Through the drape at that location the stomach is digitally palpated to confirm appropriate puncture site. (G) The needle is used to puncture the gastric wall at a 45 degree angle, penetrating the gastric lumen (I, J).

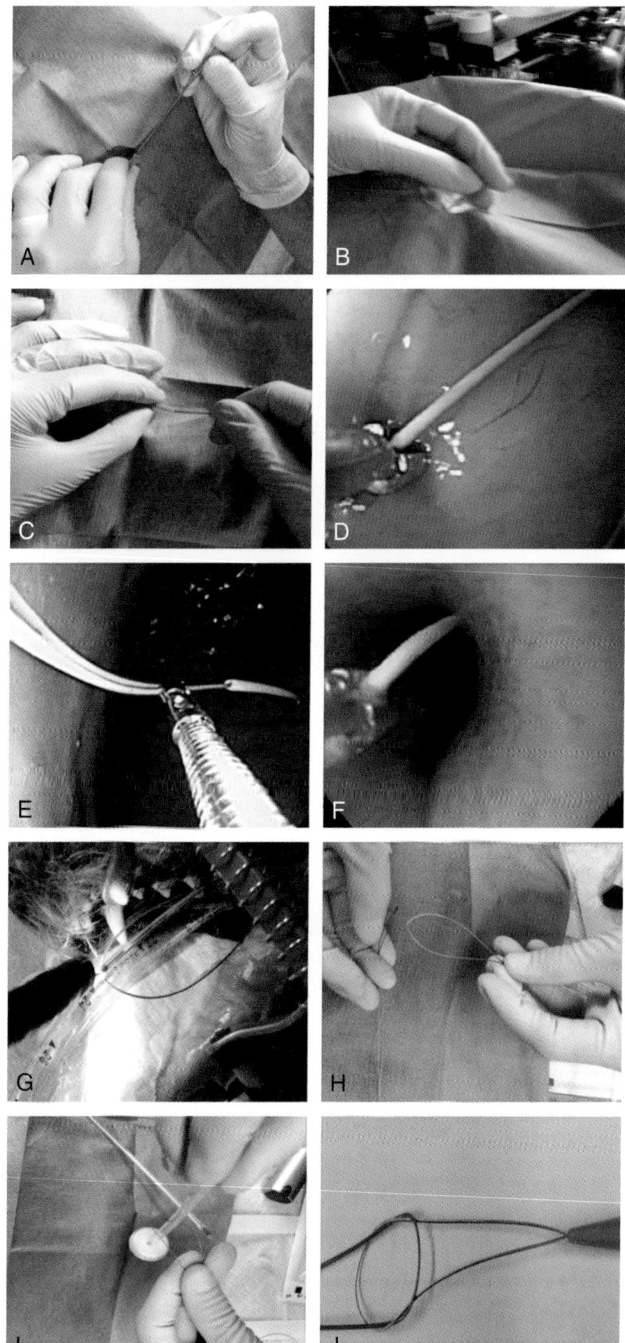

Figure 16.7 Placement of the snare through the introducer catheter for PEG tube placement. (A) Removal of the stylet from the catheter. (B) Illumination from the endoscope seen through the drape. The catheter tip is covered to prevent air escape. (C) Guide wire/snare being advanced through the catheter and into the stomach. (D) Wire entrapped with an endoscopic grasper in the stomach and pulled into the esophagus (E, F) and out of the mouth (G). (H–J) the swaged wire on the PEG tube is attached to the wire loop that is coming from the mouth. This can be accomplished by placing the wire loop through the swaged wire, then advancing the distal end of the PEG tube through the wire loop. This will interlock the two.

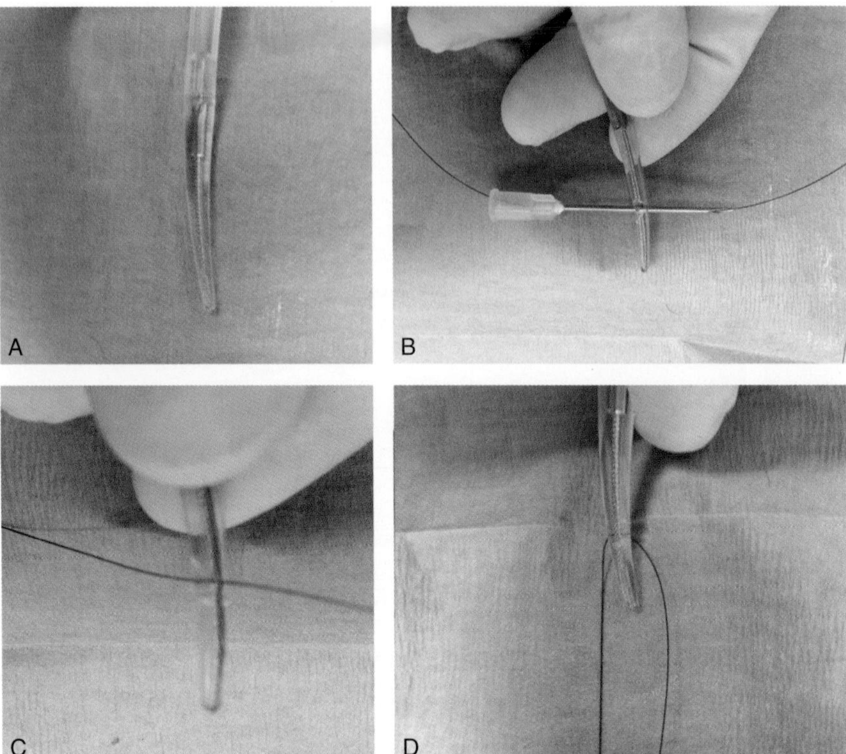

Figure 16.8 PEG tube without wire snare (A–D); the PEG tube is secured with suture before pulling the PEG tube through the body wall.

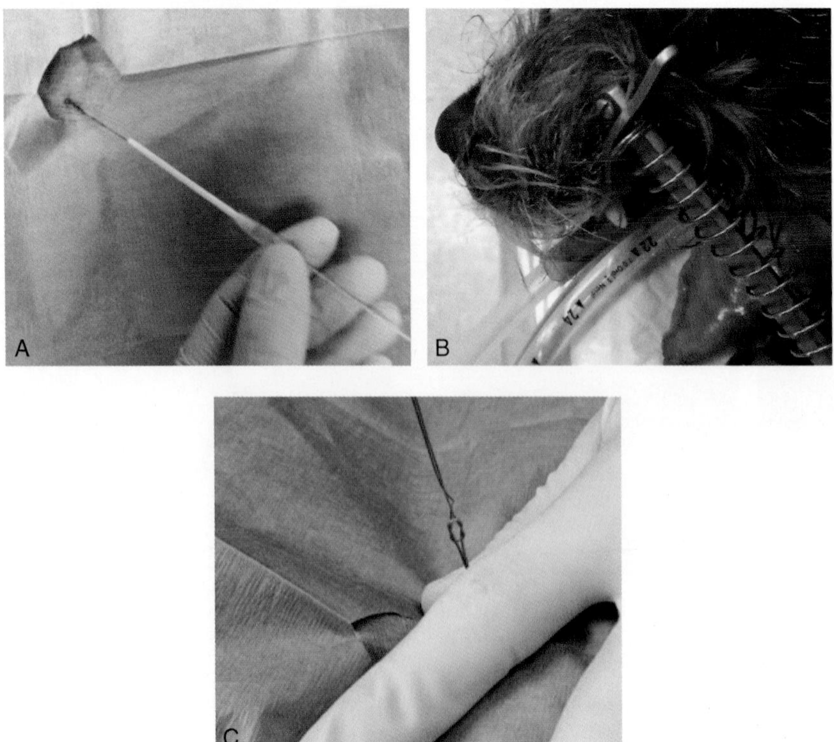

Figure 16.9 Pulling the PEG tube into the stomach. (A) The catheter is removed from the wire externally. (B) The tube is well lubricated and slowly retracted and assisted into the mouth and down the esophagus carefully, as the assistant provides tension on the wire outside the body. Note that the catheter has been removed at this time. (C) The junction of the two wires connecting the PEG tube and the snare wire guide are pulled through the body wall as the tapered end of the PEG tube reaches the body wall.

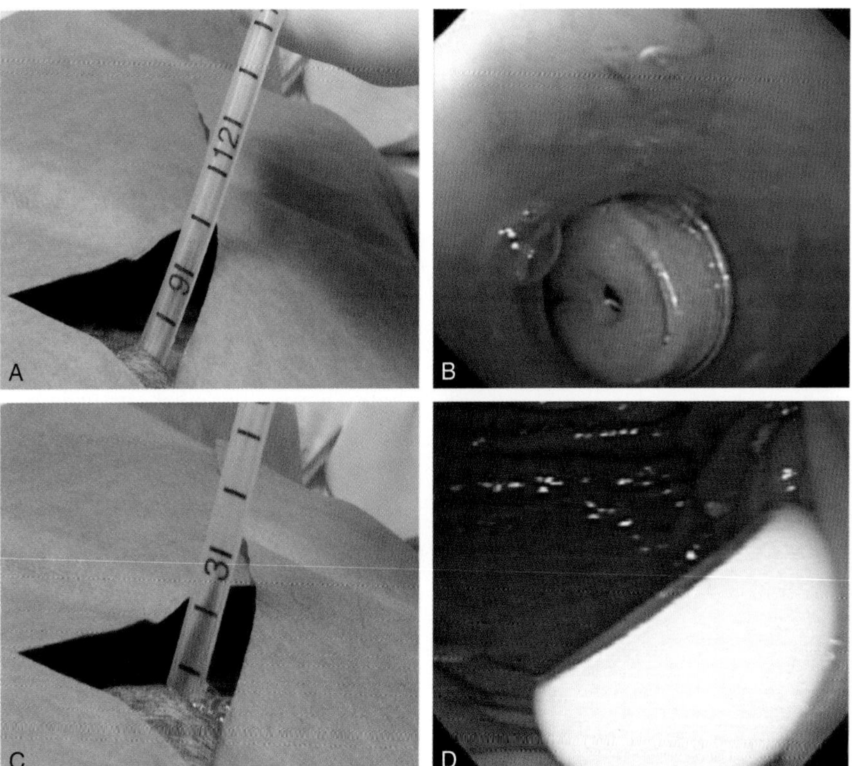

Figure 16.10 Pulling the PEG tube through the body wall. (A) Once the tapered end comes through the body wall the measuring units on the PEG tube can be visualized. The tube is pulled gently. (B) The endoscope can be used to monitor the location of the button to wnsure it is being appropriately passed through the lower esophageal sphincter. (C) Once the 2–3 cm marks are seen the tube is usually against the gastric lumen as visualized and confirmed endoscopically (D).

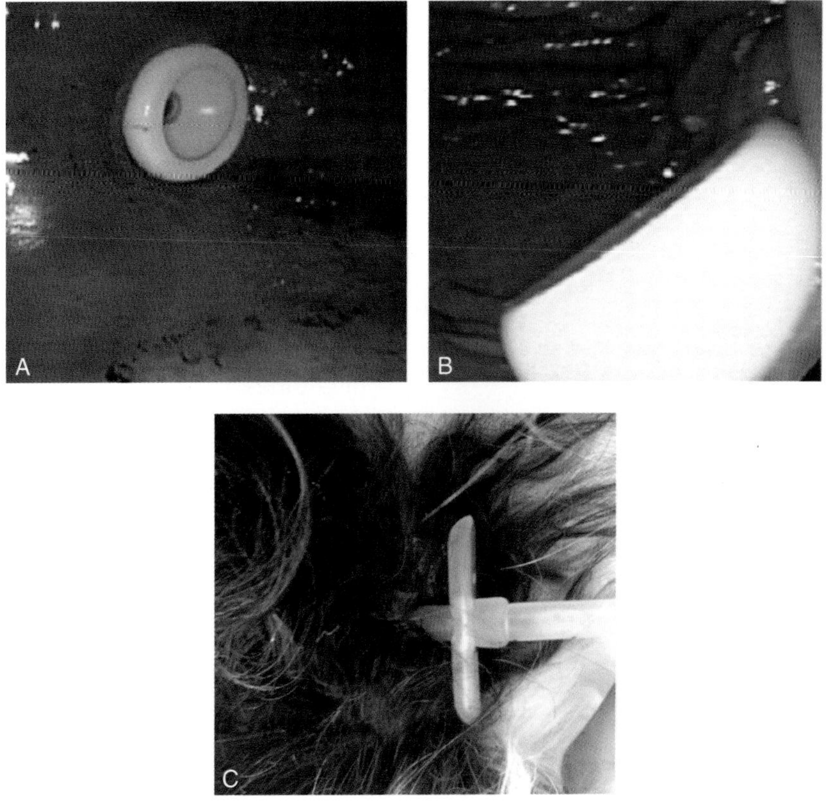

Figure 16.11 The button of the PEG tube making appropriate contact with the gastric mucosa.

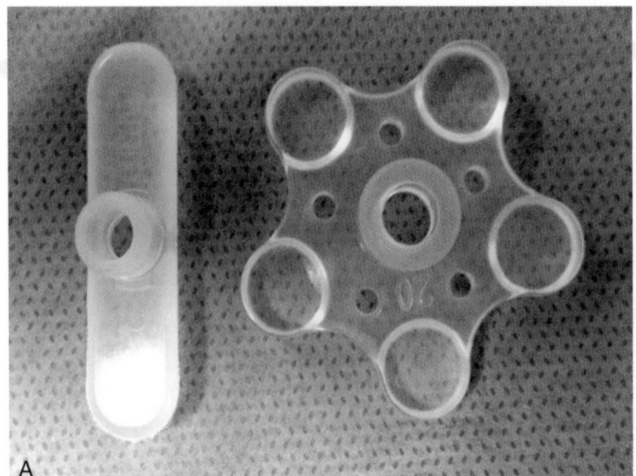

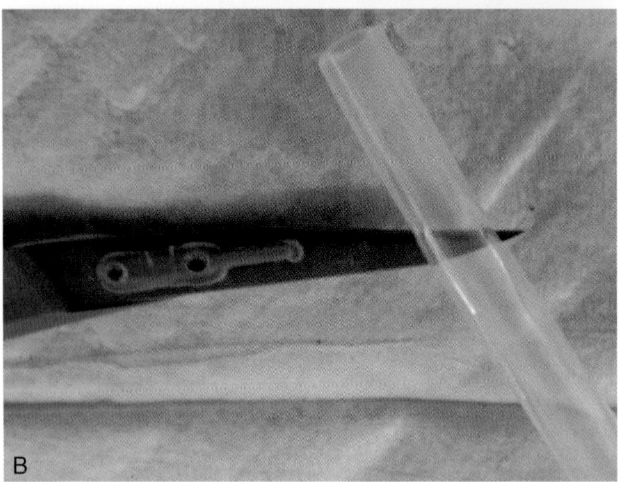

Figure 16.12 (A) Different external bolsters provided with the PEG tube kit. (B) A makeshift bolster from feeding tube

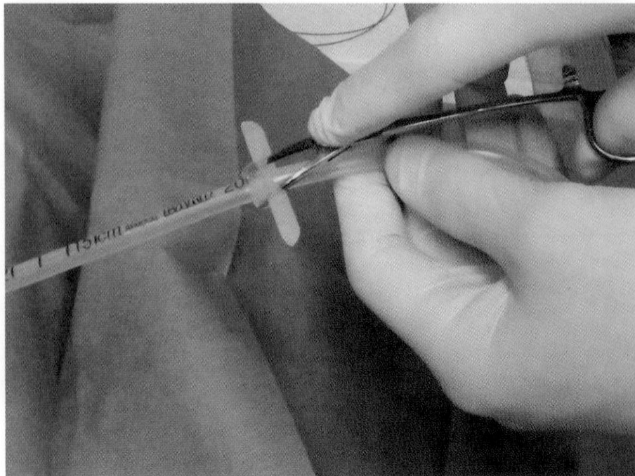

Figure 16.13 The bolster is advanced down the PEG tube to the body wall.

Post-Procedural and Follow-Up Care

The patient is typically discharged the same day of the procedure. The stoma site is allowed to form a seal for 12–24 hours before initiating feeding through the tube. Controversial evidence in human medicine is advocating early enteral feeding after PEG tube placement (6–12 hours), versus the standard-of-care, which is 24 hours after tube placement. The tube is kept covered at all times, to prevent iatrogenic trauma with either a belly wrap, Tee-shirt, or Velcro band. The client is instructed to monitor for discharge, redness or pain at the stoma site, and the site should be cleaned with warm water, hydrogen peroxide, and then triple antibiotic ointment, daily for the first week. The owner is instructed to observe the PEG tube daily for migration/dislodgement.

If any abnormalities are noted at the tube site, migration of the tube is observed, or if pain, redness or discharge is noted, feedings should be withheld, and the patient should be evaluated immediately (Figure 16.14). The author frequently uses prophylactic antibiotics on insertion of the tube to reduce postoperative infection but does not discharge patients with continued antibiotic therapy.

Tube Removal

The PEG tube can be removed at 2–6 weeks after placement, following the formation of a secure stoma (seal between the stomach and body wall). The tubes can be removed by one of three methods: (1) External traction, (2) cutting and recovering, (3) cutting and release. The author only advises the first two techniques. The patient should be fasted for 12 hours prior to and after tube removal. For external traction, it is important that you know the type of tube that was placed, to ensure it can be removed this way. Not all PEG tubes are recommended to be extracted by traction, and some require endoscopic assistance. External traction involves firm back tension on the externalized portion of the tube with your dominant hand while simultaneously pushing the body wall away with your non-dominant hand. Generally, gauze is held in your non-dominant hand to prevent gastric contents from becoming extruded during removal. This should be done quickly, as this can occasionally be uncomfortable to patients (Figure 16.15).

While commonly recommended for children, cutting and recovering of the tube is rarely necessary in our patients, and is reserved for those that require a second endoscopic evaluation. The rubber stopper is backed

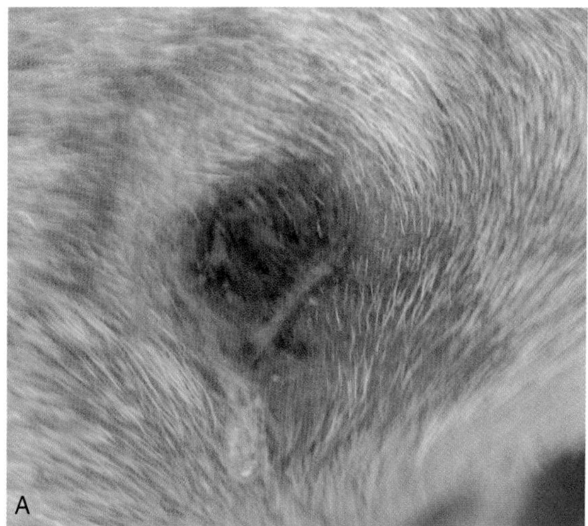

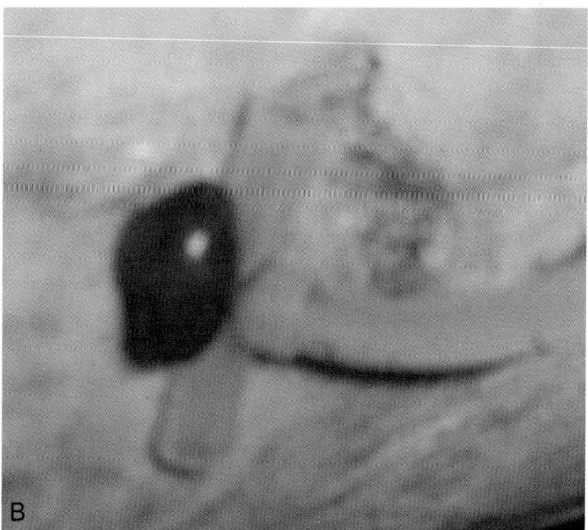

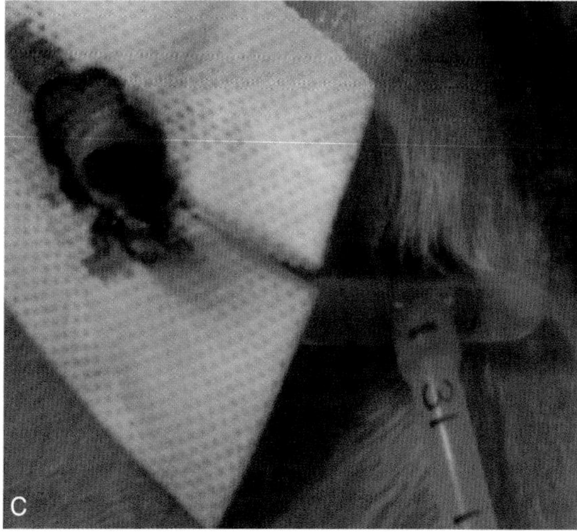

Figure 16.14 PEG tube stomas in three dogs. (A) A mature stoma site. Pigmentation at the site is common. In this case discharge is minimal, the area is non-painful and flat.(B) Abnormal tissue seen at the stoma site. This tissue migrated through the body wall between the feeding tube and gastric lumen. (C) Excessive discharge and a localized infection at a stoma site.

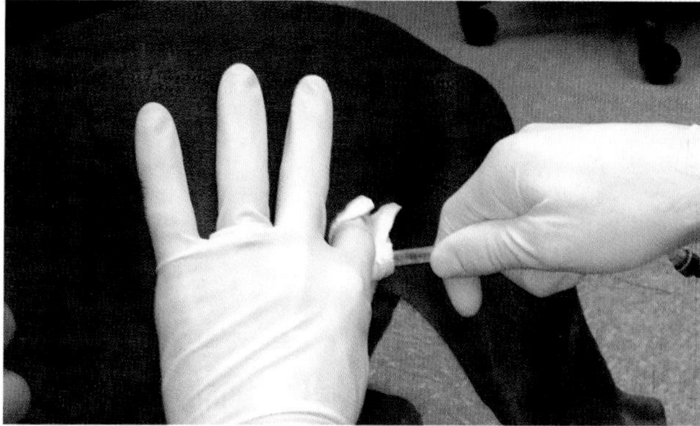

Figure 16.15 PEG tube removal. The stoma site is covered with gauze with the non-dominant hand and the feeding tube is grasped with the dominant hand. As the body wall is pushed inward and the PEG tube pulled outward, the mushroom collapses and is removed.

up to allow for tube movement. The stomach is insufflated and the tube is identified. The tube is pushed into the stomach to facilitate grasping. The endoscopist uses a standard polypectomy snare or grasping instrument to either encircle or grab the base of the mushroom tip. When the loop or instrument is engaged, the tube is cut between the body wall and the rubber stopper. The loop is retracted to the distal end of the endoscope and both are removed out of the mouth.

The cut and release technique involves cutting the tube at its base and allowing movement throughout the intestinal tract. This could be utilized in larger dogs, though concerns regarding gastrointestinal obstructions make this technique ill-advised in most patients.

Following tube removal a non-occlusive bandage is applied and a gentle abdominal wrap is placed for 24–48 hours, after which time it is removed. This is to reduce gastric contents from leaking, allowing time for a seal to occur. Food can be given per os 12 hours after PEG tube removal.

Low Profile Tubes

These tubes are flush with the body wall, giving a more cosmetic appearance, and decreasing the risk of tube dislodgment by entrapment on exterior objects (Figure 16.3 and Figure 16.16). These tubes are generally reserved for patients requiring long-term enteral demands. They have a low complication rate and have a high owner satisfaction. They should only be placed percutaneously after a secure gastropexy and stoma have been accomplished with a traditional PEG or surgically placed G-tube. Feedings are completed by attaching the detachable tubing to the low profile port (Figure 16.17).

The stoma tract (between the stomach and body wall) begins to mature in 1–2 weeks and is well formed

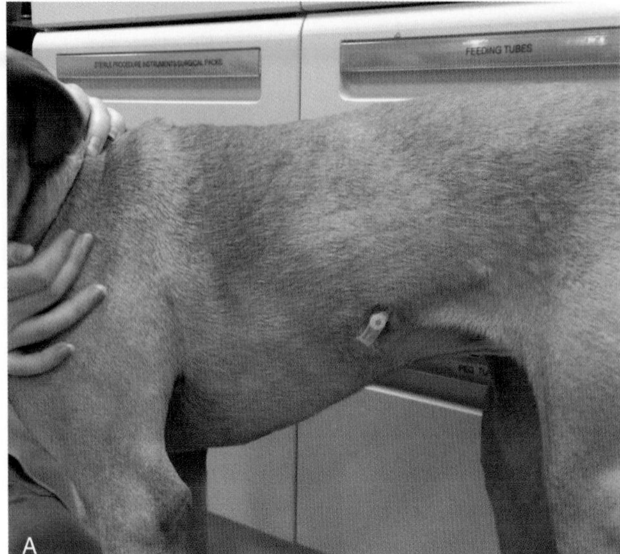

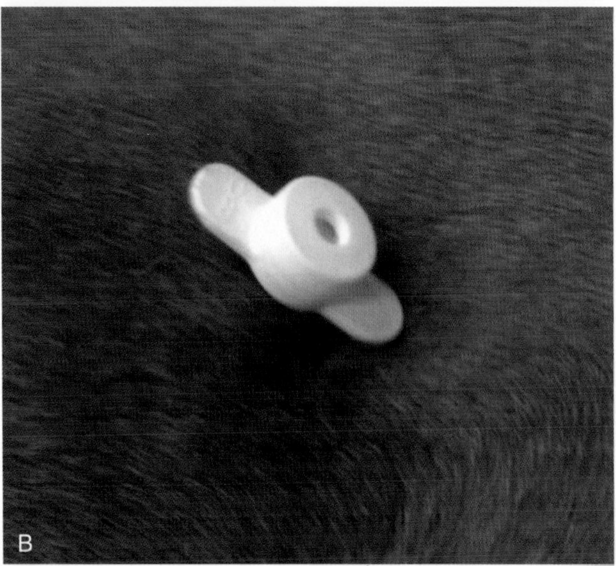

Figure 16.16 Low-profile feeding tube in a dog.

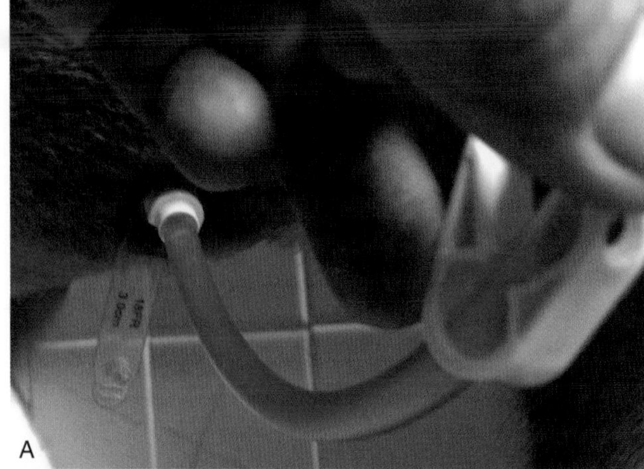

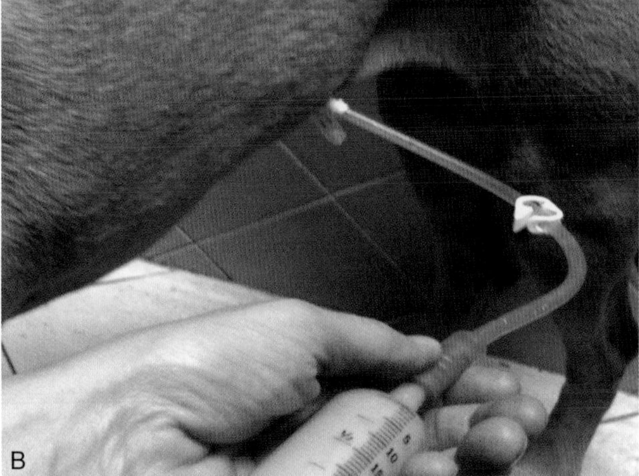

Figure 16.17 Attaching tubing to low profile feeding tube for feeding administration.

in 4–6 weeks (Lohsiriwat, 2013). The author recommends waiting a minimum of 1 month prior to removal of a traditional PEG tube and replacement with a low profile feeding tube. This will ensure a well formed stoma tract prior to insertion.

A tube of the same external diameter, or slightly smaller, should be used. The tube length is chosen based on the length between the skin surface and the gastric mucosa. This is measured with a measuring device or Foley catheter. Most dogs and cats need a 1.5–2.5 cm tube length. Once the PEG tube is removed, the measuring catheter can be inserted into the gastric lumen, through the stoma, engaged at the gastric wall by dilating the balloon, and retracted until resistance is met. The external measurements on the measuring device are used to recorded the stoma length, and an appropriate low profile tube is chosen (Figure 16.4). Different manufacturers have different measuring devices, each will engage the gastric mucosa differently (i.e., inflatable balloon, expandable basket, etc.). If a Foley is used, the balloon is engaged and the external tube is marked at the body wall, then the balloon is deflated, catheter is removed and a ruler is used to measure the distance between the balloon and mark made.

Placement of low profile tubes through the stoma differ with tube manufacturer. Some low profile tubes require an internal blunt stylet. This is typically a Malecot type of tube (Figure 16.18). The stylet is pushed into the closed ended tube and the mushroom tip will elongate and straighten, for passage through the stoma. Once it has entered the stomach, the stylet is removed and the mushroom tip forms, effectively securing the tube in place. Non-styleted tubes generally have a balloon tip for security, which is inflated with air once in place (Figure 16.19). This balloon should be

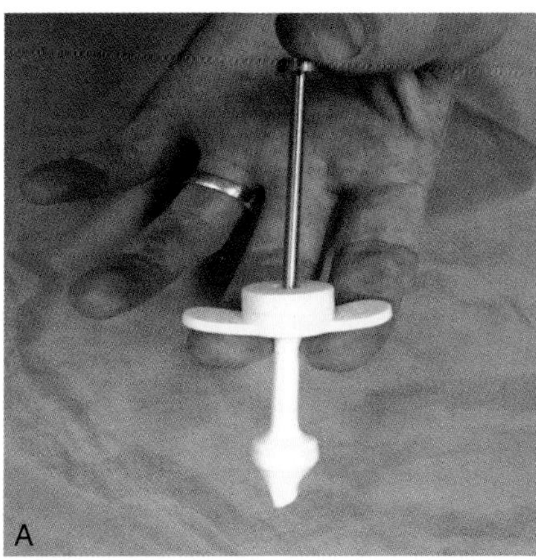

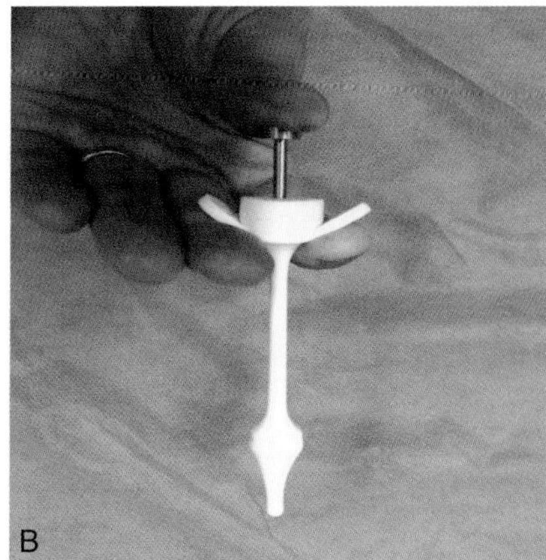

Figure 16.18 Insertion of the stylet into the low-profile tube results in elongation and collapse of the malecot button for placement across an intact stoma.

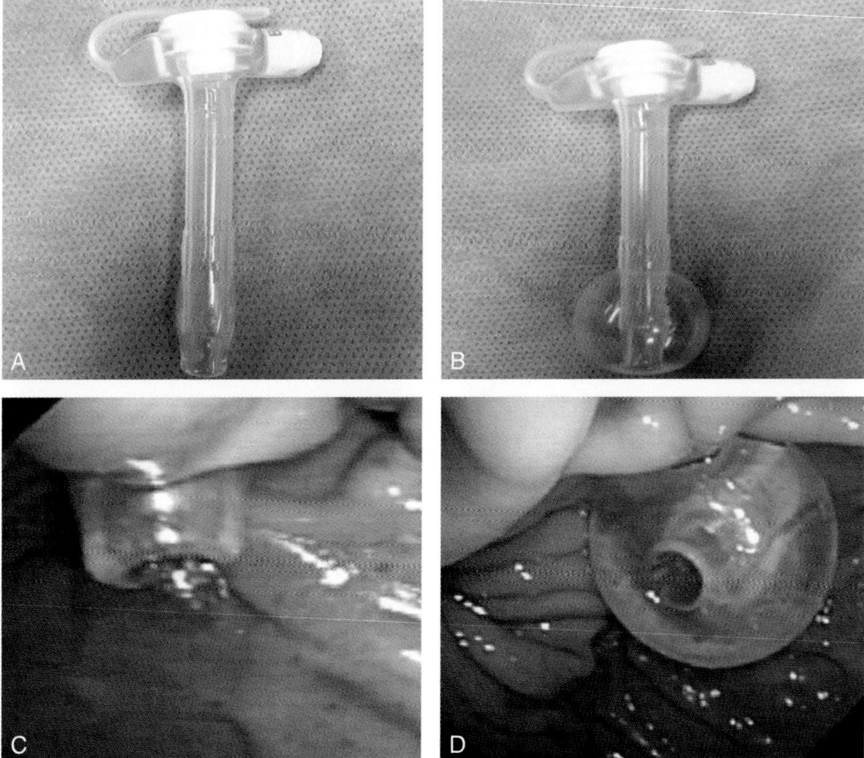

Figure 16.19 Balloon low-profile feeding tube. (A, B) The tube outside of the dog before and after balloon dilation. (C, D) The same tube inside the dog during gastroscopy.

leak tested two to three times prior to placement, as the biggest problem with this type of tube is that the balloon can deflate or pop, and ultimately fall out. The tube should be gently retracted to ensure the balloon is effective. The owner should always have an extra low-profile tube on hand for immediate replacement if needed. Another manufacturer makes a compressed mushroom tip with an outer plastic capsule cover.[9] The capsule and stoma are well lubricated and pushed through the stoma. When entering the gastric lumen the obturator is held firmly while the pull tab is retracted and the suture is removed. This acts to shed the external capsule and allow for mushroom tip expansion and deployment (Figure 16.20).

It is critical that the appropriate feeding tube size is selected for passage. Angulation and slight pressure of the tube may be necessary to pass through a slightly curved stoma tract. However, the tube should never

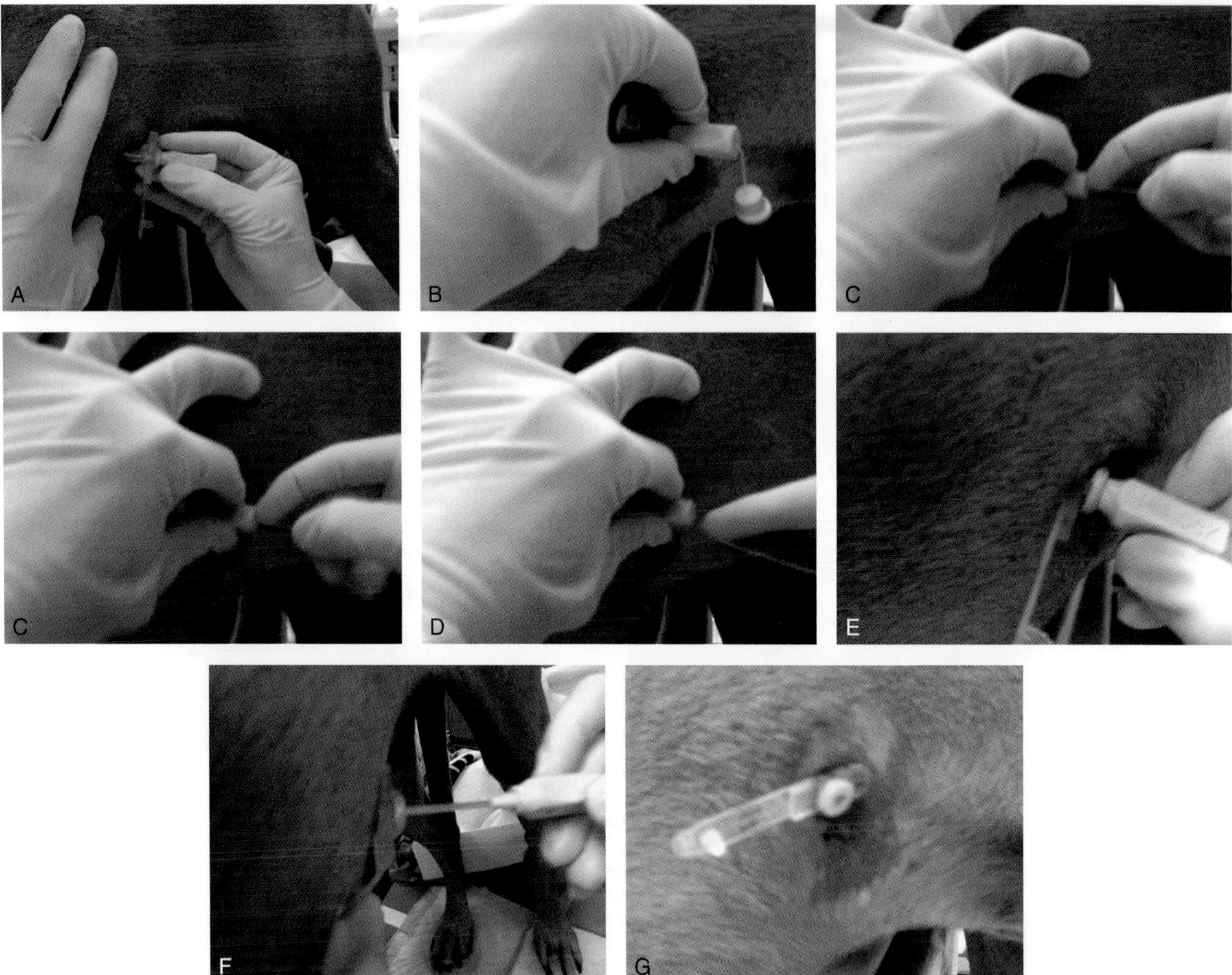

Figure 16.20 Placement of the AMT Mini-One Button Low profile tube, which uses a stiff stylet and a string to aid in flange deployment.

be forced if there is resistance, as the stoma may tear and direct communication with the peritoneal cavity can occur. In these cases, general anesthesia is required to facilitate passage, and endoscopy is often helpful to get through-and-through guide wire access to straighten out the stoma. Dilation of the stoma tract has been achieved in some patients by passing a red rubber tube of equal to slightly larger diameter than the previous tube size. Radial forces will help to dilate the tract and pass the low profile tube successfully (Figure 16.21). Balloon inflation can be performed, but this should be done with great caution. If this is to be performed a balloon diameter is selected that is only slightly larger than the stoma tract diameter and of adequate length extending from the skin to the gastric lumen.

Occasionally, even under anesthesia, the low-profile tube cannot be visualized entering the gastric lumen. When the "lumen cannot be found", the author has used a red rubber catheter (8–10 French) to cannulate the stoma. The distal end of the red rubber is visualized endoscopically and the distal end of the low profile tube is placed within the flanged end of the red rubber catheter (Figure 16.22) and they are both advanced into the gastric lumen coaxially. As the red rubber is introduced into the stomach, it acts as a guide to introduce the low profile without resistance. The red rubber is then snared with a polypectomy snare device or grasping instrument, and removed from the mouth.

It should be noted that one manufacturer make a tube that can be transformed into low profile tubes without the need for an intact stoma.[10] Placement requires normal PEG tube pull technique and has been described in small animals (Campbell et al, 2006). The gastric lumen is distended, the appropriate placement site is identified and the

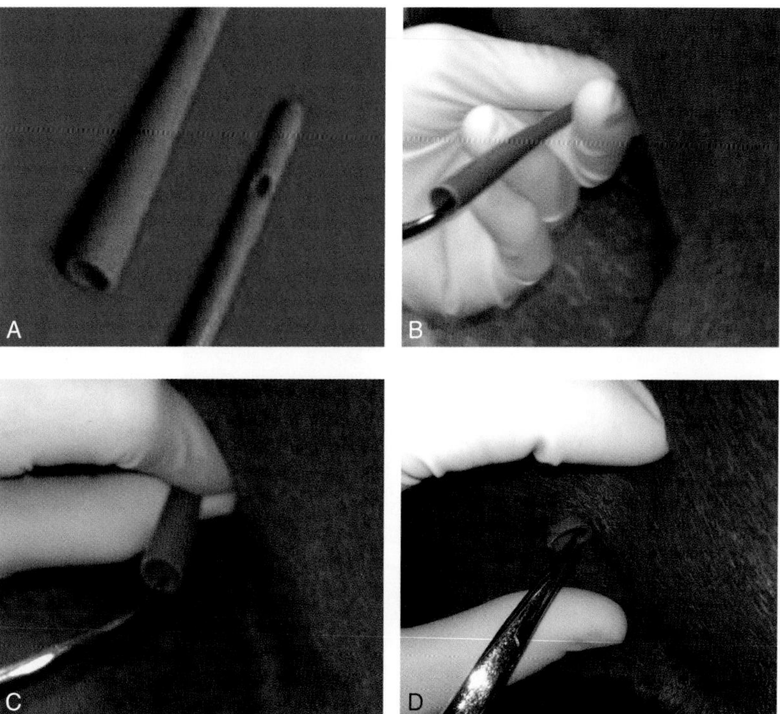

Figure 16.21 Cannulating a stoma with a red rubber catheter to maintain patency and dilate the tract for a low profile tube (A–C) a polypropylene catheter is grasped with hemostats and advanced through a mature stoma tract to provide dilation for passage of a low profile tube. The flared portion of a 14 F catheter generally will provide enough gentle pressure for easier passage. Additionally, this allows the clinician to understand the orientation of the tract.

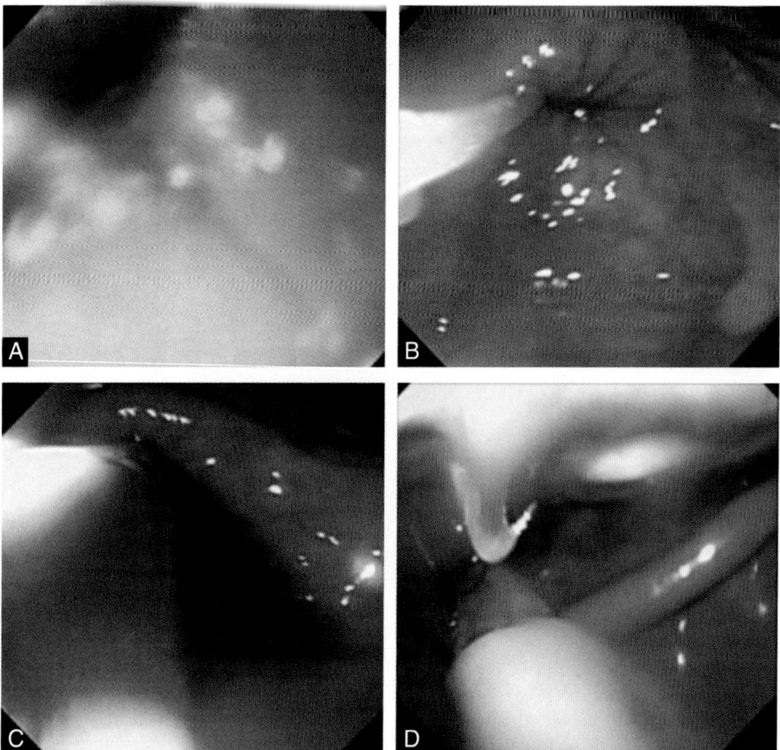

Figure 16.22 Endoscopic assistance of re-wiring a stoma for low profile tube placement. The red rubber catheter is used as a guide for placement across a tortuous stoma tract. (A) Note that the internal aspect of the stoma tract endoscopically. (B) A guide wire is inserted into the gastric lumen under visualization. (C) A soft, slightly stiff polypropylene catheter (generally 8 F) is passed over the guide wire and through the stoma tract and visualized in the gastric lumen. (D) The low profile tube is inserted into the flared end of the catheter externally and advanced together into the lumen. The catheter is grasped internally, while the assistant holds tension external on the low profile tube.

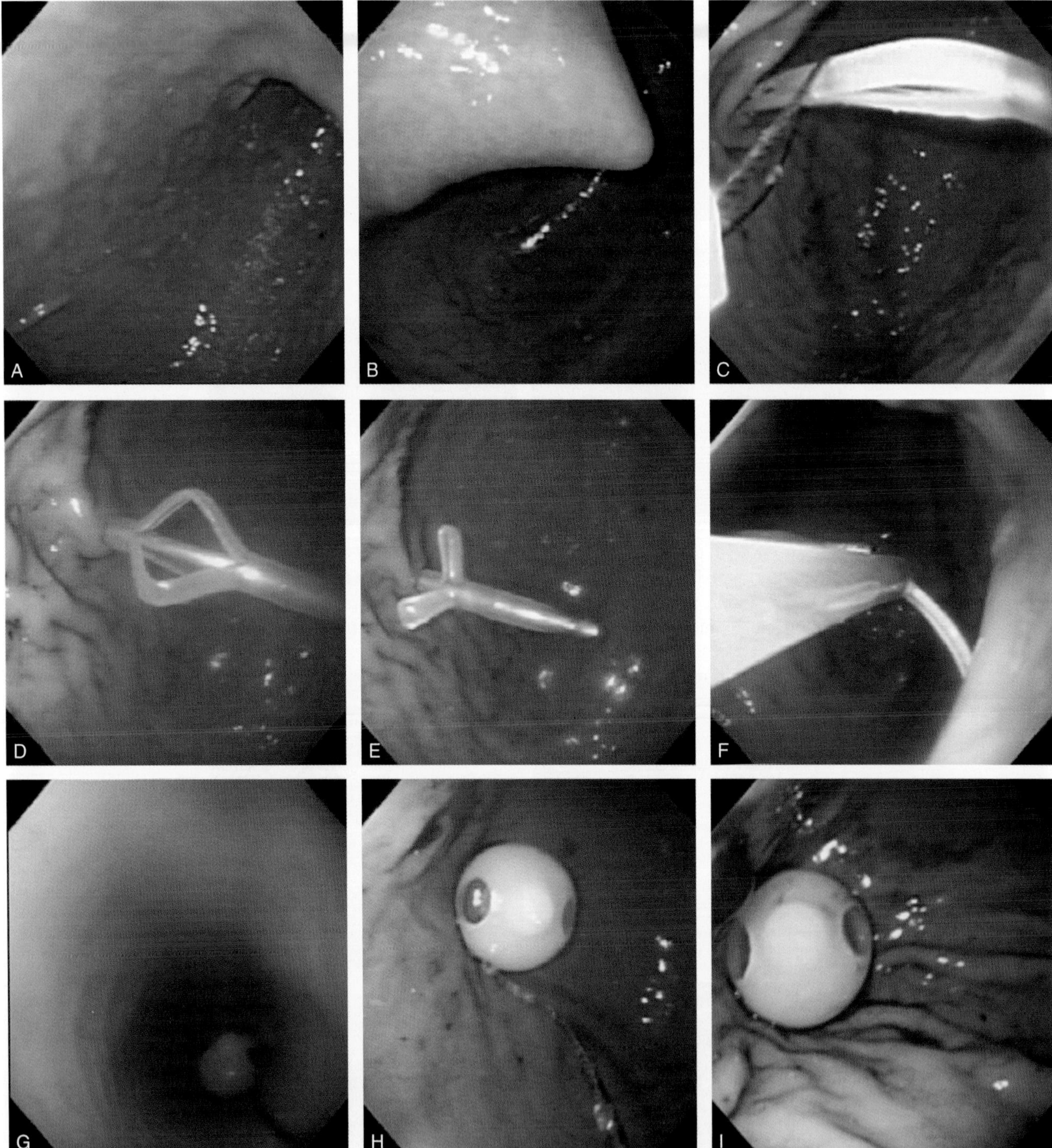

Figure 16.23 Endoscopic images showing the use of the One-Step low profile gastrostomy tube in a dog. (A–C) Percutaneous measuring device is inserted with the stomach distended. (D–E) Following insertion the external basket is deployed and retracted against the wall for appropriate tube selection. (F) The snare is passed through the measuring device chamber after removal of the stylet. (G–H) The PEG tube is placed in the standard pull fashion. (I) Note that the string noted on the previous image has been pulled by the assistant externally.

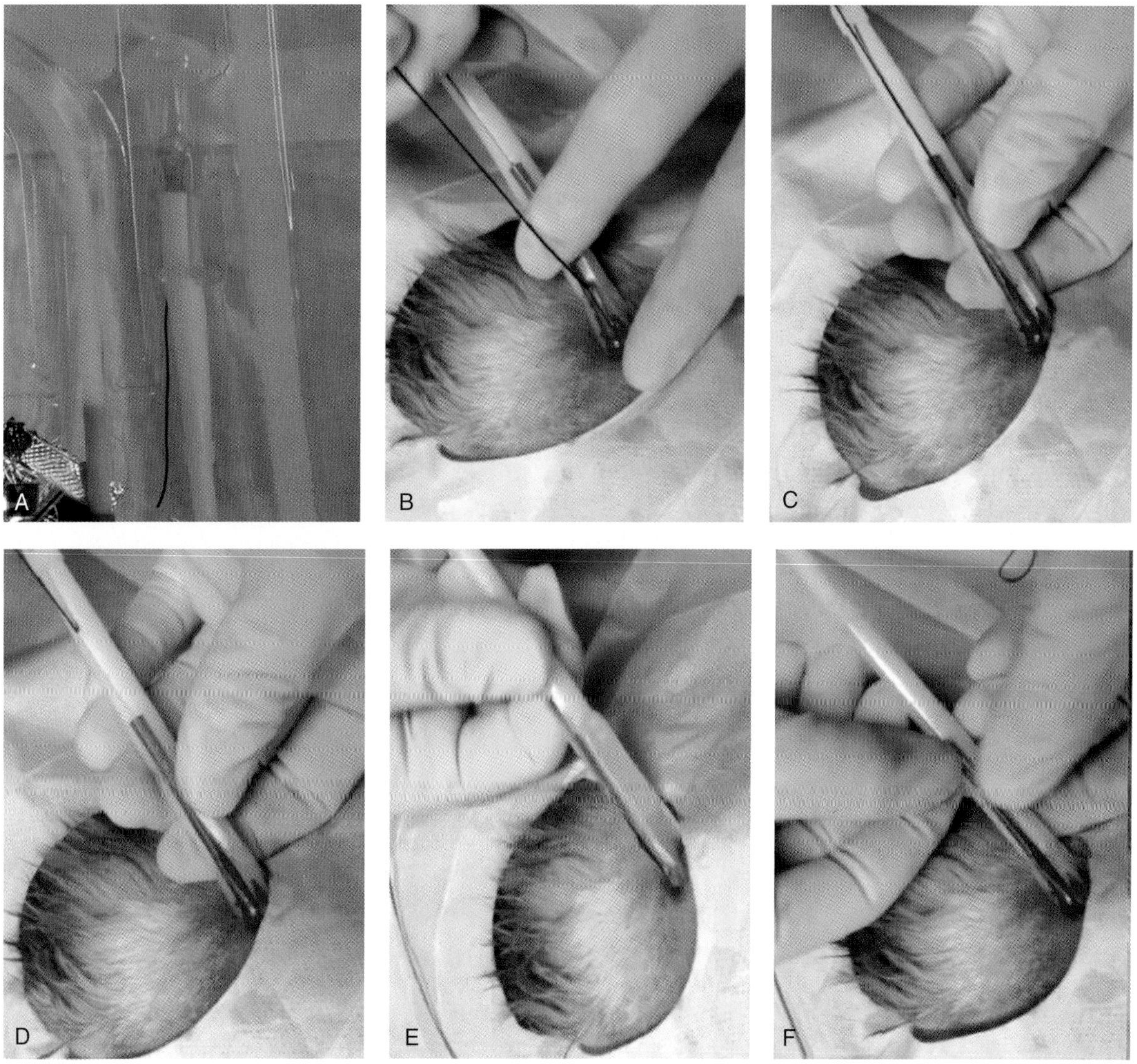

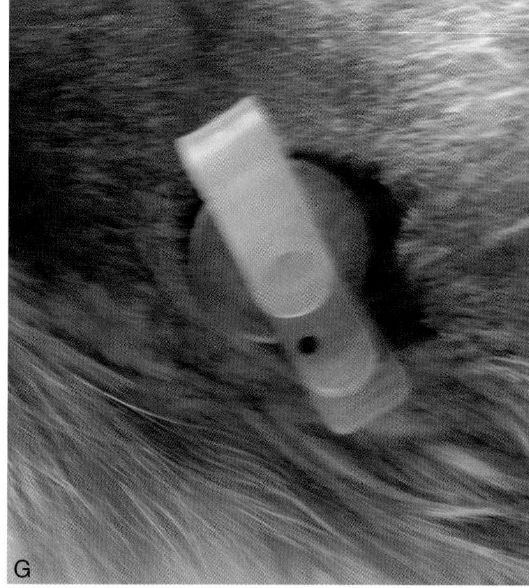

Figure 16.24 The patient in the prior image showing the formation of the low profile tube externally. (A–D) One-Step button placement involves placement of a PEG in traditional fashion as a low profile device. Then an external suture is noted on the outer aspect of the tube. This external suture is pulled, cutting between the outer plastic casing of the tube and exposing the low profile feeding tube. (E, F) The sheath is peeled off and in (G) the button remains.

manufacturer's measuring device is introduced into the gastric lumen (PSMD; percutaneous stoma measuring device). The external plastic basket is expanded in the gastric lumen and pulled up against the body wall for selection of the appropriate low profile tube (based on external measurements). Without removing the measuring device, the stylet is removed and a wire is introduced into the lumen for endoscopic retrieval as noted above (Figure 16.23). The measuring device is removed from the body wall and the snare end of the wire is connected to the snare end of feeding tube. The tube is lubricated and pulled to the body wall as described previously. When the tube exits from the body wall, an external suture located on the tube is pulled and this aids in the removal of an external plastic covering that converts the longer tube into a traditional low profile tube that is flush with the body wall (Figure 16.24).

Prognosis

The prognosis following the placement of a PEG tube is determined by the patient's underlying disease process, but the procedure is met with rare complications and should be considered safe and effective.

Notes

1. Endovive® enteral access Initial placement gastrostomy device, 20Fr Safety PEG Kit, Pull, Boston Scientific, Natick, MA.
2. Flow-20-Pull-S, Cook Medical, Winston-Salem, NC.
3. MIC PEG Feeding Tubes/Kits, Pull method 20F, Kimberly-Clark, Roswell, Ga.
4. 20 Fr PEG20, Mila International, Erlanger, KY.
5. 24 Fr Low Profile Button, Boston Scientific, Natick, MA.
6. Passport-20® Low Profile Gastrostomy Device, Cook Medical, Winston-Salem, NC.
7. BARD Button Gastrostomy Tube, 24F, Bard Access Systems, Inc., Salt Lake City, UT.
8. Cubby – Low Profile Gastrostomy Device, Mila International, Erlanger, KY.
9. AMT Mini-One Button, Applied medical technology, Brecksville, OH.
10. One-Step button™ Low Profile PEG Kit, Pull, Boston Scientific, Natick, MA.

References

Campbell SJ, Marks SL, Yoshimoto SK, et al (2006) Complications and outcomes of one-step low-profile gastrostomy devices for long-term enteral feeding in dogs and cats. *J Am Anim Hosp Assoc* 42(3), 1972–6.

Lohsiriwat V (2013) Percutaneous endoscopic gastrostomy tube replacement: A simple procedure? *World J Gastrointest Endosc* 16;5(1), 141–8.

Suggested Reading

Schrag SP, Sharma R, Jaik NP, et al (2007) Complications related to percutaneous endoscopic gastrostomy (PEG) tubes. *Comp Clin J Gastrointest Liver Dis* 16(4), 4074–18.

Yoshimoto SK, Marks SL, Struble AL, et al (2006) Owner experiences and complications with home use of a replacement low profile gastrostomy device for long-term enteral feeding in dogs. *Can Vet J* 47(2), 1441–50.

CHAPTER SEVENTEEN

Stenting for Gastrointestinal Obstructions

Allyson Berent
The Animal Medical Center, New York, NY

Background/Indications

Gastrointestinal (GI) obstructions can occur secondary to strictures or tumors and occur most commonly in the descending colon or proximal duodenum/pylorus. In humans GI obstructions from tumors are common, and stenting is considered for endoluminal decompression, especially for colonic neoplasia. Various studies in humans have shown that colonic stenting is an effective treatment option for malignant obstructions, but the long-term success is higher when definitive surgery is performed, making stenting a "bridge to surgery" for de-obstipation. Stents decrease the need for a stoma or colostomy bag during this transitional period and have shown to improve a patient's quality of life. In cases where palliation is required, and aggressive surgery is contraindicated, than stenting is considered a good long-term solution. In humans with malignant obstructions the technical success rate after palliative stenting is reported to be as high as 92–100%, with a clinical success rate of 88%. The complication rate is typically low (<10%), and these include re-obstruction, migration and perforation.

There are a few reports in the veterinary literature utilizing stents to palliate gastrointestinal obstructions. Feline GI adenocarcinoma is commonly found at the colorectal junction, and over 75% of cases have evidence of distant metastasis at the time of diagnosis. After colectomy, cats with and without metastasis had a median survival time of 49 days and 259 days, respectively. In dogs, colorectal neoplasia is uncommon, and these lesions are typically adenocarcinoma (~60%), adenomatous polyps (~20%), or carcinoma in situ (~15%). Colorectal polyps can undergo a malignant transformation (~18%), like that seen in humans. These have been reported in a small handful of dogs, but it is important to realize that endoscopic biopsies of the mucosal tissue may not be deep enough to definitively represent the lesion, and a malignant tumor may ultimately be underdiagnosed. If a lesion is focal in nature and the biopsy is suggestive of a benign inflammatory polyp then endoscopic polypectomy with mucosal resection (using a saline lift technique) can be recommended. This is described in more detail in Chapter 16. If the lesion is progressing, atypical (i.e., ulcerated, eroded, indiscrete, or "napkin-ring" in nature), does not "lift" with saline injection, or is histopathologically malignant, then surgical resection should be recommended (transanal rectal pull-through, colorectal resection and anastomosis, excision by mucosal eversion, etc.). If there is concurrent distant metastasis, surgery is declined or considered contraindicated, and the tumor is causing signs of obstipation, and/or GI obstruction, than a stent can be considered for palliative relief over more aggressive surgical options. Many owners will pursue palliative stenting over pelvic osteotomy and colonic resection and anastomosis due to the outpatient nature, minimal morbidity, and low complication rates. If surgery has a high chance of clean margins and no metastasis is present than surgery should always be considered prior to stenting. Outcomes in dogs with malignant colorectal adenocarcinoma undergoing surgical excision have a longer survival than those without surgical excision (22 months versus 15 months, respectively). Dogs with single pedunculated masses, versus dogs with annular "napkin-ring" masses, had survival times of 32 versus 1.6 months, respectively.

Colonic strictures are another indication for GI stenting. In humans this is most commonly seen secondary

Veterinary Image-Guided Interventions, First Edition. Edited by Chick Weisse and Allyson Berent.

Companion website: www.wiley.com/go/weisse/vet-image-guided-interventions

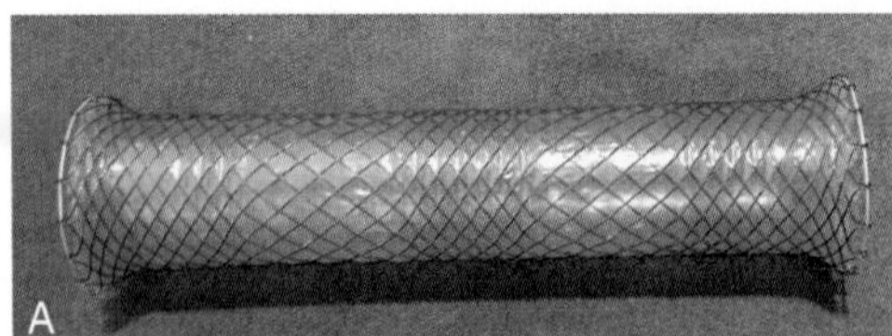

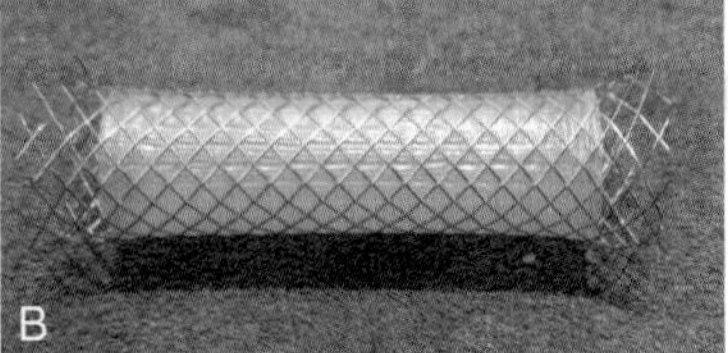

Figure 17.1 Colonic stents. (A) This is a covered retrievable colonic stent. Notice the dumb-bell appearance of the end to prevent migration. (B) This is a partially covered woven self-expanding colonic stent.

to radiation therapy, post-anastomosis, or post-ischemic damage. The most common type of stent used with colonic strictures are covered self-expanding metallic stents (SEMS) (Figure 17.1), which are ultimately removed 4–6 weeks post-placement. These stents are reported to provide 80% clinical success. The covering prevents the metal of the stent from incorporating into the intestinal mucosa, which also prevents the strictured tissue from growing through the mesh of the stent. The most common complications with covered stents are migration (>60%) and stricture recurrence after stent retrieval (~50%).

Upper tract gastrointestinal stenting is typically performed for obstructive lesions involving the stomach, duodenum, and pancreas. It has been used in human medicine for inoperable strictures, fistulas, and intra- and extraluminal tumors. Stents are most useful when the lesion is obstructive causing vomiting and malnutrition. The clinical success, defined by adequate oral feedings and palliation of symptoms, is reported in about 85–90% of patients after stenting. In humans, upper GI stents have shown advantages to more invasive surgery when metastatic disease is present including: shorter hospital stays, lower cost, and complications (such as less intestinal perforation/dehiscence). The median duration of patency for tumors in humans is approximately 6 months, so this is ideal for patients whose life expectancy is similar. For benign strictures, retrievable SEMs are recommended but have similar limitations to that seen with colonic stents. They are typically not recommended for a long-term solution. Re-obstruction and migration are the major complications. Re-obstruction is typically due to tumor or stricture ingrowth through the mesh or around the distal edges of the stent (3–15% with covered stents and 10–42% with uncovered stents). Migration is reported to occur in 10–25% of covered and 2–6% of uncovered stents. Double-layered stents have been developed to try and prevent this problem. Clipping or suturing the end of the covered stent to the GI wall has been recommended in both people and veterinary patients to help prevent migration, and has been successful.

Patient Preparation

Prior to considering GI stenting a patient should have a histopathologic diagnosis of the obstructive lesion. A stent should not be considered if the patient is not obstructed, and if medical management has not been attempted (lactulose, low residue diet, non-steroidal anti-inflammatory drugs and chemotherapy), when indicated. An upper GI obstruction is often more emergent than a colonic obstruction. An endoscopy should be performed to ensure the location, length, and characteristics of the tumor. If a polypoid mass is in the colon, this should be biopsied and a polypectomy could be performed to avoid the need for a stent, pending the biopsy results. Laser ablation of GI tumors/lesions have been considered but are typically of low yield unless they are benign in nature. "Napkin-ring" lesions may not be amenable to endoscopic mucosal resection, but sessile and polypoid lesions that can be lifted with saline injections respond well (see Chapter 16).

Once a diagnosis is obtained, the remainder of the intestinal area of interest is deemed patent, and there is no evidence of distant metastasis (thoracic radiographs, abdominal ultrasound with or without computerized tomography scan) than surgical resection should be recommended. If this is contraindicated, declined, or deemed inappropriate, than a stent can be considered.

Prior to stenting, each patient should have full blood work (complete blood count, serum biochemical profile), a thorough physical examination including rectal and anal sac palpation, and body cavity imaging. For colonic stenting the patient does not need to be de-obstipated. The risk of colonic perforation during enema administration is too high and having feces orad to the stent allows one to see efficacy of the stent after the procedure. For polypectomy, than cleansing is needed.

The patient should be pretreated with broad-spectrum antibiotics, covering for intestinal microflora (anaerobes, Gram-negative bacteria). The author uses cefoxitin (30 mg/kg IV first dose, than 20 mg/kg IV q 4–6 hours) or metronidazole (10 mg/kg BID PO or IV) and enrofloxacin (10 mg/kg IV or PO q 24 hours in dogs and 5 mg/kg IV or PO q 24 hours in cats).

Potential Risks/ Complications/Expected Outcomes

Gastrointestinal stenting is met with few major complications. The most common concerns are tissue ingrowth with uncovered stents, and stent migration with covered stents. Stents in the upper GI tract involving the gastroesophageal junction can cause significant gastroesophageal reflux disorder (GERD), which can be quality of life limiting. There are stents available with one-way antireflux valves, but these have never been used in the author's practice clinically. Other possible complications include GI perforation, irritation, intractable tenesmus (for colonic stents), fecal incontinence (for colonic stents), vomiting (upper GI stents), stent shortening requiring another stent, and hemorrhage. Most of these complications have not been seen in the small number of veterinary patients to date.

In the author's practice colonic stents have been placed for both malignant and benign obstructions in a small number of dogs and cats (~10). Stent migration only occurred in one case, and this was a dog with a postsurgical anastomotic stricture that had a covered stent placed. After the stent was replaced and sutured to the rectal mucosa it remained in place for over 9 months. All other colonic stents placed in feline and canine patients were well tolerated, did not exhibit ingrowth, migration, excessive tenesmus, or fecal incontinence. Nearly all of the cases stented for malignancy had evidence of distant metastasis at the time of placement, so surgery was declined, and one patient developed a colonic stricture postresection of a colonic adenocarcinoma, at which time a second surgery was declined. This patient had tenesmus both before and after stent placement and was mildly fecally incontinent. The clinical success for benign colonic stenting is good with over 4-year followup in one patient, with no failures. For malignancies and the median survival time was approximately 6 months (range, 19–274 days). All patients with tumors died of distant tumor effects (metastasis, cachexia, chemotherapy toxicity, etc.), and none of local disease.

It is important to realize that stents placed for obstructions will only be of benefit if the patient is obstructed from the lesion. Tumors and strictures at surgical sites, or near nerves (pelvic canal) can be irritating, causing signs of pain, tenesmus and dyschezia. A stent will not improve these signs. It will open the lumen of the intestine so that feces and ingesta can more easily pass and the tenesmus associated with the lesion, unrelated to the obstructive component, will likely remain static.

Equipment

Gastrointestinal stents are typically metallic and of a self-expanding nature. They are either uncovered, partially covered or fully-covered.[1–3] The advantages of a covered stent is a lower rate of re-obstruction, especially with strictures, but a higher rate of migration, due to the failure of tissue ingrowth. Biodegradable stents[4] are available but these are not typically used for gastrointestinal stenting as they are weak and can easily migrate. These are discussed in more detail in Chapter 13. Some of the currently available colonic stents have a dumb-bell shape at each, or one, end, to aid in preventing migration (Figure 17.1), and the covered stents, since they are intended for short-term use, have a string around each end so that they can be removed endoscopically with a grasping instrument.

Self-expanding metallic stents are discussed in great detail in other chapters. This specific stent is a woven SEMS, so that is it longer on the delivery system than it is once within the patient, and as it opens up over time with have a tendency to foreshorten.

A standard flexible endoscope is needed for this procedure. The author prefers the video gastroduodenoscope.[5,6] If the stent is to be placed through the working channel of the endoscope than the larger scope is necessary. A 0.035″ hydrophilic angle-tipped guide wire[7] that is long enough to be exchanged through the endoscope should be used (260 cm) (Figure 17.2). A marker catheter[8] is used to estimate colonic diameter and obstruction length to aid in stent sizing (Figure 17.3). The author prefers a pigtail marker catheter.

A traditional fluoroscopic C-arm is sufficient for visualization. Fluoroscopy entails the risk of radiation exposure so care must be taken to reduce exposure through beam collimation, reducing dose, and wearing standard radiation protection gear.

Procedure

Colonic Stenting

Patients should be treated with perioperative broad-spectrum antibiotics. Routine colonoscopy is performed. If the lumen of the mass can be cannulated with the endoscope than the entire colon should be

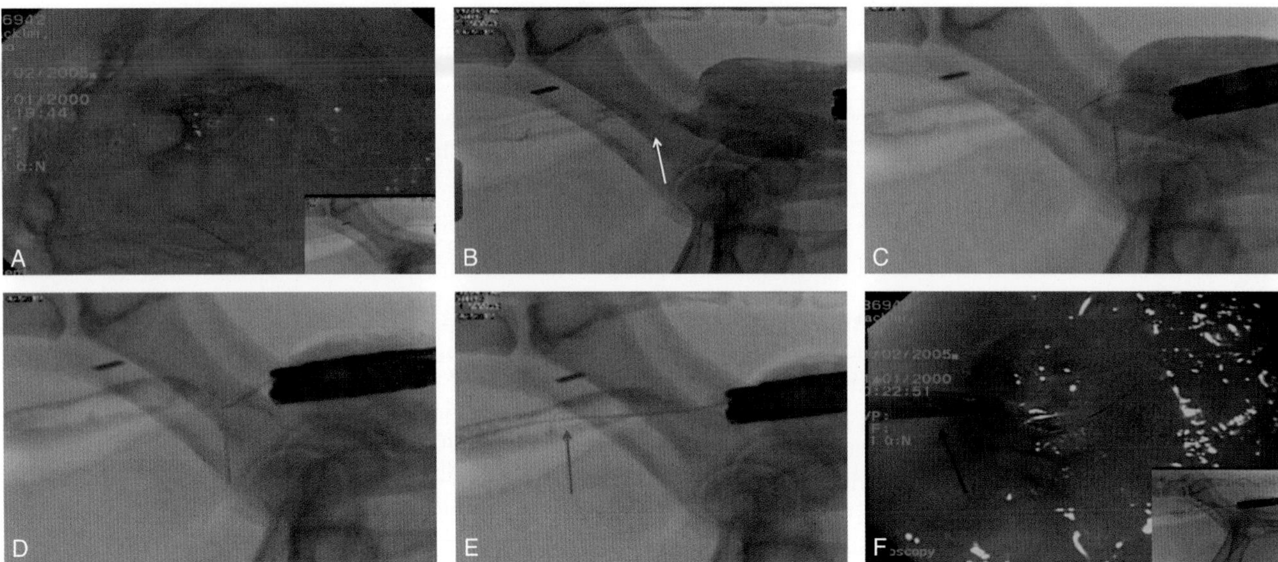

Figure 17.2 Colonic stricture in a dog. (A) Endoscopic image of a colonic stricture in a dog that occurred after a colectomy for colorectal adenocarcinoma. There is a small fluoroscopic image in the right corner as showing the endoscope entering the distal colon. (B) Fluoroscopic image of the colonic stricture during a contrast colongram. White arrow is the small opening through the stricture where contrast is seen entering the area orad to the stricture. (C) Fluoroscopic image of a guide wire (red arrow) passing through the stricture via the working channel of the endoscope where it is directed using both endoscopic and fluoroscopic guidance. (D) The guide wire (red arrow) passing through the stricture. (E) The guide wire (red arrow) once it is orad to the stricture in the normal descending colon. (F) Endoscopic image of the guide wire (black arrow) through the colonic stricture.

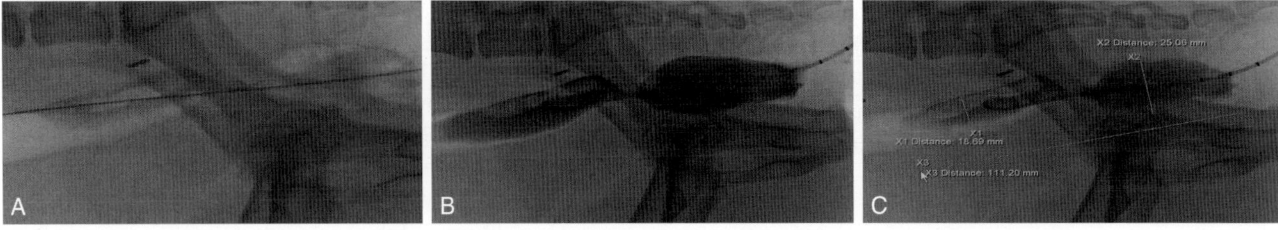

Figure 17.3 Measuring of the colon for stent sizing. (A) Fluoroscopic image of the stricture cannulated with the guide wire. (B) Pigtail marker catheter across the stenosis so a contrast study can be performed. Note this is a multifenestrated catheter so holes are strategically placed on each side of the stenosis to allow contrast to fill both sides and demarcate the stricture length accurately. (C) Using the marker catheter to adjust for magnification (distance from beginning of one mark to the beginning of another mark is 10 mm), the diameter of the colon in front and behind the stenosis is measured. The length of the stent is also shown to mark the location where the stent will sit.

carefully evaluated to make sure there are no other masses. Once the mass is found and the rest of the colon is biopsied (normal colon beyond the mass), a guide wire and marker catheter should be placed across the stenosis (Figure 17.2). This can either be done passing the guide wire through the working channel of the endoscope to monitor as the wire passes, or all done using a contrast colonogram under fluoroscopic guidance (Figure 17.2 and Figure 17.3). Once the wire is through the lumen of the obstruction, and the marker catheter is passed over the wire (Figure 17.3), the wire is removed. Since the marker catheter is multifenestrated the holes on the catheter are placed so that some are oral to and some are aboral to the obstruction. The anus is held off manually to prevent contrast leakage and allow distal colorectal distension. The catheter is then injected to distend the colon and demarcate the obstructive lesion (Figure 17.3). The marker catheter is then used to measure the diameter of the colon and length of the obstruction in order to adjust for magnification, and a stent size is chosen. The colonoscopy aids in measuring obstruction length as well if both sides can be visualized. The wire is re-advanced through the catheter and the catheter is then removed over the wire, so that the stent can be advanced over the wire using fluoroscopic guidance (Figure 17.4).

Once a stent size and type are chosen, typically based on the cause of the obstruction (covered, uncovered,

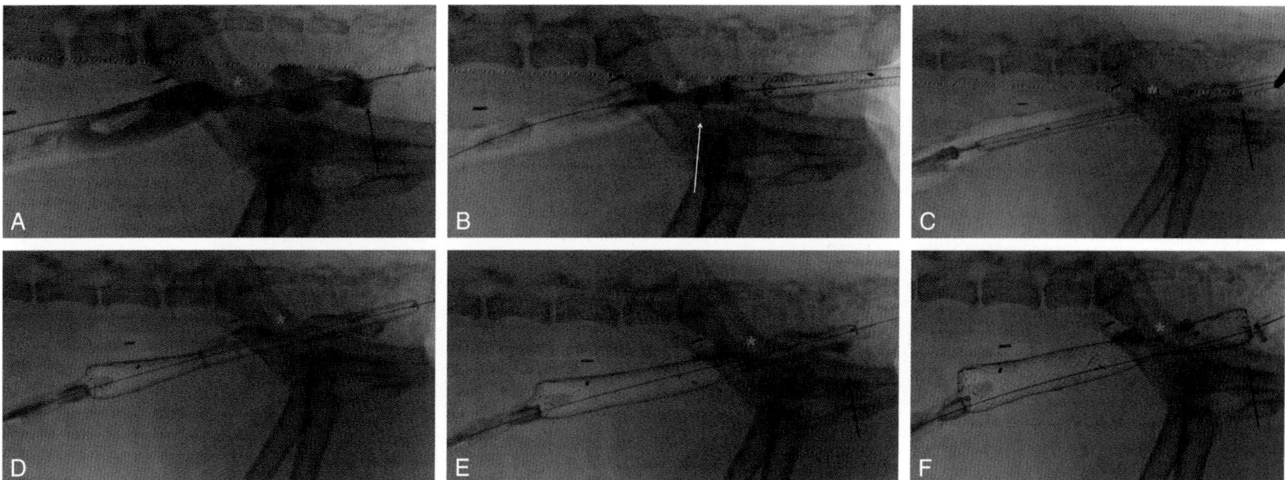

Figure 17.4 Fluoroscopic image of colonic stent placement. (A) Guidewire through the stenosis after colonogram. The red asterisk is the stenosis and the black arrow is the location of the anorectal junction. (B) The stent delivery system is advanced over the guide wire. The tip of the delivery system is tapered to the wire and this is called a nose cone (white arrow). (C) The stent is advanced through the stenosis compressed in the delivery system. A hemostat is sitting against the anus to ensure the caudal end is appropriately placed. The black arrow is marking the anorectal junction, which is where the caudal end of the stent should end. (D) The stent is being deployed and the red asterisk is marking the stenosis. (E) The stent being deployed across the stenosis (red asterisk) as the caudal end is carefully placed at the anorectal junction (black arrow). (F) The stent once it is fully deployed across the stenosis (red asterisk), with the caudal end just orad to the anorectal junction (black arrow).

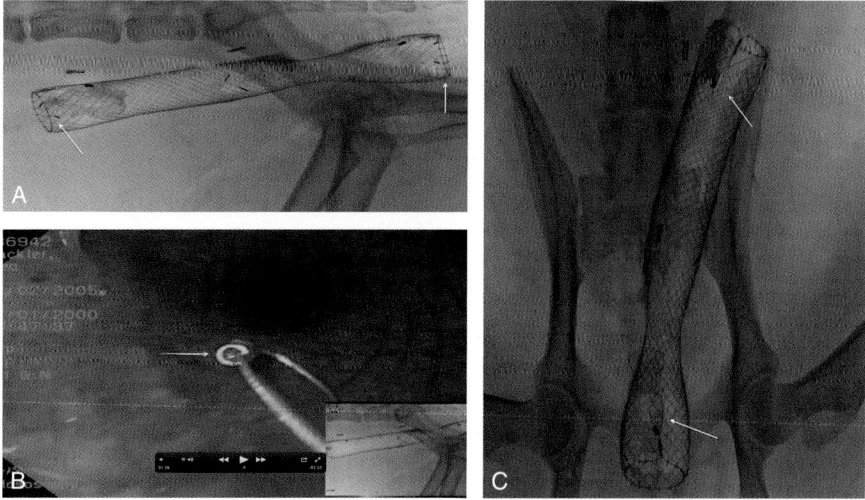

Figure 17.5 Images of colonic stent after deployment and expansion. (A) Colonic stent is in place across the stenosis. This is a covered stent so the retrieval string is seen on each end (white arrows). (B) Endoscopic image of colonic stent after deployment. Notice the retrieval string (white arrow) at the distal end. The colon is now patent. (C) A ventrodorsal image of the colonic stent after deployment with the retrieval strings (white arrows).

biodegradable, etc.), the stent is flushed through the central lumen and around the sheath. The stent is then advanced over the guidewire using fluoroscopic guidance across the obstruction. The contrast outlines the obstructive lesion to ensure the stent is appropriately placed (Figure 17.4). The obstruction does not usually require balloon dilation, the stent slowly opens the narrowed region over time by a constant outward radial force. This has been shown to help prevent colonic perforation and stent migration. Care should be taken to cross the obstruction without placing the end of the stent within in anus. The caudal end is usually up to the rectal/anal junction (Figure 17.4F and Figure 17.6). Once the stent is in place the scope is replaced to assess stent location and ensure the entire obstructive region is spanned (Figure 17.5 and Figure 17.6). For covered stents the distal end can be sutured to the colonic mucosa to prevent stent migration.

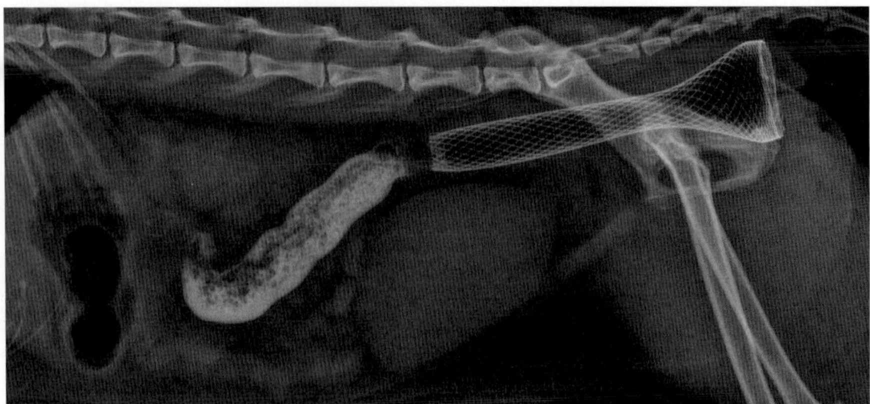

Figure 17.6 Lateral radiograph of a colonic stent in a feline patient for colonic adenocarcinoma. Notice the distal flare of the stent to prevent migration at the anorectal junction.

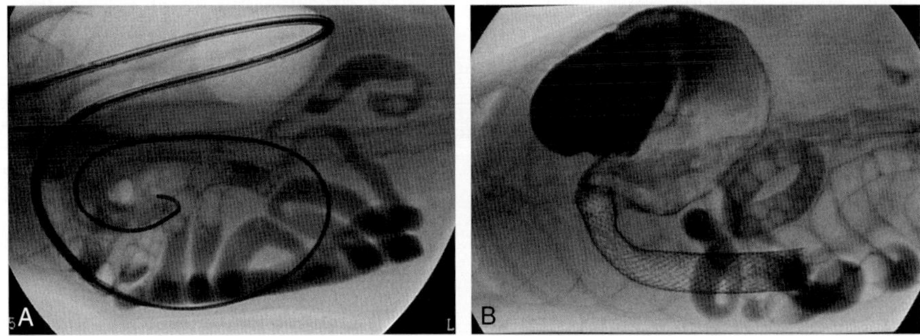

Figure 17.7 Ventrodorsal fluoroscopic images of a ferret with a pyloric/duodenal adenocarcinoma causing a gastric outflow obstruction during stent placement. (A) A guide wire is advanced from the mouth, into the stomach, across the pylorus and duodenum and into the proximal jejunum. Over the wire is the delivery system with a non-deployed self-expanding woven metallic stent placed across the obstruction. (B) The SEMS after deployment documenting patency of the proximal duodenum and pylorus. (Courtesy of Dr. Chick Weisse.)

Gastroduodenal Stenting

Stenting of the stomach or descending duodenum is not very common, but has been performed (Figure 17.7). This has been necessary for malignant obstructions of the gastric cardia, pyloric outflow tract, and duodenum. Traditional surgical resection should be recommended when possible, but for cases where palliation is desired, and surgery is either declined or contraindicated, than a stent can be considered. If the obstructive lesion is in the area of the major duodenal papilla care should be taken to avoid covering the opening to the common bile duct, which could ultimately result in a biliary obstruction. If needed a biliary stent can be placed to open the common bile duct (see Chapter 24) prior to duodenal stent placement.

Gastroduodenal stenting is performed similarly to that described above for colonic stenting. A gastroduodenoscope is used to assess the obstructive lesion and biopsies are taken if needed. Then a guidewire is used to cannulate the lumen of the obstruction and is passed down the duodenum using fluoroscopic guidance. Next the marker catheter can be used to measure the diameter of the obstructive lesion to choose a stent size. The appropriately sized SEMS can then be placed. This can either be done through the working channel of the endoscope (must have a delivery system over 150 cm long), or over the wire, using fluoroscopic guidance alone. A stiffened guide wire is recommended if a scope is not used. Once the stent is deployed the endoscope is used to assess the stent location and document the obstruction has been appropriately spanned with the stent length and size being appropriate.

Post-Procedural and Follow-Up Care

Patients with colonic stents should be placed on a low residue diet and treated with stool softeners (lactulose 0.2–1 ml/kg BID to TID PO) to effect. The goal is soft stool that is easy to pass without creating diarrhea, which could be irritating. Patients should be treated with appropriate chemotherapy and non-steroidal anti-inflammatory drugs when necessary for their tumor type and should always consult with an oncologist. Patients with upper gastrointestinal stents should be fed small amounts of soft food often for the first few days and should not be given hard bones or treats. Gastroesophageal or gastroduodenal reflux is possible so proton pump inhibitors, and antiemetic drugs should be used initially. These may not need to be continued. Post-stent radiographs are usually taken 24 hours after stent placement to assess stent location and degree of stent expansion. Then the stent location and length can be monitored after 1 month to ensure the stent has not migrated or shortened excessively.

Prognosis

The prognosis for dogs and cats with obstructive, non-resectable, colonic adenocarcinoma is not readily available. In the author's practice, feline patients with colonic stents placed for malignant obstructions and distant metastasis lived between 3 and 9 months (median 6 months), most of which had evidence of carcinomatosis or distant metastasis at the time of diagnosis. This compares to a 49-day median survival without stenting in the historical literature. None of the stented cats died of colonic re-obstruction and all were stented with uncovered SEMS. One cat was stented for a colonic stricture, unrelated to any neoplasia, and this cat is still alive after 4.5 years. Also, an uncovered SEMS was placed in this patient. No cat was fecally incontinent. Fewer canine patients have been stented for colonic neoplasia. One dog stented for a primary tumor survived over 7 months and was fecally continent, and another dog stented for a colonic stricture, secondary to a colonic resection and anastomosis for a colorectal adenocarcinoma, survived over 9 months. This dog was minimally fecally incontinent but also continued to have tenesmus post-stent placement. This was a covered stent, due to the risk of stricture in-growth. This stent migrated after 24 hours and was defecated out. It was replaced and sutured in place within the rectum using 3–0 monofilament absorbable suture material and remains in place 9 months later.

Other potential complications that should be considered include: tumor ingrowth, stent migration, colonic perforation, stent fracture, fecal incontinence, and pain associated with the stent. In the author's limited experience these are not commonly seen.

Upper gastrointestinal stenting has not been performed in many patients, so a prognosis is unavailable. One dog with a stent placed across the cardia of the stomach did not do clinically well. This dog continued to have GERD and was ultimately euthanized. A ferret with a pyloroduodenal adenocarcinoma had a pyloroduodenal stent placed and this patient tolerated the stent very well.

Special Considerations

Animals with colonic neoplasia typically present for tenesmus and dyschezia, regardless if they are fecally obstructed. This is likely due to the presence of the tumor and the possible invasion of the tumor to the pelvic nerves. A stent should not be expected to relieve the tenesmus unassociated with fecal obstruction. Owner expectations should be appropriate after this procedure.

Notes

These are only a few of the possible options for this procedure:

1. WallFlex Colonic Stent (covered or uncovered), Boston Scientific, Natick, MA.
2. VetStent-Colorectal, Infiniti Medical, LLC, Menlo Park, CA.
3. Covered SEMS (silicone), Infiniti Medical, Menlo Park, CA.
4. Biodegradable SEMS, Infiniti Medical, Menlo Park, CA.
5. 9.9 mm gastroduodenoscope, Olympus, Southborough, MA.
6. 6 mm gastroduodenoscope, Olympus, Southborough, MA.
7. Weasel wire 0.035″ 260 cm, Infiniti Medical, Menlo Park, CA.
8. Marker Catheter, Merit Medical UHF, South Jordan, UT.

Suggested Reading

Bonin EA and Baron TH (2010) Update on the indications and use of colonic stents. *Curr Gastroenterol Rep* 12(5), 374–82.

Boškoski I, Tringali A, Familiari P, et al (2010) Self-expandable metallic stents for malignant gastric outlet obstruction. *Adv Ther* 27(10), 691–703.

Church EM, Mehlhaff CJ, and Patnaik AK (1987) Colorectal adenocarcinoma in dogs: 78 cases (1973–1984). *J Am Vet Med Assoc* 191, 727–30.

Culp WTN, MacPhail CM, Perry JA, et al (2011) Use of a nitinol stent to palliate a colorectal neoplastic obstruction in a dog. *J Am Vet Med Assoc* 239(2), 222–7.

Hume D, Solomon J, and Weisse C (2006) Palliative use of a stent for colonic obstruction caused by adenocarcinoma in two cats. *J Am Vet Med Assoc* 228, 392–6.

Kim SG and Yang CH. (2012) Upper gastrointestinal stent. *Clin Endosc* 45, 386–91.

Small AJ, Young-Fadok TM, and Baron TH (2008) Expandable metal stent placement for benign colorectal obstruction: outcomes for 23 cases. *Surg Endosc* 10, 901–6.

Valerius KD, Powers BE, McPherron MA, et al (1997) Adenomatous polyps and carcinoma in situ of the canine colon and rectum: 34 cases (1982–1994). *J Am Anim Hosp Assoc* 33, 156–60.

CHAPTER EIGHTEEN

IMAGE-GUIDED NUTRITIONAL SUPPORT TECHNIQUES

Matthew W. Beal
College of Veterinary Medicine, Michigan State University, East Lansing, MI

BACKGROUND/INDICATIONS

Nutritional support plays a critical role in the management of the hospitalized small animal patients (Remillard et al, 2001, Chan 2004, Michel and Higgins, 2006, Chan and Freeman, 2006, Holahan et al, 2010). However, considerable debate still exists in both human and veterinary medicine as to the significance of the benefits that enteral nutritional (EN) support may impart over parenteral nutritional (PN) support (Heyland et al, 2003, Gramlich et al, 2004, Peter et al, 2005, Altintas et al, 2011). In humans, EN is associated with shorter lengths-of-stay, and significantly fewer infective complications than PN. EN may also directly promote gastrointestinal mucosal health and is consistently less expensive than PN (Gramlich et al, 2004, Altintas et al, 2011). Placement of nasoesophageal, nasogastric, or esophagostomy feeding tubes usually occurs without the need for image guidance. Radiography is used to confirm accurate placement. However, clinical problems encountered in some patients may necessitate the placement of a gastrostomy or postpyloric feeding tube. This can be accomplished with various forms of image-guided technology.

INDICATIONS FOR GASTROSTOMY TUBE PLACEMENT

Gastrostomy tubes (G-tubes) are indicated in animals that are in need of long term (months to years) nutritional support, provided they are tolerant of gastric feeding. Contraindications include persistent vomiting, altered levels of consciousness, the presence of peritoneal fluid, or other reasons that would prevent the apposition of the stomach to the body wall. The rise in popularity of esophageal feeding tubes (E-tubes) has decreased the frequency of G-tube placement over the last 15 years. However, G-tubes are well tolerated and offer specific advantages over E-tubes in animals with esophageal disease/dysfunction or dysphagia. Because G-tubes are relatively large, like E-tubes, they allow for blenderized commercial diets to be fed, as well as liquefied medications to be administered. In some conditions, gastric decompression may be necessary, and this can easily be accomplished with a G tube. These tubes may be placed via a percutaneous endoscopic approach (PEG) (see Chapter 16), a percutaneous radiologic approach (PRG), or surgically. The former is used most commonly, however, the latter are useful in animals where endoscopic access to the stomach is not feasible due to the presence of an esophageal stricture or neoplasia. Blind placement techniques are well described (Han 2004, Mauterer et al, 1992), but may be associated with significant risk of visceral injury and severe complications. As a result, image-guided interventions are preferred. Surgical gastrostomy is generally safe and appropriate if the patient is undergoing a concurrent abdominal surgical procedure.

INDICATIONS FOR POSTPYLORIC FEEDING

Postpyloric feeding methods are indicated in animals that are intolerant of, or have contraindications to gastric feeding. This intolerance may manifest as persistent nausea, vomiting, regurgitation, or large gastric residual volumes due to poor motility (Abood and Buffington, 1992, Holahan et al, 2010). Contraindications to gastric feeding may include an altered level of consciousness, altered laryngeal function or other

Veterinary Image-Guided Interventions, First Edition. Edited by Chick Weisse and Allyson Berent.

Companion website: www.wiley.com/go/weisse/vet-image-guided-interventions

TABLE 18.1
Abbreviations for image-guided nutritional support techniques

PEG	Percutaneous endoscopic gastrostomy
PEGJ	Percutaneous endoscopic gastrojejunostomy
PRG	Percutaneous radiologic gastrostomy
PRGJ	Percutaneous radiologic gastrojejunostomy
NJT	Nasojejunal tube
RNJT	Radiologic nasojejunal tube
EndoNJT	Endoscopic nasojejunal tube
EJT	Esophagojejunal tube

conditions that put the patient at a high risk of aspiration. Postpyloric feeding for pancreatic disease, particularly pancreatitis, is considered controversial, and a trend toward "feeding the pancreas", rather than "resting the pancreas" is now being employed in the veterinary and human community if gastric feeding is tolerated. In the current veterinary literature, the most common conditions that necessitate the placement of post-pyloric feeding tubes included pancreatitis, septic peritonitis, acute renal failure, parvoviral enteritis, and those with neurologic abnormalities (Jennings et al, 2001, Wohl 2006, Beal and Brown, 2011, Campbell and Daley, 2011). Although surgical options for placement of postpyloric feeding tubes exist (Crowe and Devey, 1997, Swann et al, 1997, Hewitt et al, 2004, Yagil-Kelmer et al, 2006), most veterinarians favor minimally invasive techniques that prevent the need for enterotomy or gastrotomy, thus helping to minimize the likelihood of complications such as septic peritonitis. Minimally invasive techniques for achieving jejunal access utilizing the nasojejunal (NJ), esophagojejunal (EJ), and gastrojejunal routes (GJ) with either fluoroscopic or endoscopic guidance are well established (Jennings et al, 2001, Heuter 2004, Wohl 2006, Jergens et al, 2007, Papa et al 2009, Beal et al, 2007, 2009a,b, Beal and Brown, 2011, Campbell and Daley, 2011). In the animal with critical illness and poor wound healing that requires post-pyloric feeding, the NJ tube (NJT) and EJ tube (EJT) may be associated with a lower risk of complications than GJ techniques because they do not penetrate the peritoneal cavity, and thus do not put the patient at risk of septic peritonitis. See Table 18.1 for a list of abbreviations of the various techniques.

Patient Preparation

Prior to elective image-guided placement of feeding tubes, a full diagnostic workup focused on identifying major problems and potential contraindications to feeding tube placement is recommended. Assessment for hemostatic abnormalities should be performed when indicated (platelet count, activated partial thromboplastin time, prothrombin time, ± buccal–mucosal-bleeding time or platelet function testing, von Willebrand factor antigen assay, etc.) to help minimize the chance of significant hemorrhage during feeding tube placement. If poor gastric motility is associated with large volumes of gastric fluid, gastric decompression is recommended prior to the procedure. This may be accomplished pre-induction via nasogastric, or postinduction via orogastric routes (once the airway is protected).

General anesthesia with endotracheal intubation is recommended for all image-guided nutritional support techniques to minimize pharyngeal stimulation, emesis, and the risk of aspiration pneumonia. The use of local anesthetics with general anesthesia is recommended for NJ tube placement. Prior to beginning, the author instills approximately 1 mg/kg of lidocaine[1] intranasal every 5 minutes for three doses.

Prophylactic antibiotic therapy (perioperative and 5 days postoperative) and preprocedural oropharyngeal decontamination are recommended to decrease stoma infection rates (in all but NJ tubes). Although definitive evidence in veterinary medicine is currently lacking, human medical experience is supportive of these measures (Cantwell et al, 2008, Lipp and Lusardi, 2009, Horiuchi et al, 2008). An investigational veterinary protocol (Mack et al, 2013) involves placement of a sterile gauze pharyngeal pack to occlude the larynx prior to irrigation and decontamination. A 0.12% chlorhexidine solution is applied with either a spray bottle (approximately 20 pumps) or a 20-gauge catheter attached to a syringe with 6mls of 0.12% chlorhexidine solution. This should be equally applied to all dental, buccal, and lingual surfaces. A 5-minute wait period should be allowed for bactericidal effects to ensue. The laryngeal / pharyngeal pack should be removed at the end of the five minute wait period. Early clinical research supports the reduction of oropharyngeal bacteria post decontamination in veterinary patients (Mack et al, 2013).

Potential Risks/ Complications/ Expected Outcomes

Although risks and complications can be mitigated through careful patient preparation, clinicians and clients alike must be aware of the potential risks and complications associated with placement of feeding tubes via image guidance.

General risks include anesthesia and the risk of aspiration pneumonia. Much of the time, nutritional support techniques are utilized in animals that are not eating and/or demonstrate vomiting or regurgitation. These same indications to place the feeding tube also predispose to risks of aspiration pneumonia.

PEG, PRG, percutaneous endoscopic gastrojejunostomy (PEGJ), and percutaneous radiologic gastrojejunostomy (PRGJ) tubes all traverse the stomach through the left lateral abdominal wall. As a result, acute complications may include gastric hemorrhage, pneumoperitoneum, and splenic injury. The latter injury can be minimized by insufflating adequately and transilluminating the stomach through the body wall when using endoscopic techniques. When placing a PRG or PRGJ, insufflating the stomach and using ultrasound to ensure that the spleen is not interposed between the stomach and body will minimize this complication. The most catastrophic risk of PEG, PRG, PEGJ, and PRGJ tubes involves the development of septic peritonitis. This complication may develop due to the tube pulling through the stomach wall due to patient size (most do not advocate placement of PEG or PEGJ if >30 kg), gastric pressure necrosis, or removal of the tube prior to formation of a mature gastrostomy (by the patient or the veterinarian). In one case series of animals undergoing gastrostomy, severe complications requiring an intervention occurred in approximately 10% of patients (Salinardi et al, 2006).

Minor complications, including gastrostomy site infection and discomfort, are common and can generally be treated utilizing local wound care coupled with systemic antibiotics and pain medications (if needed).

Complications of NJT and EJT are generally minor in nature and include sneezing (potentially resulting in loss of the tube) and epistaxis (NJT), or esophagostomy site infection/inflammation (EJT).

Complications of jejunal tubes (PEGJ, PRGJ, NJT, EJT) include oral migration and tube occlusion. With appropriate jejunal placement and proper flushing of the tube, these are uncommon.

All of the aforementioned image-guided nutritional support techniques are likely to be successful from both a placement and utilization perspective. Placement of the distal aspect of NJT and EJT in the jejunum appears to be somewhat operator dependent, but overall success is still expected to be >90% in various studies (Beal et al, 2007, 2009a,b, Beal and Brown, 2011, Papa et al, 2009; Campbell and Daley, 2011). Nutritional support may be initiated when the patient's stability allows it. In general, feeding may commence within 24 hours of placement of PEG and PRG tubes. Postpyloric feeding via PEGJ, PRGJ, NJT, and EJT can be initiated once the patient has recovered from anesthesia. Postpyloric feeding should be performed via a constant rate infusion as the jejunum is not a reservoir organ like the stomach. The author usually initiates feeding of a commercially available liquid diet[2] at approximately 25% of resting energy requirement (RER) and increases 25% every 12 hours until RER is attained (total 36 hours).

Equipment

A list of equipment can be found in Table 18.2. PEG, PRG, PEGJ, and PRGJ equipment is best purchased in a commercially available kit that contains most everything needed for a given procedure.

Procedures

Percutaneous Endoscopic Gastrostomy

See Chapter 16 for a complete discussion of this technique.

Percutaneous Endoscopic Gastrojejunostomy

Equipment needed for PEGJ tube placement may be found in Figure 18.1. The PEGJ technique (Jergens et al, 2007) is very similar to that of the PEG. Routine PEG placement is performed as described in Chapter 16. Choosing a PEGJ kit that allows interdigitation between the jejunal tube and the gastrostomy tube is important. Most kits fulfill this requirement. A gooseneck snare is advanced through the gastrostomy tube and into the stomach. The endoscope is directed through the loop in the snare and into the duodenum. A 0.035″ × 260 cm standard stiffness hydrophilic guide wire (HGW) is then advanced into the jejunum, and the endoscope is removed over the HGW. This leaves the HGW coursing through the snare. The snare is activated and withdrawn, exteriorizing the HGW via the PEG tube. The oral side of the HGW is pulled down from the mouth and exteriorized via the PEG tube. The jejunal segment of the GJ tube is then advanced over the wire, through the PEG tube, and into the jejunum. This is secured within the lumen of the PEG tube. The HGW is then removed. An alternative technique combining both endoscopic and fluoroscopic guidance involves advancing the

TABLE 18.2
Equipment commonly utilized for image-guided nutritional support techniques

Technique	Imaging required	Major equipment/supplies needed
PEG	Endoscopy	1. Numerous commercial PEG kits are available[3–5] 2. Gastrointestinal suture anchors (optional)[6,7] See Chapter 16
PEGJ	Endoscopy	Figure 18.1 1. Numerous commercial PEGJ kits are available[8,9] 2. Gastrointestinal suture anchors (optional)[6,7] 3. 0.035 in × 260 cm standard stiffness or stiff hydrophilic guidewire[10] 4. Gooseneck snare[11]
PRG	Fluoroscopy	Figure 18.2 1. Percutaneous introducer kit[6] 2. Iodinated contrast medium[12] 3. Gastrointestinal suture anchors[6,7] 4. Gastrostomy tube kit[8]
PRGJ	Fluoroscopy	Figure 18.3 1. Percutaneous introducer kit[6] 2. 0.035 in × 150 cm straight-tip standard stiffness or stiff hydrophilic guidewire[10] 3. Gastrointestinal suture anchors[6,7] 4. Iodinated contrast medium[12] 5. 4–5 F 65 cm Berenstein[13] or similar seeking catheter (included in most percutaneous introducer kits) 6. Gastro-enteric feeding tube[14]
RNJT	Fluoroscopy	Figure 18.4 1. Lidocaine Injectable 2%[1] 2. Feeding tube and urethral catheter (8 Fr) with tip removed[15] 3. 0.035 in × 260 cm straight-tip standard stiffness hydrophilic guidewire[10] 4. 100 cm 4–5Fr Berenstein catheter[13] 5. Nasogastric feeding tube 8 Fr × 137.5 cm[16] 6. Sterile lubricant[17] 7. Iodinated contrast medium[12] 8. 3-0 Nylon suture[18]
EndoNJT	Endoscopy	Figure 18.5 1. 0.035 in × 260 cm straight-tip standard stiffness hydrophilic guidewire[10] 2. Nasogastric feeding tube 8 Fr × 137.5 cm[16] 3. Sterile lubricant[17] 4. 3-0 Nylon suture[18]
EJT	Fluoroscopy	Figure 18.6 1. Right-angle forceps for esophagostomy tube placement 2. Feeding tube and urethral catheter (10 Fr) with tip removed[15] 3. 0.035 in × 260 cm straight-tip standard stiffness hydrophilic guidewire[10] 4. 10 F Peel-away sheath[19] 5. 100 cm 4–5 Fr Berenstein catheter[13] 6. Nasogastric feeding tube 8 Fr × 137.5 cm[16] 7. Sterile lubricant[17] 8. Iodinated contrast medium[12] 9. 3-0 Nylon suture[18]

HGW into the lumen of the stomach via the PEG. Then, using endoscopic guidance, a grasping instrument entraps the wire and advances it across the pylorus and it is then advanced into the jejunum using fluoroscopic and/or endoscopic guidance. Subsequently, the jejunal segment of the tube is advanced over the HGW and interdigitated with the gastrostomy tube. The HGW is then removed.

Percutaneous Radiologic Gastrostomy

Equipment for PRG tube placement may be found in Figure 18.2. PRG is performed with the patient in right lateral recumbency. Following routine surgical preparation and draping of a wide area caudal to the last rib, the stomach is insufflated with air via a nasogastric or orogastric tube. Ultrasound may be utilized to ensure that the spleen is not interposed between the insufflated stomach and the body wall. The insufflated stomach is palpated behind the last rib. Three to four gastrointestinal suture anchors are placed in a triangular or square pattern spaced approximately 3–4 cm apart (Figure 18.3 and Figure 18.4). Fluoroscopic guidance is used to ensure that the anchors penetrate all layers of the gastric wall (Videos 18.1 and 18.2). Intraluminal placement can also be confirmed through injection of 1–2 ml of a dilute, sterile, iodinated contrast agent through the suture anchor deployment needle. Different brands of gastrointestinal suture anchors deploy using different techniques. Although unnecessary for the completion of the procedure, concurrent gastroscopy (if possible) can be

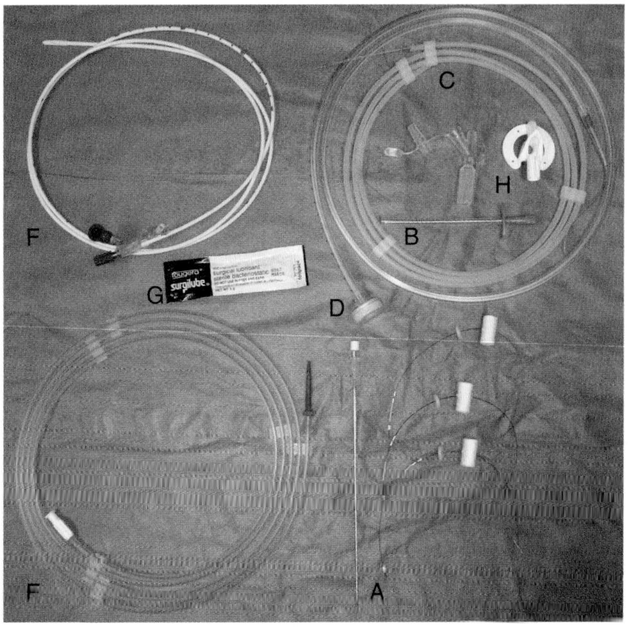

Figure 18.1 Equipment for PEGJ tube placement. (A) Gastrointestinal suture anchors and deployment needle (optional). (B) Gastric puncture needle. (C) Looped insertion wire (pull method). (D) PEG tube. (E) 260 cm 0.035 in straight tip, hydrophilic guide wire. (F) Jejunal component of PEGJ tube. (G) Sterile lubricant. (H) PEG accessories. Not pictured: Gooseneck snare (optional equipment based on technique utilized.

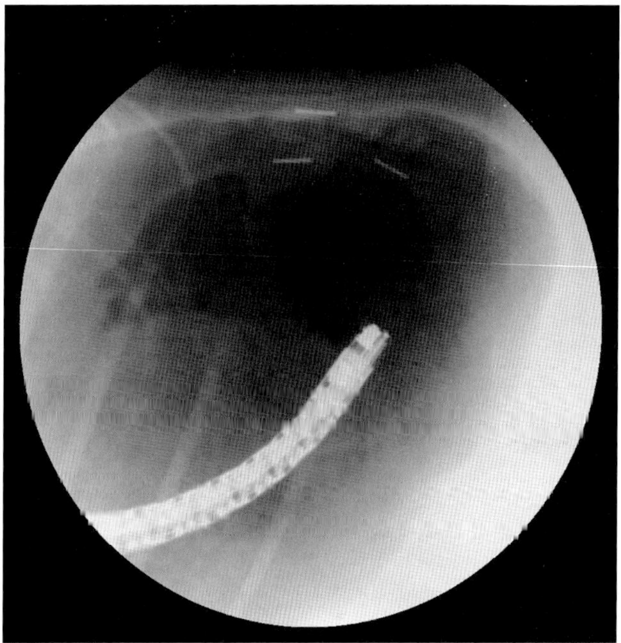

Figure 18.3 Fluoroscopic image from a dog with three gastrointestinal suture anchors[5] placed in a triangular pattern. The endoscope visible in the image was unnecessary for this procedure.

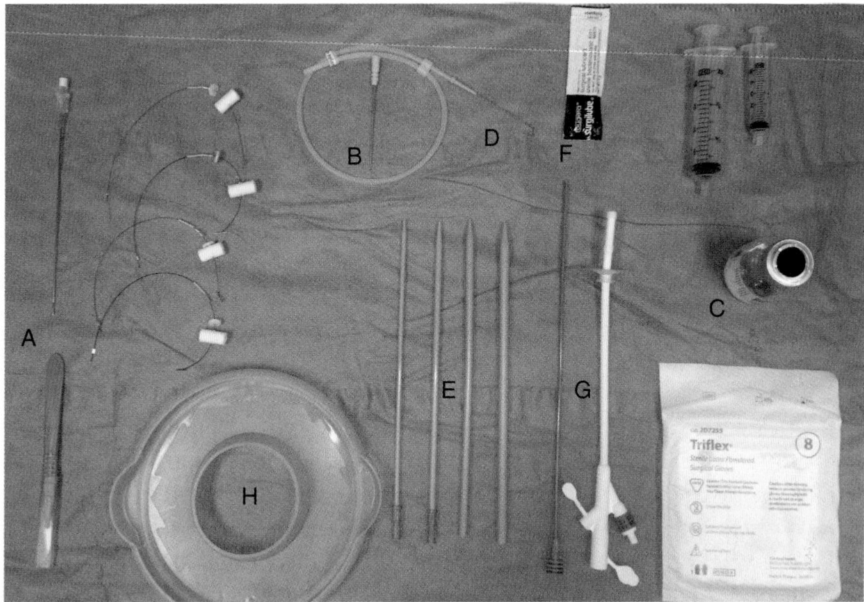

Figure 18.2 Equipment for PRG tube placement. (A) Gastrointestinal suture anchors and deployment needle. (B) Gastric puncture needle. (C) Iodinated contrast media. (D) J-tip guide wire. (E) Serial dilators. (F) Sterile lubricant. (G) PRG tube and stylet for over-the-wire insertion. (H) Wire basin. Note: Other PRG kits utilize serial dilators that transition to a peel-away sheath as described in the text.

utilized to further optimize positioning. Gastrointestinal suture anchors create a gastropexy and help ensure that the stomach remains apposed to the body wall throughout the procedure and the immediate postprocedural period. A 5mm skin incision is made at the center of the anchors and blunt dissection is utilized to reach the abdominal wall. A puncture needle is then introduced into the stomach via this incision. Confirmation of entry into the stomach can be made via aspiration of air and injection of a small volume (2–5ml) of sterile, iodinated contrast medium. A J-tip PTFE guide wire is then introduced through this puncture needle and into the stomach. The "J-tip" prevents injury to the stomach wall. The puncture needle is then removed. A 2–3mm stab incision can then be made through all layers of the abdominal wall along the path of the wire. This incision will facilitate serial dilation of the gastrostomy tract (Figure 18.5) (Video 18.3). Intermittent fluoroscopy should be utilized to ensure penetration of the body wall and stomach with the dilators. The tract is enlarged through progressive dilation until a large peel-away sheath can be advanced into the gastric lumen, or until the PRG (with stylet/stiffener) can be introduced directly. The peel-away sheath should be large enough to accommodate the diameter of the proposed gastrostomy tube. The well lubricated gastrostomy tube is then advanced over the wire, through the sheath, and into the stomach. The peel-away sheath is removed and the internal balloon/bolster is inflated or the retention device is activated, and gentle outward tension is applied to the tube to ensure a snug fit. The external bolster is advanced to a level approximately 0.5cm from the surface of the skin and the tube is secured in place (Figure 18.6). The guide wire is then removed. The position of the external bolster may need to be adjusted outward initially to accommodate swelling within the first few days. Later, it may need to be lowered closer to the skin. Numerous commercially available introducer and placement kits are available for these procedures (Table 18.2).

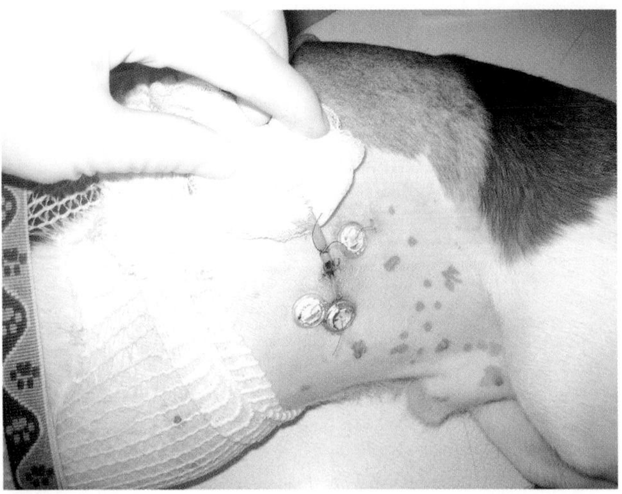

Figure 18.4 External view of a dog with three gastrointestinal suture anchors[5] placed in a triangular pattern.

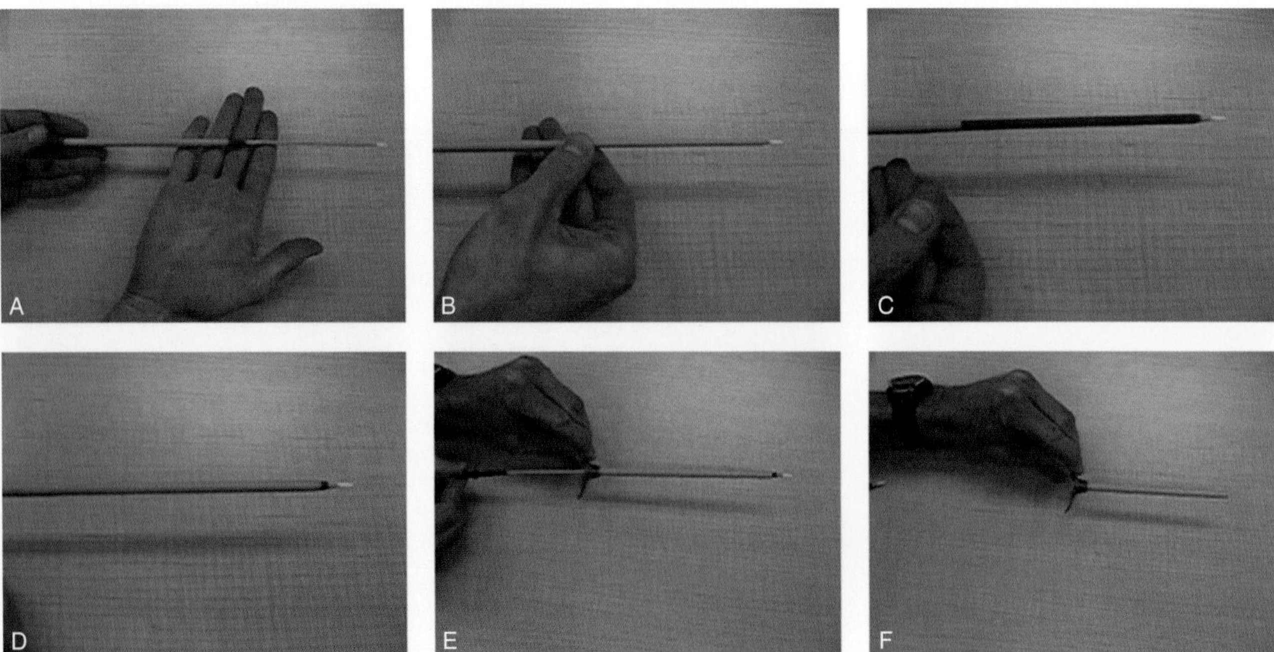

Figure 18.5 (A–F) In vitro images demonstrating use of an over-the-wire coaxial serial dilation (A–E) system[5] allowing for introduction of a peel-away sheath (F).

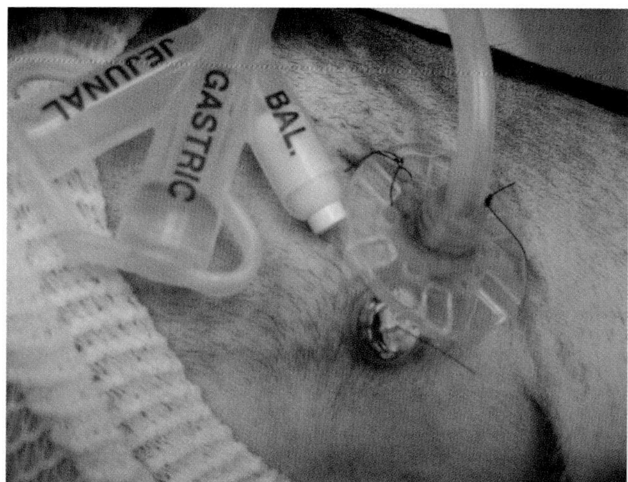

Figure 18.6 External bolster of a percutaneous radiologic gastrostomy/gastrojejunostomy tube. Note the separate ports for jejunal feeding and gastric decompression. GJ Parts004.

Percutaneous Radiologic Gastrojejunostomy Tube

Equipment for PRGJ tube placement may be found in Figure 18.7. The PRGJ tube placement is almost identical to the PRG technique described above (Beal et al, 2009a). The only difference is the need to advance a 0.035in × 150cm standard stiffness or stiff, straight tip hydrophilic guide wire (HGW) through the gastric puncture needle. The needle is removed and a Berenstein catheter is used to navigate through the pylorus, allowing the HGW to be advanced into the jejunum. This step is challenging because the patient may need to be repositioned to facilitate identification of the pylorus. Once the wire is positioned in the jejunum and the peel-away sheath is in place, the GJT is advanced over the wire (Figure 18.8). An injection of 3–5mL of a sterile, dilute iodinated contrast material

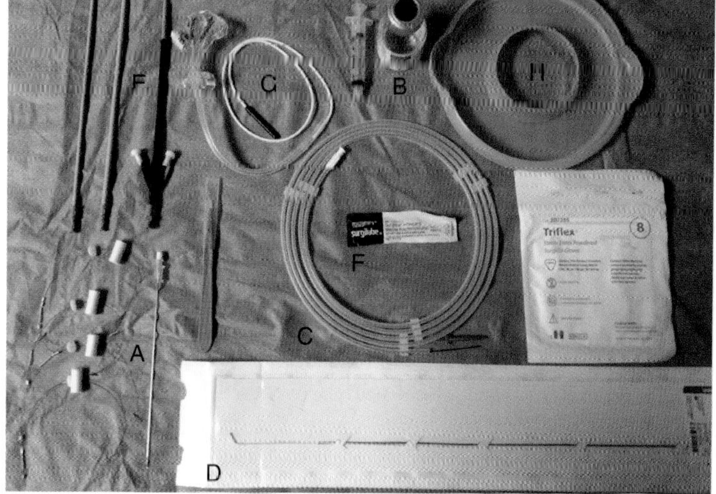

Figure 18.7 Equipment for PRGJ tube placement. (A) Gastrointestinal suture anchors and deployment needle. (B) Iodinated contrast media. (C) 0.035in × 260 cm straight tip standard stiffness hydrophilic guidewire. (D) 4–5 Fr × 65–100 cm Berenstein catheter. (E) Serial dilators and peel-away sheath (large enough to accommodate GJ tube passage). (F) Sterile lubricant. (G) PRGJ tube (H) Wire basin. Not pictured: Gastric puncture needle.

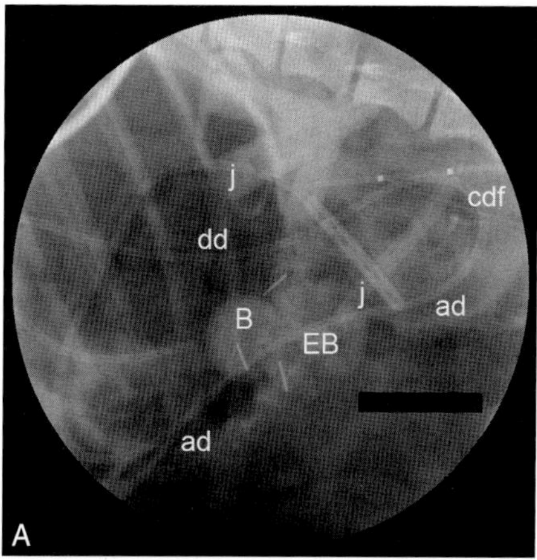

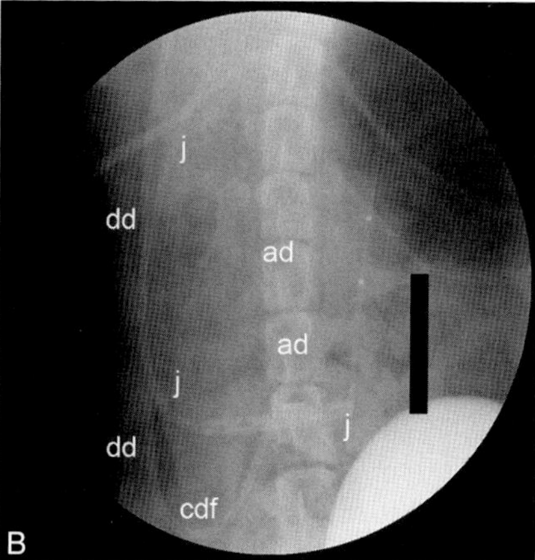

Figure 18.8 (A) Lateral radiograph of a dog with a percutaneous gastrojejunostomy in place. (B) Ventrodorsal radiograph of a different dog with a percutaneous gastrojejunostomy in place. EB, External bolster. B, Balloon. dd, descending duodenum. cdf, caudal duodenal flexure. ad, ascending duodenum. j, jejunum.

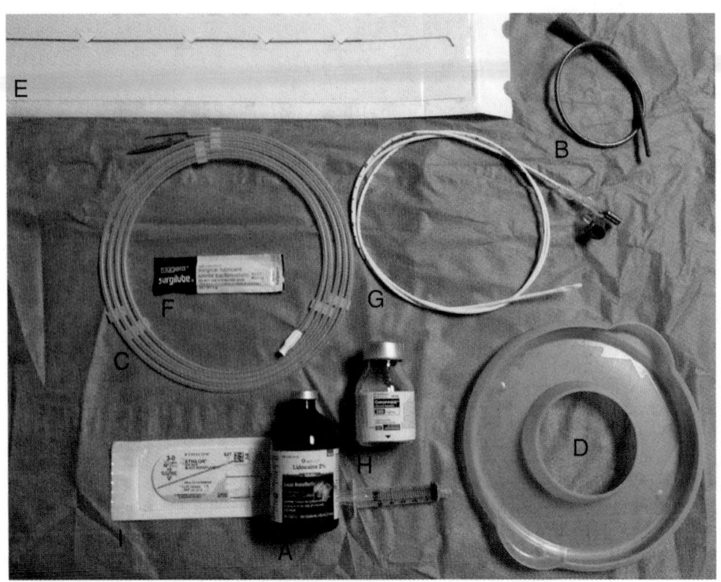

Figure 18.9 Equipment for RNJT placement. (A) Lidocaine injectable 2%. (B) 8 Fr Feeding tube and urethral catheter (requires tip removal). (C) (C) 0.035 in × 260 cm straight tip standard stiffness hydrophilic guidewire. (D) Wire basin. E) 4–5 Fr × 100 cm Berenstein catheter. (F) Sterile lubricant. (G) 8 Fr × 137.5 cm NJ tube (requires tip removal). (H) Sterile iodinated contrast agent. (I) 3–0 nylon suture material.

will confirm intraluminal placement. Most of these tubes have a port for jejunal feeding and another for gastric decompression/feeding (Figure 18.6). Based on design, some of the available GJT tubes' jejunal segment can be disarticulated from the gastrostomy tube while others are permanently joined.

Nasojejunal Tube

Equipment for RNJT tube placement may be found in Figure 18.9. Radiologic nasojejunal tube (RNJT) placement techniques are well described (Wohl, 2006, Beal et al, 2007, 2009b, Beal and Brown, 2011, Heuter, 2004). The following description is that of the technique developed by the author (Figure 18.10, Video 18.4). The patient is positioned in left lateral recumbency. This positions the pylorus such that it will fill with air. A local anesthetic is utilized as described above. A well-lubricated 8 Fr Red rubber catheter, with the tip removed, is advanced in an antegrade manner from the nares, through the ventral nasal meatus and nasopharynx, into the proximal esophagus. Positioning is confirmed fluoroscopically. A moistened 0.035″ × 260 cm standard stiffness, straight tip hydrophilic guide wire (HGW) is advanced down the 8 Fr catheter and into the esophagus and stomach. The 8 Fr catheter is removed and a 100 cm 4–5 F Berenstein catheter is advanced over the HGW and into the stomach (Figure 18.10A). The angle on the Berenstein catheter will allow the HGW to be directed into the pyloric antrum. Throughout all manipulations, the HGW should "lead" the catheter to prevent gastrointestinal injury. If the pyloric antrum is not air-filled, 5–15 mL of air may be introduced into the Berenstein catheter to help illustrate its exact location (Figure 18.10B). The pylorus is then serially probed with the HGW until it crosses into the descending duodenum. The Berenstein catheter is then advanced over the HGW and the HGW and Berenstein catheter are serially advanced until the HGW is well within the jejunum (Figure 18.10C). The jejunum can be identified as a ventrocaudal or dorsocaudal deviation in the bowel aboral to the ascending duodenum (Figure 18.10C). Efforts should be made to position the tip of the tube 5–10 cm into the jejunum. The Berenstein catheter is then removed and the 8 Fr open-ended 137.5 cm feeding tube is well lubricated and advanced over the HGW into the jejunum (Figure 18.10D). The HGW is removed and any "slack" in the tube is removed from the stomach with gentle traction. The tube is sutured adjacent to the alar fold of the nose. Occasionally, the feeding tube will not advance over the HGW due to the numerous turns in its path. In these situations, exchanging the standard stiffness HGW for a stiff HGW will sometimes allow the feeding tube to be advanced with greater ease. An injection of 3–5ml of a sterile, dilute iodinated contrast agent will confirm intraluminal placement.

Endoscopic NJT (EndoNJT) techniques have also been described (Papa et al, 2009, Campbell and Daley, 2011). Equipment for EndoNJT tube placement may be found in Figure 18.11. One technique (Campbell and Daley, 2011) utilizes endoscopic guidance, coupled with the use of grasping forceps via the working channel, to grasp a feeding tube in the stomach and manually advance it through the pylorus incrementally, and into the duodenum and jejunum. Radiography can be utilized to optimize final positioning of the tube within the jejunum. This technique may be useful for those without fluoroscopic capabilities. If endoscopic

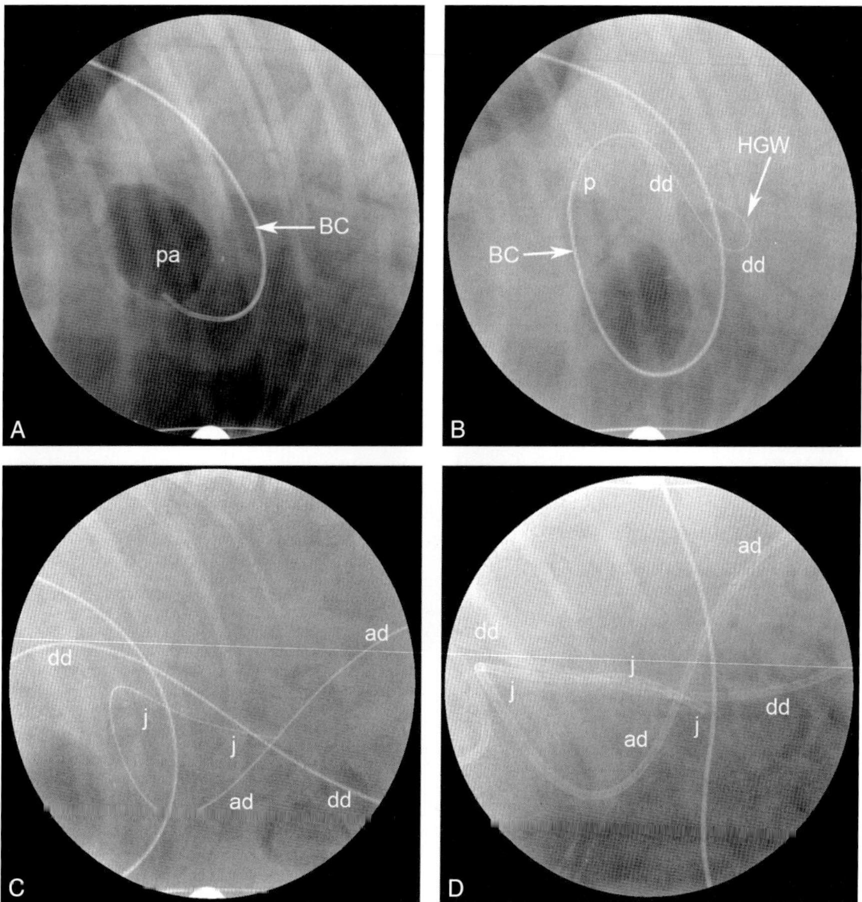

Figure 18.10 (A) The Berenstein catheter (BC) is positioned in the pyloric antrum (pa). The angle of the Berenstein catheter is used to direct the guide wire into the pyloric antrum. (B) In left lateral recumbency air will fill the pyloric antrum and help illustrate the location of the pylorus (p). The 0.035in 260 cm straight tip, standard stiffness hydrophilic guidewire (HGW) has been advanced across the pylorus and is in the descending duodenum (dd). The berenstein catheter (BC) has been advanced to the pylorus c) The HGW has been advanced down the descending duodenum (dd), up the ascending duodenum (ad), and into the jejunum (j). The Berenstein catheter is in the descending duodenum (dd). (D) The 8 Fr × 137.5 cm feeding tube has been advanced over the HGW and the HGW has been removed.

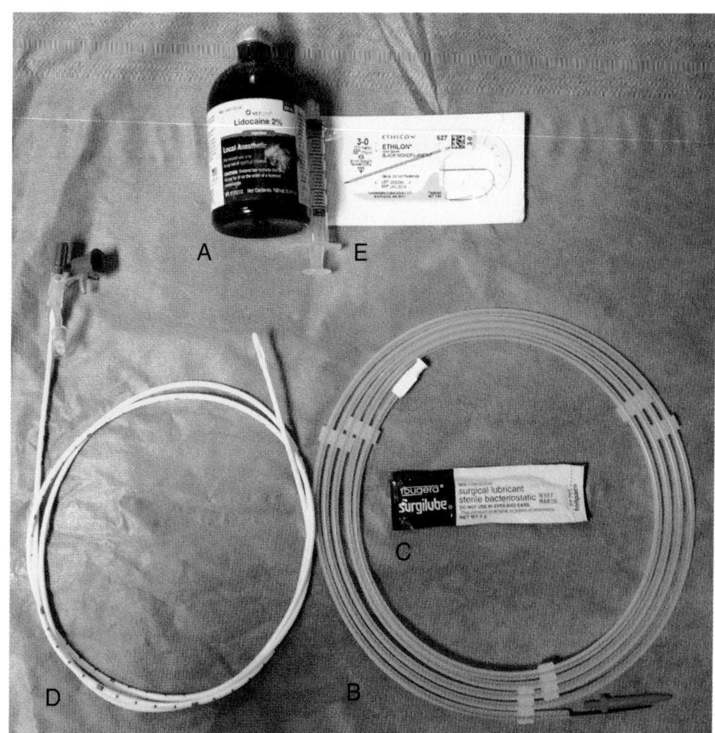

Figure 18.11 Equipment for EndoNJT placement. (A) Lidocaine injectable 2%. (B) 0.035 in × 260 cm straight tip standard stiffness hydrophilic guidewire. (C) Sterile lubricant. (D) 8 Fr × 137.5 cm NJ tube (requires tip removal). (E) 3 0 nylon suture material.

and fluoroscopic capabilities are both available, a hybrid technique utilizing endoscopy to direct a HGW across the pylorus is performed. The HGW is directed across the pylorus via the working channel of the endoscope or it is grasped via an endoscopic grasping instrument and passed across the pylorus as described above. Fluoroscopy is then utilized to complete the procedure as describe for RNJT above.

Esophagojejunal Tube

Equipment for EJT tube placement may be found in Figure 18.12. EJT placement is very similar to NJT placement. Following routine placement of an esophagostomy (E) tube using oropharyngeal decontamination (please see above) and aseptic technique externally, the HGW is advanced down the E-tube and into the stomach. The E-tube is removed and a 10 Fr peel-away sheath is advanced over the HGW. The patient is then positioned in left lateral recumbency and the Berenstein catheter is advanced over the HGW and into the stomach. The remainder of the procedure is performed in identical fashion to the NJT technique described above. Once the tube is in position (Figure 18.13A, B; Video 18.5), the peel-away sheath is removed and the tube is sutured in place using a purse string and finger trap pattern. Alternative techniques using nearly identical methodology involve

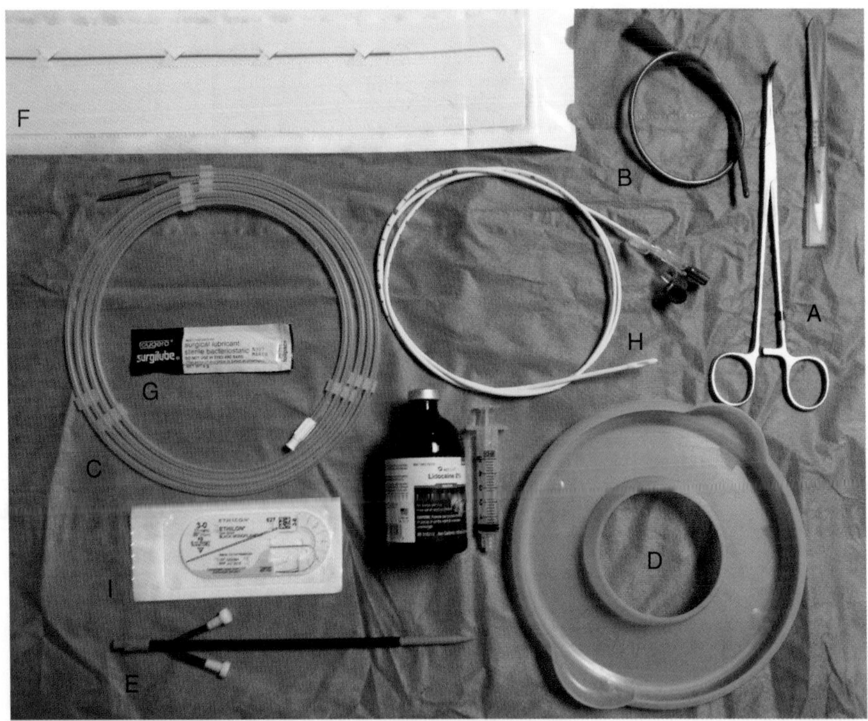

Figure 18.12 Equipment for EJT placement. (A) right-angle forceps. (B) 10F Feeding tube and urethral catheter (requires tip removal). (C) 0.035 in × 260 cm straight tip standard stiffness hydrophilic guidewire. (D) Wire basin. (E) 10F Peel-away sheath. (F) 4–5 Fr ×100 cm Berenstein catheter. (G) Sterile lubricant. (H) 8 Fr × 137.5 cm NJ tube (requires tip removal). (I) 3–0 nylon suture material. Not pictured: Sterile iodinated contrast agent.

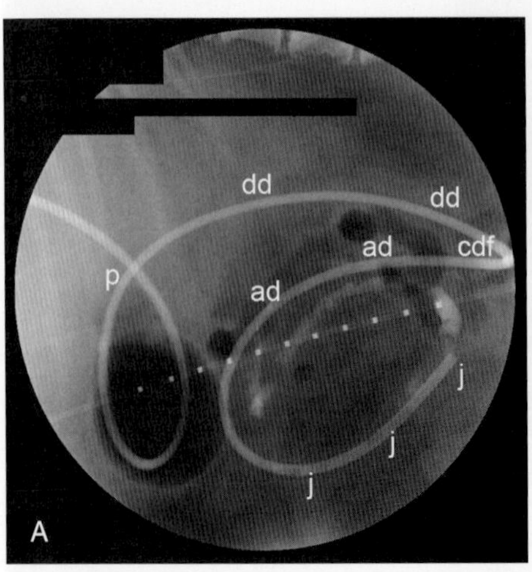

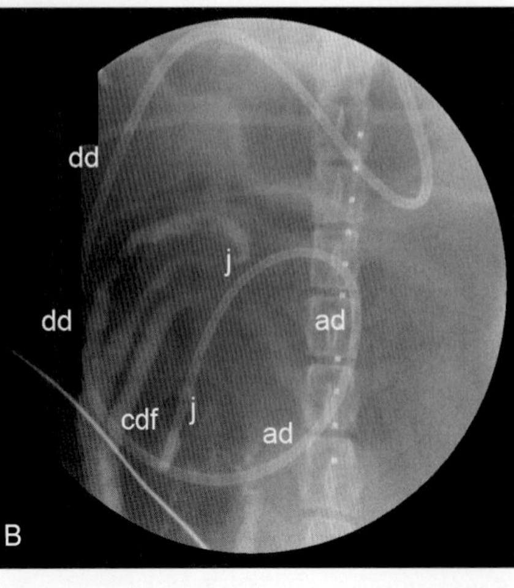

Figure 18.13 (A, B) Lateral and ventrodorsal radiographs illustrating final positioning of an EJT in a dog. p, pylorus. dd, descending duodenum. cdf, caudal duodenal flexure. ad, ascending duodenum. j, jejunum.

placing the jejunal segment through the esophagostomy tube, such that when postpyloric feeding is no longer necessary, gastric feeding and medication administration may be performed. Commercially produced kits may be available for this technique.[20]

Follow-Up

Nutritional support devices with exception of the NJT must have their access site evaluated daily for redness, swelling, or discharge and the dressing must be changed. Access site infection is not uncommon and systemic antibiotic therapy coupled with local wound care may be necessary.

NJT and EJT may be removed at any time; however, gastrostomy tubes should remain in place for approximately 4–6 weeks to allow the adhesion between the stomach and body wall to mature. Animals with critical illness or other conditions that could predispose to poor wound healing may require additional time for adhesion maturation.

Notes

1. Lidocaine Injectable 2%; Sparhawk Laboratories Inc. Lenexa, KS.
2. Clinicare; Abbott Animal Health, Abbott Park, IL.
3. PEG Kit; Mila International Inc. Erlanger, KY.
4. Flow 20 (Pull or Push Method); Cook Medical Inc. Bloomington, IN.
5. MIC Safety PEG; Kimberly-Clark Worldwide Inc. Roswell, GA.
6. MIC, MIC-KEY Introducer Kits. Kimberly-Clark Worldwide Inc. Roswell, GA.
7. Cope Gastrointestinal Suture Anchors; Cook Medical Inc. Bloomington, IN.
8. MIC Gastrostomy Feeding Tube. Kimberly-Clark Worldwide Inc. Roswell, GA.
9. Flow 20 Jejunal; Cook Medical Inc. Bloomington, IN.
10. Weasel Wire Hydrophilic Guide Wire; Infiniti Medical LLC. Menlo Park, CA.
11. Amplatz Goose Neck Snare Kit, ev3 Endovascular Inc. Plymouth, MN.
12. Omnipaque 300; GE Healthcare Inc. Princeton, NJ.
13. Performa 5 French, 65–100cm Berenstein 1; Merit Medical Systems Inc. South Jordan, UT.
14. MIC Gastro Enteric Feeding Tube; Kimberly-Clark Worldwide Inc. Roswell, GA.
15. Feeding Tube and Urethral Catheter; Tyco Healthcare Group LP. Mansfield, MA.
16. Nasogastric Feeding Tube 8 French × 55in (137.5cm); Mila International Inc. Erlanger, KY.
17. Fougera Surgilube; E. Fougera & Co. Melville, New York.
18. 3–0 Ethilon; Ethicon LLC. San Lorenzo, PR.
19. Peel-Away Sheath Introducer Set; Cook Medical Inc. Bloomington, IN.
20. Mila International Inc. Erlanger, KY.

References

Abood SK and Buffington CA (1992) Enteral feeding of dogs and cats: 51 cases (1989–1991). *J Am Vet Med Assoc* 201, 619–22.

Altintas ND, Aydin K, Turkoglu MA et al (2011) Effect of enteral versus parenteral nutrition on outcome of medical patients requiring mechanical ventilation. *Nutr Clin Pract* 26, 322–9.

Beal MW, Jutkowitz LA, Brown AJ (2007) Development of a novel method for fluoroscopically-guided nasojejunal feeding tube placement in dogs (abstr). 2007 IVECC Symposium Abstracts. *J Vet Emerg Crit Care* 17, S1.

Beal MW, Mehler SJ, Staiger BA et al (2009a) Technique for percutaneous radiologic gastrojejunostomy in the dog (abstr). 2009 ACVIM Forum Abstracts. *J Vet Intern Med* 23, 713.

Beal MW, Mehler SJ, Staiger BA et al (2009b) Technique for nasojejunal tube placement in the dog (abstr). 2009 ACVIM Forum Abstracts. *J Vet Intern Med* 23, 713.

Beal MW and Brown MA (2011) Clinical experience utilizing a novel fluoroscopic technique for wire guided nasojejunal tube placement in the dog: 26 cases (2006–2010). *J Vet Emerg Crit Care* 21, 151–7.

Campbell SA and Daley CA (2011) Endoscopically assisted nasojejunal feeding tube placement: technique and results in five dogs. *J Am Anim Hosp Assoc* 47, e50–e55.

Cantwell CP, Perumpillichira JJ, Maher MM, et al (2008) Antibiotic prophylaxis for percutaneous radiologic gastrostomy and gastrojejunostomy insertion in outpatients with head and neck cancer. *J Vasc Interv Radiol* 19, 571–5.

Chan DL and Freeman LM (2006) Nutrition in critical illness. *Vet Clin N Am Small Anim Pract* 36, 1225–41.

Chan DL (2004) Nutritional requirements of the critically ill patient. *Clin Tech Small Anim Pract* 19, 1–5.

Crowe DT and Devey JJ (1997) Clinical experience with jejunostomy feeding tubes in 47 small animal patients. *J Vet Emerg Crit Care* 7, 7–19.

Gramlich L, Kichian K, Pinilla J, et al (2004) Does enteral nutrition compared to parenteral nutrition result in better outcomes in critically ill adult patients? A systematic review of the literature. *Nutrition* 20, 843–8.

Han E (2004) Esophageal and gastric feeding tubes in icu patients. *Clin Techn Small Anim Pract* 19, 22–31.

Heuter K (2004) Placement of jejunal feeding tubes for post-gastric feeding. *Clin Tech Small Anim Pract* 19, 32–42.

Hewitt SA, Brisson BA, Sinclair MD et al (2004) Evaluation of laparoscopic-assisted placement of jejunostomy feeding tubes in dogs. *J Am Vet Med Assoc* 225, 65–71.

Heyland DK, Dhaliwal R, Drover JW, et al (2003) Canadian clinical practice guidelines for nutrition support in mechanically ventilated, critically ill adult patients. *J Parent Ent Nutr* 27, 355–73.

Holahan M, Abood S, Hauptman J et al (2010) Intermittent and continuous enteral nutrition in critically ill dogs: a prospective randomized trial. *J Vet Intern Med* 24, 520–6.

Horiuchi A, Nakayama Y, Kajiyama M, et al (2006) Nasopharyngeal decolonization of methicillin-resistant Staphylococcus aureus can reduce PEG peristomal wound infection. *Am J Gastroenterol* 101, 274–7.

Jennings M, Center SA, Barr SC et al (2001) Successful treatment of feline pancreatitis using an endoscopically placed gastrojejunostomy tube. *J Am Anim Hosp Assoc* 37, 145–52.

Jergens AE, Morrison JA, Miles KG et al (2007) Percutaneous endoscopic gastrojejunostomy tube placement in healthy dogs and cats. *J Vet Intern Med* 21, 18–24.

Lipp A and Lusardi G (2009) A systematic review of prophylactic antimicrobials in PEG placement. *J Clin Nursing* 18, 938–48.

Mack RM, Moon LT, Fritz MC, et al (2013) Efficacy of pre-operative oropharyngeal decolonization procedure for placement of esophageal feeding tubes in cats. In *Proceedings of the 13th Annual American Academy of Veterinary Nutrition*, Seattle, WA.

Mauterer JV, Abood SK, Buffington CA, et al (1994) New techniques and management guidelines for percutaneous and nonendoscopic tube gastrostomy. *J Am Vet Med Assoc* 207, 574–9.

Michel KE and Higgins C (2006) Investigation of the percentage of prescribed enteral nutrition actually delivered to hospitalized companion animals. *J Vet Emerg Crit Care* 16, S2–S6.

Papa K, Psader R, Sterczer A et al (2009) Endoscopically guided nasojejunal tube placement in dogs for short-term postduodenal feeding. *J Vet Emerg Crit Care* 19, 554–63.

Peter JV, Moran JL, and Phillips-Hughes J (2005) A metaanalysis of treatment outcomes of early enteral versus early parenteral nutrition in hospitalized patients. *Crit Care Med* 33, 213–20.

Remillard RL, Darden DE, Michel KE et al (2001) An investigation of the relationship between caloric intake and outcome in hospitalized dogs. *Vet Ther: Res Appl Vet Med* 2, 301–10.

Salinardi BJ, Harkin KR, Bulmer BJ et al. (2006) Comparison of complications of percutaneous endoscopic versus surgically placed gastrostomy tubes in 42 dogs and 52 cats. *J Am Anim Hosp Assoc* 42, 51–6.

Swann HM, Sweet DC, and Michel KE (1997) Complications associated with use of jejunostomy tubes in dogs and cats: 40 cases (1989–1994). *J Am Vet Med Assoc* 210, 1764–7.

Wohl JS (2006) Nasojejunal feeding tube placement using fluoroscopic guidance: technique and clinical experience in dogs. *J Vet Emerg Crit Care* 16, S27–S33.

Yagil-Kelmer E, Wagner-Mann C, and Mann FA (2006) Postoperative complications associated with jejunostomy tube placement using the interlocking box technique compared with other jejunopexy methods in dogs and cats:76 cases (1999–2003). *J Vet Emerg Crit Care* 16, S14–S20.

Video 18.1 In vitro deployment of gastrointestinal suture anchors.[5]

Video 18.2 Fluoroscopic deployment of gastrointestinal suture anchors.[5]

Video 18.3 In vitro demonstration of a co-axial dilation system for serial dilation of the percutaneous radiologic gastrostomy tract.[5]

Video 18.4 Nasojejunal tube placement in a dog.

Video 18.5 Final positioning of an esophagojejunal tube in a dog.

These video clips can be found in the online material at **www.wiley.com/go/weisse/vet-image-guided-interventions**

SECTION FOUR

Hepatobiliary System

Edited by Chick Weisse

CHAPTER NINETEEN

Hepatobiliary Imaging

Allison Zwingenberger
School of Veterinary Medicine, University of California – Davis, Davis, CA

Imaging Protocols

Cross-sectional imaging of the hepatobiliary system has rapidly developed into the gold standard method for diagnosis of liver disease and for treatment planning. Computerized tomography (CT) has particularly emerged as a valuable technique for angiography due to the widespread availability of multislice CT scanners which provide rapid imaging and very high spatial resolution. Magnetic resonance imaging (MRI) is also used for angiography and for providing detailed information on tissue characteristics, but is currently not as widely used as CT. Both modalities acquire a 3D volume that can be displayed in multiple planes for best depiction of the abnormality in question. Ultrasonography is also widely used to diagnose masses and vascular anomalies. Ultrasound can be insensitive to the extent of nodular and mass lesions, however the character of visible lesions can be used to rank differential diagnoses. Doppler ultrasonography is valuable for evaluating flow in the hepatic vessels and portal veins, such as pulsatile flow in arteriovenous fistulas, hepatofugal flow in portal hypertension, and directional flow in following shunt vessels.

Protocols for CT and MRI studies can be performed with the animal in dorsal or ventral recumbency. General anesthesia is recommended for control of respiratory motion artifacts to obtain the highest quality scans. Thin slice collimation (0.6–2.5 mm) is necessary to trace the vasculature, and less than 1 mm slice thickness produces the best resolution for multiplanar reformatting and 3D modeling. In very small dogs (<10 kg) the thinnest collimation possible is recommended due to the small scale of the vasculature.

Parenchymal Imaging

Imaging of the liver parenchyma is usually performed with precontrast and postcontrast images to provide high contrast images of nodules or masses that may be present. Precontrast images are acquired in a soft tissue algorithm during a breath hold or a period of apnea. Non-ionic contrast medium is injected intravenously, preferably into a cephalic vein to avoid pooling in the caudal vena cava with resultant high-density streak artifacts. The injection may be done by hand or using a power injector at 2–3 ml/s injection rate. The standard dose is 2 ml/kg of nonionic contrast medium at 300–370 mg I/ml concentration. Postcontrast images should be acquired 60–180 seconds after injection for maximal tissue enhancement. This protocol will allow the characterization, localization, distribution, and measurement of hepatic lesions such as nodules, masses, and inflammatory lesions. The gallbladder and bile duct are also visible and may be evaluated for abnormalities.

CT Angiography

CT angiography is a method of timing the CT scans to coincide with the contrast bolus as it travels though the hepatic arterial system, the portal system, and the hepatic venous system (Table 19.1). Single slice scanners are capable of performing this protocol with meticulous planning, however multislice scanners make it much easier to acquire the desired images in the correct time frame. A precontrast series from the diaphragm to the pelvic inlet is acquired first in a soft tissue algorithm to define the margins of the anatomy in question. To determine the time of arrival of contrast in the vasculature, either a timing bolus or an automatic detection protocol can be used. A power injector with 3–5 ml/s injection rate provides the most consistent results with regard to timing and a tightly formed bolus. Contrast medium should be high concentration (>350 mg I/ml) and non-ionic, as the injection is rapid and the contrast will be diluted before reaching the portal vein. Timing boluses allow the planning of delays for both the arterial and portal phases of the scan, while the automatic detection protocol only

Veterinary Image-Guided Interventions, First Edition. Edited by Chick Weisse and Allyson Berent.

Companion website: www.wiley.com/go/weisse/vet-image-guided-interventions

TABLE 19.1
Protocols for CT angiography

Series	Phase	Start	End	Direction	Collimation	Algorithm	Contrast medium	Delay
Survey abdomen	Precontrast	Diaphragm	Pelvic inlet	Cr-Cd	0.6–2.5 mm	Soft tissue	none	0
Dynamic	Timing	Porta hepatis	n/a	Stationary	2–5 mm	Soft tissue	0.25 ml/kg, 5 ml/s, 1 s rotation, 60 s duration	0 (start scan and injection simultaneously)
Dual-phase	Arterial	Porta hepatis	Diaphragm	Cd-Cr	0.6–2.5 mm	Soft tissue	2 ml/kg, 3–5 ml/s	(TA) Peak arrival in aorta (from dynamic)
	Portal	Diaphragm	Pelvic inlet	Cr-Cd	0.6–2.5 mm	Soft tissue		(TA+TAPS+Delay) Plateau of portal (from dynamic)
Multiphase	Delayed	Diaphragm	Pelvic inlet	Cr-Cd	0.6–2.5 mm	Soft tissue		60–180 s post injection
Single-phase	Portal	Diaphragm	Pelvic inlet	Cr-Cd		Soft tissue	2 ml/kg, 3–5 ml/s	(TP) Plateau of portal (from dynamic). Estimate method 20–30s post injection, increasing with body weight

Choose whether to perform a single phase or dual-phase protocol. The most thinly collimated images are appropriate for very small dogs (<10 kg) and multislice scanners. Timing is determined from the dynamic CT scan by creating a graph with regions of interest, or by counting the number of images (at 1 slice/second) until peak vessel enhancement. TA = time to peak contrast in aorta (s), TAPS = total time of arterial phase scan (s), Delay = time delay between arterial and portal phase scans. Pre-delay (TA) and interscan delay (Delay) are programmed into the dual phase scan at setup. The portal phase scan should begin at plateau of portal enhancement, which can be estimated at 20–30 s depending on body weight, with moderate individual variability. Contrast medium used should be non-ionic and high concentration.

determines when contrast reaches the arteries to trigger the scan. Experience with each method will allow the operator to fine tune the protocols. A single-phase study can also be acquired, omitting the arterial phase, for simple portosystemic shunts. If estimating the timing of a single-phase portal scan, the delay should be 20–30 s, increasing with body weight. There is moderate variability with estimation and the portal phase can be missed. The portal phase lasts for approximately 60–90 s, so a longer delay is more likely to be successfully timed than a shorter delay.

CT angiography is useful for vascular anomalies such as intrahepatic, extrahepatic, and acquired portosystemic shunts. Dual-phase angiography is necessary to diagnose arterioportal fistulas/arteriovenous malformations, however these are uncommon. Dual-phase scans are also recommended when the clinician is considering embolization of a hepatic mass, as the arterial supply to the tumor can be accurately mapped.

MR Angiography

Techniques for MR angiography of the hepatic vasculature may either be performed without contrast (phase contrast, time of flight) or using gadolinium as a contrast agent. Contrast enhanced MR angiography has a greater likelihood of high contrast of the vasculature and good anatomic detail than the time of flight technique. This technique uses a 3D volume acquisition and a fast spoiled gradient recalled echo (3D FSPGR) pulse sequence. Timing of the bolus is not required as the arterial and portal phases are captured in one of four sequential acquisitions. This method has been successfully used to diagnose a variety of hepatic vascular disorders.

CT versus MR angiography

CT is advantageous for fast scan speeds and excellent vascular detail. The volumetric MR technique allows for fast scan speeds as well, and provides excellent 3D images as the background tissues are subtracted from the vasculature. Both methods require technical expertise, though MR is more challenging and has particular coil and software requirements.

Outcome Measures

CT is an excellent anatomic imaging modality, but there are several uses that allow outcome measures of hepatic function. Hepatic volume is a determinant of hepatic function, and is being used successfully to measure the pre- and post-treatment change following surgical and minimally invasive interventions. It has good correlation with the attenuation of extrahepatic portosystemic shunts. The dynamic CT acquisition used for scan timing can also be used to measure the flow of contrast through the hepatic tissue. Hepatic arterial fraction, blood flow, and blood volume are being investigated as measures of blood flow alteration after shunt attenuation and tumor embolization. There is very good potential for evaluating the results of novel techniques being developed in the field of interventional radiology.

Hepatic Anatomy

Hepatic Arteries

The hepatic artery originates from the celiac artery, and divides into one to five branches as it enters the liver. The hepatic artery is normally visible in cross section at the level of the porta hepatis, in close association with the portal vein. The arterial branches travel into the hepatic parenchyma along the walls of the portal veins. They are best evaluated during the arterial phase of a dual-phase scan, and are most apparent in the caudal portion of the liver (Figure 19.1).

Portal Tributaries and Branches

The portal vein forms at the junction of the cranial and caudal mesenteric veins and travels cranially toward the liver (Figure 19.2). The two main additional tributaries are the splenic vein from the left, and the gastroduodenal vein from the right side (Figure 19.3). The left gastric vein drains into the splenic vein just before its junction with the portal vein. The transverse portal vein diameter increases with each additional tributary. At the porta hepatis, the portal vein is at its largest diameter and gives off a small branch to the right lateral liver lobe (Figure 19.4A). The largest branch is the left divisional branch that curves to the left lateral and medial lobes. A smaller branch divides from the left branch to supply the right medial lobe of the liver (Figure 19.4B).

Hepatic Veins

Hepatic veins originate in the central portions of each liver lobe and drain into the caudal vena cava (Figure 19.5). The most visible veins on angiographic scans include the small branch draining the caudate lobe, and the large left hepatic vein, with a branch draining the right medial and quadrate lobes, at the

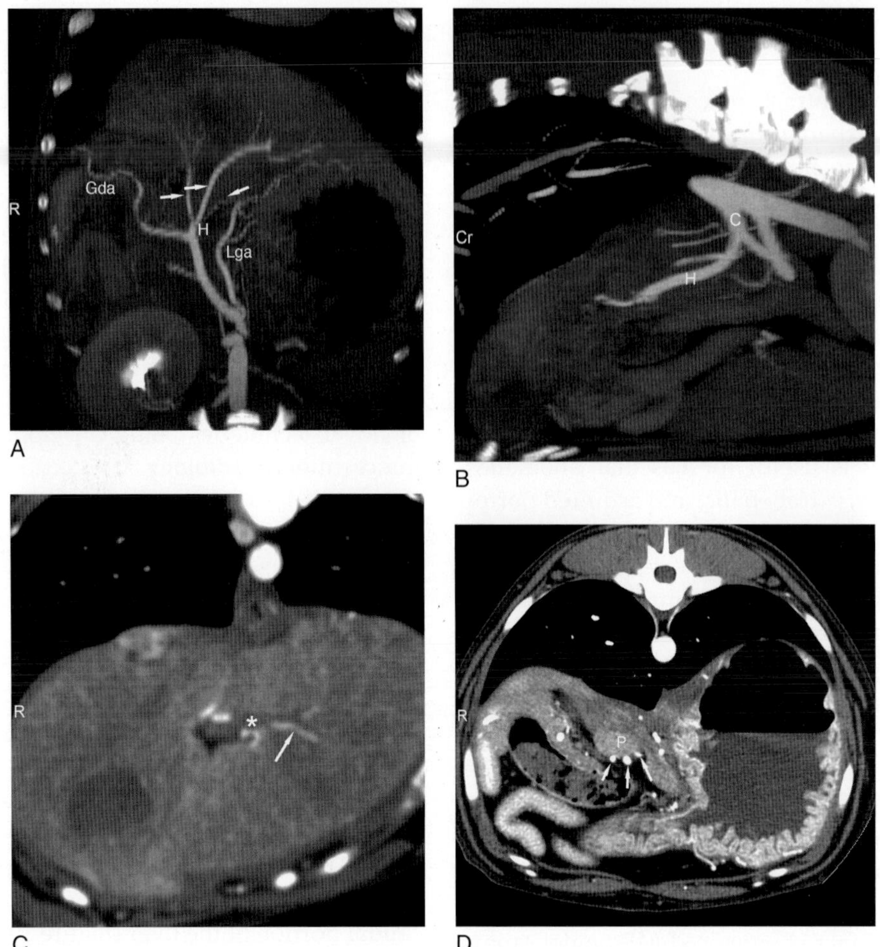

Figure 19.1 Reformatted CT angiographic arterial phase images of the hepatic artery. (A) Dorsal reformatting shows three main branches originating from the hepatic artery and supplying the divisions of the liver (arrows). (Gda) Gastroduodenal artery, (Lga) left gastric artery. (B) A sagittal image shows the celiac artery (C) giving rise to the hepatic artery (H). (C) The small hepatic arteries (arrow) run parallel to the portal veins (*). The liver enhances in a heterogeneous fashion during the arterial phase. (D) In the transverse image, the three portal branches are visible in cross section (arrows) ventral to the portal vein (P).

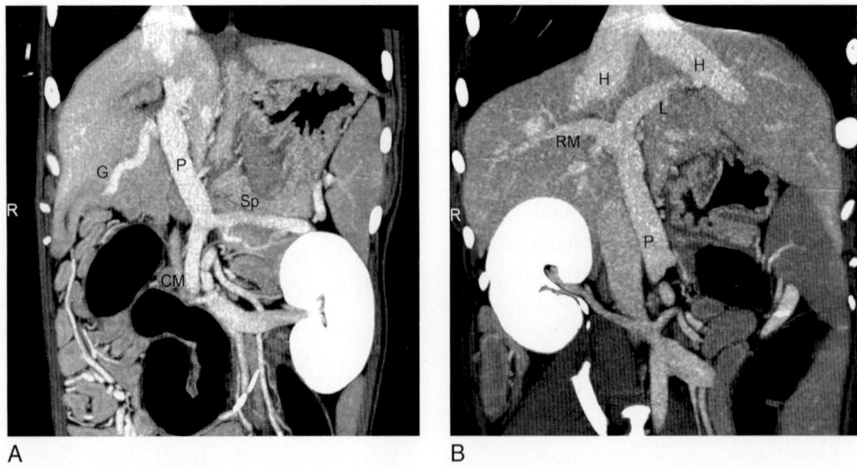

Figure 19.2 Dorsal reformatted CT maximum intensity projection (MIP) images of the portal tributaries and branches. (A) The cranial mesenteric vein (CM) and the caudal mesenteric vein (smaller, not shown) join to form the portal vein (P). The splenic vein is the first tributary from the left side (Sp), and the gastroduodenal vein joins the portal vein from the right lobe of the pancreas, on the ventral aspect (G). (B) The left portal vein branch divides into branches supplying the right medial lobe (RM) and left liver lobes (L) cranial to the porta hepatis, and interdigitates with the hepatic veins (H).

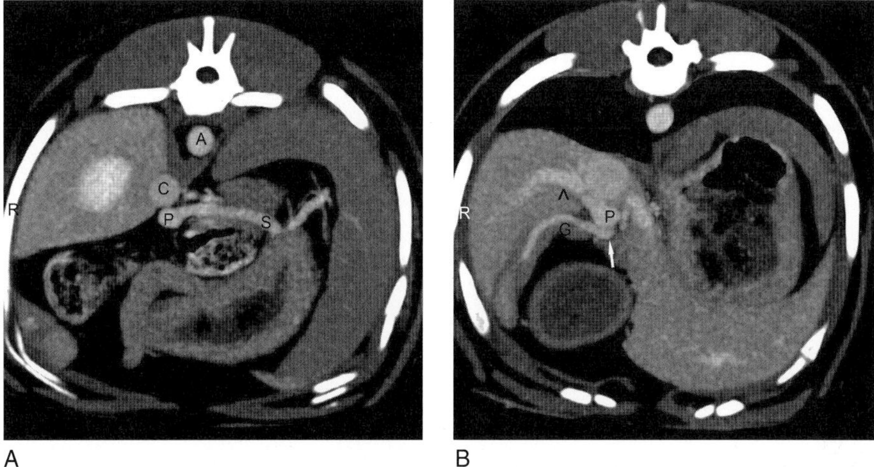

Figure 19.3 Transverse CT MIP images of the portal tributaries. (A) The splenic vein joins the portal vein (P) from the left side, parallel to the dorsal axis. It is a large vein with several splenic tributaries. (B) The gastroduodenal vein (G) travels along the right pancreatic lobe, and enters the portal vein from the ventral aspect. The right portal branch is visible dorsal to it (^). Caudal vena cava (C), aorta (A).

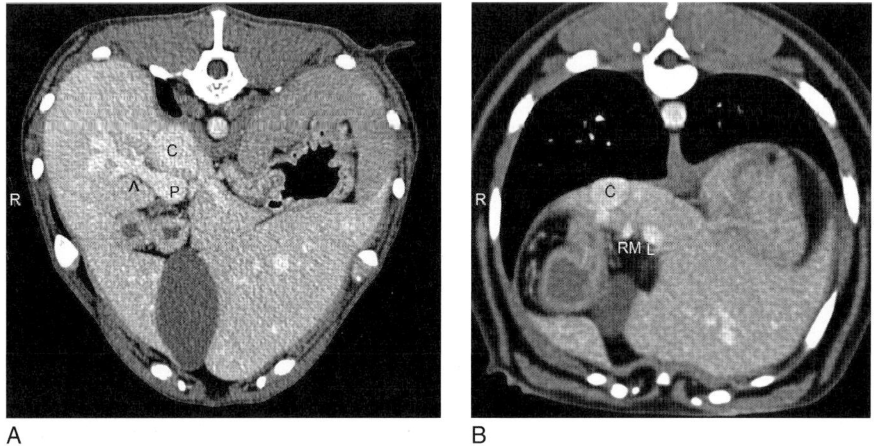

Figure 19.4 Transverse CT images of the portal branches. (A) The right divisional portal branch (^) exits the portal vein (P) shortly after the junction of the gastroduodenal vein, and travels dorsally to the right lateral liver lobe. (B) The left branch then divides to supply the right medial lobe (RM) and the left liver lobes (L). The right medial lobe branch is smaller in diameter than the left lobe branch. Caudal vena cava (C).

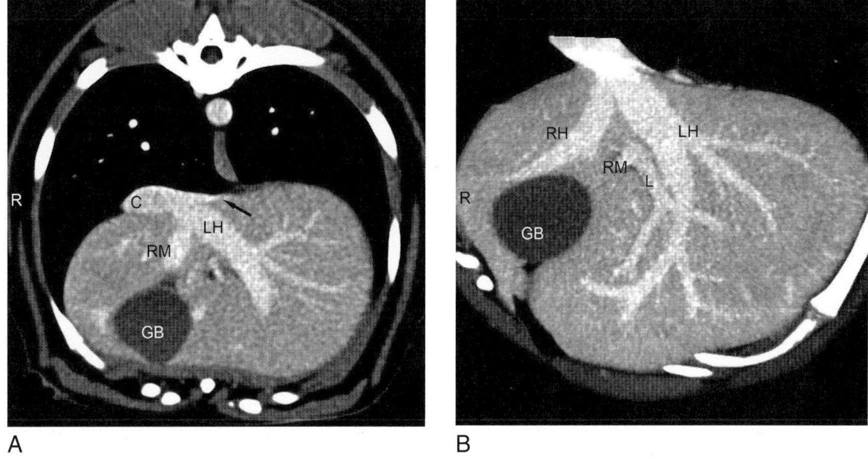

Figure 19.5 Transverse and oblique CT images of the hepatic veins. (A) The left hepatic vein (LH) is the largest, and drains the left hepatic division. The large branch joins it from the right medial and quadrated lobe (RM) and the common trunk enters into the caudal vena cava (C) ventrally and on the left side. The small phrenic vein (black arrow) travels parallel to the diaphragm and enters at this same location. (B) On this transverse oblique image, the right and left hepatic veins are seen to interdigitate with the right medial (RM) and left lobar (L) portal vein branches. Gall bladder (GB).

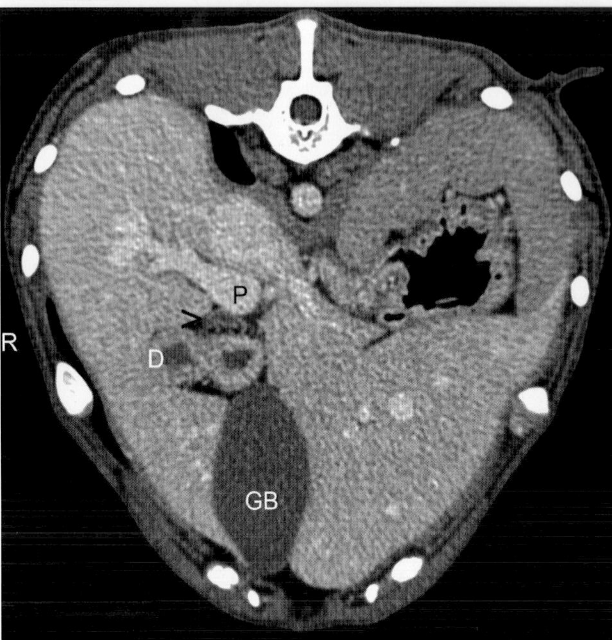

Figure 19.6 Transverse CT image of the liver and biliary system. The gallbladder (GB) is visible as a non-contrast enhancing, fluid attenuating structure. The common bile duct (>) travels dorsally and to the right at the level of the porta hepatis ventral to the portal vein (P). The walls are mildly contrast enhancing. The duct joins the duodenum (D), which is seen in two cross sections at the level of the proximal descending duodenum.

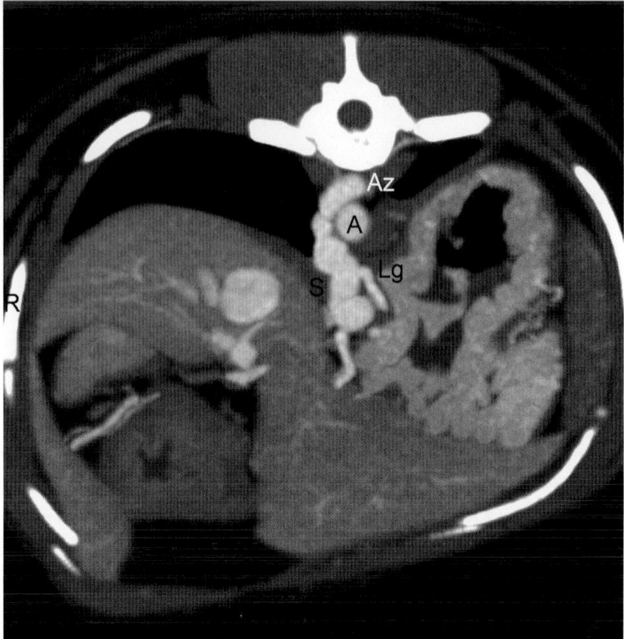

Figure 19.7 Transverse CT MIP portal phase image of a dog with a portoazygous shunt. The shunt vessel (S) travels dorsally in a tortuous fashion to join with the azygous vein (Az). Note that the left gastric vein (Lg) joins the shunt vessel after it exits the portal vein, which affects the planned placement of ligatures or ameroid constrictors to avoid postoperative shunting.

level of the diaphragm. The phrenic vein is often visible traveling in the transverse plane to join the left hepatic vein.

Hepatic Parenchyma and Biliary Structures

The hepatic parenchyma is uniform, and the liver lobes are not visible individually except for using certain landmarks. The gallbladder is located between the right medial and quadrate lobe, and the portal vein branches can be followed to their respective divisions. The common bile duct is visible as a small structure at the porta hepatis that travels to the right to join the duodenum (Figure 19.6). Intrahepatic bile ducts are not normally visible.

Imaging of Hepatic Disorders

The two most common indications for hepatic imaging are evaluation of hepatic vascular anomalies and hepatic masses. Dual-phase or multiphase

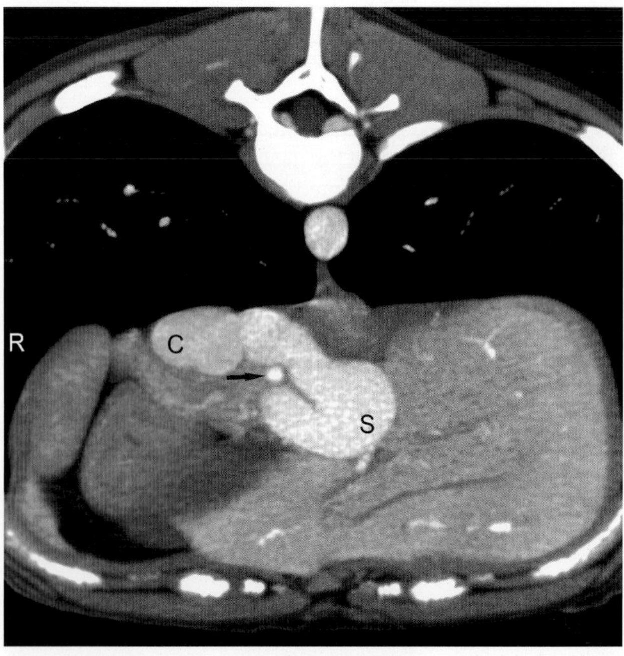

Figure 19.8 Transverse CT MIP portal phase image of a dog with a left divisional intrahepatic portosystemic shunt. The left divisional shunt travels from the left side of the portal vein (not shown) through the left hepatic division, and meets the caudal vena cava (C) on the left side. The cross section of vessel in the curve of the shunt (black arrow) is a hepatic vein.

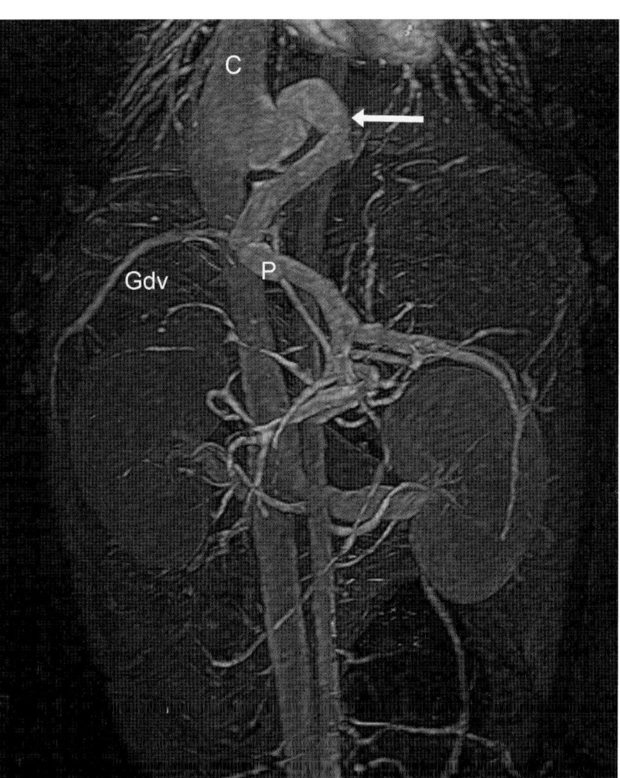

Figure 19.9 3D MR angiographic image of a dog with a left divisional portosystemic shunt. The shunt (arrow) exits the portal vein (P) and curves to the left within the liver, forming a loop that joins with the left hepatic vein and caudal vena cava (C). Image courtesy of Dr. Wil Mai.

scans are recommended when possible, as they can add valuable information to the diagnostic study. For vascular anomalies, the arterial phase is indicated to rule out arteriovenous fistulas or malformations.

CT angiograms should be approached by first identifying the portal vein, the tributaries, and then the size and presence of the portal branches. Anomalous vessels can be recognized arising from the portal vein or its tributaries and branches (Figure 19.7, Figure 19.8, and Figure 19.9). Other vessels, such as splenic vein branches and left gastric veins may enter the shunt vessel itself, and should be noted for surgical planning (Figure 19.7).

Hepatic parenchymal disease should be characterized by its pre- and postcontrast attenuation characteristics and enhancement patterns. The precise localization of a mass to certain liver lobes may not always be reliable. Proximity to the gall bladder and bile duct should also be noted. Dual-phase scans are also useful in detecting hepatic metastatic disease which is occasionally only visible during the arterial phase, and later is indistinguishable from the enhanced liver parenchyma (Figure 19.10). This is presumed to be due to the arterial neovascularization of the tumor tissue.

Other disorders such as hepatic cysts, abscesses, biliary inflammation, and obstruction can be evaluated well with CT. These disorders have enhancement patterns consistent with their tissue vascularization. For example, cysts are of fluid attenuation (0–10 HU) and

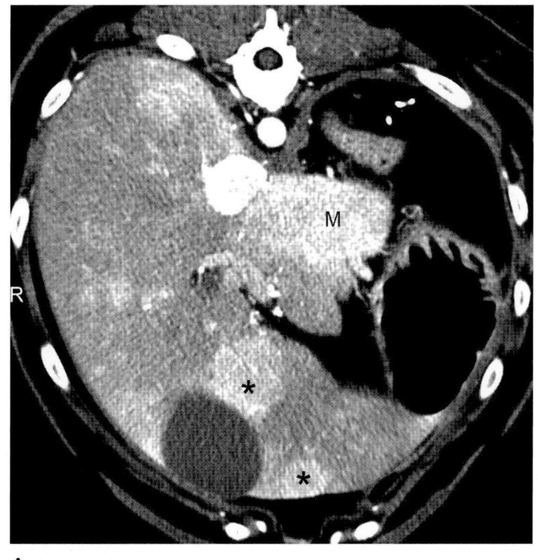

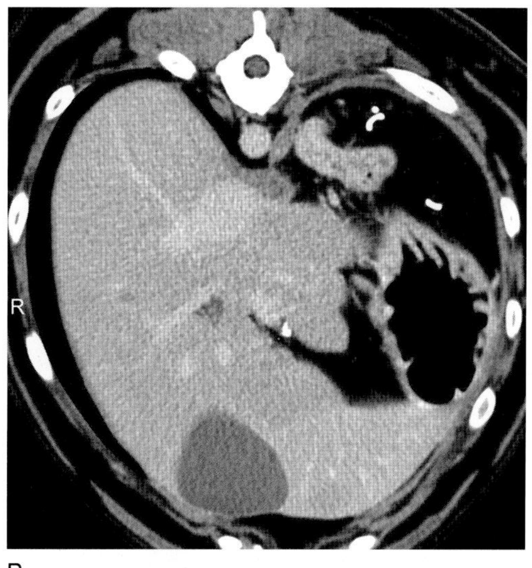

Figure 19.10 Transverse CT dual phase scan images of a dog with hepatocellular carcinoma and intrahepatic metastases. (A) On the late arterial phase images, the main mass (M, incompletely shown) and the intrahepatic metastases (*) are contrast enhancing compared to the normal liver parenchyma. (B) On the delayed phase images, the mass and metastases are isoattenuating to the normal liver parenchyma.

do not contrast enhance, while hepatic abscesses often have a contrast enhancing rim and non-enhancing center. Bile ducts, when enlarged, are non-contrast enhancing linear structures that are parallel to the portal veins.

Suggested Reading

Fukushima K, Kanemoto H, Ohno K et al. (2012) CT characteristics of primary hepatic mass lesions in dogs. *Vet Radiol Ultrasound* 53(3), 252–7.

Jones AC, Hornof WJ, London CA, Wisner ER et al. (2003) Multiple phase computed tomography of the canine liver: protocol for contrast injection and scan timing. In American College of Veterinary Radiology. Chicago, Illinois..

Mai W and Weisse C (20111) Contrast-enhanced portal magnetic resonance angiography in dogs with suspected congenital portal vascular anomalies. *Vet Radiol Ultrasound* 52(3), 284–8.

Seguin B, Tobias KM, Gavin PR and Tucker RL (1999) Use of magnetic resonance angiography for diagnosis of portosystemic shunts in dogs. *Vet Radiol Ultrasound* 40(3), 251–8.

Stieger SM, Zwingenberger A, Pollard RE, Kyles AE and Wisner ER (2007) Hepatic volume estimation using quantitative computed tomography in dogs with portosystemic shunts. *Vet Radiol Ultrasound* 48(5), 409–13.

Zwingenberger A (2009) CT diagnosis of portosystemic shunts. *Vet Clin N Am Small Anim Pract* 39(4), 783–92.

Zwingenberger AL and Schwarz T (2004) Dual-phase CT angiography of the normal canine portal and hepatic vasculature. *Veterinary Radiol Ultrasound* 45(2), 117–24.

Zwingenberger AL, McLear RC and Weisse C (2005) Diagnosis of arterioportal fistulae in four dogs using computed tomographic angiography. *Veterinary Radiol Ultrasound* 46(6), 472–7.

CHAPTER TWENTY

Vascular Anatomy

Fei Sun[1] and Rafael Latorre[2]

[1]*Jesús Usón Minimally Invasive Surgery Centre, Caceres, Spain*

[2]*Department of Anatomy and Comparative Pathological Anatomy, University of Murcia, Murcia, Spain*

Introduction

The liver receives a dual blood supply from the hepatic artery and portal vein. The hepatic artery carries blood rich in oxygen while the portal vein supplies the blood draining from the gastrointestinal tract, spleen, pancreas, and gallbladder. The blood in the portal vein contains nutrients, toxins, as well as oxygen. Blood leaves the liver through the hepatic veins into the caudal vena cava.

Arterial System

Celiac Artery

The celiac artery is the first ventral branch of the abdominal aorta, arising at the level of the 1st lumbar vertebral body (Figure 20.1). It is approximately 2 cm long and 4 mm in diameter depending on the dog size. It gives off three major branches, including the hepatic artery, splenic artery, and left gastric artery. The caudal phrenic arteries and small pancreatic branch may also arise from the celiac artery.

Hepatic Artery

The hepatic artery runs cranioventrally and to the right toward the hilus of the liver (Figure 20.2 and Figure 20.3). When reaching the liver, the hepatic artery sends two or three major branches entering the hilus of the liver in accompaniment to the branches of the portal vein. In the most common variation (~50%), a small right lateral branch and a large left branch arise from the hepatic artery (see Figure 20.6A). The right lateral branch supplies the right lateral lobe, caudate process, and part of the right medial lobe. The left branch gives off the cystic artery, right medial branch, and branches to the quadrate lobe, papillary process and the two left lobes. In another frequent variation (~45%), the right medial branch directly arises from the hepatic artery and gives off the cystic artery and branches to right medial and quadrate lobes. Occasionally, the branch to the papillary process can emerge directly from the hepatic artery. The hepatic artery bifurcates into two terminal arteries outside the

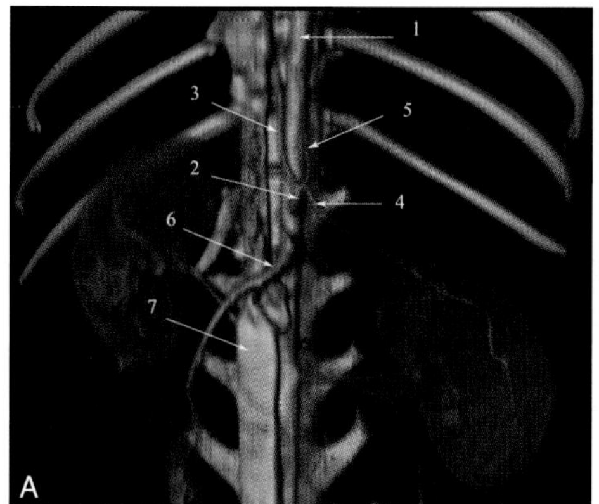

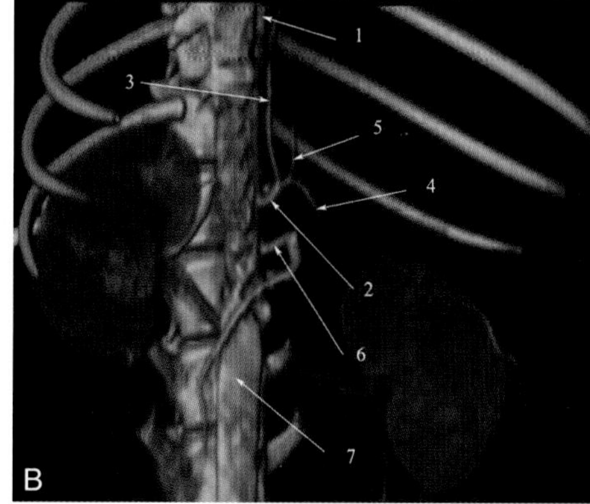

Figure 20.1 CT-Angiography of the abdominal aorta and its branches. Note the origin of the celiac artery at the level of L-1. (A: VD view; B: RAO view) 1 – abdominal aorta, 2 – celiac a., 3 – hepatic a., 4 – splenic a., 5 – left gastric a., 6 – cranial mesenteric a., 7 – caudal vena cava.

Veterinary Image-Guided Interventions, First Edition. Edited by Chick Weisse and Allyson Berent.

Companion website: www.wiley.com/go/weisse/vet-image-guided-interventions

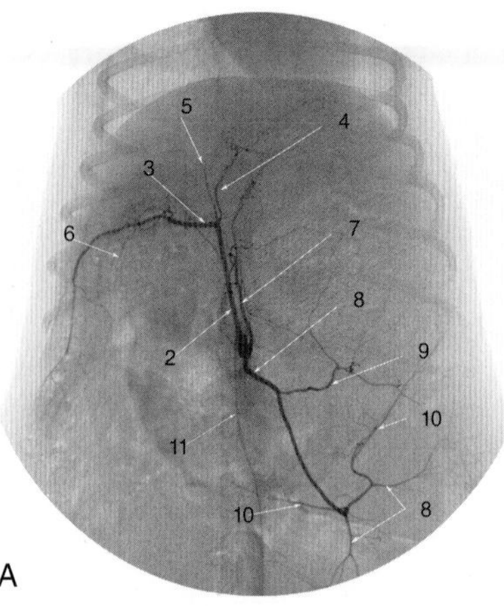

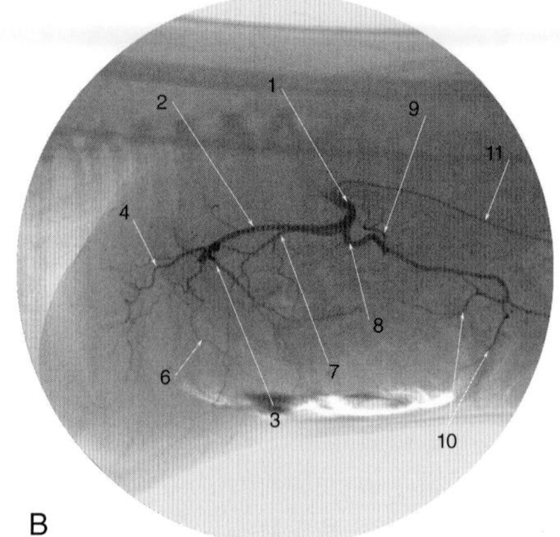

Figure 20.2 Angiography of the celiac artery in VD view (A) and lateral view (B) shows: 1 – celiac artery, 2 – hepatic artery, 3 – gastroduodenal artery, 4 – left branch of the hepatic artery, 5 – right branch of the hepatic artery, 6 – right gastroepiploic artery, 7 – left gastric artery, 8 – splenic artery, 9 – short gastric artery, 10 – left gastroepiploic artery and 11 – angiographic catheter.

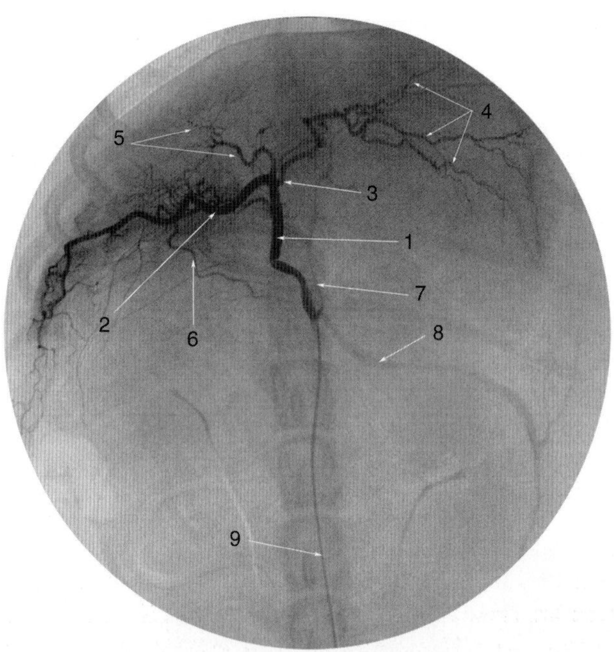

Figure 20.3 Selective angiography of the hepatic artery (VD view) shows: 1 – hepatic artery, 2 – gastroduodenal artery, 3 – left branch of the hepatic artery, 4 – branches to the left lobes, 5 – right branch of the hepatic artery, 6 – right gastroepiploic artery, 7 – left gastric artery, 8 – splenic artery and 9 – angiographic catheter.

liver – the small right gastric artery and the larger gastroduodenal artery (Figure 20.2 and Figure 20.3).

Splenic Artery

The splenic artery runs to the left and slightly caudally toward the hilus of the spleen (Figure 20.2). The splenic artery terminates as the left gastroepiploic artery that runs along the greater curvature of the stomach and anastomoses with the right gastroepiploic artery. The major branches of the splenic artery include the short gastric artery, the splenic branch and some pancreatic branches.

Left Gastric Artery

The left gastric artery originates from the cranial surface of the celiac artery and runs cranially in the lesser omentum to the fundus of the stomach (Figure 20.1 and Figure 20.2). It anastomoses with the short gastric artery, the right gastric artery, and esophageal branches from the thoracic aorta.

Portal Venous System

The portal system includes all veins that carry blood from the gastrointestinal tract (except the caudal part of the rectum), spleen, pancreas and gallbladder (Figure 20.4). The portal vein originates by the confluence of the cranial and caudal mesenteric veins in the root of the mesojejunum and dorsally to the junction of the right and left lobes of the pancreas. It runs cranially toward the hilus of the liver, and ventrally to the caudal vena cava. The normal portal pressure is about 10–15 cmH_2O (8–12 mmHg). At the hepatic porta, the portal vein is approximately 12 mm in diameter in a medium sized dog and divides into a short, small right portal branch and a long left portal branch (see Figure 20.6B). The right portal branch sends branches to the right lateral lobe and the caudate process of the caudate lobe. The left portal branch gives off more branches to the left and central hepatic segments.

The major tributaries include the cranial mesenteric vein, caudal mesenteric vein, splenic vein and

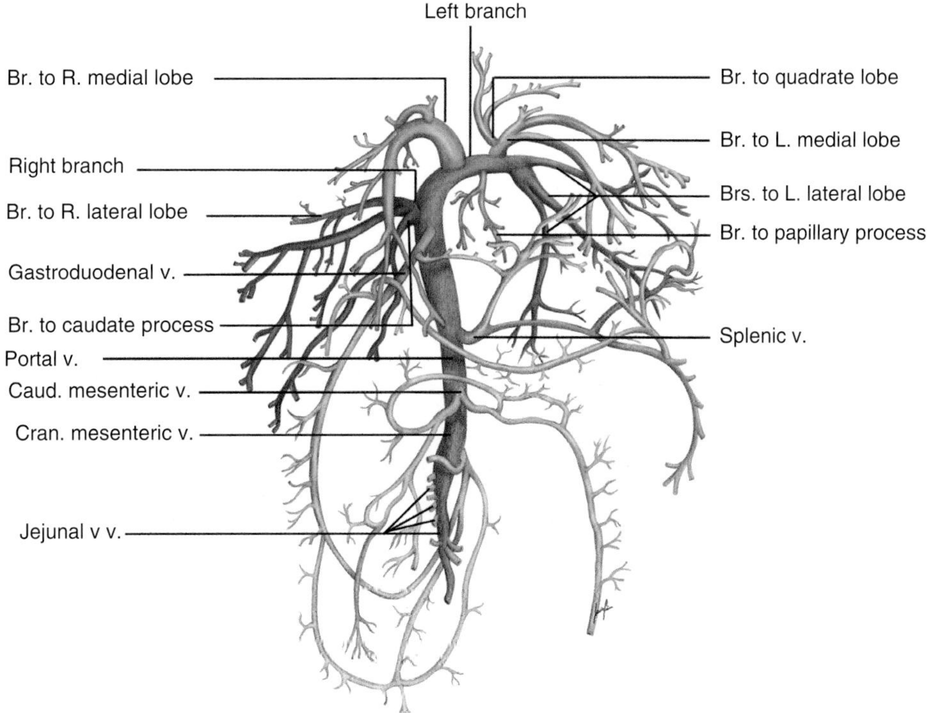

Figure 20.4 Schema of the portal system in VD view. (Modified with permission from Kalt DJ, Stump JE (1993). Gross anatomy of the canine portal vein. *Anat Histol Embryol* 22(2), 191–7.)

gastroduodenal vein (Figure 20.4 and Figure 20.5). The cranial mesenteric vein is always the largest vein, collecting 12 jejunal and ileal veins. The caudal mesenteric vein begins as the cranial rectal vein and receives blood primarily from the ileocolic vein. The splenic vein enters the portal trunk at the left, dorsal surface and receives the blood from the left gastric vein, pancreatic veins and left gastroepiploic vein. The gastroduodenal vein empties blood into the portal vein about 1.5 cm from the hilus of the liver. Its major tributaries include the cranial pancreaticoduodenal vein and the right gastroepiploic vein. In the fetus the left umbilical vein from the placenta enters the liver and communicates with the caudal vena cava via the ductus venosus. Two to six days after birth the ductus venosus closes and then gradually becomes the ligamentum venosum. The left umbilical vein finally becomes the round ligament of the liver.

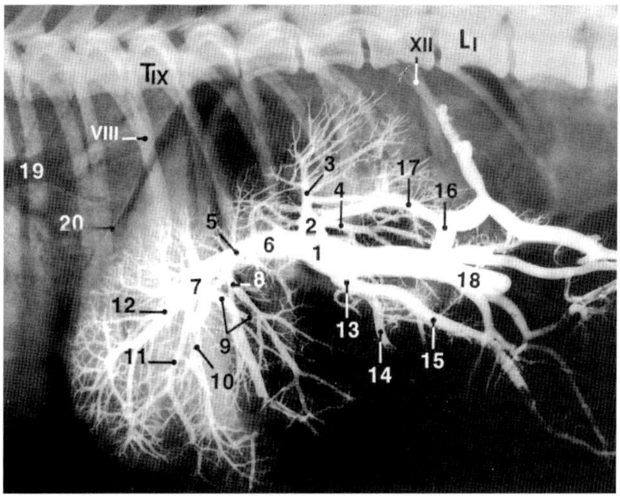

Figure 20.5 Venogram of the portal vein (left lateral view) by injection of contrast medium in the cranial mesenteric vein. 1 – portal vein, 2– right branch, 3 – branch to the right lateral lobe, 4 – branch to the caudate process, 5 – left branch, 6 – transverse part of left branch of portal vein, 7 – umbilical part, 8 – branch to the right medial lobe, 9 – branch to the papillary process, 10 – branch to the quadrate lobe, 11 – branch to the left lateral lobe, 12 – branch to the left medial lobe, 13 – gastroduodenal vein, 14 – right gastroepiploic vein, 15 – cranial pancreaticoduodenal vein, 16 – splenic vein, 17 – left gastric vein, 18 – cranial mesenteric vein, 19 – caudal lobe bronchus, 20 – diaphragm. (Reproduced with permission from Ruberte J, Sautet J. (1998) *Atlas de Anatomía del Perro y del Gato* (Vol. 3). Universitat Autónoma de Barcelona, Barcelona.)

Hepatic Veins and Caudal Vena Cava

There are three main hepatic veins emptying into the caudal vena cava. The left hepatic vein is the largest and most cranial and drains blood from the left lateral, left medial, quadrate, and part of the right medial lobe. It enters the caudal vena cava at the foramen venae cavae. Two hepatic veins (right hepatic and middle

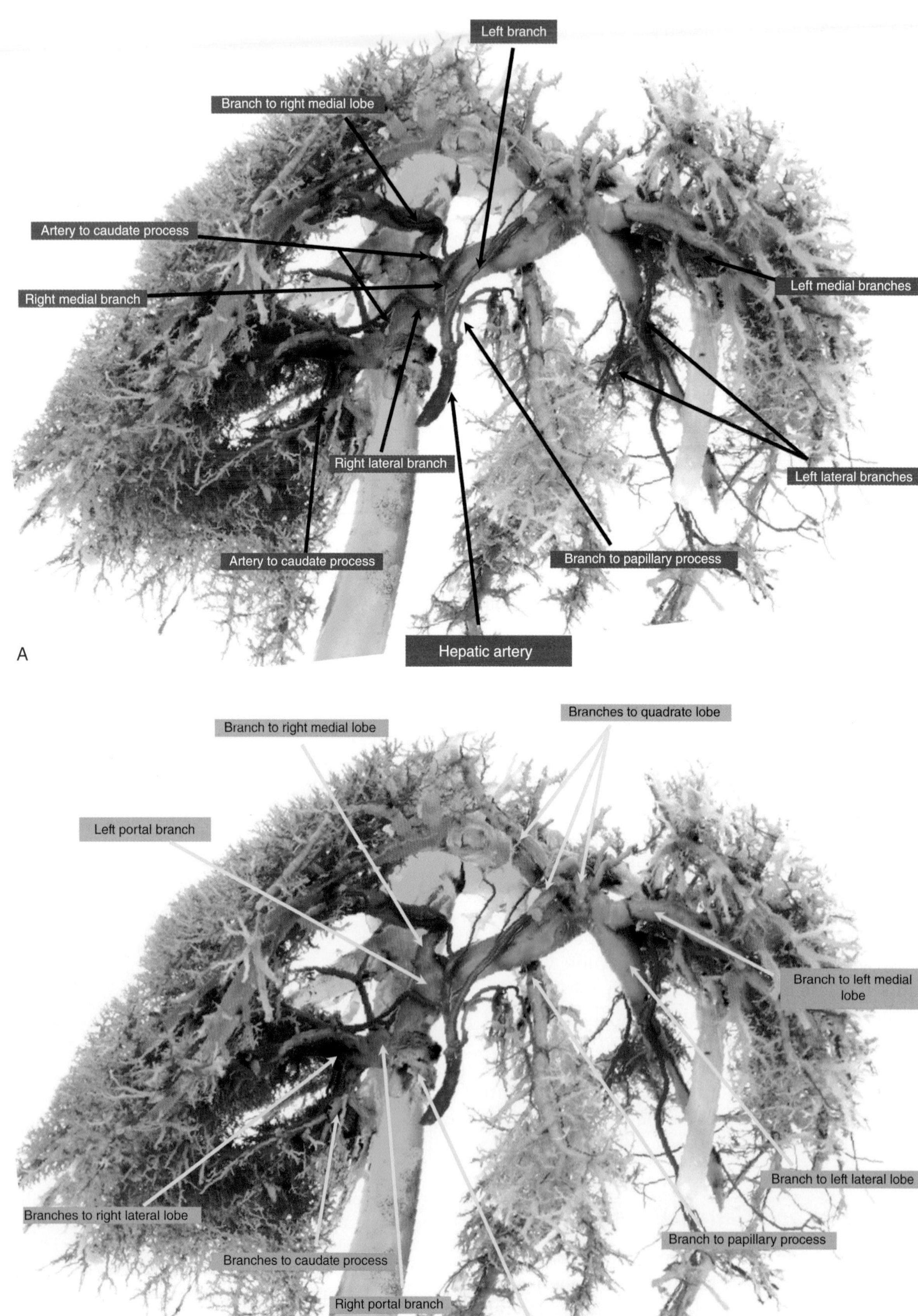

Figure 20.6 Corrosion cast of (A) the hepatic artery, (B) the portal vein, and (C) the hepatic veins (VD view).

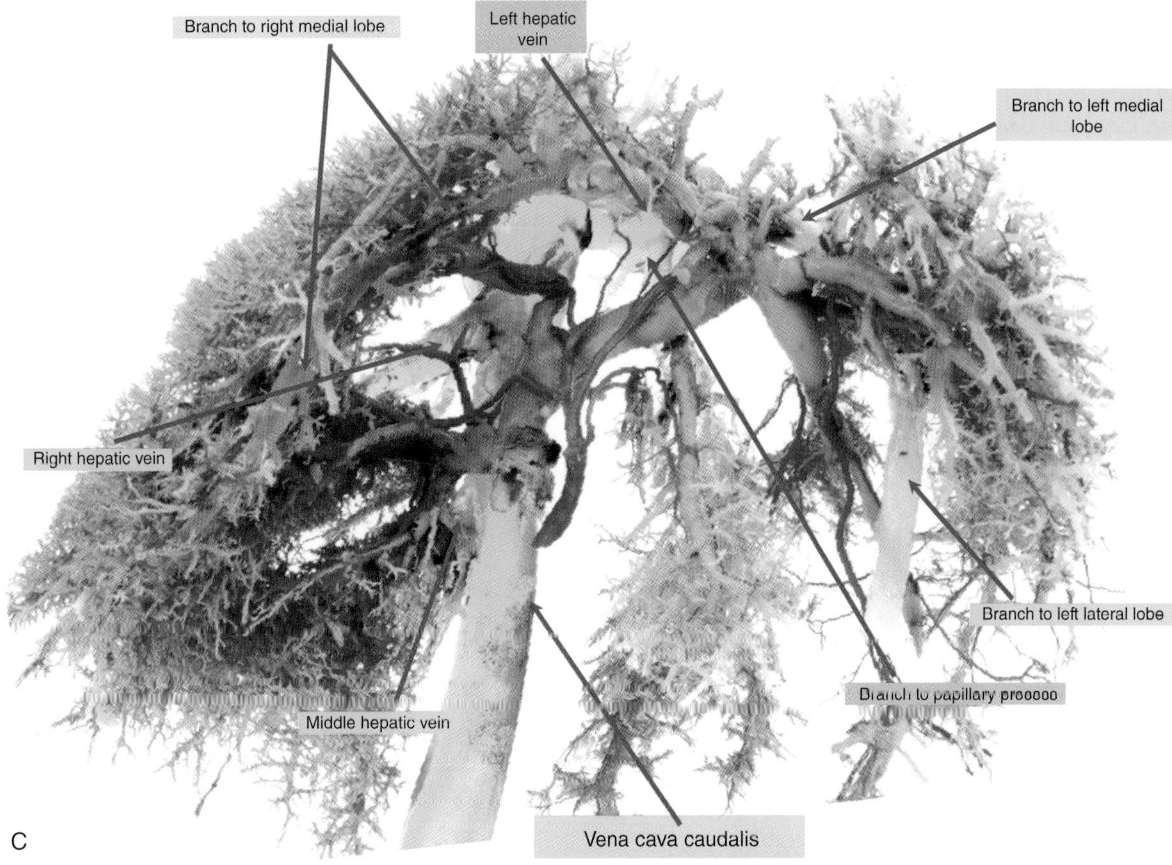

Figure 20.6 (*Continued*)

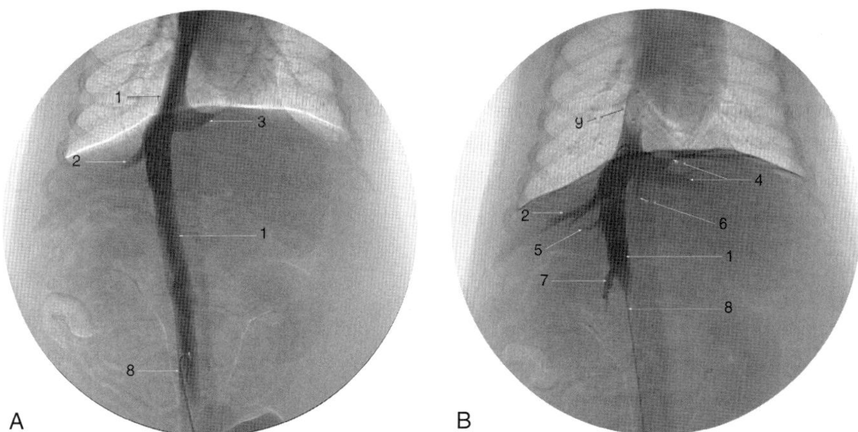

Figure 20.7 Caudal vena cavography with hepatic veins (VD view) during a positive pressure breath hold (A) and by balloon occlusion (B) shows: 1 – caudal vena cava, 2– right hepatic vein, 3 – left hepatic vein, 4 – branches to the left lobes, 5 – middle hepatic vein, 6 – branch to papillary process, 7 – right renal vein, 8 – angiographic catheter and 9 – occlusion balloon.

hepatic veins) drain the right lateral lobe and the caudate lobe, opening at the caudal vena cava slightly caudally to the orifice of the left hepatic vein (Figure 20.6C and Figure 20.7). Anatomic studies by gross dissection in large dogs document that the diameter of the caudal vena cava is at least 10 mm and the length of the intrathoracic caudal vena cava is approximately 4 cm long. However, in live dogs, the caudal vena cava is much larger in size. In vena cavography during a positive pressure breath hold, the diameter of the caudal vena cava is measured between 16–28 mm in large breed puppies.

Suggested Reading

Evans HE (1993) The heart and arteries. In: *Miller's Anatomy of the Dog*, 3rd edn (ed. Evans HE), pp. 586–681. WB Saunders, Toronto.

Evans HE (1993) The veins. In: *Miller's Anatomy of the Dog*, 3rd edn (ed. Evans HE), pp. 682–716. WB Saunders, Toronto.

Kalt DJ and Stump JE (1993) Gross anatomy of the canine portal vein. *Anat Histol Embryol* 22(2), 191–7.

Nomenclature World Association of Veterinary Anatomists (WAVA) Nomina anatomica veterinaria, 5th Editorial Committee, Hannover, Columbia, Gent, Sapporo: International Committee on Veterinary Gross Anatomical Nomenclature, 2005.

Richter KP (2003) Diseases of the liver and hepatobiliary system. In: *Handbook of small animal gastroenterology*, 2nd edn (ed.Tams TR), pp 286–352. Saunders, St. Louis.

Ruberte J and Sautet J (1998) *Atlas de Anatomía del Perro y del Gato* (Vol. 3). Universitat Autónoma de Barcelona, Barcelona.

Ursic M, Ravnik D, Hribernik M, et al (2007) Gross anatomy of the portal vein and hepatic artery ramifications in dogs: corrosion cast study. *Anat Histol Embryol* 36(2), 83–7.

White RN and Burton CA (2000) Anatomy of the patent ductus venosus in the dog. *Vet Rec* 146(15), 425–9.

CHAPTER TWENTY-ONE

Portosystemic Shunt Embolization: IHPSS/EHPSS

Chick Weisse
The Animal Medical Center, New York, NY

Background/Indications

Portosystemic shunts (PSS) are vascular anomalies connecting the portal and systemic venous systems that result in varying degrees of biochemical and clinical abnormalities. Growing evidence supports conventional wisdom that the treatment of choice is to attenuate the abnormal vessel in order to restore or improve portal perfusion and ultimately maximize hepatic function. Unfortunately, due to diminished portal perfusion, only a minority of intrahepatic PSS (IHPSS) can be completely occluded acutely without resulting in life-threatening portal hypertension (Figure 21.1) (Kyles et al, 2001, Papazoglou et al, 2002). Surgical treatment of IHPSS has been associated with perioperative complication rates as high as 77%, peri-operative mortality rates up to 28%, and overall mortality rates as high as 64% (Bostwick and Twedt, 1995, Komtebedde et al, 1995, Smith et al, 1995, White et al, 1998, Hunt et al, 2004). More recently, endovascular management of portosystemic shunts has been described (Weisse et al, 2014). These techniques can be used to provide partial or complete endovascular attenuation of IHPSS or EHPSS, achieve similar clinical results, and result in fewer perioperative complications and mortalities compared to those reported following traditional surgery.

Patient Preparation

Following diagnosis, all dogs are treated medically (Table 21.1) for a period of weeks to months in order to improve body condition score and allow clinical signs of hepatic encephalopathy (HE) to resolve. In addition, to prevent placing undersized implants, it is best that the patient have time to grow to more closely achieve its ultimate size. The patients are typically at least 5 months of age at the time of the procedure when possible.

Approximately 15% of IHPSS dogs demonstrate signs of gastrointestinal (GI) ulceration prior to treatment (Weisse et al, 2011). It is imperative a careful history, rectal examination, and evaluation of recent bloodwork be performed to identify any evidence of GI hemorrhage. Concurrently raising portal blood pressure in these patients can be life threatening. If present, these patients are aggressively treated for GI ulceration for a period of weeks to months prior to shunt attenuation.

Anti-seizure medications are not routinely prescribed unless the animal has persistent neurological symptoms following appropriate treatment with the previous medications (Table 21.1). When possible, CT or MR angiography is performed to delineate the shunt anatomy and obtain caval and shunt measurements under a separate anesthetic episode (Zwingenberger, 2005 et al, Mai and Weisse, 2011). When possible, these cross-sectional imaging studies are performed as closely as possible to the time of the procedure so that measurements are accurate for the patient size at the time of the procedure.

Potential Risks/Complications/Expected Outcomes

Little information exists for EHPSS embolization so the following information pertains to that reported for IHPSS percutaneous transvenous embolization (PTE) in 100 dogs. Perioperative mortality rates of 5% and perioperative complications of 13% have been reported with half of the complications being postoperative seizures/neurological sequelae (similar to previously

Veterinary Image-Guided Interventions, First Edition. Edited by Chick Weisse and Allyson Berent.

Companion website: www.wiley.com/go/weisse/vet-image-guided-interventions

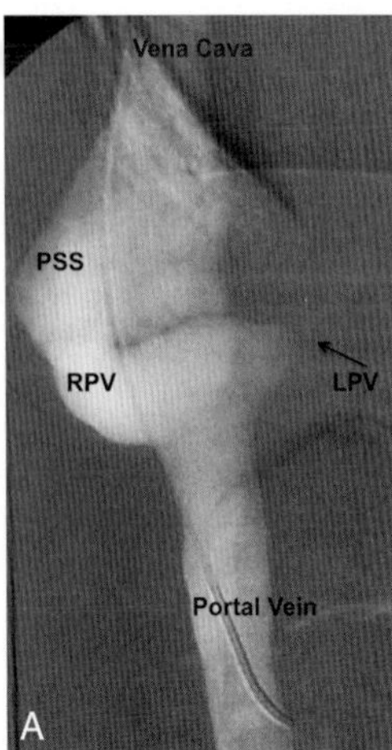

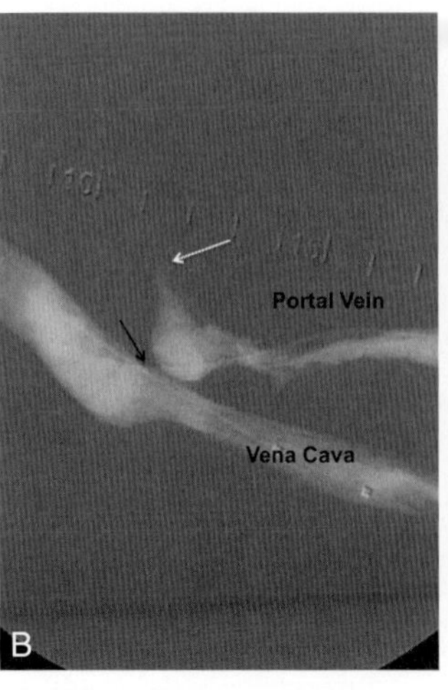

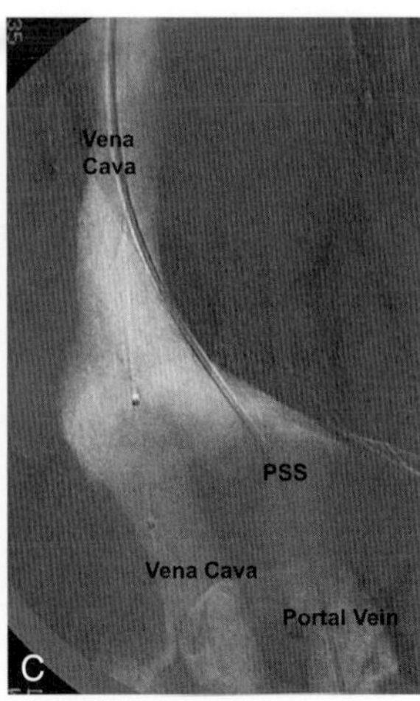

Figure 21.1 Transjugular DSA portograms of dogs with various IHPSS anatomies. (A) Right divisional IHPSS (PSS) DSA portogram performed in dorsal recumbency with the patients head at the top of the image. This demonstrates minimal left portal vein (LPV) perfusion and large right portal vein (RPV) entering the PSS and then continuing to enter the vena cava on the right side. (B) Lateral DSA cavagram and portogram of a dog with a central divisional IHPSS. The portal vein enters the vena cava at a shunt "window" (black arrow) and narrows as it travels towards the liver (white arrow). The head is to the left of the image. (C) Left divisional IHPSS (PSS) DSA portogram and cavagram performed in dorsal recumbency with the head to the top of the image. This image demonstrates no evidence of right portal perfusion and large left portal vein entering the PSS and then continuing to enter the left hepatic vein and vena cava on the left side.

TABLE 21.1
Pre- and post-procedural medical management

- Antibiotics:
  - Pre- and postoperative: metronidazole: 7.5 mg/kg PO q12 hr until weaning
  - Intraoperative: cefoxitin (30 mg/kg IV once, then 20 mg/kg IV q2 hr)
- Laxatives:
  - Pre- and postoperative: Lactulose: 0.1–0.2 ml/kg PO q8–12 hr (dosed to form soft but formed stools) until weaning
- Gastroprotectants:
  - Pre- and postoperative: omeprazole: 1 mg/kg PO q12 hr for life
- Low-protein diet:
  - Pre- and postoperative: Hill's L/D, Royal Canin Hepatic LS or similar
- Anticonvulsants (for use in dogs with persistent neurological dysfunction while on appropriate medical management or if feline patient):
  - Pre- and postoperative: levetiracetam (Keppra): 40 mg/kg at 0 and 2 hr, then 20 mg/kg q8 hr until weaning
- Analgesics (Not standardly necessary):
  - Post-operative: tramadol (2–4 mg/kg PO q8–12 hr × 3 days)

reported rates) (Tisdall et al, 2000, Weisse et al, 2014). Portal hypertension occurs uncommonly following PTE, likely due to the post-sinusoidal location of the shunt attenuation favoring the development of intrahepatic venous collaterals over portal hypertension (Figure 21.2G, H, I). Approximately 20% of dogs may require or benefit from additional coils to further attenuate the shunt (Weisse et al, 2014). In addition, approximately 20% of dogs demonstrate signs consistent with GI bleeding post-treatment; Severe GI bleeding complications have been identified years following treatment and mortality rates in these patients have been greatly reduced by maintaining lifelong proton-pump inhibition therapy (Weisse et al, 2014).

Considerable variation exists in IHPSS patients for which clients should be informed. Approximately 10% of these dogs have multiple shunts (Figure 21.3) and approximately 5% have elevated portal pressures (or elevated portal:CVP gradients) possibly preventing the embolization procedure (Weisse et al, 2014). Alternatively, approximately 5% may have sufficient portal vein perfusion to allow acute total IHPSS occlusion (Weisse et al, 2014). Options for performing complete acute shunt occlusion include vascular plugs, covered caval stents (stent grafts), or the standard stent-supported coil technique.

When performed by someone familiar with IR procedures, PTE is a safe, fast, and effective therapy for canine intrahepatic portosystemic shunts associated with lower morbidity and mortality rates, and equal (or even improved) long-term outcomes when compared to historical surgical techniques. Pet owners should be warned that these dogs have an increased risk of gastrointestinal hemorrhage prior to, and following, treatment for the IHPSS, both in the short and the long term. Overall, PTE results in fair to excellent outcomes in 81% of patients (15% fair and 66%

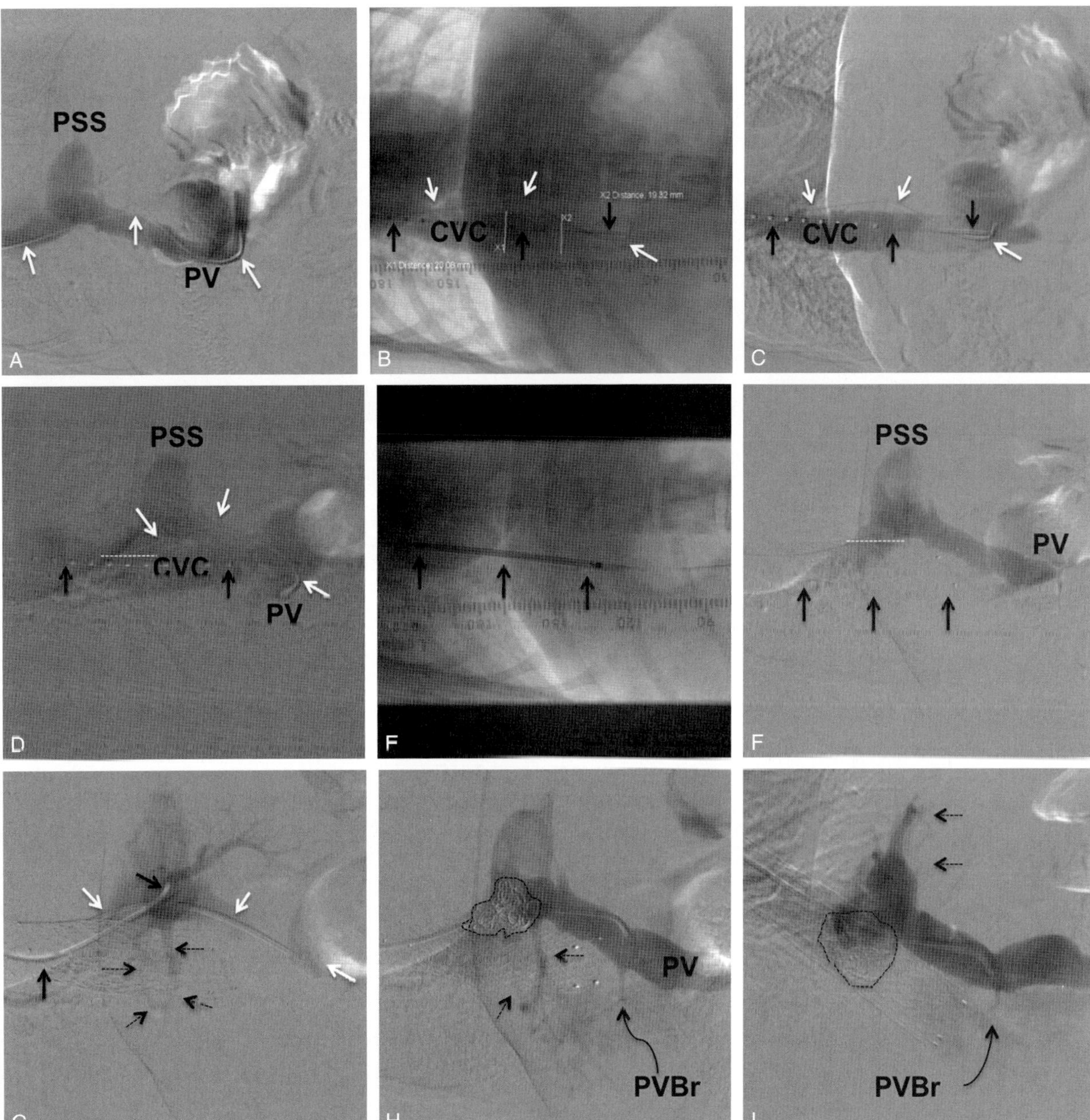

Figure 21.2 Serial images of a dog with a left divisional IHPSS receiving coil embolization with multiple collateral intrahepatic shunting vessels. The dog is in dorsal recumbency and the head is to the left in each image. (A) Transjugular portogram with 4 Fr Cobra catheter (white arrows) demonstrating portal vein (PV) with large left divisional intrahepatic shunt (PSS). B/C. Transjugular caudal vena cava (CVC) angiogram (B) and digital subtraction angiogram (C) through 5Fr marker catheter (black arrows) performed under positive pressure ventilation for maximal abdominal cava diameter. (D) Dual portogram and cavagram demonstrating junction of PSS entering the CVC (white dotted line). The anatomical location of the line is matched with the stent guide beneath the patient to assist with stent deployment that is easily visualized in figure E. This is best seen in the native view and not this DSA image. (E) Constrained stent within the delivery system (black arrows) positioned across the shunt (~175–155=mouth of shunt) by using the numbers on the stent guide (~205–135=ends of stent). (F) Repeat DSA portogram after stent deployment (black arrows) demonstrating proper positioning across the entire shunt entrance (white dotted line). (G) One Cobra catheter (white arrows) in the portal vein to measure portal pressures and another Cobra catheter (black arrows) in shunt for coil deployment. A digital subtraction angiogram through the shunt catheter demonstrates the presence of intrahepatic venous collaterals already present (black dotted arrows). (H) Following placement of a number of coils (black dotted line) with subsequent portal pressure increase, a repeat DSA portogram demonstrates improved portal perfusion through a right portal vein branch (PVBr). (I) Orthogonal DSA portogram showing coils (black dotted line), intrahepatic venous collaterals (black dotted arrows), and improved portal perfusion (PVBr).

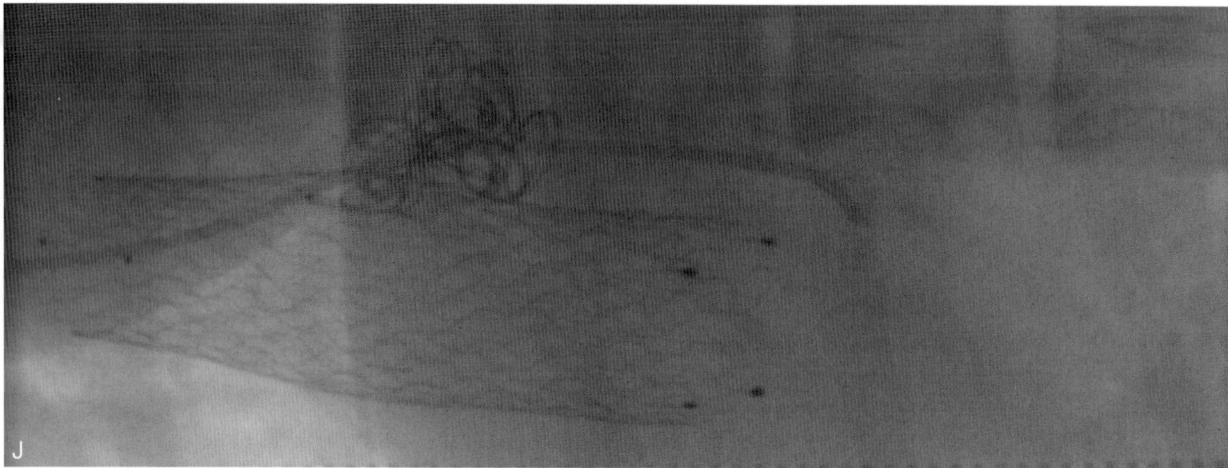

Figure 21.2 (*Continued*) (J) Final radiographic image with caval stent and coils in place.

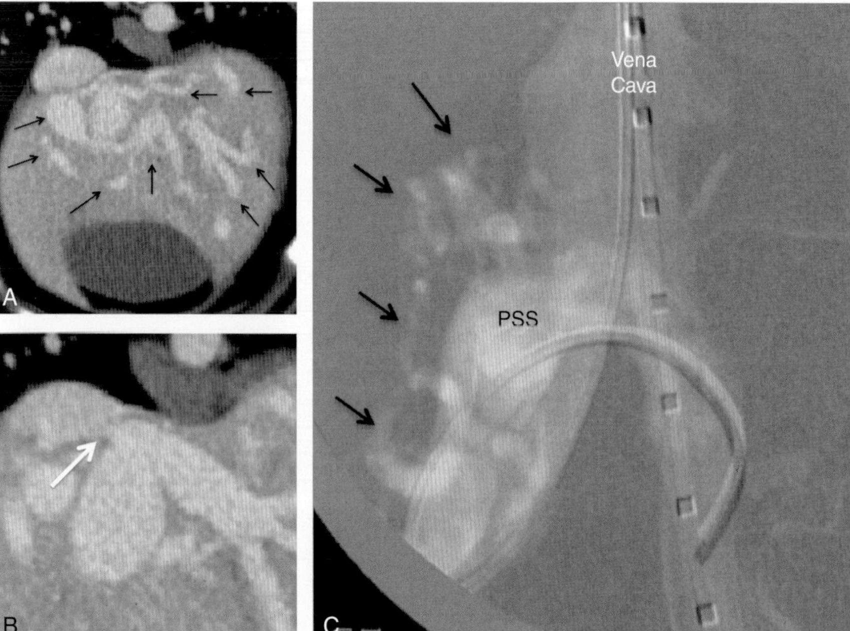

Figure 21.3 Two dogs with multiple IHPSS. (A) Axial CTA demonstrating multiple intrahepatic shunting vessels (black arrows) mostly on the left side of the liver prior to any therapy. (B) Close-up axial CTA of the same dog showing the narrow shunt opening (white arrow) that often signifies a pressure gradient exists or existed prior to the development of the intrahepatic venous collaterals. These dogs seem often to also have some portal perfusion present as well. (C) DSA portogram in a different dog in dorsal recumbency with the head to the top of the image. There are multiple IHPSS (black arrows) evident, mostly on the right side, prior to any therapy.

excellent) with a median survival time over 6 years and under 5% perioperative mortality rate (Weisse et al, 2014). Preoperative bloodwork values are not statistically correlated with patient outcome or survival; however changes in these values postoperatively are significant, so following biochemical trends is recommended.

Equipment

Recommended equipment is shown in Figure 21.4. Digital subtraction angiography is highly recommended when performing the PTE procedure. A number of different self-expanding metallic stents (SEMS) can be used; however, the author prefers laser-cut stents due to the lack of foreshortening that occurs during deployment providing precise and predictable stent placement. The author routinely uses a standard coil size being 0.035″ 8 mm diameter and 5 cm length.

Fluoroscopic Procedure

All PTE procedures are performed under general anesthesia using standard liver dysfunction protocols and occasionally neuromuscular blockade, in order to minimize respiratory artifact during digital subtraction angiography. Perioperative cefoxitin[1] is administered at 30 mg/kg once, followed by 20 mg/kg q2 hours during the procedure.

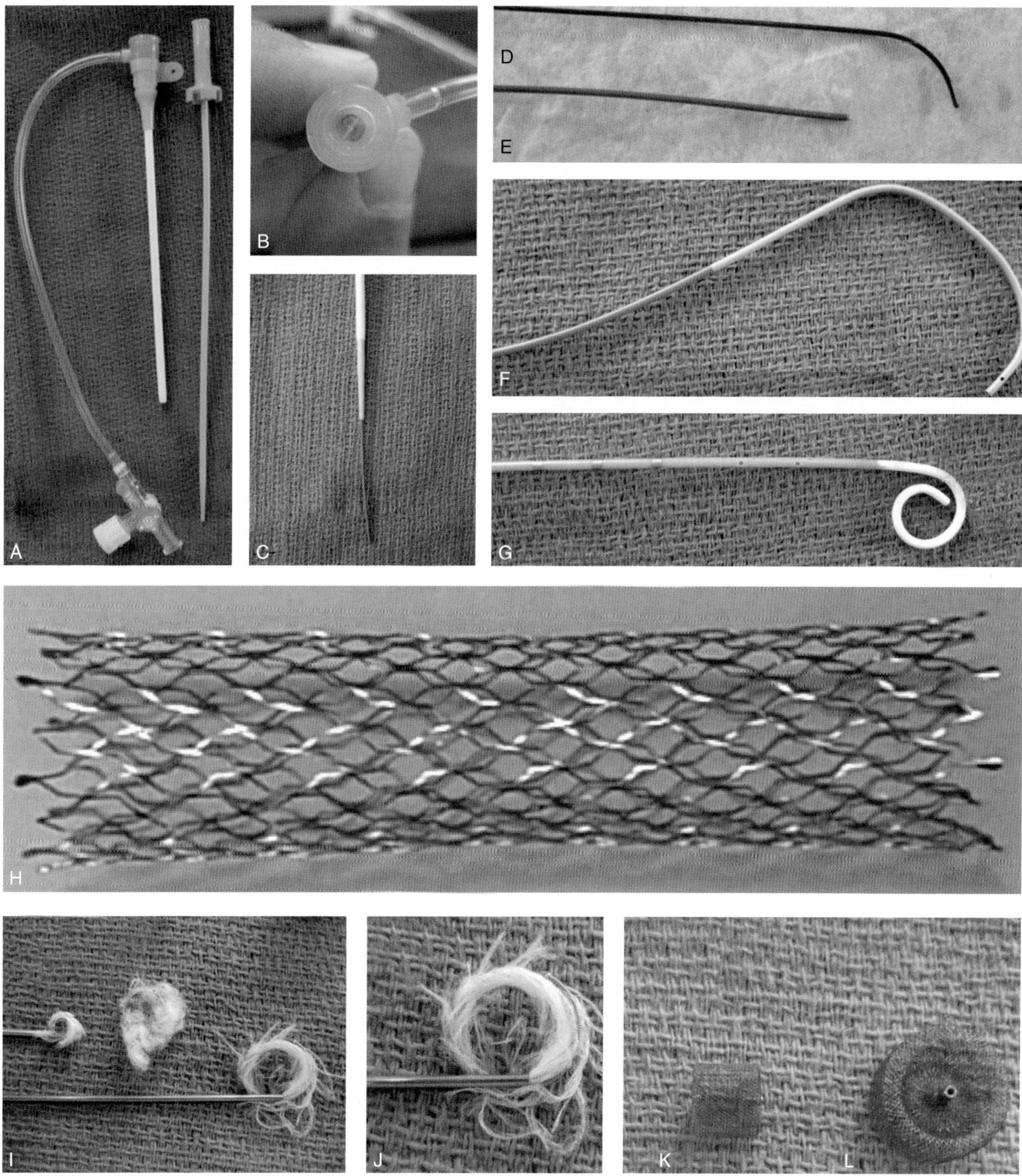

Figure 21.4 Equipment used for PSS embolization procedures. 12 Fr vascular introducer sheath and dilator (A) with hemostasis valve (B) and smooth transition from sheath to dilator to 0.035″ guide wire (C). (D) 0.035″ angled hydrophilic guide wire, typically 150 or 180 cm in length. (E) Floppy tip PTFE guide wire, typically 260 cm long. (F) 4 Fr Cobra catheter. (G) Pigtail (shown here) or straight tip marker catheter. Straight catheter more commonly used. The radio-opaque marks are 10 mm from the beginning of mark to the beginning of the next. (H) Appropriate-sized, laser-cut nitinol self-expanding metallic stent (shown here) preferred to the mesh self-expanding stents. Various stainless steel embolization coils (I) and close-up (J) showing the interwoven thrombogenic Dacron fibers. The most common sized used are 0.035″ 8 mm diameter and 5 cm length. (K, L) Vascular plugs of various sizes knitted from fine nitinol wire used for acute, complete occlusion of EHPSS.

Patients are placed in dorsal recumbency, neck extended, with a radio-opaque stent guide[2] placed between the patient and the tabletop. The stent guide is ideally positioned adjacent to the vena cava contralateral to the side of the shunt (e.g., the guide is just to the right of the vena cava for left-divisional shunts). The ventral cervical region is clipped, scrubbed, and draped, exposing the right jugular vein (preferred over the left jugular vein because of the straight path into the vena cava). A 3–5 mm skin incision facilitates percutaneous placement of an 18-gauge over-the-needle catheter into the right jugular vein. A 0.035″ angled, hydrophilic guide wire[3] is advanced through the catheter and into the caudal vena cava. The catheter is removed over-the-wire and replaced with either a 10 Fr or 12 Fr vascular introducer sheath,[4] depending upon the anticipated caval stent delivery system size. The sheath is secured in place with a single nylon suture and the dilator is removed over the guide wire.

For left (Figure 21.2 and Figure 21.5) and right (Figure 21.6) divisional shunts the animal remains in dorsal recumbency. For central divisional shunts (Figure 21.7), the animal (or c-arm) is rotated to lateral recumbency (or lateral imaging) following sheath placement and caudal vena cava access in order to facilitate angiographic identification of the shunt (Figure 21.1). A 4 Fr Cobra catheter[5] and 0.035″ angled hydrophilic guide wire combination are used under fluoroscopic guidance to selectively access the shunt and/or portal vein. If access is difficult, the use of a Berenstein catheter or hydrophilic catheters can facilitate advancement over the guide wire to access the portal vein. Digital subtraction portal venography is then performed to confirm appropriate catheter placement, delineate shunt anatomy and identify the presence or absence of portal perfusion. Angiograms are performed using a 50:50 iohexol[6]:saline mixture in order to reduce the total contrast load, standardly maintained below 3 ml contrast/kg of bodyweight total for the entire procedure. If considerable portal perfusion is present (second generation portal vessels or more), balloon occlusion can be performed to assess whether complete shunt attenuation could be tolerated. If so, alternate complete shunt embolization techniques are considered (vascular plug or covered caval stent [stent graft]). Next, a 5 Fr marker catheter[7] and 0.035″ angled hydrophilic guide wire combination are advanced into the sheath beside the Cobra catheter and down the caudal vena cava. A digital subtraction caudal vena cavagram is performed under 20 cmH_2O positive pressure ventilation in order to compress the thoracic caudal vena cava and maximally distend the abdominal vena cava. The maximal abdominal vena cava diameter is then calculated using the marker catheter to determine radiographic magnification to measure for stent diameter. Next, a combination digital subtraction portogram and caudal vena cavagram is performed without PPV, to identify the precise location and length of the shunt entrance into the caudal vena cava, as well as to determine the maximal intrathoracic caudal vena cava diameter (non-PPV). Caval diameters and shunt opening lengths are used to choose an appropriately sized, self-expanding metallic stent; typically at least 10–25% greater in diameter than the maximal caval diameters measured and at least 20 mm longer cranially and caudally to the shunt opening into the vena cava when possible (Figure 21.8). Care should be taken to monitor the location of the right atrium, especially when a left divisional IHPSS is being treated. Portal pressures are then recorded through the end-hole Cobra catheter and central venous pressures (CVP) measurements are recorded through the marker catheter before stent placement. If resting portal pressures are greater than 16 mmHg (21 cmH_2O) or the pressure gradient between the portal vein and CVP is greater than 6 mmHg (8 cmH_2O), the embolization procedure may be reconsidered, and repeat angiography recommended, in approximately 3 months.

The Cobra catheter is then removed from the portal vein, a 0.035″ exchange-length (260 cm) floppy-tip PTFE (Teflon) guide wire[8] is advanced down the marker catheter and the marker catheter removed over the wire. The stent delivery system[9] (containing the stent) is advanced over the PTFE guide wire and deployed under fluoroscopic guidance (during a pause in respiration) to ensure that the entire mouth of the shunt is spanned by the stent. Marks on the underlying stent guide are used to assist in stent positioning in reference to the previous angiogram to ensure the stent is deployed in the proper location, avoiding the right atrium and covering the entire mouth of the shunt. Following self-expanding metallic stent deployment, the delivery system is removed and the 4 Fr Cobra catheter and 0.035″angled hydrophilic guide wire combination are used again to select the portal vein or shunt through the stent interstices. Following portal vein or shunt access a repeat digital subtraction venogram is performed to confirm the stent is placed appropriately across the entire shunt orifice, otherwise coils can migrate after deployment. Repeat pressure measurements of the portal vein/shunt are obtained to determine if the stent placement has raised the pressure within the portal vein. While leaving this Cobra catheter in place within the portal system and recording real-time portal pressures, another 4 Fr Cobra catheter

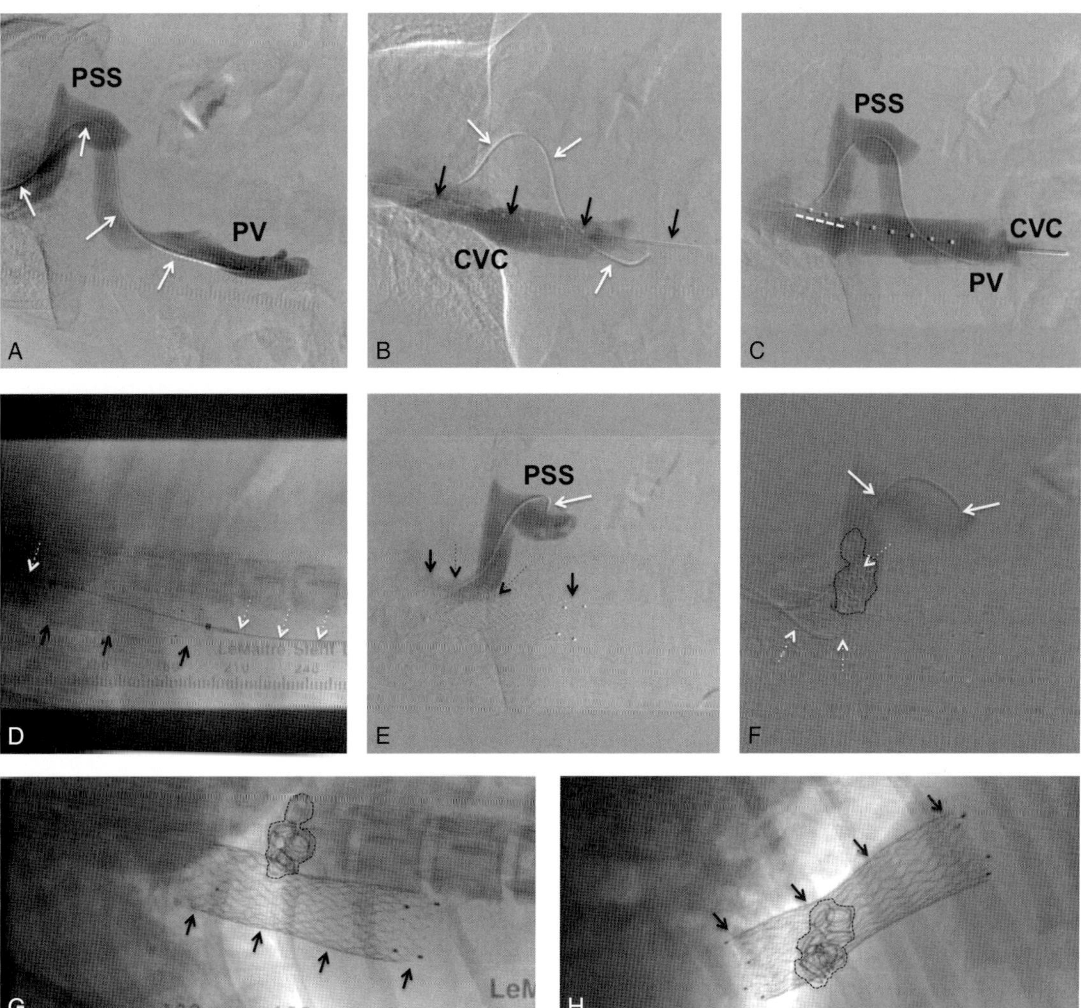

Figure 21.5 Serial fluoroscopic and radiographic images of a dog with a left divisional IHPSS during the PTE procedure. The head is to the left of each image. (A) DSA portogram through a 4Fr Cobra catheter (white arrows) passing from the caudal vena cava, through the left hepatic vein, the shunt (PSS) and into the portal vein (PV). No portal perfusion is evident. (B) Positive pressure DSA cavagram through 5 Fr straight marker catheter (black arrows) for maximal abdominal caudal vena cava (CVC) distension. (C) Dual DSA portogram and cavagram demonstrating the location of the shunt entrance (white dotted line) into the vena cava at the level of the left hepatic vein and diaphragm. This line is used in reference to the stent guide underneath the patient to help guide caval stent placement that is more easily seen on the native image. (D) Following caval stent placement (black arrows) over a 0.035″ floppy-tip exchange length Teflon guide wire (white dotted arrows). (E) Repeat DSA study through Cobra catheter placed through stent (black arrows) interstices with the tip (white arrow) located in PSS. The angiogram demonstrates that the stent has been placed across the entire shunt entrance marked by the black dotted arrows so embolization can proceed safely without risk of coil migration. (F) Repeat DSA study through same Cobra catheter (white arrows) after multiple thrombogenic coils (black dotted line) within the shunt through a separate Cobra catheter (white dotted arrows) just through the stent interstices. The shunt Cobra catheter is attached to continuous pressure measurements while the coils are being placed through the latter cobra catheter to identify portal pressure increases. There is still no portal perfusion evident; this is not uncommon immediately after the procedure. Final radiographs in ventrodorsal (G) and lateral (H) projections demonstrating final caval stent (black arrows) and coil (black dotted line) locations. Notice the advantage of performing left divisional IHPSS embolization in ventrodorsal position rather than lateral positioning in which coil deployment within the shunt would be much more difficult as the shunt is directly overlying the vena cava (H) rather than adjacent (G) to it.

and 0.035″ angled hydrophilic guide wire combination is used to select the shunt through the interstices of the stent at the level of its communication with the caudal vena cava. At this location, thrombogenic stainless steel coils[10] (usually 8 mm diameter × 5 cm length) are advanced through this second, more proximal, Cobra catheter and deployed into the shunt at the junction of the stent and the hepatic vein, so that the stent can

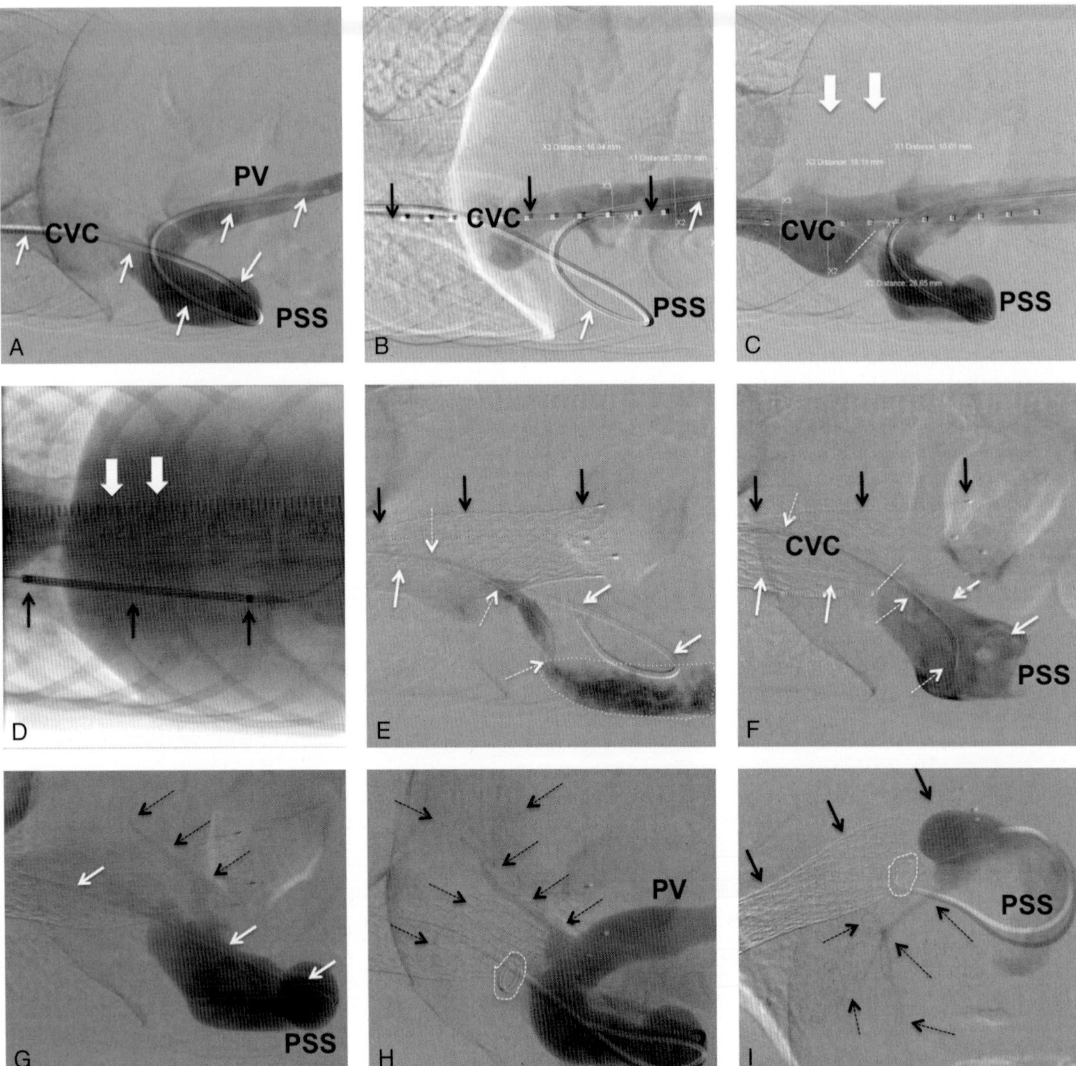

Figure 21.6 Serial fluoroscopic and radiographic images of a dog with a right divisional IHPSS during coil embolization. The head is to the left. (A) DSA portogram through a 4 Fr Cobra catheter (white arrows) passing from the caudal vena cava, through the right hepatic vein, the shunt (PSS) and into the portal vein (PV). (B) Positive pressure DSA cavagram through 5 Fr marker catheter (black arrows) for maximal abdominal caudal vena cava (CVC) distension. (C) Dual DSA portogram and cavagram demonstrating the location of the shunt entrance (white dotted line) into the vena cava at the level of the right hepatic vein. This line is used in reference to the stent guide (white block arrows) underneath the patient to help guide caval stent placement. The dilated vena cava at the level of the diaphragm is not uncommon. (D) Constrained caval stent (black arrows) within the delivery system passed over 0.035″ exchange-length floppy-tip guide wire centered across the location of the shunt entrance into the vena cava as identified by the numbers on the stent guide (white block arrows). (E) Following stent (black arrows) placement two Cobra catheters placed through the stent interstices; one within the portal vein (white arrows) used for continuous pressure measurements while coils will be placed through the other (dotted white arrows) placed at the shunt entrance. A DSA study is performed to make certain the catheter is positioned appropriately before adding coils. During this injection, the catheter appears inappropriately positioned within a small hepatic vein branch demonstrating parenchymal staining (white dotted line). This catheter needs to be repositioned prior to adding coils. (F) Following repositioning, a repeat DSA study reveals the catheter (white dotted arrows) is appropriately placed within the shunt lumen. (G) DSA portogram through portal vein Cobra catheter (white arrows) demonstrates improved portal perfusion through left portal vein (black dotted arrows) as compared to before stent placement. (H) Following placement of a single coil (white dotted line) further enhanced portal perfusion is clearly seen (black dotted arrows) via DSA portogram. (I) Orthogonal DSA portogram demonstrating alternate view of improved portal perfusion.

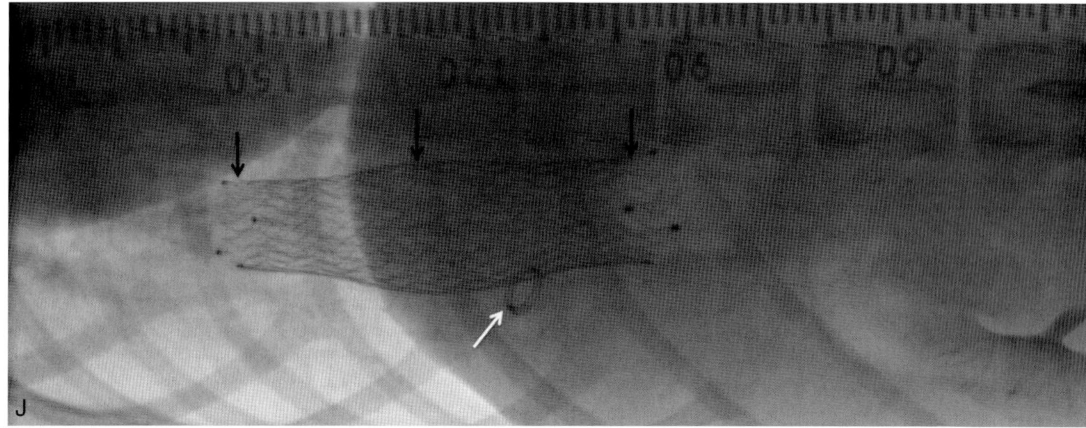

Figure 21.6 (*Continued*) (J) Final radiograph with stent (black arrows) and single coil (white arrow).

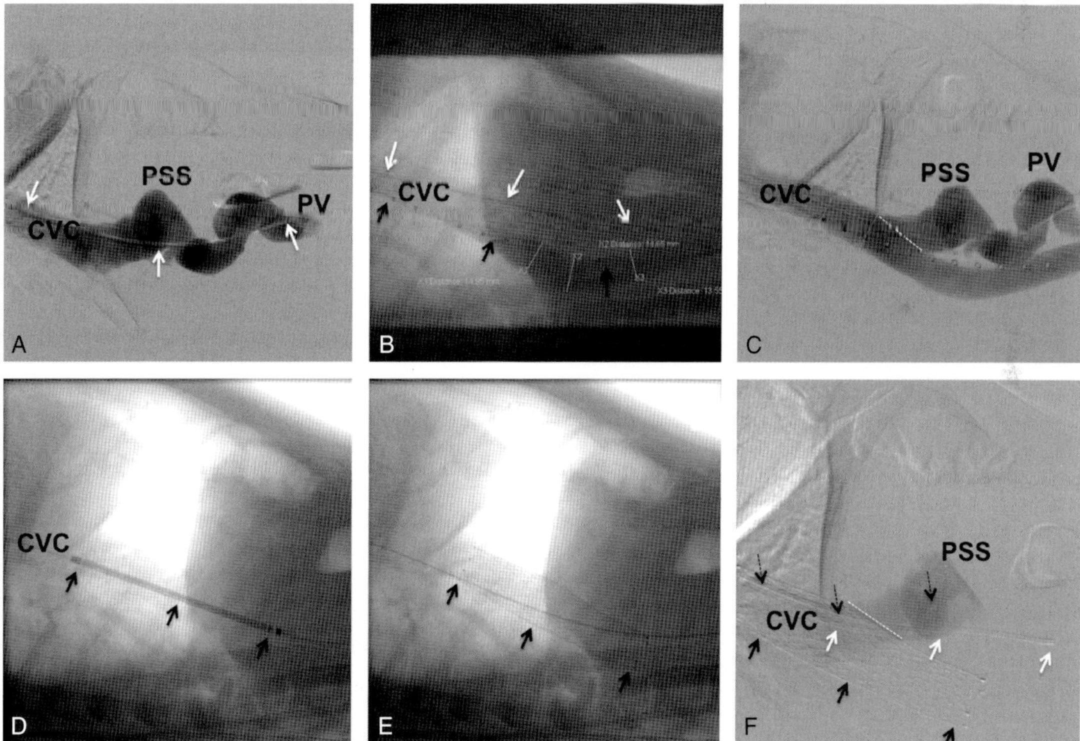

Figure 21.7 Serial fluoroscopic and radiographic images of a dog with a central divisional IHPSS during coil embolization. The head is to the left for all images and viewed in lateral projection in images (A) DSA portogram through a 4 Fr Cobra catheter (white arrows) passing from the caudal vena cava (CVC), the shunt (PSS) and into the portal vein (PV). (B) Positive pressure cavagram through 5 Fr marker catheter (black arrows) for maximal abdominal caudal vena cava (CVC) distension. (C) Dual DSA portogram and cavagram demonstrating the location of the shunt entrance (white dotted line) into the vena cava just caudal to the diaphragm. This line is used in reference to the stent guide (white block arrows) underneath the patient to help guide caval stent placement. The dilated vena cava at the level of the diaphragm is not uncommon. (D) Constrained caval stent (black arrows) within the delivery system passed over 0.035″ exchange-length floppy-tip guide wire centered across the location of the shunt entrance into the vena cava. (E) Immediately following caval stent deployment. (F) Following stent (black arrows) placement two Cobra catheters placed through the stent interstices; one within the portal vein (white arrows) used for continuous pressure measurements while coils will be placed through the other (dotted black arrows) placed at the shunt entrance. A DSA study confirms appropriate stent placement completely across the shunt entrance (white dotted line) and catheter positioning (black dotted arrows) within the shunt lumen.

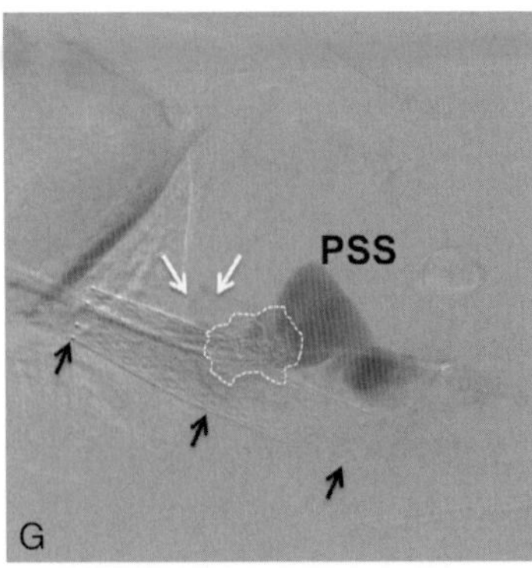

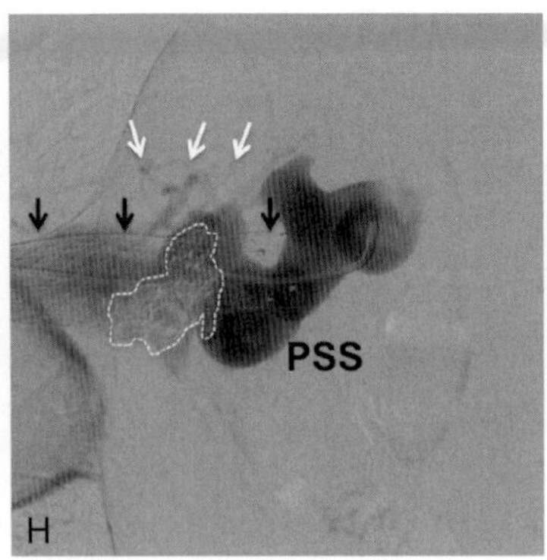

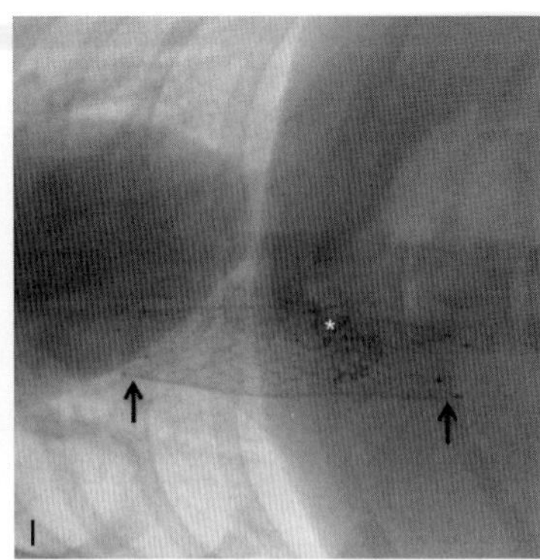

Figure 21.7 (*Continued*) DSA portograms in lateral (G) and VD (H) projections after multiple coils placed (white dotted line) demonstrating the development of intrahepatic venous collaterals (white arrows) secondary to post-hepatic shunt attenuation. This is not unexpected and has not been associated with a worse prognosis. I. Final radiograph with caval stent and coil nest (*). Notice that performing the central divisional IHPSS procedure is facilitated by lateral (G) versus VD (H/I) projection; Central divisional IHPSS directly overly the CVC in the VD projection.

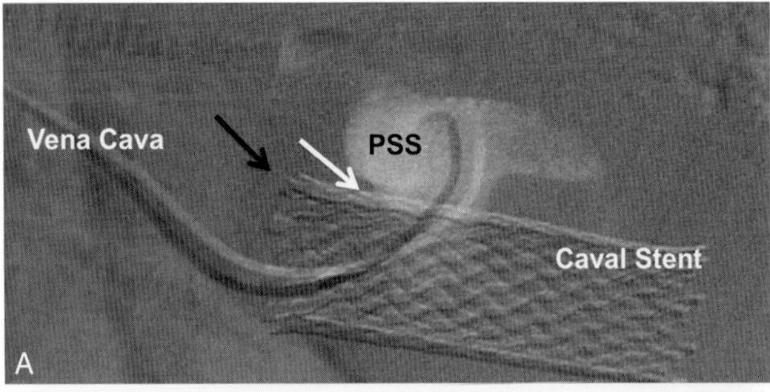

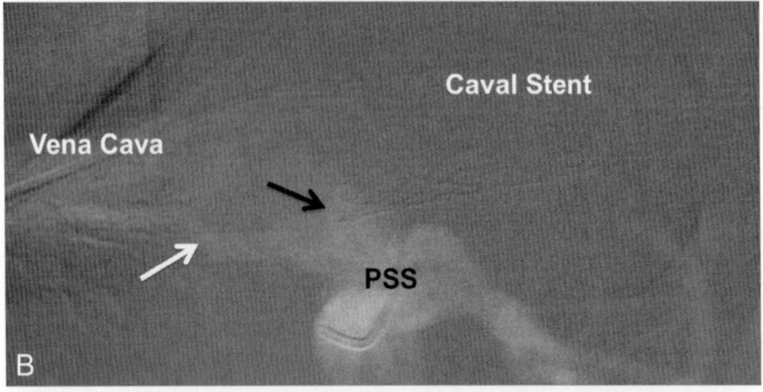

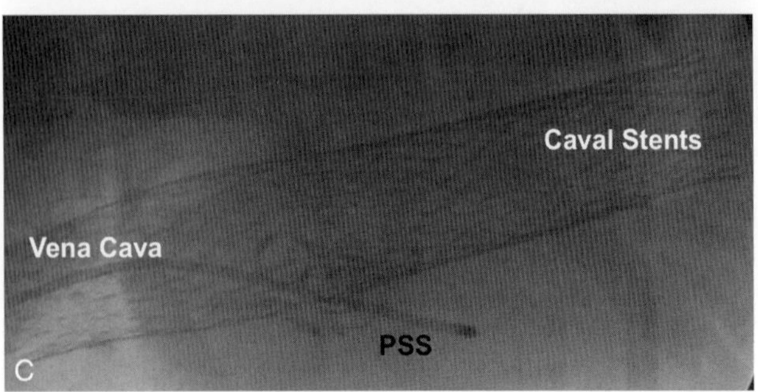

Figure 21.8 Serial images in a dog with a central divisional IHPSS undergoing coil embolization. The dog's head is to the left. (A) Lateral DSA portogram through Cobra catheter in shunt entrance (white arrow) following caval stent (black arrow) placement demonstrating what appears to be appropriate spanning across the shunt entrance. (B) Orthogonal (ventrodorsal) DSA portogram demonstrating the cranial aspect of the caval stent (black arrow) does not sufficiently span the entire shunt entrance cranially (white arrow). (C) Lateral radiograph following second caval stent placement within the first more cranially to prevent coil migration. This image is following coil placement.

prevent the coils from migrating into the caudal vena cava. This should all be done carefully and slowly under fluoroscopic guidance. Coils are subsequently added during portal pressure measurements until the shunt mouth is covered or the shunt pressures increase by approximately 6–7 mmHg [~8–9 cmH_2O] or maximal pressures approach 16 mmHg [~21 cm H_2O]. Repeat angiography is performed at the completion of the procedure, ultimate shunt and caval pressures are recorded, the jugular sheath is exchanged for a 7 Fr multi-lumen catheter[11], and the animal is recovered from anesthesia. The multilumen catheter is present for 1–2 days and allows time for the relatively large hole in the jugular vein to partially close while also facilitating repeat access should it be necessary emergently.

For repeat procedures, the patients are positioned as above and vascular access is achieved the same way. Typically, a 10 Fr vascular introducer sheath is used in order to have two 4—5 Fr angiographic catheters in place simultaneously: one within the portal vein measuring portal pressures and the other in the shunt for coil deployment. The same guidelines for portal pressure and portal:CVP gradient are used when performing repeat procedures. In some cases, dramatic improvement in portal perfusion permits complete (or near complete) shunt attenuation without reaching the limits of the pressure guidelines. In other cases, acquired intrahepatic venous collaterals may be identified that can be embolized as well.

Animals recover in the intensive care unit on intravenous fluid therapy (3–4 ml/kg/hr until awake and eating or longer if excessive contrast volumes administered), lactulose, antibiotics, low-protein diet, and proton-pump inhibitors (Table 21.1). Analgesics are not routinely necessary.

Follow-Up

Patients are typically discharged 2 days postoperatively and owners are instructed to continue all previous medications (as well as 10–14 days of an additional broad-spectrum antibiotic) for 1 month, at which time repeat chemistry panel and complete blood count are obtained. At that time, medications can be slowly weaned (except the proton-pump inhibitor) and the dog transitioned to a normal dog food over the next 2–4 weeks. If clinical signs do not return following discontinuation of medications or special diet, no further treatment is recommended. Repeat chemistry panel, a protein C level, and complete blood count are again recommended at three months post procedure and then encouraged every 6–12 months for the first year, and yearly thereafter. If clinical signs return, medications are reinstituted and an additional embolization procedure is recommended.

Special Considerations/ Alternative Uses/ Complication Examples

The same procedure described above has been used in cats with IHPSS and dogs with EHPSS (Figure 21.9). When performing these procedures in smaller patients, laser-cut stents can still be used but smaller thrombogenic coils may be necessary to avoid complete acute attenuation of these often smaller shunt vessels. Additionally, vascular plugs have been used when the portal perfusion is excellent and the patient can tolerate complete shunt occlusion based on testing with an occlusion balloon prior to device deployment.

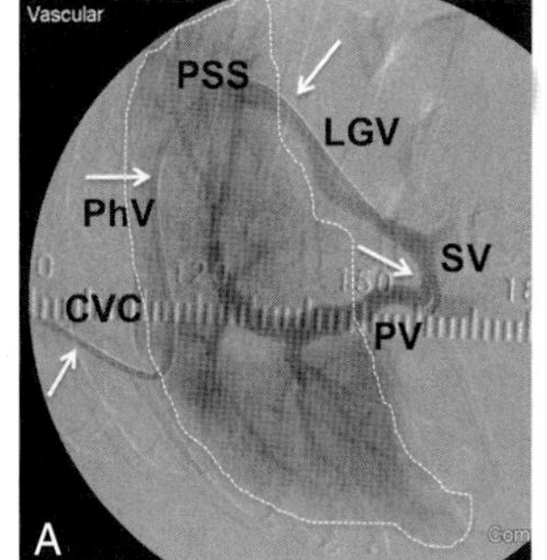

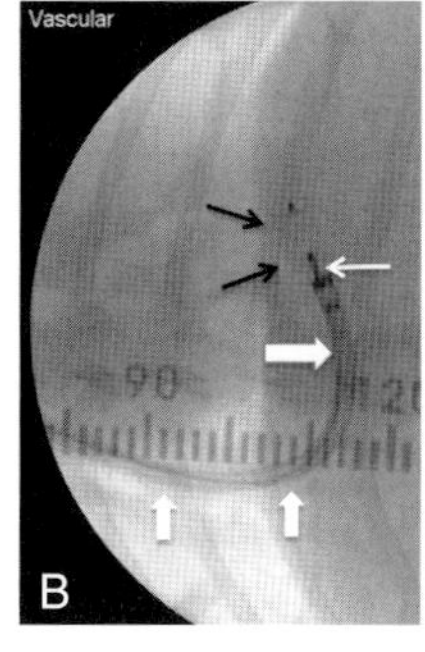

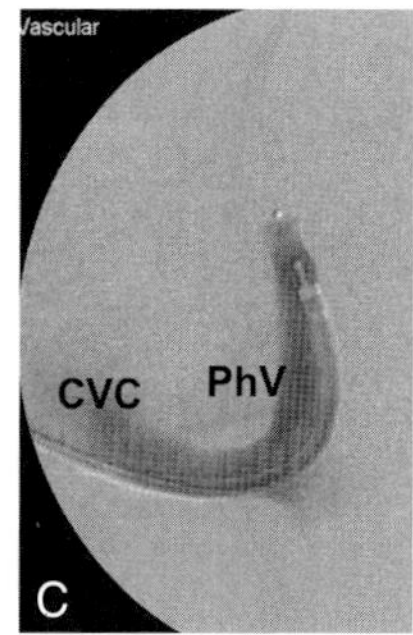

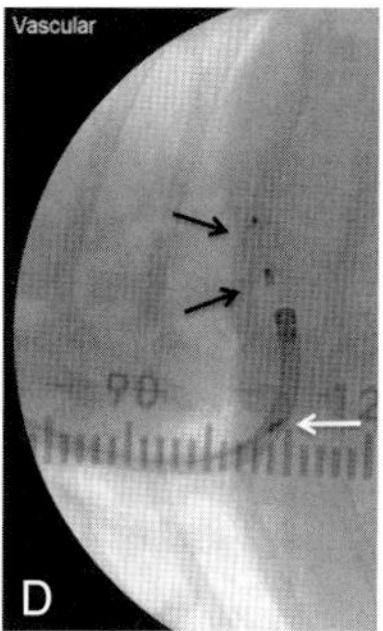

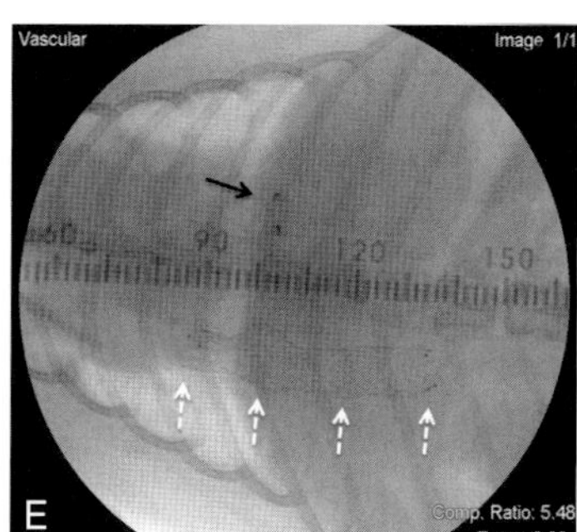

Figure 21.9 Serial fluoroscopic images of a dog with an EHPSS during embolization. The is in the VD projection and the head is to the left of each image. (A) A 4 Fr Berenstein catheter (white arrows) and guide wire combination were placed through the jugular vein and advanced down the caudal vena cava (CVC), into the phrenic vein (PhV), through the shunt (PSS), into the left gastric vein (LGV), the splenic vein (SV), and ultimately into the portal vein (PV). The guide wire has been removed and a DSA portogram demonstrates excellent portal perfusion to the entire liver (white dotted line). (B) A long, angled vascular sheath (white block arrows) has been advanced into the phrenic vein. A vascular (black arrows) attached to the delivery wire (white arrow) has been deployed to acutely and completely occlude the EHPSS. (C) A repeat DSA study through the sheath confirms complete occlusion of the vessel. (D) The delivery wire (white arrow) has been unscrewed to deploy the vascular (black arrows) that remains in place. (E) Final image with the in place (black arrow) and after a caval stent (white dotted arrows) has been placed in case the dislodges. This is not routinely necessary.

Notes

(Samples; Multiple vendors available)

1. Cefoxitin (Mefoxin), Merck & Co., Whitehouse Station, NJ.
2. Le Maitre Stent guide, Infiniti Medical, Menlo Park, CA.
3. Weasel wire, Infiniti Medical, Menlo Park, CA.
4. 10 Fr or 12 Fr Vascular introducer sheath, Infiniti Medical, Menlo Park, CA.
5. Cobra head catheter, Infiniti Medical, Menlo Park, CA.
6. Omnipaque (iohexol) injection, Amersham Health Inc., Princeton, NJ.
7. Measuring catheter, Infiniti Medical, Menlo Park, CA.
8. Bassett wire, Infiniti Medical, Menlo Park, CA.
9. Vet Stent-Cava, Infiniti Medical, Menlo Park, CA.
10. Cook embolization coils, Cook Medical Inc., Bloomingdale, IN.
11. Triple-lumen catheter, Infiniti Medical, Menlo Park, CA.
12. Amplatzer vascular plug, AGA Medical Corp, Golden Valley, Minn.

References

Bostwick DR and Twedt DR (1995) Intrahepatic and extrahepatic portal venous anomalies in dogs: 52 cases (1982–1992). *J Am Vet Med Assoc* 206, 1181–5.

Hunt GB, Kummeling A, Tisdall PLC, et al (2004) Outcomes of cellophane banding for congenital portosystemic shunts in 106 dogs and 5 cats. *Vet Surg* 33, 25–31.

Komtebedde J, Koblik PD, Breznock EM, et al (1995) Long-term clinical outcome after partial ligation of single extrahepatic anomalies in 20 dogs. *Vet Surg* 24, 379–83.

Kyles AE, Gregory CR, Jackson J, et al (2001) Evaluation of a portocaval venograft and ameroid ring for the occlusion of intrahepatic portocaval shunts in dogs. *Vet Surg* 30, 161–9.

Mai W and Weisse C (2011) Contrast-enhanced portal magnetic resonance angiography in dogs with suspected congenital portal vascular anomalies. *Vet Radiol Ultrasound* 52(3), 284–8.

Papazoglou LG, Monnet E, Seim HB, et al (2002) Survival and prognostic indicators for dogs with intrahepatic portosystemic shunts: 32 cases (1990–2000). *Vet Surg* 31, 561–70.

Smith KR, Bauer M, Monnet E (1995) Portosystemic communications: follow-up of 32 cases. *J Small Anim Pract* 36(10), 435–40.

Tisdall PL, Hunt GB, Youmans KR, et al (2000) Neurological dysfunction in dogs following attenuation of congenital extrahepatic portosystemic shunts. *J Small Anim Pract* 41, 539–46.

Weisse C, Berent A, Todd K, et al. (2014) Endovascular evaluation and treatment of intrahepatic portosystemic shunts in dogs: 100 cases (2001–2011). *J Am Vet Med Assoc* 244, 78–94.

White RN, Burton CA, McEvoy FJ, et al (1998) Surgical treatment of intrahepatic portosystemic shunts in 45 dogs. *Vet Rec* 142, 358–65.

Zwingenberger A, Schwarz T, and Saunders HM (2005) Helical computed tomographic angiography of canine portosystemic shunts. *Vet Radiol Ultrasound* 46(1), 27–32.

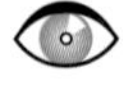

Video clips to accompany this chapter can be found in the online material at **www.wiley.com/go/weisse/vet-image-guided-interventions**

CHAPTER TWENTY-TWO

Hepatic Arteriovenous Malformations (AVMs) and Fistulas

Chick Weisse
The Animal Medical Center, New York, NY

Background / Indications

The WSAVA liver study group has recently reclassified circulatory disorders of the liver (Cullen, 2009). One of the less common congenital vascular anomalies present within the liver previously termed, "arteriovenous fistula (AVF)," is more appropriately termed "hepatic arteriovenous malformation (HAVM)" due to more recent evidence and a better understanding of the anatomy of such lesions. Little veterinary information exists on the nature of AVMs so much of the information presented here is based upon human experiences (Chanoit, 2007, Legendre, 1976, Whiting, 1986). Although both forms are "high-flow" vascular anomalies, an AVF is a single communication between an artery and vein and can typically be easily identified using cross-sectional imaging or angiography. A more common example of such a lesion could be considered a patent ductus arteriosus. On the other hand, an AVM is composed of multiple small communications involving a "nidus", or nest, of vessels and can be more difficult to identify and treat. Treatment is often much more complicated, aimed at embolizing the nidus rather than the feeders, and inappropriate treatment can exacerbate the lesion by stimulating growth and making future treatments more difficult. In addition, treatment of AVMs is often considered more palliation than cure as repeat treatments can be anticipated in the human experience. AVMs are believed to be congenital lesions in veterinary patients even though the diagnosis may not be made until later in life depending upon the location. AVFs can be congenital or acquired following trauma (bite wound or biopsy), ligation of an artery to a vein, etc.

HAVMs are most often diagnosed in young dogs (or less often cats) and typically involve too numerous to count communications between the hepatic artery and portal vein in the right or central divisions of the liver. Consequently, arterialization of the portal vein (rather than the substantially lower venous pressures of 7–9 mmHg) results in development of multiple acquired extrahepatic portosystemic shunts (Figure 22.1D). This often results in similar clinical signs of hepatic encephalopathy, gastrointestinal disturbances, etc, as seen with with IHPSS/EHPSS. Alternatively, HAVM will often have concurrent ascites, whereas a congenital IHPSS/EHPSS will not. In the author's experience of about 20 cases, a direct communication has not been seen between the hepatic artery and hepatic vein, but instead it has always been between the hepatic artery and the portal vein. Clinical signs are typically associated with ascites (75% of dogs; Figure 22.1) and/or hepatoencephalopathy (less common than with PSS). As such, these patients are often misidentified as having an IHPSS as the bloodwork changes and clinical syndrome is similar, and a large intrahepatic vessel is identified on ultrasonography. The presence of ascites should raise suspicion (rare in IHPSS cases as shunt patients have portal hypotension while HAVM dogs have portal hypertension). While 25% of dogs will not have ascites presumptively due to the acquired EHPSS decompressing the portal system, a reliable diagnostic tool seems to be identification of hepatofugal (retrograde) portal blood flow that is always present. Other clinical signs include gastrointestinal signs (diarrhea, vomiting), stunted growth, lethargy, and heart murmurs (present in ~20% of dogs) (Chanoit, 2007). The author has rarely appreciated the reportedly identified audible "bruit" when the AVM is ausculted.

Veterinary Image-Guided Interventions, First Edition. Edited by Chick Weisse and Allyson Berent.

Companion website: www.wiley.com/go/weisse/vet-image-guided-interventions

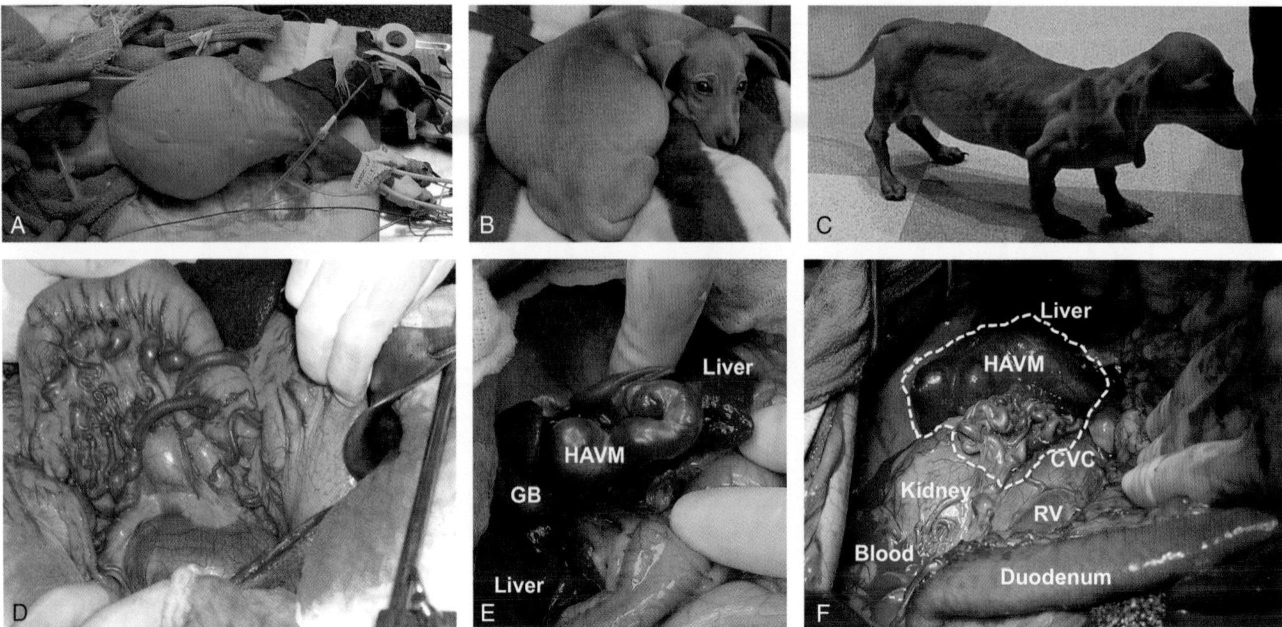

Figure 22.1 (A) Anesthetized HAVM Boxer puppy with massive ascites. Dachshund puppy with HAVM prior to embolization (B) and a few weeks after embolization (C) demonstrating dramatically reduced ascites but also the often underestimated cachexia that accompanies this condition due to portal hypertension and reduced gastrointestinal absorption. (D) HAVM intraoperative picture demonstrating too numerous to count acquired extrahepatic shunts secondary to the HAVM portal hypertension. (E, F) Intraoperative pictures of HAVMs demonstrating the vascular dilation present throughout the affected liver lobes(s), multiple shunts with distended renal veins and vena cava, and often some associated bleeding.

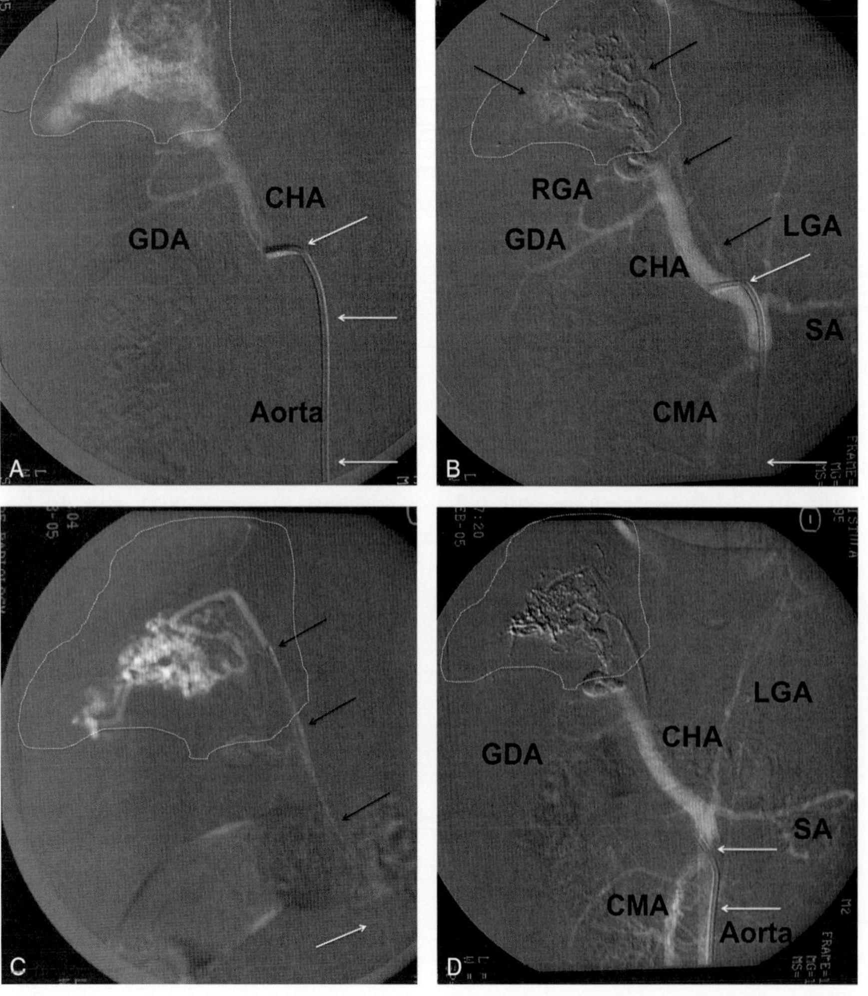

Figure 22.2 Serial digital subtraction angiograms (DSA) in dog with HAVM glue embolization in a ventrodorsal projection. The head is to the top of each image. (A) Catheter (white arrows) from groin, up aorta, and into common hepatic artery (CHA) with angiogram demonstrating HAVM (white dotted outline). The gastroduodenal artery (GDA) does not appear to be involved. (B) Repeat DSA after initial glue injection demonstrating less flow through HAVM and more through other vessels previously under-perfused such as the splenic artery (SA), left gastric artery (LGA) and some reflux into cranial mesenteric artery (CMA). The right gastric artery (RGA) can also be seen. There is now another feeding vessel not previously identified (black arrows). A surgical ligation of the hepatic artery would have missed this vessel. (C) Microcatheter (black arrows) access of this feeding vessel with HAVM perfusion. (D) Repeat DSA after glue embolization of the additional feeding vessel demonstrating complete embolization with no further HAVM perfusion (white dotted line).

Potential treatment options for HAVM have included nutrient artery ligation, surgical resection (liver lobectomy or lobectomies), and more recently transarterial embolization (TAE) with glue (cyanoacrylate). It is the author's opinion that nutrient artery ligation should not be performed for AVMs as there are numerous contributing vessels and this limits access to the AVM in the future if necessary (Figure 22.2). Ligation is a reasonable option for AVFs, although this form of vascular anomaly is exceedingly rare in the animal liver and embolization would likely be easier. The latter two treatments are both reasonable options for discussion with the owner.

As the majority of HAVMS are located in the right and central divisions of the liver (often surrounding or involving the gall bladder or caudal vena cava), and approximately 25% involve more than one lobe, surgery can be challenging (Figure 22.1). In addition, keep in mind the entire portal circulation is arterialized so there are no "minor bleeds" from the omentum or mesentery and strict hemostasis is required. When surgery is performed, temporary vascular occlusion has been recommended (Whiting, 1986), but the author has found that the cranial mesenteric artery needs to be temporarily attenuated along with both the celiac artery and portal vein. This will help to limit otherwise substantial intra-operative hemorrhage that has been reported in 39% of cases during surgery (Chanoit, 2007). Other reported surgical complications besides hemorrhage include portal hypertension, systemic hypotension, bradycardia, and portal or mesenteric vein thrombus formation (Chanoit, 2007). In dogs undergoing surgical therapy alone, perioperative survival rates were 77% and long-term outcome was fair or good for 38% to 57% (Chanoit, 2007). Overall 75% of dogs continue to require dietary or medical management of clinical signs due to patent acquired EHPSS that will always persist (Chanoit, 2007). These multiple acquired EHPSS may be amenable to caval banding but this remains an uncommonly performed procedure. Transcatheter therapies typically involve cyanoacrylate glue, or more recently "Onyx", (ethylene-co-vinyl alcohol [(EVOH] in dimethyl sulfoxide [DMSO]) a slower polymerizing agent. While sclerosants such as alcohol and particles such as PVA or microspheres have been described, these are less typically used for high-flow lesions such AVMs.

Patient Preparation

Preoperative medical management should be similar to that used for portosystemic shunts, however diuretics may be indicated if ascites is massive, resulting in patient morbidity (Table 22.1). A cardiac evaluation is recommended prior to the procedure as high-output cardiac failure is a perceived sequela to AVMs (although the author has only seen this in one cat with a chronic (>10 years) peripheral hindlimb AVM). Routine bloodwork (complete blood count and chemistry panels) is performed prior to the procedure as are liver function tests (bile acids and protein C) to monitor improvements or worsening of function over time. The author tries to avoid abdominocentesis unless the ascites is massive and the patient is uncomfortable, having respiratory issues, or perceived anesthetic difficulties (decreased cardiac venous return when in dorsal recumbency). When required, abdominocentesis should be performed under ultrasound guidance to avoid puncture of the spleen or other organ that could result in substantial hemorrhage due to (1) severe portal hypertension, and (2) diminished ability of blood to coagulate when surrounded by fluid.

Cross-sectional imaging has greatly enhanced pre-surgical planning and is highly recommended whether surgical or interventional treatment will be pursued. While human interventionalists often prefer MRI due to the reduced radiation exposure, dual-phase CT angiograms are the author's diagnostic cross-sectional imaging of choice (Figure 22.3 and Figure 22.4). The arterial phase is the most important for identification of feeders, however multiple venous phases are recommended to evaluate the often-diminished portal perfusion recently identified in these dogs that may have prognostic significance in the future. As HAVMs likely change over time, the imaging should be performed as close to the procedure as possible. Embolization is typically performed under a separate anesthetic event as the contrast load will be reached when performing the CTA precluding subsequent arteriography. Maintenance intravenous fluids may be administered overnight for mild diuresis and the procedure is typically performed the following day. Although termed "hepatic" AVMs, the author has identified contributions from many other arteries including the left gastric, phrenic, gastroduodenal, and other neighboring arteries. An extensive knowledge of the hepatic vascular anatomy is required and becoming comfortable reading cross-sectional imaging on such cases greatly facilitates the procedure (see Chapter 20). The radiologists will often make the diagnosis using the cross-sectional imaging but will often not be able to discern the precise vascular anatomy required to ensure no contributing vessels are missed during the procedure. This is more easily determined via angiography. In addition, the CTA will often underestimate the degree of vessel contributions that will

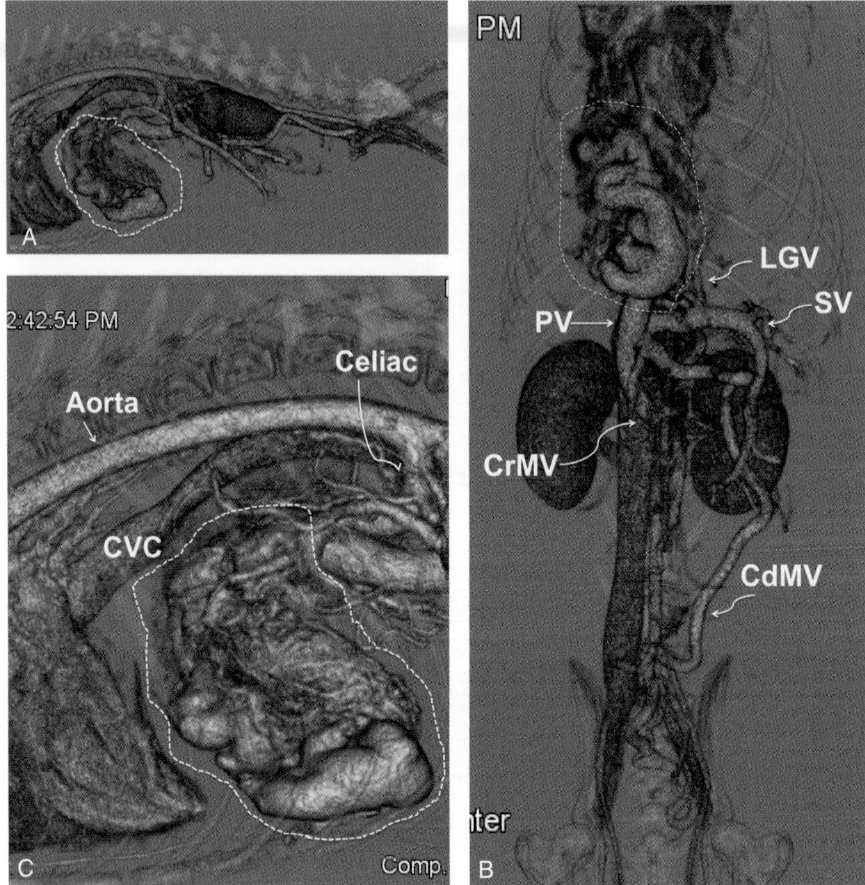

Figure 22.3 3-D dual-phase CTA reconstructions of a dog with an HAVM. (A) Sagittal reconstruction demonstrating large HAVM (white dotted line). The aorta can be seen to narrow beyond the origin of the celiac artery. (B) Coronal reconstruction demonstrating large HAVM (white dotted line) as well as arterialization (same color as aorta) of portal vein (PV) and tributaries including cranial (CrMV) and caudal (CdMV) mesenteric, splenic (SV), and left gastric veins (LGV). (C) Close-up sagittal reconstruction with aorta, celiac artery, HAVM (white dotted line) and caudal vena cava (CVC).

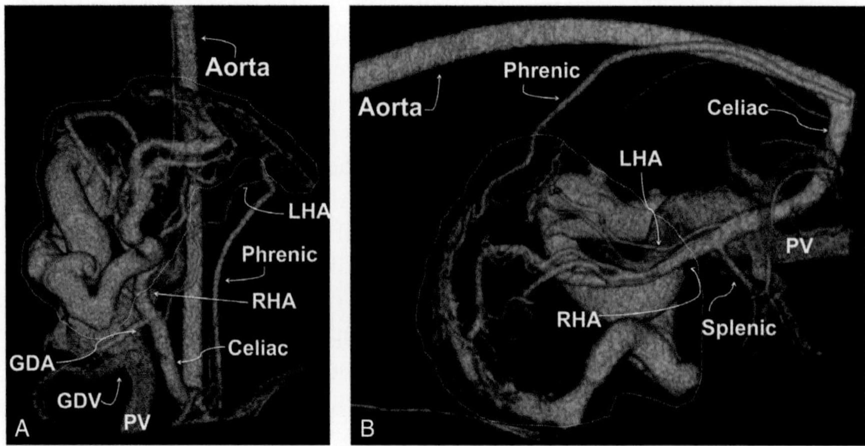

Figure 22.4 3-D dual-phase CTA reconstructions of a dog with an HAVM. Coronal (A) and sagittal (B) reconstructions demonstrating that the HAVM (white dotted line) is being fed from multiple branches including the right hepatic (RHA) and left hepatic (LHA) arteries as well as the phrenic artery. Notice the hypertrophy of the RHA, the major feeding vessel. The gastroduodenal artery (GDA) and splenic artery are not contributing to the HAVM. The portal vein (PV) and gastroduodenal vein (GDV) are also identified.

become more evident during embolization of the major feeding branches and subsequent angiography. In addition, recording portal blood flow direction and velocity prior to, and immediately following, the embolization procedure may be helpful in identifying completeness of embolization as well as early recurrence of the HAVM.

Prior to performing HAVM glue embolization, discussions about surgical resection (historical standard-of-care) should occur and owner consent obtained. Diuretics (if used preoperatively) are discontinued a week or two prior to the procedure in order to monitor the patients response prior to, and following, the embolization procedure. Pre-medications include broad-spectrum antibiotic coverage for common liver organisms (Table 22.1). Post-embolization syndrome, as seen with liver tumor embolization, has not been appreciated in the author's practice following HAVM embolization.

Potential Risks/Complications/Expected Outcomes

One potential major complication associated with HAVM glue embolization includes non-target embolization. This involves distal glue migration and embolization beyond the HAVM nidus and into the draining venous systems including the portal system, the acquired extrahepatic shunts, and/or the pulmonary circulation (Figure 22.5). Non-target

TABLE 22.1
Pre- and postprocedural medical management

- Antibiotics:
  - Preoperative: metronidazole (7.5 mg/kg PO q12 hr)
  - Intraoperative: cefoxitin (30 mg/kg IV once, then 20 mg/kg IV q2 hr)
  - Postoperative: clavamox (13.75 mg/kg PO BID × 14 days)
- Laxatives: (often for life)
  - Lactulose (~0.1–0.2 ml/kg PO q8–12 hr. Dosed to form soft but formed stools)
- Gastroprotectants: (for life)
  - Omeprazole (1 mg/kg PO q12 hr for life)
- Diuretics (Uncommonly very helpful):
  - Spironolactone (1–4 mg/kg PO q12 hr)
  - Furosemide (0.5–2 mg/kg PO q8–12 hr)
- Low-protein diet: (often for life)
  - Hill's L/D, Hepatic LS, or similar
- Anticonvulsants (if clinical signs not regulated with other medications-uncommon):
  - Levetiracetam [Keppra] (20 mg/kg PO q8 hr)
- Analgesics:
  - Perioperative: opioid premedications
  - Post-operative: tramadol (2–4 mg/kg PO q8–12 hr × 3 days)

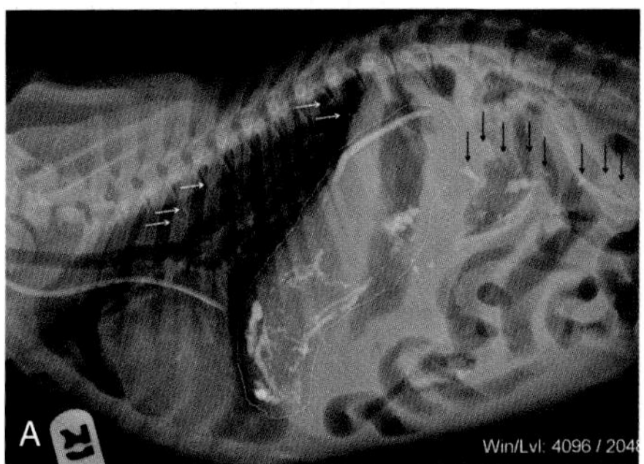

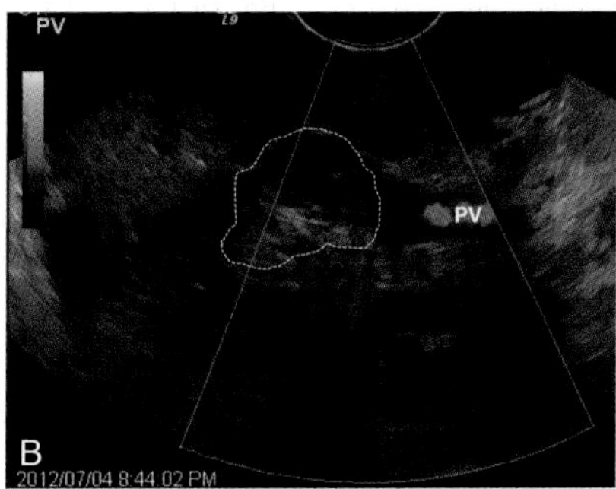

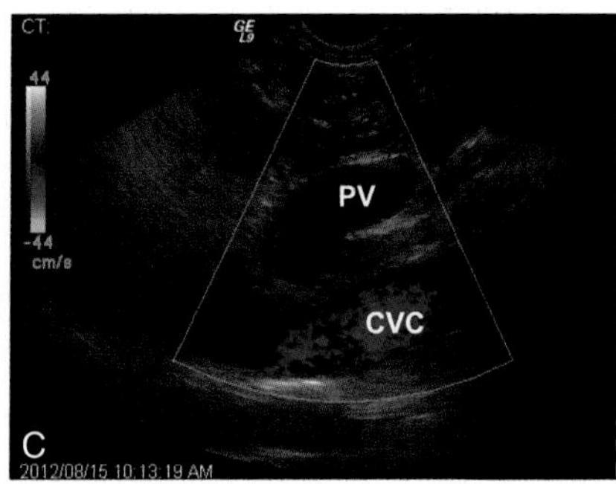

Figure 22.5 Several potential complications (all clinically inconsequential) following HAVM glue embolization in three different dogs. (A) Lateral radiograph following HAVM (white dotted line) glue embolization demonstrating non-target embolization of small pieces of glue within pulmonary circulation (white arrows) and within multiple acquired extrahepatic portosystemic shunts (black arrows). (B) Ultrasonographic image of large portal vein (PV) thrombus (white dotted line) likely composed of glue mixture and blood components. C. Ultrasonographic image of the portal vein (PV) and caudal vena cava (CVC) demonstrating normal flow through the CVC but stagnant flow within the PV.

embolization can also include glue occlusion of proximal vessels such as the common hepatic artery, gastroduodenal artery, and/or splenic or left gastric arteries. In addition, the glue can polymerize between the catheter tip and vessel wall locking it in place; this would be considered a technical error and while glue has become attached to the catheter tip in the author's experience, the catheter has always been able to be removed. While some non-target embolization has occurred in the author's experience, there have been no appreciated deleterious consequences as a result.

Another complication identified in a small number of patients is (partial) portal vein thrombosis (Figure 22.5). The goal of the embolization procedure is to completely occlude arterial supply to the portal system; if performed completely it is conceivable that the hepatofugal portal blood flow will reverse and become hepatopetal (towards the liver). In between these two possibilities includes the potential of creating stagnant portal blood flow; this is often close to what is appreciated ultrasonographically immediately after the embolization procedure. While un-nerving to see, the author has not had to intervene in any of the cases; the body accommodates over the next few days as the shunting is diminished and rerouted. The ascites may temporarily worsen within the first week but this should resolve quickly without treatment.

It remains unclear if HAVM recurrence should be considered a true procedural complication. The author typically warns the owner that there is an approximate 30% recurrence rate (requiring future interventions). In addition, as reported with surgery, all of these patients have acquired extrahepatic portosystemic shunts that will not regress so the majority will require some degree of lifelong medical management. Caval banding can be considered in certain cases but the author has not performed this yet in one of these cases. Unless the HAVM recurs, the diuretics should not be necessary after the procedure.

Lastly, historical complications associated with general anesthesia, seizures, arterial access site hemorrhage/infection, and contrast allergies/nephropathy must be discussed.

In the four reported cases of HAVM glue embolization, perioperative survival was 100% and long-term outcome fair or good in all four even though one required surgery after the HAVM recurred following glue embolization (early case). The author has not had to perform surgery on any other case in approximately 15 HAVM patients treated.

Human interventionalists typically undergo special training in the use of glue prior to performing these procedures. It is recommended by the author to have someone with such training present prior to performing these procedures for the first time, as the potential for causing irreversible harm to the patient exists.

Equipment

A list of recommended equipment can be found in Figure 22.6. Glue embolization procedures require very little equipment but the fluoroscopy unit must provide adequate imaging detail to identify very small caliber vessels using digital subtraction angiography and the ability to obtain orthogonal imaging when necessary. Failure to identify collateral vessels could lead to non-target embolization and severe consequences or continued HAVM flow. A cut-down set is required for non-percutaneous vascular access. Everyone in the room MUST wear eye protection during handling of glue to prevent contact with the cornea. It is important that the cyanoacrylate glue never comes into contact with the iohexol contrast material or any saline, as it can polymerize, and should only be in contact with sterile water in 5% dextrose (D5W) (see below). The operator should have a separate embolization table that prevents contamination of the supplies with the rest of the angiography materials. A short list of the supplies needed includes: a vascular access sheath (4 Fr),[1] a micropuncture set[2] for smaller dogs or cats, a 4 Fr Cobra head catheter[3], a hydrophilic guide wire[4] (0.035"), contrast material (iohexol)[5], a Touhy–Borst adaptor[6] and flow switch[7], a few microcatheter/microwire combinations[8–11], 1 mL polycarbonate syringes[12], cyanoacrylate glue[13], iodized poppy seed oil (ethiodol or lipiodol),[14] and tantalum,[15] when necessary for improved contrast enhancement (see details below).

Fluoroscopic Procedure

Following induction of general anesthesia, hair on the caudoventral aspect of the abdomen, the inguinal area, and on the medial aspects of both thighs is clipped. The animal is placed in dorsal recumbency with the chosen hind limb extended, abducted, and secured in place to allow access to the inguinal area. The skin over the inguinal area is aseptically prepared and draped, and the femoral artery pulse identified. Femoral artery access is described in Chapter 20 using a standard vascular access sheath (4 or 5 Fr)[1] that is typically no larger than the catheter being used (4–5 Fr). When small caliber femoral arteries are encountered, micropuncture sets[2] are used for initial access. Typically a 4Fr cobra catheter[3] and 0.035" angled hydrophilic guide

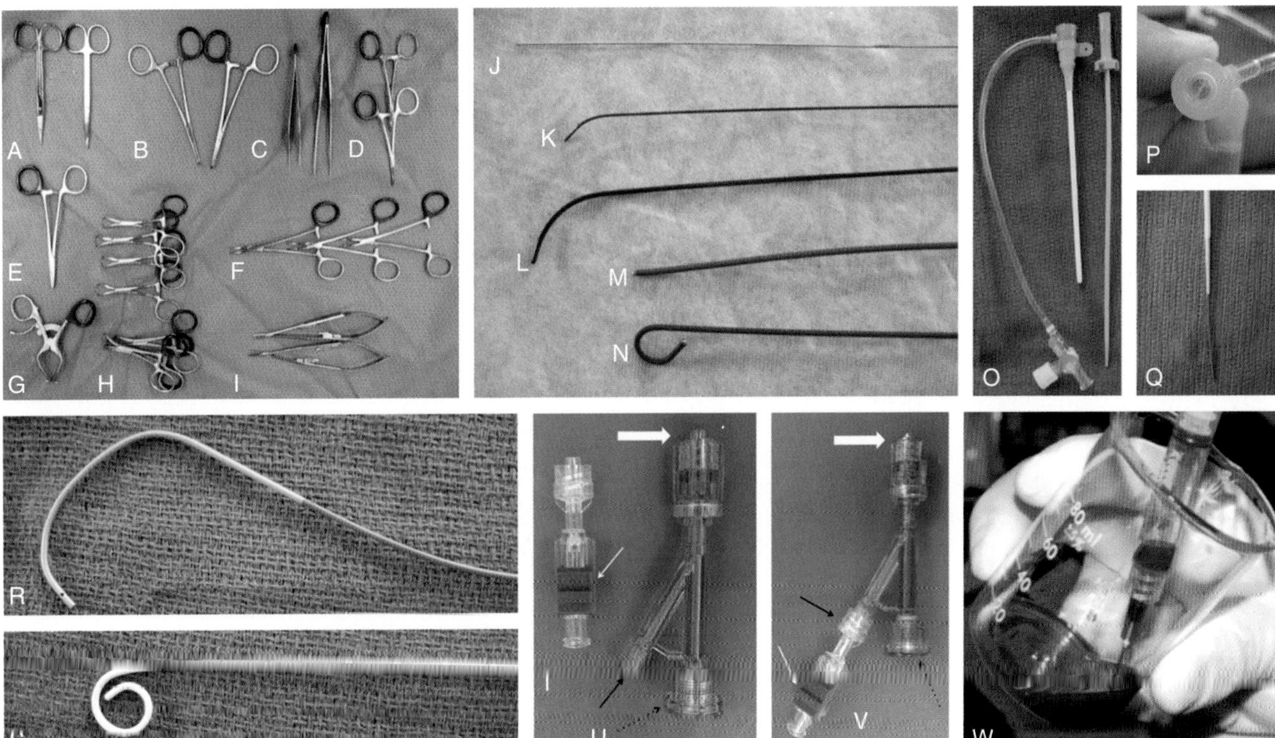

Figure 22.6 (A–I) Sample surgical cut-down set. (A) Sharp sharps and small Metzenbaum scissors. (B) Right-angled forceps. (C) Brown–Adson and Debakey forceps. (D) Mosquito hemostats. (E) Needle drivers. (F) Kelly hemostats. (G) Small Gelpi retractors. (H) Small Babcock towel clamps. (I) Castrovlejo needle drivers for vessel repair. (J–N) Guide wires. (J) 0.018″ microwire; (K) 0.018″ angled, hydrophilic guide wire; (L) 0.035″ angled, hydrophilic guide wire; (M, N) 0.035″ straight PTFE wire (M) and 0.035″ Rosen PTFE wire (N), both of which uncommon used for this procedure. (O–Q) Vascular introducer sheath. 4 Fr vascular introducer sheath made up of shaft (white) with 4 Fr inner diameter, hemostasis valve (P) to prevent bleeding, three-way stop-cock (yellow cap) to flush and/or aspirate, and 4Fr dilator (blue) to make smooth transition from sheath down to 0.035″ guide wire (Q). (R) 4Fr Cobra catheter. (S) 4 Fr marker pigtail catheter for aortogram and measurements if needed. (T–V) Flo-switch (T) and Touhy–Borst adapter (U), which connect (V) to form a hemostasis valve (dotted black line) and side-port that can be switched on or off (white arrow) for flushing or aspirating. This device is attached to the hub of the 4 Fr catheter (at white block arrow) and allows coaxial passage of a microcatheter/microwire through the 4 Fr catheter. (W) Glue (cyanoacrylate), iodinated poppy-seed oil, and tantalum mixture prepared prior to injection.

wire[4] are used in combination to select the celiac artery and common hepatic artery (Figure 22.7). A diagnostic arteriogram is performed using 50:50 iohexol[5]:saline mixture. All contrast studies should be performed under digital subtraction angiography (DSA) and respiratory pause in order to identify small caliber vessels (Figure 22.8). In addition, for very high-flow HAVMS, using higher frame rates (>15 fps) will permit improved identification of vessels but also higher radiation exposure. All non-critical personnel should leave the room during the acquisition of these images. The author tries to limit total iohexol administration to 3 ml/kg for the entire procedure when possible. As these patients have often received diuretic therapy, care to avoid contrast nephropathy must be taken.

The 4Fr catheter remains in position in the proximal common hepatic artery and a Touhy–Borst adapter[6] and Flo-switch[7] are attached to permit a 1.9 to 3 Fr microcatheter[8,9] to be coaxially introduced. The microcatheter/microwire[10,11] combination is used to superselect the particular vessel supplying the HAVM. The primary vessels are substantially hypertrophied so access is typically straightforward as it is the preferential path the microcatheter will take. Due to the vascular "stealing" of the HAVM, the standard tributaries of the hepatic artery such as the other hepatic artery branches and gastroduodenal artery may not be clearly visible. This makes identification of the catheter location more difficult for those not well-versed in hepatic vascular anatomy. Repeat DSA is performed through the microcatheter using 100% iohexol via a 1 ml Luer-lock polycarbonate syringe[12] as needed to identify the HAVM anatomy and target the nidus if possible. Once the proper location is

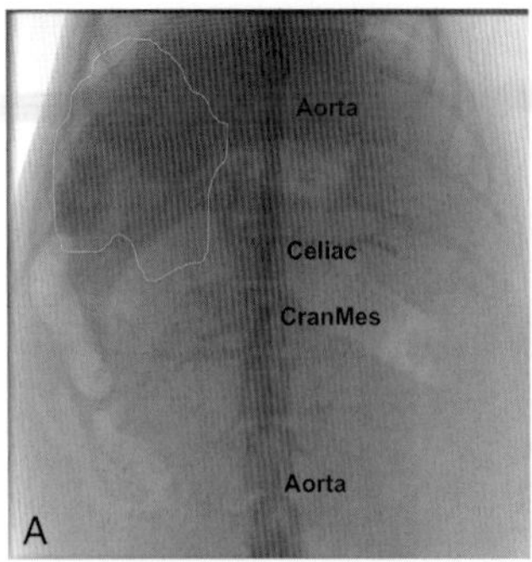

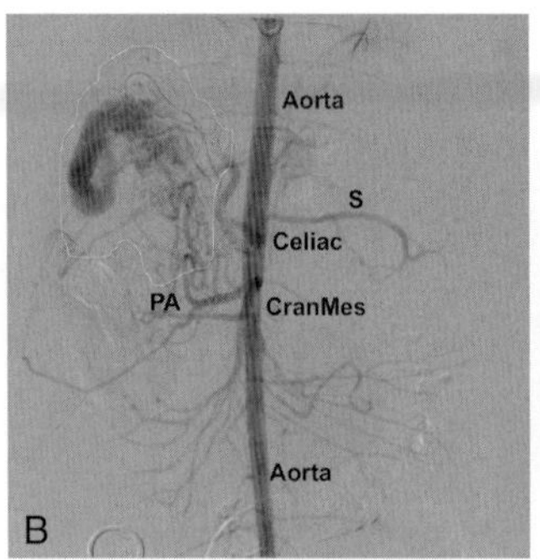

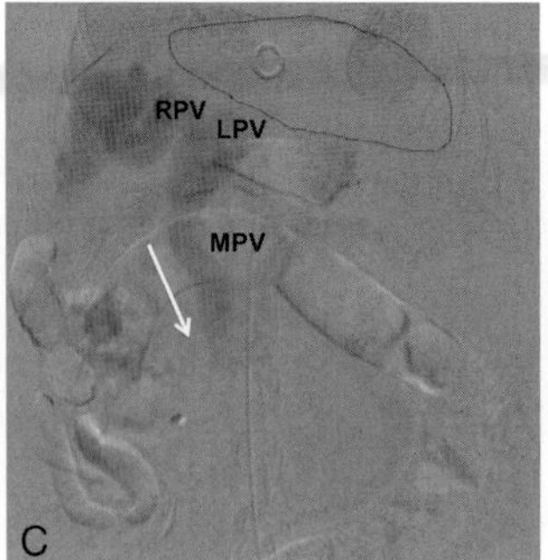

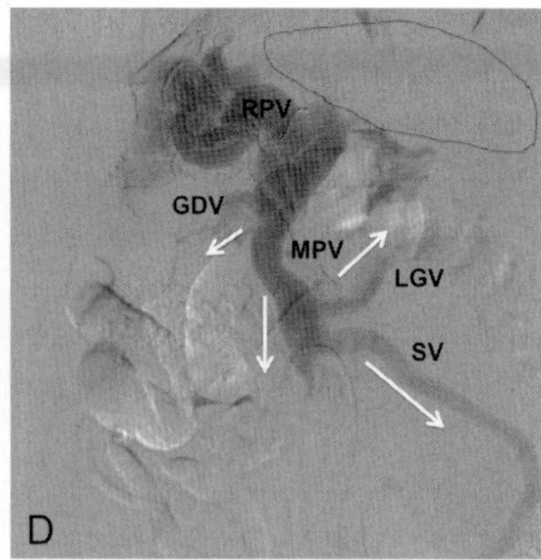

Figure 22.7 Serial angiograms in a dog with an HAVM. The head is to the top of each image. Aortogram (A) and digital subtraction (DSA) aortogram (B) demonstrating numerous tangled vessels (HAVM-white dotted line) identified in right cranial abdomen. Identified vessels include the celiac, cranial mesenteric (CranMes), splenic (S) and hypertrophied phrenicoabdominal (PA) arteries. (C) The venous phase of the DSA becomes evident overtime demonstrating hepatofugal (reverse/retrograde) filling of the right portal vein (RPV) and main portal vein (MPV). Notice the lack of filling of the left portal vein (LPV) and absent perfusion of the left division of the liver (black dotted line). (D) As the DSA finishes, hepatofugal bloodflow continues in reverse (white lines) filling the gastroduodenal (GDV), left gastric (LGV), and splenic (SV) veins with persistent lack of perfusion to the left division. This lack of portal perfusion may contribute to patient deterioration (liver failure) following resection of HAVMs. Glue embolization does not involve liver resection, therefore attempting to maximize hepatic function.

identified, the microcatheter is flushed and glue preparation can begin.

A dry, unused area on the surgical table is isolated and surgical gloves are changed. Any contact with ionic liquid will cause premature glue polymerization. Separate syringes are used. 5% dextrose in water (D5W) is poured into a basin; this will be used for catheter flushing as this non-ionic liquid will not lead to glue polymerization in the catheter but saline or contrast will. One ml of n-butyl-cyanoacrylate glue[13] (nbca) is mixed with iodized poppy seed oil[14] (ethiodol or lipiodol) in a 1:1 to 1:3 mixture of glue to oil inside a sterile shot glass (round bottom and convenient, easily cleaned glass container). If necessary, a small amount of tantalum powder can be added to the mixture to lend radio-opacity to the mixture (not often necessary as the oil is radio-opaque enough). The oil slows polymerization time and the tantalum delays the start of polymerization; the ratio of the mixture is based upon personal experience and the rate of flow through the HAVM. Once mixed, approximately 0.1 to 0.5 ml of the glue mixture is drawn up into each of two or three different 1 cm polycarbonate syringes and two or three 1 cm syringes are filled with D5W as well. Time is now important as the longer the glue is exposed to the environment the more likely polymerization will begin. While one person is preparing this glue mixture, another is washing the hub of the microcatheter with D5W to remove any saline and contrast. They then flush the microcatheter with a 1 cm syringe of D5W to clear out the lumen to prevent glue polymerization within the microcatheter. The anesthetist is asked to hyperventilate to avoid breathing during the glue delivery (avoid motion artifact during fluoroscopy). The glue syringe is attached to the microcatheter and under fluoroscopic guidance the glue is injected into the catheter. The empty syringe is removed and the full 1cc syringe with D5W is attached and injected while watching under fluoroscopy. During the slow D5W injection, the small volume of glue will begin to be visualized exiting the microcatheter. The rate of injection is commensurate with the flow through the HAVM in order to fill the nidus if possible. Once injected, the microcatheter is removed as an assistant is holding the 4 Fr catheter to prevent it from moving during microcatheter removal. Care must be taken to avoid injecting the D5W as the microcatheter is being removed. Now a repeat DSA run can be performed through the 4 Fr catheter in the common hepatic artery to identify the remaining perfusion to the HAVM. Sometimes the microcatheter can be reused before removing it but this adds the risk of potentially gluing the catheter in place or the glue polymerizing within the catheter and losing a substantial amount of expensive glue mixture. The procedure is repeated as necessary with subsequent selective and super-selective arteriograms to evaluate the success of the procedure. The author has used as many as eight separate microcatheters for a single glue embolization procedure when many vessels were involved. Alternatively, "Onyx"[16] can be used to embolize the HAVM; see package insert for special handling instructions as this is beyond the scope of this chapter.

Ideally, the procedure is completed when there is no longer any flow identified to the HAVM; Multiple vessels should be interrogated including a final aortogram to make sure embolization is complete. It is

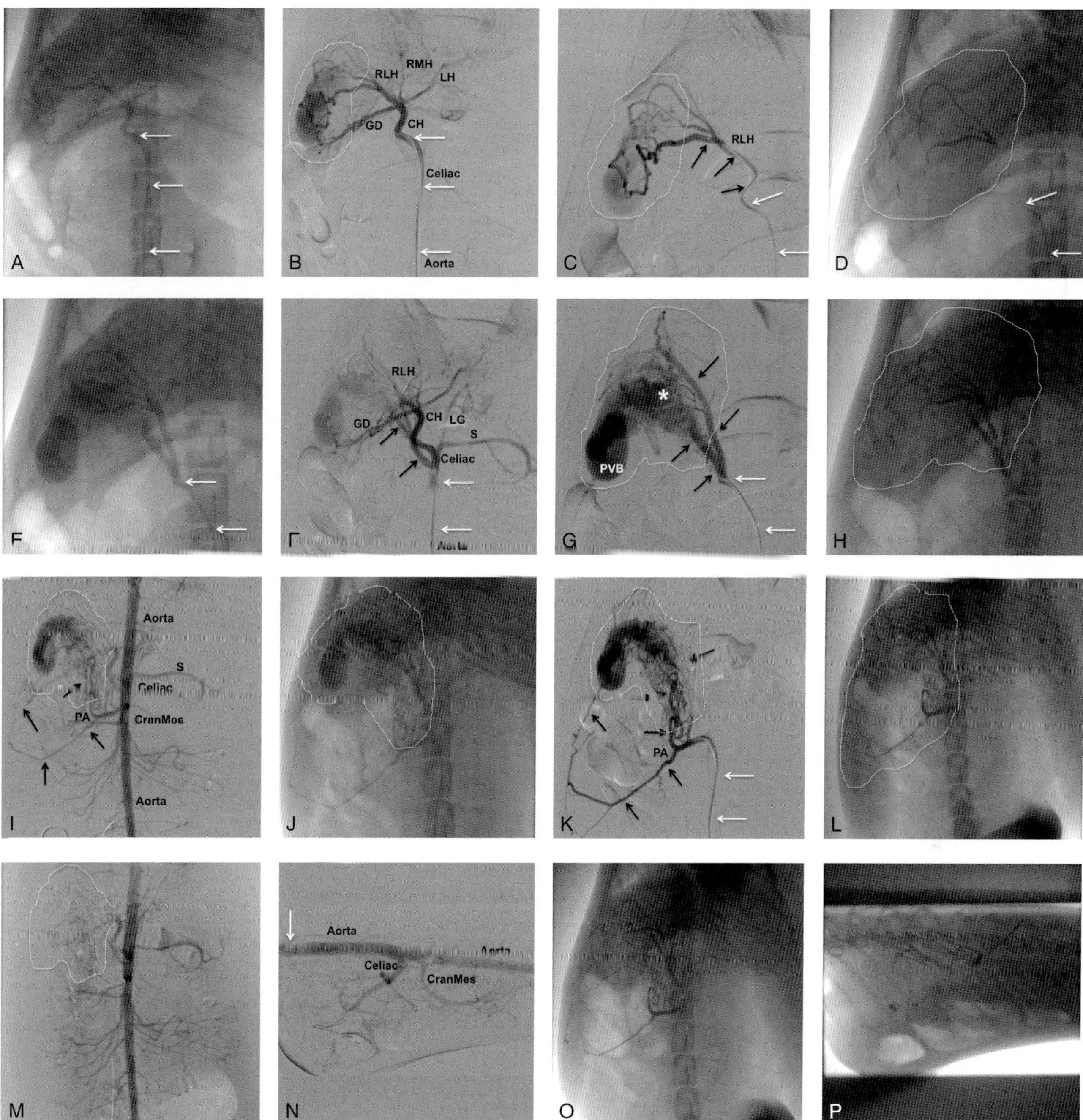

Figure 22.8 HAVM glue embolization. The dog's head is to the top of each VD image or the left in each lateral image. Angiogram (A) and DSA (B) through 4 Fr Berenstein catheter (white arrows) with tip in the common hepatic artery (CH). With DSA, the left (LH), right medial (RMH), and right lateral (RLH) hepatic arteries can be identified, as well as the gastroduodenal artery (GD). The HAVM (white dotted line) is identified in the right lateral quadrant of the liver. (C) Close-up DSA through microcatheter (black arrows) in RLH artery demonstrating multiple feeders. (D) Radio-opaque glue cast in RLH artery immediately postembolization. Repeat angiogram (E), DSA (F), and close-up DSA (G) demonstrating additional newly identified feeders (black arrows), improved bloodflow to the celiac axis including the splenic (S) and left gastric (LG) arteries, and the distended right portal vein branch (PVB) receiving the HAVM (*) bloodflow. (H) Radio-opaque glue cast in both feeders immediately after second embolization. DSA aortogram showing cranial mesenteric artery (CranMes) (I), angiogram (J), and close-up DSA (K). Branches of the right phrenicoabdominal (PA) artery (black arrows) can be seen contributing to the HAVM. (L) Radio-opaque glue cast immediately after third embolization. VD (M) and lateral DSA (N) aortograms demonstrating no filling of the HAVM. VD (O) and lateral (P) radiographs post glue embolization demonstrating glue vascular casts in vessels.

not uncommon to identify more and more feedings vessels as previous vessels are occluded. In addition, care must be taken to avoid excessive contrast loads in these often young patients that have sometimes received diuretics; the owners should be warned about the possibility of staged procedures being necessary. The author has found this often involves completely embolizing the hepatic artery such that there is no visible arterial blood flow to the liver. The author has not seen acute liver failure develop following any of these procedures.

Following embolization, all catheters and sheaths are removed. Hemostasis is typically achieved with femoral artery ligation. All animals recover from anesthesia in an intensive care unit for monitoring. Perioperative medical management is standard for these patients (Table 22.1).

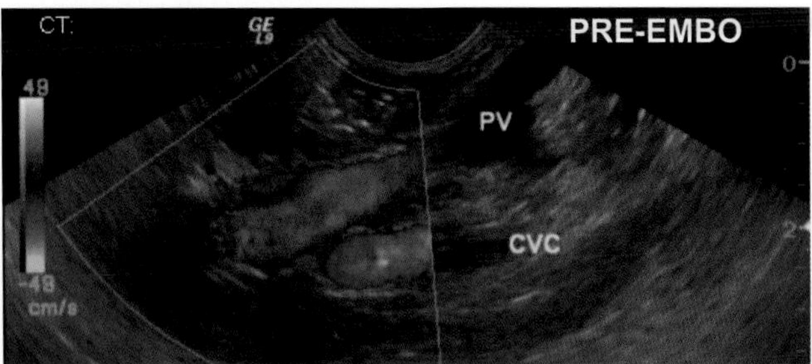

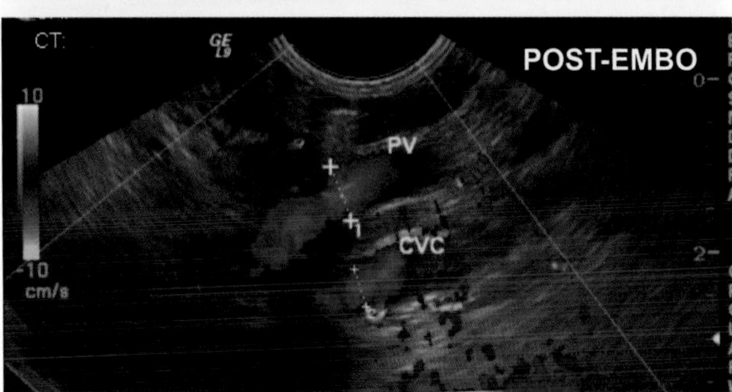

Figure 22.9 Abdominal ultrasonography in a dog prior to (PRE-EMBO) and the day following (POST-EMBO) glue embolization of an HAVM. The PRE-EMBO image demonstrates hepatofugal bloodflow in the portal vein (PV), and therefore in the opposite direction of the caudal vena cava (CVC). The following day, the POST-EMBO ultrasonography image demonstrates hepatopetal (forward) direction of the PV bloodflow, and therefore the same direction as the CVC.

Follow-Up

Patients are typically discharged the following day with a standard protocol to minimize signs associated with the presence of multiple EHPSS (Table 22.1). Instructions also include limited activity and an Elizabethan collar with regular monitoring of the groin incision for two weeks. Although ascites sometimes develops, the portal hypertension should now be dramatically diminished; the ascites is likely due to fluid shifts taking place and possible presence of portal thrombosis that can be evaluated using ultrasonography (which is recommended the following day regardless to record portal flow direction and velocities; Figure 22.9). Blood work including complete blood count and chemistry panel is usually repeated the day after the procedure as well. Liver function tests (bile acids and protein C) are repeated at 1 month; These values will unlikely ever be normal as the acquired EHPSS will never go away but worsening should raise a concern for re-establish HAVM flow. Repeat treatments are typically recommended if ascites persists or liver function is worsening; these are usually performed within a few weeks to months (or years) later.

Special Considerations/ Alternative Uses/ Complication Examples

Examples of potential non-target embolization and stagnant portal vein blood flow can be seen in Figure 22.5. Each of these complications was inconsequential in these patients but possible significant morbidity could result in other patients.

Notes

(Examples; multiple vendors available)

1. Vascular access sheath (4–5 Fr), Infiniti Medical, Menlo Park, CA.
2. Micropuncture set, Infiniti Medical, Menlo Park, CA.
3. Cobra head catheter, Infiniti Medical, Menlo Park, CA.
4. Weasel wire, Infiniti Medical, Menlo Park, CA.
5. Omnipaque (iohexol) injection, Amersham Health Inc., Princeton, NJ.
6. Touhy–Borst adapter, Cook Medical, Bloomington, IN.
7. Flo-switch, Boston Scientific, Natick, MA.
8. Renegade or Tracker microcatheter, Boston Scientific, Natick, MA.
9. Microcatheter, Infiniti Medical, Menlo Park, CA.
10. 0.018 Transend or V-18 microwire, Boston Scientific, Natick, MA.
11. 0.014 Microwire or 0.018 Weasel wire, Infiniti Medical, Menlo Park, CA.
12. 1 ml polycarbonate syringes, Merit Medical, South Jordan, UT.
13. TRUFILL n-BCA liquid embolic system, Cordis Neurovascular, Miami Lakes, FL.
14. Lipiodol/Ethiodol, Guerbet LLC, Bloomington, IN.

15. TRUFILL Tantulum powder, Cordis Neurovascular, Miami Lakes, FL.
16. Onyx liquid embolic system, Micro Therapeutics, Inc., Irvine, CA.

REFERENCES

Butler-Howe LM, Boothe HW, Boothe DM, et al (1993) Effects of vena caval banding in experimentally induced multiple portosystemic shunts in dogs. *Am J Vet Res* 54, 1774.

Chanoit G, Kyles AE, Weisse, C, et al (2007) Surgical and interventional radiographic treatment of dogs with hepatic arteriovenous fistulae. *Vet Surg* 36, 199.

Cullen JM (2009) Summary of the world small animal veterinary association standardization committee guide to classification of liver disease in dogs and cats. *Vet Clin N Am Small Anim Pract* 39, 395–418.

Legendre AM, Krahwinkel DJ, Carrig CB, et al (1976) Ascites associated with intrahepatic arteriovenous fistula in a cat. *J Am Vet Med Assoc* 168(7), 589.

Whiting PG, Breznock EM, Moore P, et al (1986) Partial hepatectomy with temporary hepatic vascular occlusion in dogs with hepatic arteriovenous fistulas. *Vet Surg* 15, 171.

SUGGESTED READING

Taksawa C, Seiji K, Matsunaga, K, et al (2012) Properties of n-butyl cyanoacrylate-iodized oil mixtures for arterial embolization: In vitro and in vivo experiments. *J Vasc Interv Radiol* 23(9), 1215–21.

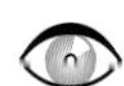

Video clips to accompany this chapter can be found in the online material at **www.wiley.com/go/weisse/vet-image-guided-interventions**

CHAPTER TWENTY-THREE

Liver Tumors/Metastases (TAE/cTACE/DEB-TACE)

Chick Weisse
The Animal Medical Center, New York, NY

Background/Indications

Solitary massive hepatocellular carcinoma (HCC) in dogs carries a good prognosis following complete excision with median survival times greater than 3 years, less than 5% surgical mortality, and a minority of patients having metastatic disease at the time of diagnosis (Liptak, 2004). In this same study, right-sided solitary HCC (~12%) had a reported 40% surgical mortality rate and approximately 10% of the HCC resections had dirty margins (Liptak, 2004). Unfortunately, nodular (~30% of HCC cases) or diffuse (~10% of HCC cases) forms are not amenable to surgery (Patnaik, 1981). The relatively limited efficacy of routine (intravenous) chemotherapy for macroscopic disease, and the cost and potential deleterious side effects associated with radiation therapy have resulted in a substantial portion of HCC dogs receiving only conservative and symptomatic treatment as the tumor grows. In one report including six dogs with HCC not receiving surgery, median survival times were 270 days with supportive care (Liptak, 2004). A number of regional tumor therapies have recently been developed to improve local tumor control without increasing systemic toxicities and side effects.

Intravascular techniques such as intra-arterial (IA) delivery of chemotherapy and transarterial chemoembolization (TACE) have been developed in order to increase local chemotherapy concentrations and dwell times within the tumor, reduce subsequent systemic toxicities, reduce tumor blood supply and oxygenation, and improve local tumor control rates in those cancers that have demonstrated otherwise poor responses following systemic chemotherapy. IA chemotherapy is not routinely performed in dogs with nonresectable HCC. IA infusions without embolization results in a lower percentage of tumor necrosis, particularly large HCCs, but may also lead to reduced toxicity to the surrounding liver (Brown, 1999). For this reason, this technique may be preferred in debilitated patients. While local delivery of certain chemotherapy drugs in humans has been demonstrated to result in elevated intratumoral drug concentrations, and even improved biological tumor responses, improved survival times are not necessarily routinely achieved. More recently, hepatic arterial ports have been placed providing sustained local delivery of chemotherapy into the liver tumors over time. Routine use of these devices would be difficult and expensive in animals. The author has preferred the use of TACE in these cases.

Transarterial embolization (TAE) without chemotherapy has been performed by the author instead of TACE in debilitated patients, dogs with benign liver tumors, and dogs with diffuse liver neoplasia resulting in hemorrhage. TACE involves superselective intra-arterial chemotherapy delivery in conjunction with subsequent particle embolization and has been shown to result in a 10- to 50-fold increase in hepatic intratumoral drug concentrations when compared to systemic intravenous chemotherapy administration (Dyet, 2000). Subsequent particle embolization results in tumor cell necrosis and paralyzes tumor cell excretion of chemotherapy resulting in minimized systemic toxicity. This procedure is most commonly used in the treatment of diffuse hepatocellular carcinoma or metastatic liver disease in humans due to the unique dual hepatic blood supply. Most hepatic tumors depend upon hepatic arterial blood supply (up to 95%) for growth in contrast to the normal liver parenchyma that receives the majority of its blood supply via the portal vein (only ~20% from the hepatic artery) (Breedis, 1954). This anatomy favors the use of these arterial directed therapies. More recently, drug-eluting beads (DEB) are being evaluated in veterinary patients with non-resectable liver tumors.

In humans, a number of randomized controlled trials have demonstrated significantly improved survival

Veterinary Image-Guided Interventions, First Edition. Edited by Chick Weisse and Allyson Berent.

Companion website: www.wiley.com/go/weisse/vet-image-guided-interventions

times with TACE versus symptomatic treatment. In addition, DEB and oily TACE have similar tumor response outcomes at 6-month endpoints but patients with limited hepatic reserve, massive tumors, or worse performance status had better outcomes with DEB TACE as well as a significantly longer time to tumor progression compared to bland embolization (TAE).

Percutaneous tumor ablation techniques performed in the liver of humans tend to be most effective in those patients with a few (less than three), small (<4 cm diameter) lesions. As these circumstances are rarely encountered in the author's clinical experience in veterinary medicine, our patients are more commonly candidates for chemoembolization for the palliative treatment of nonresectable and metastatic liver neoplasia.

Patient Preparation

Prior to performing TACE, tumor biopsy and staging should be performed. Cross-sectional imaging has greatly enhanced presurgical planning but care should be taken concerning conclusions about "tumor resectability" based on imaging alone; Ideally, these patients will have surgical exploration when possible as complete tumor resection (when possible) remains the preferred treatment for isolated HCC in dogs. Consultation with an oncologist is critical for developing a treatment plan and ensuring standard-of-care therapies have been discussed. Full bloodwork screening is recommended, as well as liver function tests prior to embolization in those dogs with very large tumors or minimal normal remaining liver. Careful history taking helps identify pelvic limb osteoarthritis that may result in limited hip extension for vascular access. Ideal patients are those with liver tumors identified incidentally on physical examination or via routine bloodwork. Similar to humans, the patient's performance status often indicates how well a patient will tolerate the procedure. Dual phase CT angiography is the pre-operative (and follow-up) diagnostic imaging modality of choice for the author (Figure 23.1A, B). Arterial phase studies help determine

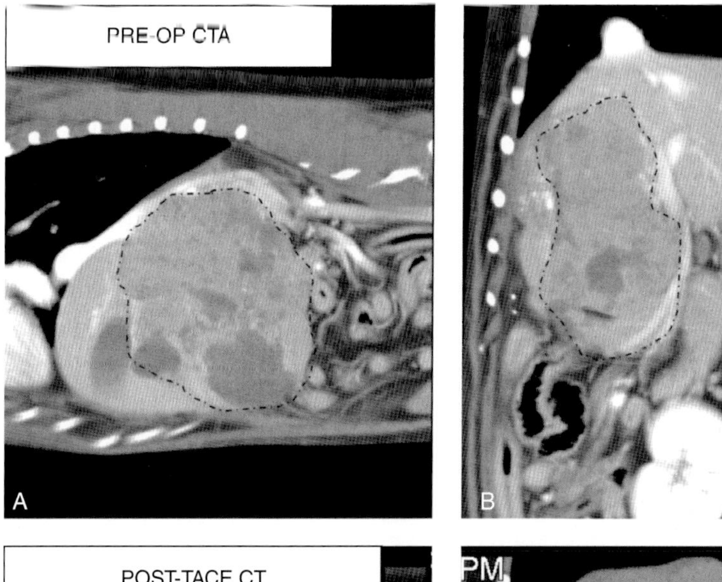

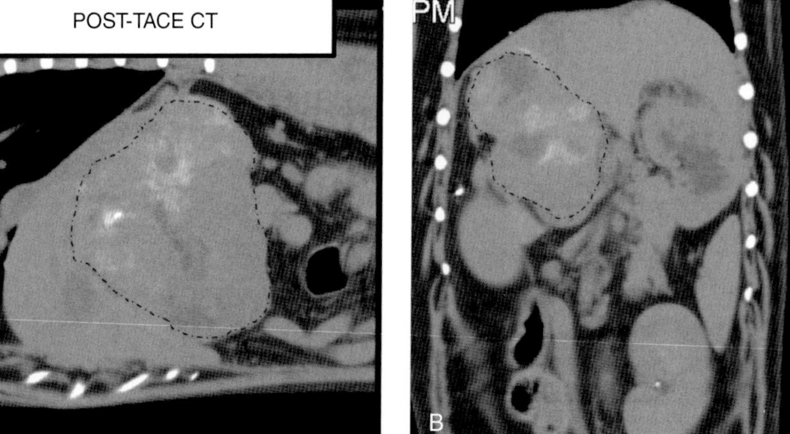

Figure 23.1 Sagittal (A) and coronal (B) reconstructions of liver tumor CT both pre-operatively (PRE-OP CTA) and ~6 week post-TACE, non-contrast follow-up (POST-TACE CT). PRE-OP demonstrates large right-sided liver tumor. POST-TACE CT demonstrates staining of tumor after TACE with no non-target staining as well as tumor shrinkage.

TABLE 23.1
Procedural and post-procedural medical management

- Antibiotics:
  - Intraoperative: cefoxitin (30 mg/kg IV once, then 20 mg/kg IV q2 hr)
  - Postoperative: clavamox (13.75 mg/kg PO BID × 14 days)
- Anti-inflammatories:
  - Intraoperative: dexamethasone SP (0.01 mg/kg IV once at induction)
  - Postoperative: prednisone (1 mg/kg/day PO × 5 days, then 0.5 mg/kg/day PO × 5 days, then 0.5 mg/kg/q2 days PO × 5 days)
- Gastroprotectants:
  - Postoperative: omeprazole (1 mg/kg PO q12 hr × 7 days)
- Antiemetics:
  - Perioperative: dolasetron (0.5 mg/kg IV once)
  - Perioperative: maropitant citrate (1 mg/kg IV once (dog), 0.5 mg/kg once (cat))
  - Postoperative: ondansetron (0.1–1 mg/kg PO q8–12 × 7 days)
- Analgesics:
  - Perioperative: opioid premedications
  - Postoperative: tramadol (2–4 mg/kg PO q8–12 hr × 3 days)

primary feeding vessels as well as the presence of dual/multiple blood supplies. An intimate knowledge of the hepatic arterial supply is an absolute necessity prior to performing the procedure to avoid embolization of the gastroduodenal artery, gall gladder, or other non-target organs (Ursic, 2007). In addition, proximity to the gall bladder is useful information in order to avoid inadvertent non-target embolization. Multiple venous phases are performed as well to help identify early venous filling (arteriovenous fistulas or venous lakes present, or other lesions not identified in the arterial phase).

Premedications include broad-spectrum antibiotic coverage for common liver organisms, anti-inflammatories (corticosteroids), and antinausea medications (Table 23.1).

Potential Risks/Complications/Expected Outcomes

Contraindications to TACE in dogs are relative; however, in humans with greater than 50% liver replacement with tumor, bilirubin levels > 2 mg/dl, LDH > 425 mg/dl, and AST > 100 IU/l have been associated with increased post-procedural mortality rates. In the author's experience, every animal has had AST > 100 IU/l, and many have >50% liver replacement with tumor with no apparent increased mortality risk appreciated.

Reported TACE complications in the human literature consensus statement suggest an overall major complication threshold of 15% (highest tolerated). The more common complications might include post-embolization syndrome (a collection of clinical signs characterized by malaise, fever, and pain), non-target embolization complications (damage to normal parenchyma, cholecystitis), hepatic failure/infarction/abscessation, acute renal failure, and septicemia (Hemingway, 1988). The author's experience with HCC chemoembolization suggests similar risks in veterinary patients may be anticipated as well as reduced systemic exposure to chemotherapy, minimal morbidity, and improved tumor response rates when compared to systemic chemotherapy. The worst complications experienced by the author have been acute gall bladder infarction with bile peritonitis in two dogs, acute renal failure in one dog, hemoabdomen in two dogs, and hepatic abscess and subsequent peritonitis in one dog. In humans, chemoembolization of the gall bladder is reportedly tolerated (with subsequent cholecystitis developing) but that may not be the case with dogs. Improved fluoroscopy hardware, more distal catheter superselection, better vascular anatomy understanding, and perhaps technical improvement with practice seem to have eliminated this early encountered problem in the author's cases. In humans, supcapsular, cystic, and exophytic tumors are more likely to rupture (hemoabdomen) after TACE, and these are the typical veterinary HCC encountered. Neither veterinary case that developed a hemoabdomen required surgical intervention, in the author's experience, but red blood cell transfusions were necessary for stabilization.

The operator should appreciate that the arterial supply to the gall bladder can be variable, and in 50% of dogs has its major contribution from the left hepatic artery. During common hepatic arteriography careful attention should be paid to the location of this blood supply to ensure it does not get embolized during any hepatic embolization procedure when it is possible to avoid it.

Most of the expectations described below are those following DEB-TACE in dogs, as the author has the most experience using this modality. Chemotherapy (doxorubicin) side effects should not be anticipated in these dogs and blood count nadirs have not been appreciated. Intravenous chemotherapy results in up to 40 times higher systemic exposures to doxorubicin compared with DEB-TACE in dogs depending upon the technique used for administration. In general, the clients can anticipate "stable" disease while receiving chemoembolization treatments every 5 or 6 weeks. The tumors do tend to shrink but typically not more than 10–30% in size; however, the tumor parenchyma often becomes cavitated as it undergoes necrosis. As World Health Organization (WHO) or RECIST imaging measurement criteria are typically used in tumor staging, these changes would be characterized as stable disease even though necrosis often encompasses larger portions of the tumor.

Equipment

Recommended equipment is shown in Figure 23.2. Additionally, a microcatheter (1.7–3.0 Fr) and microwire (0.010–0.018″), of various shapes and sizes are needed for most cases. TACE procedures require very little equipment, but the fluoroscopy unit must provide adequate imaging detail to identify very small caliber vessels using digital subtraction angiography and the ability to obtain orthogonal imaging when necessary. Failure to identify collateral vessels could lead to non-target embolization and severe consequences.

Fluoroscopic Procedure

Following induction of general anesthesia, hair on the caudoventral aspect of the abdomen, in the inguinal area, and on the medial aspects of both thighs is clipped. The animal is placed in dorsal recumbency with the chosen hind limb extended, abducted, and secured in place to allow access to the inguinal area. The skin over the inguinal area is aseptically prepared and draped, and the femoral artery pulse identified. Femoral artery access is described in Chapter 44. When

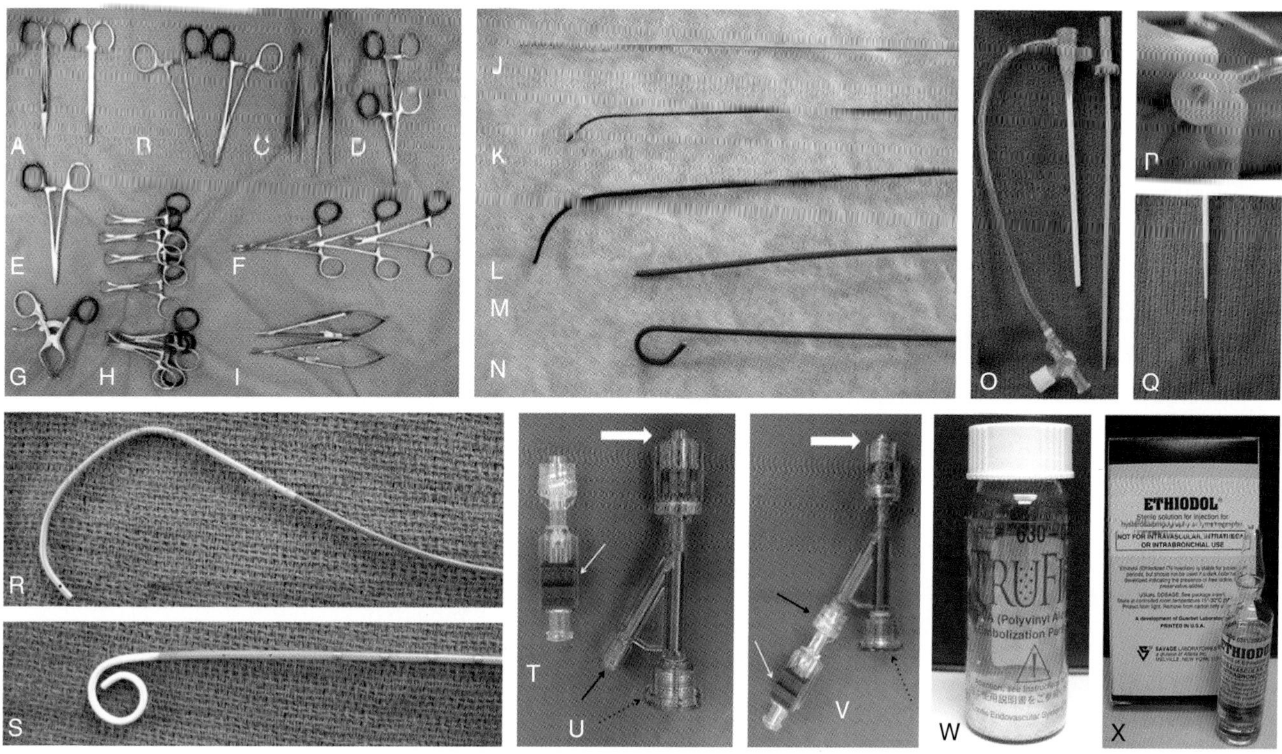

Figure 23.2 A-I. Sample surgical cut-down set. (A) Sharp-sharps and small Metzenbaum scissors. (B) Right-angled forceps. (C) Brown–Adson and Debakey forceps. (D) Mosquito hemostats. (E) Needle drivers. (F) Kelly hemostats. (G) Small Gelpi retractors. (H) Small Babcock towel clamps. (I) Castroviejo needle drivers for vessel repair. (J–N) Guide wires (J) 0.018″ microwire. (K) 0.018″ angled, hydrophilic guide wire (L) 0.035″ angled, hydrophilic guide wire. (M, N) 0.035″ straight PTFE wire (M) and 0.035″ Rosen PTFE wire (N), both of which uncommonly used for this procedure. (O–Q) Vascular introducer sheath. 4 Fr vascular introducer sheath made up of shaft (white) with 4 Fr inner diameter, hemostasis valve (P) to prevent bleeding, three-way stop-cock (yellow cap) to flush and/or aspirate, and 4 Fr dilator (blue) to make smooth transition from sheath down to 0.035″ guide wire (Q). (R) 4 Fr Cobra catheter (S). 4Fr marker pigtail catheter for aortogram and measurements if needed. (T–V) Flo-switch (T) and Touhy–Borst adapter (U), which connect (V) to form a hemostasis valve (dotted black line) and side-port that can be switched on or off (white arrow) for flushing or aspirating. This device is attached to the hub of the 4 Fr catheter (at white block arrow) and allows coaxial passage of a microcatheter/microwire through the 4 Fr catheter. (W) Poly-vinyl alcohol particles. (X) Iodinated poppy-seed oil.

small-caliber femoral arteries are encountered, micropuncture sets are used for initial access. An introducer sheath[1] no larger than the catheter used is selected. Typically a 4 Fr Cobra catheter[2] and 0.035″ angled hydrophilic guide wire[3] are used in combination to select the celiac artery and common hepatic artery. In humans, superior mesenteric artery and celiac artery angiograms are recommended to identify variant anatomy, retrograde gastroduodenal artery bloodflow, and portal venous bloodflow/occlusion (which had been, but is no longer, considered a contraindication to TACE). These studies are not routinely performed by the author due to contrast load issues in the considerably smaller veterinary population. The author tries to limit total iohexol administration to 3 ml/kg (240 mg/ml iodine) for the entire procedure. During common hepatic arteriography using a 50:50 dilution of iohexol[4]:saline, monitor for arteriovenous shunting or venous lakes (uncommonly identified) and tumor blushing.

The 4 Fr catheter remains in position in the common hepatic artery and a Touhy–Borst adapter[5] and Floswitch[6] are attached to permit a 1.7 to 3 Fr microcatheter[7,8] to be introduced into the Cobra catheter. The microcatheter/microwire[9,10] combination are used to superselect the particular vessel supplying the tumor bed ensuring catheter placement is not occlusive within the often very small caliber vessels. Repeat angiography is performed using 100% iohexol via a 1 ml luer-lock polycarbonate syringe.[11] When performing TACE, superselection is the goal to minimize non-target embolization. Some recommend intra-arterial lidocaine infusion at this time in order to provide immediate analgesia and reduce post-procedural clinical signs.

Bland Embolization (TAE)

The appropriate size of polyvinyl alcohol (PVA) or other embolization particles (see Chapter 1) are chosen on the basis of vascular architecture. Use of undersized particles carries the risk of extreme distal vascular occlusion and increases the risk of necrosis and tissue sloughing. On the other hand, use of inappropriately large particles carries the risk of proximal vessel thrombosis, which may allow for development of collateral vessels that bypass the proximal occlusion and re-establish perfusion to the tumor. In cases with spontaneous arteriovenous or arterioportal shunting, proximal occlusion may be preferred to mitigate the risk of embolization of particles to the lungs. The author has used PVA-200 particles[12] (180–300 μm) or 100–300 μm PVA hydrogel microspheres[13] for liver embolization. HCC intratumor vessels have been described to be in the 40–140 μm range. The chosen embolic is primed for delivery by preparing it as a slurry with iodinated contrast material. To do so using PVA, the embolic is loaded into a syringe, the plunger replaced, and all of the air evacuated to densely compact the material. This syringe is connected with a three-way stopcock to a second syringe filled with contrast material and the contents are vigorously mixed together through the stopcock to form the slurry. The viscosity is adjusted by additional dilution with sterile saline of the PVA as necessary to match the caliber of the delivery catheter and the flow in the vessel to be embolized. Relatively dilute concentrations are required to prevent occlusion of microcatheters or clumping within the small caliber vessels and subsequent proximal embolization.

Embolization is performed by injecting the slurry through a selectively placed microcatheter under fluoroscopic visualization using digital roadmapping software. The slurry is radio-opaque and can be seen perfusing the tumor. Care is taken to prevent reflux of particles into non-target vessels. As embolization proceeds, flow decreases (Figure 23.3). Prior to complete bloodflow stasis (and periodically during the embolization procedure), the catheter is flushed of slurry by injecting saline solution. Selective arteriography is performed to evaluate the success of the procedure after all particles are flushed out. If embolization is successful, no flow is seen in the target artery feeding the tumor. The microcatheter is withdrawn and repeat common hepatic (or other) angiography is performed through the 4 Fr catheter to identify other feeding vessels that are subsequently catheterized, and confirm the patency of the gastroduodenal artery. If more vessels are found the procedure is repeated.

Chemoembolization (TACE)

A similar technique is used for oily (conventional or cTACE) or DEB-TACE; however, refer to manufacturer instructions for information regarding handling, drug loading, and administration of DEBs.[14] Diagnostic arteriography is performed and the proper vessel to be treated is selected (Figure 23.4). The dose of chemotherapeutic agent to be used is selected on the basis of the animal's total body surface area and is historically equivalent to the maximum dose administered systemically. The author uses single agent powdered doxorubicin at a dose of 30mg/m^2 (or if body weight is under 10 kg, then dosed at 1 mg/kg).

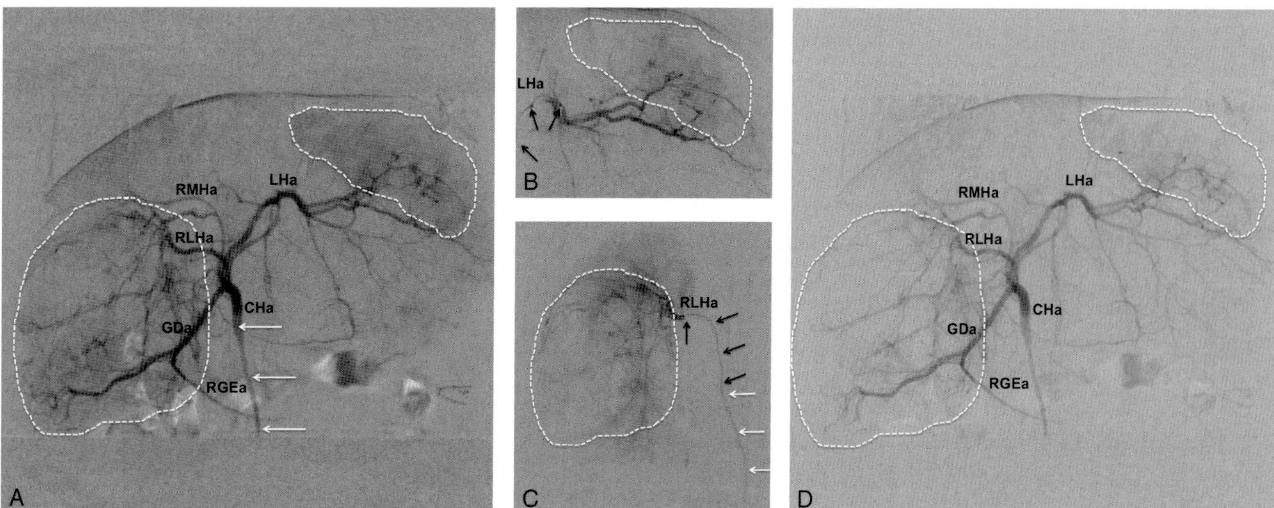

Figure 23.3 DSA during TAE in a dog with two HCCs; large right lobe and smaller left lobe. Dog's head is to the top of each VD image. (A) Common hepatic DSA (CHa) through 4 Fr Cobra catheter (white arrows) demonstrating left hepatic artery (LHa) feeding left tumor (white dotted line) and right lateral hepatic artery (RLHa) feeding right tumor (white dotted lines). Also visible are the right medial hepatic artery (RMHa), gastroduodenal artery (GDa), and right gastroepiploic artery (RGEa). (B) Superselective microcatheterization (black arrows) of the LHa with DSA showing perfusion of left tumor prior to TAE. (C) Microcatheterization (black arrows) of the RLHa with DSA showing perfusion of right tumor prior to TAE. (D) Post-TAE CHa DSA demonstrating similar hepatic perfusion (no non-target embolization) with absent perfusion/embolization of both tumors (white dotted lines).

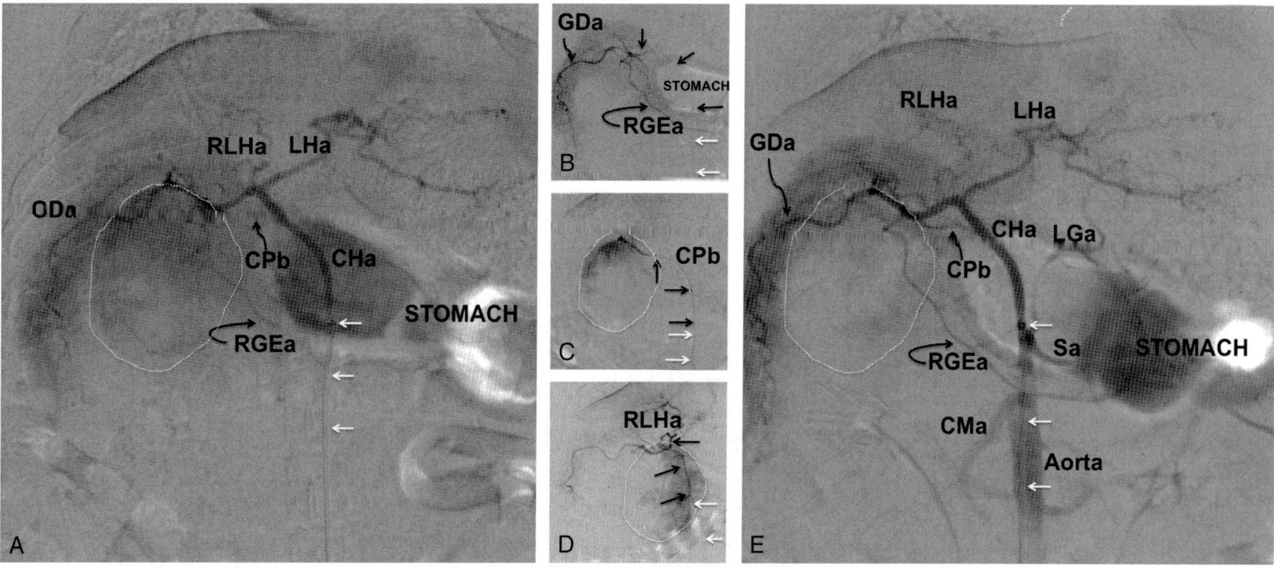

Figure 23.4 DSA during TACE in a dog with a right-sided HCC. Dog's head to the top of each VD image. (A) Common hepatic DSA (CHa) through 4 Fr Cobra catheter (white arrows) demonstrating left hepatic artery (LHa), right lateral hepatic artery (RLHa), gastroduodenal artery (GDa), right gastroepiploic artery (RGEa), and caudate process branch (CPb) with tumor opacification (white dotted lines). (B) Superselective microcatheterization (black arrows) of GDa demonstrating no contribution to tumor blush. (C) Superselective microcatheterization (black arrows) of CPb demonstrating cranial and lateral contribution to tumor blush prior to TACE. (D) Superselective microcatheterization (black arrows) of RLHA branch demonstrating medial contribution to tumor blush prior to TACE. (E) Celiac axis DSA pot-TACE demonstrating splenic artery (Sa), left gastric artery (LGa) and reflux into aorta and cranial mesenteric artery (CMa) filling. Notice lack to tumor blush (white dotted lines) following TACE compared to prior (A).

cTACE

In order to perform cTACE, it is imperative that the emulsion used be created appropriately. In order to do so, the oil and contrast/chemotherapy mixture must be the same specific gravity in order to permit an emulsion to form. The chosen contrast agent is mixed with sterile water to achieve the same specific gravity as the oil. The chemotherapy is then dissolved into this mixture. This contrast/chemotherapy mixture is then mixed with a varying amount of iodinated poppy-seed oil[15] to form the oily suspension. The goal is to create an emulsion in which oil and aqueous drops do not separate; this has been described as "making mayonnaise, not oil and vinegar". The former allows the chemotherapy to be dissolved into the oil and elute over time rather than the chemotherapy dissolved in aqueous form, which will wash out. Small aliquots of the mixture are then delivered or first mixed with appropriately sized PVA. The amount of PVA added is titrated so that complete stasis to flow coincides with delivery of the total volume of the chemotherapeutic agent–contrast material mixture (if complete embolization is the goal). Again, embolization is performed during fluoroscopy to ensure that there is no reflux into non-target vessels. cTACE has historically been performed until stasis or near-stasis of the feeding artery has been achieved. In the author's experience, very little oil should be added to the mixture or else premature embolization will occur before the total chemotherapy dose is adminstered.

DEB-TACE

In order to perform DEB-TACE, individual manufacturer guidelines must be followed carefully. The procedure is similar; however, superselective catheterization may be more important with DEB-TACE as the delivered drug-eluting beads are highly potent in comparison to TAE or cTACE (which may be better tolerated when lobar or segmental delivery is performed). In addition, the angiographic endpoint when performing DEB-TACE is not completely clear; Currently it seems most are recommending delivering the total systemic chemotherapy dose in the DEBs only (do not add additional beads after dose is administered), or stopping once the tumor blush is no longer apparent (but flow through the feeding artery remains).

Once delivery of slurry or DEBs has been completed or stasis has occurred, the catheter is flushed with saline solution, and selective and nonselective arteriography is performed. If possible, the author likes to perform a post-procedural, non-contrast enhanced computerized tomography (CT) prior to recovery (Figure 23.1C, D). Contrast (or iodinated oil) is often identified within the tumor and helps confirm correct catheter placement, degree of tumor bed filling, and lack of non-target embolization. This information is particularly helpful when repeat procedures are performed in order to treat the same vessel if perfusion persists, or identify other vessels feeding the tumor that may have been missed during previous treatments.

Following embolization, all catheters and sheaths are removed. Hemostasis is typically achieved with femoral artery ligation. All animals recover from anesthesia in an intensive care unit for monitoring. Perioperative medical management is standard for these patients (Table 23.1).

Follow-Up

Patients are routinely discharged the following day with a standard protocol to minimize signs associated with possible post-embolization syndrome (Table 23.1). Instructions also include limited activity and an Elizabethan collar with regular monitoring of the groin incision for two weeks. As with standard chemotherapy treatment, complete blood counts are recommended at 7 and 14 days post-treatment although systemic levels are so low following TACE changes are unlikely to be identified. Repeat treatments are typically recommended every 5 to 6 weeks but likely can be performed sooner if only one side of the liver treated (for diffuse hepatic disease for instance). Follow-up dual phase CTA can be performed at 5–6 week intervals to determine tumor response and arterial supply if additional treatments are being considered (Figure 23.1).

Special Considerations/ Alternative Uses/ Complication Examples

Although an established procedure, there is not only discrepancy between bland versus chemoembolization and cTACE versus DEB-TACE, many technical differences exist among interventionalists routinely performing these techniques. One technical aspect worthy of discussion is the technical end-point of the procedure. Historically, blood flow stasis for tumor bed ischemia was the goal, but more recently, reduced bloodflow (without stasis) has been recommended to prevent rapid chemotherapy washout and permit future access to the target vessel (which may not be possible if complete stasis is achieved) (Figure 23.5). This is not a theoretical concern; the author has

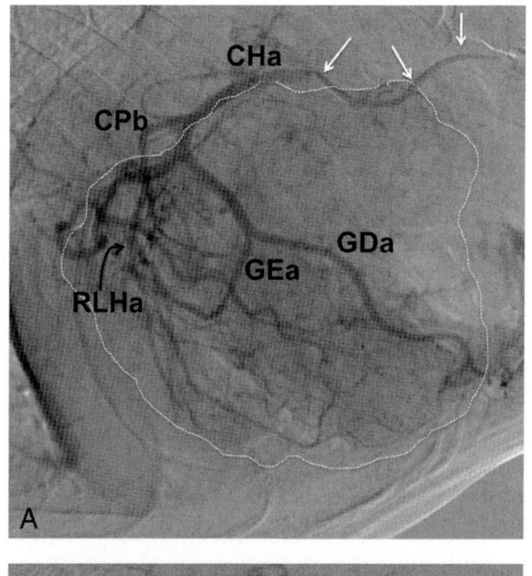

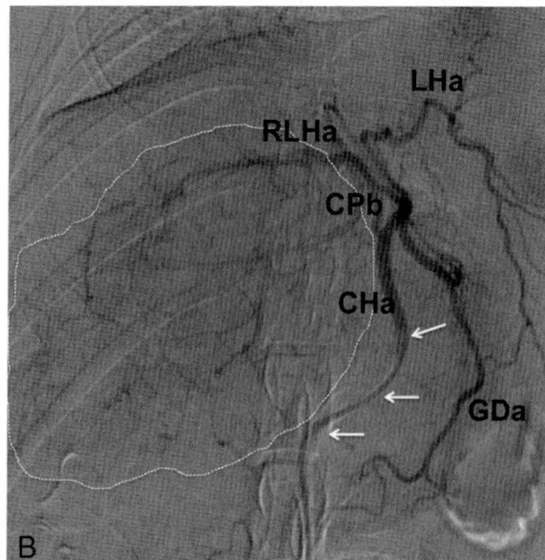

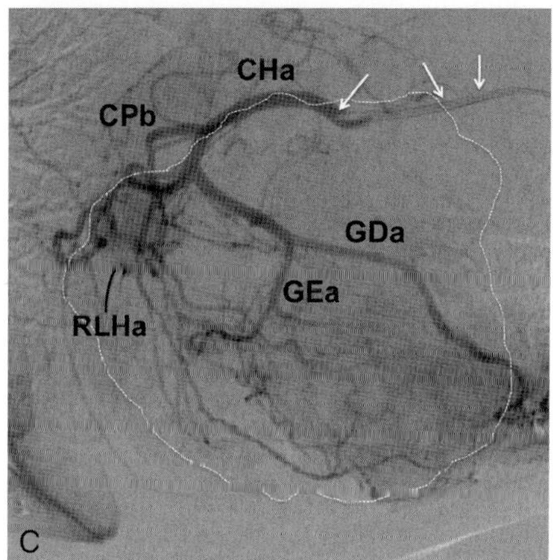

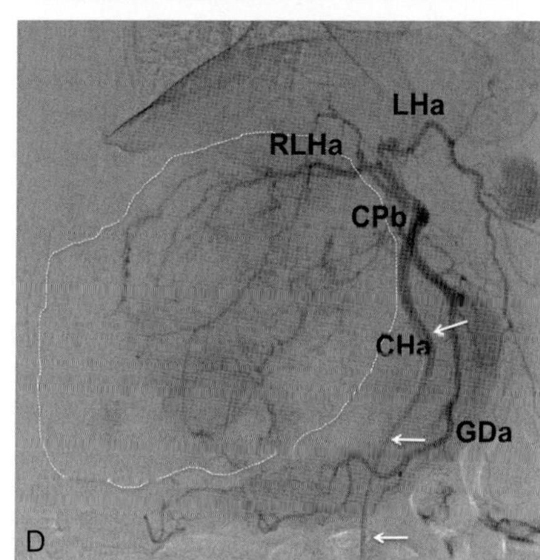

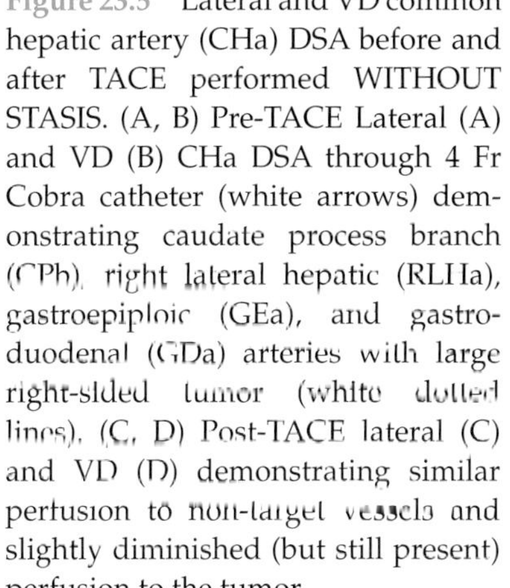

Figure 23.5 Lateral and VD common hepatic artery (CHa) DSA before and after TACE performed WITHOUT STASIS. (A, B) Pre-TACE Lateral (A) and VD (B) CHa DSA through 4 Fr Cobra catheter (white arrows) demonstrating caudate process branch (CPb), right lateral hepatic (RLHa), gastroepiploic (GEa), and gastroduodenal (GDa) arteries with large right-sided tumor (white dotted lines). (C, D) Post-TACE lateral (C) and VD (D) demonstrating similar perfusion to non-target vessels and slightly diminished (but still present) perfusion to the tumor.

repeated TACE procedures in some dogs initially treated to bloodflow stasis only to find the original target vessel no longer patent and therefore limiting subsequent treatments. At this time, there is no clear consensus on the preferred technical procedure but treating to stasis has resulted in less systemic chemotherapy exposure (and presumably more intratumoral chemotherapy) than the same patients treated without stasis in a small number of dogs. There is also a trend to use better calibrated and smaller size beads (70–150 µm) when performing TACE to better target the tumor vasculature.

Notes

(Examples; Multiple vendors available)

1. 5 Fr Vascular introducer sheath, Infiniti Medical, Menlo Park, CA.
2. Cobra head catheter, Infiniti Medical, Menlo Park, CA.
3. Weasel wire, Infiniti Medical, Menlo Park, CA.
4. Omnipaque (iohexol) injection, Amersham Health Inc., Princeton, NJ.
5. Touhy–Borst adapter, Cook Medical, Bloomington, IN.
6. Flo-switch, Boston Scientific, Natick, MA.
7. Renegade or Tracker microcatheter, Boston Scientific, Natick, MA.
8. Microcatheter, Infiniti Medical, Menlo Park, CA.
9. 0.018 Transend or V-18 microwire, Boston Scientific, Natick, MA.
10. 0.014 Microwire or 0.018 Weasel wire, Infiniti Medical, Menlo Park, CA.
11. 1 ml polycarbonate syringes, Merit Medical, South Jordan, UT.
12. PVA-200 particles, Cook Medical Inc., Bloomington, IN.
13. Beadblock 100–300 µm PVA hydrogel microspheres, Biocompatibles UK Limited, Farnham, UK.
14. LC/DC Bead 100–300 µm hydrogel microspheres, Biocompatibles UK Limited, Farnham, UK.
15. Lipiodol/Ethiodol, Guerbet LLC, Bloomington, IN.

References

Breedis C and Young G (1954) Blood supply of neoplasms of the liver. *Am J Pathol* 30, 969–72.

Brown KT, Koh BY, Brody LA, et al. (1999) Particle embolization of hepatic neuroendocrine metastases for control of pain and hormonal symptoms. *J Vasc Interv Radiol* 10, 397–403.

Dyet J, Ettles D, Nicholson A, et al (2000) *Textbook of Endovascular Procedures.* Churchill Livingstone, Philadelphia, 357–67.

Hemingway AP and Allison DJ (1988) Complications of embolization: Analysis of 410 procedures. *Radiology* 166(3), 669–72.

Liptak JM, Dernell WS, Monnet E, et al (2004) Massive hepatocellular carcinoma in dogs: 48 cases (1992–2002). *J Am Vet Med Assoc* 225, 1225–30.

Patnaik AK, Hurvitz AI, Lieberman PH, et al (1981) Canine hepatocellular carcinoma. *Vet Pathol* 18, 427–38.

Ursic M, Ravnik D, Hribernik M, et al (2007) Gross anatomy of the portal vein and hepatic artery ramifications in dogs: corrosion cast study *Anat Histol Embryol* 36, 83–7.

Suggested Reading

Barone M, Ettorre GC, Ladisa R, et al (2003) Transcatheter arterial chemo- embolization (TACE) in treatment of hepatocellular carcinoma. *Hepato-gastroenterology* 50, 183–7.

Lammer J, Malagari K, Vogl T, et al (2010) Prospective randomized study of doxorubicin-eluting-bead embolization in the treatment of hepatocellular carcinoma: results of the PRECISION V study. *Cardiovasc Interv Radiol* 33, 41–52.

Llovet JM, Real MI, Montana X, et al (2002) Arterial embolisation or chemoembolisation versus symptomatic treatment in patients with unresect- able hepatocellular carcinoma: a randomised controlled trial. *Lancet* 359, 1734–9.

Lo CM, Ngan H, Tso WK, et al (2002) Randomized controlled trial of trans-arterial lipiodol chemoembolization for unresectable hepatocellular carcinoma. *Hepatology* 35, 1164–71.

Malagari K, Pomoni M Kelekis A, et al (2010) Prospective randomized comparison of chemoembolization with doxorubicin-eluting beads and bland embolization with BeadBlock for hepatocellular carcinoma. *Cardiovasc Interv Radiol* 33, 541–51.

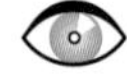 Video clips to accompany this chapter can be found in the online material at **www.wiley.com/go/weisse/vet-image-guided-interventions**

CHAPTER TWENTY-FOUR

Endoscopic Retrograde Cholangiopancreatography (ERCP) and Biliary Stent Placement

Allyson Berent
The Animal Medical Center, New York, NY

Background/Indications

Endoscopic retrograde cholangiopancreatography (ERCP), first described in humans in 1970, is a minimally invasive technique that combines endoscopy and fluoroscopy to image the biliary system and pancreatic ducts. This imaging can detect irregularities or filling defects in the biliary and pancreatic ducts, localize and facilitate removal of gallstones, identify and access neoplastic lesions for biopsy, culture bile, and diagnose and relieve bile and pancreatic duct obstructions with stenting. This procedure has more recently been described in children as the size of the instruments has become smaller. In humans, this modality is considered the best option for improving the diagnosis of biliary and exocrine pancreatic tract diseases, as well as therapeutically relieving an obstruction when present.

Traditional therapy in veterinary patients involves surgical manipulation of the common bile duct/pancreatic duct via choledochotomy, re-routing surgeries, or surgical stent placement. Surgical biliary diversion techniques in dogs and cats have been associated with a 25–73% and 50–75% mortality rate, respectively. Prolonged anesthesia times and manipulation of the pancreatic and biliary system in unstable patients can lead to excessive morbidity. In humans, similar problems have resulted in the use of interventional radiology techniques (e.g., cholecystostomy tubes or percutaneous biliary stenting) or interventional endoscopy techniques (ERCP and biliary stenting) to minimize complications and provide improved outcomes when compared to open surgery.

Since 1974 healthy research dogs were used as models for ERCP showing the success rate in cannulating the common bile duct (CBD) improved with experience. Stents have been shown to be well tolerated in the CBD of dogs in various studies (polyurethrane, bare balloon expandable metallic stents (BEMS), covered BEMS stent grafts, etc.). Spillmann et al reported on diagnostic ERCP in 7 normal beagle dogs and 30 clinical dogs with vague GI signs. Diagnostic cholangiopancreatography in cats was recently reported in abstract form. (Spillman et al, 2012) Endoscopic biliary stenting has not been reported in veterinary medicine, other than in an abstract form by the author in 2008. In that study the ERCP was done using an adult side-view duodenoscope (11.3 mm) in 7 terminal research dogs. Cannulation of the duodenum and identification of the CBD with the side-view scope was successful in six of seven dogs; however, two required balloon dilation to pass the large endoscope through the pylorus. ERC was performed successfully in five of seven dogs (71%) (10.5–14.6 kg). The placement of a biliary stent was possible in four of seven dogs (57%) with a 5 Fr ($n=3$) or 7 Fr ($n=1$) polyurethane stent, and a sphincterotomy was done in all four dogs. All stents were easily removed upon completion. On post-mortem examination there were no signs of duodenal or CBD perforation. We performed the first clinical case of ERCP and biliary stenting in a dog with a stricture of the common bile duct secondary to severe pancreatitis. The dog has been followed-up for over 685 days and the stent has been well tolerated, and the biliary obstruction resolved immediately. Since that time, ERCP and biliary stenting has been successfully performed in another 2 dogs (3.1 and 28 kg) and one cat (3.9 kg), and was successful in

Veterinary Image-Guided Interventions, First Edition. Edited by Chick Weisse and Allyson Berent.

Companion website: www.wiley.com/go/weisse/vet-image-guided-interventions

resolving the biliary obstruction immediately after stent placement in all patients. All 3 patients had a plastic stent placed. The plastic stent in the cat was found in the stool 3 months after ERCP at which time there was resolution of the obstructive pancreatitis.

This chapter will introduce the theory of ERCP and stent placement in veterinary patients and to describe the steps necessary to perform this procedure. Keep in mind this procedure is considered very difficult, and should ideally be done in stable patients under the supervision of a human gastrointestinal (GI) interventionalist that has experience with adult and pediatric ERCP. Other minimally invasive options for biliary obstruction, including cholecystostomy tube placement, are described in Chapter 25.

Potential Risks/Complications/Expected Outcomes

An experienced interventional endoscopist comfortable cannulating the CBD with a guide wire and catheter, performing endoscopic electrocautery, and maneuvering guide wires and stents should perform this procedure. The most substantial risk, aside from general anesthesia in these debilitated patients, is inducing pancreatitis during retrograde pancreatic filling with contrast (occurs in 5–20% of humans). In addition, perforating the duodenum or CBD during cannulation of the major duodenal papilla (MDP), bleeding, and refluxing infected bile into the intrahepatic bile ducts or pancreatic ducts can occur. During the learning the process, there is the added risk of delaying surgical decompression of the biliary system during a failed endoscopic attempt; A presurgical, agreed-upon, endoscopic procedure time should be determined, at which point surgical decompression will be pursued.

In a dog model, ERCP was performed in an attempt to induce pancreatitis as a model for human disease. Interestingly, iatrogenic pancreatitis was found to be clinically difficult to create. In another dog model various interventions were performed during ERCP (pancreatic acinarization, pancreatic duct sphincterotomy, and pancreatic duct stenting to induce reflux) and it was found that manipulation of the pancreatic duct could induce pancreatitis. However, since the CBD and pancreatic duct in dogs have separate openings into the duodenum, routine ERC (versus ERP) holds a lower risk for pancreatitis than it does in people who have an anatomy similar to cats in which the CBD and pancreatic duct have a common opening into the duodenum (see anatomy section below).

This procedure is still currently under investigation in veterinary medicine. Owners need to be aware of the limited experience with this procedure in clinical veterinary patients and conversion to alternative decompression methods must be available.

Anatomy

The common bile duct in dogs and cats enters the proximal duodenum at the MDP and travels intramurally. The accessory pancreatic duct is the major secretory duct in dogs and terminates in the duodenum at the minor duodenal papilla. There is a small branch that exits at the MDP, though it has a separate opening from the CBD (Figure 24.1A). This makes cannulation of the CBD, without excessive manipulation of the pancreatic duct, easier in dogs than in cats (Figure 24.1) or humans.

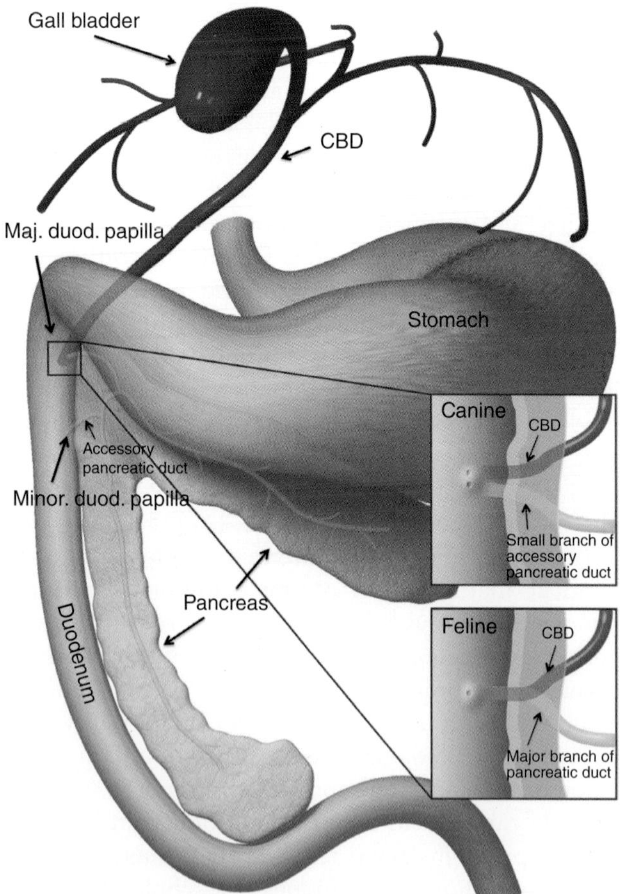

Figure 24.1 Anatomy of the excretory biliary and pancreatic tracts in dogs and cats. Notice the common bile duct (CBD) enters the major duodenal papilla (MDP) with a pancreatic duct. In dogs this is a minor branch of the accessory pancreatic duct that enters next to the CBD at the MDP. In cats this is the major branch of the pancreatic duct that enters a common branch with the CBD before entering the MDP. In dogs the minor duodenal papilla is where the major accessory pancreatic duct drains.

In dogs, two duodenal papillae are nearly always present, and the MDP is typically orad to the minor and found 3–7 cm aborad to the pylorus in the proximal descending duodenum. The CBD and small branch of the accessory pancreatic duct terminate in the MDP forming the sphincter of Oddi. The minor papilla, which is where the larger accessory pancreatic duct terminates, is typically 1–4 cm aborad to the MDP.

In cats and humans, the CBD and major branch of the pancreatic duct terminate together before exiting the MDP. An accessory duct (which is not the main branch in cats) is only found occasionally in cats and terminates in the minor duodenal papilla, aborad to the major papilla. In people the minor papilla is orad to the major papilla. The pancreas is divided into the right (duodenal) and left (gastric) lobe.

Equipment

Endoscopy is performed with a side-view duodenoscope[1,2] (Figure 24.2). This is available in two sizes: 11.3 mm and 7.5 mm (pediatric). The smaller scope has a smaller working channel (2.0 mm versus 3.2 mm) so it only accommodates small devices (6 Fr versus 9 Fr) complicating manipulations during cannulation and stent placement of the CBD. A traditional fluoroscopic C-arm is sufficient for visualization during the cholangiogram and pancreatogram, as well as during stent placement. Care must be taken to reduce fluoroscopic radiation exposure through beam collimation, dose reduction, and standard radiation protection gear.

The pylorus of smaller dogs and cats (<10–12 kg) may be too small to accept the adult duodenoscope. If a pediatric scope is not available a balloon dilation catheter (12 mm) may be necessary for pyloric dilation. This has not yet been performed in a cat to know the safety. The operator should be aware of the risk of perforation. The sphincterotome catheter[3] (Figure 24.3) must be appropriately sized for the working channel of the endoscope. Iodinated contrast material will be necessary for imaging. An exchange-length, soft-tipped guide wire is needed, typically 480 cm long[4] (Figure 24.4). An electrocautery unit, the adaptor for the sphincterotome catheter (Figure 24.3), and a foot pedal is required to perform the sphincterotomy.

Various sized polyurethane biliary stents[5–7] are available, typically provided in a set with a pusher catheter so that the stent can be pushed over the guide wire through the entire length of the endoscope (~125 cm) working channel (Figure 24.5). These stents come with either flanges on each end to prevent migration or a double pigtail, like ureteral stents. These are temporary stents that can easily be retrieved when the obstructive lesion resolves (i.e., pancreatitis). A permanent stent is also available;

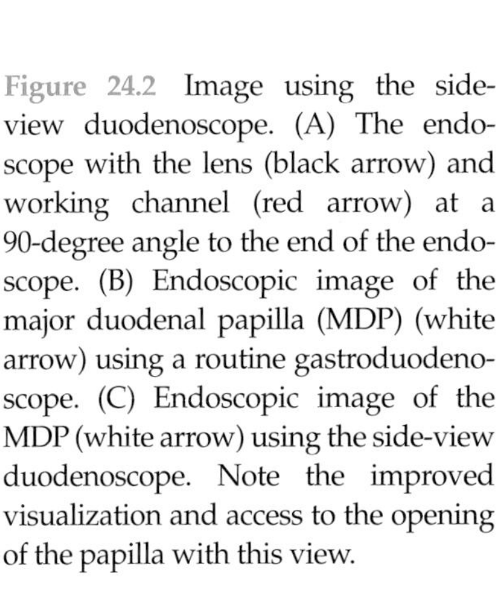

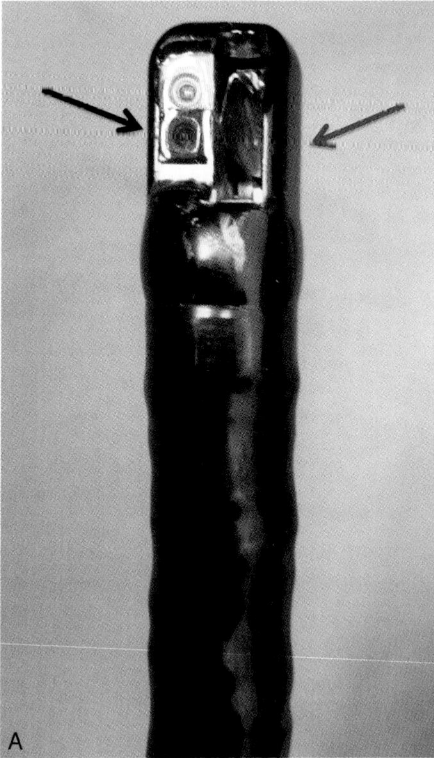

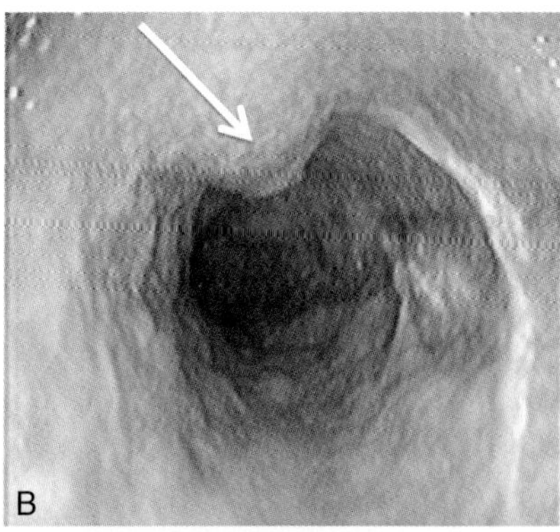

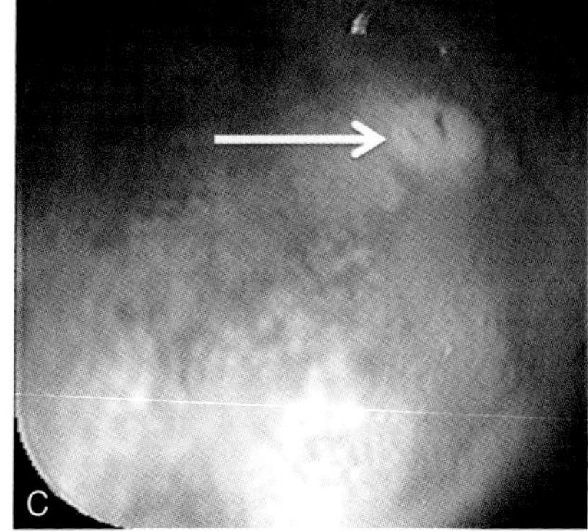

Figure 24.2 Image using the side-view duodenoscope. (A) The endoscope with the lens (black arrow) and working channel (red arrow) at a 90-degree angle to the end of the endoscope. (B) Endoscopic image of the major duodenal papilla (MDP) (white arrow) using a routine gastroduodenoscope. (C) Endoscopic image of the MDP (white arrow) using the side-view duodenoscope. Note the improved visualization and access to the opening of the papilla with this view.

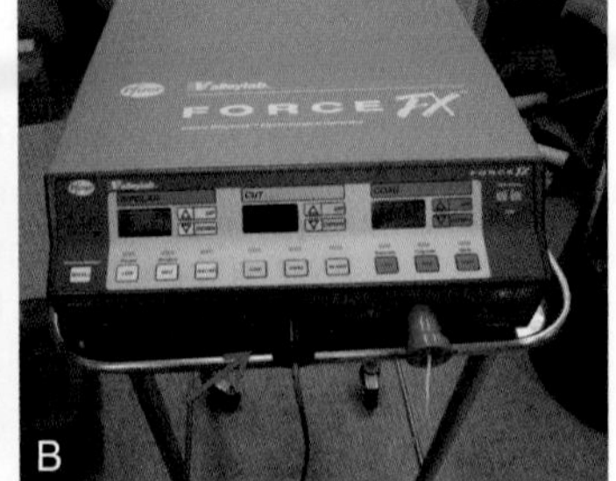

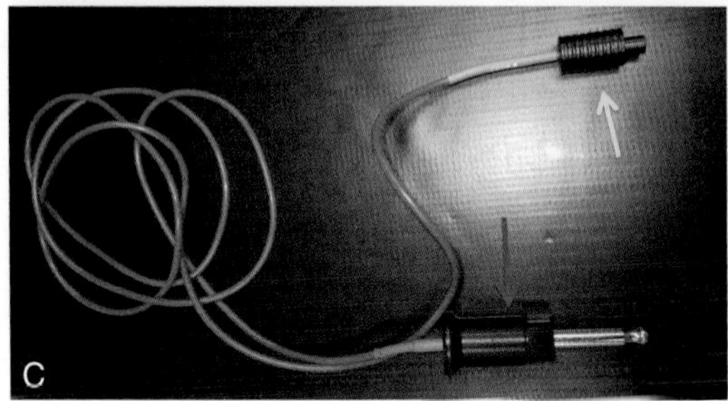

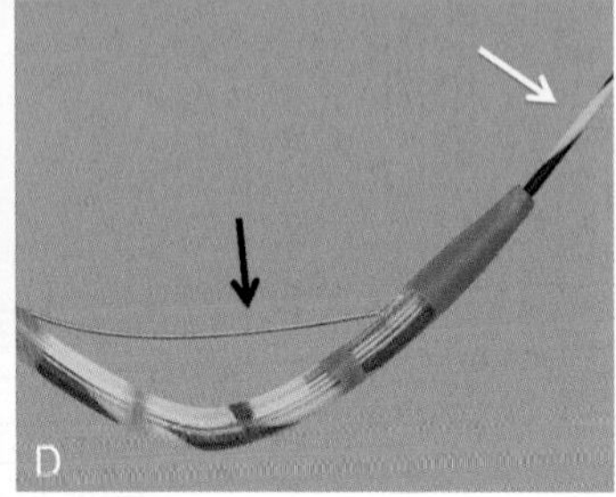

Figure 24.3 Sphincterotome catheter for common bile duct cannulation. (A) Hand-piece of catheter where electrocautery adaptor is connected (yellow arrow). (B) Electrocautery unit showing where the male adaptor of the cable is connected (red arrow). (C) Female adaptor where the hand-piece attaches to the cable (yellow arrow) and the male adaptor (red arrow) where the cable attaches to the electrocautery unit. (D) Sphincterotome catheter. Notice the electrocautery wire (black arrow) that allows the sphincterotomy to be performed.

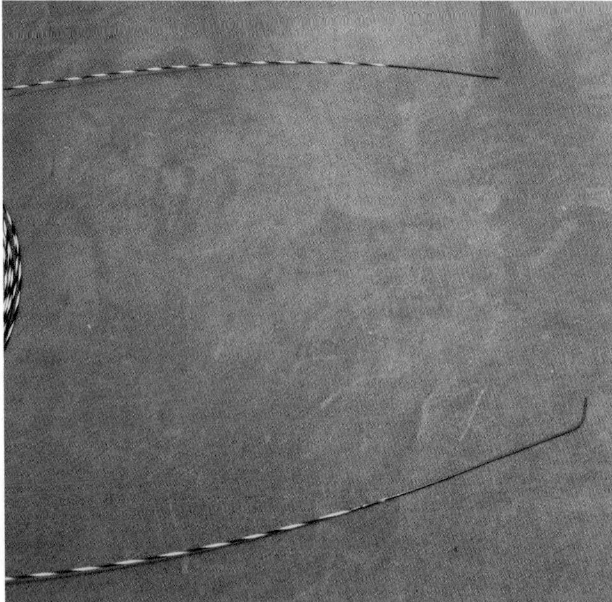

Figure 24.4 Guide wires. Notice the "zebra-striped" design. This allows the endoscopist to appreciate movement of the wire during catheter and stent manipulations. The tip of the wire comes either straight or angled and has a hydrophilic coating.

classically a mesh or laser-cut SEMS[8] mounted on a delivery system long enough to fit through the duodenoscope (>180 cm). Some stents are covered so they can be removed (Figure 24.5).

A retrieval/grasping instrument that fits through the working channel of the scope and a regular end-view gastroduodenoscope should also be available so that the stent can be removed if necessary.

Patient Preparation

All patients should have a CBC, serum biochemical profile, urinalysis, coagulation profile, spec PLI, and abdominal ultrasonography performed prior to any biliary intervention. If a biliary obstruction is diagnosed the cause should be elucidated. Benign pancreatitis may be managed medically and serial blood and ultrasound monitoring should be performed. Please refer to other resources concerning the medical management of pancreatitis-induced biliary obstruction.

If ERCP is elected the entire abdomen should be clipped in the event surgical conversion is necessary. All patients should be administered broad-spectrum antibiotics, including a fluoroquinolone, covering both aerobic and anaerobic intestinal microflora prior to any procedure (Cefoxitin or enrofloxacin and metronidazole is typically used). The patient should be appropriately hydrated, provided appropriate pain medications, and treated with vitamin K1. Hepatically metabolized drugs should be avoided, especially those used for anesthesia (i.e., benzodiazepines). The patient should be fasted for 12 hours prior to anesthesia. Endoscopy and fluoroscopy should be available simultaneously.

Procedure

The animal is placed under general anesthesia and atropine may be needed to slow GI mobility during cannulation of the duodenum with the scope. Alternatively, glucagon is commonly used in people for this problem. Dogs are initially placed in sternal recumbency but may need to be rotated into left lateral or dorsal recumbency to facilitate access. This is the recommendation of Dr. Spillman, who has done a great

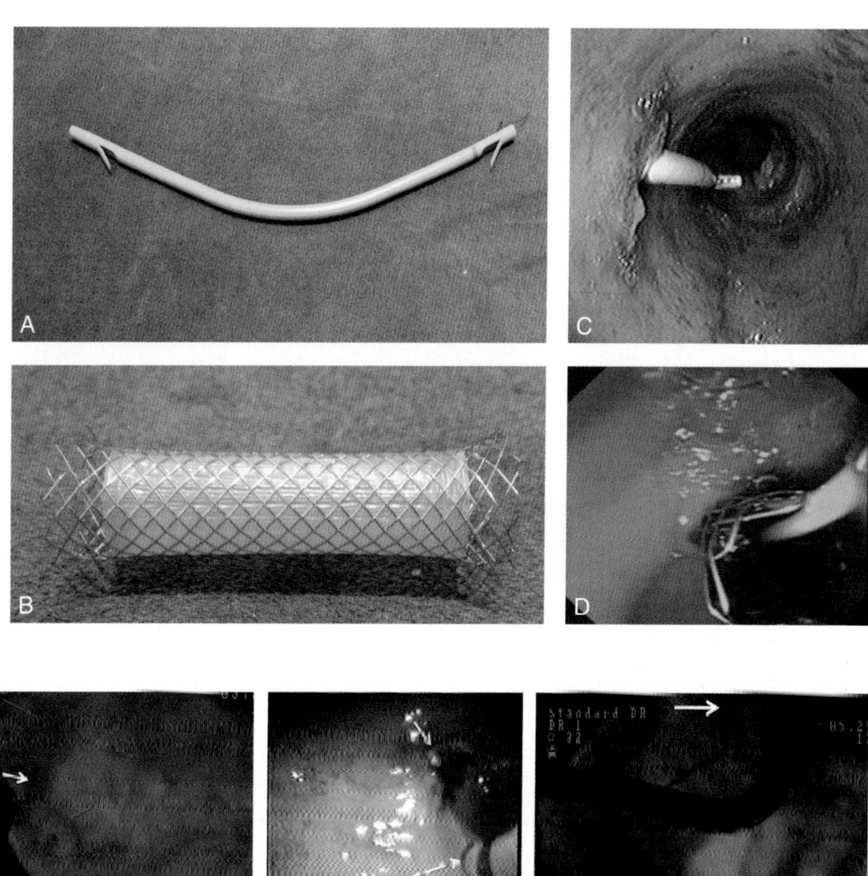

Figure 24.5 Biliary stents. (A) Polyurethane biliary and pancreatic duct stent used for temporary drainage of either the common bile duct or the pancreatic duct. (B) Endoscopic image of a temporary polyurethrane stent in a dog after ERCP and sphincterotomy. (C) Mesh partially covered self-expanding metallic stents (SEMS). Note the woven design. (D) Endoscopic image of an SEMS exiting the CBD through the MDP following deployment.

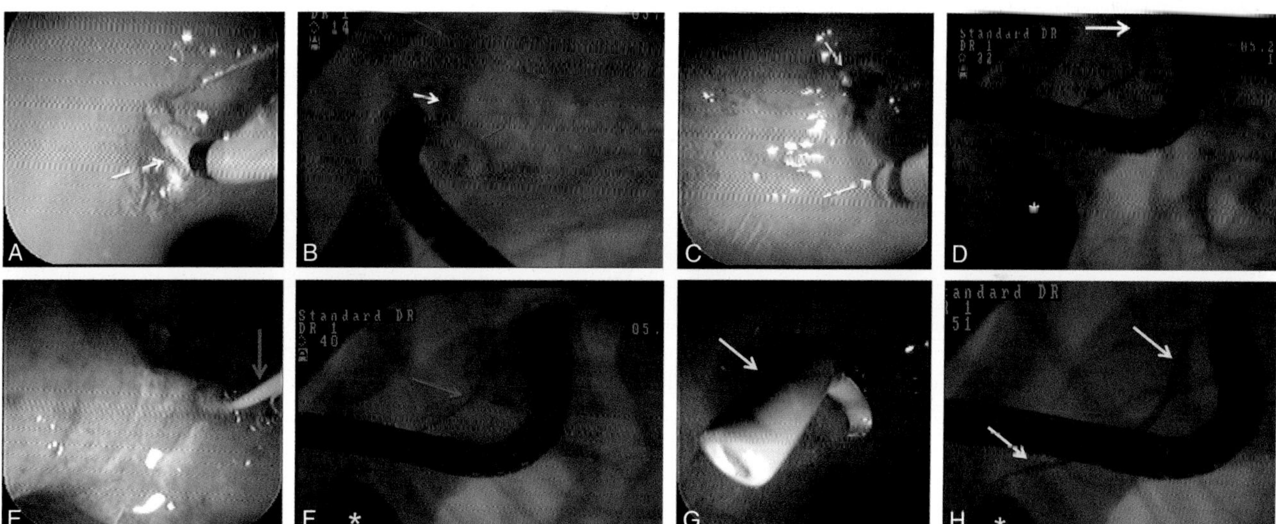

Figure 24.6 ERCP in a dog with a temporary biliary stent. (A) Endoscopic image using the side-view duodenoscope of the sphincterotome catheter (white arrow) in the major duodenal papilla (MDP) cannulating the minor pancreatic duct. (B) Fluoroscopic image during endoscopic retrograde pancreatography (ERP). Red arrows show contrast in the pancreatic ducts. White arrow is catheter in duct under fluoroscopic guidance. (C) Endoscopic image after sphincterotome (white arrow) cannulating common bile duct (CBD) through MDP. Notice the sphincterotomy (yellow arrow) with bile coming out of the MPD. (D) Fluoroscopic image of the sphincterotome catheter (white arrow) in the CBD and a retrograde cholangiogram (ERC). The gallbladder is filled with contrast (yellow asterisk). (E) Endoscopic image of the guide wire (red arrow) within the CBD through the MDP. (F) Fluoroscopic image of the guide wire (red arrow) within the CBD up to the gallbladder (yellow asterisk). (G) Endoscopic image of the polyurethane biliary stent (yellow arrow) exiting the MDP. (H) Fluoroscopic image of the stent (yellow arrows) within the CBD, over the guide wire.

deal of work on ERCP in dogs and cats. In the author's experience dogs in left lateral recumbency has worked well. The limited experience in cats would suggest that dorsal recumbency is easiest (Spillman et al, 2012).

A mouth gag is placed for routine GI endoscopy and using the side-view duodenoscope the gastric lumen is entered. The pylorus is cannulated with the side-view scope and the duodenum is entered (Figure 24.6, Figure 24.7). Once within the duodenal lumen the MDP is identified (Figure 24.1, Figure 24.6, and Figure 24.7). A sphincterotome catheter[3] is then used to cannulate the common bile duct (Figure 24.6 and Figure 24.7). This requires gentle manipulation of the endoscope and control of the working channel lever to direct the catheter

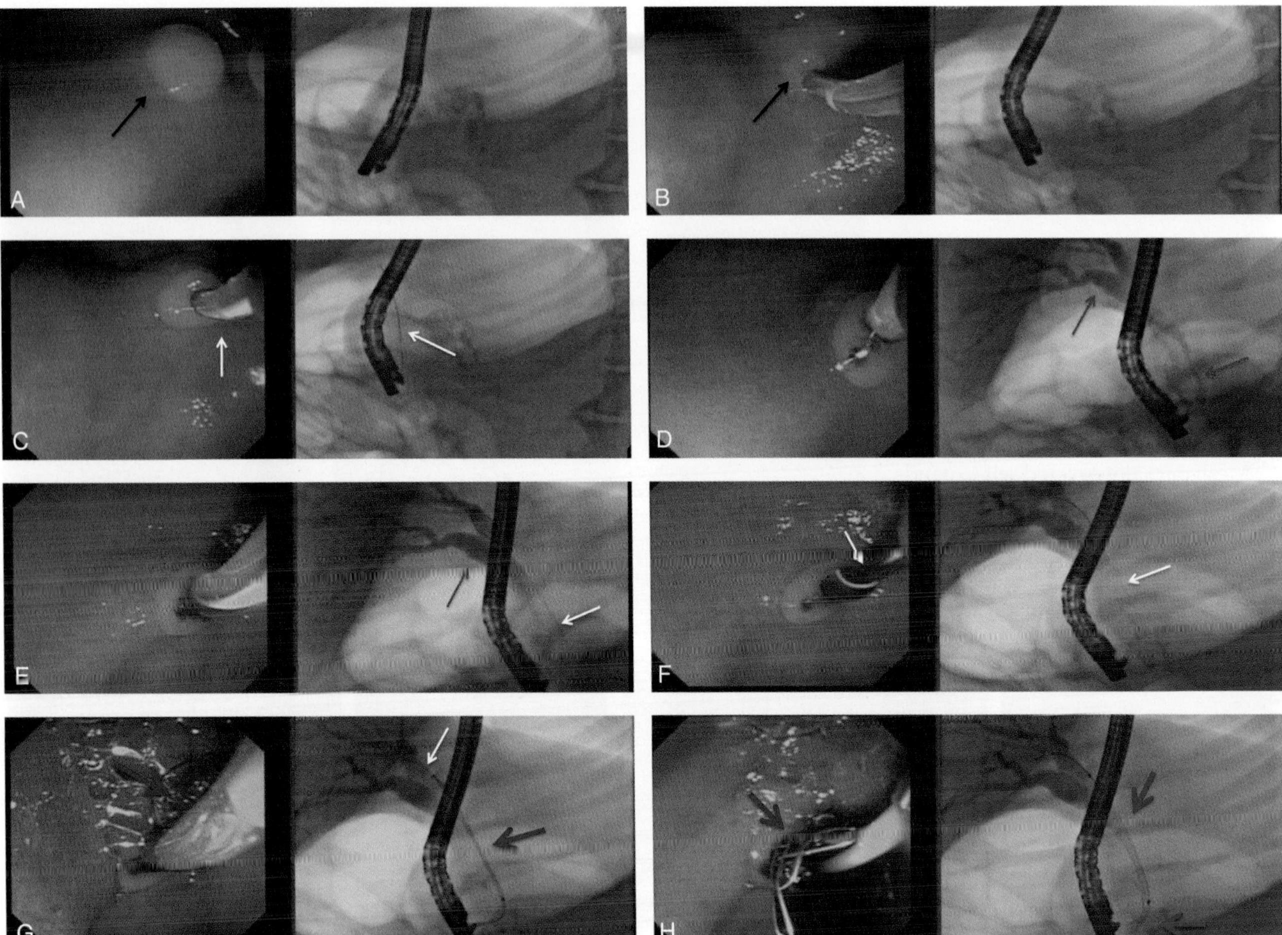

Figure 24.7 ERCP in a dog with a distal stricture of the common bile duct (CBD) after pancreatitis. In each picture there is an endoscopic image on the left and the same fluoroscopic image on the right. (A) Endoscopic image of the major duodenal papilla (black arrow) using the side-view duodenoscope. The fluoroscopic image is showing the endoscope in the proximal duodenum. (B) The sphincterotome catheter cannulating the MDP (black arrow). You can see the tip of the catheter entering the CBD in the fluoroscopic image. (C) The guide wire is passed through the catheter (white arrow), and up the CBD using both endoscopic and fluoroscopic guidance. (D) The guide wire is removed and a contrast study (red arrows) is performed documenting severely dilated intrahepatic bile ducts and the CBD. (E) The guide wire is replaced (white arrows) and advanced up to the intrahepatic bile ducts (red arrows) using fluoroscopic guidance. (F) The catheter is removed and the guide wire is seen entering the MDP and remains up the CBD (white arrows). (G) A SEMS is advanced on its delivery system (blue arrows) through the working channel of the endoscope, over the guide wire, and into the CBD. (H) The stent (blue arrows) is deployed using both endoscopic and fluoroscopic guidance, opening the CBD and exiting into the duodenum, through the MDP.

into the orifice. A combination of gentle lever lift, sphinctertome wire manipulation, and catheter advancement is used in tandem to advance the sphincterotome once in position. Gentle tension to the metallic wire of the sphincterotome aids in directing the catheter as well.

Using a 50:50 mixture of 0.9% saline and iodinated contrast material, approximately 1–3 mL of contrast are injected through the catheter slowly to identify the CBD or the pancreatic duct (Figure 24.6A–C and Figure 24.7). Once CBD cannulation is confirmed, a guide wire[4] is advanced through the sphincterotome and into the CBD using fluoroscopic and endoscopic guidance (Figure 24.6 and Figure 24.7). The catheter is then advanced into the CBD just enough that the wire of the sphincterotome is able to perform a sphincterotomy using blend mode on the electrocautery unit (Figure 24.6), if needed. This is not done in every case, and should be reserved for patients with a very tight opening. In human medicine controversy exists on whether or not this is additional procedure is routinely necessary. Care should be taken not to advance the catheter too deep or perforation of the CBD can occur during sphincterotomy. Once the wire is beyond the obstruction and within the cystic duct, gallbladder,

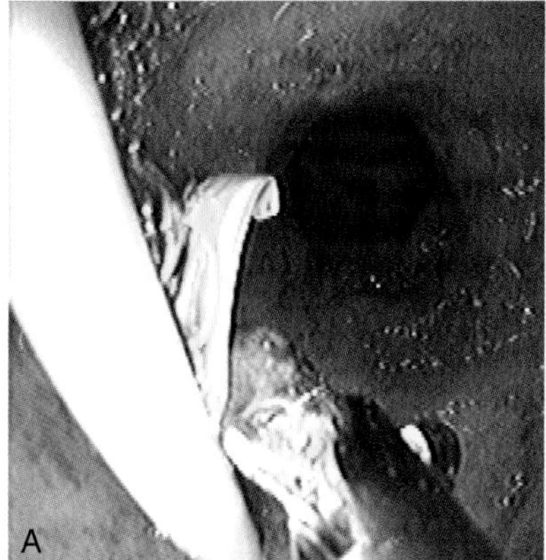

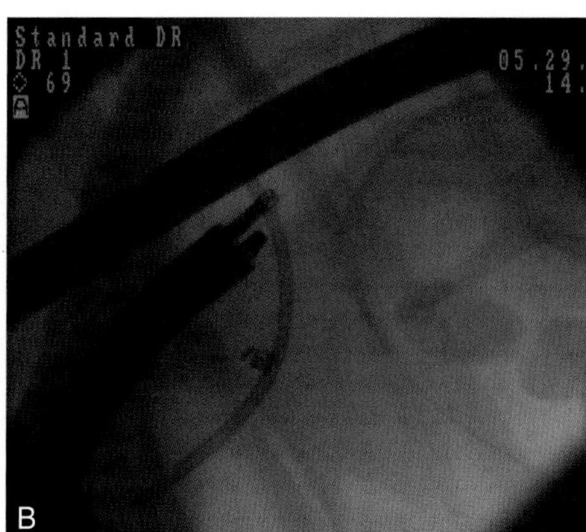

Figure 24.8 Endoscopic biliary stent retrieval. (A) Endoscopic grasping instrument through a regular gastroduodenoscope in a dog. (B) Fluoroscopic image after the stent is grasped endoscopically while it is being retracted for removal.

or proximal CBD the sphincterotome is removed over the wire (Figure 24.6 and Figure 24.7) using endoscopic and fluoroscopic guidance with the wire remaining in the CBD. The "barber-pole" or "zebra-striped" design on the wire allows the operator to watch endoscopically and make certain the wire is not moving as the sphincterotome is removed. Finally, the appropriately sized biliary stent[5–7] is advanced over the guide wire through the working channel of the scope and pushed into the common bile duct to traverse the opening at the MDP, beyond the obstruction. The endoscope needs to remain in close association with the MDP during stent placement to avoid being pushed orad as the stent enters the CBD. This should all be carefully monitored under fluoroscopic guidance simultaneously (Figure 24.6 and Figure 24.7). When placing polyurethane stents[5,6], a pusher catheter is needed to advance the stent through the scope and into the CBD. Once the obstruction is passed the scope is gently withdrawn as the stent is pushed out and the distal flange is placed within the duodenum (Figure 24.6). For a metallic SEMS[7] the entire delivery system is passed through the scope, over the guide wire, and then deployed appropriately (Chapter 1, Chapter 7, and Chapter 34) (Figure 24.7). Once the stent is in place and bile is seen to drain, the scope and wire are removed. The plastic/polyurethane (removable) stent should remain in place until there is complete resolution of the pancreatitis (approximately 6–8 weeks). The risk of leaving the stent in place is occlusion, dislodgement and reflux. The metallic stent is permanent and cannot be removed unless it is covered. The plastic stent can be removed easily with a grasping instrument (Figure 24.8).

Other interventions, aside from sphincterotomy and biliary stenting, are mechanical lithotripsy for biliary stones. In humans, the stones have a large cholesterol component making them relatively soft, so a biliary basket device[9] can be used to crush the stones and remove the pieces. In dogs and cats biliary stones are typically firm and this may not be possible, though has not been attempted. Extracorporeal shockwave lithotripsy (ESWL), commonly used for urinary tract stones, has been used for biliary stones in human and dog models and may be a good alternative in clinical veterinary patients (Chapter 27).

Postprocedural and Follow-Up Care

Following ERCP most patients will need standard therapy for pancreatitis and EHBDO. Pain medications may be indicated for pancreatitis (buprenorphine 0.01–0.02 mg/kg IV QID or a fentanyl CRI (3–5 μg/kg/hr)) if present. The procedure itself should not be painful and pain medications are not routinely necessary after standard ERCP in people. Patients should be treated with liver-supportive medications such as ursodeoxycolic acid, vitamin E supplementation, broad-spectrum antibiotics, typically including a fluoroquinolone (options: cefoxitin [20–30 mg/kg IV q4–8 hr]; enrofloxacin [10 mg/kg/day – dog; 5 mg/kg/day – cat] with ampicillin [22 mg/kg IV q 8 hr] and/or metronidazole [7.5 mg/kg IV BID]). Intravenous fluid therapy, with vitamin B-complex supplementation, is recommended. If there is any component of encephalopathy than oral or rectal lactulose can be considered. If a coagulopathy is present then Vitamin K1 can be administered at recommended doses, and plasma transfusions might be necessary. Please see other sources for detailed management of post-hepatic cholestasis.

Once the patient is discharged and all blood work and ultrasonographic inflammatory changes have resolved, the stent can be endoscopically removed (if the plastic/polyurethane or covered metallic stent was placed). The antibiotics should be continued at home until 1–2 weeks after stent removal to prevent ascending cholangitis. If a permanent stent is placed (SEMS) than metronidazole and ursodeoxycolic acid therapy should be continued.

Patients should be monitored while hospitalized daily post-stent placement with serial liver and complete blood counts to ensure improvement is occurring. Once discharged, liver values should be monitored weekly, then monthly. A spec PLI should also be done before the procedure and at 1 day, 1 week, 2 weeks and 6 weeks post procedure to ensure pancreatitis is resolving prior to removal of the stent.

Prognosis

There is not enough data on ERCP in canine and feline patients to discuss the ultimate prognosis. In our practice an ERCP was performed in seven research animals and three clinical dogs, and one clinical cat. These procedures were performed with the help of a human gastroenterologist who is considered an expert in ERCP. The first clinical patient presented with a total bilirubin of 26.5 mg/dl. The procedure was successful and took 26 minutes. An uncovered metallic stent was placed and the dog's total bilirubin was 3.1 mg/dl 48 hours later and was normal within 5 days. The dog has continued to tolerate the stent well (>24 months) and has not re-obstructed to date. A permanent stent was placed in this case due to the presence of a stricture. This is the recommendation in people, though a covered stent is often considered. Due to the location of the extrahepatic bile ducts, and the risk of blocking them with a covered stent, an uncovered stent was chosen in this case.

Knowing the morbidity and mortality with re-routing surgery is high, and may be associated with excessive pancreas manipulation, enterotomy-related sepsis, or depth and length of the anesthesia, stents are a promising alternative. Stents have been placed surgically and may have improved mortality rates slightly (30–50% versus 25–75%), but still require an enterotomy with pancreatic manipulation. Additionally, when ERCP is unsuccessful, we have had high success rates with metallic stenting using antegrade access through the CBD rather than performing an enterotomy.

Special Considerations

Care should be taken when considering ERCP in veterinary patients; all of those performed in the author's practice were guided by a human interventional gastroenterologist who performs hundreds of ERCPs/year in people and still found the procedure difficult in the small dog and cat population. The use in cats is possible but this will require the use of pediatric scopes and more research is necessary before this is recommended. This procedure should only be performed if immediate surgical conversion and/or the placement of a cholecystostomy tube is available if this procedure fails.

Notes

Please note these are only a few of the possible sources for each piece of equipment.

1. Side-view duodenoscope, TF-160VF, 11.3mm, Olympus.
2. Side-view duodenoscope, pediatric, PJF-160, 7.5mm, Olympus.
3. Sphincterotome catheter, 5–6 Fr., Autotome™ Sphincterotome Flexed, Boston Scientific, Natick, MA.
4. Hydra Jagwire® Guide wire, 0.035", 0.021" 480mm, Boston Scientific, Natick, MA.
5. Cotton-Huibregtse Biliary Stent Set, 7 Fr., Cook Medical, Bloomington IL.
6. Zimmon Biliary Stent, 5,6,7 Fr., double pigtail, Cook Medical, Bloomington, IL.
7. Pancreatic Stent, 5–7 Fr., Cook Medical, Bloomington, IL.
8. WALLSTENT® RX Biliary Endoprosthesis, Boston Scientific, Natick, MA.
9. Mini Basket, 5 Fr, Cook Medical, Bloomington, IL.

Reference

Spillman T, Willard MD, Ruhnke I, et al (2012) Endoscopic retrograde cholangiopancreatotograpy (ERCP) in healthy cats – a feasibility study. European College of Veterinary Internal Medicine, Maastricht, NL.

Suggested Reading

Buote NJ, Mitchell SL, Penninck D, et al (2006) Cholecystoenterosctomy for treatment of extrahpatic biliary tract obstruction in cats: 22 cases (1994–2003). *J Am Vet Med Assoc* 228(9), 1376–82.

Herman B, Brawer R, Murtaugh R, et al (2005) Therapeutic percutaneous ultrasound-guided cholecystocentesis in 3 dogs with EHBDO and pancreatitis.). *J Am Vet Med Assoc* 227(11), 1782–6.

Mayhew P and Weisse C (2008) Treatment of pancreatitis-associated extrahepatic biliary tract obstruction by choledochal stenting in seven cats. *J Small Anim Pract* 49, 133–8.

Mayhew P, Richardson R, Mehler S, et al (2006) Choledochal tube stenting for decompression of the extrahepatic portion of the biliary tract in dogs: 13 cases (2002–2005).). *J Am Vet Med Assoc* 228(8), 1209–14.

Mehler S, Mayhew PD, Drobatz KJ, et al (2004) Variables associated with outcome in dogs undergoing extrahepatic biliary surgery: 60 cases. *Vet Surg* 33(6), 644–6.

Murphy SM, Rodriguez JD, McAnulty JF (2007) Minimally invasive cholecystostomy in the dog: evaluation of placement techniques and use in extrahepatic biliary obstruction. *Vet Surg* 36(7), 675–83.

Spillmann T, Happonen I, Sankari S, et al (2004). Evaluation of serum values of pancreatic enzymes after endoscopic retrograde pancreatography in dogs. *Am J Vet Res* 65(5), 616–19.

Spillmann T, Schnell-Kretschmer H, Dick M, et al (2005) Endoscopic retrograde cholangio-pancreatography in dogs with chronic gastrointestinal problems. *Vet Radiol Ultrasound* 46(4), 293–9.

Spillmann T, Happonen I, Kähkönen T, et al (2005) Endoscopic retrograde cholangio-pancreatography in healthy Beagles. *Vet Radiol Ultrasound* 46(2), 97–104.

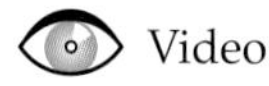 Video clips to accompany this chapter can be found in the online material at **www.wiley.com/go/weisse/vet-image-guided-interventions**

CHAPTER TWENTY-FIVE

Cholecystostomy

Sean Murphy
Westvet Emergency and Specialty Center, Garden City, ID

Background/Indications

Surgery for extrahepatic biliary obstruction (EHBO) carries a high risk for mortality ranging from 28–64% in veterinary patients. High mortality rates are likely related to the emergent requirement for involved surgical repairs in the face of significant patient comorbidities. Temporary biliary drainage via cholecystostomy has been used for stabilization of such patients prior to definitive surgical repair and may be indicated in those with known risk factors for perioperative mortality such as elevated serum creatinine, prolonged clotting times, and hypotension. Additionally, cholecystostomy allows for hepatobiliary drainage during temporary obstructions, such as pancreatitis, which can resolve and eliminate the need for an open, surgical procedure.

Patient Preparation

Patients should undergo complete abdominal ultrasonography and medical workup to ensure that a post-hepatic cause of biliary obstruction is present. For successful cholecystostomy, the obstructing cause must be distal to the cystic duct, the bile viscosity amendable to catheter drainage, and the gallbladder wall healthy enough for catheter maintenance (Figure 25.1). Preoperative blood chemistry, complete blood count, coagulation times and blood pressures are recommended. Debilitated patients will require careful anesthetic monitoring and protocols that minimize hypotension.

Overview/Risks/Outcomes

Options for gallbladder drainage include cholecystocentesis and cholecystostomy tube placement. Regardless of the method chosen, the technique must have a high level of success as it is typically performed in patients with substantial comorbidities. Ultrasound (U/S) guided cholecystocentesis has been reserved for treatment of temporary obstructions such as pancreatitis. It usually requires several aspirations to decompress the biliary tract until the obstruction resolves. Approaches described have used an 18–22g needle directed subxyphoid through the falciform to puncture the gallbladder fundus. A trans-hepatic puncture has also been described and may minimize gallbladder leakage.

For cholecystostomy, the gallbladder is drained via placement of a Foley or locking-loop catheter inserted via ultrasound, fluoroscopic, laparoscopic or open surgical guidance. U/S and fluoroscopic guidance accomplish insertion with a locking-loop catheter via a modified-Seldinger technique or direct puncture of the gallbladder using the internal trocar of the catheter. These methods allow the catheter to traverse hepatic tissue when an intercostal puncture is used, but up to 100% of such insertions traversed the pleural cavity in a cadaver study; laparoscopic placement traversed the pleural cavity in 0% of cases. In the same study, placement using fluoroscopy or U/S also had significantly lower chances for successful catheter insertion when compared to laparoscopy-guided catheter placement. Thus, fluoroscopic or ultrasound-guided placement may be associated with higher risk. The failure mode of such catheter insertions is not guide wire access but rather failure to insert the catheter successfully over the wire. Operator experience level with IR methods, individual patient anatomy, and gallbladder size may allow for higher success rates with percutaneous image-guided techniques, however at least one veterinary study suggests laparoscopic-guided catheter placement is currently the preferred technique.

The definitive benefit of preoperative biliary drainage in veterinary patients is unknown. Experimental study in dogs undergoing partial hepatectomy after 3 weeks of simulated biliary obstruction had 100% perioperative mortality while those with 3 weeks of drainage prior to hepatectomy had 0%. The theoretical advantages of preoperative drainage include improved reticuloendothelial function of the liver, enhanced portal endotoxin clearance, restoration of the GI barrier, correction of comorbidities such as coagulopathy and hypovolemia, reduction in circulating bile acids, establishment of a port for cholangiography, and

Veterinary Image-Guided Interventions, First Edition. Edited by Chick Weisse and Allyson Berent.

Companion website: www.wiley.com/go/weisse/vet-image-guided-interventions

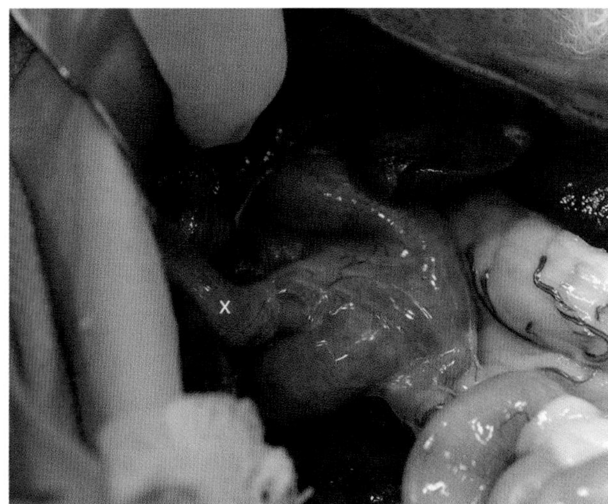

Figure 25.1 Surgical image of a distal bile duct obstruction. The cystic duct "X" remains patent proximal to the obstruction making cholecystostomy possible in this case.

potential avoidance of an open procedure for a temporary obstruction. An individual comfortable with laparoscopy can perform cholecystostomy with minimal anesthetic and surgical time.

The potential risks of cholecystostomy include bowel or organ puncture during catheter insertion, pneumothorax, catheter leakage or premature dislodgment, bile peritonitis, establishment of biliary infection, catheter obstruction, and prolonged hospitalization. Use of preoperative drainage prior to resection of neoplastic obstructions within human medicine remains controversial. In such cases endoscopic drainage with ERCP and biliary stenting (see Chapter 24) is typically preferred to percutaneous drainage in distal obstructions but requires expertise and specialized endoscopes. Preoperative drainage may be more indicated in malnourished, hypoalbuminemic, and long-term jaundice patients. The author currently considers cholecystostomy in cases with high ASA status, prolonged biliary obstruction, and those patients with known perioperative risk factors. Once a catheter is placed, hospitalization time likely increases thus financial considerations should be made as well.

Equipment for Laparoscoic Cholecystostomy

- Laparoscopic tower and insufflator, two laparoscopic 5 mm portals and 5 mm telescope
- 5 mm laparoscopic Babcock forceps
- Locking pigtail catheter 8–10 Fr (Figure 25.2). The author has solely used the Abscession Catheter™ (Angiodynamis, Queensbury, NY) as pressure testing and insertion of these catheters was examined in cadavers.
- Sterile collection system
- Diluted contrast medium for cholangiography and fluoroscopy.

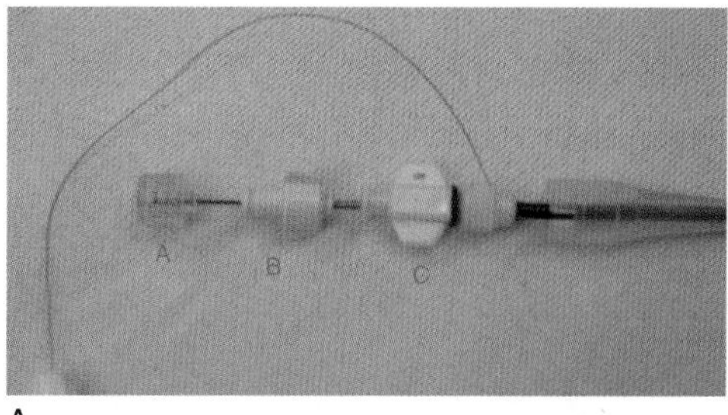

A

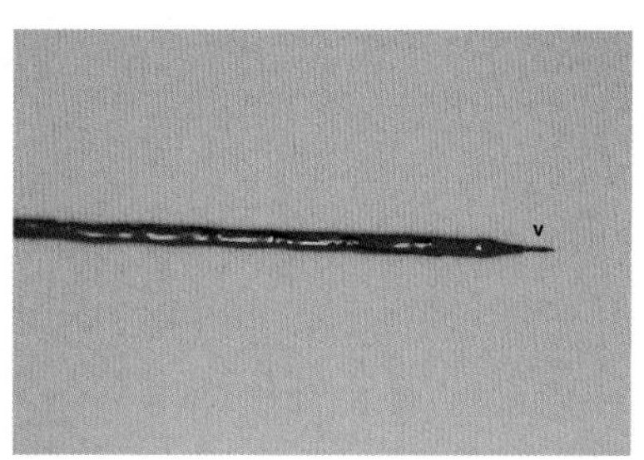

B

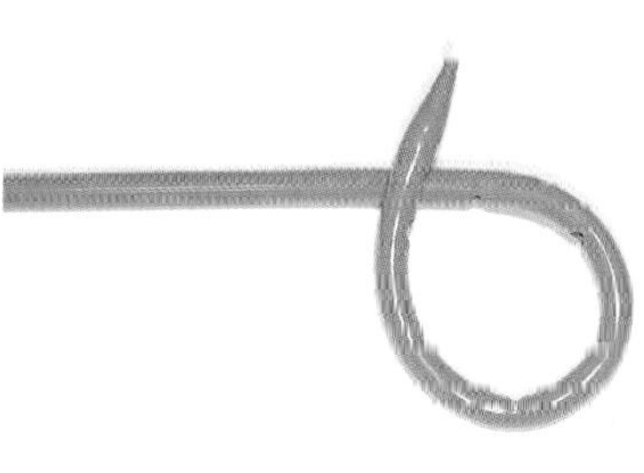

C

Figure 25.2 (A) A locking-loop catheter end showing the internal sharp trocar "A", stainless steel cannula "B" and hub for connection to a sterile drainage set "C". (B) The catheter tip with the cannula in place and sharp trocar extended (open arrowhead). (C) The catheter tip in a locked configuration which is accomplished by tensioning the internal suture. Note the catheter fenestrations positioned on the interior of the loop to limit obstruction.

Laparoscopic Procedure

The patient is placed in dorsal recumbency and prepared for a full abdominal exploratory surgery. A telescope portal is placed 1 cm cranial to the umbilicus using a Hassan or equivalent technique (Figure 25.3). Carbon-dioxide insufflation pressures can generally be kept low as the gallbladder is easily visualized; pressures should not exceed 15 mmHg. An optional right paramedian instrument portal for a laparoscopic Babcock forceps

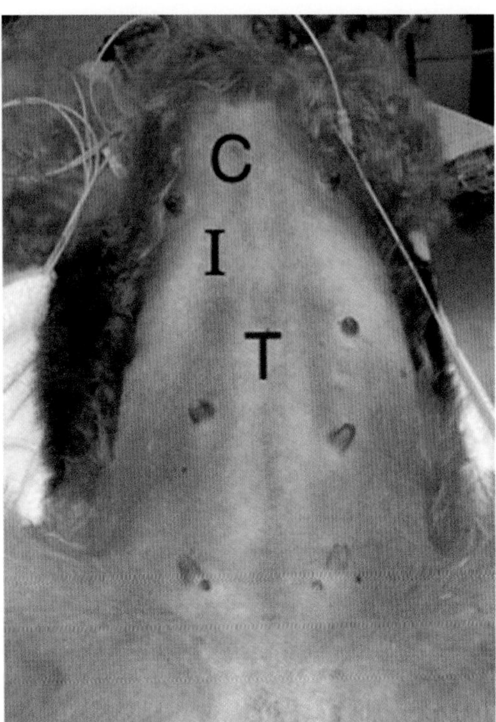

Figure 25.3 Positioning for laparoscopic cholecystostomy with telescope "T" and instrument "I" portal locations. The right paraxyphoid region for catheter insertion is labeled "C".

allows for stabilization of the GB. This instrument is especially helpful to reinsert the catheter through a puncture hole in the case of a failed attempt. The drainage catheter is placed through a right stab incision (Figure 25.3). The incision must be kept caudal to the diaphragm insertion to avoid a pneumothorax, which happens rapidly when the abdomen is insufflated. Transcutaneous illumination is helpful in directing the stab incision.

A locking-loop catheter is inserted through the stab incision with the cannula and sharp trocar in place. The trocar is then internalized and the apex of the gallbladder is pushed with the blunt catheter tip. This practice insertion allows one to see how the gallbladder will displace when pressure is applied. The angle of insertion is planned and should be in line with the central lumen and long axis of the gallbladder when possible. If liver parenchyma can be traversed safely then it should be considered. The catheter's internal trocar is advanced and the gallbladder is punctured inserting the catheter 1–2 cm. The trocar is again retracted to prevent "double-walling" the gallbladder (perforating the opposite side during advancement). The catheter is freed from the internal cannula and trocar then slid over the stabilized cannula until the string of the locking-loop is completely within the gallbladder. This is much like threading a standard IV catheter into a vein. An alternative placement technique is performed over a guide wire placed through a percutaneously placed 18-gauge Chiba needle (or renal

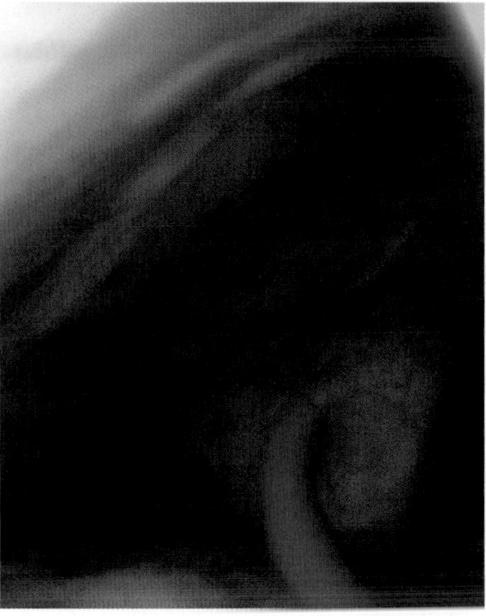
A

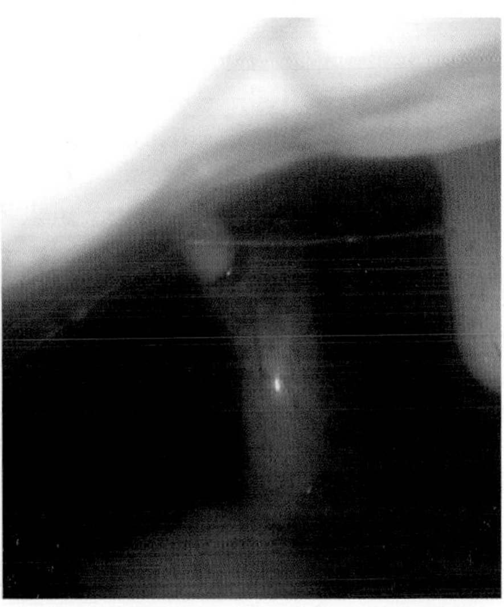
B

Figure 25.4 Laparoscopic view of a cholecystostomy catheter. (A) A shorter catheter length is preferred to minimize the eventual tract length that will form. (B) The catheter must not be over tensioned when secured to the body wall as this could lead to premature catheter pullout. When possible, transhepatic catheter placement should be attempted to minimize leakage.

puncture set). The catheter is then advanced over the guide wire without the sharp trocar.

The catheter's locking-loop is engaged and checked for security (see Video 25.1)

The gallbladder is drained, samples are collected for culture and cytology, and then it is flushed with sterile saline. A laparoscopic liver biopsy is obtained if indicated. The free segment of the inta-abdominal catheter should be kept as short as possible but without excessive tension. Limiting length helps to keep the eventual tract that will form between the gallbladder and abdominal wall shorter (Figure 25.4). The catheter is secured with 0 or 2–0 nylon

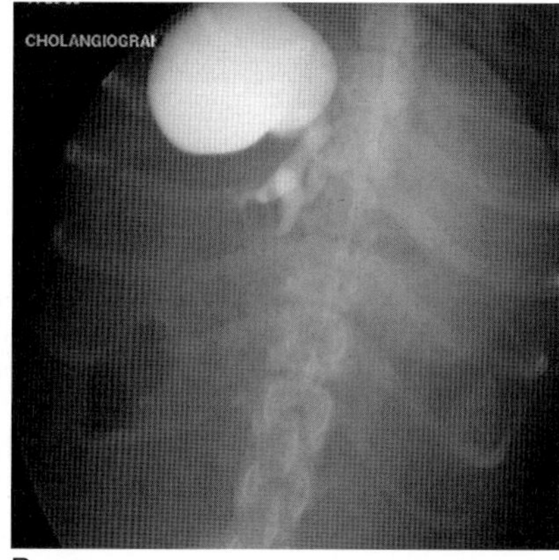

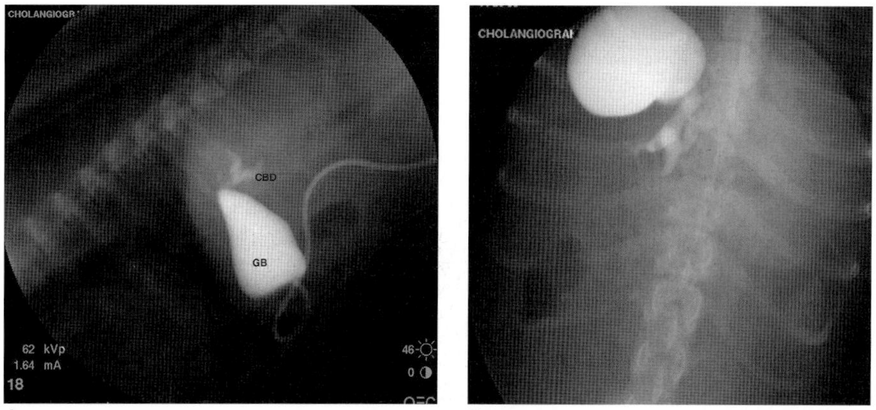

Figure 25.5 (A, B) Lateral and ventral-dorsal fluoroscopic cholangiograms demonstrating obstruction of the common bile duct "CBD". Note the gallbladder "GB" is dilated with contrast injected under mild pressure.

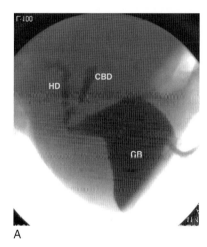

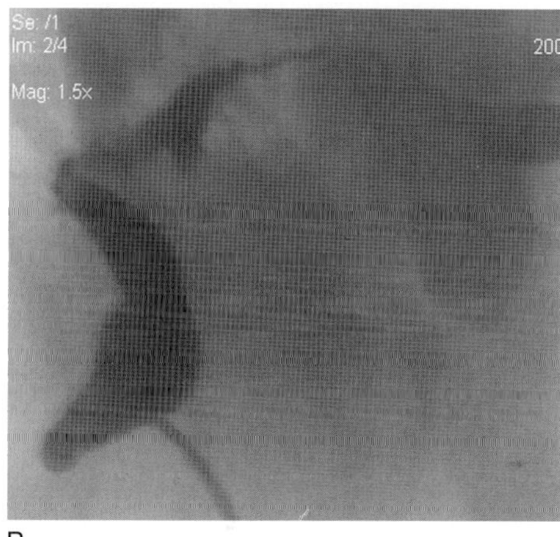

Figure 25.6 (A) A cholangiogram showing common bile duct "CBD" and hepatic duct "HD" obstruction secondary to pancreatitis. (B) Repeat cholangiogram 4 days post catheter placement shows a patent duct and contrast within the small intestine. The catheter was capped in this case and the dog discharged to allow catheter tract maturation prior to removal.

suture in a finger-trap fashion. The anchoring bite of suture should purchase the abdominal wall adjacent to the site of puncture; skin purchase only allows excessive movement and pull on the catheter. A second fingertrap suture is often placed 4cm distal to limit tension on the primary anchor. A cholangiogram with diluted contrast may be performed to assess the level of biliary obstruction. The authors have typically utilized fluoroscopic evaluation during injection to examine the biliary tract from multiple angles (Figure 25.5).

Follow-Up

Animals are recovered in the intensive care unit. An esophagostomy or nasoesophageal feeding tube should be placed to provide early enteral nutrition. A portion or all of the drained bile may be replaced with enteric feedings. The catheter is bandaged and hooked to a closed collection system with the extension tubing secured to the bandage creating a third point of attachment. Sterile saline may be used as needed to flush or check the patency of the catheters. Antimicrobial therapy may be considered to limit biliary sepsis.

After establishing temporary biliary drainage, the length of time required to improve patient status ranges from 24 hours to several weeks. The optimal time to obtain patient stabilization before surgery is unknown and likely depends on factors such as duration of obstruction, pre-existing hepatic disease, and other co-morbidities. During this time oral lactulose, early enteral feeding, and enteric bile replacement may be used as such therapies have been shown to improve intestinal permeability and lower serum endotoxin levels within 5–21 days. In five clinical cases performed by the author, greater than 50% reduction in serum bilirubin occurred within 48 hours, at which time all dogs resumed oral food intake. The average duration of drainage was 6 days prior to an open biliary diversion procedure or capping of the catheter for an additional 10–21 days (prior to removal) in cases with temporary obstruction.

Close monitoring of patients is essential. Catheter leakage and peritonitis must be identified quickly. This has not been a problem in the author's experience despite not traversing the liver parenchyma prior to gallbladder insertion. Catheter obstruction has presented as reduction in output and elevating serum

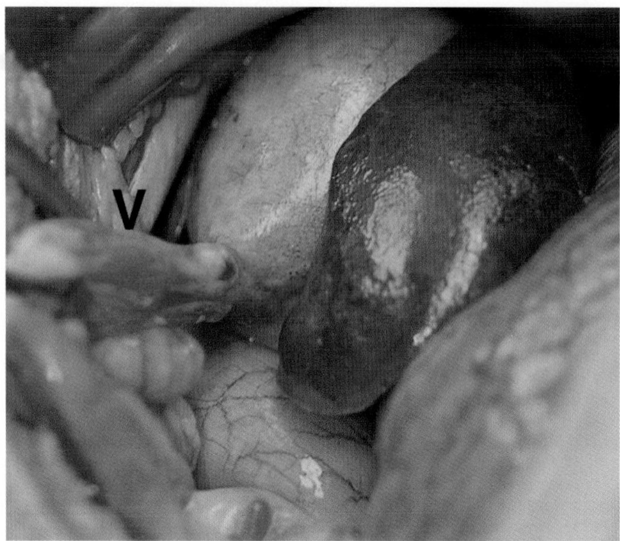

Figure 25.7 Cholecystostomy tract at 25 days post placement. This dog prematurely removed the catheter in its locked configuration causing rupture of the tract. The tract (open arrowhead) was dissected and two sutures placed to seal the stoma.

bilirubin requiring an emergency rerouting procedure. A cholangiogram may be performed at any time to evaluate patency of the catheter and biliary tract. If an obstruction resolves during drainage (Figure 25.6) the catheter is capped and bandaged. Maturation of the catheter tract (Figure 25.7) must occur prior to percutaneous catheter removal. Tract development was not considered complete in two clinical cases at 9 and 25 days postoperatively. This differs from some veterinary textbook recommendations of 5–10 day catheter residence requirements for adequate tract maturation and removal. In humans at least 21–28 days is required when hepatic parenchyma is not traversed.

Catheter Removal

Fluoroscopy is used and the catheter is injected with dilute contrast to lightly opacify the gallbladder. The end of the catheter is cut or the locking mechanism is opened to disengage the locking-loop. An appropriately sized guide wire is advanced down the catheter prior to gentle removal. Next, a sheath with similar size to the drainage catheter is placed into the stoma and a fistulogram with undiluted contrast material is performed through the side-port during withdrawal with the guide wire remaining in place. If no contrast material leaks then the guide wire is removed and the site bandaged. If contrast leakage is noted then a new catheter is inserted over the guide wire and left in place for an additional period. Alternatively, the site can be closed in an open procedure.

Suggested Reading

Hatjidakis A, Karampekios S, Prassopoulos P, et al (1981) Maturation of the tract after percutaneous cholecystostomy with regard to the access route. *Cardiovasc Intervent Radiol* 21, 36–40.

Herman BA, Brawer RS, Murtaugh RJ, et al (2005) Therapeutic percutaneous ultrasound-guided cholecystocentesis in three dogs with extrahepatic biliary obstruction and pancreatitis. *J Am Vet Med Assoc* 227, 1782–6.

Hewitt S, Brisson B, Sinclair M, et al (2007) Comparison of cardiopulmonary responses during sedation with epidural and local anesthesia for laparoscopic-assisted jejunostomy feeding tube placement with cardiopulmonary responses during general anesthesia for laparoscopic-assisted or open surgical jejunostomy feeding tube placement in healthy dogs. *Am J Vet Res* 68, 358–69.

Iacono C, Ruzzenente A, Campagnaro, et al (2013) Role of preoperative biliary drainage in jaundiced patients who are candidates for pancreatoduodenectomy or hepatic resection: highlights and drawbacks. *Ann Surg* 257, 191–204.

Kamiya S, Nagino M, Kanazawa H, et al (2004) The value of bile replacement during external biliary drainage: an analysis of intestinal permeability, integrity, and microflora. *Ann Surg* 239, 510–17.

Kawarada Y, Higashiguchi T, Yokoi H, et al (1995) Preoperative biliary drainage in obstructive jaundice. *Hepatic Gastroenterol* 42, 300–7.

Lawrence D, Bellah JR, Meyer DJ, et al (1992) Temporary bile diversion in cats with experimental extrahepatic bile duct obstruction. *Vet Surg* 21, 446–51.

Mehler SJ, Mayhew PD, Drobatz KJ, et al (2004) Variables associated with outcome in dogs undergoing extrahepatic biliary surgery: 60 cases (1998–2002). *Vet Surg* 33, 644–9.

Murphy S, Rodriguez D, and McAnulty J (2007) Minimally invasive cholecystostomy in the dog: evaluation of placement techniques and use in extrahepatic biliary obstruction. *Vet Surg* 36, 675–83.

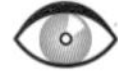
Video 25.1 Laparoscopic placement of a cholecystostomy catheter. The cutaneous stab for catheter entrance should have been directed more caudally to avoid a pneumothorax (seen as caudal bulging of the diaphragm toward the end of the video clip). Also note the placement of the catheter in line with the long axis of the gallbladder. This video clip can be found in the online material at **www.wiley.com/go/weisse/vet-image-guided-interventions**

SECTION FIVE

Urogenital System

Edited by Allyson Berent

CHAPTER TWENTY-SIX

Imaging of the Urinary Tract

Amy M. Habing and Julie K. Byron
Department of Veterinary Clinical Sciences, The Ohio State University, Columbus, OH

Introduction

Imaging, plain and contrast-enhanced, and uroendoscopy is essential to interventional evaluation and treatment of the urinary tract, and are often best used in combination. Here we review the indications, procedures, complications, and interpretation of some of the most common imaging studies performed for the urinary tract. Table 26.1 offers a quick reference to various non-endoscopic imaging techniques and specific considerations of each study are discussed in the following sections.

Excretory Urography

Indications

Excretory urography (EU) is of use in a variety of diagnostic scenarios. The study allows for examination of kidney morphology and subjective assessment of renal function. Assessment of the renal pelves and a suspicion of the presence of masses, hematomas, or nephroliths is a frequent indication for EU.

EU may assist in the differentiation between acute kidney injury, chronic renal dysfunction, and renal dysplasia based on the timing and persistence of renal opacification, as well as the morphologic characteristics of the kidneys. Its use in this diagnostic capacity may be limited, however, by the concern around contrast-induced kidney injury and further morbidity in an already compromised patient. Ultrasound-guided percutaneous pyelography is particularly useful in patients that are being evaluated for ureteral disease, avoiding contrast-induced nephropathy. This procedure does not allow evaluation of the renal parenchyma, however due to ureteral opacification, aids in the diagnosis of ureteral obstruction. In a normal animal, only regions of ureteral peristaltic contraction are not opacified. These regions may be examined with repeat static images or fluoroscopy. It is important to note that in order to safely perform a percutaneous pyelogram, the renal pelvis must be dilated. Typically, the renal pelvis should be at least 4–5 mm dilated; however this varies depending on clinician experience and comfort level.

A common use of the EU, with or without computed tomography, is the investigation of ureteral abnormalities. One indication for EU in veterinary patients is to assess the patency of the renal pelvis and ureters. Animals with acute onset of azotemia are often imaged for post-renal obstruction. Ultrasound may indicate dilation of the renal pelvis and ureter proximal to the obstruction, but the location and size of the obstructing agent may be difficult to determine. EU may assist in determining its location within the renal pelvis or along the ureter, which can influence the options available for treatment (medical vs. interventional [stent or subcutaneous ureteral bypass device] vs. surgical [resection/reimplantation or ureterotomy]) (see Chapters 30 and 31). If a nephrotomy or nephrectomy is necessary, the EU may provide some qualitative information about the function and patency of the contralateral kidney and ureter. Renal scintigraphy is recommended for assessment of differential renal function over EU due to the risk of contrast load and the subjectivity of this test. Care should be taken not to overinterpret renal function based on either EU or differential glomerular filtration rate (GFR) studies when a complete ureteral obstruction is present. Excessive backpressure from a ureteral obstruction will result in decreased GFR, and therefore decreased positive contrast or radiopharmaceutical within the collecting system, resulting in an underestimated renal function.

Ectopic ureters are a common differential diagnosis in patients with urinary incontinence prior to neutering. Cystoscopy and computed tomographic EU (CTEU) are considered superior to standard EU in the diagnosis of

Veterinary Image-Guided Interventions, First Edition. Edited by Chick Weisse and Allyson Berent.

Companion website: www.wiley.com/go/weisse/vet-image-guided-interventions

TABLE 26.1

Procedure	Patient preparation	Contrast	Dose/Volume	Technique	Additional considerations
EU (fluoroscopy/ radiography)	• 12–24 hr fast • +/– Enema • Sedation/ general anesthesia • IV catheter	Aqueous iodinated (non- ionic preferred)	• 600–880 mgI/kg • Inc. dose by 20% if renal azotemia is present	1. Survey RT and VD 2. Rapid IV bolus injection 3. RL and VD time 0, 5, 20, 40 minutes 4. Repeat RT and LT OBL as needed starting at 5 minutes for UVJ	• Concurrent negative contrast cystogram may be performed for ectopic ureter evaluation • If poor filling of the renal pelves, caudal abdominal compression may be applied using a tight elastic bandage after the 5 minute image. Images are made after 5–10 minutes and the bandage is removed. Caudal abdominal compression should not be performed with negative contrast cystogram.
CT EU[8]			• 400–880 mgI/kg • Inc. dose by 20% if renal azotemia is present	1. Position in sternal recumbency with pelvis elevated 2. Survey CT (cranial to kidneys to caudal urethra) 3. Rapid IV bolus injection 4. Repeat scan at time 0, 3 minutes 5. Repeat scans from mid bladder to caudal urethra as needed for UVJ	
Ultrasound guided percutaneous pyelogram	• 12–24 hr fast • +/–Enema • General anesthesia/ heavy sedation • Surgical scrub of skin	Aqueous iodinated	• Replace 50–100% of renal pelvic fluid with positive contrast media	1. Survey RL and VD 2. Using ultrasound guidance, aseptically advance a 22 gauge spinal needle through the renal cortex, and into the dilated renal pelvis 3. Remove approximately 50% renal pelvic fluid and replace with positive contrast 4. RT and V/D time 0, 15 minutes	• Repeat bolus injections and images as needed for diagnosis

Procedure	Patient preparation	Contrast	Dose/Volume	Technique	Additional considerations
Positive contrast cystogram	• 12–24 hr fast • +/– Enema • Sedation/ general anesthesia	20 % aqueous iodinated (diluted with sterile saline/ sterile water)	• 5–10 ml/kg (dog) • 2–5 ml/kg (cat)	1. Survey RT and VD 2. Inject positive contrast through urinary catheter. 3. LL, VD, RT and LT OBL	• Terminate injection if bladder feels turgid and/or back pressure is felt on the syringe plunger
Negative contrast cystogram	• Aseptic urinary bladder catheterization with urine removal	Nitrogen or CO2 (preferred), or room air	• 5–10 ml/kg (dog) • 2–5 ml/kg (cat)	1. Survey LL and VD 2. Inject negative contrast through urinary catheter. 3. LL, VD, RT and LT OBL	
Double contrast cystogram	• +/– 2% lidocaine (2–5 ml) injected into urinary bladder to reduce bladder pain/ spasm	Aqueous iodinated	• 5–10 ml (dog) • 3 ml (cat)	1. Survey LL and VD 2. Inject positive contrast through urinary catheter 3. Rotate patient to allow adequate coating of the bladder mucosa 4. Place in LEFT lateral recumbency 5. Inject negative contrast through urinary catheter 6. LL, VD, RT and LT OBL	
		Nitrogen or CO2 (preferred), or room air	• 5–10 ml/kg (dog) • 2–5 ml/kg (cat)		
Urethrogram	• Sedation/ general anesthesia • Aseptic distal urethral catheterization • +/– 2% lidocaine (2–5 ml) injected into urethra to reduce spasm	Aqueous iodinated	• 10–15 ml (dog) • 5–10 ml (cat)	1. Survey RL and RL with legs pulled forward (male dogs) 2. Inject 50% of contrast media 3. RL with legs forward (image made at end of injection) 4. Inject remaining contrast 5. RL, RL and LT OBL	• Urinary bladder should be fully distended to facilitate urethral distension • Terminate injection if back pressure is felt on the syringe plunger • Foley catheter is preferred in male dogs • Red rubber or Tomcat catheter is used in cats and females
Vaginourethrogram	• General anesthesia • Aseptic vestibule foley catheterization	Aqueous iodinated	• 10–15 ml (dog) • 5–10 ml (cat)	1. Survey RL and VD 2. Inject 50% of contrast media 3. RL (image made at end of injection) 4. Inject remaining contrast 5. RL and VD	• Plastic hemostats are used to clamp vulvar lips around the catheter to prevent contrast leakage • The tip of the catheter should be cut to prevent it from extending into the vagina • Terminate injection if back pressure is felt on the syringe plunger

*CT technique may vary and should be optimized based on machine (generation), size of patient and question to be answered. At the author's institution, helical imaging is performed using 125 mAs and 130 kVp. and a pitch of 1.25. Slice thickness ranges from 2.5 mm – 5 mm for both pre and post contrast acquisition, depending on size of patient. Transverse images from the mid urinary bladder through the urethra are obtained using 1.25 mm slice thickness to document ureteral termination. If multi-detector CT is used, images may be reconstructed in thinner slices.

ectopic ureters with reported sensitivities of 100% and 91% compared to 80%, respectively (Samii et al, 2004). The determination of the intramural and extramural course of ectopic ureters, however, is best performed with either antegrade pyelography, or a cystoscopic-guided retrograde ureterogram. Ureteroceles and ureteral strictures can also be assessed with these techniques.

Contraindications/ Complications

Excretory urography may be performed using traditional radiography, fluoroscopy, or computed tomography. Contraindications of these techniques are related to the use of intravenous injection of iodinated contrast media and the need for sedation or general anesthesia. The most common adverse reaction to iodinated contrast media is retching and/or vomiting, and changes in heart rate and blood pressure. These reactions are usually transient and most frequently occur immediately or soon after injection (Heuter, 2005). Although uncommon, other possible reactions include hives, facial and pharyngeal/ laryngeal edema and hypotension (Heuter, 2005, Wallack, 2003). Contrast induced nephropathy (CIN) is a well-known cause of hospital-associated kidney injury in human medicine (Jorgensen, 2013). Although uncommon, acute kidney injury (AKI) has been reported in dogs following intravenous administration of ionic iodinated contrast media (Ihle and Kostolich, 1991, Margulies et al, 1990). The mechanism of CIN AKI is not well understood; however, it is believed to occur secondary to renal vasoconstriction, preexisting hypotension, and direct renal cellular toxicity by the contrast agent (Wallack, 2003). Contraindications for IV iodinated contrast administration (and therefore excretory urography) include previous adverse reaction to iodinated contrast, dehydration, and severe renal compromise. Dehydration must be corrected before IV iodinated contrast administration. Atopic patients may also be at increased risk of an anaphalactoid reaction (Schabelman and Witting, 2010). In general, adverse reactions are more severe and more frequent with the more hypertonic contrast agents; therefore non-ionic contrast media is preferred for all intravascular studies. At the authors' institution, Iohexol [1](240 mg I/ml) is used routinely for all intravascular and urinary positive contrast studies.

Iodinated contrast media has been proven to increase urine specific gravity and also inhibit bacterial growth. It may also falsely elevate urine protein, alter cellular morphology and create atypical urine crystals. For these reasons, it is important to collect urine samples for evaluation prior to injecting any contrast into the urinary tract (Feeney et al, 1980, Ruby et al, 1983).

Specific Advantages of CT Excretory Urography

Compared to radiography and fluoroscopy, CTEU allows the entire urinary tract to be evaluated without superimposition of other structures. CTEU has proven to be more sensitive than radiographic/ fluoroscopic EU in diagnosing ectopic ureters in dogs (Samii et al, 2004). Enemas prior to CTEU may be useful; however, they may not be as crucial as compared to conventional EU. In addition, diagnostic studies may be made with a lower contrast dose of 400 mg I/kg. Multi-planar and 3D reconstructions can be created to further aid in diagnosis, surgical or interventional planning, as well as depicting disease for educational purposes. Although beyond the scope of this chapter, dynamic contrast enhanced CT of the kidneys has been used as an alternate method to calculate GFR.

Interpretation

Normal

There are three phases of the excretory urogram: vascular, nephrogram, and pyelogram (Figure 26.1). The vascular phase occurs approximately 5–7 seconds after contrast injection, and is often not documented. Beginning at approximately 10 seconds, contrast agent enters the glomerular vessels and filtration begins within the nephrons, indicating the nephrogram phase. The normal nephrogram phase is characterized by homogeneous enhancement of the renal parenchyma, with the cortical enhancement occurring first. In addition to evaluation of renal opacification, kidneys should also be assed for normal size, location and margination. The canine kidney should measure 2.5–3.5 times the length of L2 (as measured on the ventrodorsal view); width should be approximately 2 times the length of L2. Normal feline kidneys are 2.4–3.0 times the length of L2 or 4–4.5 cm. The width of the kidney in the cat should measure 3–3.5 cm. At approximately 2 minutes post injection, the nephrogram phase begins to fade and the pyelogram phase begins. The nephrogram phase should continue to fade; in most dogs it is undetectable by 2 hours (Feeney et al, 1980). Differentials for alterations in nephrogram opacifiation and wash out patterns are shown in Figure 26.2. During the pyelogram phase, contrast media is concentrated in the renal tubules, and excreted in the renal pelvis, diverticula, and ureters. In dogs, renal pelvic width should be less than 2 mm. Diverticula should measure less than 1 mm. Normal ureteral peristalsis causes intermittent opacification

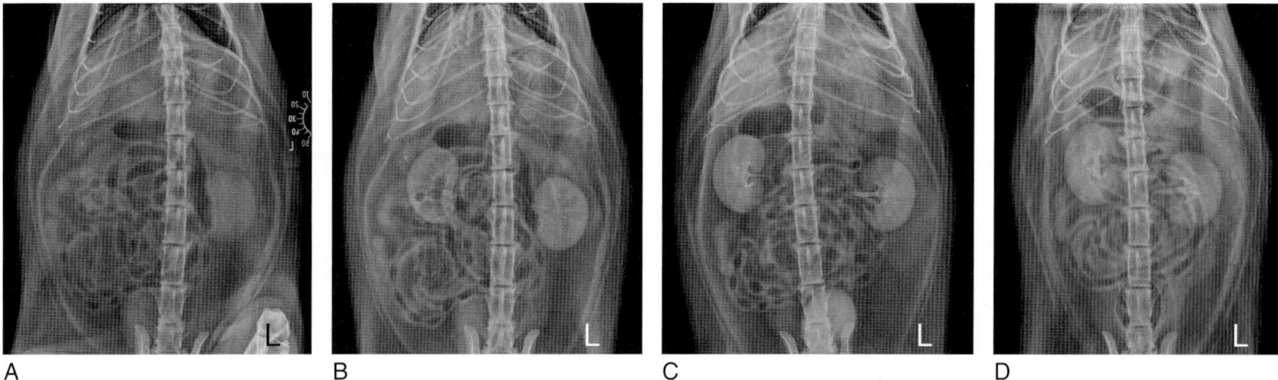

Figure 26.1 Normal phases of the excretory urogram. (A) VD image of the kidneys before IV iodinated contrast administration. (B) Vascular and early nephrogram phases: VD image made approximately 12 seconds after the start of injection. Note the diffuse increase in opacity within the abdomen and numerous contrast enhanced vessels within the peritoneal space, representing the vascular phase. Opacifaction of the renal parenchyma is homogeneous secondary to contrast material within the renal capillaries and tubules, representing a normal nephrogram. (C) Pyelogram phase: VD image made at approximately 5 minutes post IV contrast administration. Positive contrast is now present within the renal pelves, diverticula, and proximal ureters. The pyelogram is more opaque than the nephrogram secondary to water resorbtion within the renal tubules. Note the proximal left ureter is minimally dilated. (D) Pyelogram phase: VD image made at 30 minutes post IV contrast administration. Note the persistent pyelogram and decreased opacification of the nephrogram.

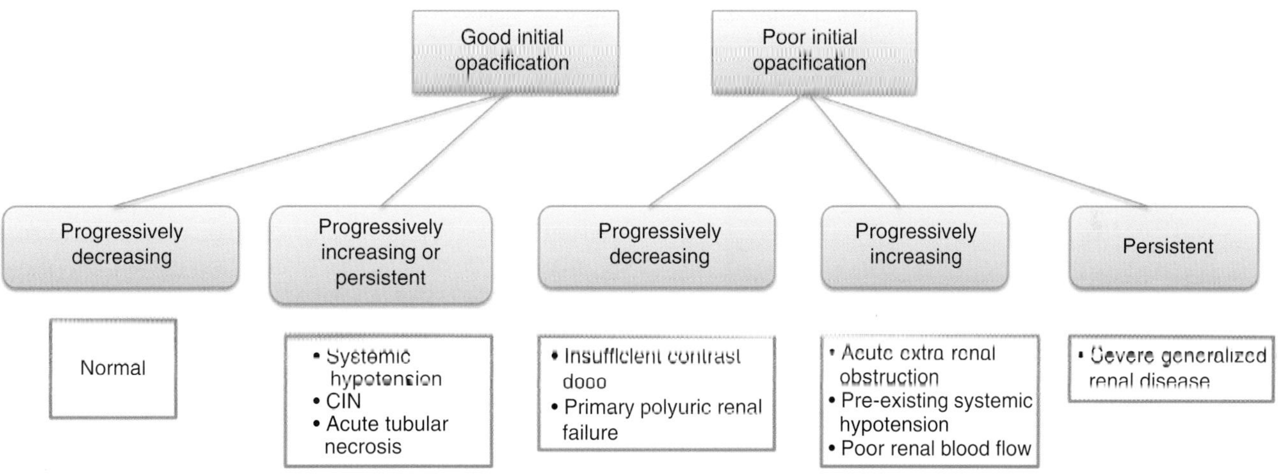

Figure 26.2 Differentials for possible nephrographic opacification patterns.

which often necessitates serial imaging to evaluate their entirety. Normal canine ureters measure less than 2–3 mm. The normal width of the feline renal pelvis and ureter has not been reported but in the author's experience, should measure less than 1.5 mm.

Abnormalities

Absent nephrogram

Diffuse lack of renal opacification may be caused by renal aplasia, renal artery obstruction, non- functioning renal tissue, nephrectomy, or insufficient contrast dose (Figure 26.3).

Non-uniform nephrogram

Non-uniform opacification of the renal parenchyma may be caused by neoplasms, hematomas, cysts, infarcts, or abscess (Figure 26.4). Multifocal non-uniform opacification may also be seen with chronic generalized glomerular or tubulointerstitial disease and feline infectious peritonitis (Seiler, 2012).

Renal pelvic and ureteral dilation

Renal pelvic and ureteral dilation is caused by inflammation (pyelonephritis and ureteritis) or obstruction (hydronephrosis and hydroureter). Although mild renal pelvic dilation may occur secondary to diuresis or

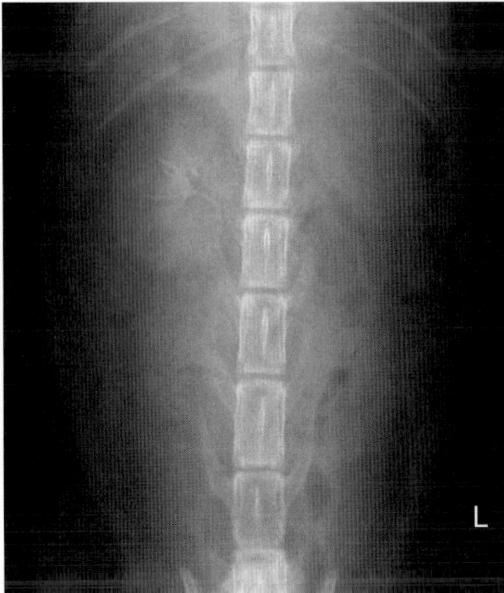

Figure 26.3 A feline patient with renal vascular compromise. VD image during an excretory urogram of a cat presenting for renal failure following vehicular trauma. Notice the lack of nephrogram and pyelogram opacification of the left kidney. Lack of blood flow to the left kidney was confirmed with abdominal ultrasound, presumed secondary to renal artery thrombosis and/or avulsion.

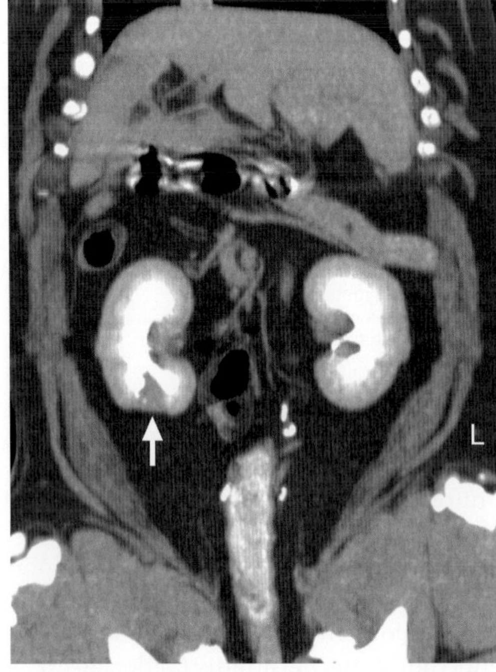

Figure 26.4 Chronic renal infarct as seen with CTEU in a dog. Dorsal maximum intensity projection (MIP) of an excretory urogram in a dog. There is a triangular non- contrast enhancing region within the caudal pole of the left kidney and an associated flattening of the caudal cortex (arrow), consistent with a chronic renal infarct.

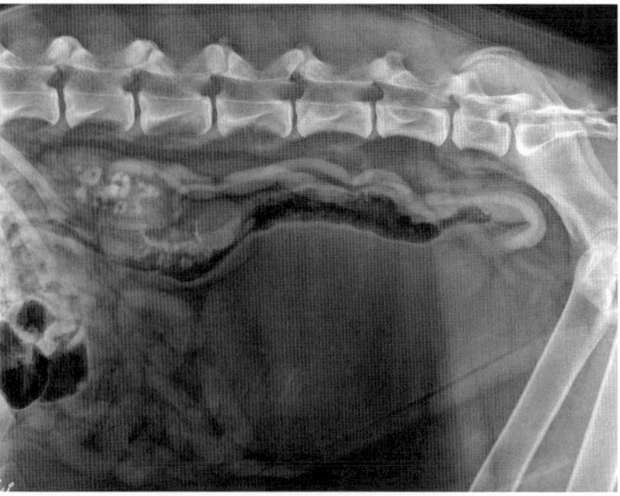

Figure 26.5 Lateral radiograph of a male dog after excretory urogram with bilateral hydroureter. The renal diverticula are mild to moderately distended and blunted with rounded margins. Both ureters are also moderately dilated to the level of the ureterovesicular junctions, measuring greater than 3 mm wide, likely secondary to associated ureteritis or a ureteral obstruction. Note the normal "J hook" of the caudal ureters.

renal insufficiency, pelvic dilation greater than 3 mm should raise concern for pyelonephritis and/or obstruction. Pyelonephritis alone typically causes renal pelvic dilation less than 8 mm in dogs and 5 mm in cats and may cause mild proximal ureteral dilation. Early or partial ureteral obstruction, however, may also cause a similar degree of dilation. In addition to dilation of the renal pelvis and proximal ureter, as seen with acute pyelonephritis, chronic pyelonephritis may cause irregularity of the renal pelvis and blunting of the renal diverticula. Obstructive disorders secondary to calculi, blood clots, neoplasms, or strictures often result in renal pelvic dilation greater than 8 mm (greater than 5 mm in cats), and may result in concurrent hydroureter. In both dogs and cats, a renal pelvis measuring greater than 13 mm is indicative of obstruction (with or without concurrent infection) (D'Anjou et al, 2011) (Figure 26.5). It is important to remember that a normal pyelogram phase does not rule out acute pyelonephritis. Various degrees of renal pelvic dilation are shown in Figure 26.6.

Renal pelvic or ureteral filling defects

Filling defects within the renal pelvis can be caused by calculi, blood clots, or neoplasms (Figure 26.7). Radiopaque calculi may appear either radiolucent or mineral opaque when surrounded by positive contrast material (Figure 26.8). Blood clots and neoplasia will appear radiolucent.

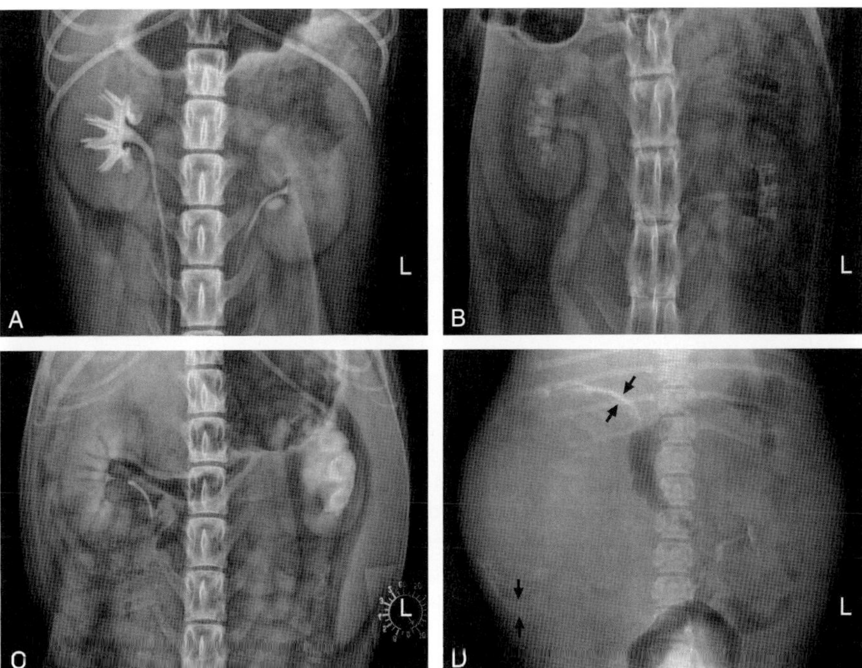

Figure 26.6 VD radiographic images of various degrees of renal pelvic dilation as seen with EU in the dog. (A) Mild to moderate dilation of the right renal pelvis with mild dilation of the diverticula. (B) Moderate dilation of the right renal pelvis, diverticula and ureter and mild dilation of the left diverticula and proximal ureter. Note the blunted diverticula, bilaterally. (C) Marked dilation of the left renal pelvis causing effacement of the diverticula. (D) Severe hydronephrosis of the right kidney causing severe renomegaly and thinning of the renal cortex (black arrows).

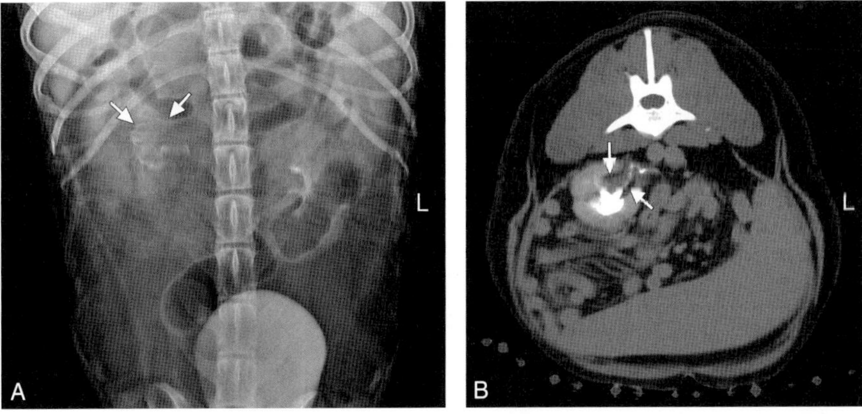

Figure 26.7 Renal pelvic filling defects as seen with excretory urography in a dog. (A) Ventrodorsal image of the pyelogram phase in a dog with chronic hematuria. The right renal pelvis is expanded and there is a poorly defined, irregular filling defect (arrows) in the cranial and medial aspect, extending into the proximal ureter. (B) CTEU showing the pyelogram phase of the right kidney of a different dog with chronic hematuria. A triangular hypoattenuating filling defect (arrows) is located within the dorsal aspect of the renal pelvis and extending into the proximal ureter. The pelvis is moderately dilated. Differentials for both of these cases include renal pelvic blood clot or neoplasia. Blood clots were confirmed with surgery in both patients.

Ectopic ureters

Ectopic ureters may be normal in size; however, 50% are dilated and associated with hydronephrosis (Berent et al, 2012; Reichler et al, 2012). They may terminate within the bladder neck, urethra, vestibule, or vagina. Additional abnormalities that can be seen with ureteral ectopia include abnormal accumulation of positive contrast within the urethra, vagina, or vestibule, and ureterocele (Figure 26.9). Distinguishing between extramural and intramural ectopic ureters can be

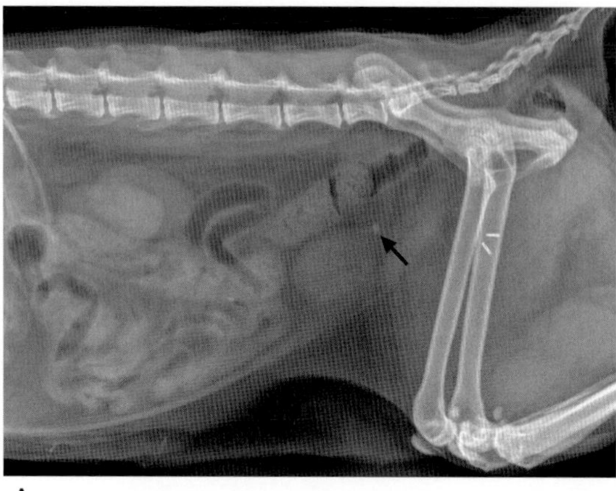

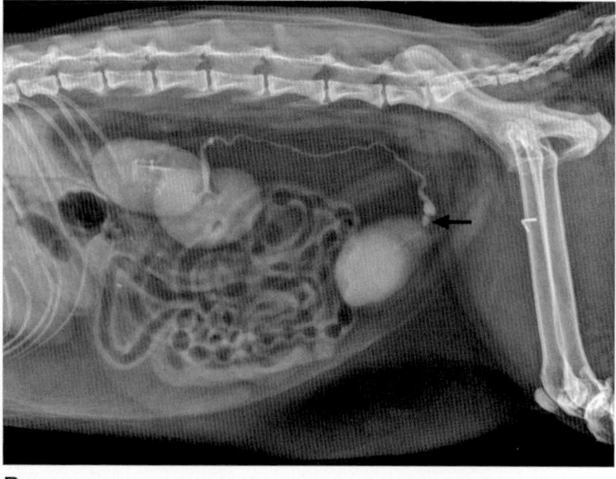

Figure 26.8 Ureterolith in a cat. (A) Lateral survey image of a cat with a history of chronic urinary bladder and urethral calculi. There is a small oval mineral opacity (arrow) along the dorsal aspect of the trigone of the urinary bladder. (B) Lateral image of the same patient during the pyelogram phase of an excretory urogram. The mineral opacity seen on survey images represents a calculus in the distal left ureter (arrow). Notice the focal dilation of the ureter immediately proximal to the calculus, the diffuse ureteral opacification, indicating decreased peristalsis, and the mild dilation of the proximal left ureter secondary to partial ureteral obstruction.

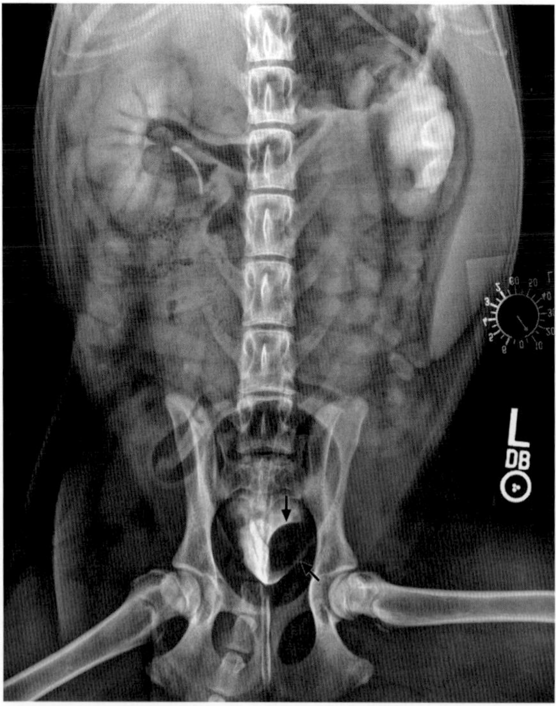

Figure 26.9 Ureterocele. Excretory urogram in a dog with chronic urinary incontinence. There is an ovoid, well defined, filling defect (arrows) along the left caudal aspect of the urinary bladder, secondary to focal dilation of the left ureter. Notice the moderate dilation of the left renal pelvis. The right ureter can be seen along the medial aspect of this filling defect, extending caudal to the trigone, and lacks a normal "J hook". Bilateral ectopic ureters and left ureterocele were confirmed with cystoscopy.

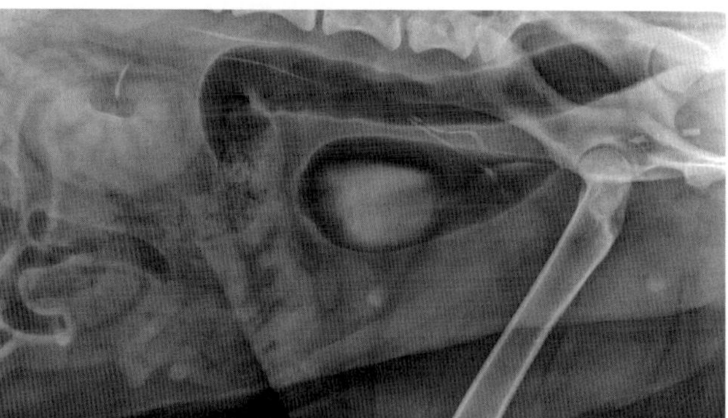

Figure 26.10 Excretory urogram of intramural ectopic ureters. Oblique image of an excretory urogram in a female dog with chronic urinary incontinence. The distal right ureter approaches the trigone, however continues caudally, conforming to the dorsolateral wall of the urinary bladder neck. The left ureter has a similar course but cannot be seen caudal to the trigone on this image. Notice the lack of the normal "J hook" of the caudal ureters, bilaterally. Both ureters have intermittent opacification, indicating normal peristalsis. Bilateral intramural ectopic ureters were confirmed with cystoscopy.

difficult; however, in a study comparing the use of radiography/fluoroscopy and CTEU, more dogs were correctly diagnosed with intramural tunneling using CTEU (Samii et al, 2004) (Figure 26.10 and Figure 26.11). Severe hydroureter and hydronephrosis, to the level of the ureterovesicular junction, is commonly seen in male dogs with ectopic ureters, and many may be

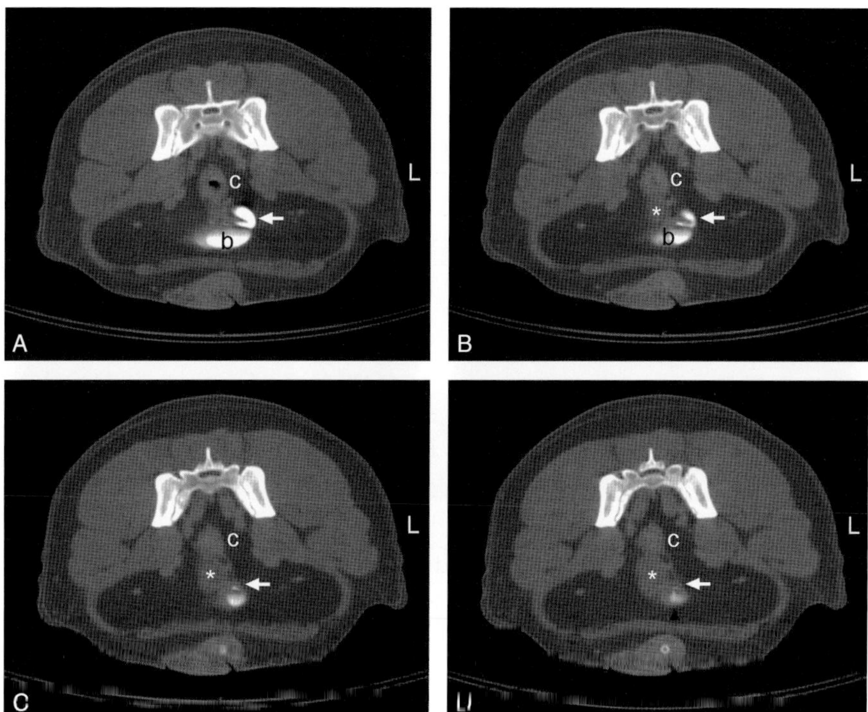

Figure 26.11 CTEU of left intramural ectopic ureter. Sequential (cranial to caudal) transverse images of the termination of the left ureter of an incontinent male dog during excretory urography. (A) The caudal left ureter (arrow) is mild to moderately dilated and turning medially to form a normal "J hook" as it nears the caudal trigone. A small amount of positive contrast is in the urinary bladder (b). (B) The positive contrast media within the caudal left ureter courses within the wall of the dorsal urinary bladder neck. (C) A focus of positive contrast material is in the dorsal wall of the urinary bladder neck, representing tunneling of the left ectopic ureter. (D) The focus of positive contrast within the dorsal wall of the proximal urethra is confluent with intraluminal urethral contrast material (arrow), indicating the ectopic ureteral opening. (b = urinary bladder, c = colon, * = prostate)

completely continent. This finding should instigate a thorough investigation of the location of the UVJ by cystoscopy or CTEU.

Focal ureteral abnormalities

Focal, persistent ureteral narrowing may be secondary to ureteral stricture or extra-luminal compression, secondary to an adjacent mass. Ureterocele and ureteral diverticulum are seen as focal ureteral dilations (Figure 26.9).

Percutaneous Antegrade Pyelography

Indications

Percutaneous pyelography using ultrasound guidance is indicated in patients who produce inadequate excretory urograms, or those in which intravenous iodinated contrast administration is contraindicated. Percutaneous pyelography gives no information about the nephrogram phase; however, it is more useful than an EU to evaluate the renal pelvis, ureters, and ureteral termination, particularly in cases of suspected partial or complete ureteral obstruction. Better contrast may be achieved, and each ureter can be evaluated individually, allowing increased sensitivity to subtle changes. Interpretation is similar to the pyelogram phase of the excretory urogram (Figure 26.12).

Contraindications/Complications

Possible complications of percutaneous antegrade pyelography include direct damage from needle placement, renal hemorrhage, renal pelvic laceration, and renal pelvic clot formation. Leakage of positive contrast from the renal pelvis can occur (Figure 26.12), and if severe may lead to a non- diagnostic exam. In a study of 18 antegrade pyelograms in cats with suspected ureteral obstruction, leakage of contrast occurred in 44% of exams, preventing interpretation in 28% (5/18) (Adin et al, 2003; Heuter, 2005).

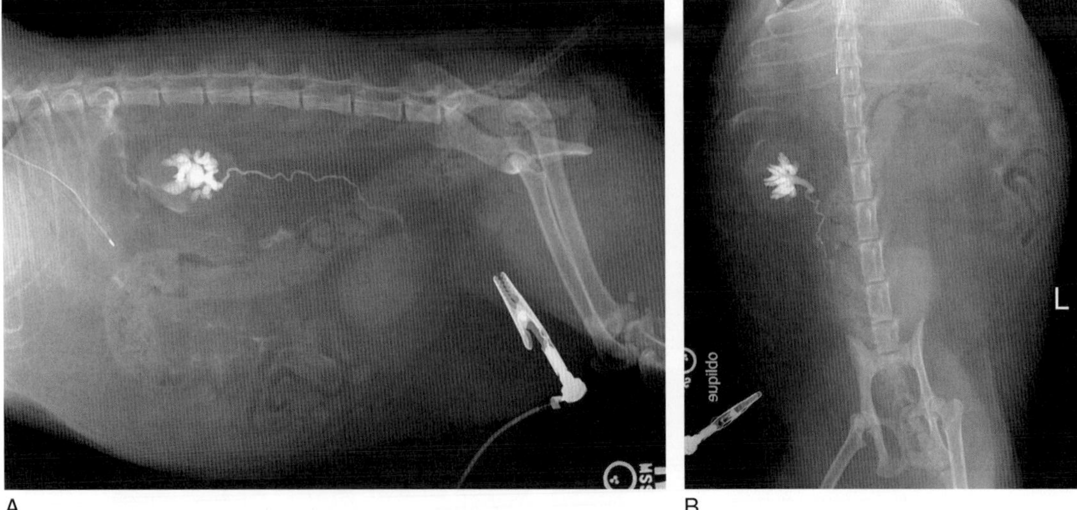

Figure 26.12 Percutaneous pyelogram in a cat. Lateral (A) and ventrodorsal (B) images after ultrasound guided percutaneous injection of iodinated contrast media into the right renal pelvis. The right renal pelvis and diverticula are mild to moderately dilated and the proximal ureter is mildly dilated. The right ureter is entirely opacified and slightly tortous. Notice the lack of positive contrast media within the urinary bladder. There is a small amount of positive contrast media within the retroperitoneal and peritoneal spaces, secondary to leakage at the injection site. Wet hair is also along the right abdominal body wall. A stricture of the distal right ureter was confirmed with surgery.

Cystography

Indications (Positive, Negative, Double)

Contrast cystography allows for visualization of the bladder, assessment of bladder wall integrity, thickness and contour, and the investigation of intraluminal abnormalities such as cystoliths and masses. Negative contrast cystography is primarily useful for the determination of bladder wall thickness (Figure 26.13) and to provide a negative contrast to the ureters in EU investigation of ectopic ureters. Positive and double contrast cystography are more sensitive for mucosal and luminal abnormalities which may be associated with clinical signs of dysuria, as well as for bladder rupture. These may also be used to assess patients for urachal diverticulae. Double contrast cystography is often used to detect radiolucent cystoliths, and appears to be more accurate than ultrasonography in determining their size regardless of radiopacity (Byl et al, 2010).

Ultrasonography and plain radiography may not clearly determine the position of the bladder in a patient with an intra-abdominal, perineal, or retroperitoneal mass, particularly if it is fluid-filled (Figure 26.14). Contrast cystography will clearly distinguish the urinary bladder, and assess any luminal communication between it and the mass.

Contraindications/Complications

Complications of cystography are uncommon; however, they are usually associated with catheterization. Possible adverse events include iatrogenic urinary bladder or urethral trauma, bacterial contamination, and intramural contrast medium accumulation (Figure 26.15). Although rare, fatal gas embolization has been reported as a complication of pneumocystography in dogs and cats (Thayer et al, 1980, Ackerman et al, 1972). Risk of death by gas embolization is reduced by use of nitrogen or carbon dioxide. Imaging in left lateral recumbency during negative contrast cystography may also prevent death from embolism by trapping gas emboli in the right ventricle thus preventing release into the pulmonary arterial system (Wallack, 2003).

Interpretation

The urinary bladder should be evaluated for normal margination, shape, location, and lack of contrast media extravasation. With positive and negative cystography, contrast media should be homogeneous and evenly distributed throughout the urinary bladder. During double contrast cystography, positive contrast media should pool in the dependent portion of the urinary bladder. Abnormalities may appear as mucosal

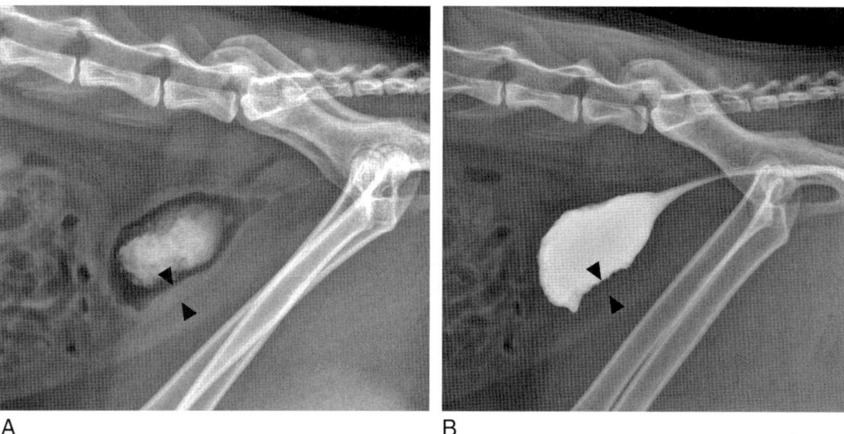

Figure 26.13 Double contrast (A) and positive contrast (B) cystograms in a cat with chronic cystitis. The bladder wall is diffusely thickened, most severe cranioventrally (arrows) with an irregular mucosal margin. Notice the improved visualization of the bladder wall with the double contrast study. The small out-pouching of the cranioventral wall may represent irregularity secondary to cystitis or a small diverticulum. Although the urinary bladder appears incompletely distended, adequate distension was determined based on manual palpation. Further distension was not possible in this patient due to non- compliance of the chronically diseased bladder wall.

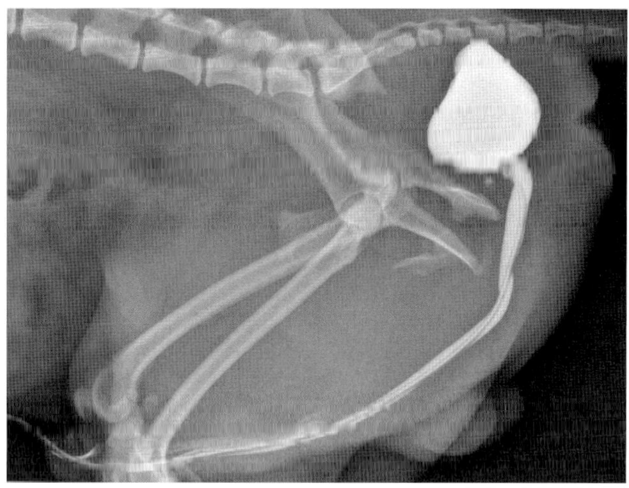

Figure 26.14 Traumatic perineal urinary bladder herniation in a dog. A positive contrast cystogram was performed to confirm the location of the urinary bladder, which is retroflexed and herniated into the perineal region. Extravasation of contrast media is not seen, however complete distension of the bladder was not attempted. Note the multiple pelvic fractures and loss of serosal detail within the retroperitoneal space, secondary to hemorrhage and/or urine.

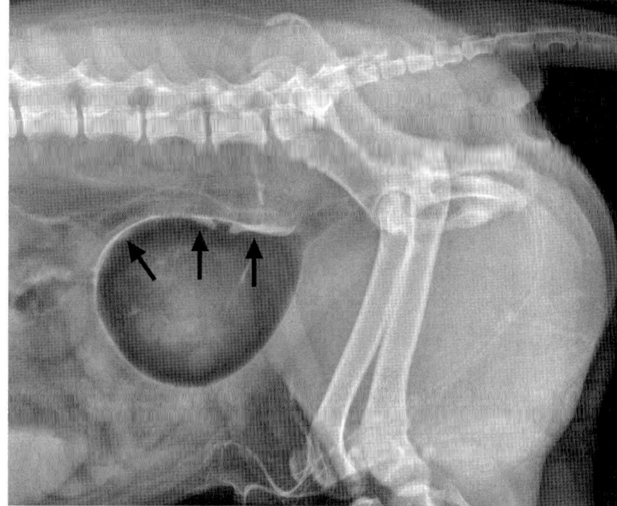

Figure 26.15 Intramural contrast accumulation secondary to double contrast cystogram. Lateral image of a double contrast cystogram in a dog. There is a small amount of positive contrast material and a gas bubble conforming to the dorsal wall of the urinary bladder (arrows), consistent with intramural contrast media accumulation. Note the several small gas bubbles along the periphery of the positive contrast pool. A small amount of positive contrast media is on the patient's fur.

irregularity, intramural thickening, filling defects, and extravasation.

Abnormalities

Mucosal irregularity

Mucosal irregularity can be focal or diffuse and may be seen with cystitis, neoplasms, or hematoma. Cystitis, including polyploid cystitis, is often located cranioventrally (Figure 26.13). Regions of ulceration can be diagnosed with double contrast cystography as focal contrast adherence along the bladder mucosa. Contrast dissection into the bladder wall as a result of high contrast injection pressures and/or disease of the bladder wall is also best seen with a double contrast study (Figure 26.15).

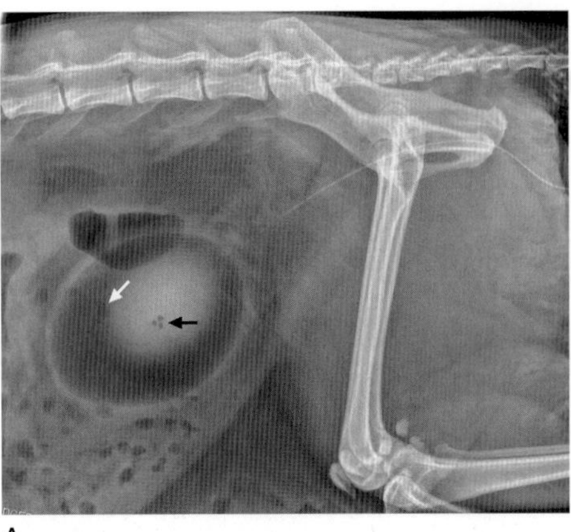
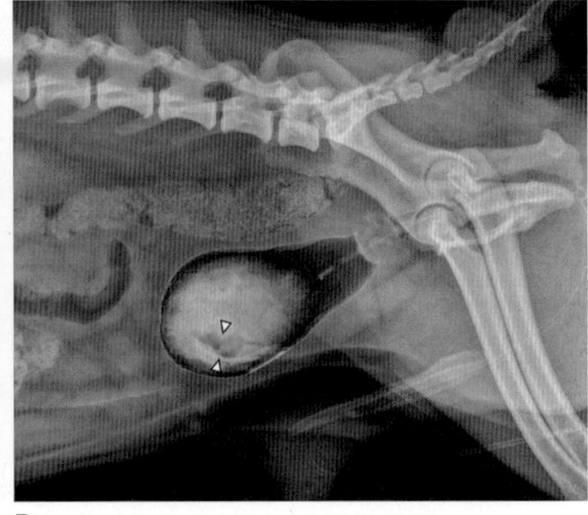

A B

Figure 26.16 Filling defects seen with double contrast cystography. (A) Lateral view of a double contrast cystogram in a cat. There are three small round, smoothly margined filling defects (black arrow), consistent with calculi, located within the central region of the pool of positive contrast. Several gas bubbles are seen along the periphery of the positive contrast pool (white arrow). (B) Lateral view of a double contrast cystogram in a male dog with hematuria. The central pool of positive contrast media is not homogeneous and there is a fusiform filling defect within the ventral periphery of the contrast pool (arrow heads), consistent with a blood clot.

Intramural thickening

Although bladder wall thickening may be seen with all forms of cystography, it is best evaluated using a negative or double contrast study (Figure 26.13). The normal canine bladder wall has been reported to measure approximately 1 mm thick on double contrast cystogram (Mahaffey et al, 1984). Thickening may be focal or diffuse and is seen with inflammation, fibrosis, hemorrhage/hematoma, and neoplasia. Because mild wall thickening may be masked by over-distension and thickening may be artifactual due to inadequate distension, the importance of appropriate bladder distension is stressed. The typical urinary bladder can hold 5–10 ml/kg and 2–5 ml/kg in dogs and cats, respectively. A non-compliant bladder wall secondary to disease may tolerate much less, therefor it is recommended that the bladder be palpated during injection to prevent overdistension and rupture. It should be distended until palpably turgid.

Filling defects

Filling defects may be mobile or attached and always appear radiolucent when surrounded by positive contrast media. Mobile filling defects are caused by calculi, gas bubbles and blood clots (Figure 26.16). Using double contrast cystography, gas bubbles can be distinguished by their peripheral location along the pool of contrast. Unless adhered to the bladder mucosa, calculi are centrally located on all contrast studies. Blood clots may be located anywhere within the lumen (Essman, 2005). The margination and shape of these filling defects are also useful identifiers. Gas bubbles will be round, well defined, and smoothly margined. Blood clots are often poorly defined, and irregularly margined. Calculi can vary in margination and shape and often have ill-defined borders. Attached (non-mobile) filling defects may be created by bladder wall neoplasia, polyps, inflammation or hematoma, adhered blood clots, adhered calculi, or ureteroceles.

Bladder diverticulum

Urinary bladder diverticuli may be congenital or acquired secondary to trauma. They appear as a focal outward extension of the cranioventral bladder lumen (Figure 26.17).

Contrast extravasation

Loss of integrity of the urinary bladder wall will lead to leakage of positive or negative contrast into the peritoneal cavity (Figure 26.18). When adequate bladder distension is achieved, contrast media leakage usually occurs simultaneously with injection, therefore fluoroscopic examination during injection is useful. Small bladder tears may require additional images to be made after 5–10 minutes to document delayed leakage of contrast media (Marloff and Park, 2012). Contrast extravasation may also be caused by congenital or acquired fistulas. Rectovesicular and vaginovesicular are most common.

Vesicoureteral reflux

Reflux of contrast media into the ureters can be seen in normal animals, most commonly less than 3 months of age (Thrall, 2012). Occasionally iatrogenic vesicoureteral

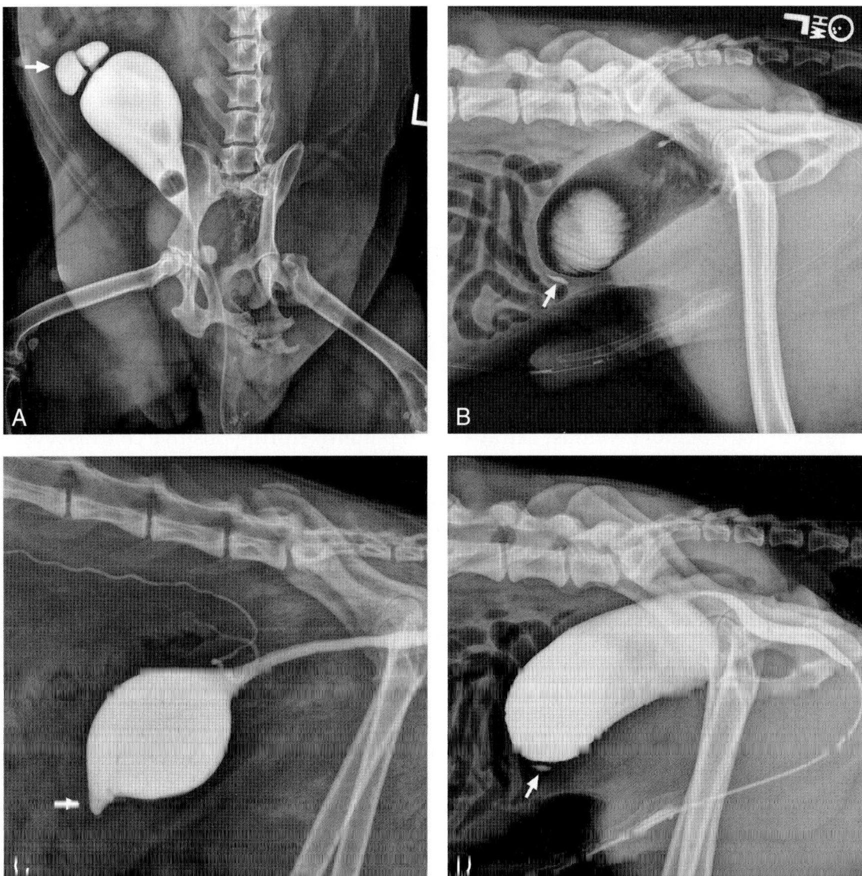

Figure 26.17 Urinary bladder diverticula. (A) Positive contrast cystogram with a dog in VD showing a large, septated diverticulum arising from the cranial bladder wall. Note the gas within the Foley catheter balloon and the gas bubbles within bladder lumen, seen as eccentrically located, smoothly margined filling defects. (B) A double contrast cystogram in a dog in lateral recumbency with a small diverticulum. A small amount of positive contrast is retained within the diverticulum or adhered to the mucosa. Notice the pelvic location of the caudal urinary bladder (pelvic bladder). (C) Positive contrast cystogram in a cat with a urinary bladder diverticulum and chronic cystitis. Notice the mild irregularity of the mucosa adjacent to the diverticulum, secondary to chronic cystitis. There is bilateral vesicoureteral reflux. Notice the location of the UVJ in the feline patient is in the proximal urethra, rather than the bladder trigone as seen in dogs. (D) Positive contrast cystogram in the same dog as (B) in lateral recumbency. Notice the small separate accumulation of positive contrast within the diverticulum. The urinary bladder is partially intra-pelvic with lack of a bladder neck (pelvic bladder).

reflux occurs in older animals, especially with increased intravesicular pressures. Vesicoureteral reflux secondary to disease may be seen with cystitis, urinary tract obstruction, neurologic disease, and congenital ureteral anomalies (Essman, 2005) (Figure 26.19).

Urethography/Vaginourethrography

Indications

Urethrography in the male and vaginourethrography in the female are generally performed to assess the integrity of the urethral wall or to look for filling defects that may indicate urethral calculi, stricture, polyps, or neoplasia. The most common indication is an animal with difficulty passing urine or with a palpably abnormal urethra or prostate on rectal examination. Animals that have sustained trauma can be assessed for urethral or vaginal rupture using these techniques. In male dogs with functional obstruction of the urethra due to urethrospasm, transient narrowing of the urethra may be seen using contrast urethrography. Although rare, the visualization of urethrovaginal or urethrorectal fistulas may also be diagnosed with this technique. This procedure combined with urethroscopy is often ideal in the diagnosis of urethral lesions, allowing the potential for biopsy and/or treatment concurrently (see subsequent sections).

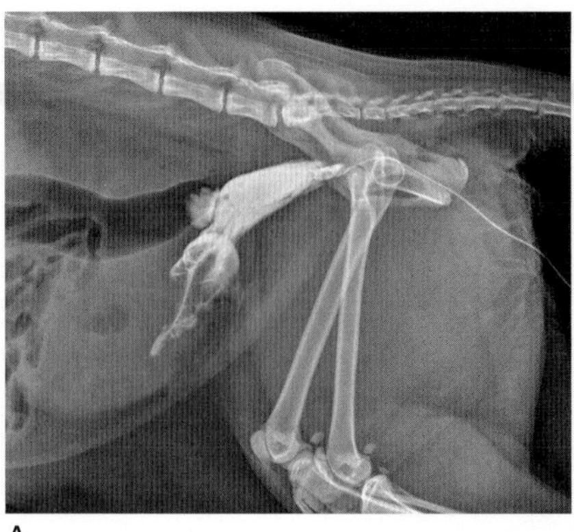
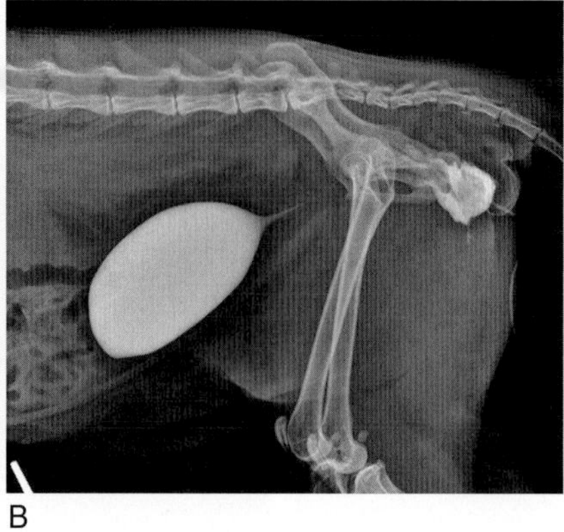
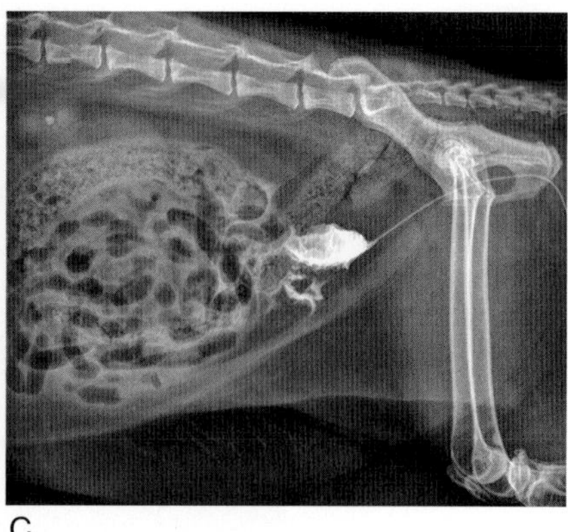

A B C

Figure 26.18 Urethral and urinary bladder contrast extravasation patterns during positive contrast cystourethrogram studies in three different cats in lateral recumbency. (A) Positive contrast cystourethrogram in a cat with recent urethral obstruction. The urinary bladder neck and proximal urethra are not defined and positive contrast material is extending into the caudal peritoneal space, secondary to a tear in the bladder neck and proximal urethra. Notice the lack of positive contrast within the urinary bladder and the mild loss of serosal detail. The urinary catheter is coiled on itself in the membranous urethra. (B) Positive contrast cystourethrogram in cat with recent urethral obstruction and repeated catheterization. Positive contrast is extending into the soft tissues in the region of the penile and caudal membranous urethra. A defined urethra in this region is not identified. Note the increased soft tissue opacity and loss of serosal detail within the retroperitoneal space, secondary to urine tracking cranially from the intrapelvic periurethral tissues. (C) Positive contrast cystogram in a cat with uroabdomen after recent cystotomy. The urinary bladder is minimally distended and there is extension of positive contrast into the adjacent peritoneal space, secondary to leakage at the cystotomy site. Notice the mild loss of serosal detail. A nephrolith is located within the right kidney and the right kidney is small and misshapen, secondary to chronic renal disease.

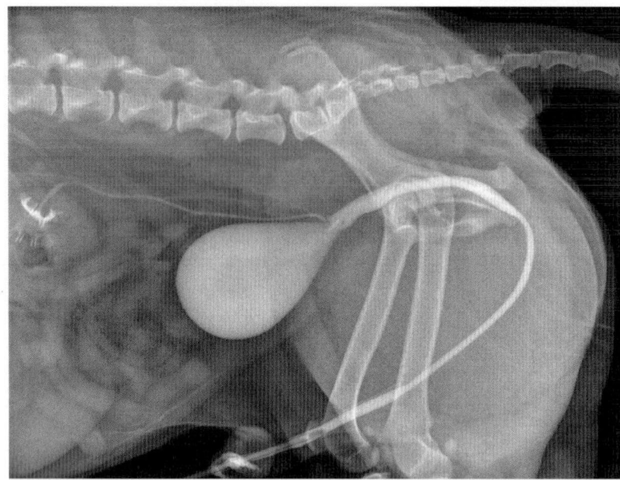

Figure 26.19 Cystourethrogram in a male dog with ectopic ureters. Lateral image of a positive contrast cystourethrogram with ureterovesicular reflux. The ureters enter caudally at the junction of the bladder neck and proximal urethra, indicating bilateral ectopia. The urethra and bladder are otherwise normal.

Contraindications/Complications

Complications of urethrography include trauma, rupture, or tearing of the urethra, vagina, and vestibule. In addition, sterile technique should be employed to prevent bacterial contamination.

Interpretation

The normal urethra should be smoothly margined and well defined along its entire length. The diameter of the normal male urethra can vary slightly depending on anatomic region and degree of distension. Not to be confused with urethral narrowing secondary to prostatic enlargement, the prostatic urethra may be narrower than the membranous portion when incompletely distended. This is often confused for a urethral obstruction (Figure 26.20). During maximum distension, the prostatic urethra has a greater diameter than the membraneous portion and longitudinal striation may be seen dorsally representing the urethral crest (Ticer et al, 1980). The colliculus seminalis is located at the center of the urethral crest and may be seen as a focal small filling defect along the dorsal wall of the prostatic urethra (Figure 26.20). Varying degrees of urethroprostatic reflux (Figure 26.21) and mild tapered narrowing of the penile urethra at the ischial arch may be seen in normal dogs. Otherwise, the diameter of the penile urethra should be uniform (Ticer et al, 1980).

During vaginourethrography, positive contrast media preferentially fills the vagina and vestibule and extends cranially to the cervix. If performed during estrus, contrast media may pass through the cervix into the uterus (Thrall, 2012). A normal mild narrowing is present at the junction between the vagina and vestibule (cingulum).

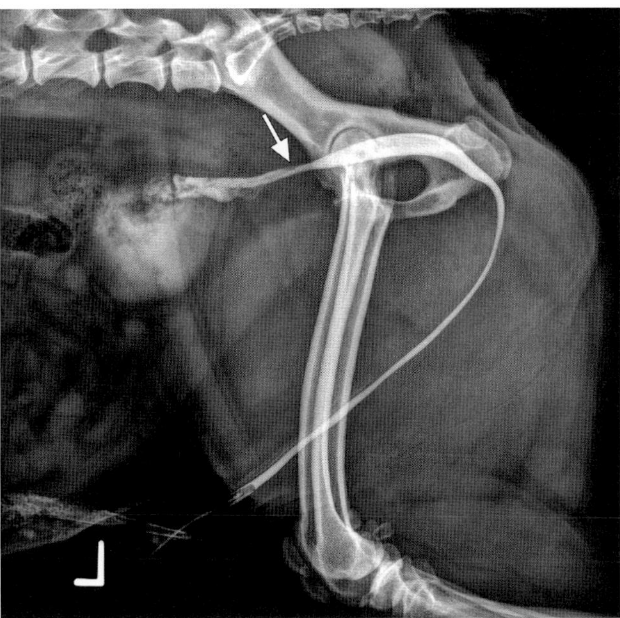

Figure 26.20 Normal urethrogram in a dog. The colliculus seminalis is variably seen as a small filling defect along the dorsal aspect of the prostatic urethra (arrow).

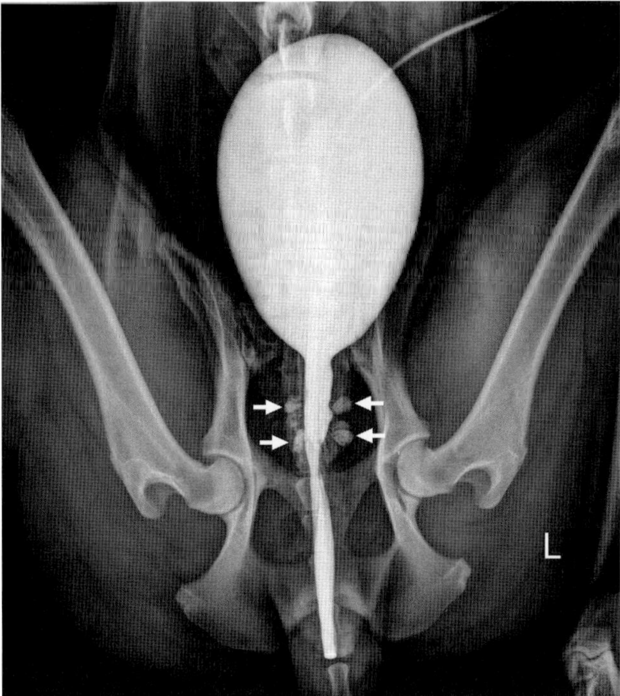

Figure 26.21 Urethroprostatic reflux. Ventrodorsal urethrogram image of a male intact dog. There are several rounded accumulations of positive contrast material (arrows) within the central aspect of the prostate, adjacent to the prostatic urethra. Cystic benign prostatic hypertrophy was confirmed with ultrasound examination and cytology.

Vestibulovaginal stenosis has been reported as a possible contributor to urinary incontinence and recurrent urinary tract infection. Dogs with a vestibulovaginal ratio of < 0.20–0.25 were reported to have increased incidence of lower urinary tract disease (Crawford and Adams, 2002, Kieves, 2011); however, not all dogs with a narrowed cingulum have clinical signs of disease (Wang et al, 2006). More study is needed to understand the contribution of the vestibulovaginal junction to lower urinary tract disease. With increased pressure during contrast media injection, retrograde filling of the urethra will occur. The female urethra should be smoothly margined, well defined and uniform in diameter (Figure 26.22).

Intraluminal filling defects

Intraluminal filling defects may represent calculi, blood clots, or gas bubbles. The most common locations for urethral calculi in male dogs are at the base of the os penis and at the ischial arch. Calculi appear as persistent filling defects that are variable in shape and indistinctly margined (Figure 26.23). They may be associated with focal widening of the urethral lumen. Gas bubbles are smooth, round to oval filling defects that do not persist with subsequent injections. Blood clots are often poorly margined and may either be mobile or fixed.

Mucosal irregularity and mural filling defects

Filling defects originating from the urethral wall and mucosal irregularity may be caused by either inflammation or neoplasia. These lesions may be associated with urethral luminal narrowing; however expansion can also be seen if a luminal mass is present (Figure 26.24).

Urethral stricture

Strictures appear as a repeatable focal luminal narrowing and must be differentiated from incomplete urethral distention or spasm. To confirm the presence of a stricture, adequate distension may be ensured by placing the tip of the urinary catheter immediately distal to the narrowing and making images during contrast media injection (Figure 26.25).

Contrast extravasation

Extravasation of positive contrast into the adjacent soft tissues occurs with urethal rupture occurring secondary to obstruction, neoplasia, trauma, or catheterization (Figure 26.18). Urethroprostatic reflux can be normal; however, contrast media should be confined to the prostatic ducts. Large regions of positive contrast within the prostate or pooling of contrast within the prostate is abnormal and may be associated with neoplasia, cystic benign prostatic hypertrophy, or prostatic abscess (Dennis et al, 2001) (Figure 26.21).

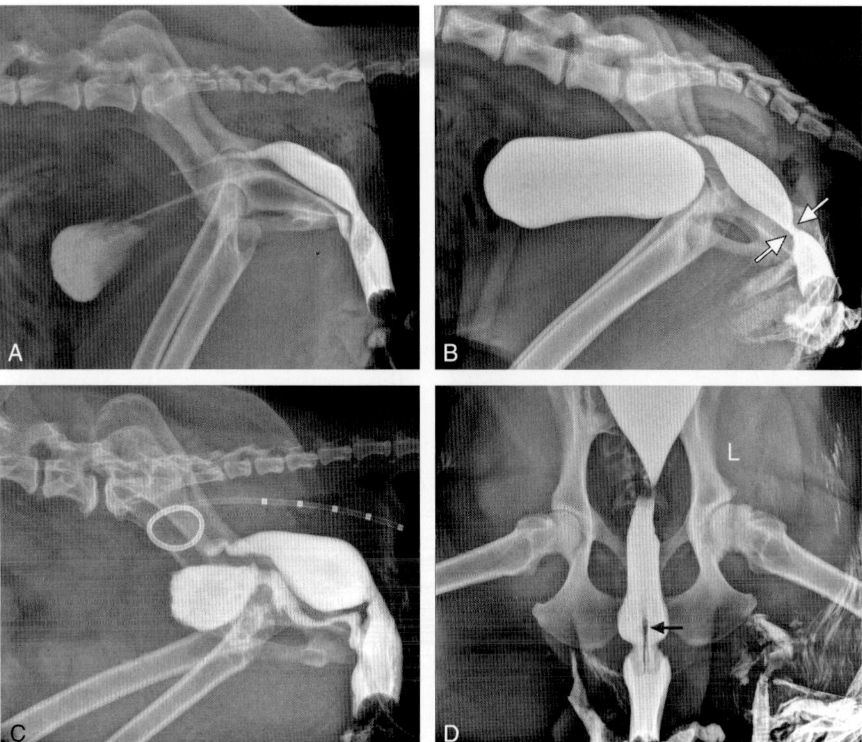

Figure 26.22 Normal and abnormal vagionourethrogram studies. (A) Normal vagiourethrogram. Aside from the Foley catheter and intravestibular gas bubbles, positive contrast media in the vestibule, vagina, and urethra is homogeneous and mucosal margins are smooth. (B) Vagiourethrogram in a dog with recurrent urinary tract infections. Notice the mild narrowing at the vestibulovaginal junction (white arrows) and partially intra-pelvic bladder. (C) Vagiourethrogram of a dog with urethral and bladder transitional cell carcinoma. The mucosal margins of the mid to proximal urethra and entire urinary bladder are irregular and there is a focal mural filling defect along the ventral aspect of the caudal bladder neck/proximal urethra. Note the lack of urinary bladder distension and compensatory vaginal dilation, secondary to non- compliance of the urinary bladder and/or partial urethral obstruction. Note the radiopaque measuring catheter within the rectum. (D) Ventrodorsal view of a vagiourethrogram in a dog with a vaginal septum. There is a linear filling defect (black arrow) in the region of the vestibulovaginal junction and extending into the vagina.

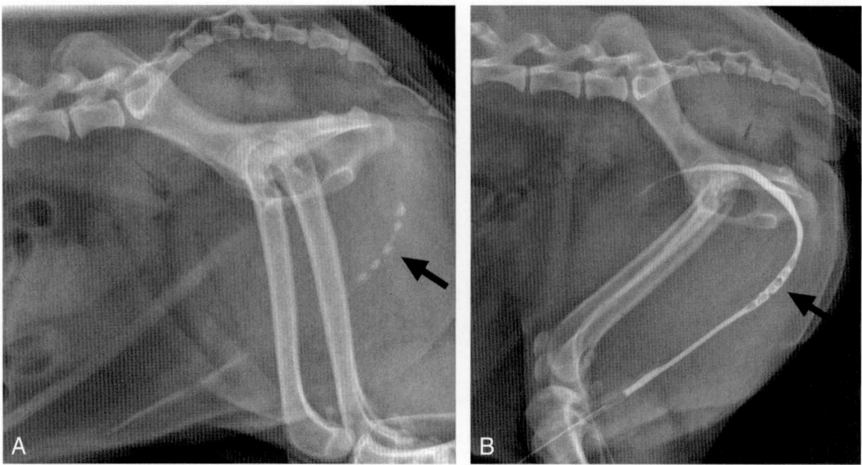

Figure 26.23 Urethral calculi in a male dog. (A) Lateral survey image of a dog presenting for pollakiuria and hematuria. There are several oval mineral opacities (arrow) within the mid penile urethra, representing calculi. (B) Lateral urethrogram image of the same patient. The calculi are seen as numerous radiolucent filling defects (arrow) within the penile urethra with associated mild urethral expansion. Note the tip of the urinary catheter in the distal penile urethra, at the level of the os penis.

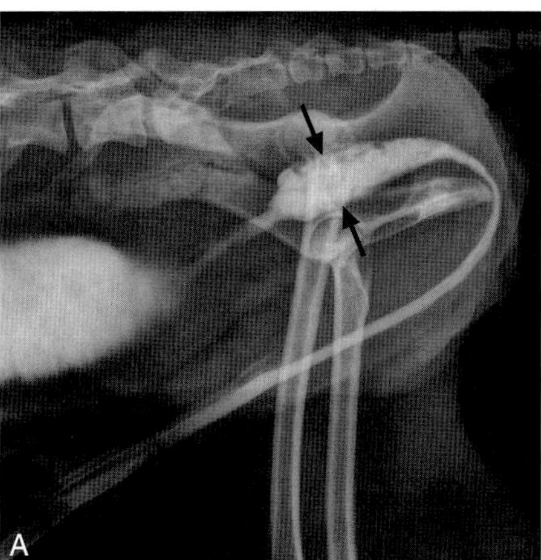

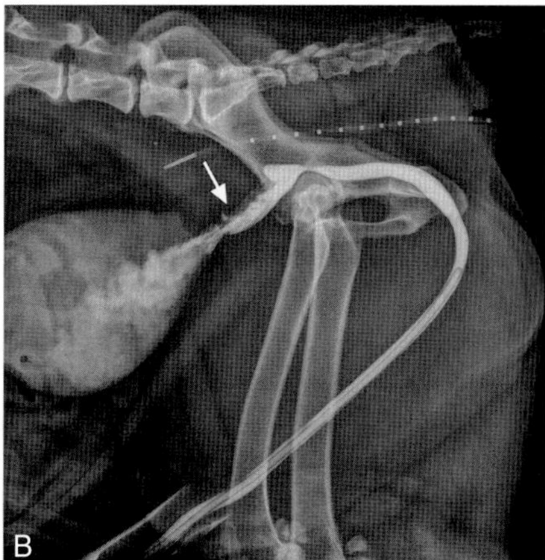

Figure 26.24 Urethral and prostatic neoplasia. (A) Urethrogram in a male dog in lateral recumbency with transitional cell carcinoma of the membraneous urethra. The membraneous urethra is dilated (black arrows) and the intraluminal positive contrast has a heterogeneous appearance secondary to numerous poorly defined filling defects. (B) Urethrogram in a male dog in lateral recumbency with prostatic adenocarcinoma. There is a large irregularly margined mural filling defect (white arrow) along the dorsal aspect of the prostatic urethra, extending cranially into the dorsal bladder neck and trigone. Note the radiopaque measuring catheter in the rectum and caudal colon.

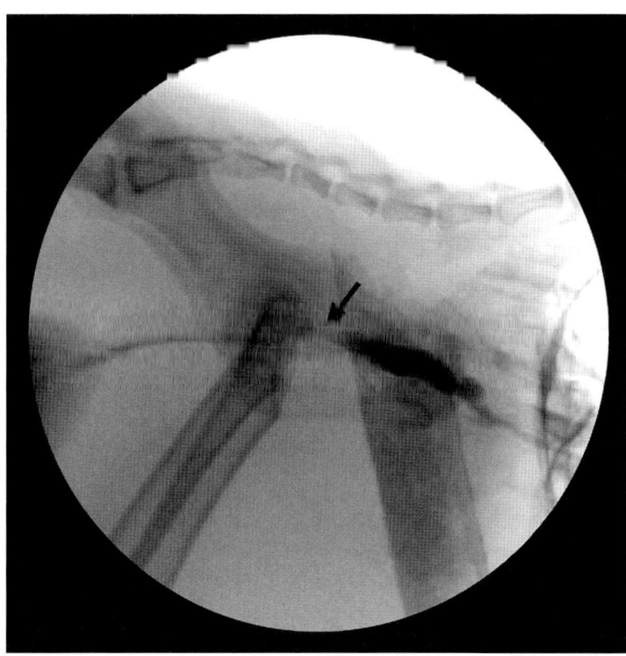

Figure 26.25 Urethral stricture. Urethrogram in a cat with recent onset of recurring lower urinary tract obstruction. The focal narrowing of the membranous urethra (arrow) was persistent throughout this fluoroscopic exam and represents a stricture. The tip of the urinary catheter is located caudal to stricture. Notice the dilation of the membranous urethra caudal to the stricture secondary to high pressure during contrast injection. There is a small focal urethral dilation cranial to the stricture, possibly representing a site of previous obstruction.

Uroendoscopy

Endoscopic evaluation of the lower urinary tract is an important tool when performing interventional therapy of the lower urinary tract. Uroendoscopy does not replace contrast imaging but complements it by providing additional detail about the lower urinary tract. It also provides an opportunity to biopsy lesions and perform therapeutic interventions such as laser ablation of ectopic ureters or lithotripsy of embedded urethral calculi (see other chapters)

Uroendoscopy of female dogs and cats, and some male cats with a perineal urethrostomy is performed using rigid cystoscopes which consist of a telescope and operating sheath. These are available in a variety of sizes and lengths (see Chapter 2). The most common telescopes used in a well-equipped urologic service are 4.0 mm × 30 cm, 2.7 mm × 18 cm, and 1.9 mm × 18 cm.[2–5] Male dogs with a urethra large enough to accommodate an 8 Fr urinary catheter can be evaluated with a 7.5 Fr × 45 cm flexible endoscope.[6] Urethroscopy of male cats and very small dogs can be performed using a 1.1 mm flexible endoscope; however, due to its small size it is not useful for assessing the bladder and does not have an instrument channel.[7] All uroendoscopes have an irrigation channel, which allows for infusion of 0.9% NaCl or sterile water to facilitate dilation and visualization of the lower urinary tract. In male dogs a perineal approach can be taken to provide rigid endoscopic imaging, allowing excellent visualization and ease of therapeutic cystourethroscopy. This is described in detail in Chapter 39.

Female Dog and Cat

Uroendoscopy can be performed in dorsal, sternal or right lateral recumbency with the animal under general anesthesia. Care should be taken in understanding the urogenital anatomy before performing cystoscopy (Figure 26.26 and Figure 26.27). Anecdotally, sternal recumbency has been associated with a higher rate of urethral tearing, so this is not recommended. Dorsal recumbency is recommended for therapeutic cystourethroscopy, especially during ureteral interventions. Each operator has their own personal preferences. The external genitalia are clipped and aseptically prepared. The patient should ideally be draped, especially during therapeutic endoscopy. The operator should wear a sterile gown and gloves. With slow fluid irrigation, the lubricated scope is gently inserted into the vestibule, taking care not to enter the clitoral fossa, which sits ventral to the vestibule (Figure 26.28, Figure 26.29, and Figure 26.30). The vulva is secured gently around the scope to allow the irrigation fluid to distend the vestibule. This allows optimal visualization. The scope is typically passed into the vagina after the investigation of the urethra since this is less

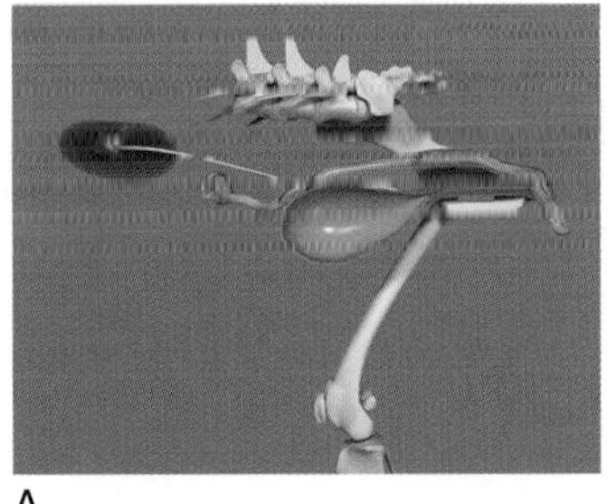

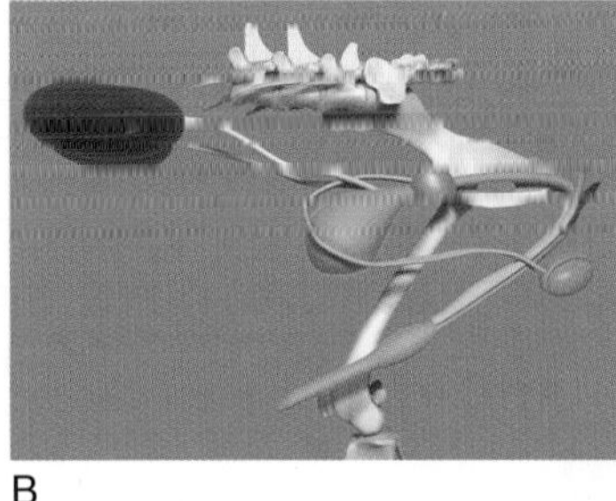

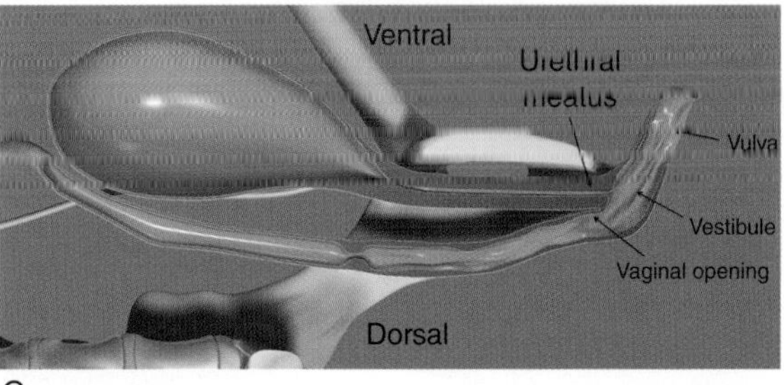

Figure 26.26 Schematic of canine urogenital tract anatomy. (A) Female canine anatomy in a ventrodorsal projection. (B) Male canine anatomy in a ventrodorsal orientation. (C) Feline canine anatomy as seen during cystoscopy in a dorsoventral orientation. Used with permission from The Ohio State University.

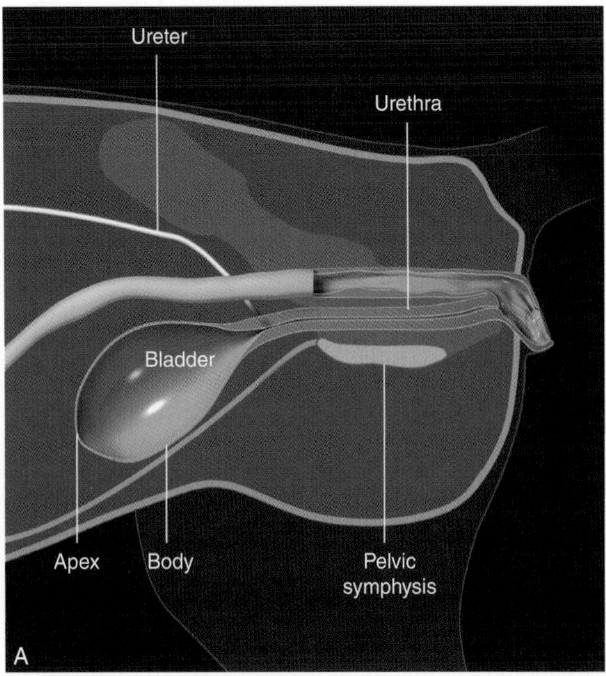

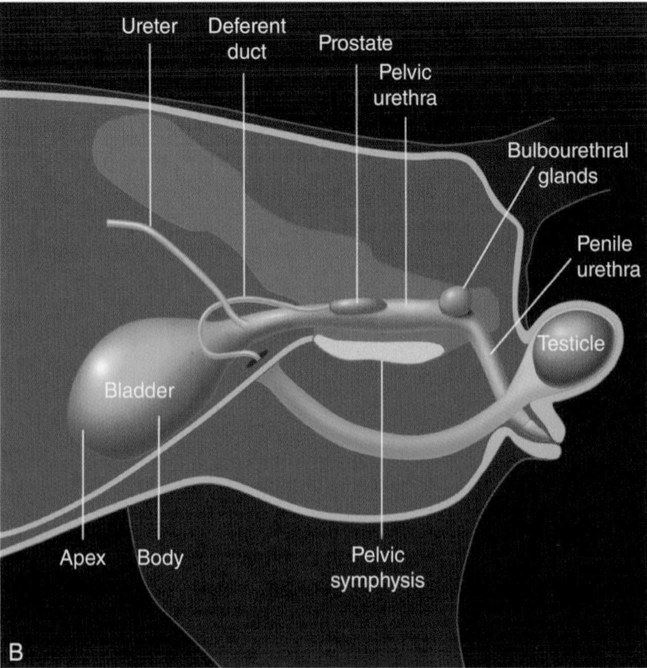

Figure 26.27 Schematic of feline urogenital tract anatomy. (A) Female feline anatomy in a ventrodorsal orientation. Notice the feline ureters enter the proximal urethra/bladder neck rather than the urinary bladder as seen in the canine patient. (B) Male feline anatomy in a ventrodorsal orientation. Used with permission from The Ohio State University.

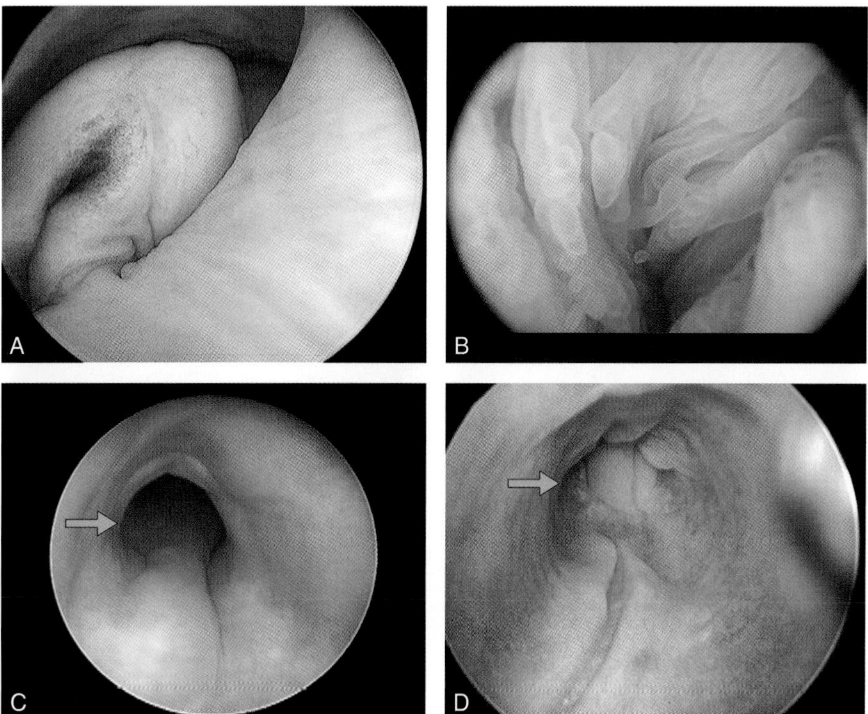

Figure 26.28 Endoscopic images of the normal canine female genitalia with the patient in dorsal recumbency with dorsal to the bottom of each image. (A) Clitoris; (B) fibrous bands within the clitoral fossa; (C) vagina, dorsal vaginal ridge, arrow indicates the caudal aspect of the cervix; (D) vagina, arrow indicates the caudal aspect of the cervix.

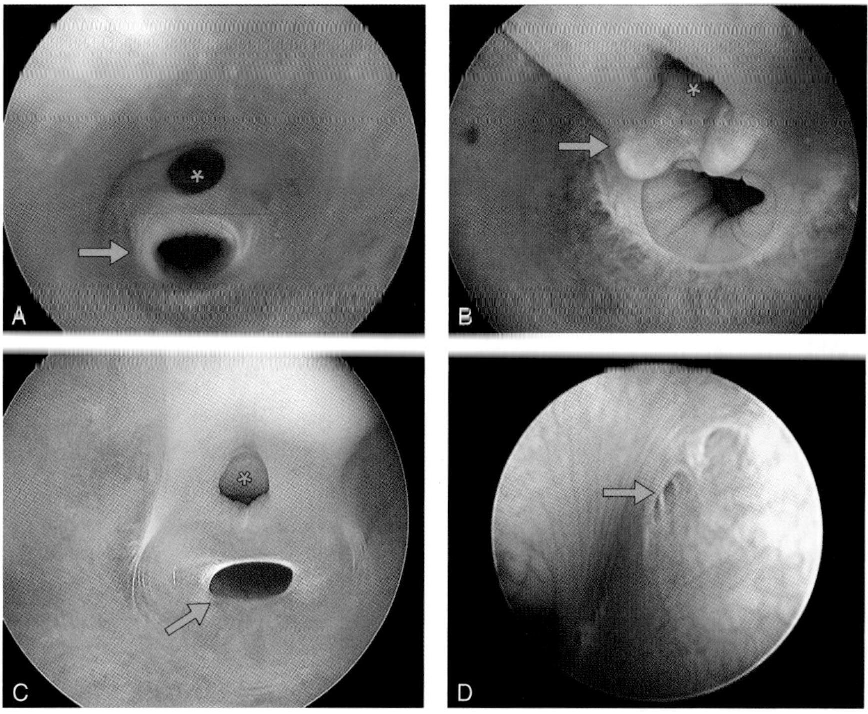

Figure 26.29 Endoscopic images of a normal canine female vestibule imaging the patient in dorsal recumbency. (A) Neutered female dog. The vagina (arrow) and external urethral meatus (asterisk) can be seen in this view. The band around the vaginal opening is called the cingulum and is a normal structure. (B) Intact female dog. The arrow indicates the urethral papilla which is seen in intact females but appears to regress in the neutered female. Asterisk indicates the external urethral meatus. (C) Narrowed cingulum in a neutered female dog. The arrow indicates the vaginal opening. Note the small diameter of the cingulum. The asterisk indicates the urethral meatus. (D) Vestibular fossae. These fossae are often seen in the ventrolateral vestibular walls and can be of variable size. They should not be mistaken for ectopic ureters. They are most commonly seen on the lateral margins of the vaginal orifice.

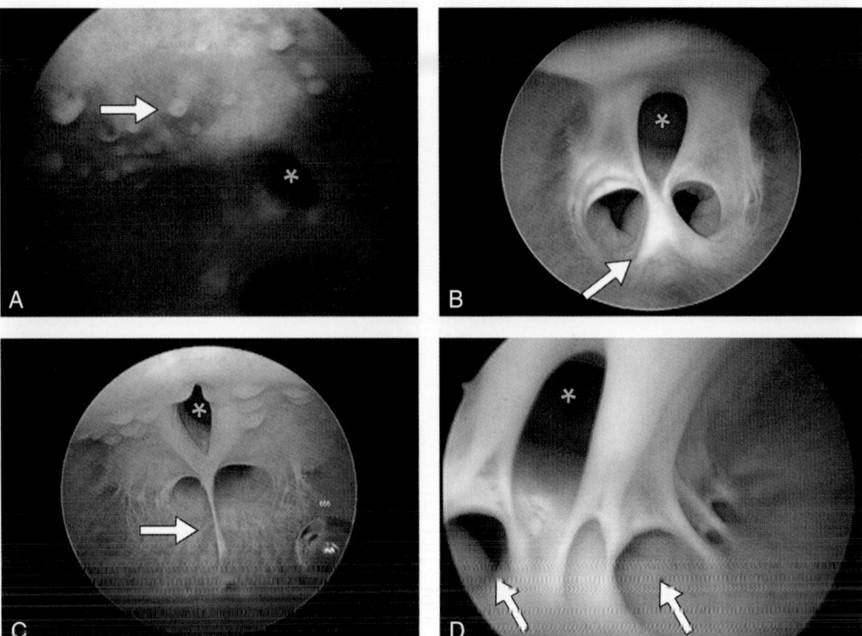

Figure 26.30 Abnormalities of the vestibular structures in 4 different female dogs in dorsal recumbency. (A) Lymphoid follicles. These are commonly seen with chronic inflammation or infection of the lower urinary tract. The asterisk indicates the external urethral meatus. (B) Paramesonephric remnant (arrow). The urethral meatus is indicated by an asterisk. (C) Thin paramesonephric band or hymenal remnant (arrow). (D) Thick paramesonephric band and bifid vagina. The arrows indicate the divided vaginal opening. The asterisk indicates the urethral meatus. The other openings may be mistaken for ectopic ureteral openings, but are actually blind fossae.

sterile than the urethra. In animals with a thick paramesonephric remnant, or bifid vagina, investigation of the vagina may be limited or require switching to a smaller diameter scope (see Chapter 42). After evaluation of the vaginal orifice, the scope is directed into the urethra and passed slowly to the neck of the bladder. Continuous irrigation during its passage will reduce the risk of trauma to the urethra by the endoscope and reduce artifact lesions from the procedure. Care must be taken when using a 30 degree cystoscope to maintain appropriate orientation so that the urethral lumen is maintained appropriately angled. During dorsal cystoscopy, if the light cable is angled down than the urethral lumen should be maintained in the bottom 70% of the screen (Figure 26.31). Observation of the condition of the urethra during initial advancement of the scope as well as on withdrawal is important to distinguish pathologic from iatrogenic lesions (Figure 26.32 and Figure 26.33D). As the tip of the scope reaches the neck of the bladder and enters the trigone care should be taken to prevent trauma of this lip of tissue. Once within the urinary bladder the endoscopist should evaluate the ureteral openings. This is best done by angling the 30 degree endoscope (Figure 26.31 and Figure 26.33) toward the ureteral openings on the dorsal surface of the bladder (down if the patient is in dorsal recumbency, and laterally if in lateral recumbency). These are normally two C-shaped slits facing each other in the dorsal wall. Pulsatile jets of urine should be observed from each of them (Figure 26.33). The bladder is drained and refilled with irrigation fluid to improve visibility. The bladder is explored by either manipulating the scope or manually manipulating the bladder by external palpation. Careful and thorough evaluation of the bladder apex, urachal remnant, body (dorsal, ventral and lateral), trigone and UVJs should be done assessing vascularity, masses, or any lesions (Figure 26.34 and Figure 26.35). This is best done by utilizing the 30 degree angle of the cystoscope to get a full 360 degree view. Care must be taken not to over distend the bladder with irrigation fluid since this will cause hemorrhage and make visualization difficult. If hemorrhage does occur, the infusion of cold saline may reduce it by causing vasoconstriction. Uroliths, mass lesions, and other debris are noted (Figure 26.35). If a lesion is seen a biopsy instrument can be used through the working channel of the endoscope. The bladder is then drained and any additional interventional procedures are performed.

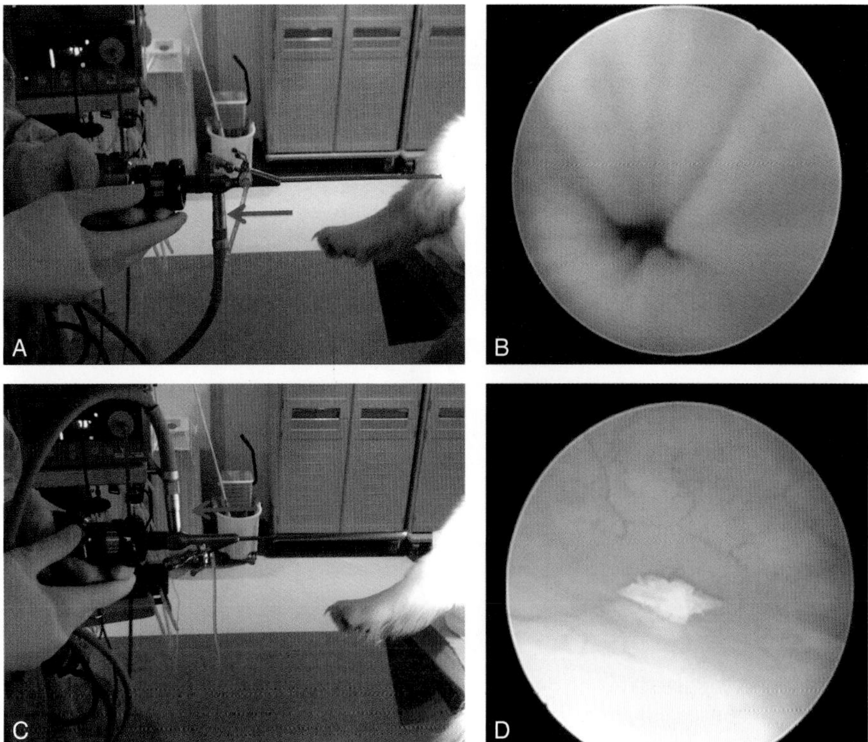

Figure 26.31 Cystoscopic angles when using a 30 degree endoscope. (A) The endoscope with the 30 degree angle facing up, resulting in imaging of the top of an image when the endoscope is straight. (B) During urethroscopy the urethral lumen should be seen on the bottom of the screen (bottom 30%) which allows the rigid endoscope to be straight within the urethral lumen, preventing trauma to the dependent urethral wall. (C) If the 30 degree lens angle is facing down than the bottom of the image is more easily seen. (D) Once within the urinary bladder the operator turns the endoscope as seen in (C) so that the dependent portion of the bladder is easily imaged using the angle of the lens. Notice the cystolith on the floor of the bladder which is easy to see when the endoscope is used appropriately. (Images courtesy of Dr. Allyson Berent)

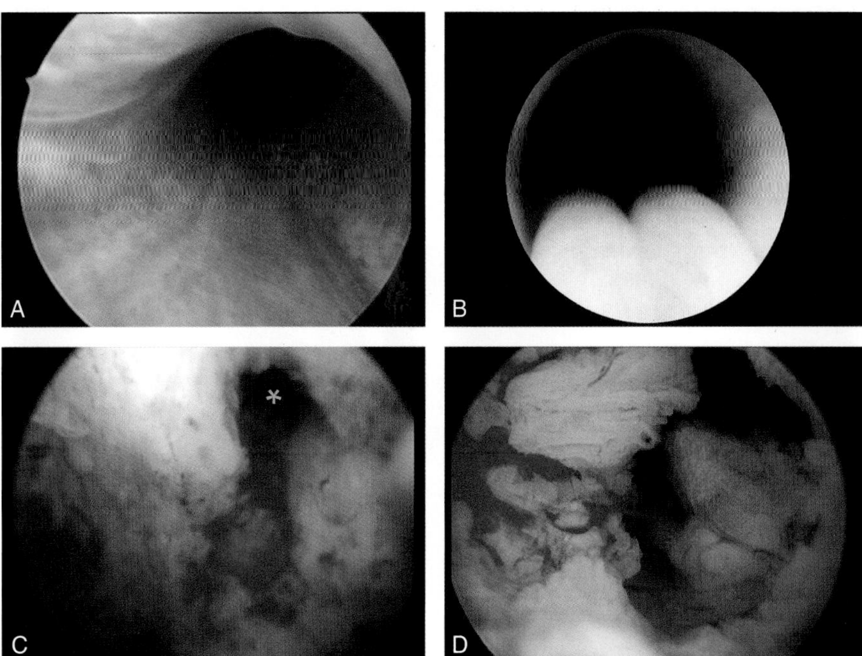

Figure 26.32 Endoscopic images of the urethra during cystourethroscopy. (A) Normal female dog urethra; (B) normal female cat urethra. Notice the two ureteral papilla; they are in the proximal urethra rather than the urinary bladder. (C) Canine proliferative urethritis. This is an inflammatory process that can only be differentiated from neoplasia with histopathology. The asterisk indicates the urethral lumen. (D) Transitional cell carcinoma in the urethra and bladder of a female dog.

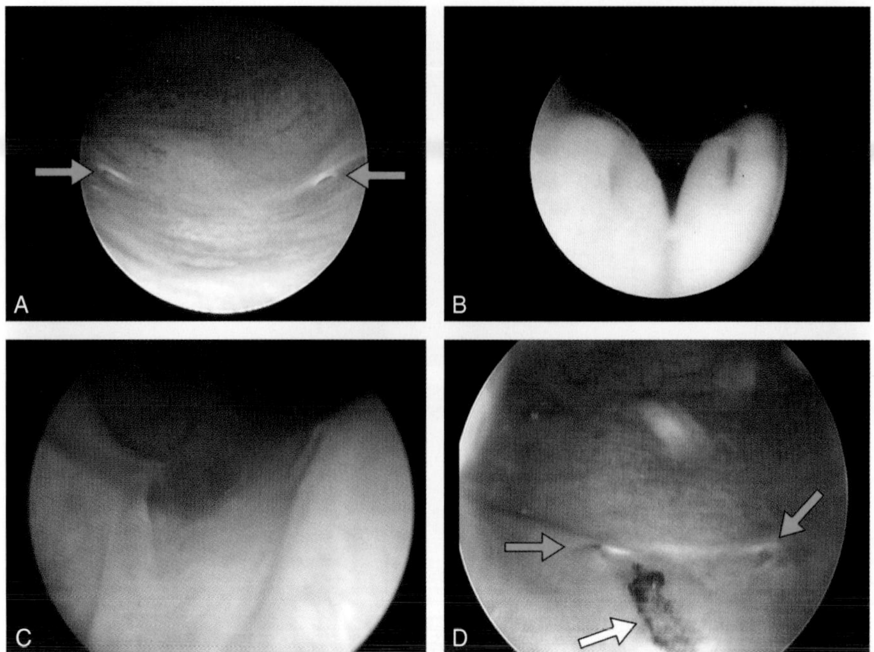

Figure 26.33 Ureteral openings visualized during dorsal cystoscopy. (A) Normal female dog with a distended urinary bladder resulting in flattening of the ureteral openings. These openings are slightly stenotic. (B) Normal female cat. Notice the ureteral openings sitting on the top of each papilla that is sitting in the proximal urethra, rather than the urinary bladder as in dogs. (C) Normal pulsatile urine stream seen from the right UVJ in a female dog. (D) Scope-induced artifact (white arrow), between normal ureters (blue arrows).

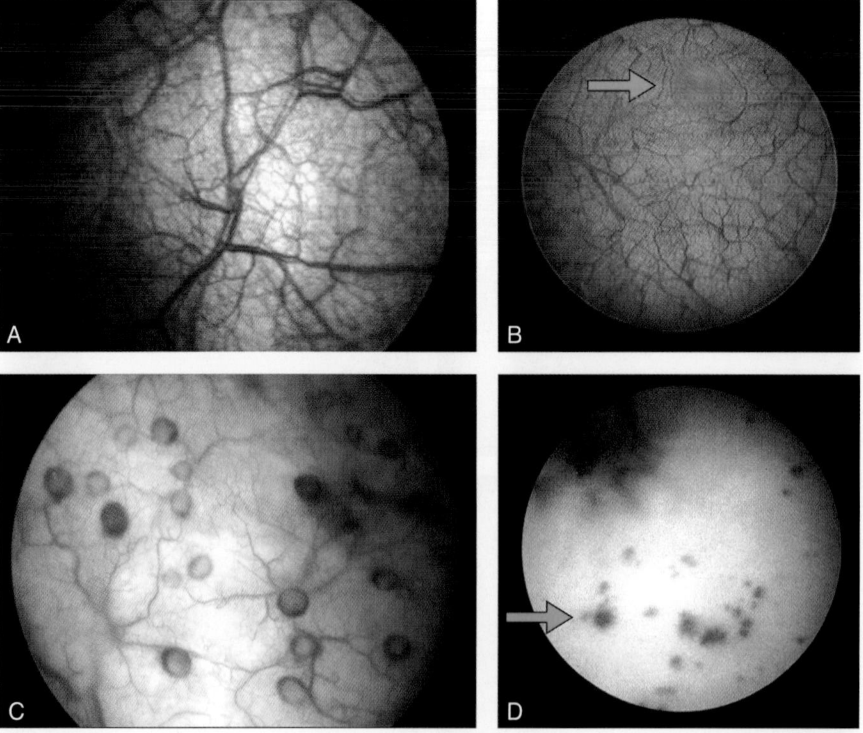

Figure 26.34 Bladder wall abnormalities seen during cystoscopy. (A) Increased vascularity in the canine bladder wall. There is a slight transparent quality to the wall which is normal. (B) Increased vascularity in the canine bladder wall. A small diverticulum is noted at the apex of the bladder (blue arrow). (C) Inflammatory lesions in the bladder wall with a typical "fried egg" appearance. These are usually associated with chronic relapsing urinary tract infections and biopsy as neutrophilic lymphoplasmacytic, or lymphocytic inflammation. (D) Bladder wall hemorrhages (blue arrow), "glomerulations", in a female cat with feline idiopathic cystitis.

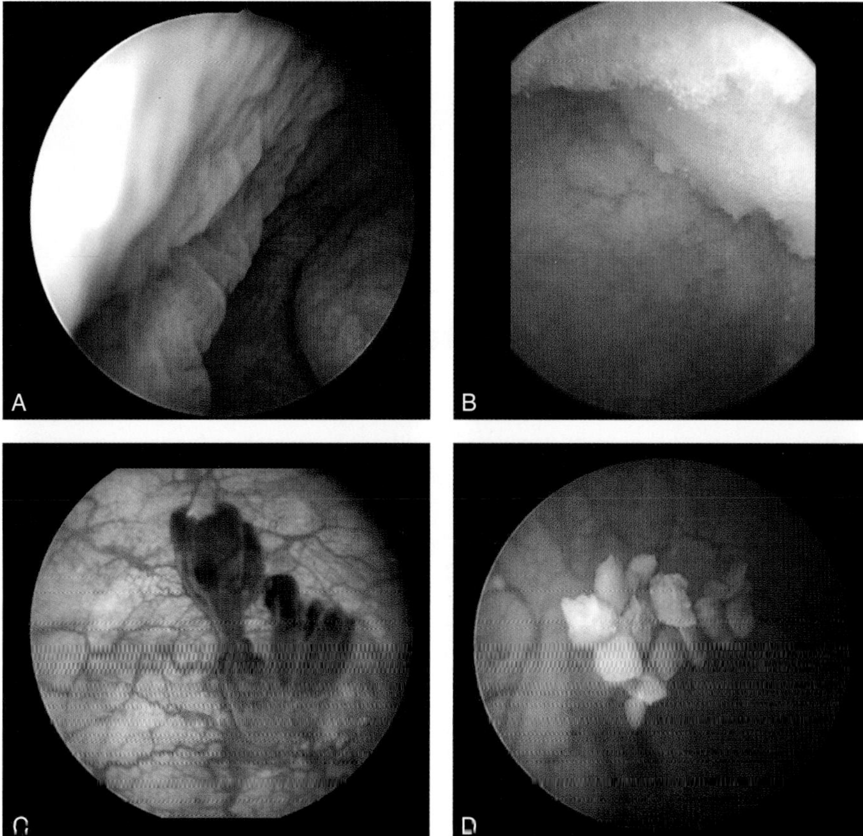

Figure 26.35 Endoscopic images of various canine urinary bladder lumens. (A) Normal appearance of the undistended bladder wall. (B) Crystalloid material settling in the bladder. The distended wall behind it has a normal appearance. (C) Inflammatory polyps. These may be seen singly or clustered together. Histopathology is necessary to differentiate these lesions from neoplasia. The bladder wall has significantly increased vascularity. (D) Uroliths in the bladder. There is a mild increase in the vascularity of the bladder wall.

Male Dog

The patient is positioned in right lateral or dorsal recumbency under general anesthesia. The hair around the prepuce is clipped and the prepuce is flushed with diluted chlorohexidine solution. The prepuce is then scrubbed and draped. The lubricated flexible scope is passed into the urethra after penis extrusion, with sterile saline fluid irrigation. Some resistance may be encountered as the scope passes the proximal end of the os penis and again at the level of the ischial arch. The male urethroscope is a zero degree scope, so maintaining the lumen of the urethra in the center of the screen is appropriate to avoid urethral trauma. This may require gentle endoscope manipulation, being careful to avoid excessive torque on the endoscope to avoid fiberoptic damage. As with the rigid scopes, the continuous irrigation with fluid will help distend the urethra, improve the visualization, and reduce damage and artifact lesions. The scope is passed through the perineal urethra and up to the prostatic urethra. At this level several structures may be noted. The colliculus seminalis is a dorsal ridge of tissue which sits at the level of the openings of the ductus deferens along the dorsal urethral wall (Figure 26.36 and Figure 26.37). It should not be mistaken for a mass lesion. In addition, the ductus openings should not be mistaken for ectopic ureters (Figure 26.38). Proximal to this, at the level of the prostate, numerous small openings may be seen over the circumference of the urethral wall. These are normal prostatic ducts and are also often mistaken for ureteral ectopia (Figure 26.37 and Figure 26.38). The quality of the endoscope and camera/light source equipment can have a significant impact on the image quality of each of these structures. The bladder and ureteral openings are evaluated in a similar manner to the female dog and cat and appear similarly, though are more difficult to find with the flexible endoscope (Figure 26.38).

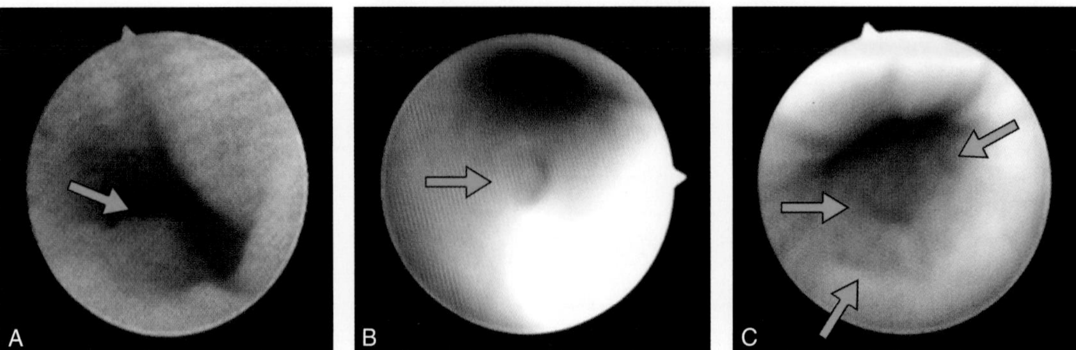

Figure 26.36 Normal male canine urethra visualized during flexible urethroscopy. (A) Colliculus seminalis. This short ridge in the pelvic urethra is located at the level of the ductus deferens openings and is a normal structure. (B) Ductus deferens opening in the male dog urethra (arrow). This normal structure should not be mistaken for an ectopic ureter. (C) Prostatic ducts (arrows). These small openings are normally seen at the level of the prostate.

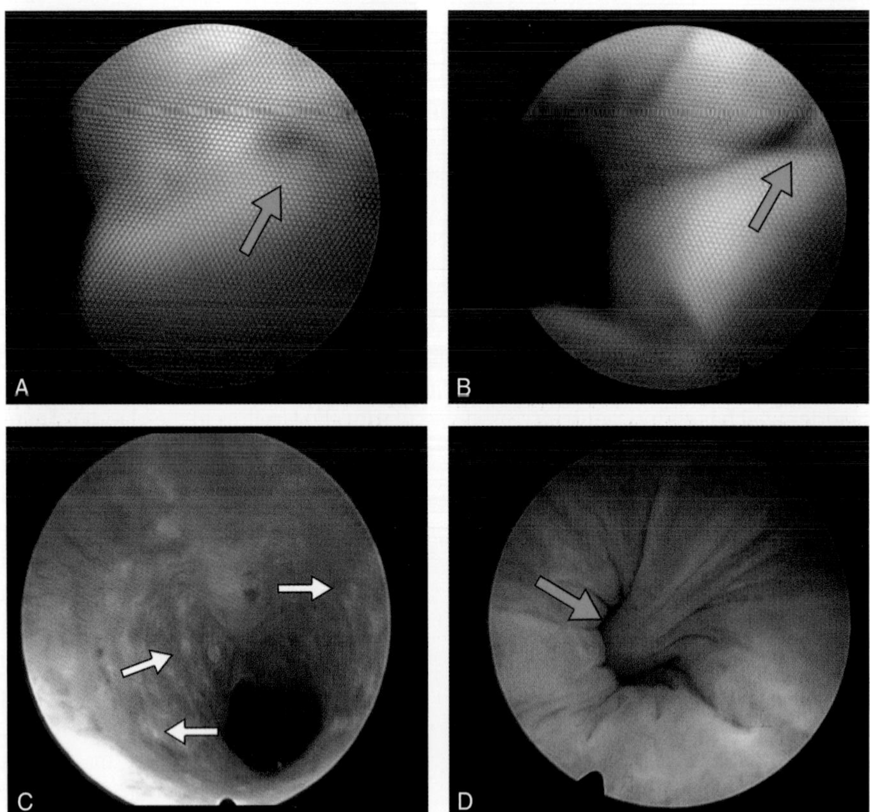

Figure 26.37 Urethroscopic images in a male canine urethra. (A) Ectopic ureter opening (arrow). (B) Same dog as A with a guide wire in the ureter. (C) Normal prostatic urethra with prostatic ducts (arrows). (D) Normal urethra showing colliculus seminalis (arrow) and prostatic ducts. (Images courtesy of Allyson Berent.)

Ectopic Ureters

Ectopic ureter openings may be seen in the proximal, middle, or distal urethra, and in the vestibule or vagina (Figure 26.39). It is important to visualize urine emerging from the ectopic stoma to confirm its identity. There are many other small fossae and blind openings that can easily be mistaken for an ectopic ureter, so care must be taken when investigating these (Figure 26.30D). Passage of a guide wire and injection of contrast into the opening can be very useful in these cases. In male dogs the openings are often very small, narrow and stenotic, and very difficult to find (Figure 26.37A, B).

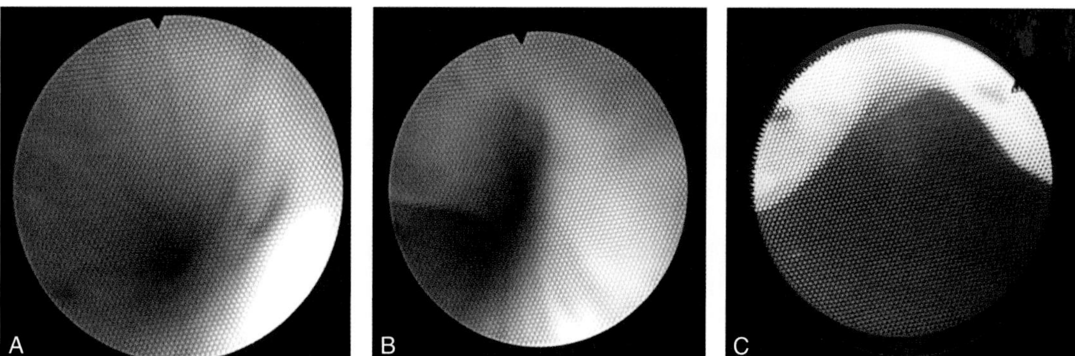

Figure 26.38 Endoscopic images using a male fiberoptic cystoscope. (A) prostatic ducts; (B) Colliculus seminalis; (C) ureteral openings.

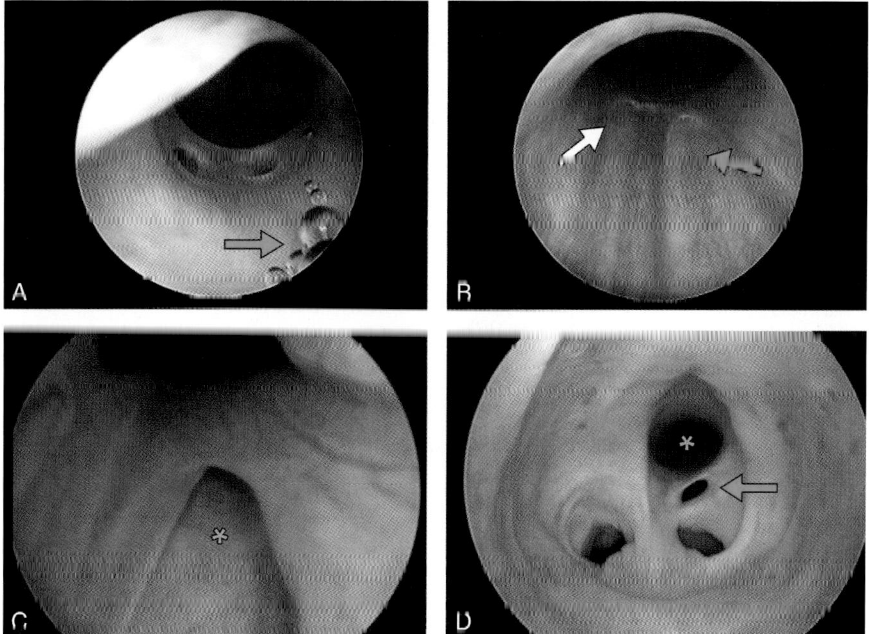

Figure 26.39 Endoscopic images of various ectopic ureters in the female dog. (A) Proximal ectopic ureteral openings in the proximal urethra. Small gas bubbles are indicated by the blue arrow. (B) Proximal ureteral openings (white arrow) with shallow troughs (blue arrow) ecoptically positioned in the proximal urethra. (C) Deep trough (asterisk) leading from an ectopic ureter. (D) Distal ectopic ureter (arrow), opening into the vestibule. Note the thick paramesonephric remnant. The urethral meatus is indicated by an asterisk.

Complications

Two of the complications of uroendoscopy are rupture of the bladder and perforation of the urethra. Animals with abnormal bladder and urethral walls have an increased risk. Appropriate lubrication, gentle manipulation, and care not to overinflate the bladder will minimize these complications. If you can not visualize the urethral lumen (i.e., when there is a urethral tumor), it is advised to avoid advancing the endoscope blindly, as this is the most common cause for perforation. Bacterial urinary tract infection can also occur post-uroendoscopy so sterile preparation, gowning, and draping the patient is recommended. Most animals receive a prophylactic course of antibiotics during, and for several days after the procedure (3–5 for diagnostic cystoscopy and 10–14 for therapeutic cystoscopy). Vesicoureteral reflux can occur in any animal but is more likely in those with ectopic ureters. This can lead to pyelonephritis if an infection is already present. If possible, the clinician should try to clear a patient's urinary tract infection prior to performing uroendoscopy.

Summary

Imaging provides valuable diagnostic and therapeutic information about the upper and lower urinary tract in dogs and cats, and is best when used in combination (i.e., cystoscopy and excretory urography). Lower urinary tract endoscopy provides details of disease that other imaging modalities can not, but does not provide the imaging needed for the upper urinary tract. Selection of the proper technique and positioning can give the clinician invaluable data for diagnosis and treatment planning. This is often best used in combination with endoscopic images, especially in the lower urinary tract.

Notes

1. Omnipaque, Nycomed Inc., Princeton, NJ.
2. Rigid endoscope, 1.9-mm 30° lens, Karl Storz Endoscopy, Culver City, CA.
3. Rigid endoscope, 2.7-mm integraded sheath 30° lens, Richard Wolf, Vernon Hills, IL.
4. Rigid endoscope, 2.7-mm 30° lens, Karl Storz Endoscopy, Culver City, IL.
5. Rigid endoscope, 4-mm 30° lens, Karl Storz Endoscopy, Culver City, IL.
6. Flex X^2 Flexible ureteroscope, Karl Storz Endoscopy, Culver City, CA.
7. 1 mm, 6-inch Semi-Flexible Micro-Endoscope, MDS Inc., Brandon, FL.

References

Ackerman N, Wingfield WE, and Corley E A (1972) Fatal air embolism associated with pneumourethrography and pneumocystography in a dog. *J Am Vet Med Assoc* 160(12), 1616–8.

Adin CA, Herrgesell EJ, Nyland TG, et al (2003) Antegrade pyelography for suspected ureteral obstruction in cats: 11 cases (1995–2001). *J Am Vet Med Assoc* 222, 1576–81.

Brown J (2012) The urethra. In: *Textbook of Veterinary Diagnostic Radiology*, 6th edn (Thrall DE, ed.). Elsevier, St. Louis, MO, pp 744–748.

Berent AC, Weisse C et al (2012) Evaluation of cystoscopic-guided laser ablation on intramural ectopic ureters in female dogs. *J Am Vet Med Assoc* 240, 716–25.

D'Anjou, M., Bedard, A., and Dunn, M., et al (2011). Clinical significance of renal pelvis dilatation on ultrasound in dogs and cats. *Vet Radiol Ultrasound* 52(1), 88–94.

Dennis R, Kirberger RM, Wrigley RH, et al (2001) *Handbook of Small Animal Radiological Differential Diagnosis*. WB Saunders Ltd., Philadelphia.

Essman SC (2005) Contrast cystography. *Clin Tech Small Anim Pract* 20(1), 46–51.

Feeney DA, Barber DL, Culver DH, Prasse KW, Thrall DE, and Lewis RE (1980) Canine excretory urogram: correlation with base-line measurements. *Am JVet Res* 41(2), 279–83.

Feeney DA, Osborne CA, and Jessen CR (1980) Effects of radiographic contrast media on results of urinalysis, with emphasis on alteration in specific gravity. *J Am Vet Med Assoc* 176(12), 1378–81.

Heuter KJ (2005) Excretory urography. *Clin Techn Small Anim Pract* 20(1), 39–45.

Ihle SL and Kostolich M (1991) Acute renal failure associated with contrast medium administration in a dog. *J Am Vet Med Assoc* 199(7), 899–901.

Jorgensen AL (2013) Contrast-induced nephropathy: pathophysiology and preventive strategies. *Crit Care Nurse* 33(1), 37–46.

Lattimer J and Essman S (2012) The prostate gland. In: *Textbook of Veterinary Diagnostic Radiology*, 6th edn (Thrall DE, ed.). Elsevier, St. Louis, MO, pp 749–756..

Mahaffey MB, Barber DONL, Barsanti J, and Cowell W (1984) Simotaneous double- contrast cystography and cystometry in dogs. *Veterinary Radiology and Ultrasound*, 25(6), 254–259.

Margulies, K. B., Mckinley, L. J., Cavero, P. G., and Burnett, J. C. (1990). Induction and prevention of radiocontrast-induced nephropathy in dogs with heart failure. *Kidney International*, 38(6), 1101–1108.

Marlolf A and Park R (2012) The urinary bladder. In: *Textbook of Veterinary Diagnostic Radiology*, 6th edn (Thrall DE, ed.)., Elsevier, St. Louis, MO, pp 726–741.

Reichler IM, Specker CE, Hubler M et al (2012) Ectopic ureters in dogs: Clinical features, surgical techniques and outcome. *Vet Surg*, 41(4), 515–22.

Ruby AL, Ling GV, and Ackerman N (1983) Effect of sodium diatrizoate on the in vitro growth of three common canine urinary bacterial species. *Vet Radiol* 24(5), 222–5.

Samii VF, McLoughlin MA, Mattoon JS, et al (2004) Digital fluoroscopic excretory urography, digital fluoroscopic urethrography, helical computed tomography, and cystoscopy in 24 dogs with suspected ureteral ectopia. *J Vet Intern Med* 18(3), 271–81.

Schabelman E and Witting M (2010) The relationship of radiocontrast, iodine, and seafood allergies: a medical myth exposed. *J Emerg Med* 39(5), 701–7.

Seiler G (2012) The kidneys and ureters. In: *Textbook of Veterinary Diagnostic Radiology*, 6th edn (Thrall DE, ed.). Elsevier, St. Louis, MO, pp 705–723.

Thayer GW, Carrig CB, and Evans AT (1980) Fatal venous air embolism associated with pneumocystography in a cat. *J Am Vet Med Assoc* 176(7), 643–5.

Ticer J, Spencer C, and Ackerman N (1980) Positive contrast retrograde urethrography: a useful procedure for evaluating urethral disorders in the dog. *Vet Radiol* 21(1), 2–11.

Wallack ST (2003) *Handbook Of Veterinary Contrast Radiography*. San Diego Veterinary Imaging, Inc, Solano Beach, CA.

CHAPTER TWENTY-SEVEN

Interventional Management of Complicated Nephrolithiasis

Allyson Berent[1] and Larry G. Adams[2]
[1]The Animal Medical Center, New York, NY
[2]Department of Veterinary Clinical Sciences, Purdue University, West Lafayette, IN

Background/Indications

Most canine and feline nephroliths remain clinically silent for years. Some controversy exists as to whether non-obstructive kidney stones worsen underlying kidney disease. Since their removal is often met with excessive morbidity and mortality, few indications exist in which removal is recommended. The criteria for a complicated nephrolith and possible removal of nephroliths in dogs would be the following: if there is a partial or complete ureteropelvic junction (UPJ) obstruction resulting in progressive hydronephrosis, renal parenchymal loss is occurring due to stone growth, severe chronic hematuria is occurring, pain associated with the kidneys is appreciated, or if recurrent urinary tract infections are occurring despite appropriate medical management of an infected nephrolith. The main indication for removal of upper tract uroliths in cats is when the nephrolith moves into the ureter and becomes an obstructive ureterolith (see Chapter 30).

In small animals, traditional surgical treatment of nephrolithiasis involves a nephrotomy, pyelotomy, or a salvage ureteronephrectomy. Complications can be severe resulting in hemorrhage, diminished renal function, nephrolith, or edema-induced ureteral obstructions, and urinary leakage. In a study of normal cats, there was a 10–20% decrease in the glomerular filtration rate (GFR) of the ipsilateral kidney after a nephrotomy. Though clinically insignificant in normal cats, a patient who has maximally hypertrophied the remaining nephrons due to prior nephrolith induced damage, may have a more severe decline in renal function. Also, knowing that over 30% of adult cats will develop chronic kidney disease in their lifetime, resulting from more than 75% loss of overall renal function, they cannot tolerate a 10–20% decline in GFR from a nephrotomy. A pyelotomy is not as easy in cats and dogs, compared to humans, due to the intrarenal location of the renal pelvis. Pyelotomy has the risk of severe hemorrhage, urinary leakage, failure to remove all stones due to the lack of visibility, and stricture formation at the UPJ. In the authors' opinion, these surgical options should be avoided whenever possible.

In humans, minimally invasive treatment of problematic nephroliths is always recommended. This typically involves extracorporeal shockwave lithotripsy (ESWL) for nephroliths smaller than 1–1.5 cm and percutaneous nephrolithotomy (PCNL) for nephroliths larger than 1.5 cm. For stones between 1–1.5 cm, if ESWL is attempted, then concurrent ureteral stenting should be considered. Open surgery and laparoscopy is only considered necessary after other less invasive options have failed or have been deemed inappropriate. Various human studies have shown ESWL and PCNL to have minimal effect on the GFR of clinical stone forming patients. These procedures, particularly PCNL, have been shown to be highly effective (90–100%) in removing all stone fragments, as endoscopic calyceal inspection is superior for visualization and fragment retrieval. PCNL has been shown to be best procedure in children to preserve renal function.

ESWL involves the delivery of high-energy shock waves to the nephrolith(s) resulting in fragmentation

Veterinary Image-Guided Interventions, First Edition. Edited by Chick Weisse and Allyson Berent.

Companion website: www.wiley.com/go/weisse/vet-image-guided-interventions

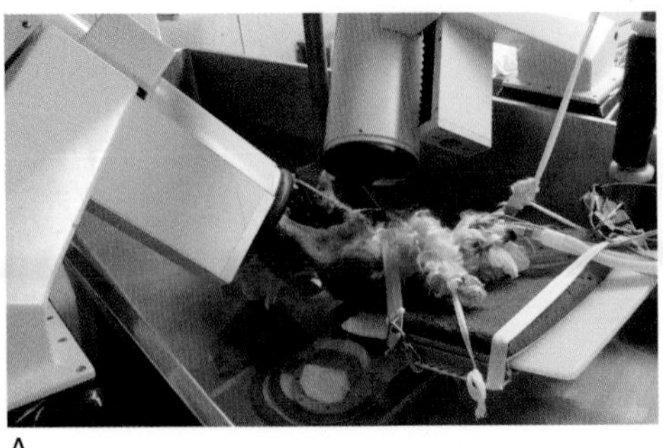
A

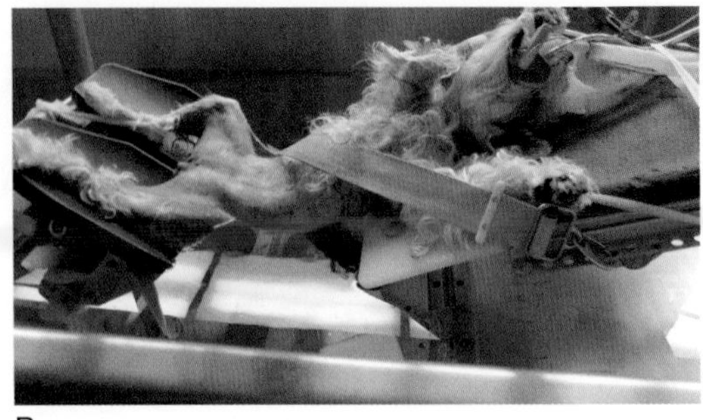
B

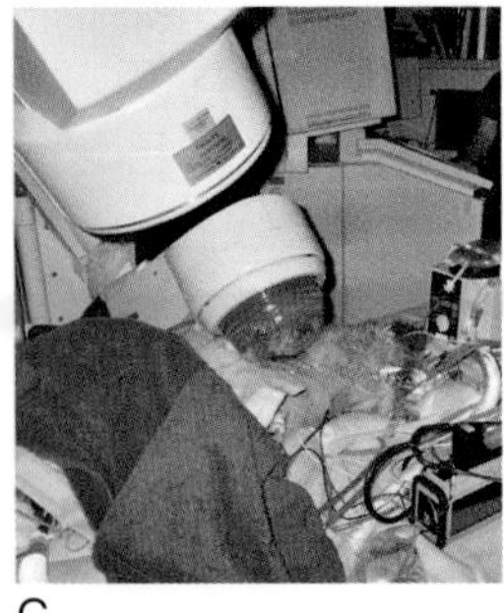
C

Figure 27.1 (A) Dog positioned in Dornier HM-3 lithotripter for ESWL treatment. Note biplanar fluoroscopic image intensifiers above patient. (B) Dog suspended in gantry for support and positioning in water bath during ESWL using the Dornier HM-3. (C) Dog positioned for dry ESWL treatment. Note the treatment head is positioned in apposition to the patient's skin to permit shock wave transmission. Also note C-arm fluoroscopy used to target the urolith.

of the stone into small pieces that pass down the ureter and into the urinary bladder. Shock waves are high amplitude sound waves generated by electrohydraulic, electromagnetic or piezoelectric energy sources. Shock waves are generated outside the body (extracorporeal) and must be transmitted into the body by coupling the shock wave generator to the patient. The initial ESWL devices, such as the Dornier HM3, utilized a water bath for coupling and required the patient to be partially submerged in a large water bath (Figure 27.1A–B). Newer ESWL devices are referred to as dry lithotriptors because the shock wave generator is incased in silicone-covered, water-filled coupling device eliminating the need for the large water bath (Figure 27.1C).

In a series of 140 dogs with nephroliths or ureteroliths treated by ESWL, the most common complication was ureteral obstruction by nephrolith fragments passing through the ureter, which occurred in approximately 10% of dogs treated with ESWL. With the addition of ureteral stent placement for larger nephroliths (>10–20 mm, depending on stone type and dog size) prior to ESWL, the risk of ureteral obstruction has declined. The presence of the ureteral stent facilitates the passage of the stones due to passive ureteral dilation, and also helps to improve fluoroscopic identification of small ureteral stones during the ESWL treatment.

ESWL is not recommended for treatment of nephroliths in cats for several reasons. One is that the feline ureter is only 0.3 mm in diameter with a typical nephrolith fragment after ESWL being approximately 1 mm. Therefore, fragmentation of nephroliths in cats is likely to result in ureteral obstruction. In addition, feline kidneys may have a tendency to hemorrhage more with ESWL and cause substantial reduction in renal function. Calcium oxalate uroliths from cats are more resistant to ESWL fragmentation than calcium oxalate uroliths from dogs even for similar size and similar composition uroliths. Over 98% of upper tract stones in cats are calcium oxalate, most of which are monohydrate. Calcium oxalate monohydrate stones have been shown to be more difficult to fragment with ESWL, and they break into larger pieces rather than sand, making fragment passage more difficult.

Ureteral stents have been placed to improve stone fragment passage after ESWL. This has been found to be very effective in dogs. Stent-induced passive ureteral dilation is beneficial in cases with large nephroliths, as the risk of developing a ureteral obstruction during passage of nephrolith fragments is the major concern. Animals with ureteral stents in place often require shorter hospital stays, as the concern for post ESWL ureteral obstruction is diminished. There is some evidence in research dog models that ureteral stenting may diminish ureteral peristalsis, which may ultimately result in slower stone passage after ESWL. In the authors' experience ureteral stents typically accelerate the passage rate after ESWL when compared to non-stented dogs.

In small animals, if ESWL fails, is not available, there are cystine stones (ESWL resistant), or the stone is larger than 15–25 mm (pending on patient's size, stone type, and the presence of a ureteral stent), then a PCNL (or endoscopic nephrolithotomy [ENL]) is considered. This is where intracorporeal lithotripsy is performed on a large nephrolith, so that all fragments can be removed, preventing the need for multiple procedures or the risk of ureteral obstruction. Typically, this is done using a combination of ultrasonographic, endoscopic and fluoroscopic guidance. The authors perform this procedure either percutaneously (PCNL) or surgically assisted (SENL). The benefit of SENL to PCNL is that a nephrostomy tube does not need to remain in place while the renal access point heals.

When a laparotomy is performed the renal tract is primarily closed once the procedure is complete remaining minimally invasive to the kidney, but opening the abdomen for closure of the tract.

The authors recently reported an abstract of nine dogs and one cat (12 renal units) in which ENL was performed. Indications included recurrent UTIs, worsening azotemia with stone growth, and ureteral-outflow obstructions. The median stone size was 2 cm (0.7–5 cm) and the median pre- and 3-month postoperative creatinine was 1.3 (0.8–9.1) and 1.1 mg/dl (0.6–6.1), respectively. Successful removal of all stones was documented in 92% of renal units with one procedure, and no patient died from the ENL procedure. This suggests that ENL can be safely performed in dogs and cats, yielding similar success rates to that seen in people. For this procedure, advanced endourologic experience is highly recommended.

This chapter will focus on the use of ESWL and ENL for the treatment of complicated nephrolithiasis in dogs and cats.

Patient Preparation

A full diagnostic work-up is necessary, including a complete blood count, serum biochemical profile, urinalysis and urine culture, coagulation profile, abdominal radiographs and an abdominal ultrasound prior to considering ESWL or ENL. If struvite stones are suspected based on a high urine pH and a positive culture of urease-producing bacteria, then medical dissolution using an appropriate dissolution diet and antibiotic therapy should first be considered for a minimum of 3–9 months (and possibly longer). If after 3 months the stone is getting bigger, despite a negative urine culture and neutral or acidified urine pH, then ESWL or ENL can be considered. Serial radiographs and urine cultures (with urine pH) should be performed monthly to ensure appropriate treatment.

Potential Risks/ Complications

Anesthetic risks should be considered for each patient, as renal compromise is commonly present prior to any procedure. For ESWL the main risks are transient hemorrhage, shock wave-induced pancreatitis, arrhythmias, and the potential to exchange a non-obstructive nephrolith for an obstructive ureterolith. Owners should be made fully aware that 15–30% of patients will require more than one ESWL procedure to make them stone free and the stone fragments can take weeks, and sometimes months, to pass. They should also be aware that stone recurrence could occur. If a concurrent ureteral stent is to be placed then the main risk of this would be similar to that outlined in Chapter 34, including stent migration, ureteral perforation, stent encrustation, and bladder wall irritation. Pancreatitis is an uncommon complication of treatment of right nephroliths in dogs because of the close proximity of the right kidney to the right limb of the pancreas. In over 200 ESWL treatments by one of the authors (LGA), clinical pancreatitis has occurred in less than 2% of dogs. Asymptomatic elevations of amylase, lipase and cPLI occur in some dogs following ESWL without any clinical evidence of pancreatitis. Arrhythmias rarely occur during ESWL treatment with the older water-bath lithotriptors. Therefore, these ESWL units have integrated ECG-gaiting mechanism to only allow the unit to discharge the spark and generate shock waves between patient heartbeats. Each author (L.G.A. and A.B.) observed an ESWL-induced arrhythmia in one dog when ESWL (water-bath and dry unit) was performed without the ECG-gaiting mechanism; therefore, ECG-gaiting is required for ESWL treatments.

For ENL the main risks are hemorrhage and urine leakage from the renal access point. If the procedure is done percutaneously (PCNL), than a nephrostomy tube is typically left indwelling for a minimum of 4 weeks (capped and wrapped) to create a nephropexy, otherwise urine leakage can occur while the nephrostomy site heals. If this is left in place, the risk of nephrostomy tube dislodgement and urinary tract infections should be considered and carefully monitored for these complications. This is why most owners prefer the SENL procedure because the access point is closed with a suture once the procedure is complete. During the ENL procedure ureteral perforation is possible and this should be carefully monitored for as well. If there are bilaterally large nephroliths, the authors typically recommend staging each procedure, so that one kidney can heal prior to considering treatment of the other side (4–8 weeks later), though bilateral treatment has been performed in certain circumstances. After ENL a ureteral stent is usually placed to prevent any ureteral edema induced ureteral obstruction. This can be removed endoscopically 2–4 weeks later.

Regardless of the procedure being performed, the owners should be fully aware of the risk of stone recurrence. The exact percentage of nephrolith recurrence for each stone type is not known but urate, cystine and calcium oxalate stone formers should be medically managed to try and help prevent stone recurrence. For many calcium oxalate stone formers the author (AB) will consider leaving the ureteral stent indwelling long-term to prevent future ureteral obstructions, if it is well tolerated, monitoring carefully for encrustation. If the patient is hypercalcemic, this is not recommended.

Equipment

For ESWL there are many different machines that are available. The original shock wave lithotripsy unit introduced in the 1984 was the Dornier HM-3 lithotripter[1] that is still in use in some human hospitals; although this device has not been sold as a new unit since 1987. This water bath lithotripter has advantages of excellent shock wave transmission through the water bath, large treatment focal spot, and high efficiency of urolith fragmentation. The disadvantages include the fact that the procedure is painful and requires general anesthesia, high maintenance costs, use of disposable spark gap generators, and lack of mobility. The patient is positioned such that the nephrolith or ureterolith is targeted with the treatment focal spot (or F2) of the lithotripter. The patient is supported in a hydraulic gantry that is lowered into the water bath and positioned using biplanar fluoroscopy (Figure 27.1A–C). Newer dry lithotriptors come in a variety of designs with single or dual treatment heads. Dry lithotriptors are less painful than the Dornier HM-3, permitting the human patients to be awake or sedated, thereby avoiding general anesthesia. The efficiency of urolith fragmentation is lower with the newer dry lithotriptors compared to the Dornier HM-3 (Lingeman et al, 2002). Dry lithotriptors[2] also have the advantages of being less expensive, more mobile permitting transportation to different hospitals, and easier to maintain than water bath units.

The ENL procedure requires renal access with an 18 gauge renal access needle,[3] an angle-tipped hydrophilic 0.035″ guide wire,[4] and an open-ended ureteral catheter.[5] After through-and-through access is obtained, a percutaneous renal access sheath set (18, 24, 30 Fr) is used to balloon dilate or bougienage a tract over the guidewire.[6,7] This must be an appropriate size based on the nephroscope and lithotrite being used.

The lithotrite the author prefers for ENL is a device made by ACMI/Gyrus called the Cyberwand,[8] which is a dual probe ultrasonic lithotrite. This device, inside the working channel of the nephroscope,[9] can fit through a 24 Fr renal access sheath. If a Hol:YAG laser[10] is to be used, this can fit through a small cystoscope,[11,12] making the size of the renal access sheath much smaller (15 or 18 Fr). The pre-made access set comes with an appropriate balloon dilation catheter and sheath, but this can also be made with an appropriate sized balloon (5, 6, 8, 10 mm × 8–15 cm long)[13] and peel-away sheath (15, 18, 24, 30 Fr),[14] respectively. Once the stones are removed, an appropriately sized ureteral stent is placed (4.7 Fr typically).[15,16] If a PCNL is done then a 6 Fr locking loop pigtail nephrostomy tube[17] is placed, as described in Chapter 29.

A traditional fluoroscopic C-arm is sufficient for visualization during the ENL procedure. Fluoroscopy may be associated with radiation exposure, but this is usually minimal during urinary interventions. Regardless, care must be taken to reduce exposure through beam collimation, reducing dose, and wearing standard radiation protection gear. Ultrasonography is useful for percutaneous renal access in order to cannulate the renal pelvis and ureter in an antegrade manner. This is needed for PCNL.

Procedure ESWL

For ESWL in dogs, the patient must be anesthetized to permit accurate positioning and minimizing patient movement during the procedure. The hair overlying the entry point of the shock waves should be clipped to prevent trapping of air bubbles under the hair that could attenuate the shock wave at the skin surface. With dry lithotriptors, the treatment head of the lithotripter must be carefully coupled to the body wall with ultrasonic coupling gel to assure transmission of the shock waves into the body. Air bubbles should be avoided between the coupling cushion and the skin because even small air bubbles can dramatically impair shock wave transmission and reduce efficiency of stone fragmentation.

For accurate targeting and treatment with ESWL, the urolith must be accurately identified by fluoroscopy, ultrasonography or both (Figure 27.2). The patient is positioned such that the urolith is placed within the focal spot of the lithotripter utilizing the integrated targeting system of the lithotripter. Accurate targeting is essential to fragment uroliths and prevent damage to other organs. The Dornier HM-3 has integrated biplanar fluoroscopy such that once the urolith is targeted in both fluoroscopic images, the urolith is located within the treatment focal spot (Figure 27.1C). For dry lithotripsy units, targeting is based on C-arm fluoroscopy that is integrated with the unit and may also be assisted by ultrasonography for some lithotriptors.

Once the patient is anesthetized and positioned with the urolith in the treatment focal spot, shock waves are

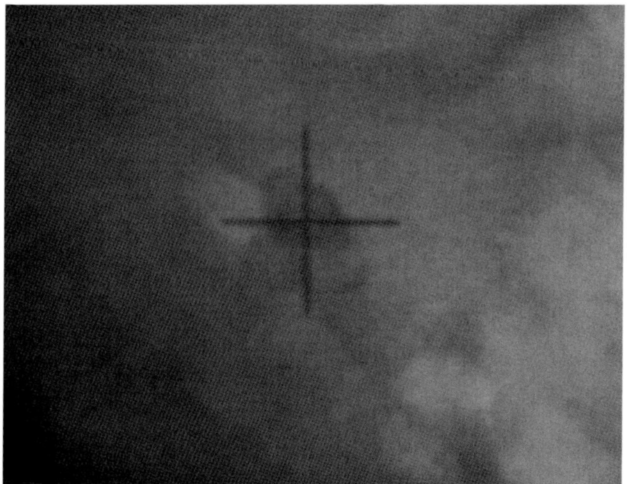

Figure 27.2 Fluoroscopic image of targeted left nephrolith immediately prior to ESWL treatment.

delivered to the urolith to induce fragmentation. Voltage stepping is the term used to describe ESWL protocols that begin with low voltage settings per shock wave and progressively increase the voltage during treatment as compared to setting the lithotripter at a constant voltage for the entire duration of shock wave therapy. Voltage stepping (e.g., increasing voltage from 16 to 18 kV) results in improved fragmentation of uroliths compared to using the same voltage (18 kV) for all shock wave administered.(Zhou et al, 2004) Patient tolerance of ESWL therapy is also improved with voltage stepping allowing for lighter planes of anesthesia during ESWL (Lingeman et al, 2002). Therefore, ESWL protocols for dogs should include voltage stepping by increasing the shock wave voltage from a lower initial setting up to a maximum safe dose during ESWL. For the Dornier HM-3, the initial shock waves are generated at 14 kV and gradually increased to a maximum of 16 kV in step-wise fashion throughout the treatment.

Shock wave treatment may cause injury to the kidney, therefore the total dose delivered to the kidney and/or proximal ureter must be below the threshold for inducing clinically relevant renal injury. Shock wave induced renal injury occurs primarily by formation and collapse of microscopic air bubbles within the kidney tissues, especially within the blood vessels (Evan et al, 2002, Pishchalnikov et al, 2003, Sapozhnikov et al, 2002). Severity of the renal injury is influenced by the rate of shock wave administration such that slower rates (60/min) are less damaging to renal parenchyma that more rapid rates (120/min) (Sapozhnikov et al, 2002). Furthermore, the efficacy of urolith fragmentation is improved by slower rates of shock wave administration compared to faster rates (Pace et al, 2005). Given this information, ESWL treatment for dogs with uroliths should include using slower treatment rates (60–80 shocks per minute) and maintaining total shock wave dose delivered to the kidney below 1500 shock waves at a maximum power setting of 16 kV for the Dornier HM-3 (or equivalent dose for other lithotriptors).It is important to remember that the shock waves are delivered with a EKG gated system, so if the heart rate is too high the rate of shock waves will be affected. With EKG gating, if the rate is too fast, then shock waves are delivered after every other heartbeat.

The urolith is monitored periodically during treatment to monitor the urolith fragmentation and confirm accurate targeting. For larger nephroliths, several areas within the urolith should be targeted with conformation of accurate positioning by fluoroscopy. This is particularly important for lithotriptors with small focal spots.

ENL

The entire abdomen, vulva/prepuce should be clipped and ascetically prepared.

For a *percutaneous nephrolithotomy (PCNL)* the patient is placed in lateral recumbency with the affected kidney up. This procedure is performed using ultrasonographic, fluoroscopic and endoscopic guidance (Figure 27.3). The renal pelvis is accessed through the greater curvature of the kidney with ultrasound guidance using a renal access needle (18 g) until the large nephrolith is hit or urine is obtained in the needle. Subsequently, using fluoroscopic guidance, a pyeloureterogram is performed using a 50% mixture of contrast material. Then a 0.035″ angle-tipped hydrophilic guidewire is advanced through the catheter, around the stone, down the ureter, and into the urinary bladder. Once within the bladder it is advanced out the urethra to obtained through-and-through access.

Next, a 5 Fr (or appropriate catheter for the specific sized patient) open-ended ureteral catheter is advanced over the guidewire in a retrograde manner to the level of the ureteropelvic junction (UPJ) (Figure 27.4). This catheter has a few purposes: to see where the UPJ is during nephroscopy, to ensure the lithotrite is not within the ureter, to block the ureteral lumen from stone fragment passage during lithotripsy, and to allow retrograde irrigation to keep stones fragments from travelling down the ureter. Then, the renal access sheath is loaded behind the un-inflated balloon dilation catheter (Figure 27.3D). It is important to use an appropriately sized access set to ensure that the nephroscope will fit through the sheath, with enough

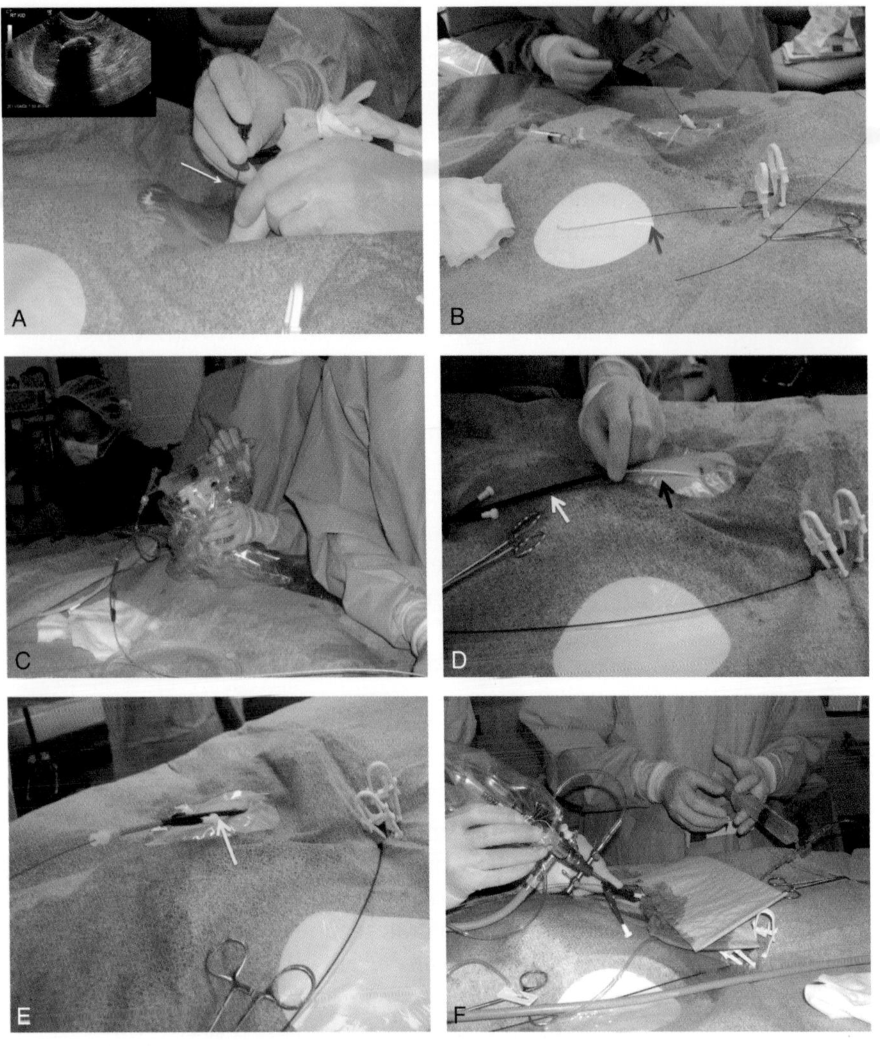

Figure 27.3 Renal access in a dog during PCNL. Dog is in left lateral recumbency. The head is to the left of the image. (A) Ultrasound guidance (white arrow) during renal puncture onto the stone. Notice the ultrasound image in he top left of the image showing a large shadowing stone. (B) Once renal access is obtained with the needle a guide wire (red arrows) is advanced from the renal pelvis, down the ureter, into the bladder and out the urethra. (C) Dilating the renal tract for the access sheath with a balloon insufflator. (D) The sheath (yellow arrow) being advanced over the inflated balloon (black arrow), into the renal pelvis. (E) The sheath (yellow arrow) within the renal pelvis. (F) The nephroscope being advanced through the sheath for intracorporeal lithotripsy to be performed.

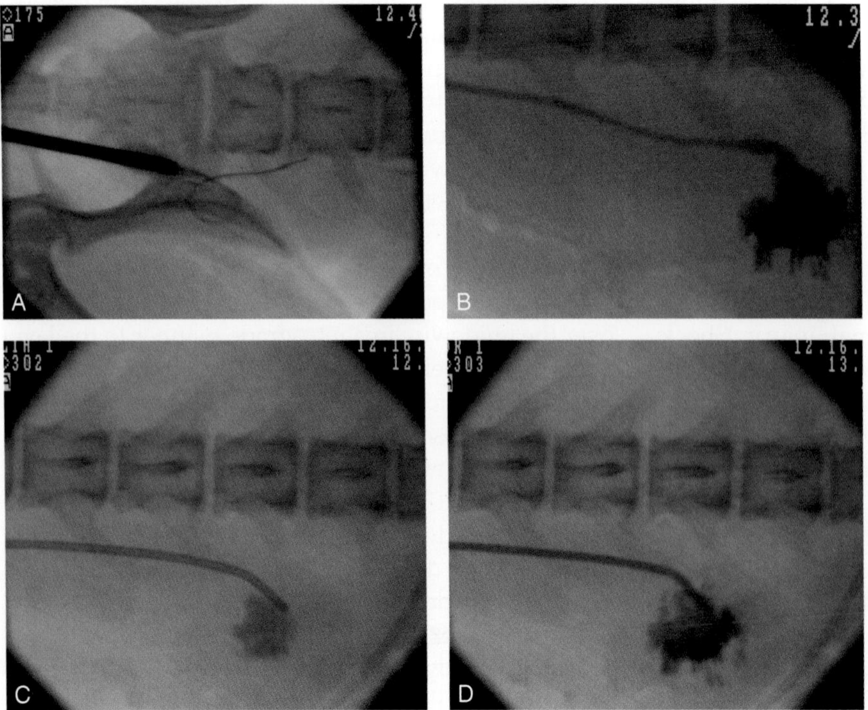

Figure 27.4 Fluoroscopic images of a female dog during a retrograde ureteropyelogram. This assisted in obtaining renal access for PCNL. The head is to the right of the image. (A) Cystoscopy being performed to assist in placement of a guide wire up the ureterovesicular junction. Notice the distal "J" of the wire in the canine ureter at the UVJ. (B) Retrograde ureteropyelogram being performed once the ureteral catheter is in the distal ureter. (C) The open ended ureteral catheter advanced up the ureter to the renal pelvis where the large nephrolith is seen. (D) Contrast injected around the nephrolith to assist in percutaneous renal access using fluoroscopic guidance.

room. This is typically a 24 Fr sheath over an 8 mm × 15 cm balloon. Once this is loaded the balloon dilation catheter is advanced over the guide wire, through the skin, into the renal parenchyma, and onto the stone (Figure 27.3C–E). Care must be taken to avoid advancing the balloon into the proximal ureter, as this will easily perforate the ureter during balloon dilation. The most proximal radiopaque marker should be seen in the center of the stone, and not in front of the stone. Another option is to use serial renal access dilators in a bougienage fashion. The author prefers the balloon dilation approach. The goal of either balloon dilation or serial bougienage is to dilate a tract between planes of the renal parenchyma, rather than cut the tissue, which stretches the renal tissue, but does not transect it, as with a nephrotomy. This is why this procedure has minimal to no effect on renal function and is considered renal sparing. Because you are dilating a hole that is 8 mm wide it can bleed and the balloon provides a tamponade effect. If the bleeding becomes excessive when the balloon is retracted it should be replaced and dilated again until the bleeding stops. Once the balloon is dilated (Figure 27.3) the sheath is advanced over the inflated balloon, into the renal parenchyma until it is touching the stone. Now the sheath will maintain the tamponade as the balloon is deflated and withdrawn over the wire.

The through-and-through wire is considered a safety wire, and should not be removed until the procedure is complete. The endoscope and lithotrite are advanced through the sheath until the stone is visualized (Figure 27.3F and Figure 27.5). Saline irrigation should be maintained in order to have good visibility. As long as there is enough space for the fluids to egress around the scope within the sheath this is not a problem. If the scope is tight within the sheath, then a larger diameter sheath should be used to avoid over-distension of the renal pelvis. The benefit of the dual probe ultrasonic lithotrite is that is can fragment any type of stone material with a jackhammer effect, while it simultaneously suctions out the fragments being created. The Hol:YAG laser lithotrite can also be used (Figure 27.6C). The benefit of this is that the fiber is smaller (200–600 µm options), allowing a smaller endoscope to be used (2.7 mm rigid cystoscope). This allows for a smaller renal access sheath (5 or 6 mm balloon and 15 or 18 Fr sheath), which is ultimately a smaller hole. The disadvantage is that the laser will fragment any stone type into thousands of pieces and each fragment needs to then be removed with a stone retrieval basket or grasping instrument, which can take an extended period of time and result in fragments passing down the ureter during irrigation. Another option for single stones, especially in cats, is to use a sheath that is slightly larger than the stone itself. This allows basket retrieval of the stone without fragmentation using a cystoscope (Figure 27.6B). Endoscopic and fluoroscopic guidance are used to monitor stone location and fragment size during the procedure (Figure 27.6A,B), and will ensure all stone fragments are retrieved from each renal calix and the entire renal pelvis prior to completion (Figure 27.5F).

Once all stone fragments are removed the ureter is carefully flushed in a retrograde manner. To do this without losing the safety wire access a second wire is advanced through the sheath, down the ureter, into the bladder, and out the urethra. Now the wire that is through the open ended ureteral catheter can be removed and this catheter can be flushed in a retrograde manner so that the saline solution flushes out of the renal access sheath while the fluid is suctioned. Once no stone fragments are seen in the ureter (using fluoroscopic guidance), a retrograde ureteropyelogram is performed to ensure the entire ureter is intact and stone free. Then the guide wire is advanced up the open-ended catheter, in a retrograde manner so that the soft angled tip is coiled within the renal pelvis. The open-ended ureteral catheter is removed over the guidewire monitoring under fluoroscopic guidance and an appropriately sized 4.7 Fr double pigtail ureteral stent is then placed. To measure the appropriate ureteral length the open-ended ureteral catheter is used. Under fluoroscopic guidance the catheter is marked at the prepuce or vulva when the tip of the catheter is at the UPJ, and then again when it is at the UVJ. The distance between these two marks is the length of the ureter. This is explained in more detail in Chapter 30. The stent is then advanced over the guidewire and once a curl is need in the renal pelvis under fluoroscopic guidance the wire is withdrawn into the proximal urethra. The distal loop of the ureteral stent is then pushed into the urinary bladder. When this procedure is done in cats a ureteral stent is not placed post ENL due to the risk of prophylactic stenting in cats with the small ureteral diameter (0.3 mm).

Once the stent is in place a locking-loop nephrostomy tube is placed through the renal access sheath, into the renal pelvis. This can be accomplished by taking the angle-tipped 0.035″ hydrophilic guidewire, advancing it through the sheath, and into the renal pelvis. Once it is curled within the pelvis, using fluoroscopic guidance the sheath is removed over the wire. Next, the 6 Fr locking-loop pigtail catheter is advanced over the guidewire and placed within the pelvis, as

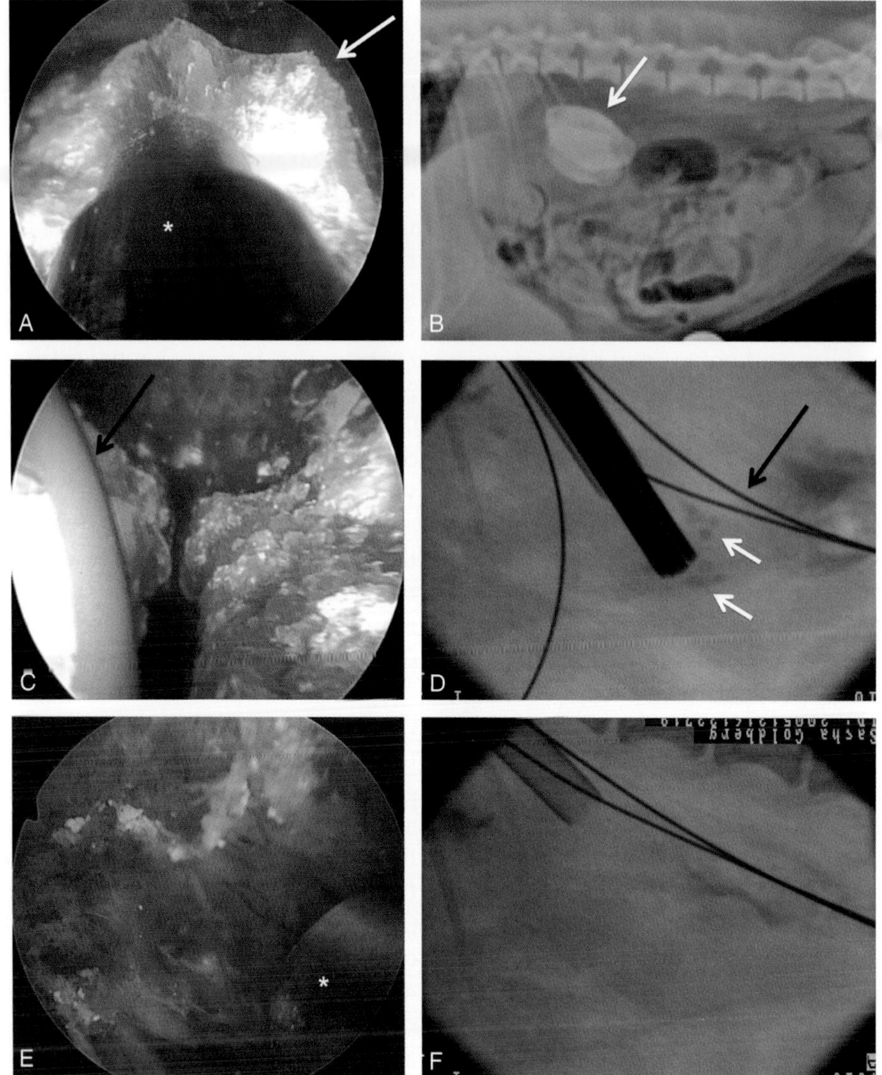

Figure 27.5 Intracorporeal lithotripy using the ultrasonic lithotripter in a dog with a large nephrolith. (A) Nephroscopy being performed through a sheath with the lithotripter (white asterisk) through the working channel of the scope, which is in contact with the large nephrolith (white arrow). (B) Lateral radiograph of the dog with large bilateral nephroliths (white arrow). (C) Nephroscopic image during lithotripsy showing the large stone broken into fragments. Notice the guide wire (black arrow) within the renal pelvis (safety wire). (D) Fluoroscopic image of the dog during lithotripsy showing the broken stone fragments (white arrows), and the safety wire (black arrow) down the ureter. (E) Nephroscopic image after the stone is removed, showing a clean renal pelvis with no stone fragments. The lithotripter is seen with the white asterisk. (F) Fluoroscopic image after all stone fragments are removed.

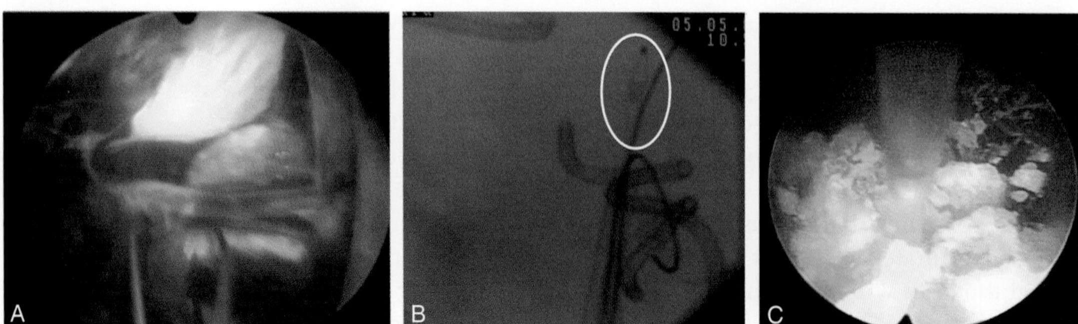

Figure 27.6 Various ways to perform a nephrolithotomy. (A) Nephroscopic image of a dog with the stone being removed en-bloc using a stone retrieval basket. (B) Fluoroscopic image in a cat showing the stone being removed with a stone retrieval basket (white circle) using fluoroscopy alone. (C) Nephroscopic image of a dog during laser lithotripsy of a nephrolith.

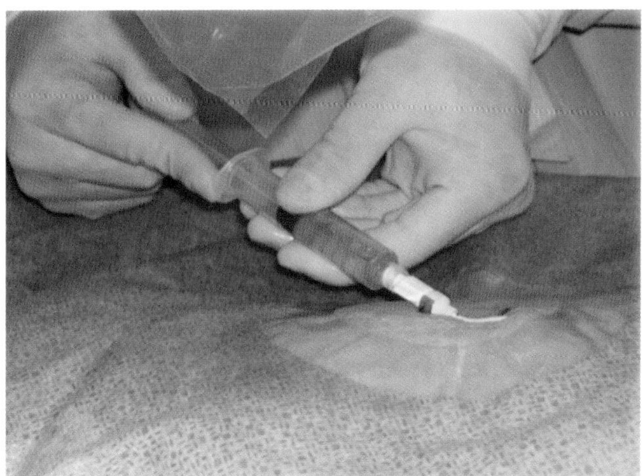

Figure 27.7 Percutaneous nephrostomy tube placed after PCNL in a dog.

described in Chapter 29 (Figure 27.7). Once the nephrostomy tube is in place it is securely sutured to the body wall using a purse-string suture and a Chinese-finger trap pattern. The tube should be left to gravity drain for 24 hours, and then it can be capped and covered to prevent inadvertent removal. The nephrostomy tube should remain in place for 4 weeks while a nephropexy forms.

A *surgically assisted endoscopic nephrolithotomy* (SENL) is performed as described above, though ultrasound is not needed to gain renal pelvis access. Instead the patient is placed in dorsal recumbency and an abdominal incision is made from the xiphoid to the bladder. The affected kidney is isolated and an 18 gauge over-the-needle catheter is advanced from the renal capsule onto the affected stone using only fluoroscopic guidance. This is typically done from the caudal pole of the kidney because this makes use of the scope intra-operatively easier. The rest of the procedure is done the same as above other than there is no nephrostomy tube placed. Instead the hole is primarily closed using 3–0 PDS using a horizontal mattress suture pattern. Because there is no nephrostomy tube these patients are monitored carefully for 12 hours to ensure there is no evidence of a uroabdomen post-operatively.

Postoperative and Follow-Up Care

After ESWL dogs are treated with IV fluid therapy for 12 to 36 hours. Pain medications are usually not required unless nephrolith fragments cause partial to complete ureteral obstruction during initial passage down the ureter. Abdominal radiographs are performed 24 hours after ESWL to evaluate the degree of nephrolith fragmentation and observe for any problems with passage of urolith fragments through the ureter (Figure 27.8). If there is a large fragment in the ureter with multiple fragments located proximally to the "lead" fragment, then the patient should be evaluated for ureteral obstruction and renal pelvic dilation. Abdominal ultrasound should be performed if ureteral obstruction or pancreatitis is suspected. Dogs are typically discharged within 24–48 hours after ESWL. Dogs with preplaced ureteral stents may be discharged sooner since the stent eliminates the risk of ureteral obstruction post ESWL. Follow-up evaluation with abdominal radiographs and ultrasound are performed within 1 month to evaluate if all nephrolith fragments have passed down the ureter and into the urinary bladder. In many dogs, the urolith fragments accumulate in the urinary bladder and may need to be removed by voiding urohydropropulsion. If a ureteral stent was placed prior to ESWL, cystoscopic-assisted stent removal may be performed once the majority of the nephrolith fragments have passed into the urinary bladder. Passive ureteral dilation around the ureteral stent facilitates passage of the urolith fragments before or after stent removal.

After ENL dogs are treated with 24 hours of an opioid for pain (buprenorphine 0.01 mg/kg IV TID) and then 3 days of oral medications (tramadol 3–5 mg/kg TID PO). They are typically discharged within 24–36 hours. Prior to discharge a focal ultrasound is performed to get a measurement of the renal pelvis diameter and assess for excessive fluid accumulation in the abdomen. A radiograph is taken to asses stent location and document the absence of nephroliths and/or ureteroliths comparing pre-and post ENL (Figure 27.9). The renal pelvis will usually maintain the size of the previous stone for a minimum of a few weeks, and sometimes chronically.

After a PCNL the urine is cultured from the nephrostomy tube in 5–7 days postoperatively to ensure no infection is present. Then at 1 month, another ultrasound is performed and if no fluid is present in the abdomen the nephrostomy tube is removed. This should be done over a guidewire using fluoroscopic guidance to ensure the ureteral stent is not accidentally retracted as well. In most circumstances the ureteral stent will also be removed at this time, either endoscopically or fluoroscopically using a retrieval basket or snare device from the bladder. After a SENL the patient is started on a fluoroquinolone antibiotic for 2 weeks and the urine should be cultured 4 weeks post-procedure. At that time the ureteral stent can be retrieved from the urinary bladder.

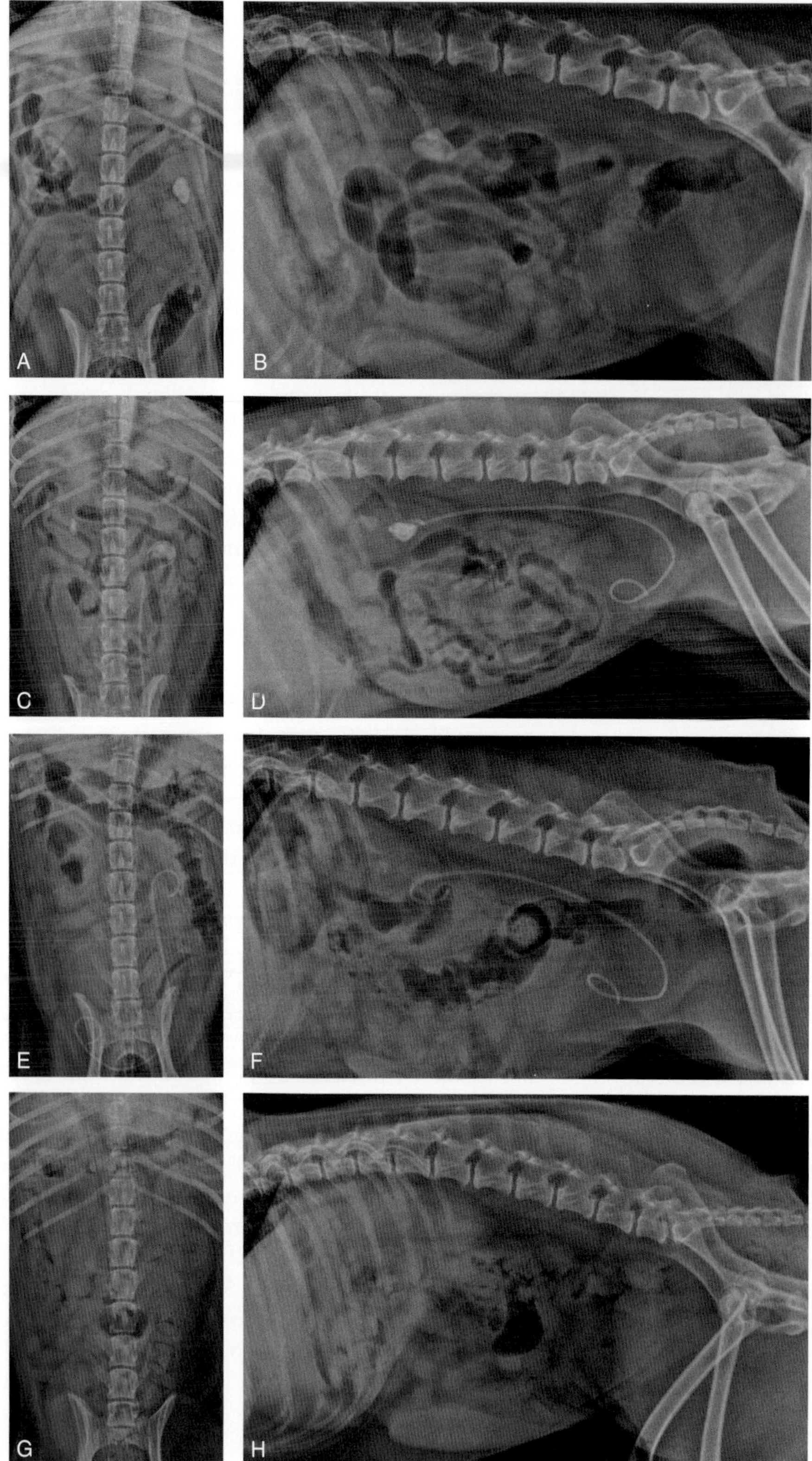

Figure 27.8 Radiographs of a dog before and after ESWL therapy. (A) VD abdominal radiograph showing large compound nephrolith (5% calcium oxalate, 80% struvite and 15% calcium phosphate) in the left kidney and small right nephroliths. Note discrete layers within the large left nephrolith. (B) Lateral abdominal radiograph showing large compound left nephrolith and smaller right nephrolith. Note discrete layers within stone visible on radiographs. (C) VD abdominal radiograph after left ureteral stent placement prior to ESWL treatment. (D) Lateral abdominal radiograph after left ureteral stent placement prior to ESWL treatment. (E) VD abdominal radiograph 24 hours after ESWL treatment showing successful fragmentation of the nephrolith. Note small sand-like nephrolith fragments around the proximal aspect of the ureteral stent. (F) Lateral abdominal radiograph 24 hours after ESWL treatment showing successful fragmentation of the nephrolith. (G) VD abdominal radiograph 1 week after ESWL and following ureteral stent removal. The nephrolith fragments were removed by voiding urohydropropulsion and the ureteral stent was extracted by cystoscopy (see Chapter 30). (H) Lateral abdominal radiograph 1 week after ESWL and following ureteral stent removal.

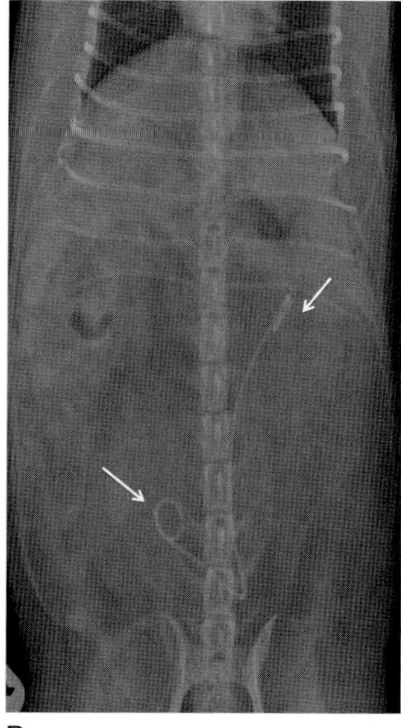

A B

Figure 27.9 Dorsoventral radiographs of a female dog before and after ENL. The head is to the top of the images. A) Large left nephrolith (black arrow) prior to the ENL procedure. B) The nephrolith is no longer present in the dog and a ureteral stent (white arrows) is in place traveling from the renal pelvis, down the ureteral lumen, and into the urinary bladder.

All patients should be aggressively treated for stone prevention with appropriate diet, chelation agents, alkylating agents (when indicated), and enzyme inhibitors (when indicated). Urine should be serially evaluated for infection and urine pH every 3 months for the first 2 years, along with serial abdominal radiographs and ultrasounds.

Prognosis

ESWL and ENL are safe, minimally invasive procedures, and can be highly effective when performed by an experienced operator. Each procedure has different indications. ENL is typically more effective (90–100%) than ESWL (70–80%) when a single treatment is desired, and has been shown in humans to have minimal to no negative effect on kidney function when compared to all other options. Though, it is important to realize that ENL is more difficult to perform and more invasive than ESWL. The benefit of ureteral stenting when performing ESWL is controversial, but should be considered for large stone burdens. The operator should not consider performing ESWL if they are not comfortable handling the consequences of a potential ureteral obstruction afterwards.

Special Considerations

Both of these procedures should only be performed by operators highly trained in endourology. It is important to realize that over 90% of canine and feline nephroliths are clinically silent, regardless of size or type (other than struvite), and nearly all pure struvite stones can be successfully dissolved with aggressive medical management over a 6–9-month period. If a suspected struvite stone is not showing evidence of dissolution by 3–6 months than it is likely to be a mixed stone with a calcium containing shell (Figure 27.8), inhibiting the dissolution. This type of stone can be successfully managed with ESWL. Also, both ESWL and ENL are contraindicated in patients that have active urinary tract infections and antibiotic therapy should be instituted for at least 48–72 hours prior to considering a procedure. For human patients that are concurrently azotemic, ENL is considered more renal sparing than ESWL. In the absence of obstruction or infection, treatment of nephroliths in dogs with stage 3–4 chronic kidney disease (CKD) is unlikely to affect progression of CKD. Therefore the benefits must be weighed against risks of nephrolith removal for dogs with advanced CKD. Removal of nephroliths that are infected associated with recurrent pyelonephritis is more likely to be beneficial. Likewise, removal of nephroliths causing obstruction of the UPJ may stabilize or improve their azotemia following nephrolith removal.

It is important to remember that much of the ENL details described above have been performed in a small number of patients, and in only a few facilities around the world, therefore many of these procedures are still considered investigational.

Minimally invasive management of nephroliths in veterinary medicine is following the trend seen in human medicine. Over the past 10 years, the veterinary community has made great strides in adapting the technology used for humans to be more applicable to small animal veterinary patients. Conditions that have traditionally been considered a major therapeutic dilemma now have new, effective, and safe options.

Notes

These are only examples of equipment used but there are other options for each device noted.

1. Dornier HM-3, Dornier MedTech, Atlanta, GA.
2. Dornier Compact Delta II, Dornier MedTech, Atlanta, GA.
3. 18 gauge renal access needle × 15 cm, Cook Medical, Bloomington, IN.

4. Weasel Wire 0.035-inch hydrophilic angle-tipped guidewire, Infiniti Medical LLC, Menlo Park, CA.
5. 5 Fr, open-ended ureteral catheter, Cook Medical Inc, Bloomington, IN.
6. Renal Access Sheath Set (18, 24, 30 Fr), Cook Medical, Bloomington, IN.
7. Amplatz Renal Dilator Set, Cook Medical, Bloomington, IN.
8. Cyberwand Dual Ultrasonic Lithotriptor, Olympus, Gyrus/ACMI, Southborough, MA.
9. OES Pro Nephroscope 30 degree, Olympus, Gyrus/ACMI, Southborough, MA.
10. Odyssey Hol:YAG laser, 30W, Convergent Laser Technology, Alameda, CA.
11. Rigid endoscope, 2.7-mm 30° lens, Richard Wolf, Vernon Hills, Ill.
12. Rigid endoscope, 2.7-mm 30° lens, Karl Storz Endoscopy, Culver City, CA.
13. Ultraxx Nephrostomy Balloon, Cook Medical, Bloomington, IN.
14. Peel-Away Introducer Sheath, Cook Medical, Bloomington, IN.
15. Ureteral stents (2.5, 3.7 and 4.7 Fr) double pigtail, Infiniti Medical LLC, Menlo Park, CA.
16. InLay double pigtail ureteral stent (4.7 Fr), Bard Medical, Covington, GA.
17. Nephrostomy tube 6 Fr Pigtail non-locking drainage catheter, Infiniti Medical LLC, Menlo Park, CA.

References

Evan AP, Willis LR, McAteer JA, et al (2002) Kidney damage and renal functional changes are minimized by waveform control that suppresses cavitation in shock wave lithotripsy, *J Urol* 168, 1556–62.

Lingeman JE, Lifshitz DA, and Evan AP (2002) Surgical management of urinary lithiasis. In Campbell's Urology (Retik AB, Vaughan ED, Jr., and Wein AJ, eds), W.B. Saunders, Philadelphia, pp 3361–451.

Pace KT, Ghiculete D, Harju M, et al (2005) Shock wave lithotripsy at 60 or 120 shocks per minute: a randomized, double-blind trial, *J Urol* 174, 595–9.

Pishchalnikov YA, Sapozhnikov OA, Bailey MR, et al. (2003) Cavitation bubble cluster activity in the breakage of kidney stones by lithotripter shockwaves, *J Endourol* 17, 435–46.

Sapozhnikov OA, Khokhlova VA, Bailey MR, et al (2002) Effect of overpressure and pulse repetition frequency on cavitation in shock wave lithotripsy, *J Acoustical Soc Am* 112, 1183–95.

Zhou Y, Cocks FH, Preminger GM, et al (2004) The effect of treatment strategy on stone comminution efficiency in shock wave lithotripsy, *J Urol* 172, 349–54.

Suggested Reading

Adams LG, William JC, McAteer JA, et al (2005) In vitro evaluation of canine and feline calcium oxalate urolith fragility via shock wave lithotripsy, *Am J Vet Res* 66, 1651–4.

Adams LG and Goldman CK (2011) Extracorporeal shock wave lithotripsy. In: Nephrology and Urology of Small Animals (Polzin DJ, Bartges JB, eds). Blackwell Publishing, Ames, IA, pp 340–8.

Adams LG (2013) Nephroliths and ureteroliths: A new stone age. *N Z Vet J* 61, 1–5.

Al-Shammari AM, Al-Otaibi K, Leonard MP, et al (1999) Percutaneous nephrolithotomy in the pediatric population. *J Urol* 162, 1721–4.

Block G, Adams LG, Widmer WR, et al (1996) Use of extracorporeal shock wave lithotripsy for treatment of nephrolithiasis and ureterolithiasis in five dogs. *J Am Vet Med Assoc* 208, 531–6.

Bollinger C, Walshaw R, Kruger JM, et al (2005). Evaluation of the effects of nephrotomy on renal function in clinically normal cats. *Am J Vet Res* 66, 1400–7.

Donner GS, Ellison GW, et al (1987) Percutaneous nephrolithotomy in the dog: an experimental study, *Vet Surg* 16, 411–17.

Lane IF (2004) Lithotripsy: an update on urologic applications in small animals. *Vet Clin N Am Small Anim Pract* 34, 1011–25.

Shokeir AA, Sheir KZ, El-Nahas AR, et al (2006) Treatment of renal stones in children: a comparison of percutaneous nephrolithotomy and shock wave lithotripsy. *J Urol* 176, 706–10.

Stone E, Robertson JL, and Metcalf MR (2002) The effect of nephrotomy on renal function and morphology in dogs. *Vet Surg* 31, 391–7.

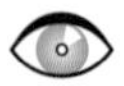 Video clips to accompany this chapter can be found in the online material at **www.wiley.com/go/weisse/vet-image-guided-interventions**

CHAPTER TWENTY-EIGHT

Interventional Treatment of Idiopathic Renal Hematuria

Allyson Berent
The Animal Medical Center, New York, NY

Background/Indications

Idiopathic renal hematuria (IRH), or benign essential renal hematuria, is a rare condition of chronic severe renal bleeding. This condition typically results in persistent port-wine colored urine that can be intermittent and may or may-not be progressive. It is not associated with trauma, nephroliths, neoplasia, coagulopathy, hypertension, or other obvious causes. Although it has been described in the human literature for decades, it is considered a rare condition. The first report in humans was in 1959, in which a small hemangioma of the kidney causing severe hematuria was described. In veterinary medicine, there have been a few cases sporadically reported. The earliest reports of the condition were in the early 1980s, and until recently a total of 17 dogs were cumulatively reported.

Typically, this is considered a condition of young, large-breed dogs, with the majority reported under 2 years of age. Cats have also been seen in the author's practice and are often found to have ureteral obstructions secondary to dried solidified blood stones. There does not seem to be a sex predilection. Historically, cases in the veterinary literature were diagnosed with ureteral catheterization during a cystotomy before the wide-spread introduction of cystoscopy. Hydronephrosis and hydroureter have been reported in nearly half of the cases, and is suspected to be due to the accumulation of blood clots resulting in a partial or complete ureteral obstruction. The condition has been reported to occur bilaterally as well (21–33% of patients reported), and when unilaterally identified there is no lateralizing preference. In a more recent series of six dogs treated in the author's practice, four were unilateral and two were bilateral, totaling eight renal units affected (five were left sided and three were right sided) with five of six patients being male dogs (Berent et al, 2013).

In humans, renal vascular abnormalities (like hemangiomas, papillary angiomas and minute venous ruptures) are typically the cause of renal hematuria (Bagley and Allen, 1990). This has been identified in dogs and cats as well (Figure 28.1). Although the long-term course appears to be benign, frequent bouts of hematuria can lead to iron deficiency anemia, ureteral colic, and ureteral/urethral obstructions. In addition, persistent hematuria is distressing to visualize grossly.

Cystoscopy for evaluation of the ureterovesicular orifice is the diagnostic method of choice for upper tract bleeding (Figure 28.2). With the advent of contemporary imaging and small ureteroscopes, endourologic treatment via ureteroscopy and electrocautery is considered the diagnostic and therapeutic modality of choice in human medicine (Tawfiek and Bagley, 1998). In ~80% of cases, ureteronephroscopy is successful in identifying the lesion in the renal pelvis. Once identified, endoscopic guided therapy is effective in over 90% of human patients.

Since the lesion(s) are not typically considered of renal parenchymal origin, and over 20–30% are, or can become, bilateral, nephrectomy is not recommended. Due to the small size of a canine and feline ureter (0.5–2.0 mm, 0.3–0.4 mm, respectively), it does not easily accommodate a ureteroscope (2.7 mm) without manual or passive dilation, which can be accomplished sufficiently in some animals with a ureteral stent. The use of retrograde sclerotherapy for hemostasis, using liquid silver nitrate and a povidone iodine solution, was recently investigated in dogs and has been shown to be effective for this condition in humans. This is performed in people with IRH in countries where

Veterinary Image-Guided Interventions, First Edition. Edited by Chick Weisse and Allyson Berent.

Companion website: www.wiley.com/go/weisse/vet-image-guided-interventions

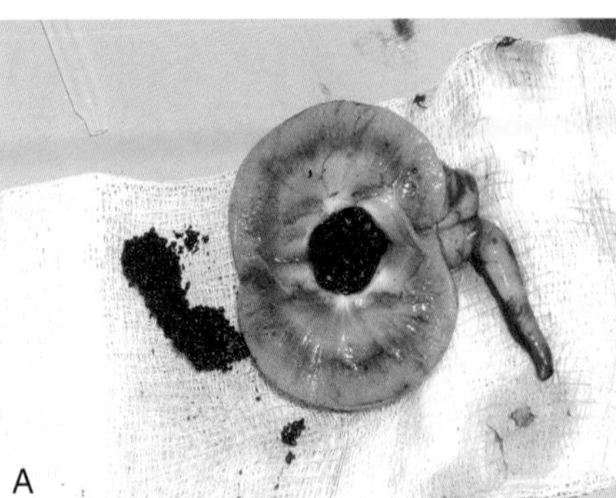

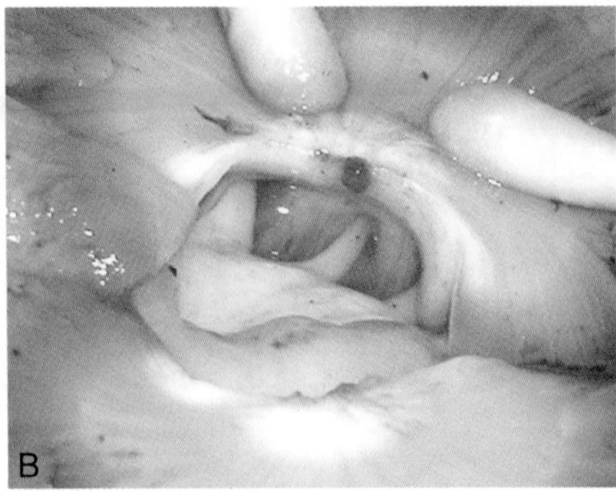

Figure 28.1 Kidney of a cat after a ureteronephrectomy was performed for persistent renal hematuria. The renal pelvis was carefully dissected and revealed numerous dried solidified blood stones. Once the stones were removed a lesion was seen on the papilla of the renal pelvis. This was histologically confirmed as a hemangioma.

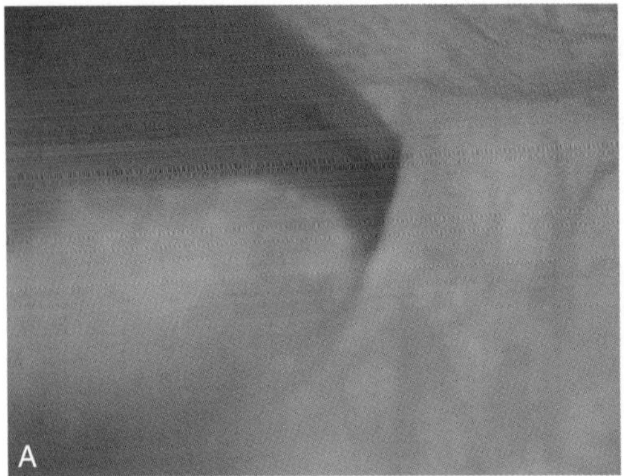

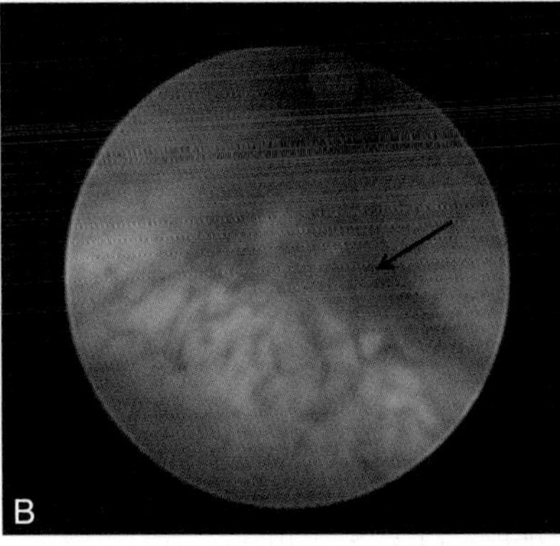

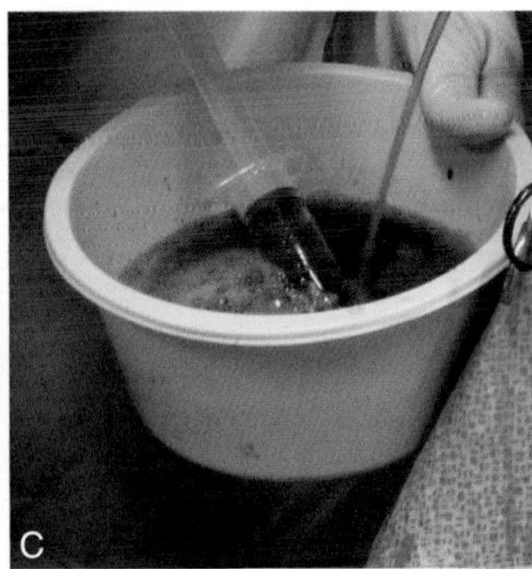

Figure 28.2 (A) Endoscopic image of a female dog in dorsal recumbency during a routine retrograde cystoscopy. There is a jet of red urine coming from the left ureteral orifice. (B) Antegrade cystoscopy in a male cat with chronic hematuria. The right UVJ (black arrow) has a jet of bloody urine coming from it, consistent with renal hematuria. There is a red rubber catheter seen in the proximal urethra. (C) Classic "port-wine" colored urine being drained from the bladder during a cystoscopy in a dog with IRH.

ureteroscopes are not available or the bleeding lesions are too numerous. In addition, this sclerotherapy treatment is commonly used for chyluria in humans in whom numerous lymphatic anastomoses to the renal pelvis are found, typically due to malarial disease.

Patient Preparation

All patients should have a CBC, serum biochemical profile, urinalysis, urine bacteriologic culture, coagulation profile, and abdominal ultrasonsography performed. Von Willebrand factor antigen testing is recommended in all patients. A platelet function test (PFA) is recommended when possible, and a buccal mucosal bleeding time (BMBT) should be considered when a PFA is not possible. A thorough history and physical examination should be obtained, assessing for concurrent illnesses or potential causes for bleeding. A rectal examination should be performed to ensure there is no vaginal, urethral, or prostatic masses. Intact male dogs could have bleeding associated with benign prostatic hyperplasia and these dogs usually only have blood at the beginning or the end of urination with normal yellow colored urine in between or when assess via cystocentesis.

The author recommends a 2-week trial with the Chinese herb Yunnan Paiyou (also written "Yunnan Baiyou"). This herb has unknown mechanisms that result in improving coagulation and platelet function. This has improved the bleeding in about 10–15% of cases. Additionally, there is a small group of dogs that have responded to treatment with an angiotensin-converting enzyme inhibitor. This is likely due to a decrease in the renal glomerular pressure resulting in diminished bleeding tendencies. This has not been beneficial in the author's practice but might be useful if the bleeding is of renal origin rather than renal pelvic origin. There is also some data in children with peripheral infantile hemangiomas that are highly responsive to propranolol therapy. This has not been used in dogs, cats, or humans for IRH, but may be worth further investigation. The mechanism of action is currently unknown but might be associated with vasoconstriction and decreasing local blood flow to the lesion(s).

If all of these findings are normal and medical management fails to control the bleeding, urinary tract imaging with cystoscopy with or without computerized tomography (CT) renal angiography, or selective renal arteriography is recommended. Rarely, a renal arteriovenous fistula or malformation can be seen with advanced imaging.

Potential Risks/Complications/Expected Outcomes

An experienced interventional endoscopist comfortable cannulating the UVJ with a wire and catheter, and ureteroscope if it is necessary, should perform these procedures. The most substantial risk is perforating the ureter during cannulation or excessive renal filling/distension resulting in nephritis or pelvic rupture. By using fluoroscopy and endoscopy together the appropriate filling volume of the renal pelvis during sclerotherapy is ensured. Also, the risk of post-sclerotherapy ureteritis and post-ureteroscopy edema is possible so the operator should be comfortable with retrograde ureteral stent placement.

In a recent study in which sclerotherapy was used for the treatment of IRH complete cessation of macroscopic hematuria occurred in four of six dogs within a median of 6 hours (range, immediately postoperatively to 7 days). Two additional dogs improved: one moderately and one substantially. None of the dogs required nephrectomy. Ureteroscopy for electrocautery has only been performed in a small number of patients, and this is typically reserved for larger patients that have failed sclerotherapy.

It is important for the reader to realize that this procedure is still currently under investigation in veterinary medicine. Based on the few cases (approximately 15 to date) treated in the author's practice, as well as hundreds in human medicine, it is presumed to be safe and effective. Owners need to be aware of the limited experience with this procedure in clinical veterinary patients.

Equipment

Endoscopy is typically performed with an appropriate diameter 30 degree rigid cystoscope for female dogs (1.9, 2.7, or 4 mm)[1–3] or a 7.5–8.1 Fr flexible ureteroscope[4] for male dogs. Perineal access (see Chapter 39) should be obtained once renal hematuria is confirmed with the flexible endoscope in males, in which the 2.7 mm cystoscope can be utilized for the remainder of the procedure. Ureteral access is obtained with an appropriately sized angle-tipped hydrophilic guide wire[5] and open-ended ureteral catheter[6] (see Table 2.1 in Chapter 2). A traditional fluoroscopic C-arm is sufficient for visualization of the upper urinary tract during the procedure.

A ureteropelvic junction balloon (UPJ) balloon[7] is used for ureteral occlusion and this is often placed over a stiffened J-tipped guide wire.[8] For sclerotherapy a sterilized liquid 0.5–1% silver nitrate solution,[9] in addition to a 1:1:3 ratio of 1 part 5% povidone iodine[10]: 1 part 76% meglumine diatrizoate (76MD):[11] 3 parts D5W is used.

Instead of saline irrigation during endoscopy, 5% dextrose in sterile water (D5W) is used. This helps to prevent red blood cell lysis, improving the visibility during cystoscopy. In addition, D5W prevents silver salt development during sclerotherapy with silver nitrate, and aids in conduction during Bugbee electrocautery, if necessary.

For ureteroscopic electrocautery a 0.035″ stiffened angle-tipped hydrophilic guide wire[12] is used, along with serial ureteral dilators[13] to assist in the advancement of the flexible ureteroscope. Irrigation is done manually through the ureteroscope using D5W. Once a lesion is found in the renal pelvis a Bugbee cautery electrode[14] (1–2 Fr) is used in either blend or coagulation mode through the working channel of the ureteroscope to ablate the lesion. This small diameter electrode maintains the flexibility of the ureteroscope within the renal pelvis. If necessary a ureteral access sheath[18] can be used to maintain ureteral patency during ureteroscopy.

Finally, after all procedures are complete a double pigtail ureteral stent[15–17] of appropriate size (typically 4.7 Fr) (see Table 34.1 in Chapter 34) is placed over the working guide wire and left in place for 2 weeks to prevent ureteral edema/ureteritis and subsequent obstruction.

Prior to cystoscopy renal angiograms are offered to owners for evaluation of gross vascular anomalies if a CT scan is not performed during the diagnostic work-up. In the few cases this has been done, no lesions were documented.

Procedure

Dogs are placed in dorsal recumbency, and the vulva or prepuce are clipped and aseptically prepared. In male dogs the entire perineum is clipped as well and a purse-string suture is placed in the anus. Periprocedural antimicrobials are given (cefazolin 22 mg/kg [10 mg/lb], IV).

Preprocedural diagnostic cystoscopy for full evaluation of the prepuce, vulva, vagina, urethra, prostatic urethra, UVJ, and bladder wall is completed on a day when gross hematuria is present. For female dogs a rigid cystoscope with a 30 degree angle is used and in male dogs a 2.7 mm flexible ureteroscope is used. In male dogs, once the hematuria is identified using flexible urethrocystoscopy, perineal urethral access is obtained to allow the use of a 2.7 mm rigid cystoscope for UVJ access (see Chapter 39).

Using the rigid cystoscope, each UVJ is identified and monitored for at least 30 seconds to see two or more urine jets in order to assess for hematuria. The urine in the bladder is typically "port-wine" color (Figure 28.2). The irrigation fluids are changed from 0.9% sodium chloride to 5% dextrose in water (D5W). Once the hematuric UVJ is identified (Figure 28.2A,B) an appropriately sized (typically 0.035") angle-tipped hydrophilic guide wire is advanced up the affected ureter using cystoscopic and fluoroscopic guidance (Figure 28.3). An open-ended ureteral catheter (typically 5 Fr), appropriately sized for the guide wire being used, is then advanced over the guide wire using fluoroscopic guidance. A urine sample is obtained for culture. Then a retrograde ureteropyelogram is performed to confirm there are no gross lesions present in the ureter or renal pelvis (Figure 28.3C).

Sclerotherapy

The contrast agent used for the retrograde ureteropyelogram is 76% MD because this is the recommended mixture with povidone iodine to accomplish appropriate sclerotherapy in humans. The guide wire is advanced into the renal pelvis and the catheter is advanced to the UPJ. The guide wire is exchanged for a J-tipped stiffened guide wire and the cystoscope is removed over the guide wire, while the wire remains inside the proximal ureter, at the UPJ. Then, over the guide wire, a UPJ balloon catheter (Figure 28.3D) is advanced to the level of the UPJ or proximal ureter (Figure 28.3D). The guide wire is subsequently removed. The balloon is filled using air to allow a compliant occlusion of the proximal ureter (typically 0.3–0.6 ml). The patient is tilted into a 20 degree Trendelenberg position to allow dwelling of material into the renal pelvis (rear legs higher than kidneys). Contrast material 76% MD is used in a 50% mixture with D5W to determine the volume it takes to fill the ipsilateral occluded renal pelvis and all associated calices without renal back filling (Figure 28.3D) This volume is then used for dwelling of the sclerotherapy materials. The contrast is then removed via passive draining.

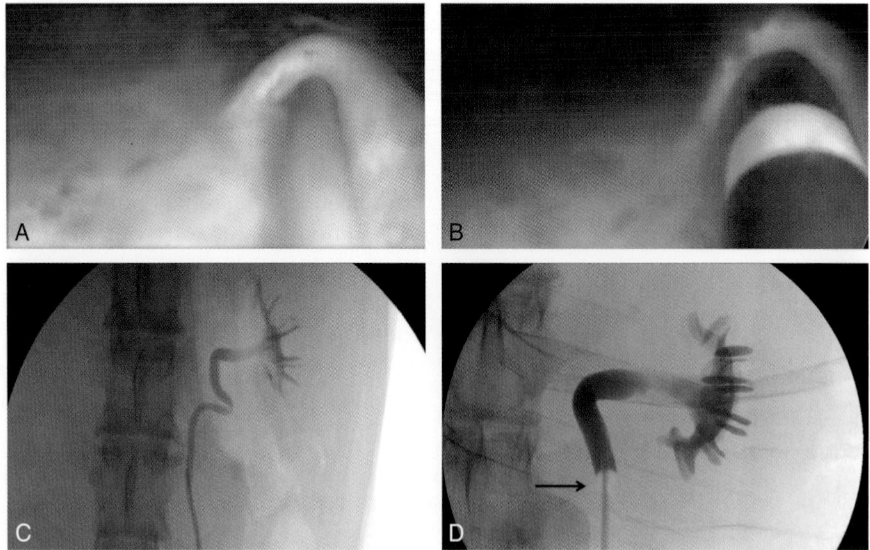

Figure 28.3 Sclerotherapy procedure in a dog with left-sided IRH. The dog is in dorsal recumbency during rigid cystoscopy. (A) A guide wire being advanced up the left UVJ using cystoscopic guidance. (B) An open-ended ureteral catheter advanced over the guide wire into the ureter. (C) The open ended ureteral catheter seen in the mid ureter using fluoroscopic guidance. A retrograde ureteropyelogram is done to ensure there are no filling defects and to mark the location of the renal pelvis. (D) The ureteral catheter is exchanged for a UPJ balloon catheter. Notice the balloon at the tip of the catheter (black arrow), which is filled with air. The renal pelvis and proximal ureter are filled with contrast to measure the volume required for sclerotherapy.

Once occlusion is obtained two dwells of the predetermined volume of the povidone iodine mixture (1:1:3) is left inside the renal pelvis for 10–20 minutes each. Then this is drained and flushed with D5W. An additional two dwells using freshly sterilized liquid 0.5–1% silver nitrate solution, at 15–20 minutes each, is then performed. This is not mixed with contrast so it cannot be monitored for backfilling. Once complete, the patient is removed from the Trendelenberg position into dorsal recumbency and the solution is passively drained. Finally, the guide wire (stiffened J-wire if the catheter is at the UPJ, or the hydrophilic guide wire if the catheter is in the proximal ureter to prevent ureteral damage) is re-introduced through the UPJ balloon catheter and curled inside the renal pelvis using fluoroscopic guidance. The catheter is removed over the guide wire and the cystoscope is advanced over the guide wire to the level of the UVJ. An appropriately sized double pigtail ureteral stent (see Chapter 34) is placed over the guide wire with one loop curled inside the renal pelvis and the other inside the urinary bladder. All fluid is drained from the urinary bladder and urethra and the cystoscope is removed while a local bupivicane infusion is given into the urethra. Male dogs with perineal urethral access have the sheath removed and the incision is left to heal by second intention.

Ureteroscopy with Electrocautery

This procedure is reserved for patients large enough for initial ureteroscopy (>20 kg), or those that had sclerotherapy performed and a ureteral stent in place >1–2 weeks, in which the stent induced passive ureteral dilation. This is typically done with rigid cystoscopy, in order to gain guide wire access to the appropriate ureter (as described above). If a stent is in place than the distal end of the ureteral stent is retrieved in the urinary bladder with a grasping instrument in the working channel. It is pulled out of the urethra and re-wired with a 0.035″ exchange length (260 cm) stiffened, angle-tipped hydrophilic guide wire under fluoroscopic guidance. Once the wire is at the UPJ the stent is removed off the guide wire. A ureteral access sheath[18] (9.5 Fr inner/11 Fr outer diameter) is advanced over the guide wire to the mid ureter and then the ureteroscope is advanced over the guide wire using endoscopic and fluoroscopic guidance (Figure 28.4). If the sheath does not fit than the ureteroscope can be placed directly over the guide wire. Once the ureteroscope is inside the

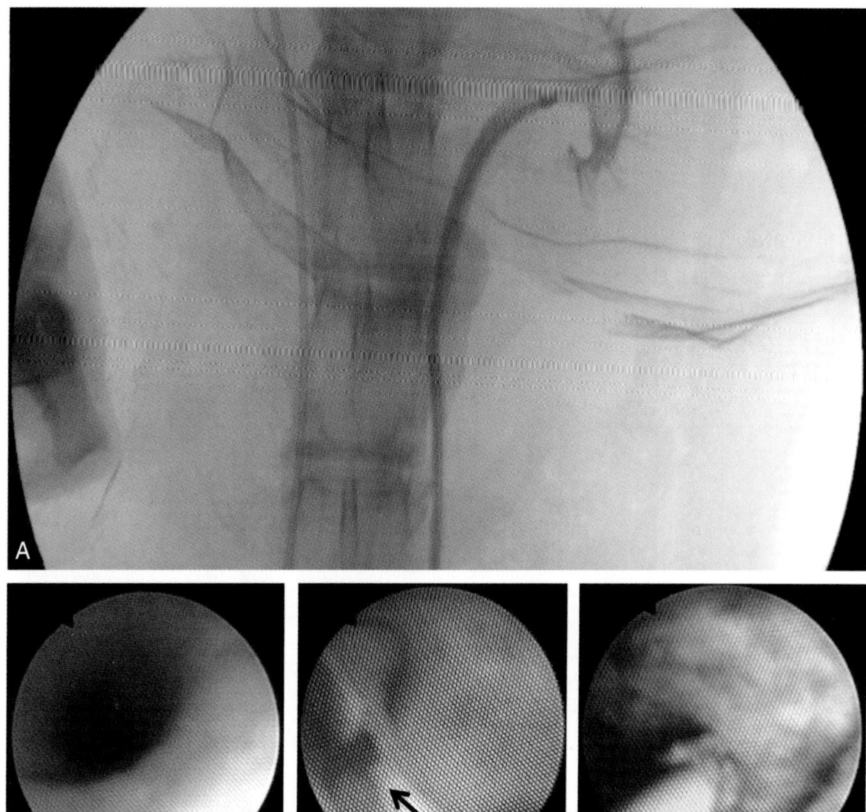

Figure 28.4 Ureteroscopy procedure in a dog with IRH. The patient is in dorsal recumbency. (A) The left ureter and renal pelvis is cannulated with a flexible ureteroscope. (B) Endoscopic image of the ureteroscope within the proximal ureter at the region of the UPJ. (C) An endoscopic image of the bleeding lesion within the renal pelvis (black arrow). (D) The Bugbee electrocautery probe through the working channel of the ureteroscope while the bleeding lesion is cauterized.

renal pelvis, providing gentle manual irrigation with D5W, the guide wire is removed. Care should be taken to try and keep the wire at the UPJ or proximal ureter rather than inside the renal pelvis while advancing the scope because the wire can cause some local trauma and result in pelvic bleeding that can be confused with the underlying bleeding lesion. Using fluoroscopic guidance the entire renal pelvis and each calix should be carefully evaluated endoscopically (Figure 28.4C). Once a bleeding lesion is seen the Bugbee cautery electrode probe (Figure 28.4D) is advanced into the working channel of the ureteroscope and the lesion is cauterized (using between 12 and 25 W in contact mode). It is important that saline solution is not the irrigant because this will not allow the electrocautery to conduct appropriately. Once the bleeding has ceased the electrode is removed and an exchange length guide wire is advanced into the ureteroscope working channel and coiled inside the renal pelvis. Once coiled, the ureteroscope is removed over the guide wire using fluoroscopic guidance and the ureteral stent is placed, as described above. If the stent is placed over the guide wire without cystoscopic guidance than it is important the urinary bladder has contrast within it to ensure the ureteral stent is not pushed up the entire ureter. The distal pigtail needs to be placed appropriately with the urinary bladder (see Chapter 34).

Other options for laser ablation include the Holmium: YAG laser (200-micron fiber) or the ND:YAG laser. For these lasers it is very important to "de-focus" the beam so that the fiber is not in direct contact with the tissue or it will cut the renal pelvic mucosa, penetrate into the parenchyma, and cause bleeding. A diode laser is typically not recommended because the fiber is too large to easily maneuver the flexible ureteroscope or provide adequate irrigation. For ablation with the YAG or diode lasers, 0.9% saline irrigation is used.

Selective Renal Arterial Embolization

A final option is selective renal arterial embolization of the branch of the renal artery that is contributing to the bleeding lesion. This has been done in only a few veterinary patients to date. This is a similar procedure to that described by Mishina et al (1997), in which ligation of a branch of the renal artery is performed via routine laparotomy, but instead of doing this surgically it can be done via angiography and cystoscopy in a minimally invasive manner. A routine cystoscopy is performed and the side of bleeding is identified and monitored. Using either femoral or carotid arterial access, an angiogram is performed of the ipsilateral renal artery, documenting the renal arterial anatomy of the affected side (Figure 28.5). Using digital subtraction angiography, each ramus of the ipsilateral renal artery is selectively catheterized. Once the six main branches of the renal arteries are identified (three dorsal and three ventral) catheterization and temporary occlusion of each is attempted. This occlusion can either be done with an occlusion balloon catheter or an angiographic catheter that is large enough to occlude blood flow. During vascular occlusion, the endoscopist is monitoring the UVJ for the cessation of bleeding over 30–60 seconds. Once bleeding has stopped, a microcoil is placed into the appropriate branch of the renal artery through the angiographic catheter and an angiogram is performed to confirm embolization. The cystoscope remains in place as the UVJ is monitored further to assure no bleeding recurs once the angiographic catheter is removed. This procedure would ultimately result in only a 1/6 loss of

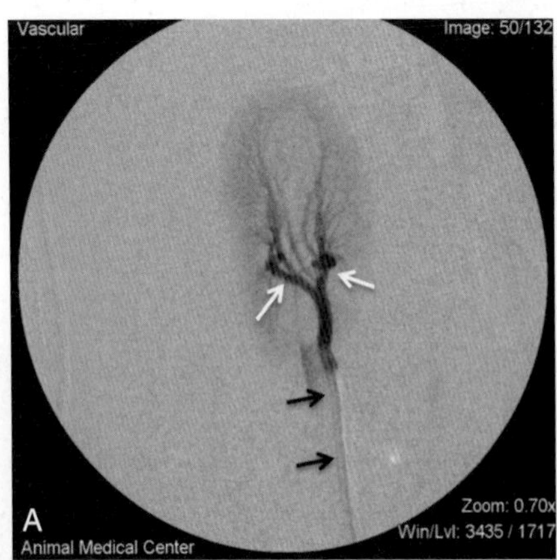

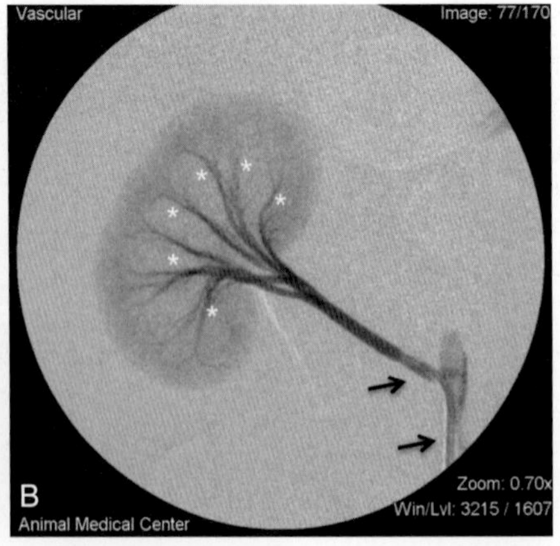

Figure 28.5 Renal angiogram of a dog with IRH using digital subtraction radiography. Renal arterial access is obtained from the femoral artery. (A) The lateral angiogram image of the right kidney that was seen to be bleeding during cystoscopy. Notice the catheter (black arrows) in the renal artery and the dorsal and ventral branches of the renal artery. (B) The angiogram being performed in VD showing the various branches of the renal artery from cranial to caudal.

renal blood flow, though collateral circulation could occur. In small dogs or cats, selective occlusion of these 6 branches is difficult and temporary iatrogenic embolization due to a clot or vascular spasm easily occurs. Therefore, dorsal or ventral occlusion, preserving only 50% of the renal tissue may be necessary and once the spasm resolves bleeding can recur. This procedure is not routinely performed in the author's practice.

Postprocedural and Follow-Up Care

Dogs are given a local urethral infusion of bupivacaine (0.6 mg/kg [0.27 mg/lb] mixed with saline in a 1:1 solution) for local urethral analgesia. Patients are discharged the same day as the procedure with oral tramadol (2 to 5 mg/kg, [1 to 2.5 mg/lb], PO, q 8 hr) for 3 days and 14 days of a fluoroquinolone antibiotic (to prevent stent biofilm formation).

For male dogs that had perineal access the site is kept clean for 3 days and monitored by the owner daily for swelling, redness or discharge. Most patients are discharged the same day as the procedure and urethral catheterization is not needed.

Microbial urine cultures, blood work (CBC and serum biochemical profile) and urinary tract ultrasonography is recommended at 2 weeks and 2 months post procedure and then every 3–6 months for 1 year. For patients in which hematuria resolves after sclerotherapy the stent should be cystoscopically removed 2–6 weeks after the procedure. For patients in whom the hematuria did not resolve, ureteroscopy with electrocautery should be considered prior to removal of the ureteral stent to maintain ureteral dilation.

If the bleeding continues despite appropriate sclerotherapy and ureteroscopy than selective renal arterial embolization is recommended if needed.

Prognosis

There is not sufficient data on ureteroscopic electrocautery or renal arterial embolization to provide a prognosis but sclerotherapy is documented to be a safe, effective, minimally-invasive and renal sparing treatment for IRH. Since nearly 33% of dogs can have bilateral bleeding, or develop bilateral bleeding over time, performing a renal sparing treatment is ideal. The documented long-term success of sclerotherapy was seen in four of six dogs (five of eight renal units), with dramatic improvements in the degree of bleeding in six of eight (75%) renal units, and some improvement seen in all renal units. The anemia and dysuria resolved in all cases, avoiding a nephrectomy. The main complications seen with sclerotherapy were migration of the ureteral stent and renal pain after the procedure in the one dog that did not receive a ureteral stent. It is important to emphasize that this was only a small case series. In humans, complications reported with silver nitrate infusions include necrotizing ureteritis with ureteral obstruction, bladder wall fibrosis, arterial hemorrhage, and hepatic dysfunction. This is not reported with povidone iodine infusion. Care should be taken to avoid overfilling the renal pelvis, as this could result in damage to the renal parenchyma and tubules. This is why using fluoroscopy for this procedure is necessary.

Special Considerations

There have been reports of the use of aminocaproic acid to treat IRH in humans (150 mg/kg divided in four doses per day). There are no known reports of using aminocaproic acid in veterinary medicine for IRH. Aminocaproic acid is a derivative and analogue of the amino acid lysine (an inhibitor of proteolytic enzymes such as plasmin) that is responsible for fibrinolysis, potentially making this effective in the treatment of bleeding disorders. Side effects that have been reported include gastrointestinal upset, fever, liver disease and thrombosis. This could be attempted in feline patients with IRH prior to considering intervention unless the dried solidified blood stones are causing a ureteral obstruction, in which case a stent or SUB device should be considered (see Chapter 34).

Notes

1. Rigid endoscope, 1.9-mm 30 degree lens, Karl Storz Endoscopy America, Culver City, CA.
2. Rigid endoscope, 2.7-mm 30 degree lens, Richard Wolf, Vernon Hills, IL.
3. Rigid endoscope, 4.0-mm 30 degree lens, Karl Storz Endoscopy-America, Culver City, CA.
4. Flexible endoscope Flex X², 2.7-mm, Karl Storz Endoscopy-America, Culver City, CA.
5. Weasel Wire 0.035-inch hydrophilic angle-tipped guidewire, Infiniti Medical LLC, Menlo Park, CA.
6. 5 French open ended ureteral catheter. Bard Medical, Covington, GA.
7. 5 French and 6 French UPJ balloon catheter. Cook Medical, Bloomington IL.
8. Amplatz super stiff J-tipped 0.035″ 150 cm guidewire, Cook Medical, Bloomington IL.
9. 0.5% silver nitrate solution, TEVA Pharmaceuticals, Sellersville, PA.

10. Povidone iodine (10%) solution, Aplicare Inc, Meriden, CT.
11. MD 76R, diatrizoate meglumine and diatrizoate sodium injection. U.S.P Mallinckrodt Inc, St. Louis, MO.
12. Weasel Wire 0.035-inch hydrophilic stiffened angle-tipped guidewire, Infiniti Medical LLC, Menlo Park, CA.
13. Serial ureteral dilators, Cook Medical, Bloomington IL.
14. Fulgurating electrode Bugbee cautery, 2 Fr, short tip, ACMI-Olympus, Southborough, MA.
15. 4.7 French × 20 cm double pigtail ureteral stent, Infiniti Medical, LLC, Menlo Park, CA.
16. 4.7 French × 22–32 cm variable length double pigtail ureteral stent, Bard Medical, Covington, GA.
17. 6 French × 26 cm double pigtail ureteral stent, Cook Medical, Bloomington IL.
18. Ureteral access sheath, 11.5 Fr. Cook Medical, Bloomington, IL.

References

Bagley DH and Allen J (1990) Flexible ureteropyeloscopy in the diagnosis of benign essential hematuria. *J Urol* 143, 549–53.

Berent A, Weisse C, Bagley D, et al (2013) Renal sparing treatment for idiopathic renal hematuria (IRH): Endoscopic-guided sclerotherapy. *J Am Vet Med Assoc* 242(11), 1556–63.

Mishina M, Watanage T, Yugeta N, et al (1997) Idiopathic renal hematuria in a dog: the usefulness of a method of partial occlusion of the renal artery. *J Vet Med Sci* 59(4), 293–5.

Tawfiek ER and Bagley DH (1998) Ureteroscopic evaluation and treatment of chronic unilateral hematuria. *J Urol* 160, 700–2.

Suggested Reading

Bahnson RR (1987) Silver nitrate irrigation for hematuria from sickle cell hemoglobinopathy. *J Urol* 137, 1194–5.

Diamond DA, Jeffs RD, and Marshall FF (1981) Control of prolonged, benign, renal hematuria by silver nitrate instillation. *Urology* 18(4), 337–41.

Dooley R and Pietrow PK (2004) Ureteroscopy of benign hematuria. *Urol Clin N Am* 31, 137–43.

Nandy P, Dwivedi US, Vyas N, et al (2004) Povidone iodine and dextrose solution combination sclerotherapy in chyluria. *Urology* 64(6), 1107–9.

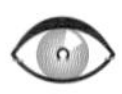

Video clips to accompany this chapter can be found in the online material at **www.wiley.com/go/weisse/vet-image-guided-interventions**

CHAPTER TWENTY-NINE

Interventional Management of Canine and Feline Benign Ureteral Obstructions

Allyson Berent
The Animal Medical Center, New York, NY

Background/Indications

Ureteral obstructions are a major clinical problem in small animal veterinary patients most commonly associated with ureteroliths, ureteral strictures, and trigonal neoplasia of the ureterovesicular junction (UVJ). With the invasiveness and morbidity associated with traditional surgical treatments, interventional options have become the mainstay of treatment in the author's practice. Using interventional radiology/interventional endoscopy (IR/IE) techniques, a clinician can simultaneously diagnose and treat various causes of ureteral obstructions in an expedient and minimally invasive manner. The main treatment options discussed in this chapter are the use of nephrostomy tubes, ureteral stents, and subcutaneous ureteral bypass devices (SUB).

Ureteral stenting is most commonly accomplished using endoscopic and fluoroscopic guidance in canine patients, and surgically-assisted with fluoroscopy in feline patients. These devices are used for a variety of obstructive disorders in both dogs and cats. The stents have a double pigtail multi-fenestrated design with one loop curled in the renal pelvis, the shaft travelling within the ureteral lumen, and the other loop curled within the urinary bladder lumen (Figure 29.1). This procedure has been performed successfully in over 250 veterinary patients to date in the author's practice. The goals of ureteral stenting are fivefold: (1) divert urine from the renal pelvis into the urinary bladder, bypassing a ureteral obstruction; (2) encourage passive ureteral dilation to prevent re-obstruction, encourage stone passage, or aid in future ureteroscopy; (3) facilitate surgery of the ureter (especially during a ureteral resection and anastomosis) and prevent postoperative leakage and edema; (4) aid in extracorporeal shockwave lithotripsy for large potentially obstructive ureteroliths or nephroliths that could result in serial ureteral obstructions, called *Steinstrasse*; and (5) prevent the migration of nephroliths resulting in future ureteral obstruction(s). The main type of ureteral stent used in veterinary medicine is an indwelling soft double pigtail ureteral stent[1,2] that can remain in place for numerous months to years if necessary. In most circumstances this is considered a long-term treatment option for various causes of ureteral obstructions in both dogs and cats.

Challenging cases for traditional ureteral surgery are those with proximal ureteral strictures, extensive ureteral injury, trauma associated with ureteral calculi in which only a short segment of proximal ureter remains, or those patients too unstable to undergo a long surgical intervention. In the past 4 years the author has been utilizing a SUB device, and over 175 of these have been placed to date, with promising results. This device typically takes 45 minutes to place, making anesthesia times predictable, and it has been proven effective in both the short and long term. This device[3] is a larger polyurethane catheter (6.5 French) that is composed of a locking-loop nephrostomy catheter, a multifenestrated cystostomy catheter, and a metallic shunting port that connects the catheters subcutaneously (Figure 29.2).

Additional information regarding the diagnostic work-up and medical management of ureteral obstructions can be found in the Suggested Reading. Management and treatment for ureteral obstructions secondary to trigonal neoplasia is addressed in Chapter 31.

Veterinary Image-Guided Interventions, First Edition. Edited by Chick Weisse and Allyson Berent.

Companion website: www.wiley.com/go/weisse/vet-image-guided-interventions

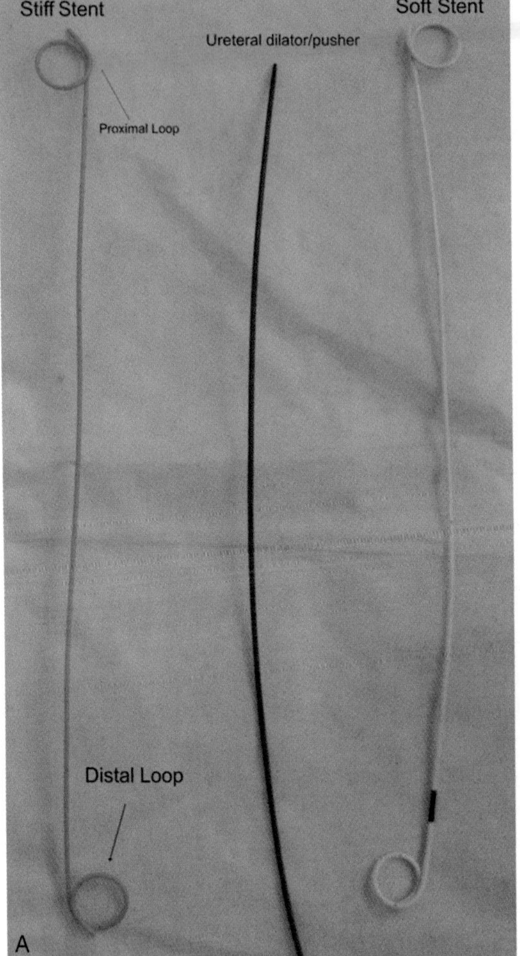

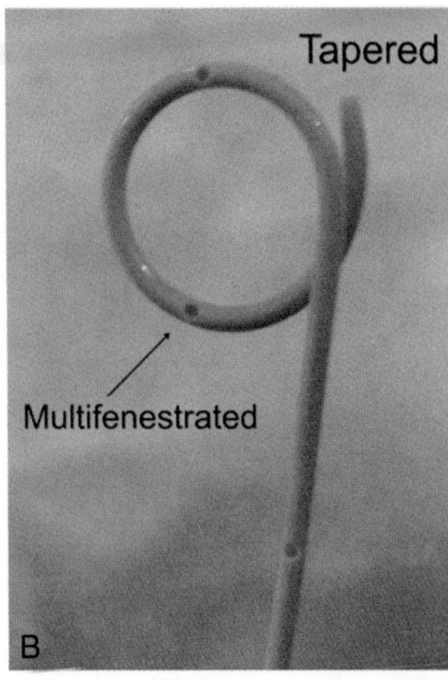

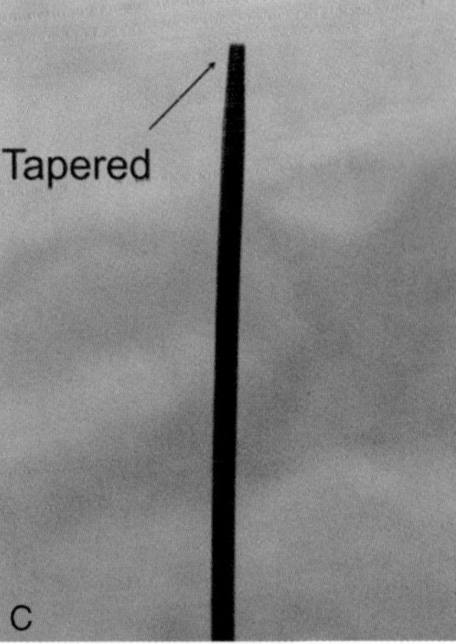

Figure 29.1 Double pigtail ureteral stents. (A) Two ureteral stents are shown, a soft and a stiff stent, that are made of different durometers, as well as a ureteral dilator/pusher. (B) The stent is tapered at the end and multifenestrated. (C) The ureteral dilator is tapered at the tip to aid in ureteral dilation over the guide wire.

Patient Preparation/ Work-Up

Prior to considering a ureteral stent or SUB device a full diagnostic work-up is necessary including full blood work, abdominal ultrasonography, abdominal radiography, a urinalysis, a urine culture, and blood pressure measurements. An obstructed ureter will have a combination of both renal pelvic dilation (>2 mm; most commonly over 6–8 mm) and hydroureter to an obstructive lesion. If a lesion is not identified on ultrasonography, a radiograph should be evaluated. Often ureteroliths (location, size, number, and shape) are best seen and quantified on radiographs. The sensitivity for abdominal radiographs for feline ureteral calculi was documented to be 81% (vs 88% in canine) and for abdominal ultrasonography 77% (vs 100% in canine). In combination, the sensitivity of both was 90%, so both are typically recommended.

When no clear obstructive lesion is seen than the cause is most commonly a ureteral stricture (>25% of cats), dried solidified blood stones (~8% of cats), or a tumor (most commonly associated with diffuse hydroureter to the level of the ureterovesical junction (UVJ) with a mass lesion seen in the dorsal aspect of the bladder trigone). Right-sided proximal ureteral obstructions without an obvious obstructive lesion can be due to a stricture associated with a circumcaval ureter, and this is most commonly seen in cats (~17% of ureteral obstructions in cats) (Figure 29.3A). Left-sided circumcaval ureters are possible as well, although less common. A diffuse hydroureter and hydronephrosis to the UVJ in male dogs is often associated with a ureteral stenosis at an ectopic ureteral opening (Figure 29.3B). This is most commonly seen in young to middle-aged male Labrador retrievers.

Basic management (Table 29.1) options include 24–48 hours of aggressive fluid therapy (5–7 ml/kg/hr), diuretic therapy (mannitol bolus 0.25–0.5 g/kg over 30 minutes, then 1 mg/kg/min CRI), and alpha-blockade (prazosin 0.25–0.5 mg/cat BID) when stone disease is present. If there are no stones seen and a stricture is suspected then the benefit of this therapy is of low yield. Broad-spectrum antibiotic therapy should also be considered as up to 34% of cats and 77% of dogs are

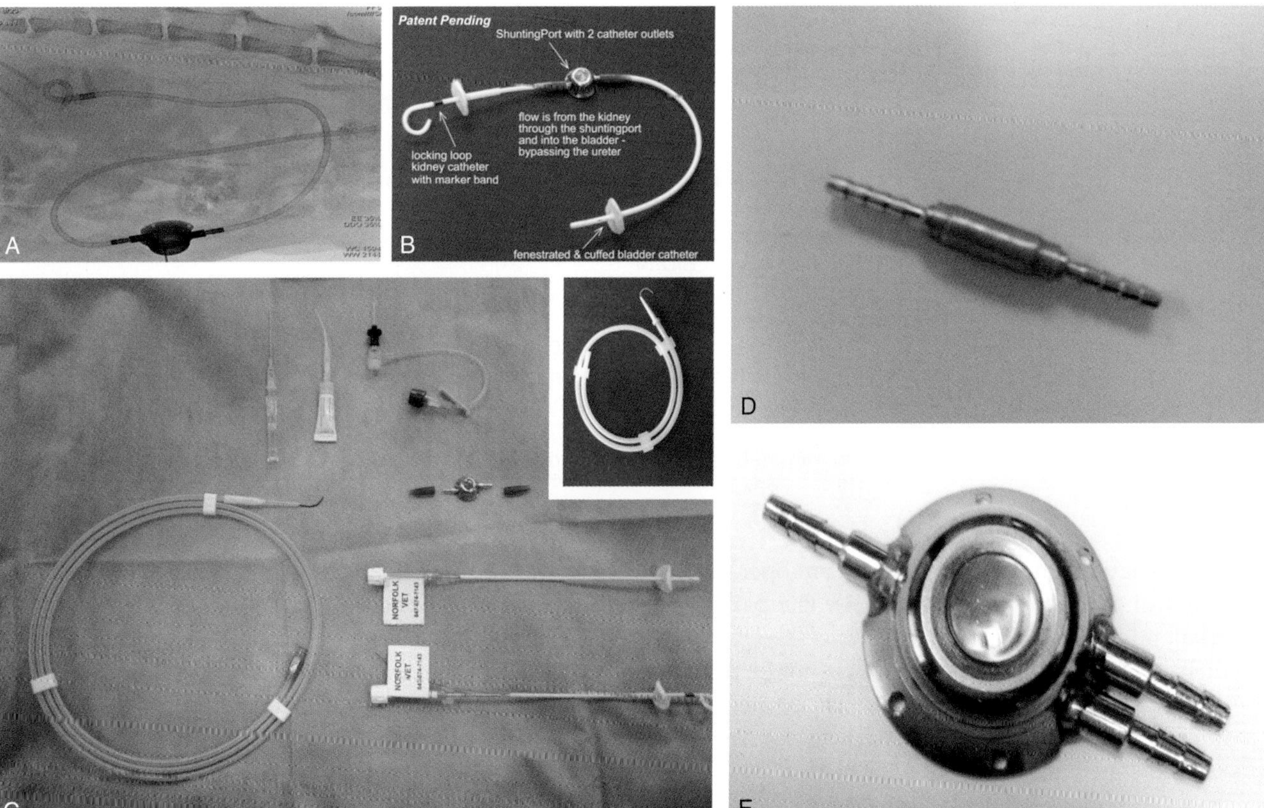

Figure 29.2 Subcutaneous ureteral bypass (SUB) device. (A) Lateral fluoroscopic image of a cat after SUB placement showing the nephrostomy catheter, cystostomy catheter, and subcutaneous shunting injection port. (B) The device assembled outside of the patient. (C) Each piece of the device and the equipment needed for SUB placement. An 18 gauge over-the-needle catheter, a 0.035″ angle-tipped hydrophilic guide wire or "J-tipped" guide wire, the nephrostomy and cystostomy catheter, sterile tissue glue (cyanoacrylate), the shunting injection port with the cuffs that secure the junction on the catheters and a Huber needle used to flush and inject the access port, connected to a T-port connector. (D) A male-to-male adaptor that can be used instead of the shunting port if the patient is unstable under anesthesia. (E) A three-way shunting port that can attach bilateral nephrostomy catheters to a single cystostomy catheter when there is bilateral obstruction and the patient is unstable under anesthesia to handle placing two subcutaneous ports.

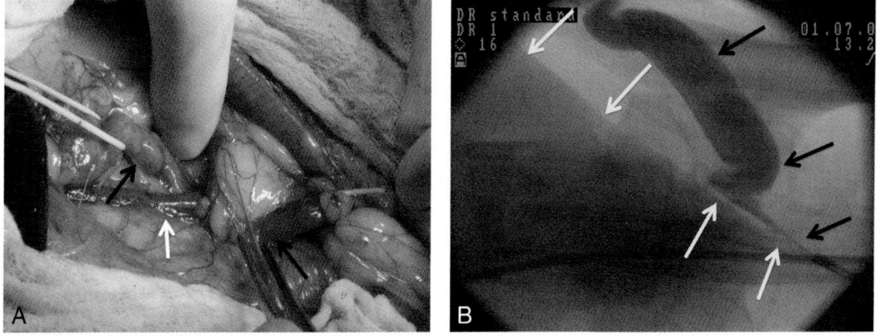

Figure 29.3 (A) A feline right circumcaval ureter. The head is to the left of the image. The caudal vena cava (white arrow) crosses the ureter (black arrows) ventrally. (B) Fluoroscopic image of a male dog with severe hydroureter and hydronephrosis. This is an intramural ectopic ureter that is most commonly associated with a distal ureteral stenosis at the ectopic orifice. The ureteral lumen (black arrows) is narrow as it enters the bladder neck (yellow arrows). The UVJ is marked by the end of the cystoscope in the proximal urethra.

TABLE 29.1
Medical management of ureteral obstructions

Medications	Dosage
Intravenous fluid therapy	90–120 ml/kg/day monitoring body weight, hydration status ± central venous pressure Author will often use 60 ml/kg/day of 0.45% NaCl with 2.5% dextrose and 30–60 ml/kg/day replacement fluid (i.e. Plasmalyte) to prevent fluid overload
Alpha-adrenergic blockage	Prazosin: 0.25 mg/cat BID or Tamsulosin 0.01 mg/kg/day monitoring blood pressure
Diuretic therapy	Mannitol 0.25 g/kg bolus over 30–60 minutes than 60 mg/kg/hour CRI for 24 hours monitor renal pelvis size, renal biochemical parameters and hydration status Author is cautious if evidence of heart disease
Amitriptyline	1 mg/kg/day There is minimal evidence to support this use and maximal effect can take a few weeks

reported to have positive urine cultures pre-operatively (Berent et al, 2013, Snyder et al, 2004). If a patient is hyperkalemic, oliguric/anuric, or is excessively painful then medical management alone should not be attempted and intervention should be immediately considered. If intermittent hemodialysis is available this can be considered as well. Nearly 15–20% of cats will be bilaterally obstructed at the time of diagnosis.

Only 8–17% of cats will have evidence of ureteral stone passage/movement following medical management alone to improve the degree of ureteral obstruction (Kyles et al, 2005a). A majority of dogs (59%; Pavia et al, 2014), in the author's experience, are infected and may have an associated pyonephrosis so immediate drainage is necessary (see Chapter 30).

Percutaneous antegrade pyelography and CT pyelography for diagnosis of ureteral obstructions is rarely performed in the author's practice prior to an intervention. Ureteropyelography is done in every case at the time of stent or SUB placement (either antegrade-cats, or retrograde-dogs). The reason for this approach is that a ureteropyelogram is only useful to diagnose a partial versus a complete ureteral obstruction. Since partial obstructions result in progressive kidney injury, as shown in various research models, we are currently recommending treatment regardless of the degree of obstruction.

Potential Risks/Complications/Expected Outcomes

The most substantial risk with ureteral interventions is the operator having appropriate training and experience. These are some of the more difficult IR/IE cases being performed. In addition, the anesthetic procedure itself should be handled with caution as these patients have renal disease and often associated heart disease. As with any procedure, complications are reduced with experience and appropriate training.

Complications are separated into four categories including: procedural (during device placement), perioperative (within the first week, typically during hospitalization), short-term (1 week to 1 month) and long-term (>1 month). These details are expanded upon further in the referenced literature and Table 29.2.

In a recent retrospective evaluation (Steinhaus et al, 2013) of 128 obstructed cats with 158 obstructed ureters treated interventionally (stent or SUB device) the median survival time was 571 days (ranging from 3 days to over 6 years) for all causes of death, and over 1500 days for those dying from renal causes. In a recent study on feline ureteral stenting (Berent et al, 2014), the survival time evaluated for renal cause of death was >1250 days with only 20% of cats dying or being euthanized for a probable or definitive renal cause of death.

Feline Stents

There are relatively few procedure-related complications when appropriate technique and equipment is used. In patients requiring a concurrent ureterotomy, leakage of urine can be seen for 1–3 days, so a closed-suction abdominal drain is typically placed. Perioperative re-obstruction is uncommon. The perioperative mortality rate is < 8%, and typically due to non-urinary causes, including congestive heart failure, pancreatitis, and/or sepsis (Berent et al, 2013). In a study looking a pre- and perioperative parameters as a predictor of renal outcome in cats after stents or SUBs (Horowitz et al, 2013), no significant factors were

TABLE 29.2
POTENTIAL OUTCOMES OF VARIOUS URETERAL INTERVENTIONS

Procedure	Operative	Post-operative (<1 week)	Short-term (1week-1month)	Long-term (>1 month)	Follow-up time
Medical Management Feline Ureteral Obstructions[1, 2] • Diuresis` • Mannitol therapy • Alpha-adrenergic blockade • Data on stones only • Will not help for the ~20% of strictures[5]		MORTALITY: 33% died or were euthanized prior to discharge[2]	Failure of renal function improvement (87%)[2]	If survived to discharge 30% had an improvement in azotemia[2]	**13% had response to medical management with 7.7% documentation of stone passage.[2]
Traditional Ureteral Surgery Feline (n=153[1, 2], 47[3]) • Ureterotomy/ Reimplantation/ • Ureteronephrectomy / Renal transplantation[1, 2] • Ureterotomy/ Re-implantation[3] • Data on ureteroliths only	• Uroabdomen Leakage (6%[3]–15%[2]) • Presence of abdominal effusion post-op (34%)[3]	• Persistent ureteral obstruction (7%)[2] due to stricture, edema, persistent stones • Failure of renal function improvement (17%)[2] • Require 2nd surgery during hospitalization (13%)[2, 3] • Other:[2] Fluid overload(3%), septic peritonitis (2%), pancreatitis (1%), MORTALITY (to discharge): 21%[2, 3] (25% with ureterotomy/ re-implant; 18% if include transplantation and ureteronephrectomy)[2]	Failure to improve renal function (17%)[2] MORTALITY (within 1 month) 25%[2]	• Re-obstruction (40%)[2] - ~1 year later - 50% mortality - in both medically and surgically managed cases[2]	Follow-up: 1->2000 days) **major issue is post-operative complications: leakage, re-obstruction, stricture formation, and long-term obstruction recurrence. There were few cases followed-up long-term (~50%)[2] **21% peri-operative mortality
Traditional Ureteral Surgery Canine (n=16)[4] • Ureterotomy/Pyelotomy • Ureteronephrectomy • Data on ureteroliths only	• Uroabdomen Leakage • Stricture	• Persistent ureteral obstruction • Failure of renal function improvement (21%)[4] • Worsening renal function (15%)[4] MORTALITY: (to discharge) 6.25%	• Re-obstruction[4] - stone or surgical site stricture Persistent renal dysfunction (43%)[4]	• Recurrent or Persistent UTI (43%)[4] • Re-obstruction (15%)[4] - stone or surgical site stricture 25% died or euthanized due to renal-related diseases[4]	Follow-up: 2-1876 days MST: 904 days (struvite MST 333 days; non-struvite MST 1238 days) **major issue is re-obstruction and worsening of creatinine long-term. There were very few cases in this series

(*Continued*)

TABLE 29.2
(Continued)

Procedure	Operative	Post-operative (<1 week)	Short-term (1week-1month)	Long-term (>1 month)	Follow-up time
Feline Ureteral Stent[5–7, 10] (n=79[5],92[7]) • Data on 71–79% ureteroliths, 21–28% strictures, 1% obstructive pyelonephritis	• Ureteral penetration with guide wire (17%) (little clinical consequence; no uroabdomen) • Leakage if concurrent ureterotomy needed (6.7%) • Eversion of ureteral mucosa during stent passage • Ureteral tear during stent passage (3.8%)	• Fluid overload during post-obstructive diuresis (17%) • Concurrent Pancreatitis (6%) • Failure for creatinine to improve (5%) • MORTALITY (to discharge) 7.5%[5] - due to non-urinary causes (pancreatitis or CHF)	• Inappetance (temporary) (25%) • Dysuria (self-limiting 7–14 days) <10%[5] • Stent Migration[7] (3%)	• Dysuria (38%)[5] • nearly all respond to prednisolone and/or prazosin (persistent 1.6% post steroid therapy) • UTI (13% post-op versus 34% pre-op)[5] • Re-obstruction (over 3.5 years) (19-26%)[5, 7] - Stricture (58% of strictures occluded the stent) - Adhesions around ureter from ureterotomy - Obstructive pyelonephritis - Proliferative ureteritis - stent encrustation • Chronic hematuria (18%)[5] • Stent migration[5] (6%) • Ureteral reflux[5] (<2%)	Follow-up: 2-1278 days MST: 498 days MST for renal cause of death >1250 days • 21% of cats died of renal related causes • Only predictor of long-term survival was the 3 month post-creatinine.[6] **major issue is need for STENT EXCHANGE in 27% of cases due to migration or occlusion of ureter and DYSURIA due to ureteral stent location in urinary bladder[5] **7.5% perioperative mortality (none related to surgical complications)
Canine Ureteral Stent (n=84[10], 14[8], 62[11]) • Data on 55% ureteroliths, 40% tumors and 5% strictures	• Endoscopic failure (~5%) • Ureteral perforation (<1%) • Leakage (<1%) • Ureteral tear (<1%)	• Hematuria (<5%) • Dysuria (<5%) • Migration (<2%) • Occlusion with debris (<2%) • MORTALITY (to discharge) <2%[11]	• Dysuria <2% • Persistent obstruction (<2%)	• Proliferative tissue at UVJ (5-25%)[8, 11] • Re-obstruction (10%)[11] • UTIs (~10–60% post-stent[8, 11]; 59% pre-stent)[11] • Migration (5%)[11] • Encrustation (2%)[11] • Hematuria (6%)[11] • Stent fracture (<2%) • Dysuria (<2%)[8, 11]	Follow-up: 30 days-6 years (median 1158 days) **major issue is re-obstruction and RECURRENT UTIs, though rate is lower than pre-stent **<2% perioperative mortality **All cases allowed for renal-sparing procedure

Feline SUB device[6, 7, 9] (n=61[9],71[7]) • Data on 20% strictures (+/-ureteroliths), 76% ureteroliths, 4% obstructive ureteritis	• Kinking of catheters (3.5%) • Inability to place SUB (<1%)	• Leakage (5%)[7] resolved with new device • Fluid overload (<5%)[7, 9] • Blockage of system (2%)[7, 9] • (blood clot, purulent material, device failure) • Failure for creatinine to improve (3%)[7, 9] • MORTALITY (to discharge) 5.8%[7]	• Dysuria <2%[7, 9] • Inappetance ~25% (temporary) • Seroma 1%[9]	• UTI[9] (15% post-op; 35% pre-op) • Re-obstruction[7] (18%) (0% strictures; 20% of stone cases); • Dysuria (<2%)[7, 9]	Follow-up time: 2 days to 4.5 years Median: 762–923 days **major issue is: 1) DEVICE OCCLUSION (10%) which requires serial flushing or exchange. Usually due to stone accumulation 2) KINKING and 3) LEAKAGE: is less of an issue with proper training **5.8% perioperative mortality (none related to surgical complications)

REFERENCES:

1. Kyles A, Hardie E, Wooden B, et al. Clinical, clinicopathologic, radiographic, and ultrasonographic abnormalties in cats with ureteral calculi: 163 cases (1984–2002). JAVMA 2005, 226(6): 932–936.
2. Kyles A, Hardie E, Wooden B, et al. Management and outcome of cats with ureteral calculi: 153 cases (1984–2002). JAVMA 2005, 226(6): 937–944.
3. Roberts S, Aronson L, Brown D. Postoperative mortality in cats after ureterolithotomy. Vet Surg. 2011; 40: 438–443.
4. Snyder D, Steffery M, Mehler S, et al. Diagnsis and surgical management of ureteral calculi in dogs: 16 cases (1990–2003). New Zealand Vet J. 2004; 53(1): 19–25.
5. Berent A, Weisse C, Bagley D, et al. Technical and clinical outcomes of ureteral stenting in cats for the treatment of benign ureteral obstruction: 2006–2010. J Am Vet Med Assoc. 2014; 244(5): 559–576.
6. Horowitz C. Berent A, Weisse C. et al. Predictors of outcome for cats with ureteral obstructions after interventional management using ureteral stents or a subcutaneous ureteral bypass device. J Feline Med Surg. 2013; 15(12): 1052–1062.
7. Steinhaus J, Berent A, Weisse C, et al. Circumcaval ureters in cats with and without ureteral obstructions. A comparative study. Abstract, American College of Veterinary Internal Medicine, Seattle WA ACVIM 2013.
8. Kuntz J, Berent A, Weisse C et al. Renal sparing treatment for obstructive pyonephrosis in dogs. Abstract, American College of Veterinary Internal Medicine, Seattle WA ACVIM 2013.
9. Berent A, Weisse C, Bagley D, et al. The use of a subcutaneous ureteral bypass device for the treatment of feline ureteral obstructions. ECVIM, Seville Spain, 2011
10. Berent A. Ureteral obstructions in dogs and cats ; a review of traditional and new interventional diagnostic and therapeutic options. J Vet Emerg Crit Care. 2011; 21(2): 86–103.
11. Pavia P, Berent A, Weisse C, et al. Canine Ureteral Stenting for benign ureteral obstruction in dogs. Abstract ACVS, 2014, San Diego, CA.

identified for short or long-term outcome. The main short-term complication in cats is dysuria, which is typically self-limiting. If necessary, low dose steroids are usually an effective treatment.

The long-term complications in cats are less serious but more common (Berent et al, 2013) including: (1) dysuria (37.7%) which resolved in all but 1.7% either spontaneously (43%), with medical management (57%), or with stent exchange (9%); (2) urinary tract infection(s) (30%), seen in 34% pre-stent and 30% post stent; (3) re-obstruction (19%) most commonly associated with ureteral stricture recurrence or at the site of a ureterotomy; (4) chronic mild hematuria (18%); and (5) stent migration (5.9%).

Variables were carefully evaluated for predictors of dysuria and the need for stent exchange. There were no significant associations with stent type, length, size, side, signalment, or surgical approach. Cats that had a ureteral stricture were more likely to re-obstruct. With the advent of the SUB device, which is now preferred in cats, especially for ureteral strictures, re-obstruction has not been a common issue (0% strictures and 14–18% stones). All of these complications were rare or minor and self-limiting, but clients should be aware of the risks prior to stent placement. Nearly all of the complications are manageable with either medical therapy or a minor out-patient procedure (stent exchange).

Stent encrustation is the major complication observed in humans, so stent exchanges are encouraged every 3–12 months; however, this has not been appreciated commonly in veterinary patients. Interestingly, the ureters remain patent in the long term in most veterinary patients without the need for stent exchange; the longest stent has been in place for over 6 years. Stent obstruction has probably occurred in many of these patients, however the ureter remains patent around the stent due to the subsequent passive ureteral dilation.

Canine Ureteral Stents

The complications observed in dogs are few in all time periods and are outlined in Table 29.2. A recent study evaluating 44 dogs (57 ureters) found ureteral perforation with a guide wire 2–4%, stent migration in 6%, stent occlusion 9%, proliferative tissue at the UVJ 5%, and intermittent hematuria 5–10%.Urinary tract infections were seen in 59% of dogs prior to stent placement, and recurrent in another 59% of dogs within the follow-up period (over 1158 days), with 76% being cleared with appropriate antibiotic therapy. Dysuria was not seen chronically in any dog. (Pavia et al, 2014).

SUBs

Some of the complications can include: (1) leakage at the nephrostomy/cystostomy tube or shunting port (<5%; this issue has been resolved with the commercially available SUB device that has the Dacron cuff design); (2) kinking of the tubing during placement (<3%); (3) hemorrhage during nephrostomy tube placement (<3%); (4) UTIs (seen 9–35% preop and 15% postop; and (5) system obstruction with blood clots, purulent debris, or stones (0% for strictures and ~15–18% for stone cases). With the new recommendation of flushing the system through the shunting port routinely (every 3–6 months), occlusion of the catheter is less common. The use of a SUB for feline and canine patients with a ureteral obstruction can be considered a functional option when other traditional therapies have failed, are contraindicated, or timely intervention is needed. At this time this device is considered to have less short- and long-term complications, and lower mortality rates, in cats than ureteral stents, and is considered the preferred treatment for feline ureteral obstructions, in the author's practice (Table 29.2).

In canine patients, stents are well tolerated and placed endoscopically, making stents the preferred device. If a surgical approach is taken in dogs then a SUB could be considered, particularly if a stricture is confirmed.

Ureteral stenting and SUBs are not meant to replace traditional surgery for ureteral obstructions, but provide alternatives when traditional surgery fails, is contraindicated, or has a high risk of failure/re-obstruction, which is often the case. Considering that over 85% of cats with ureteral stone obstructions had concurrent nephroliths and the median number of stones per ureter was four (Berent et al, 2013), a majority of cases seem to benefit from this approach. In addition, canine ureteral stenting can usually be accomplished endoscopically (85–92%) on an outpatient basis, and stone recurrence is very common, so stenting has replaced traditional surgery for dogs in the author's practice. These devices should only be placed by those trained and experienced in these techniques, as these cases can be technically challenging. The success rates are high, particularly when using the veterinary ureteral stents and SUB device, provided appropriate training has been received. Potential complications should be discussed with the owner in great detail (Table 29.2) prior to considering any surgical or interventional option.

At this time the success rate for ureteral stent placement is 100% in dogs ($n = 150$) and over 95% in cats ($n = 100$). This has improved tremendously since the development of a smaller diameter stent (2.5Fr),

TABLE 29.3
Chart of stent sizing

Ureteral stent size (French)	Guidewire size	Open-ended ureteral catheter size	Rigid cystoscope lens size (working channel diameter)	Over the needle catheter size (Gauge)
2.5-feline	0.018″	3 Fr or 0.032–0.034″ ureteral dilator	1.9 mm (3 Fr)	21 or 22
3.7-small dog	0.025″	4 Fr	2.7 mm (5 Fr)	20
4.7-medium/large dog	0.035″	5 Fr	2.7 mm (5 Fr)	18
6.0-large dog/cancer stent	0.035″	5 Fr	4 mm (6 Fr)	18

a ureteral dilator with hydrophilic material, and experience. The author has also placed 175 feline and canine SUB devices in over 5.5 years, with a placement success of 100% as well. Complications are further described in Table 29.2.

Equipment

Various rigid and flexible endoscopes are needed for retrograde ureteral stent placement in dogs, and occasionally some female cats. Ureteral access is possible in a retrograde fashion in most female patients (dog or cat) using a rigid cystoscope[4–7] and males over 6 kg using a flexible ureteroscope (7.5–8.2-Fr)[8]. In general, retrograde stent placement is not recommended in cats as surgical assistance is most often needed (>80%).

A traditional fluoroscopic C-arm is sufficient for visualization during ureteral interventions. Ultrasonography is useful for percutaneous renal access in order to cannulate the ureter in an antegrade manner when necessary (dogs with malignant obstruction or when endoscopy fails). Access to the renal pelvis can also be performed under direct fluoroscopic guidance when the renal pelvis is opacified with contrast or stones.

Various guide wires and catheters are needed for each procedure and most commonly an angle-tipped hydrophilic guide wire (0.018″, 0.025″ or 0.035″)[9] is coupled with an appropriately sized open-ended ureteral catheter (3 Fr, 4 Fr, 5 Fr),[10] respectively. This wire/catheter combination is associated with an appropriate sized ureteral stent[1,2] outlined in Table 29.3.

The SUB device[3] (Figure 29.2) is a specialized 6.5 French nephrostomy tube with a Dacron cuff and silicone sleeve, placed over a 0.035″ angle-tipped hydrophilic guide wire or a 0.035″ "J"-tip metallic guide wire. The "J"-tipped guide wire is preferred for the larger renal pelvis' (>8–10 mm). For the pelvis that is <5–6 mm a hydrophilic guide wire is used and passed down the dilated proximal ureter for nephrostomy catheter placement into the dilated ureter rather than coiled inside the renal pelvis. Guide wire access is obtained through an 18-gauge over the needle IV catheter via nephrostomy access. The cystostomy tube is a multi-fenestrated straight catheter that is also secured with a Dacron cuff (Figure 29.2). Additional options for the SUB device include a three-way port that allows bilateral treatment using one cystostomy catheter and two nephrostomy catheters (Figure 29.2) or an internalized male-to-male adaptor avoiding the need to place a subcuutaneous port. The author prefers to have a port for future system assessment, but if the patient is unstable under anesthesia the male-to-male internalized adaptor saves a substantial amount of procedure time.

A nephrostomy tube is a locking-loop pigtail catheter that is 5 Fr in cats and 6 Fr in dogs. This is placed over a 0.018″ or 0.035″ guide wire, respectively[11,12] (Figure 29.4).

Interventional Management of Benign Ureteral Obstructions

For patients that are severely uremic (cat creatinine over 8 and dog over 5 mg/dl) the author is routinely administering desmopressin (DDAVP) (1 µg/kg SQ diluted 1:9) 15 minutes before starting the procedure. This has been shown in humans to decrease the risk of procedural bleeding associated with uremic thrombocytopathia. There is no veterinary data to support this.

Nephrostomy Tube Placement

This requires fluoroscopic and/or ultrasound guidance. A nephrostomy tube (Figure 29.4, Figure 29.5, and Figure 29.6) will rapidly and effectively relieve a ureteral obstruction, as well as enable the determination of whether adequate renal function remains before subjecting a patient to a prolonged anesthesia for definitive ureteral surgery. This is either performed surgically or percutaneously. The loop on the catheter

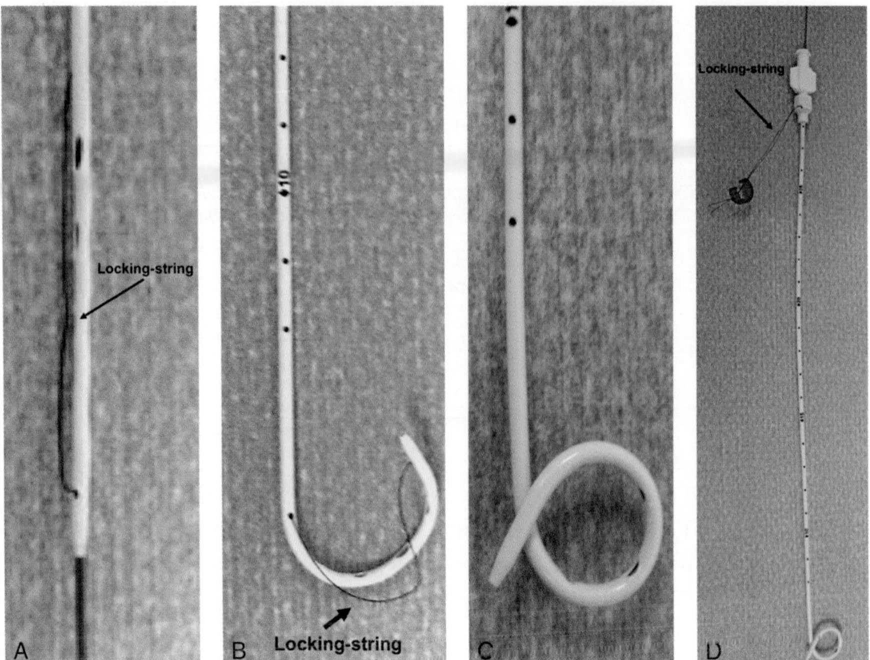

Figure 29.4 Locking-loop pigtail nephrostomy tube. (A) The loop end of the catheter is multi-fenestrated and has a string that goes from the most distal to the most proximal fenestration that aids to lock the loop in place. There is a hollow trocar inside the catheter to keep it rigid and straight as it is passed over the wire. (B) Once the guide wire and trocar are removed from the catheter the pigtail loop forms and the string is shown here to be loose and un-locked. (C) The string is pulled at the hub of the catheter curling the pigtail tight and keeping it locked. (D) The hub of the catheter showing where the locking string comes out and that is where it is secured to prevent it from loosening to keep the pigtail locked.

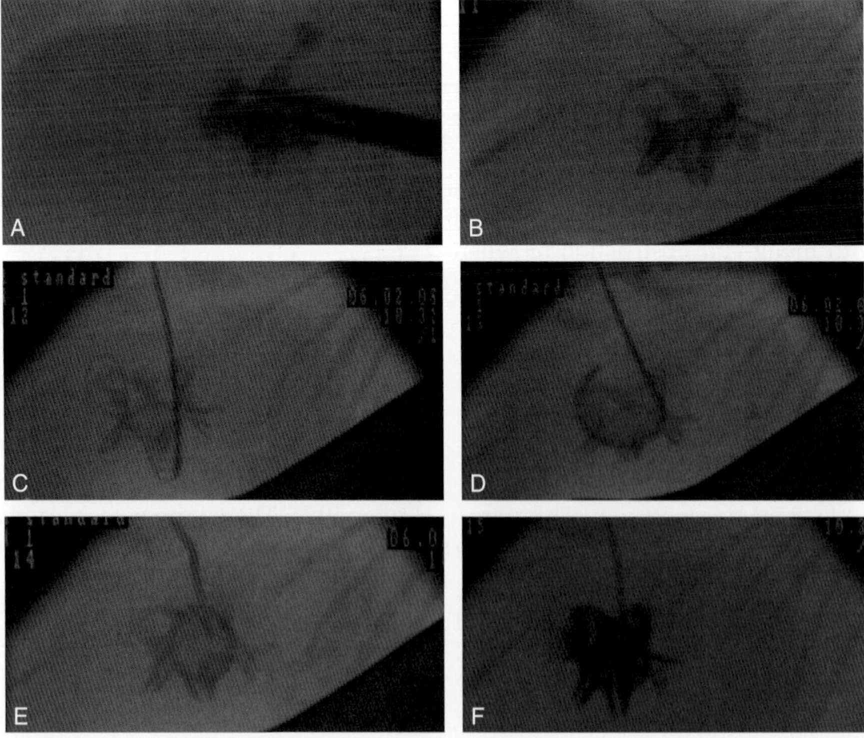

Figure 29.5 Fluoroscopic images of a cat during percutaneous locking-loop nephrostomy tube placement using the modified Seldinger-technique. (A) Renal access needle being placed into the renal pelvis using ultrasound guidance for a pyelogram. (B) A guide wire advanced through the access needle and being curled within the renal pelvis. (C) The locking-loop pigtail catheter being advanced over the guide wire into the renal pelvis. (D) The loop of the pigtail being formed in the renal pelvis. (E) Locking the string of the pigtail catheter to tighten the loop within the renal pelvis and prevent the catheter from coming out. (F) Ureteropyelogram being performed through the nephrostomy tube ensuring no leakage and appropriate drainage.

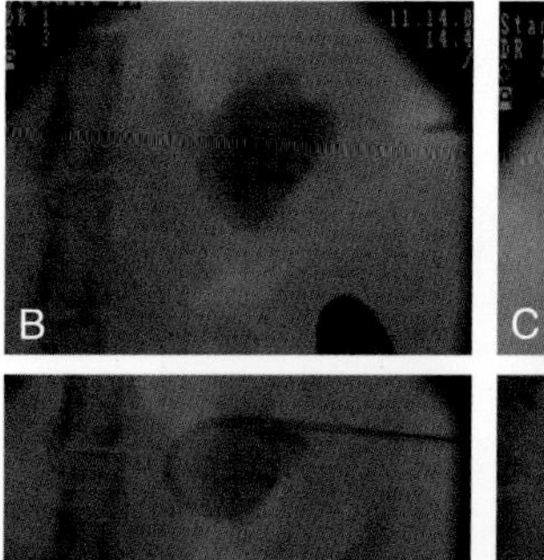
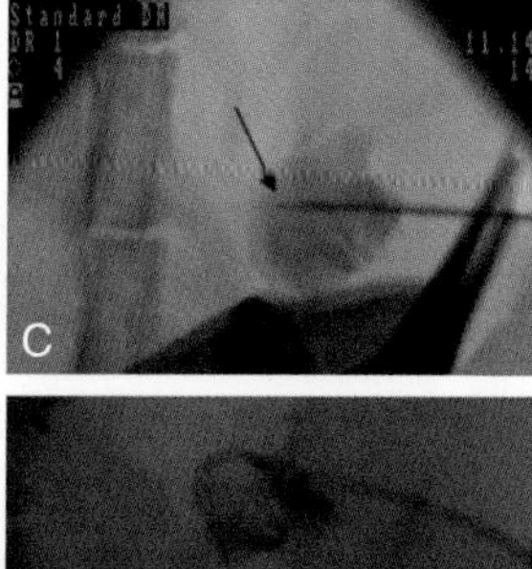
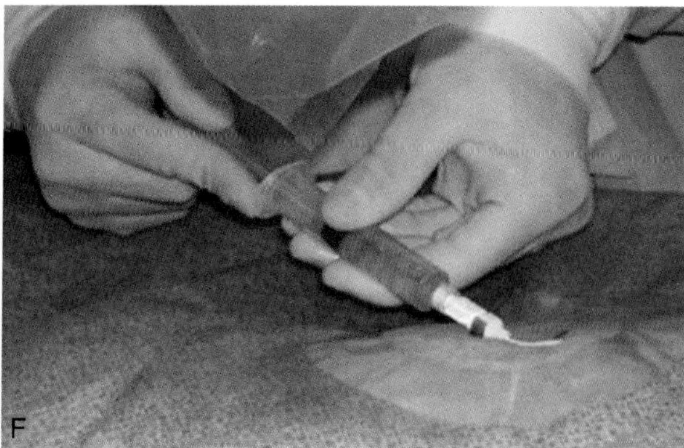

Figure 29.6 Fluoroscopic images of a cat during percutaneous locking-loop nephrostomy tube placement using the "one-stab" technique. (A) The locking-loop pigtail catheter with the sharp stylette placed within the hollow trocar. Notice the locking string and the multiple catheter fenestrations. (B) Fluoroscopic image of a cat during a pyelogram. (C) The locking-loop catheter being advanced through the greater curvature of the kidney, into the renal pelvis with the sharp stylette (black arrow). (D) The sharp stylette is removed and the catheter is advanced into the renal pelvis. (E) The locking string is pulled to tighten the catheter in place.

is approximately 10–15 mm in diameter so this procedure is reserved for dogs and cats that have a renal pelvis >10 mm. If the entire loop is not securely situated inside the renal pelvis then leakage can occur. The author typically uses a 6 Fr locking-loop catheter in dogs and a 5 Fr catheter in cats. Nephrostomy tubes are no longer commonly used since the advent of ureteral stents and SUBs.

Percutaneous Nephrostomy Tube Placement

Catheter placement is performed using either the "modified Seldinger-technique" or a "one-stab trocar introduction technique". Both techniques have been performed successfully in dogs and cats. Due to the nature of the smaller, more mobile feline kidneys, surgical placement with a nephropexy may be more appropriate and the modified Seldinger technique is preferred.

To aid in performing the percutaneous "modified Seldinger-technique", ultrasound guidance is used to perform a pyelocentesis using an over-the-needle catheter or renal access needle (Figure 29.5). This should be performed along the greater curvature of the kidney. The author recommends an 18-gauge needle for dogs and a 22-gauge needle for cats. Once the tip of the catheter or trocar is in the renal pelvis, the trocar is removed and a short extension set and three-way-stop-cock is attached to the catheter. Urine is drained for culture and an equal amount of 50% contrast material is infused to perform a pyelogram and distend the pelvis. The fluoroscopy unit is pre-aligned over the kidney. Under fluoroscopic guidance, an angle-tipped hydrophilic guide wire (dog: 0.035″ wire fits through the 18-gauge) catheter; cat: 0.018″ wire fits through the 22-gauge catheter) is advanced through the catheter and coiled (two to three loops if possible) within the renal pelvis being careful not to perforate the kidney through a renal calix or the ureter at the ureteropelvic junction (UPJ). The catheter is then removed off the wire and the locking-loop pigtail catheter is advanced over the guide wire, through the renal parenchyma, and into the renal pelvis. Once the nephrostomy tube is in the renal pelvis it is passed off the hollow trocar, onto the curl of the guide wire. When a full loop is made the locking string is pulled and the cannula and guide wire are removed. Contrast should be injected through the catheter within the renal pelvis confirming there is no leakage and the entire loop is within the pelvis. The catheter is then sutured to the body wall using a purse-string and finger-trap suture pattern and a urine collection system is attached to the catheter for gravity drainage. A secure abdominal bandage is recommended to prevent the tube from being contaminated or accidentally removed.

The "one-stab-technique" is performed using the sharp stylet through the hollow trocar inside the locking-loop catheter (Figure 29.6). A small skin incision is made in the area of the affected kidney. Using ultrasound guidance, the locking-loop catheter, with the sharp stylet, is advanced through the body wall, punctured through the greater curvature of the kidney and into the renal pelvis. A scalpel blade is needed to pierce the body wall so the sharp stylet is not blunted. Ultrasonography and fluoroscopy together aid in performing this technique. Once within the renal pelvis the sharp stylet is removed and the catheter is advanced off the hollow trocar until a curl is formed within the renal pelvis. This should never be done in a pelvis smaller than 10 mm. Once a curl is formed, the

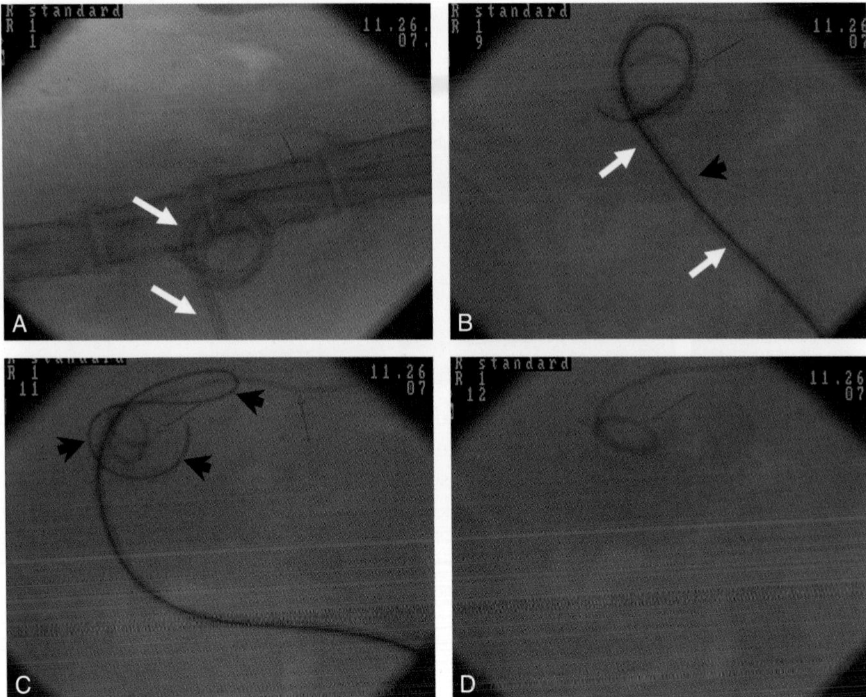

Figure 29.7 Fluoroscopic images during the removal of nephrostomy tube in a cat. (A) Within the renal pelvis is the locking-loop pigtail catheter (white arrows) and the pigtail of an indwelling ureteral stent (red arrows). (B) For removal of the nephrostomy tube the string is released and a guide wire (black arrow) is advanced through the nephrostomy tube to straighten out the loop. (C) The guide wire (black arrows) is curled within the renal pelvis and proximal ureter and the nephrostomy catheter is withdrawn. The ureteral stent (red arrows) is monitored to ensure it is not removed. (D) The ureteral stent (red arrow) is left in place.

locking-string is pulled and locked. The catheter should be leak tested with a saline/contrast infusion. Once in place the catheter can be secured as described above. This is a complex procedure and not recommended for those inexperienced with these techniques. The author does not prefer this technique over the modified-Seldinger.

Surgical Nephrostomy Tube Placement

Both techniques previously described can also be performed surgically with a standard ventral midline laparotomy. Once the catheter is in place, the hub is passed through the body wall using blunt penetration with a hemostat. A nephropexy can then be performed using 3–0 absorbable suture material. Surgical bites should include the renal capsule as well as renal parenchyma with care to avoid penetrating the renal pelvis. Nephropexy of the capsule alone is not secure.

For catheters placed percutaneously, a seal must form to the body wall prior to tube removal; This may take up to 4 weeks. If the patient is subsequently taken to surgery to relieve the obstruction, or the obstruction is addressed using other techniques before a seal is formed, (i.e., ureteral stenting, SUB, shockwave lithotripsy, etc.), the tube can either be removed with the site repaired, or capped and wrapped while left in place prior to being removed. Fluoroscopy should be used to aid in removal of the nephrostomy tube (Figure 29.7). The tube is cut (which loosens the locking suture) approximately 5 cm from the skin and aseptically scrubbed. Using fluoroscopy, a sterile hydrophilic guide wire is advanced down the tube and curled into the renal pelvis. The tube is withdrawn over the wire. Once the pigtail is straightened out the tube is removed monitoring with fluoroscopy. The site can be wrapped for a few hours thereafter to allow the site to close. Make sure the locking string does not remain in the nephrostomy tract and if it is present carefully remove this. If a stent is also in place monitor with fluoroscopy before pulling the catheter out to ensure the pigtail of the stent is not engaged in the pigtail of the nephrostomy tube, otherwise the stent can be inadvertently dislodged or removed as well.

Ureteral Stenting

Ureteral stents (Figure 29.8, Figure 29.9, Figure 29.10, and Figure 29.11) are most often placed cystoscopically in dogs and surgically in cats. In dogs this is

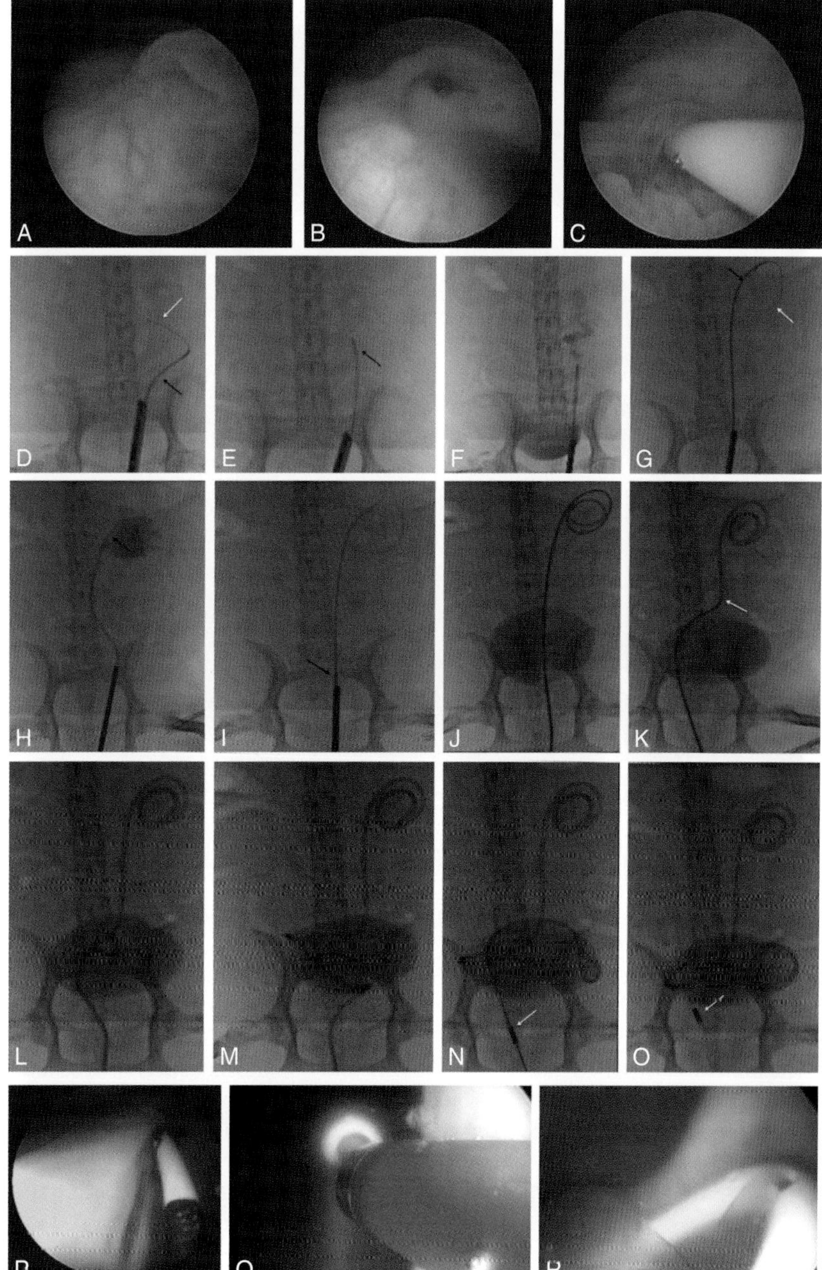

Figure 29.8 Cystoscopic and fluoroscopic-guided retrograde ureteral stent placement in a female dog. (A) Cystoscopic image of a dog in dorsal recumbency showing the left ureterovesicular junction (UVJ). (B) Guide wire being advanced into the ureteral lumen from the UVJ. (C) Open-ended ureteral catheter being advanced over the guide wire into the ureteral lumen. (D) Fluoroscopic image of the guide wire (white arrow) and open-ended ureteral catheter (black arrow) being advanced retrograde up the ureter. (E) The wire is removed and the catheter remains in the ureter for a retrograde ureteropyelogram. (F) Retrograde ureteropyelogram being performed outlining the ureteral obstruction. (G) Guide wire (white arrow) advanced back into the catheter and curled within the renal pelvis with the ureteral catheter (black arrow) advanced to the renal pelvis. (H) Contrast seen within the renal pelvis after a pyelogram was performed through the ureteral catheter (black arrow). (I) The ureteral catheter (black arrow) is pulled back over a guide wire from the UPJ in image (H) to the UVJ in image (I) allowing for measurement of the ureteral length for stent sizing. (J) The ureteral stent (blue arrow) is advanced over the guide wire and curled within the renal pelvis. The bladder is filled with contrast to be able to mark the UVJ under fluoroscopy. (K) Once the proximal loop of the stent (blue arrow) is within the renal pelvis the guide wire is retracted (white arrow). (L) The guide wire pulled back to the distal end of the stent within the urethra. Notice the distal end of the stent is folding into the bladder once the wire is not within the lumen. (M) The distal end of the stent is being pushed into the urinary bladder. (N) The pushing catheter (yellow arrow) has a radiopaque mark to mark the distal end of the stent. Notice the wire is crossing the junction between the sent (blue arrow) and pusher. The stent is coiling within the urinary bladder. (O) The entire distal end of the ureteral stent is coiled within the urinary bladder (blue arrow) and the pusher catheter is in the urethr(A) yellow arrow. (P) Endoscopic image of the ureteral stent as it exits the UVJ. The black mark seen is an endoscopic marker to alert the endoscopist when the distal loop of the pigtail is beginning. (Q) Endoscopic image of the junction of the ureteral stent and the pusher catheter as they both exit the working channel of the endoscope. Notice the guide wire is through the lumen of both catheters. (R) Once the stent is within the bladder the pushing catheter and wire are completely removed and you can see fluid draining through the fenestrations of the stent ensuring patency.

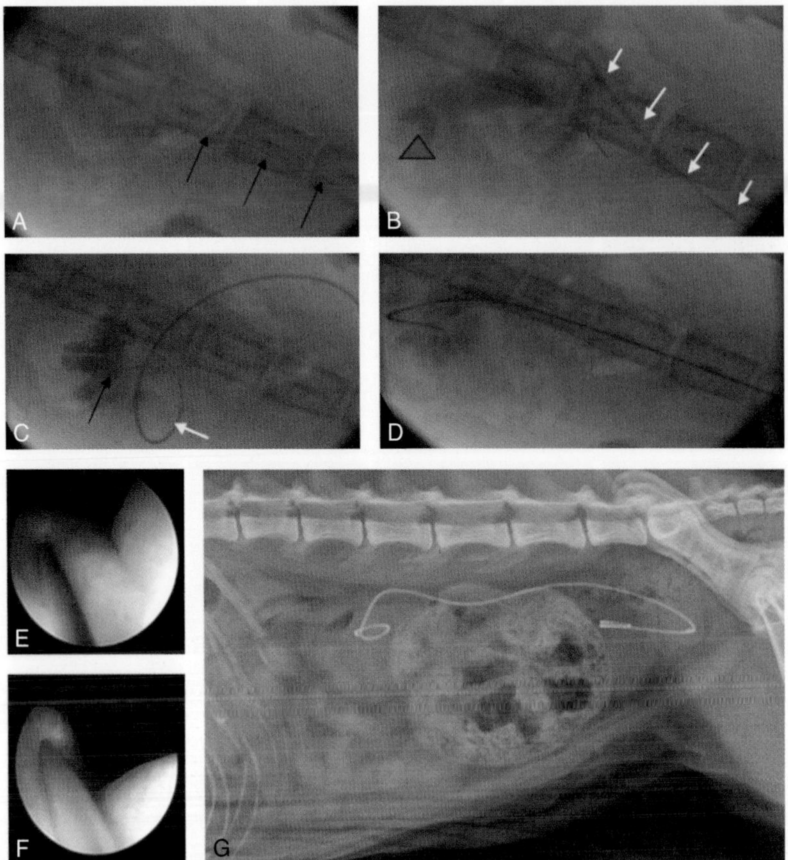

Figure 29.9 Cystoscopic and fluoroscopic-guided retrograde ureteral stent placement in a female cat. (A) Fluoroscopic image of a cat in dorsal recumbency. The head is to the left of the image. The guide wire (black arrows) being advanced up the ureteral lumen through the UVJ via endoscopic guidance (E). (B) An open-ended ureteral catheter/dilator (yellow arrows) advanced over the guide wire to the level of the stones (red arrow). The guide wire is removed and a retrograde ureteropyelogram is performed. The renal pelvis is seen filled with contrast (red arrowhea(D). (C) The guide wire (black arrow) advanced through the catheter and into the renal pelvis. (D) The ureteral catheter advanced over the wire and into the renal pelvis. (E) Guide wire advanced through the right UVJ using endoscopic guidance. (F) Ureteral dilation catheter advanced over the wire through the UVJ. (G) Lateral radiograph after the ureteral stent is in place. Notice one loop is within the renal pelvis and the other loop in the urinary bladder.

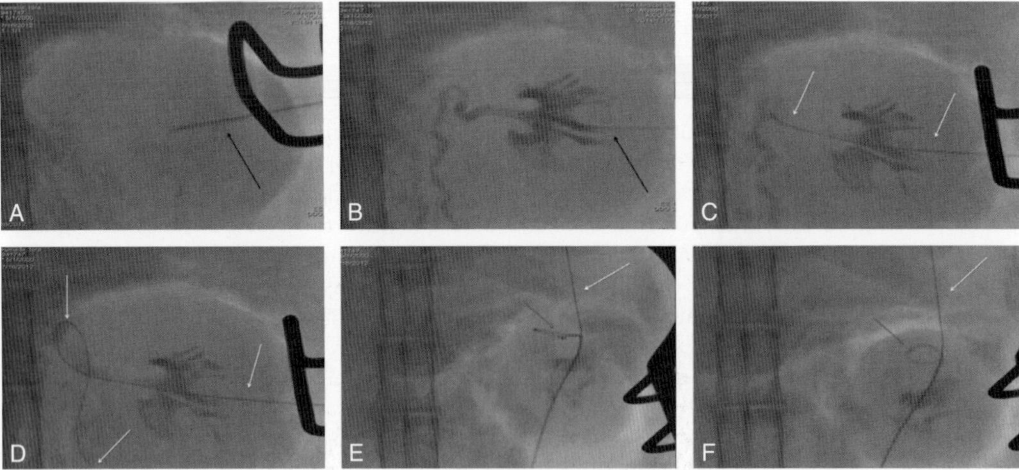

Figure 29.10 Fluoroscopic images of a feline patient during surgically-assisted antegrade ureteral stent placement. The patient is in dorsal recumbency and the head is to the top of the fluoroscopic images (A) Left renal pelvis being accessed with a 22-ga over-the-needle catheter (black arrow). (B) Ureteropyelogram being performed. Notice the dilated and tortuous ureter proximal to the more distal ureteral obstruction. (C) Guide wire (white arrow) being advanced through the catheter, into the renal pelvis and down the proximal ureter. (D) Guide wire (white arrow) advanced around the tortuous ureter and down to the obstructive lesion. (E) The ureteral stent (red arrow) being advanced over the guide wire (white arrow) in an antegrade manner after the ureteral dilator ensured the stent would fit. The wire is passed out of one of the proximal holes of the stent so the loop is not over the wire (see Figure 29.11)

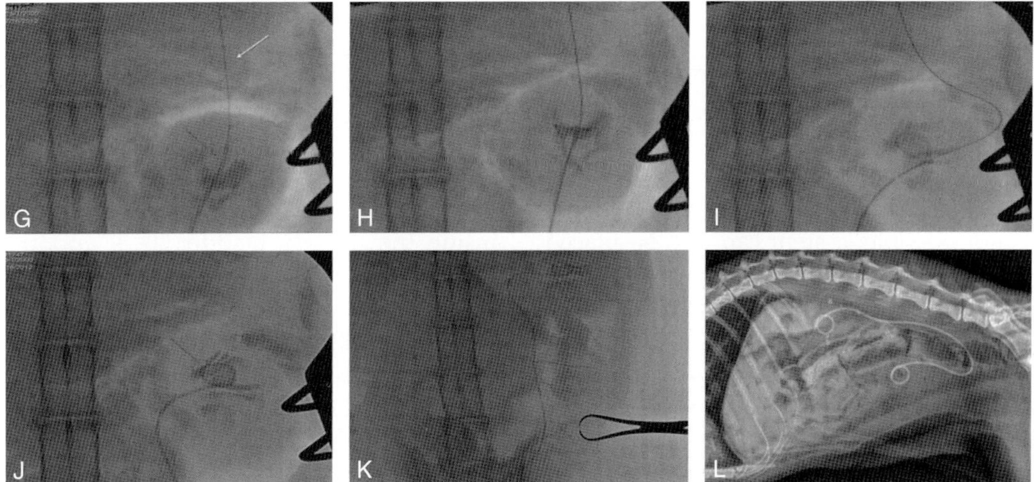

Figure 29.10 (*Continued*) (F, G) The stent (red arrow) is pulled from the bladder distally and the loop is pulled into the renal pelvis, keep the through and through wire (white arrow) access out the kidney. (H) the loop is formed within the renal pelvis and the guide wire is then removed (I). (J) The ureteral stent is coiled with one loop in the renal pelvis (red arrow). (K) The entire stent (red arrow) is seen traveling from the renal pelvis, down the ureteral lumen, and into the urinary bladder. (L) Lateral radiograph showing a double pigtail ureteral stent bypassing multiple ureteroliths.

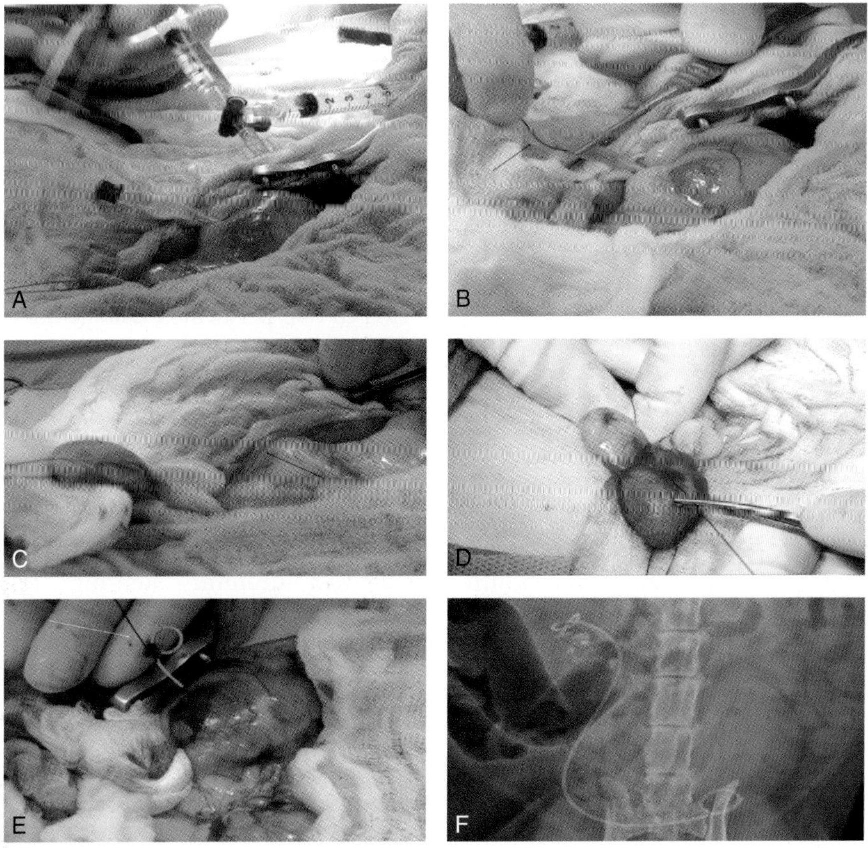

Figure 29.11 Surgical pictures during antegrade ureteral stent placement in a cat. The patient is in dorsal recumbency and the head is to the top of the image. (A) 22 gauge over-the-needle catheter advanced into the renal pelvis through the greater curvature of the kidney for a pyelocentesis and ureteropyelogram. (B) A 0.018″ hydrophilic angle-tipped guide wire (black arrow) being advanced through the catheter and into the renal pelvis. (C) Guide wire (black arrow) being advance down the ureter to the urinary bladder. (D) Guide wire being pulled out of the urinary bladder to obtain through and through access. (E) Ureteral stent being advanced over the guide wire and advanced down the ureter in an antegrade manner. Notice the guide wire is passed out one of the proximal side holes so that through and through access can be maintained while the stent is advanced into the renal pelvis. (F) A ventrodorsal radiograph after ureteral stent is in place. Notice the proximal loop is within the renal pelvis and the distal loop in the urinary bladder with the shaft within the entire ureteral lumen.

performed in a retrograde manner through the ureteral orifice at the UVJ. This is not typically possible when a trigonal tumor is causing a UVJ obstruction so they are placed percutaneously in an antegrade manner in these cases (see Chapter 31). If endoscopic placement is not possible, a stent can also be placed antegrade, through the renal parenchyma, from the greater curvature of the kidney, into the renal pelvis, either percutaneously using ultrasonography or surgically. Surgical ureteral stent placement is the most common approach in cats and is accomplished either via pyelocentesis (antegrade), through an ureterotomy (antegrade or retrograde), or via a cystostomy to access the UVJ (retrograde). The latter is no longer recommended in cats (though can be easily done in dogs) as the other techniques are preferred.

Endoscopic Retrograde Ureteral Stenting

Using cystoscopic guidance in dorsal recumbency with the endoscope turned with the 30 degree angle facing down toward the UVJ, an appropriately sized angled hydrophilic guide wire is advanced into the UVJ and up the distal ureter via the working channel of the cystoscope (Figure 29.8 and Figure 29.9). An appropriately sized open-ended ureteral catheter is advanced over the wire. The wire is removed, a urine sample obtained for analysis and culture, and a retrograde ureteropyelogram is performed. This aids in identifying any lesions, stones, or filling defects in the ureter or renal pelvis. The wire is then re-advanced up the ureter, through the catheter, and negotiated around the obstruction until it enters the renal pelvis. The wire should be curled inside the renal pelvis, being careful not to perforate the kidney through a calix. The catheter is advanced up the ureter to the level of the renal pelvis and a urine sample is obtained if one was not obtained prior. If contrast is in the sample the culture can be inaccurate. The wire is replaced and coiled within the pelvis. The catheter is withdrawn over the guide wire from the UPJ to the UVJ, under fluoroscopic guidance, obtaining a measurement of the ureteral length so an appropriate sized ureteral stent can be chosen using the 1 cm markers on the catheter (Figure 29.8). Stent lengths are described for their shaft length and the stent chosen should be a few centimeters longer than the measured shaft length (a slightly long stent is preferred to a slightly short stent). Care should be taken to ensure the guide wire is not removed as the catheter is withdrawn. Once the catheter is out, the wire is secured as the endoscope is maintained at the UVJ. Then the appropriately sized double pigtail ureteral stent is placed over the guide wire, through the working channel of the endoscope. It is very important that the endoscopist maintains the end of the cystoscope at the level of the UVJ at all times, providing the pushability necessary to advance that catheter and stent up the ureter without it buckling inside the urinary bladder. It is important that the operator understands what size stent fits in the working channel of the scope being utilized (Table 29.3). The pusher is advanced over-the-wire and used to continue to advance the stent into the renal pelvis after it has disappeared into the scope working channel. There is a black mark (Figure 29.8P) on the distal end of the ureteral stent that informs the endoscopist there is little remaining stent within the scope; this mark should not be advanced beyond the UVJ. If a curl is not inside the renal pelvis when this mark is seen then the stent is too short and a longer one should be used. Once the proximal loop is well within the renal pelvis the guide wire is withdrawn to the distal aspect of the stent that remains within the cystoscope, while monitoring under fluoroscopy. The wire remains within the pusher catheter and the distal end of the ureteral stent (Figure 29.8Q). The scope is pulled back into the proximal urethra, as the pusher catheter is advanced into the urinary bladder pushing the distal end of the stent into the bladder, and not up the ureter.

The antegrade technique (Figure 29.10) requires percutaneous or surgical pyelocentesis with a renal access needle[13] or over-the needle intravenous catheter. This can be performed using ultrasonography, fluoroscopy, or via surgical palpation for guidance. Once the catheter is within the renal pelvis a urine sample is obtained for culture and an antegrade ureteropyelogram is performed. The guide wire is passed down the ureter guided by the ureteropyelogram using fluoroscopic guidance. Once the wire is in the urinary bladder through-and-through access ("flossed") is obtained.

Feline ureteral stenting (Figure 29.10 and Figure 29.11) is typically performed with surgical assistance in an antegrade manner, as described above. Once the 0.018" guide wire is negotiated around the obstruction(s) in the ureter, and passed into the urinary bladder, a small dorsal cystotomy is done to obtain through-and-through guide wire access. If necessary a ureterotomy may be needed (~10%) to get around a large imbedded stone. More commonly this stone can be manipulated proximally so that the guide wire can pass around it, or a SUB is placed if this cannot be accomplished. The next step in cats, which is not typically necessary in dogs, is to pass a tapered feline ureteral dilator catheter (Figure 29.1). This is available in 0.032", 0.034", and 0.036" diameters. A dilator is passed in an antegrade manner over the guide wire from the kidney to the bladder. Care should be taken during passage to gently hold the area of the UPJ and UVJ to avoid trauma or avulsion of the ureter. It is very important that the wire and dilator are moist during the passage. Once the dilator is passed out of the UVJ and into the urinary bladder the ureter should be straightened out to relax for a few minutes to allow for ureteral length measurement, passive dilation, and to minimize spasm. The ureter is now measured using a sterile ruler from the center of the renal pelvis to the UVJ. Once the appropriate stent length (12, 14, 16 cm length × 2.5 Fr diameter) is chosen the stent is loaded on the moistened guide wire in an antegrade manner, with the tapered end advanced first. The stent is placed over the guide wire and advanced up to the back end of the ureteral dilator. The dilatator and stent are then passed together (piggy-back) down to ureter from the kidney to the bladder until the end of the stent passes out of the UVJ. The easiest way to pass the stent is to again have one operator gently hold the UPJ and UVJ, while the other operator has a hemostat on the guide wire (not the stent) both cranially (at the junction of the stent and wire) and distally (at the junction of the dilator and wire). This then allows the second operator to drag the stent and dilator combination antegrade through the ureteral lumen, around the obstruction and into the bladder. Once the distal end of the stent is in the bladder and the stent is through-and-through, with the proximal end of the stent out of the renal parenchyma, the dilator and guide wire are removed. The wire is then moistened and replaced inside the lumen of the stent in a retrograde manner so the angled tip is advanced retrograde up the ureteral stent, through the stent lumen, and out the stent at the level of the kidney (Figure 29.11E). Next, the wire is pulled back into the stent and the angled tip is advanced out of a cranial side hole of the stent (the first hole of the shaft after the cranial pigtail) (Figure 29.10 and Figure 29.11). The stent is retracted from the bladder side, over the wire, into the renal parenchyma. Monitoring under fluoroscopic guidance, once the stent is pulled into the renal pelvis and the curl has formed, the proximal end of the guide wire is pulled at the level of the kidney the caudal end of the stent advanced cranially up the ureter to facilitate the curl positioning inside the renal pelvis. Once this is curled appropriately in the renal pelvis the stent is secured at the level of the UVJ manually as the moistened wire is retracted slowly watching with fluoroscopic guidance to ensure the proximal end of the stent is not pulling down into the proximal ureter. Once stent location is acceptable the distal pigtail of the stent is carefully placed inside the urinary bladder through the small cystotomy incision and the incision is closed routinely. The bladder is then filled will contrast and gently expressed while the kidney and ureter are monitored fluoroscopically to ensure appropriate stent placement and no periureteral leakage. If leakage is seen (due to the need for concurrent ureterotomy or ureteral trauma), then a closed suction drain is placed for 24–48 hours.

Subcutaneous Ureteral Bypass Device

The development of an indwelling SUB device (Figure 29.2) using a combination locking-loop nephrostomy and cystostomy catheter with a shunting subcutaneous access port has simplified the treatment of feline ureteral obstructions (Figure 29.12, Figure 29.13, Figure 29.14, Figure 29.15, Figure 29.16, and Figure 29.17). This device can be serially flushed to ensure patency, is effective long-term, and eliminates the risks associated with an externalized nephrostomy tube.

A ventral midline laparotomy is performed in order to expose the bladder and affected kidney. The perirenal fat is gently and bluntly dissected off the caudal pole of the affected kidney exposing a 1–2 cm region of renal capsule (Figure 29.14). With the aid of fluoroscopy, the 6.5 Fr nephrostomy catheter is placed using the modified Seldinger-technique (Figure 29.12 and Figure 29.13). The 6.5 French locking-loop nephrostomy SUB catheter is prepared prior to renal access: The hollow trocar is placed inside the locking loop catheter (pre-loaded with the Dacron cuff and silicone sleeve) and the sharp stylet is discarded (Figure 29.2).

An 18-gauge over-the-needle catheter is used to puncture the renal pelvis through the caudal pole of the kidney where the fat was dissected off. Using a 3-way stop-cock, and empty syringe and a syringe filled with 50% contrast and pyelocentesis and antegrade pyelogram is performed. A urine sample is obtained for culture and iodinated contrast material is injected. A 0.035″ "J"-tip metallic wire (Figure 29.13A), or an angle tipped hydrophilic guide wire (Figure 29.12D), is advanced through the catheter and coiled inside the renal pelvis being careful to avoid perforation. The "J"-tip wire is ideal in a pelvis dilated over 8 mm but can be difficult to manipulate when the renal pelvis is smaller. Once the loop of the J-wire is well within the pelvis, or one to two loops of the hydrophilic wire, the 18-g catheter is removed over the wire while the wire is carefully secured to avoid losing access. If the renal pelvis is under 6 mm than a hydrophilic angle-tipped guide wire is used and passed down the ureter. The angle of renal puncture is halfway between the caudal pole and the greater curvature

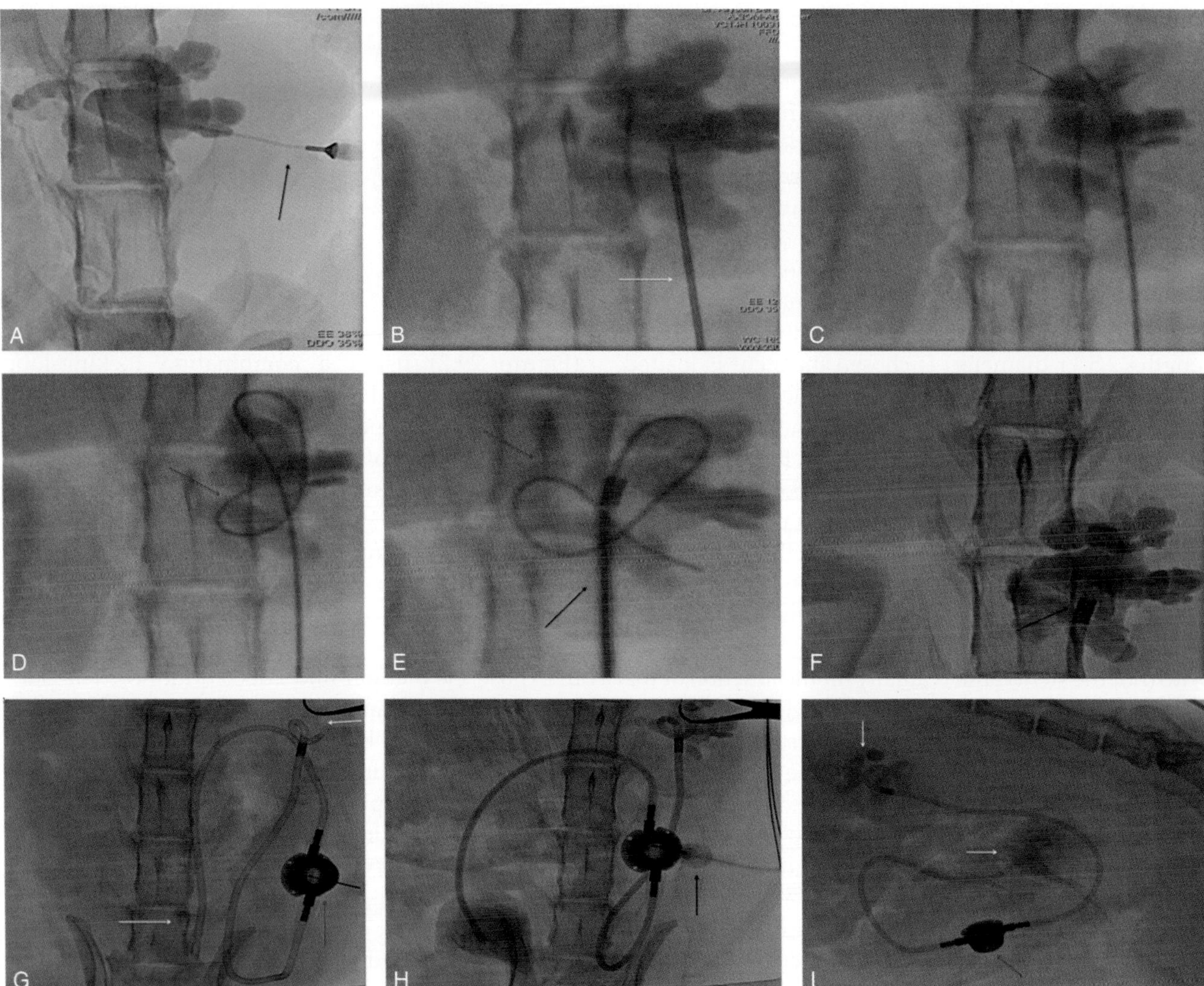

Figure 29.12 Fluoroscopic images during the placement of a subcutaneous ureteral bypass (SUB) device in a cat with a left sided ureteral obstruction. The patient is in dorsal recumbency. (A) An antegrade ureteropyelogram using a 22-gauge catheter (black arrow) from the greater curvature of the kidney showing hydronephrosis, hydroureter and then a proximal obstructive lesion. (B) An 18-gauge catheter (white arrow) advanced into the renal pelvis from the caudal pole of the kidney. This is usually how the initial pyelogram is done unless the renal pelvis is < ~6–7 mm. (C) 0.035″ angle-tipped hydrophilic guide wire (red arrow) being advanced through the catheter and into the renal pelvis. (D) Guide wire (red arrow) coiled within the renal pelvis. (E) Nephrostomy catheter (black arrow) advanced over the guide wire and coiled within the renal pelvis. (F) The radiopaque marker (black arrow) seen within the renal pelvis to ensure it is well placed. A contrast study is done to ensure no leakage is seen. (G) The cystostomy and nephrostomy tubes (white arrows) are attached to the access port (red arrow). (H) The SUB device is flushed prior to closing the abdomen with a 22-g non-coring Huber needle (black arrow). Notice the pyelogram, cystogram, and no leakage of contrast is seen from any junction of the system (port, kidney, bladder). (I) Lateral fluoroscopic image of the SUB device.

so that you are aiming down the ureter. Once the wire is down the ureter the locking string on the nephrostomy tube is cut and removed. The renal access catheter is then removed over the wire and the nephrostomy catheter is advanced over the wire and down the ureter until the radiopaque marker band is within the renal pelvis. The dacron cuff is the advanced to the renal capsule and the silicone sleeve is advanced behind that. The dacron is then glued to the renal capsule securely being careful not the dislodge the catheter, as there is no locking string. For the standard renal pelvis that is dilated over 8 mm the "J" wire is used and advanced into the renal pelvis and coiled. Once the catheter is removed off the wire the nephrostomy catheter and trocar are advanced over the guide wire into the renal parenchyma. Once it enters the renal pelvis

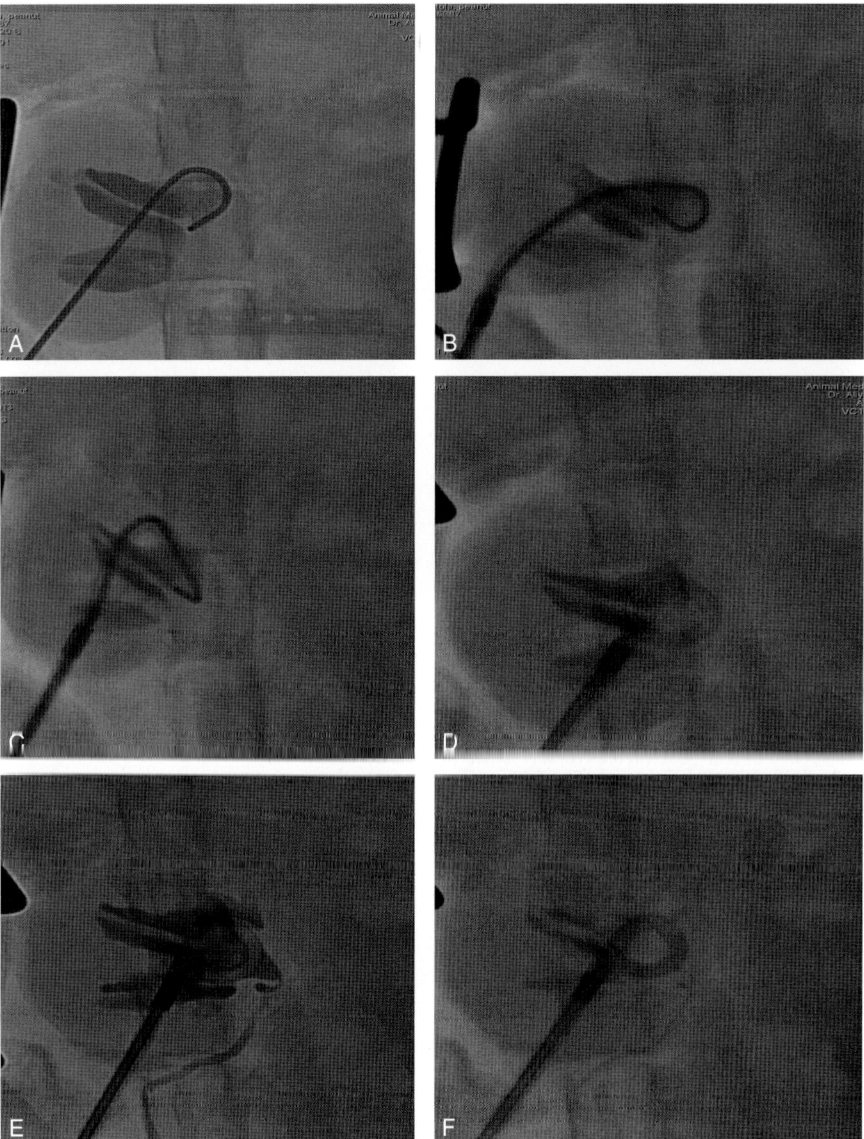

Figure 29.13 Fluoroscopy images during SUB placement in a cat. These images are showing the use of a J-wire, which is easier to use than the hydrophilic guide wire when the pelvis is over 8 mm. This wire is stiff with a very floppy end (the "J"), and the shape of the "J" prevents piercing of the renal pelvis with the wire. (A) Catheter access into the caudal pole of the renal pelvis for a pyelogram. The "J"-tipped wire is passed through the renal catheter, and allowed to bend within the renal pelvis as seen in (B). (B) The locking-loop nephrostomy catheter being advanced over the "J"-tipped wire as it is making the bend along the renal pelvis. (C) The coil of the nephrostomy catheter over the wire. (D) The wire removed as the pigtail is made by locking the loop of the nephrostomy catheter. (E) Ureteropyelogram performed showing the dilated renal pelvis and proximal tortuous ureter, which is obstructed mid ureter by stones. Notice there is no leakage at the entry point of the nephrostomy tube at the caudal pole of the kidney. (F) Draining of the renal pelvis through the nephrostomy tube showing patency.

the hollow trocar is stabilized and the catheter is carefully advanced over the wire and trocar into the renal pelvis (Figure 29.12, Figure 29.13, and Figure 29.14). The radiopaque marker on the catheter marks the location of the last fenestration of the catheter to ensure the entire loop with all fenestrations are within the renal pelvis (Figure 29.12E, F). The locking string is pulled to prevent catheter dislodgement and clamped with a hemostat to maintain tension during manipulations (Figure 29.16). This should not be tightened excessively, but just gently, to avoid kinking of the loop. Once the wire and hollow trocar are removed a contrast study is done to ensure proper placement and no leakage (Figure 29.12F). The Dacron cuff and silicone sleeve are then gently advanced down the nephrostomy catheter toward the kidney so it is snug with the renal capsule. Sterile cyanoacrylate glue is lightly applied between the Dacron and the renal capsule avoiding contact with fat to provide a secure and complete seal to prevent leakage.

The urinary bladder is then isolated. Using 3–0 monocryl suture, a purse-string is made at the apex (Figure 29.15). In the center of this purse string a #11 blade is used to puncture a small hole into the bladder lumen. Next, the loaded cystostomy catheter, with the hollow trocar and the sharp stylet, are advanced through the incision and into the urinary bladder. The sharp stylet is discarded and the catheter is advanced into the bladder lumen until the Dacron cuff is against the serosal surface of the bladder. The purse-string suture is tied and sterile cyanoacrylate glue is used to secure the Dacron cuff to the bladder serosa. Using 3–0 monocryl suture, the Dacron/silicone cuff is sutured to the bladder wall (full thickness) using three interrupted sutures. Once secured, the hollow trocar is removed.

Finally, the skin and subcutaneous tissues immediately lateral to the ventral abdominal incision on the ipsilateral side of the nephrostomy tube are dissected down to the abdominal musculature (Figure 29.16). Both catheters are passed gently through body wall. Typically the nephrostomy catheter is passed caudally and the cystostomy catheter is passed cranially to prevent kinking of the catheters (Figure 29.12 and Figure 29.18). Care should be taken to ensure there is enough space for the access shunting port with both cuffs and catheters to enter the body wall. The entry of the catheter through the body wall is a site that can kink so ensuring there is not an abrupt bend is important. Using blunt dissection with a mosquito hemostat a puncture is made from the external body wall, through the abdominal musculature, and into the abdomen. The ends of the hemostat carefully clamp the locking string just off the end of the nephrostomy catheter and the string and catheter are pulled through the body wall in unison. The catheter should not be clamped.

A blue cuff is advanced over the nephrostomy catheter (Figure 29.16), ensuring the tapered end goes down the catheter and the thicker blunt end is towards with shunting port. Finally, the shunting port is attached to the nephrostomy catheter. The pin/arm of the shunting port is used to secure the string. Once the catheter is advanced onto the first barb of the male adaptor of the port (Figure 29.16D and Figure 29.17), the string is bluntly cut using a #11 blade (Figure 29.17). The pin of the port is then completely advanced inside the lumen of the nephrostomy catheter. It is important to ensure there is no exposed string at the junction of the port and the nephrostomy catheter as this is a site of potential leakage.

The same procedure is done to the bladder catheter on the cranial aspect of the port. The distal end of the bladder catheter is clamped because there is no string. The very end of the bladder catheter is then cut flush with scissors and discarded to maintain the catheter integrity. The blue boot is advanced onto the bladder catheter as above and then the catheter is secured to the shunting port. The blue boot is advanced over the junction of the metallic pin and bladder catheter (Figure 29.16F). The location of the holes in the body wall for each catheter should be made carefully. The author typically allows at least 1 cm of white catheter after the blue boot to be exposed in the SQ before it dives down into the abdomen to ensure no kinking at the junction of the catheter and blue boot when transversing the body wall. Once this system is closed a 22 gauge Huber needle is used to flush the device while manually compressing both catheters with fingers to look for any evidence of leakage at the catheter-port junctions. Next, another flush is performed with contrast under digital subtraction fluoroscopy to ensure no leakage or kinking is seen and that both catheters flow and drain easily (Figure 29.12H, Figure 29.16H, and Figure 29.18). Once no leakage is seen the port is secured to the abdominal wall using permanent suture material (2–0 or 3–0 synthetic non-absorbable) (Figure 29.16). Care should be taken to look for leakage at the kidney, port and bladder insertion sites, and kinking of the catheter at the body wall entry site (Figure 29.19). Once patency and no leakage or kinking are confirmed than the subcutaneous tunnel is closed routinely and any dead space addressed being careful not to place sutures through the SUB catheters. Topical bupivacaine (0.3 mg/kg) is infused into the subcutaneous space prior to closure. The abdomen is flushed and closed routinely. An abdominal wrap is placed for the first 24 hours postoperatively.

Flushing of the SUB

Flushing through the port to ensure no encrustation and full patency can be done using a 22 gauge Huber needle. This can be visualized using ultrasonography or fluoroscopy. The skin over the port is clipped of fur and aseptically prepared. An extension set with a 3-way stop-cock is used with one empty syringe for urine sampling and one syringe filled with bacteriostatic saline (if being done with ultrasonography alone), or with a 1:1 dilution of iohexol and saline (if the flush is being done with fluoroscopy) (Figure 29.12H). The shunting port is palpated under the skin and the flat silicone insertion site is isolated (Figure 29.20A). Using sterile technique the Huber needle is advanced through the skin into the silicone diaphragm until metal is reached within the port. This

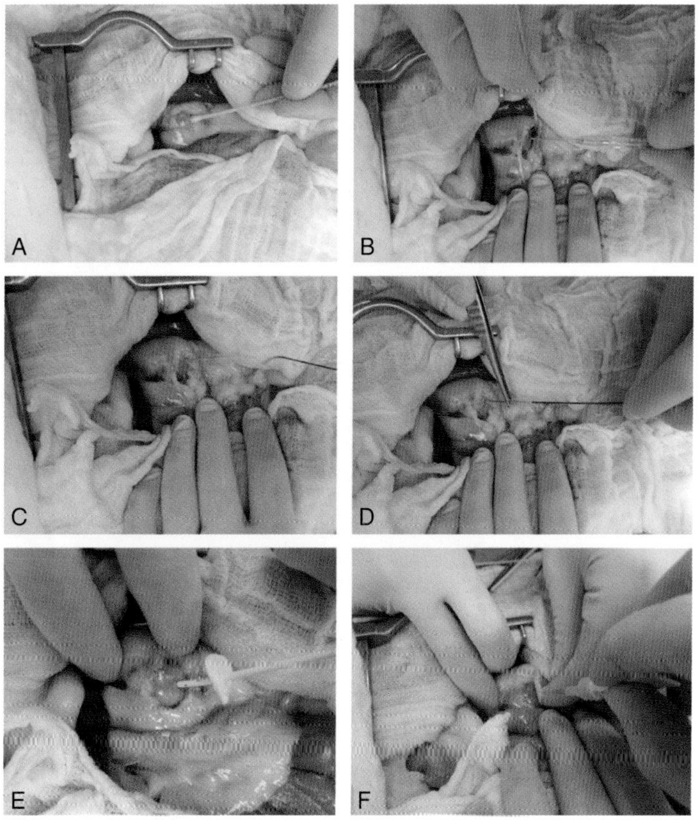

Figure 29.14 Surgical images during the placement of a SUB device. This is the nephrostomy tube access. Head is to the left of the image. (A) The retroperitoneal fat is dissected off the caudal pole of the kidney using monopolar electrocautery and blunt dissection. (B) An 18-g catheter is used to puncture the renal pelvis through the caudal pole of the kidney. (C) The 0.035″ angle-tipped hydrophilic guide wire being advanced into the catheter. (D) The wire is being coiled within the renal pelvis and the catheter is stabilized with a grasping instrument. (E) The nephrostomy catheter is advanced over the guide wire, into the renal parenchyma, and coiled over the wire in the renal pelvis. (F) Once the nephrostomy catheter is in place the Dacron cuff is glued to the renal capsule.

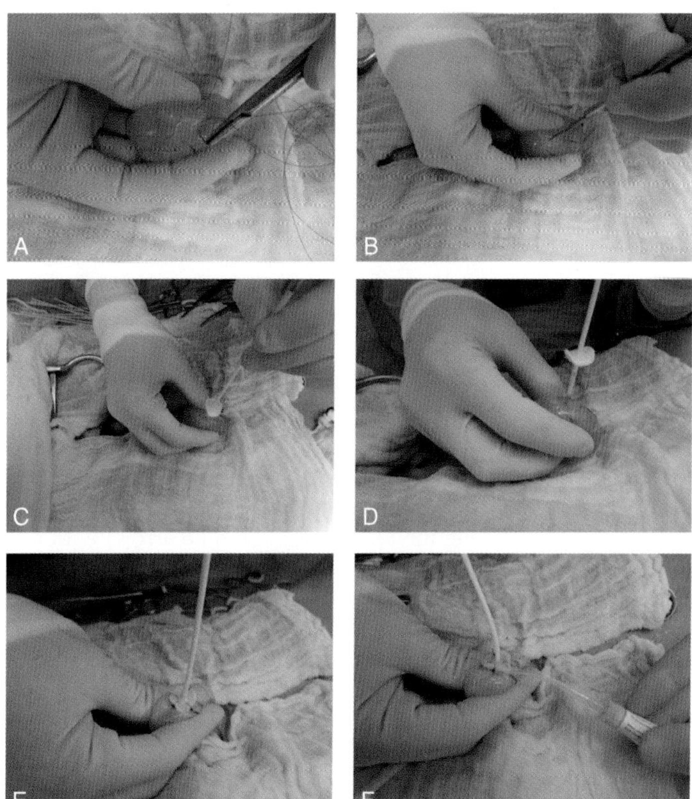

Figure 29.15 Surgical images during the placement of a SUB device. This is the cystostomy tube access. Head is to the left of the image. (A) The apex of the bladder is isolated and a purse string suture is made. (B) A #11 blade is used to make a stab incision into the bladder lumen in the center of the purse-string. C-(D) The cystostomy catheter is advanced into the bladder lumen using the sharp stylette. (E) Once the catheter is with the bladder lumen the purse-string is tightened around the catheter and the Dacron cuff is sutured using 3 interrupted sutures to the bladder wall. (F) Between the suturing, sterile tissue glue is used to secure the catheter to the bladder serosa.

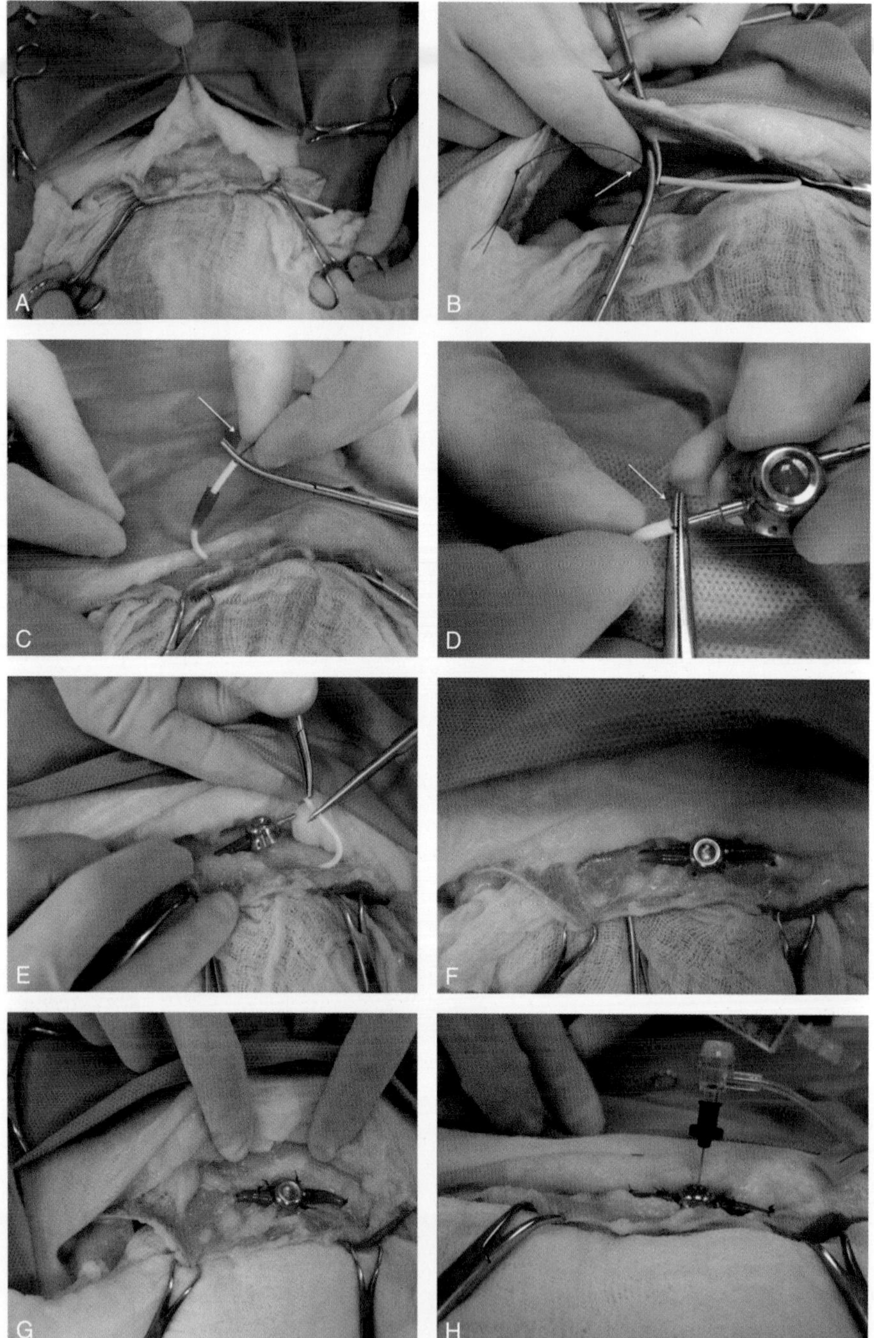

Figure 29.16 Surgical images during the placement of a SUB device. This is the subcutaneous access port placement. Head is to the right of the image. (A) The subcutaneous tissue is dissected off the ventral abdominal wall on the ipsilateral side of the obstruction just lateral to the incision. (B) The nephrostomy catheter is advanced through the body wall, at the caudal aspect of the port, by grabbing the locking string (white arrow) with hemostats, being careful not to lose the locking mechanism. (C) The catheter is pulled through the body wall and the string remains locked (white arrow). The blue cuff is advanced on the catheter. (D) The male adaptor of the shunting port is inserted into the nephrostomy catheter, entrapping the locking string (white arrow). (E) The cystostomy tube passed through the body wall cranially. (F) Both catheters through the body wall and connected to the shunting port. The blue cuffs are placed over each junction to secure the catheters and prevent leakage. (G) The shunting port gently sutured to the ventral body wall musculature to avoid tissue necrosis and port loosening. (H) The Huber needle inserted into the shunting port to test the SUB device prior to closing the abdomen and ensure there is no leakage.

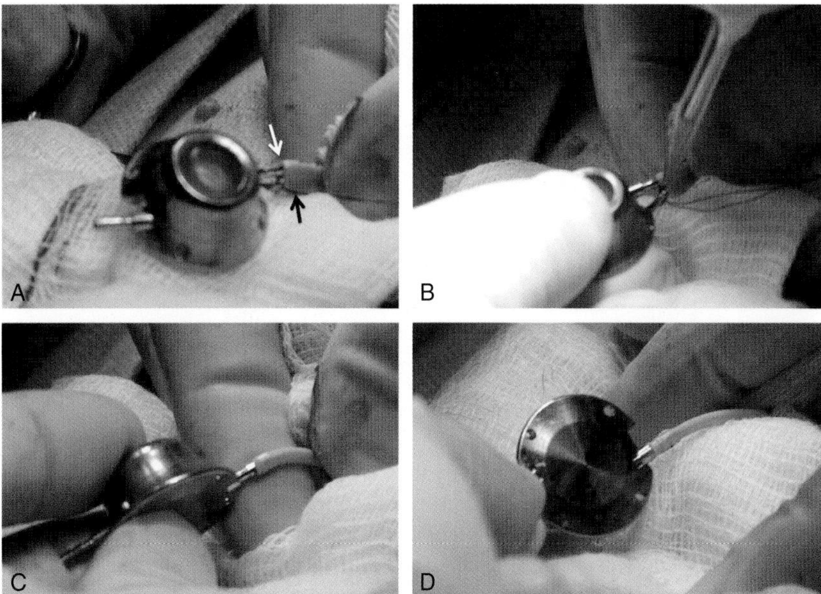

Figure 29.17 Connecting the nephrostomy catheter to the shunting port to prevent leakage. (A) The locking-loop nephrostomy catheter being connected to the pin of the shunting port (white arrow), with the locking string (black arrow) being pulled until it is entrapped. (B) The string is entrapped on the first rung of the pin and then cut flush with the pin using a #11 blade. (C) The catheter is advanced over the entire pin, locking the string but not allowing the string to break the seal between the pin and the catheter. (D) The catheter fully advanced on the pin ensuring the string is not seen.

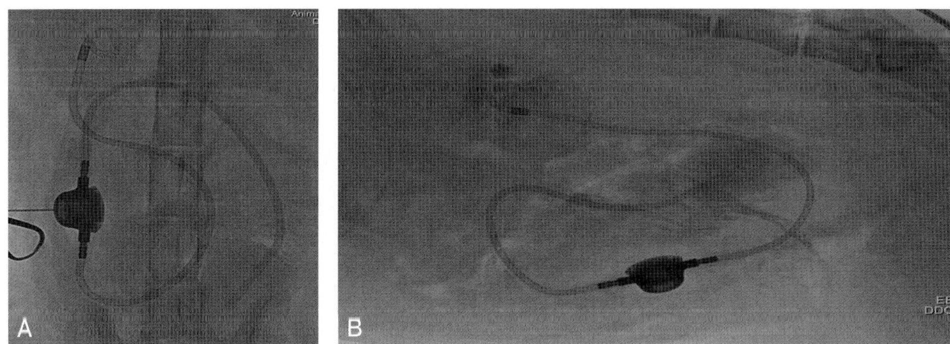

Figure 29.18 Fluoroscopic images of a cat after SUB placement. (A) Ventrodorsal image of the device traveling from the renal pelvis to the urinary bladder through a subcutaneous shunting port. (B) Lateral projection of the same patient after SUB placement. Notice that the nephrostomy tube is typically attached to the caudal aspect of the port and the bladder catheter to the cranial aspect of the port. This helps to prevent catheter kinking.

must be done in a perpendicular manner (Figure 29.20A). Once the needle is inside the shunting port a urine sample is obtained (Figure 29.20B). If no urine is able to be withdrawn than the needle is either not deep enough into the access port, at the wrong angle, or the port is blocked. Try re-directing the needle. Once urine is obtained (and submitted for urine culture and urinalysis) the syringe with saline (±contrast) is used to inject the system. The renal pelvis should always be monitored first (Figure 29.12H and Figure 29.20D) during this procedure to ensure it is not being overdistended. Never inject more fluid than the amount removed to prevent overdistension. Contrast should be seen filling both the renal pelvis and the urinary bladder equally.

If the flush is being done under ultrasound guidance (Figure 29.20) the renal pelvis should be measured prior to injection. Sterile bacteriostatic saline is used. 3–5 ml of urine is removed from the system and then, while monitoring the renal pelvis, 1 mL of the sterile saline is flushed into the port relatively hard to encourage bubbles to be seen with ultrasonography (Figure 29.20). Once saline is seen to enter the renal pelvis the fluid is withdrawn to avoid over distension. Next the ultrasound probe should be placed over the bladder apex monitoring the catheter (Figure 29.20F). The port should be flushed again with 1 mL at a time to see fluid enter the urinary bladder through the SUB cystostomy tube. Once this is seen then patency is

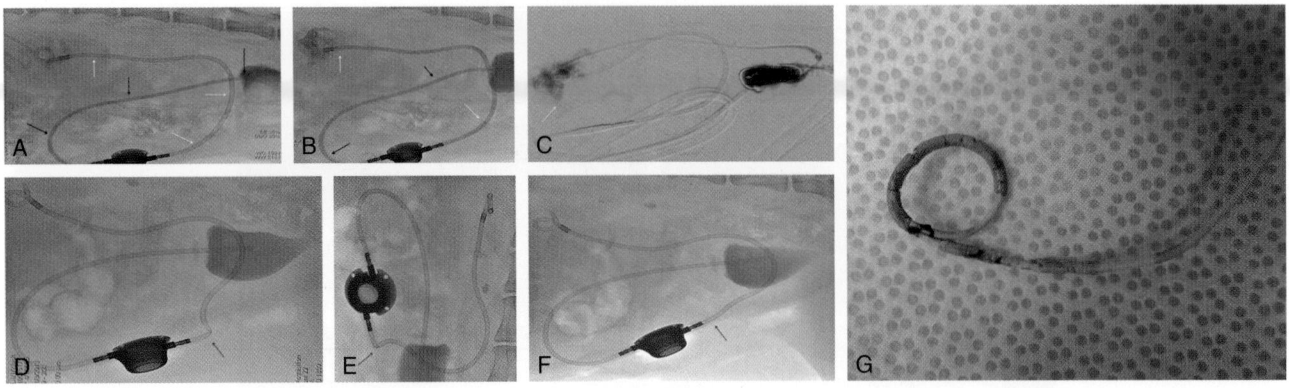

Figure 29.19 Fluoroscopic images showing some complications that can be seen with the SUB device and ureteral stents. (A) Lateral image of a cat with a SUB device. During fluoroscopic flushing at the end of the procedure the cystostomy catheter (black arrows) is seen to fill with contrast but the nephrostomy tube (white arrows) is not filling. This was due to a severe pyonephrosis and with serial flushing the catheter eventually cleared and started flowing (B). (C) A digital subtraction image of a cat with transitional cell carcinoma after ureteral and urethral diversion. During cystography, contrast is seen advancing up the ureteral stent and leaking out of the kidney (yellow arrow) at the catheter access point. (D, E) A kinked (red arrow) SUB device in a cat. (F) After digital manipulation, the kink straightened out. (G) An encrusted ureteral stent from a cat. This cat was hypercalcemic.

confirmed, urine can be drained out of the bladder, and then 1–2 ml of saline should be flushed in to ensure no stones were pulled into the catheter.

If the flush is being done under fluoroscopic guidance than a solution of iohexol:sterile saline is made in a 1:1 dilution in a 10 ml syringe. Ultrasonography is not needed for the flush but should be used prior to the flush to get an accurate renal pelvis size measurement to ensure proper function of the SUB device. The patient is placed under the fluoroscopic unit in dorsal recumbency and the port area is clipped and scrubbed aseptically as described above. The fluoroscopy image should be aligned with the patient so that the kidney, port and bladder are seen in the image. After the urine sample is obtained, to ensure proper needle placement, the contrast solution is injected into the port. Careful monitoring of the contrast should be seen using fluoroscopy traveling from the port, up the catheter, to the kidney while the renal pelvis fills. The pelvis should not get over-distended and the injection should be done slowly (1–3 ml is all that is needed). At the same time the urinary bladder should be filling with contrast. Then all of the contrast should be easily withdrawn from the bladder and renal pelvis. If contrast is used for the flushing, the author then injects 2–3 ml of sterile saline to wash the catheter of contrast material. If little urine is able to be withdrawn from the SUB system than likely the catheter(s) are blocked, which is seen in about 18% of cats with known stone disease. If the T-port and stopcock are pre-flushed with saline than 0.5–1.0 mL can be flushed into the system monitoring the renal pelvis. If bubbles are seen then withdraw that fluid and asses the bladder. If the bladder is full and you can not withdraw more than you placed in than it is likely the bladder catheter is blocked. If the bladder is draining and flushing well but nothing is seen in the renal pelvis than it is possible the nephrostomy catheter is blocked. This is when the flush can be done using contrast under either fluoroscopy or radiography.

Postoperative and Follow-Up Care

Patients with ureteral stents or SUBs need to be monitored very carefully. Feline patients are at high risk of developing a post-obstructive diuresis and potentially fluid overload. Care is taken to maintain an appropriate fluid balance using enteral hydration when possible. All cats have an esophagostomy tube placed at the time of ureteral intervention in the author's practice. Each patient should be monitored for urine leakage into the abdomen and within the subcutaneous tissues around the port. If leakage occurs in the subcutaneous space (with a SUB device) this is considered a surgical emergency and should be fixed. Two weeks of broad spectrum antibiotic therapy (typically a fluoroquinolone) is recommended once a device is placed and left indwelling. There is good evidence in humans that the use of fluoroquinolone antibiotic therapy prevents postoperative biofilm development on urinary devices and is currently considered the standard recommendation. Routine urinary tract ultrasonography focusing on the renal pelvis diameter, stent location, ureteral diameter, presence of any free fluid, and location of stent/SUB catheters in the urinary bladder, are performed to ensure there is no evidence of stent/SUB migration, occlusion,

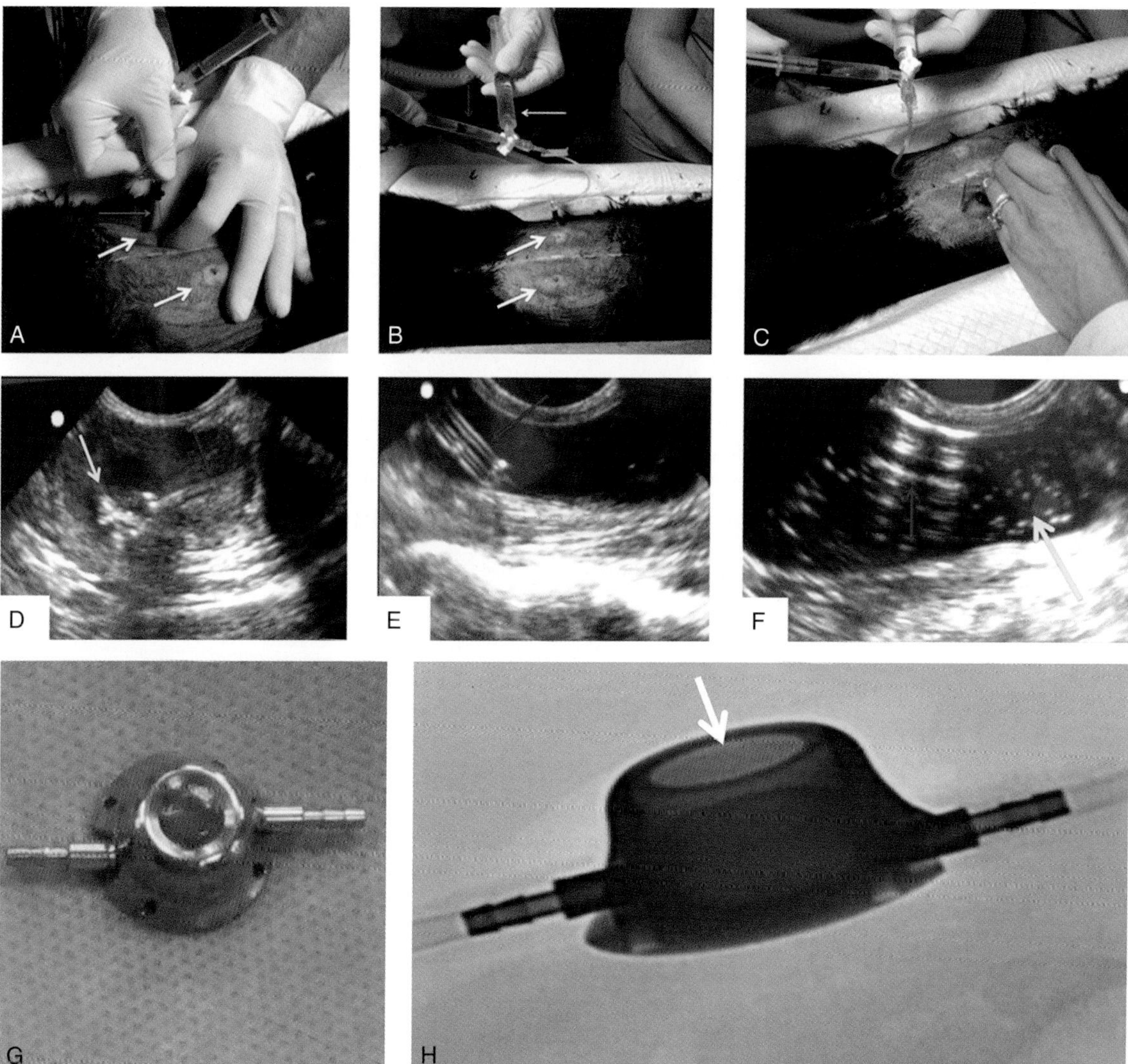

Figure 29.20 Flushing the SUB device in a cat with bilateral devices (white arrows) and renal hematuria causing dried solidified blood stones. The head is to the right of each image. (A) The right access port is being palpated and the Huber needle (blue arrow) is being advanced into the silicone diaphragm of the port in a perpendicular manner. (B) Once in place urine sample is taken for analysis and culture and to ensure access is appropriate (red arrow). Then, using a two-way stopcock and T-connector sterile saline is infused into the port. (C–F) The infusion is monitored using ultrasound guidance to ensure the renal pelvis does not overdistend and bubbles are seen in the pelvis (D) and urinary bladder (E, F) during infusion. (G, H) The SUB shunting port (G) showing the shape of the flat silicone top (H) where the needle should be perpendicularly inserted.

or encrustation. The author recommends a urine culture every 3–6 months, and a SUB flush every 3 months for 1–2 years and then every 6 months thereafter. Ureteral stents are traditionally meant to be removed in human medicine, but in veterinary medicine the author is not finding this to be necessary in a majority of cases. Stent encrustation (mineralization around the inside and outside of the stent visualized radiographically) is a common problem seen in human medicine, but has not been appreciated routinely in many clinical veterinary patients (Figure 29.19G). Ureteral stent occlusion from urinary debris and crystalline material commonly occurs within about 3 months, but with appropriate passive ureteral dilation the ureter does not typically re-obstruct. This has been appreciated on post mortem, pyelography, and ultrasound exams. Commonly, after 3–6 months, a guide wire cannot be passed up the lumen of the stent due to crystalline material accumulation, but the ureter is passively dilated so remains patent long-term. If a SUB device gets occluded with debris, stones, etc, than it can be exchanged. This requires open surgery, but is typically a relatively fast recovery. The nephrostomy catheter can be removed from the renal pelvis after the catheter is cut and the string is released.

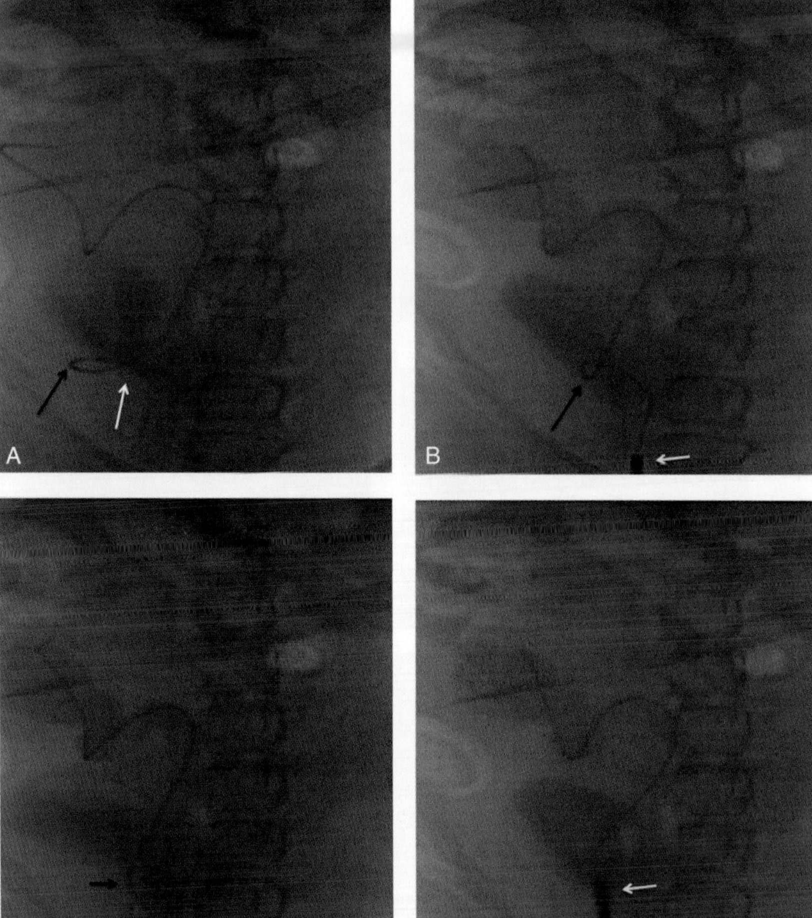

Figure 29.21 Fluoroscopic images of a female dog in dorsal recumbency during right endoscopic ureteral stent placement documenting the "J" hook the distal ureter often makes making stent placement a challenge. (A) The ureteral catheter (white arrow) coursing the "J" hook at the distal ureter (black arrow) as it advances up the ureter. (B, C) The straightening out of the ureter as the endoscope (yellow arrow) is withdrawn with the catheter/wire combination. During the process, the "J" will unwind (black arrow) and become straight (C). (D) Prior to ureteral stent placement the endoscope (yellow arrow) is re-advanced over the catheter to the level of the UVJ to maintain pushability.

The catheter is typically cut inside the abdomen, leaving the attachment to the port and the catheter through the body wall. Then the catheter is dissected to the level of the dacron cuff on the renal capsule. The catheter is pulled out of the renal pelvis, leaving the dacron in place. Next a guidewire is advanced through the hole in the dacron into the renal pelvis, as a path is likely made. Over the wire an 18 Ga IV catheter can be advanced into the renal pelvis and a contrast study can be done once the wire is removed. Once the renal pelvis is visualized the wire is replaced and the catheter removed over the wire. Next, the new nephrostomy tube is advanced over the wire. The dacron cuff is removed from the catheter but the silicone sleeve remains on the catheter. The loop is formed and the string locked. The same thing is done with the bladder side but since the catheter is adhered to the dacron the cuff is bluntly dissected off the serosal surface of the bladder and then, through the same hole, a new cystostomy catheter, with dacron cuff, is advanced into the bladder and resecured as previously, using both a pursestring suture, sterile glue and tacking sutures. Finally, once both catheters are replaced a hemostat or guide wire can be used to follow the same tunnel throug the body wall so the catheters can be passed through. The old port is then removed and a new port is attached to both new catheters in the same place.

Special Considerations/ Alternative Uses/ Complication Examples

In general, for benign canine ureteral obstructions, stents are placed endoscopically, so expertise in male and female cystoscopy is needed. It is recommended to position the dogs in dorsal recumbency as this makes ureteral access easier and more accurate. Flexible cystoscopy is possible in male dogs over 6 kg, but the working channel of a flexible scope is only 3 Fr. Ureteral access in males is typically obtained using an exchange length (260 cm) stiffened hydrophilic angled guide wire. Once access is obtained the scope is removed over the guide wire while the wire remains coiled inside the renal pelvis. The remainder of the procedure is done under fluoroscopic guidance alone using a 4 Fr Berenstein hydrophilic catheter for pyelography and ureteral length measurement. After a cystogram is performed the ureteral stent is pushed up the ureter over the guide wire using fluoroscopic guidance only, so care must be taken to ensure the caudal end of the stent is not pushed up the distal ureter, but rather appropriately curled within the urinary bladder; this is relatively difficult compared to endoscope-assisted stent placement. If needed perineal urethral access or antegrade PCCL approach can be done to make ureteral stenting easier in male dogs (Chapter 39 and Chapter 33).

In addition, during endoscopic guide wire and catheter placement, the "J" of the distal ureter can result in friction and a large curl, making stent placement difficult. The trick to getting this curl out of the ureter is to pass the wire and catheter as far cranial as possible keeping the cystoscope at the UVJ. Then the cystoscope, catheter and guide wire are all retracted together into the urethra en bloc. This typically straightens out the loop. Then the scope is passed over the catheter/wire combination back to the UVJ to maintain stability keeping the ureter straight (Figure 29.21).

Notes

1. Vet Stent ureter 2.5–4.7 Fr double pigtail ureteral stent, Infiniti Medical LLC, Menlo Park, CA.
2. Bard In-Lay ureteral stent (4.7–8.0 Fr), Bard Medical, Covington, GA.
3. Subcutaneous ureteral bypass device (SUB), Norfolk Vet, Skokie, IL.
4. Rigid endoscope, 1.9-mm 30° lens, Karl Storz Endoscopy, Culver City, CA.
5. Rigid endoscope, 2.7-mm integrated sheath 30° lens, Richard Wolf, Vernon Hills, IL.
6. Rigid endoscope, 2.7-mm 30° lens, Karl Storz Endoscopy, Culver City, IL.
7. Rigid endoscope, 4-mm 30° lens, Karl Storz Endoscopy, Culver City, IL.
8. Flex X^2 Flexible ureteroscope, Karl Storz Endoscopy, Culver City, CA.
9. 0.018"-0.035" hydrophilic angle-tipped guide wires, Weasel wire, Infiniti Medical, LLC, Menlo Park, CA.
10. 3–6 Fr open-ended ureteral catheters, Bard Medical, Covington, GA.
11. 5 Fr Dawson Mueller Locking-loop catheter, Cook Medical, Bloomington, IN.
12. 6 Fr Locking loop catheter, Infiniti Medical, LLC, Menlo Park, CA.
13. Renal access needle (0.021" or 0.018") Cook Medical, Bloomington, IN.

References

Berent A. Weisse C, Bagley D. et al Technical and clinical outcomes of ureteral stenting in cats for the treatment of benign ureteral obstruction: 2006–2010. J Am Vet Med Assoc. 2014; 244(5): 559–576.

Kyles A, Hardie E, Wooden B, et al (2005a) Clinical, clinicopathologic, radiographic, and ultrasonographic abnormalties in cats with ureteral calculi: 163 cases (1984–2002). *J Am Vet Med Assoc* 226(6), 932–6.

Kyles A, Hardie E, Wooden B, et al (2005b) Management and outcome of cats with ureteral calculi: 153 cases (1984–2002). *J Am Vet Med Assoc* 226(6), 937–44.

Snyder D, Steffery M, Mehler S, et al (2004) Diagnsis and surgical management of ureteral calculi in dogs: 16 cases (1990–2003). *N Z Vet J* 53(1), 19–25.

Steinhaus J, Berent A, Weisse C, et al (2013) Circumcaval ureters in cats with and without ureteral obstructions. A comparative study. Abstract, American College of Veterinary Internal Medicine, Seattle WA ACVIM, 2013.

Suggested Reading

Berent A (2011) Ureteral obstructions in dogs and cats: a review of traditional and new interventional diagnostic and therapeutic options. *J Vet Emerg Crit Care* 21(2), 86 103.

Berent A, Weisse C, Bagley D, et al (2011) The use of a subcutaneous ureteral bypass device for the treatment of feline ureteral obstructions. ECVIM, Seville Spain, 2011.

Berent A, Weisse C, Todd K, and Bagley D (2012) The use of locking-loop nephrostomy tubes in dogs and cats: 20 cases (2004–2009). *J Am Vet Med Assoc* 241(3), 348–57.

Horowitz C. Berent A, Weisse C et al (2013) Predictors of outcome for cats with rueteral obstructions after interventional management using ureteral stents or a subcutaneous ureteral bypass device *J Feline Med Surg* 2013 15(12), 1052–62.

Kuntz J, Berent A, Weisse C et al (2013) Renal sparing treatment for obstructive pyonephrosis in dogs. Abstract, American College of Veterinary Internal Medicine, Seattle WA ACVIM, 2013.

Lam N, Berent A, Weisse C, et al (2012) Ureteral stenting for congenital ureteral strictures in a dog. *J Am Vet Med Associ* 240(8), 983–90.

Pavia P, Berent A, Weisse C, et al (2014) Canine ureteral stenting for benign ureteral obstruction in dogs. Abstract, *American College Veterinary Surgeons*, San Diego, CA.

Roberts S, Aronson L, Brown D (2011) Postoperative mortality in cats after ureterolithotomy. *Vet Surg* 40, 438–43.

Steinhaus J, Berent A, Weisse C, et al (2013) Presence of circumcaval ureters and ureteral obstructions in cats. *J Vet Intern Med* 27(3), 604–756. *Abstract*

Zaid M, Berent A, Weisse C, et al (2011) Feline ureteral strictures: 10 cases (2007–2009). *J Vet Intern Med* 25(2), 222–9.

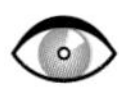
Video clips to accompany this chapter can be found in the online material at **www.wiley.com/go/weisse/vet-image-guided-interventions**

CHAPTER THIRTY

Interventional Management of Obstructive Pyonephrosis

Allyson Berent
The Animal Medical Center, New York, NY

Background / Indications

Pyonephrosis can occur when a ureteral obstruction is associated with an infection resulting in renal pelvis abscessation and potentially, sepsis. In humans, emergency decompression of the renal pelvis is recommended. This is typically accomplished with percutaneous nephrostomy tube or endoscopic ureteral stent placement. In animals the same process has been documented and seems to occur more commonly in dogs than in cats. Using IR/IE techniques the renal pelvis can be drained, lavaged, and the obstruction bypassed, without the need for aggressive and prolonged surgery.

The treatment of pyonephrosis typically requires immediate drainage, renal pelvic lavage, and then resolution of the obstruction. The recommended treatment in the author's practice is endoscopic-guided renal pelvic lavage and subsequent stenting. If this is not an option then the placement of a nephrostomy tube for lavage and drainage can be performed. This would require a second procedure when the patient has been stabilized in order to fix the inciting obstructive lesion. It is important that renal preservation is considered because most of these dogs have urolith disease and may eventually develop a nephrolith, or ureterolith, on the contralateral side even though many are not azotemic. When a ureteronephrectomy is performed, a functioning kidney is removed for a ureteral disease process that can be resolved and/or palliated. If the patient remains uninephric with systemic sepsis there is a high risk of worsening renal function (pyelonephritis still remains), and a risk of future re-obstruction of the only remaining kidney. In the author's practice ureteronephrectomy is nearly always discouraged. In addition, the severe hydronephrosis may appear as if there is little renal parenchyma that remains, but interestingly, after decompression there is often a large amount of tissue visible within a few days. Previously compression from the excessive backpressure associated with the ureteral obstruction can be deceiving (Figure 30.1).

A recent study (Kuntz et al., 2013) reported 13 dogs seen in the author's practice with pyonephrosis. All patients were septic upon presentation and had evidence of a ureteral obstruction with severely thick and purulent material in the renal pelvis and ureter, proximal to a ureteral lesion (stone, stricture, or a caseous purulent plug). Most were associated with an obstructive ureterolith. Eleven had a positive culture from the bladder and/or renal pelvis including *Escherichia coli*, *Staphylococcus* spp., and *Klebsiella* spp. Thrombocytopenia was seen in 70% of dogs, that was often severe (<30000 platelets). This encouraged a minimally invasive and fast approach for renal pelvis drainage. In animals, stents are preferred to percutaneous nephrostomy (PN) tubes due to the indwelling nature, long-term benefit, minimal risk, and concern of renal puncture with concurrent thrombocytopenia and septic luminal material. In humans PN tubes are often more comfortable and in some reports preferred to stents. Since dogs tolerate stents far better than humans with dysuria occurring in less than 2% of patients, and PN tubes are temporary, require hospitalization while present, and are met with more complications, stents are preferred in animals (92% success for pyonephrosis). Dogs typically have the stent placed endoscopically. If this is not possible, than it can be done with surgical assistance through a caudal cystotomy incision or with an ultrasound-fluoroscopic-assisted antegrade approach percutaneously.

This chapter will focus on renal pelvic lavage and endoscopic ureteral stent placement for the treatment

Veterinary Image-Guided Interventions, First Edition. Edited by Chick Weisse and Allyson Berent.

Companion website: www.wiley.com/go/weisse/vet-image-guided-interventions

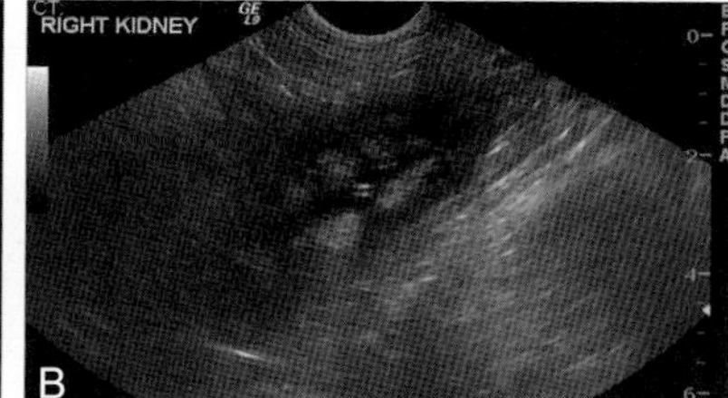

Figure 30.1 Abdominal ultrasound of a patient with right pyonephrosis and a ureteral obstruction. (A) Severe hydronephrosis of the right renal pelvis with echogenic material suspended within the renal pelvis. (B) 28 days post endoscopic ureteral stent placement showing an ultrasound image of the right kidney with complete decompression of the renal pelvis and the presence of a fair amount of renal parenchyma post decompression.

of pyonephrosis. Please refer to Chapter 29 for details of ureteral stenting and nephrostomy tube placement.

Patient Preparation

A full diagnostic work-up is necessary including a complete blood count, serum biochemical profile, urinalysis and urine culture, coagulation profile, abdominal radiography, and an abdominal ultrasonography. The urine in the hydronephrotic kidney typically is highly echogenic and a stone is most commonly seen in the ureter at the junction of the dilated and normal ureter. Looking at the urinalysis and obtaining a urine pH is recommended. If there are bacteria in the urine, consistent with *Staphylococcus*, *Proteus*, *Klebsiella*, *Corynebacterium* or *Pseudomonas* spp, in the presence of a high pH than this is most likely struvite-infected stone(s) that were formed secondary to the primary infection. If this is the case then after decompression and stent placement the stones can be dissolved with appropriate antibiotic therapy and dissolution diet. If there are bacterial rods and the pH is low than this is likely a calcium oxalate stone that caused a ureteral obstruction with a secondary urinary tract infection.

Basic management should include immediate and aggressive fluid diuresis, intravenous broad-spectrum antibiotic therapy and patient stabilization. Most of these patients are septic so care should be taken to monitor the blood pressure, blood glucose, and temperature. These patients should be decompressed immediately. Antibiotics should be continued for a minimum of 6 weeks for non-urease producing bacteria and for at least 6–9 months with a dissolution diet for suspected struvite stones.

Equipment

A traditional fluoroscopic C-arm, various flexible and rigid endoscopes, guide wires, catheters, ureteral stents and nephrostomy tubes are needed.[1–11] This is all expanded upon in Chapter 29 (benign ureteral obstruction) (Figure 30.2 and Figure 30.3).

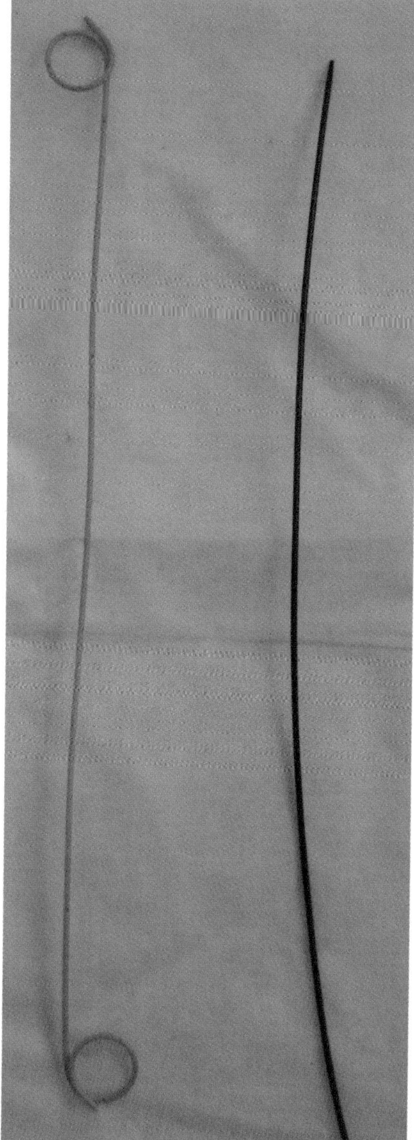

Figure 30.2 Double pigtail ureteral stent. One loop lies within the renal pelvis and the other loop in the urinary bladder. The shaft extends down the lumen of the ureter. The pusher catheter helps to push the stent into the urinary bladder when placed under endoscopic guidance.

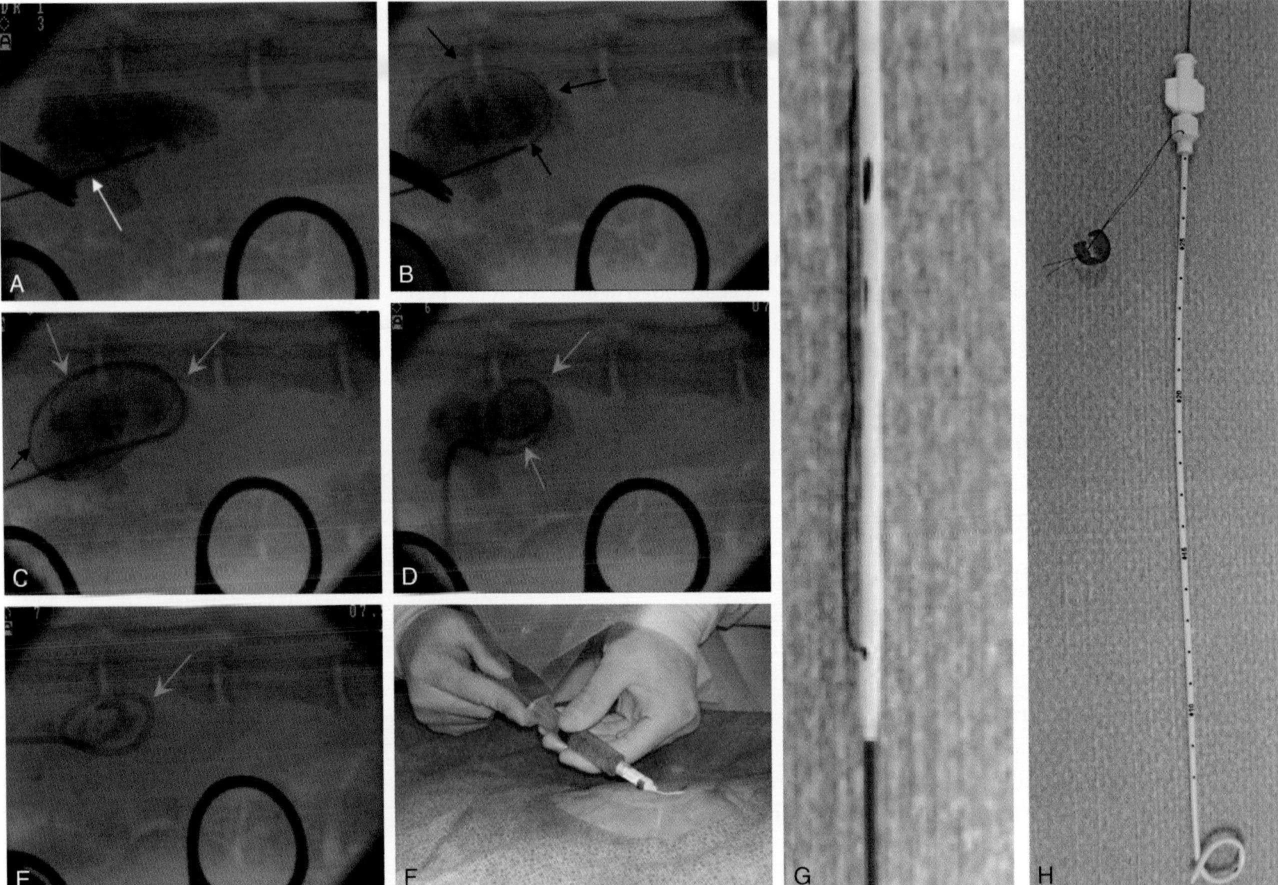

Figure 30.3 Placement of a locking-loop nephrostomy catheter percutaneously using the modified-Seldinger technique. In the fluoroscopic images the head is to the right of the image. (A) 18-g renal access needle (white arrow) being advanced into the renal pelvis using ultrasound guidance for a pyclogram. (B) Guide wire (black arrow) advanced through the access needle coiled within the renal pelvis. (C) Needle removed from the wire and the pigtail catheter (orange arrows) advanced over the wire. (D) Once the wire is removed the locking string is engaged and a tight curl is made in the pigtail to prevent migration of the catheter (orange arrows). (E) Draining of the renal pelvis to confirm the catheter (orange arrow) is in place. (F) The catheter exiting the skin after placement as the renal pelvis is drained. (G) The locking-loop pigtail catheter straight on the guide wire with the hollow trocar in place and the string taught. (H) The entire catheter showing the string at the hub and the curl in the pigtail once the string is pulled tight.

Procedure

Endoscopic Approach

Using cystoscopic guidance (Figure 30.4, Figure 30.5, and Figure 30.6), an appropriately sized angled hydrophilic guide wire is advanced into the UVJ and up the distal ureter, through the working channel of the cystoscope. The wire is advanced up the distal ureter with an appropriately sized open-ended ureteral catheter using fluoroscopic-guidance. If the wire can be carefully negotiated around the obstructive lesion than it is curled inside the renal pelvis and the catheter is advanced over the guide wire. The wire is then removed and the material in the renal pelvis is drained for culture and sensitivity (Figure 30.5). If the guide wire cannot easily be passed around the obstructive lesion than the guide wire is removed and a retrograde ureteropyelogram is performed (Figure 30.4). This aids in identifying the obstructive lesion(s), the tortuosity of the ureter, and the location and size of the renal pelvis. Care should be taken to avoid ureteral perforation with the guide wire.

Once the guide wire and catheter are within the renal pelvis than the material is drained until the pelvis is empty. Next warm saline is mixed with contrast material and the renal pelvis is lavaged carefully, using fluoroscopic guidance to avoid backfilling/overfilling, until the fluid in the pelvis is reasonably clear (Figure 30.5). A multifenestrated catheter should be

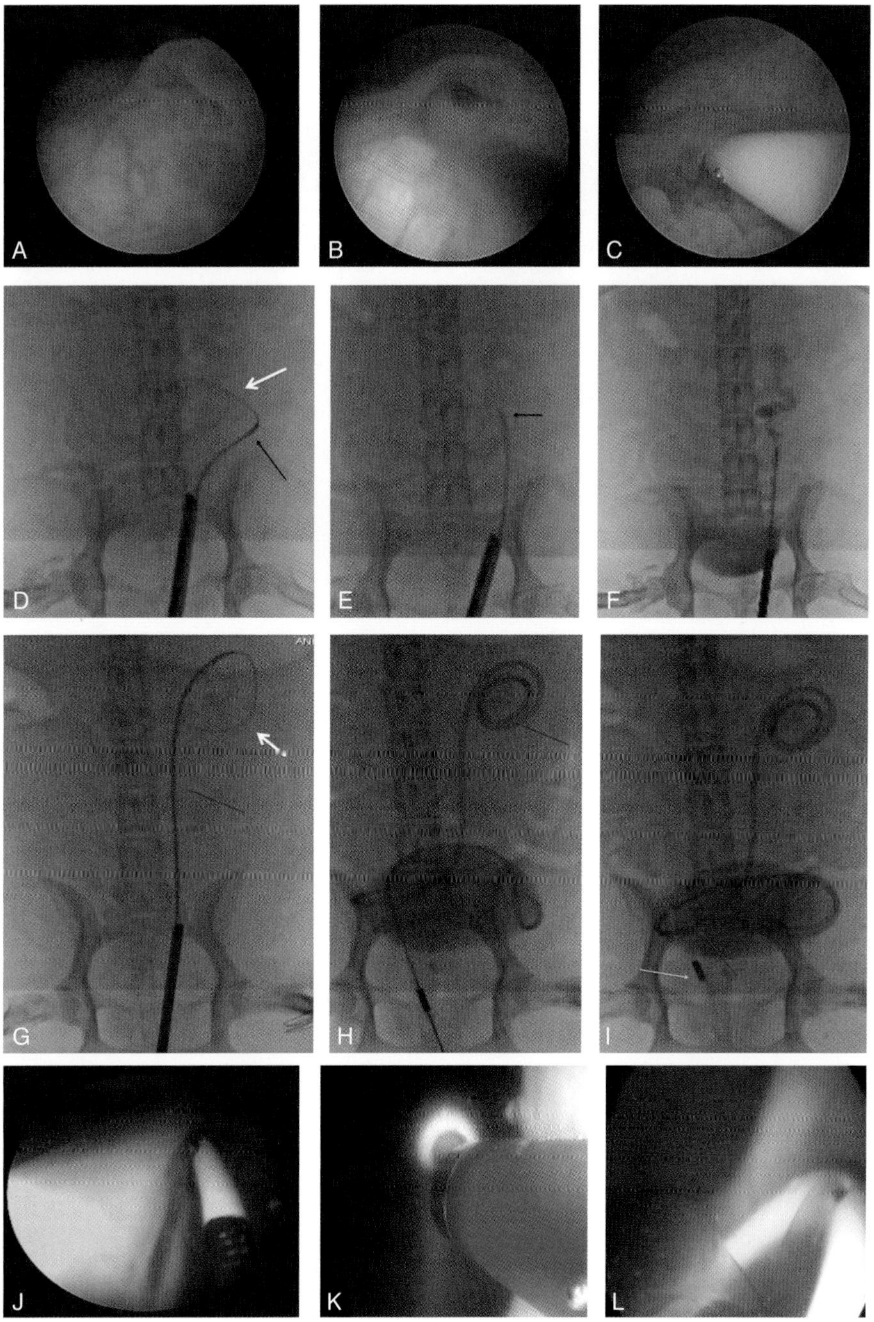

Figure 30.4 Retrograde placement of a ureteral stent for a dog with obstructive pyonephrosis using endoscopic and fluoroscopic guidance. The female dog is in dorsal recumbency with the head to the top of each fluoroscopy image. (A) Endoscopic image showing the left ureteral opening during cystoscopy. (B) Guide wire being advanced up the ureter using endoscopic guidance. (C) Open-ended ureteral catheter over the guide wire at the UVJ. (D) Fluoroscopic image of the guide wire (white arrow) and ureteral catheter (black arrow) up the distal ureter, through the endoscope. (E) Open-ended ureteral catheter (black arrow) prior to retrograde ureteropyelogram. (F) Retrograde ureteropyelogram showing the obstructive stone in the ureter. (G) The guide wire (white arrow) advance around the obstructive stone and coiled within the renal pelvis. Once the renal pelvis is drained and cleared of purulent material (Figure 30.4), the double pigtail ureteral stent (blue arrow) is advanced over the wire and coiled within the renal pelvis. (H) The ureteral stent (blue arrow) coiled within the renal pelvis as the wire is pulled into the urethra so the pushing catheter can push the distal end of the stent into the urinary bladder. (I) The pusher (yellow arrow) advancing the distal pigtail of the stent (blue arrow) into the urinary bladder. (J) The endoscopic image of the ureteral stent as the distal pigtail approaches the UVJ (black line), signaling pushing of the stent into the bladder. (K) The pusher (red catheter) and the stent engaged over the wire as the stent is pushed into the bladder, through the endoscope. (L) Urine draining from the fenestrations of the ureteral stent.

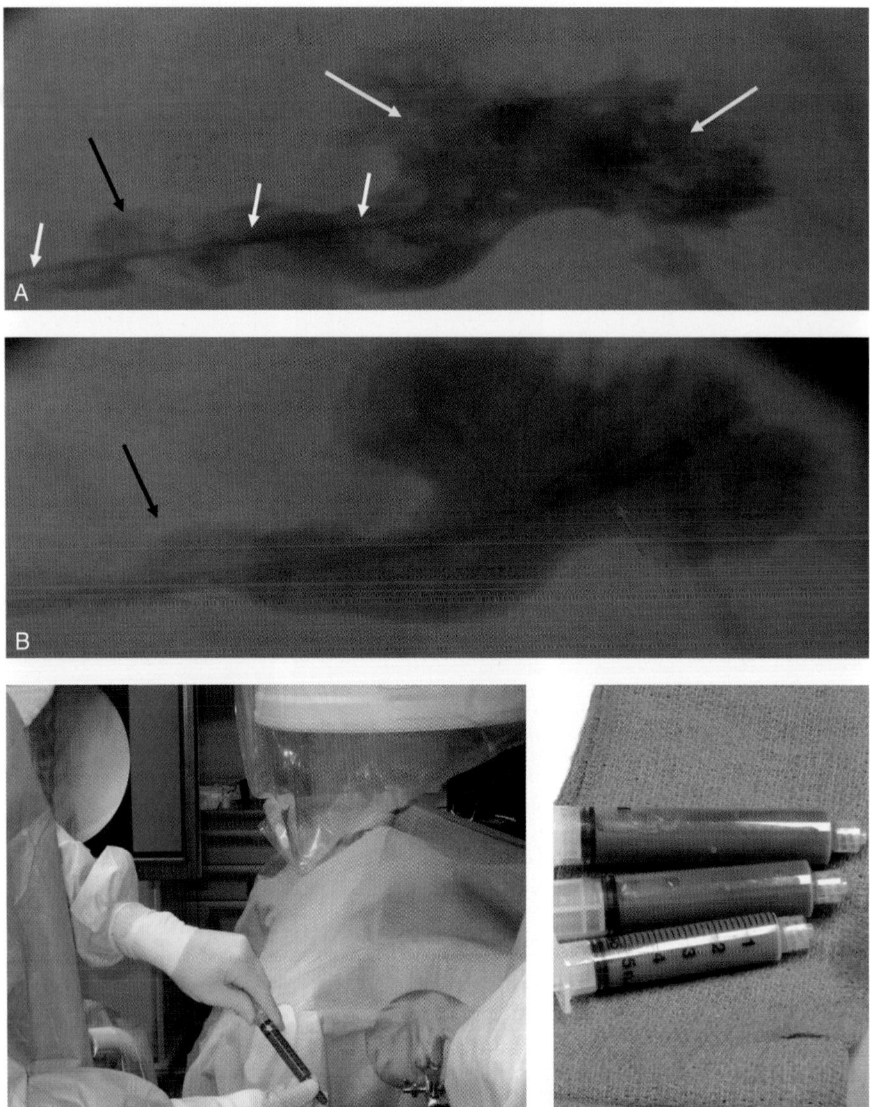

Figure 30.5 Female dog during endoscopic retrograde drainage of obstructive pyonephrosis. The dog is in dorsal recumbency. (A) Fluoroscopic image of the right renal pelvis after a retrograde ureteropyelogram using a ureteral catheter (white arrows), bypassing a stone (black arrow), showing the thick purulent material within the renal pelvis (yellow arrows). (B) After drainage of the purulent material the renal pelvis is clear of excessive purulent debris and no filling defect is seen in the large dilated pelvis. The hydroureter/nephrosis is present due to the obstructive stone (black arrow). A pigtail ureteral stent is seen in the lumen of the renal pelvis (red arrow). (C) Drainage of the purulent material through the ureteral catheter from the renal pelvis using endoscopic guidance. (D) Over 25 ml of purulent material drained from the large obstructed renal pelvis.

used. This can either but the open-ended ureteral catheter or a pigtail catheter. Once lavage is complete a guide wire is re-advanced into the renal pelvis through the catheter and curled within the renal pelvis for stent placement, as described in Chapter 29 (Figure 30.4).

For patients in whom endoscopy is not possible, lavage and stenting can all be accomplished through a small surgical approach to the bladder trigone, or with a percutaneous cystolithotomy approach (PCCL) (Figure 30.6) to the ureter, or an antegrade approach using ultrasound guidance (see Chapters 31 and 33). The author avoids renal puncture with septic fluid if possible.

Nephrostomy Tube Placement

For patients who are not stable to handle a prolonged general anesthesia, or in a facility where ureteral stenting is not possible, than a nephrostomy tube can be placed (Figure 30.3). This can be done with fluoroscopic

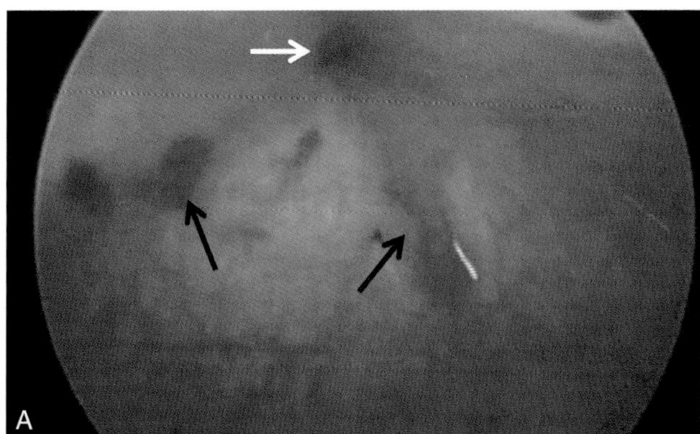

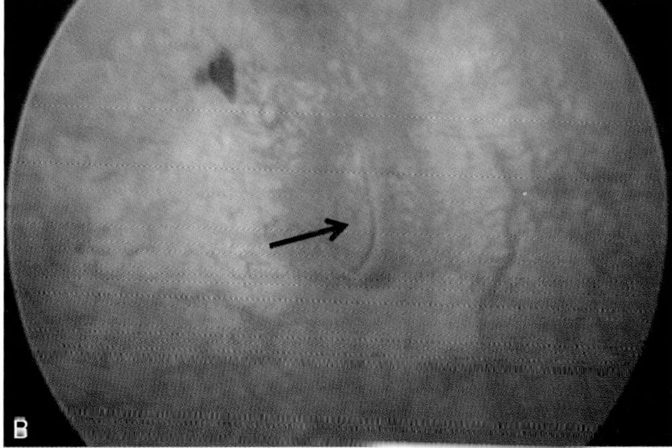

Figure 30.6 Endoscopic images of the ureterovesicular junctions (UVJ) from a percutaneous cystoscopy approach (see Chapter 41). (A) Both UVJs seen (black arrows) just dorsal and cranial to the urethra (white arrow) as viewed from the bladder apex. (B) Close up view of the right UVJ (black arrow).

and ultrasonographic guidance, with ultrasonography alone, and/or surgically assisted. This should only be performed on those comfortable with this technique. This procedure is described in more detail in Chapter 29.

Postoperative and Follow-Up Care

Patients with sepsis and a ureteral stent or nephrostomy tube need to be monitored very carefully. Experience suggests the infection is relatively easy to clear, even in the presence of a device following abscess drainage (decompressing the obstruction) and providing the appropriate antibiotics. Long-term antibiotic therapy is typically required for a minimum of 8–12 weeks. In the author's experience, infection recurrence is not a major problem.

If a nephrostomy tube is placed than a urine culture is taken from the bag 3 days post drainage to ensure clearance. The catheter is cleaned with chlorohexidine scrub four to six times per day and the bag is aseptically drained every 2–4 hours. For patients with stent placement, a urine culture is obtained via cystocentesis 3–5 days post drainage to ensure appropriate antibiotic therapy.

Once the patient is systemically stable, those stented are discharged (usually within 48 hours). Those with a nephrostomy tube require a second intervention depending on the cause of the pyonephrosis. This is typically either a ureteral stent or SUB device placement in a facility capable of this procedure, or a surgical ureterotomy, in order to re-establish patency. It is also possible (but uncommon) the obstruction may be relieved once the underlying infection has cleared.

It is important to know the type of infection, urine pH, location, and stone size. Approximately 50% of dogs with pyonephrosis have a urease-producing bacteria that is causing struvite stone formation, and these can be dissolved over 3–9 months. An appropriate diet and antibiotic should be continued until 1 month beyond resolution of the stone radiographically and ultrasonographically. The patient should have a urine culture and radiograph done monthly to monitor, and an ultrasound exam bimonthly.

For struvite stones, once the stone(s) and infection are cleared the stent can be endoscopically retrieved. For other stone types the stent remains in place long term. Ureteral stent occlusion from urinary debris and crystalline material can occur within about 3 months, but with appropriate passive ureteral dilation, the ureter does not typically re-obstruct (~9% in one study).

Stone-forming patients should remain on a neutralizing diet long term and if calcium oxalate stones are present then the author usually prescribes potassium citrate (50–75 mg/kg BID). Monitoring of urine pH, specific gravity, serum potassium and renal pelvic dilation should be routinely performed.

Prognosis

In a recent study of dogs with pyonephrosis (Kuntz et al, 2013) all patients had ureteral stents placed after retrograde ureteropelvic lavage. The double pigtail ureteral stents were placed endoscopically in 10 dogs and with surgical-assistance in 3, with a 92% success in those that had endoscopic placement attempted. The median hospitalization time was 48 hours. One dog was euthanized 2 days postoperatively for decompensating sepsis and 2 died of unrelated causes (5 months and 4 years post-stent). Long-term complications included stent encrustation requiring exchange ($n=1$), recurrent urinary tract infections ($n=2$) and tissue proliferation at the ureterovesicular junction ($n = 5$), without clinical consequence. All patients lived with their stents in place, patency was maintained long term, and none required removal. As these stents are most commonly placed endoscopically in dogs the operator must be prepared for surgical conversion if endoscopic placement fails.

Special Considerations

In general, for benign canine ureteral obstructions associated with pyonephrosis, stents are placed endoscopically, so expertise in male and female cystoscopy is needed. In humans, percutaneous nephrostomy tubes are left in place on an outpatient basis and removed after stone retrieval via ureteroscopic lithotripsy or extracorporeal shock wave lithotripsy (ESWL). Since this is not a good option in veterinary patients, and because stents are far better tolerated in dogs than in humans, ureteral stenting is the preferred technique in these patients in the author's practice.

Notes

1. Rigid endoscope, 1.9-mm 30° lens, Karl Storz Endoscopy, Culver City, CA.
2. Rigid endoscope, 2.7-mm 30° lens, Richard Wolf, Vernon Hills, IL.
3. Rigid endoscope, 4-mm 30° lens, Karl Storz Endoscopy, Culver City, CA.
4. Flex X^2 Flexible ureteroscope, Karl Storz Endoscopy, Culver City, CA.
5. Weasel Wire 0.025- or 0.035-inch hydrophilic angle-tipped guide wire, Infiniti Medical LLC, Menlo Park, CA.
6. 4 or 5 Fr, open-ended ureteral catheter, Cook Medical Inc, Bloomington, IN.
7. Ureteral stents (2.5, 3.7 and 4.7 Fr) double pigtail, Infiniti Medical LLC, Menlo Park, CA.
8. InLay Ureteral stents Bard Urological, Covington, GA.
9. Nephrostomy tube 5 Fr Pigtail non-locking drainage catheter, Infiniti Medical LLC, Menlo Park, CA.
10. Nephrostomy tube 5 Fr Dawson Mueller, Cook Medical, Bloomington, IL.
11. Nephrostomy tube 6 Fr Locking-loop pigtail catheter, Infiniti Medical LLC, Menlo Park, CA.

Reference

Kuntz J, Berent A, Weisse C (2013) Interventional renal-sparing treatment of obstructive pyonephrosis in 13 canine patients: 2008–2012. *J Vet Intern Med* 27(3), 604–756.

Suggested Reading

Berent A (2011) Ureteral obstructions in dogs and cats: a review of traditional and new interventional diagnostic and therapeutic options. *J Vet Emerg Crit Care* 21(2), 86–103.

Berent AC, Weisse CW, Todd KL, et al (2012) Use of locking-loop nephrostomy catheters in dogs and cats: 20 cases (2004–2009). *J Am Vet Med Assoc* 241(3), 348–57.

Choi J and Yoon J (2012) Primary pyonephrosis in a young dog. *J Small Anim Pract* 53(5), 304.

Mokhmalji H, Braun, PM, Martinez FJ, et al (2001) Percutaneous nephrostomy versus ureteral stents for diversion of hydronephrosis caused by stones; a prospective, randomized clinical trial. *J Urol* 165, 1088–92.

Pearle MS, Pierce HL, Miller GL, et al (1998) Optimal method of urgent decompression of the collecting system for obstruction and infection due to ureteral calculi, *J Urol* 160, 1260.

CHAPTER THIRTY-ONE

Interventional Management of Canine Malignant Ureteral Obstructions

Allyson Berent
The Animal Medical Center, New York, NY

Background/Indications

Ureteral stent placement for the management of malignant ureteral obstructions has been a mainstay of palliative treatment for humans with non-resectable tumors to preserve renal function. Ureteral stents have also been placed preoperatively for patient stabilization prior to surgical intervention. Various techniques have been described with reported success rates exceeding 90% with an antegrade approach (via percutaneous renal access) versus a 25% with a retrograde endoscopic-guided approach. This is due to the fact that the tumor is covering the UVJ so the ureteral opening is not visible endoscopically. Another interventional alternative to ureteral stent placement for malignant obstructions is using a nephrostomy tube or subcutaneous ureteral bypass (SUB) device (see Chapter 29). Predictably, long-term use of an externalized nephrostomy tube has a number of disadvantages in animals.

Urothelial neoplasia in dogs is often complicated by local tumor invasion and obstruction of the urethra, ureters, or both. Although distant metastases have been reported in 17% to 50% of patients at the time of diagnosis, clinical signs on initial examination are most often associated with the local disease, with the cause of death due to local tumor effects in over 60% of cases. Historically, once ureteral obstruction and subsequent renal compromise is identified, few management options exist. Nephrostomy tube placement or hemodialysis can provide temporary relief, but radical surgeries have traditionally been the only viable alternative for long-term management in veterinary patients. The purpose of this chapter is to describe the placement of a double pigtail ureteral stent as a minimally invasive, long-term treatment option for malignant obstructive neoplasia in dogs and cats. A recent report (Berent et al, 2011) showed this procedure to be a safe and effective option for canine patients. The author has also used this technique in a small number of feline patients with malignant obstructions, though the SUB device is generally preferred in cats. The reader is also encouraged to review Chapter 34 on urethral stent placement, because approximately 60% of dogs with malignant ureteral obstructions have concurrent urethral obstructions.

Patient Preparation

Prior to considering placement of a ureteral stent, a full diagnostic work-up is necessary including complete blood work, coagulation profile, abdominal ultrasonography, and three-view thoracic radiographs. An oncologist should be consulted. In addition, a urinalysis, urine culture, and blood pressure measurements should be obtained. An obstructed ureter will have a combination of both renal pelvic dilation and hydroureter to the level of the ureterovesicular junction (UVJ) where a large trigonal mass lesion is identified (Figure 31.1). The author has not seen malignant ureteral obstructions of the trigone without ultrasonographic evidence of a visible mass at the UVJ. In a small number of cases ureteral

Veterinary Image-Guided Interventions, First Edition. Edited by Chick Weisse and Allyson Berent.

Companion website: www.wiley.com/go/weisse/vet-image-guided-interventions

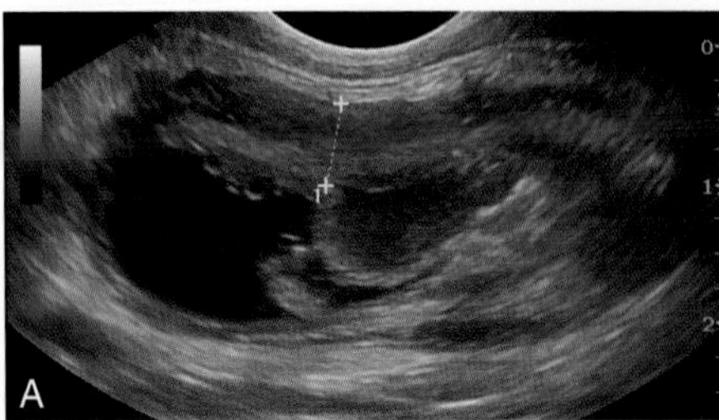

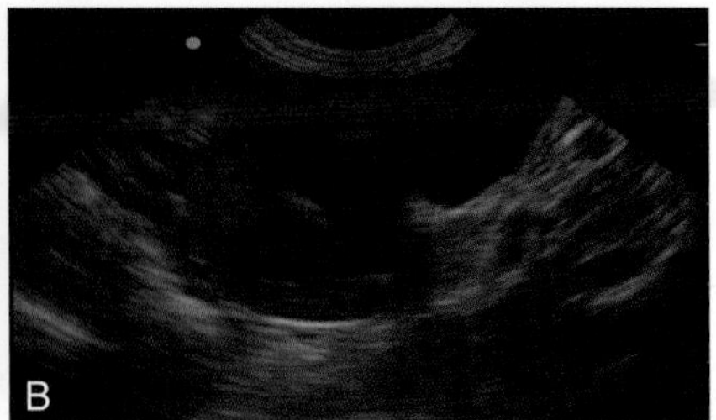

Figure 31.1 Ultrasound image of a large trigonal transitional cell carcinoma in a dog causing a ureteral obstruction at the UVJ. (A) Image of the trigonal and extensive bladder mass. (B) Renal ultrasound showing severe hydroureter and hydronephrosis.

neoplasia has been seen in the proximal ureter associated with the renal parenchyma (renal carcinoma) however this is uncommon.

The author prefers the canine renal pelvis to be dilated over 5 mm (ideally 8 mm) before considering percutaneous antegrade ureteral stenting. In cats this procedure is typically done surgically assisted as described in Chapter 29.

If a patient is azotemic, pre-anesthetic diuresis is recommended for 8–12 hours prior to the procedure. If the patient is severely azotemic (creatinine over 5 mg/dl) consider platelet function testing as uremic thrombocytopathia can result in renal hemorrhage following puncture. In this case the use of DDAVP can be considered (1 mcg/kg SQ) 15 minutes prior to renal puncture.

Potential Risks/Complications/Expected Outcomes

It is important for the operator to realize this procedure is one of the most complicated IR procedures currently performed to date and requires two to three people with an understanding of the procedure. Percutaneous ureteral stenting should only be attempted by those with advanced IR training and surgical conversion should be immediately available if the procedure is unsuccessful.

The most substantial risk is ureteral perforation resulting in uroabdomen or a puncture hole in the kidney when access across the tumor is unsuccessful. This can occur at the ureterovesicular junction just proximal to the tumor during guide wire passage antegrade, or in the proximal ureter during guide wire passage retrograde (see below). If the operator attempts this procedure and is unable to successfully place the stent, there is typically a 4–5 Fr hole in the renal parenchyma made while getting access, and if the obstruction is not relieved the risk of uroabdomen is very high, making either surgical conversion or the placement of a nephrostomy tube necessary. Another risk during antegrade ureteral stent placement is bleeding during renal puncture. Anesthetic risk is typically low since most dogs are not azotemic at the time of stent placement.

Other potential complications include stent migration, stent irritation, chronic infections and stent occlusion. All of these are rare. In a recent study looking at 12 dogs (15 ureters) that had ureteral stents placed for ureteral obstructive neoplasia, 1 dog required surgical conversion. All patients survived to discharge and the median survival time from time of cancer diagnosis was 285 days (range, 10–1571) and following stent placement was 57 days (range, 7–337).

At the time of ureteral obstruction the tumor is typically considered non-resectable, so offering a minimally invasive treatment option for palliation is ideal. The prognosis for procedural survival is excellent; No patient died from the procedure in a recent report. The long-term survival due to the cancer remains guarded, however. In the small series, patients with the longest survival times did not have azotemia at the time of initial examination, did not require urethral stent placement, did not have evidence of metastatic disease, and had a body condition score ≥4, on a scale from 1 to 9. None of these variables were significantly associated with survival time in the multivariate analysis, however the small sample size likely prevented the identification of factors associated with survival.

At this time the success rate for percutaneous antegrade ureteral stent placement is approximately 92% in the author's practice, which compares to that seen in human medicine (90%). In cats, a stent can be placed; however, the author currently recommends a SUB be placed if necessary.

Equipment

Access is typically obtained using an 18-gauge renal puncture needle.[1] This is done under ultrasound guidance in the operating room. A sterile sleeve should be placed on the curvilinear ultrasound probe.

A traditional fluoroscopic C-arm is sufficient for visualization. Sterile leaded gloves are recommended because the fluoroscopy unit is very close to the operator's hands during renal puncture. Various guide wires and catheters are needed. The most commonly used for this procedure is a stiffened angle-tipped hydrophilic guide wire (0.035″),[3] a non-stiffened angle-tipped hydrophilic guide wire (0.035″),[4] a 5 Fr vascular access sheath,[5] a 4 Fr angled angiographic catheter,[6] and a 45–55 cm 7 or 8 Fr sheath.[7] The type of stent that is typically used for this procedure is a canine cancer stent,[8] which is 6 Fr in diameter and comes in various lengths. The difference between this stent and the other ureteral stents is that the distal end of the shaft of this stent is non-fenestrated and the durometer is higher/stronger, both characteristics designed to reduce tumor ingrowth and stent compression (Figure 31.2).

A marker catheter[10] can be placed in the colon to help measure the ureteral length to know what length stent is necessary. Alternatively this is done during retraction of the ureteral sheath. Many patients have concurrent urethral obstructions and it is contraindicated to place a ureteral stent without ensuring urethral patency. Since a renal puncture is obtained, if there is resistance to outflow from the bladder urine will reflux up the stent and out the renal puncture site during urination resulting in a urine extravasation. Urethral stenting[10] is described in Chapter 34. The operator should have a locking-loop nephrostomy tube available,[11] or the ability to convert to a laparotomy, in the event the ureteral stent procedure is not successful.

Procedure

Ureteral stents are typically inserted in an antegrade direction for malignant obstructions because of the lack of visibility of the UVJ during cystoscopic examination (Figure 31.3). However, in some female patients, transurethral cystoscopy is successful for ureteral stent placement, especially in prophylactic cases in which the ureteral papilla is progressively getting covered with tumor (Figure 31.3).

The patient is placed in lateral recumbency with the affected kidney facing up (Figure 31.4). Hair is clipped on the dorsal paracostal and flank areas and the perineum (female) or prepuce (male). These areas are aseptically prepared and draped. It is generally recommended to also clip the entire abdomen so the patient does not need to be moved out of the operating room should conversion to open surgery be necessary. A marker catheter is inserted in the rectum and advanced into the descending colon to allow for ureteral length measurements which aids in choosing the appropriate stent length. A 3-mm skin incision is made over the kidney. With ultrasonographic guidance, an 18-gauge renal access needle is used and is attached to a short extension set, three-way-stopcock, one empty syringe, and one that is filled with 50% iodinated contrast

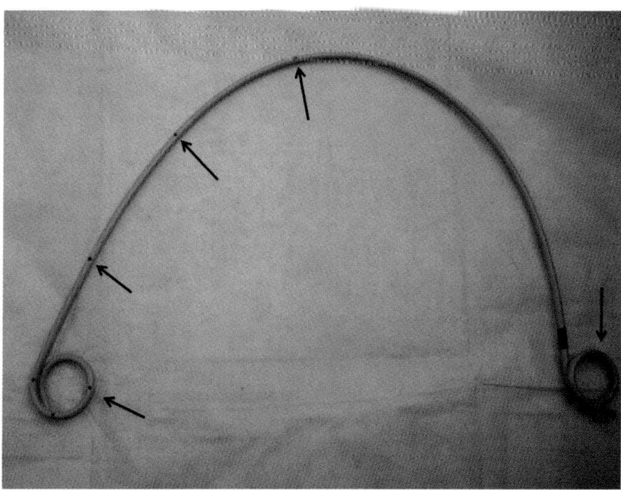

Figure 31.2 Double pigtail ureteral stent that is made for dogs with trigonal neoplasia induced obstructions. Notice the multiple fenestrations (black arrows) at each loop and along the proximal half of the shaft. The distal half is not fenestrated to prevent tumor ingrowth.

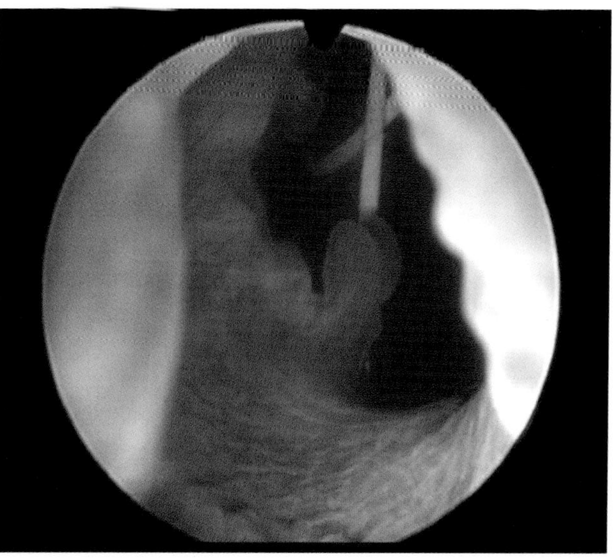

Figure 31.3 Cystoscopic image of a dog with TCC in dorsal recumbency. Notice the tumor at the right UVJ and the stent is protruding through the proliferative tissue.

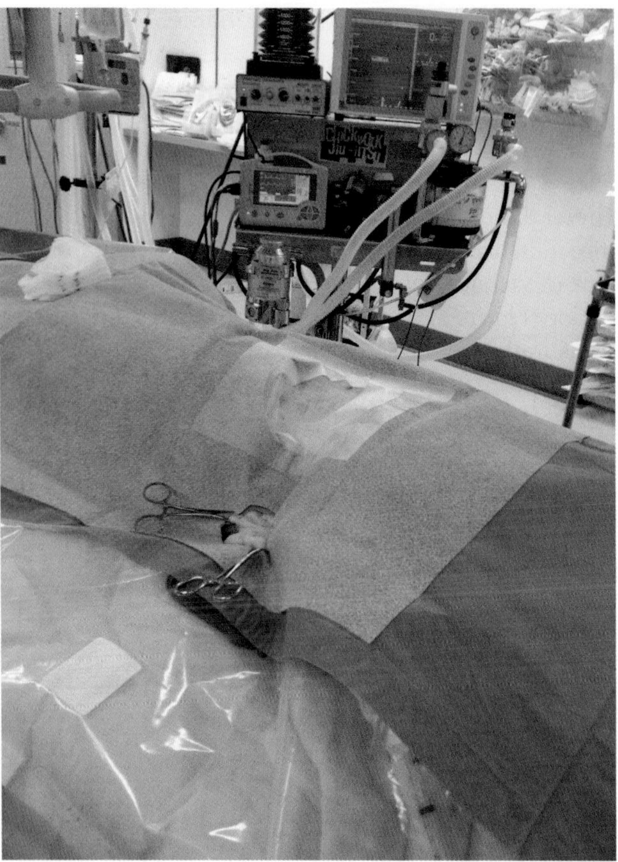

Figure 31.4 Male dog under general anesthesia in right lateral recumbency with the region of the left kidney clipped, aseptically prepared, and draped. The prepuce is clipped, scrubbed and exposed as well for through-and-through guide wire access.

material (Figure 31.5). Once access is obtained, a urine sample is obtained and submitted for bacteriologic culture and susceptibility testing. An antegrade ureteropyelogram is then performed using ultrasound and fluoroscopic guidance. The volume of iodinated contrast material injected is approximately equal to the volume of urine removed and this is monitored under fluoroscopic guidance. Once the ureter is seen to fill the injection is complete. With fluoroscopic guidance, a 0.035-inch, stiffened, angle-tipped hydrophilic guide wire is advanced through the needle, into the renal pelvis, and guided down the lumen of the ureter to the level of the ureteral obstruction at the UVJ (Figure 31.5). The guide wire is then manipulated gently and advanced into the urinary bladder. If necessary, a combination guide wire and 4 Fr angled angiographic catheter is used to achieve access across the tumor. If a catheter is need to help negotiate across the tumor a 5 Fr vascular access sheath is first advanced over the wire into the kidney and down the proximal ureter to prevent the wire from buckling in the renal pelvis. The sheath also permits performing a ureterogram during guide wire negotiations. The sheath and catheter are not placed if the guide wire access into the urinary bladder is readily achieved.

Once urinary bladder access is achieved, the wire (and catheter if used) is directed toward the bladder trigone, down the urethra caudally, and out the vulva/prepuce, until through-and-through wire access is obtained (Figure 31.5E–G). Sometimes, contrast is needed inside the bladder to identify the urethral origin when the tumor is distorting the trigone. If this is still difficult to identify, a sheath and snare device can be used in the urethra, or a cystoscope, to grasp the wire and pull it out of the urethra.

Next, a 7–8 Fr 45–55-cm introducer sheath and dilator set are advanced retrograde over the safety (through-and-through) wire within the urethral lumen, across the tumor and UVJ to the level of the UPJ (Figure 31.5G). This dilates the ureteral obstruction and allows the stent to be placed through the sheath. This is also known as "Trojan horsing". Care should be taken not to advance the dilator (which is often radiolucent) out of the renal tissue. The dilator is removed over the guide wire, leaving the sheath in place within the renal pelvis/UPJ (Figure 31.5H).

Next, a second 0.035-inch, non-stiffened, angle-tipped hydrophilic guide wire is inserted through the sheath in a retrograde manner, with the soft-angled tip advanced cranially in the ureteral lumen until it curls inside the dilated renal pelvis (Figure 31.5H). This second wire allows the stent to be placed without losing the first through-and-through wire (the safety wire) in the event that stent placement is not ideal and needs manipulation. The sheath is then removed over the two guide wires, being careful not to pull them out. During removal the ureteral length can be measured from the UPJ to the UVJ to select an appropriate stent length. The dilator is placed back through the sheath and the sheath/dilator combination is re-advanced into the ureter over the second, retrograde, soft guide wire, up near the UPJ, and the dilator removed.

The ureteral length is determined based on the ureterogram using either a marker catheter in the colon or the length of the sheath as it is removed from the UPJ to the UVJ. A double-pigtail ureteral stent of appropriate length is then advanced over the second non-stiffened guide wire, through the sheath, in a retrograde manner, bypassing the ureteral obstruction (Figure 31.5I). A pusher catheter is advanced over the same wire to continue to advance

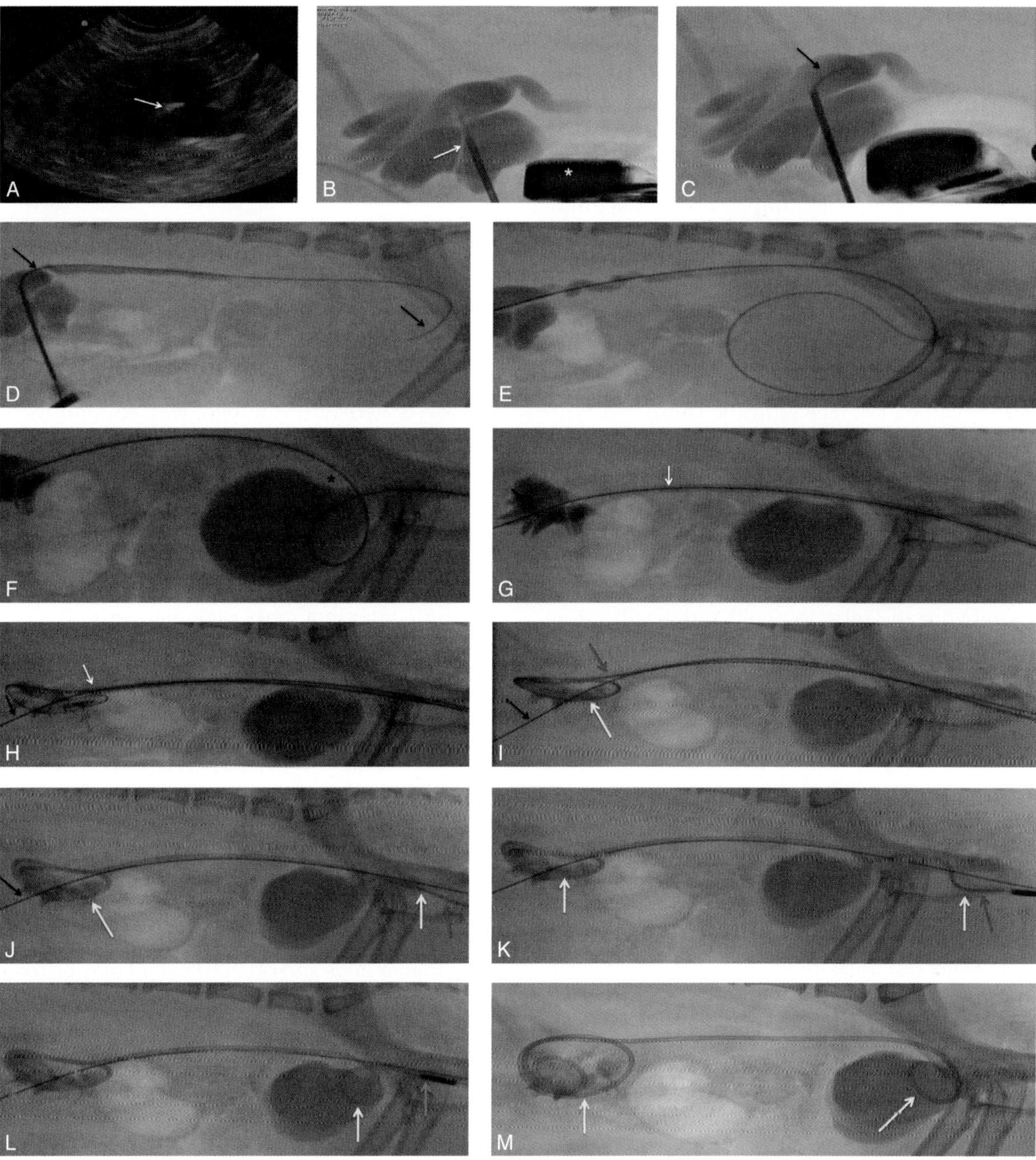

Figure 31.5 Female dog with a ureteral obstruction secondary to trigonal TCC. This patient is placed in lateral recumbency with the head to the left of each image. (A) Percutaneous renal access needle (white arrow) placed under ultrasound guidance. (B) Fluoroscopy is used to view the ureteropyelogram during contrast infusion with ultrasound guidance (yellow asterisk). (C, D) The angle-tipped hydrophilic guide wire (black arrow) is advanced down the ureter under fluoroscopic guidance to the level of the UVJ obstruction. (E) The wire is negotiated through the obstruction and into the urinary bladder. It is aimed out the urethra at the trigone. (F) The wire is passed out the urethra with the assistance of a cystourethrogram. Notice the tumor in the dorsal bladder wall at the UVJ (black asterisk). (G) A ureteral dilator and sheath (white arrow) are passed in a retrograde manner over the guide wire (black arrow) to the renal pelvis. (H) A second guide wire (red arrow) is advanced through the sheath in a retrograde manner and coiled up within the renal pelvis. Notice the initial access safety wire (black arrow) is still in place and the sheath (white arrow) remains at the UPJ. (I) The sheath is removed off both guide wires and the ureteral length is measure by marking the distance from the UPJ to the UVJ. It is then replaced only over the second wire (red arrow) and the double pigtail ureteral stent (yellow arrow) is advanced over that guide wire. The safety-wire (black arrow) remains in place. (J) Once the ureteral stent (yellow arrows) is coiled within the renal pelvis the guide wire and sheath are pulled back so that the wire is only in the part of the stent within the urethra (red arrow) and the sheath is only within the distal urethra. (K) The ureteral stent (yellow arrows) is being pushed into the urinary bladder with a pusher catheter (blue arrow). Notice the wire (red arrow) is crossing the junction of the stent and pusher to keep both together. Notice the stent starting to buckle. (L, M) The stent is then pushed into the urinary bladder (yellow arrow) and the pusher catheter (blue arrow) and safety wire are removed.

the ureteral stent into position once the stent disappears into the sheath. Once the proximal end of the stent is curled inside the renal pelvis the sheath and non-stiffened guide wire are withdrawn into the urethra (Figure 31.5 J); the long, floppy end of the guide wire remains engaging the pusher and stent, however advancement of the pusher now allows the stent to flex, bend, and flop into the urinary bladder. This last step is important as it allows the distal pigtail of the stent to be pushed into the bladder without further advancing it up the ureter (Figure 31.5 K, L). The pusher catheter comes with the stent, and typically has a radio-opaque tip so the end of the stent can be seen easily with fluoroscopy, distinguished from the pusher by the radio-opaque band. Once the stent is in place, the through-and-through safety wire is carefully removed through the urethra, leaving the double pigtail stent in place. Care should be taken when removing the wire to avoid pulling the stent caudally.

Postoperative and Follow-Up Care

Postoperatively, the urethra is infused with a 1:1 mixture of bupivacaine (1 mg/kg [0.45 mg/lb]) and saline solution for local transurethral analgesia. Patients are administered buprenorphine (10 µg/kg [4.5 µg/lb], IV, q 6 hr prn for 1 to 3 doses) following recovery from the procedure. Fluids are administered (3 to 5 ml/kg/h [1.4 to 2.3 ml/lb/hr], IV) after stent placement in all patients until discharge. At the time of discharge, owners are instructed to administer tramadol (2 to 4 mg/kg [0.9 to 1.8 mg/lb], PO, q 6 to 12 hr for 1 to 2 days) as needed to relieve signs of pain, and enrofloxacin or marbofloxacin for 14 days, unless patients are concurrently being treated with another antimicrobial based on a previously diagnosed urinary tract infection. The median hospital stay is 18 hours.

We recommend waiting a minimum of 1 week before starting, or resuming, chemotherapy. There can be a substantial post-obstructive diuresis in these patients at home and if the animal becomes dehydrated and receives chemotherapy the morbidity could increase.

Urinary tract ultrasounds and urine cultures should be obtained at 2 weeks, 6 weeks, and then every 3 months thereafter. Appropriate CBC and chemistry profiles should also be done. All patients should be encouraged to consult with an oncologist and to receive chemotherapy and NSAIDs after stent placement if they are non-azotemic, as this has shown to prolong survival times in the literature.

Special Considerations

Conversion for surgical stent placement is rare in the author's practice, but one should be prepared to do so as the tumor is often very firm and sometimes very difficult to traverse with a guide wire. If this occurs and surgery is necessary the best way to address this is using a small caudal abdominal approach and a modified Seldinger technique into the distal ureter, through the tumor and into the urinary bladder. Then the wire can be passed from the ureter and into the bladder. Once the wire is in the bladder it is retrieved via a small cystotomy. Now a 7 Fr sheath[12] can be passed over the guide wire in a retrograde manner to the ureteral access point. Once the sheath is within the distal ureteral lumen the wire is removed, turned around, and re-advanced in a retrograde manner up the ureter and into the renal pelvis. Now the stent can be passed over the guide wire into the renal pelvis, through the sheath. Once a loop is in the pelvis the sheath and wire are removed and the distal end of the stent is placed within the bladder lumen. The small puncture hole in the ureter and bladder can be closed routinely. Alternatively, if open surgery is necessary, SUBs can be considered.

In smaller dogs and cats a 6 Fr stent may be too large, and too long, in which a regular multi-fenestrated 2.5 (cat), 3.7 or 4.7 Fr ureteral stent can be used.

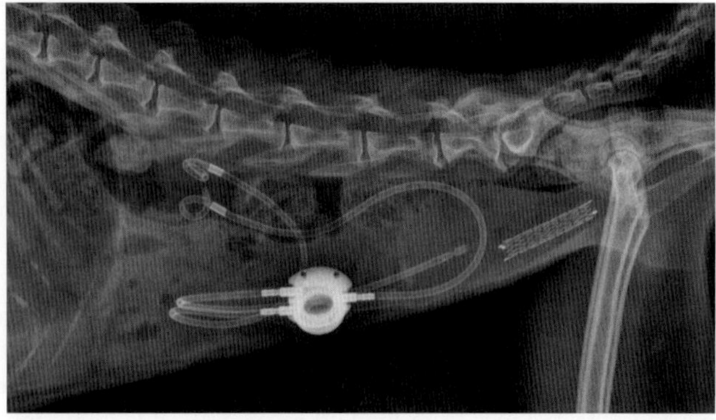

Figure 31.6 A lateral radiograph of a cat with bilateral ureteral and urethral obstructions secondary to TCC. This cat had bilateral SUB devices placed and a urethral stent. The SUB devices were placed to a three-way subcutaneous access port.

Additionally, in a few cases in which the urinary bladder is filled with cancer and there is no lumen to accommodate the distal ureteral stent pigtail, bilateral SUB devices (Figure 31.6) have been used following a radical cystectomy (Figure 31.7 and Figure 31.8). In this circumstance, the bladder catheter is instead passed down the proximal urethra and the entire bladder and distal ureters are removed en bloc. These few patients have done relatively well considering the presenting tumor burden, however the owners must understand that incontinence is guaranteed. This technique allows the surgeon to achieve complete (or near complete) excision with the potential for only microscopic disease to remain while avoiding extensive, prolonged, urinary tract reconstruction. The patients in whom this has been performed were discharged within 48 hours from the hospital without complications and complete resolution of the severe pre-operative azotemia.

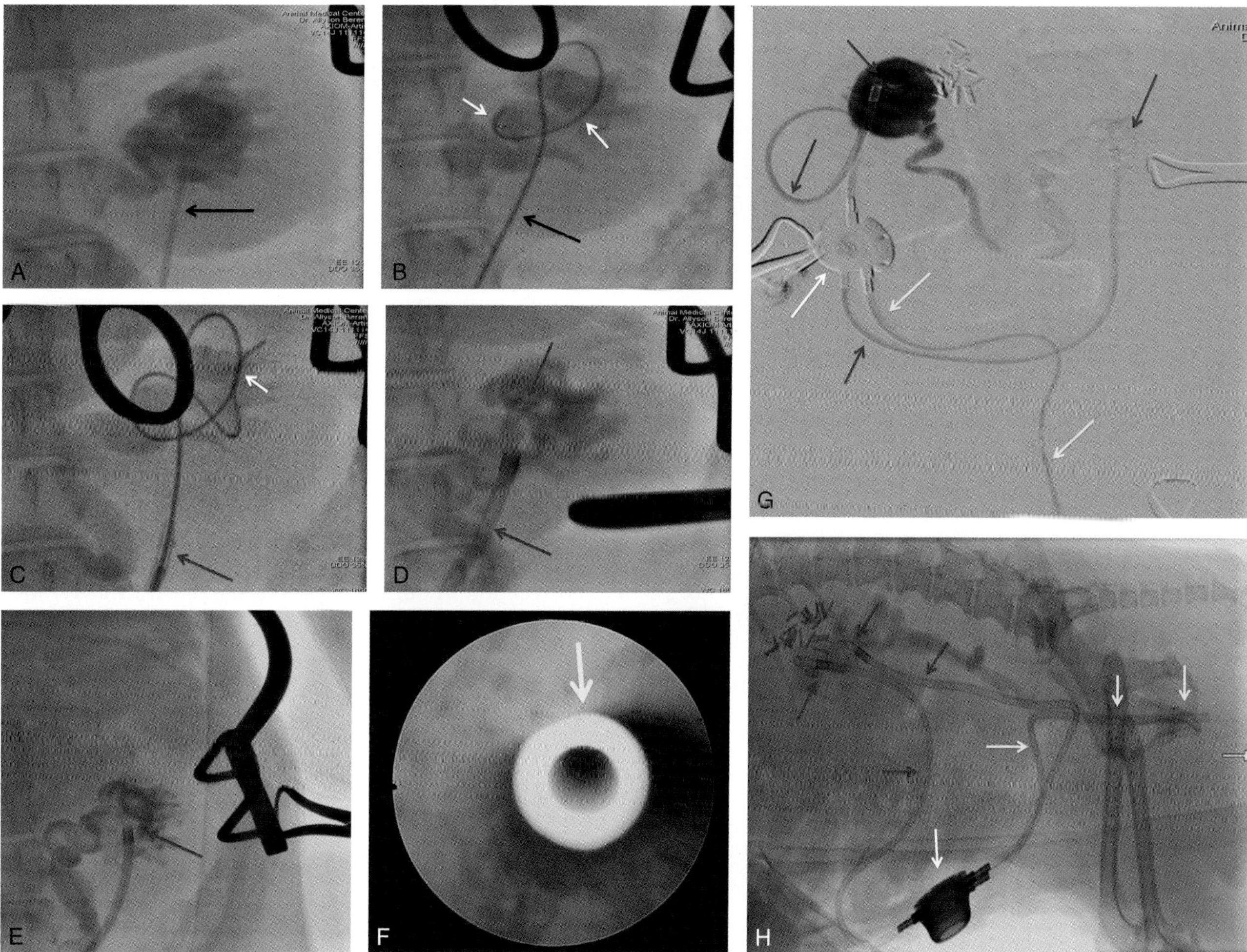

Figure 31.7 Dog with bilateral ureteral obstructions and a urethral obstruction from TCC with no bladder lumen due to tumor invasion and minimal urethral involvement. Bilateral SUBs were placed with a radical cystectomy to remove all gross disease. Fluoroscopic images A–E, and G are in dorsal recumbency during surgery. (A) Renal access using an 18-ga catheter (black arrow) into the renal pelvis from the caudal pole of the kidney. (B) Guide wire (white arrows) coiling within the renal pelvis, advanced through the catheter (black arrow). (C) Nephrostomy catheter (red arrow) being advanced over the guide wire (white arrow). (D) Locking-loop pigtail nephrostomy tube (red arrows) within the renal pelvis. (E) Contrast study through the catheter (red arrow) during a pyelogram showing patency of the catheter and no leakage. (F) Cystoscopy image of the urethral catheter (yellow arrow) coming down the urethra after radical cystectomy (Figure 31.8). (G) Dorsoventral projection during a digital subtraction image while performing a contrast study through the three-way shunting port (white arrow) showing both renal pelvises filling through the two nephrostomy catheters (red arrows) and the urethral catheter (yellow arrows). (H) Lateral fluoroscopy image showing the entire system with the red arrows outlining the two nephrostomy catheters and the yellow arrow the urethroscopy catheter after the bladder was removed. The white arrow is the three-way shunting port of the SUB device.

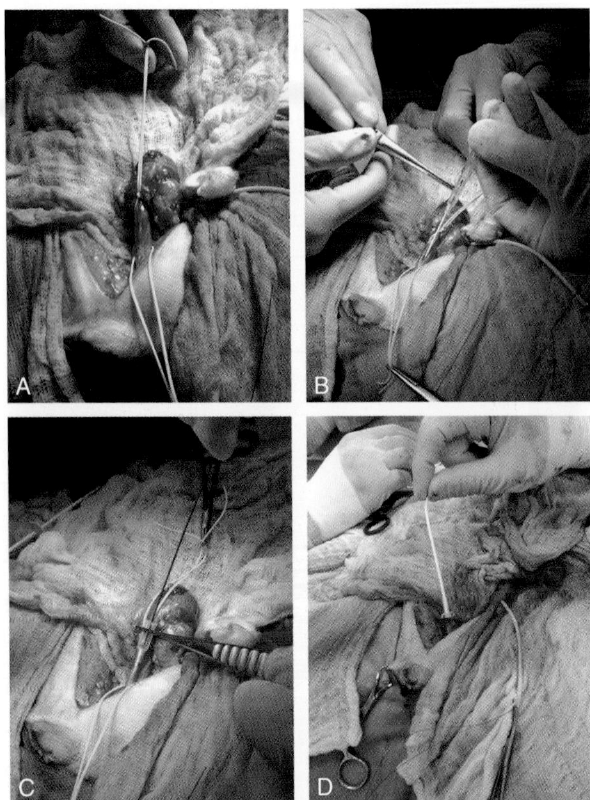

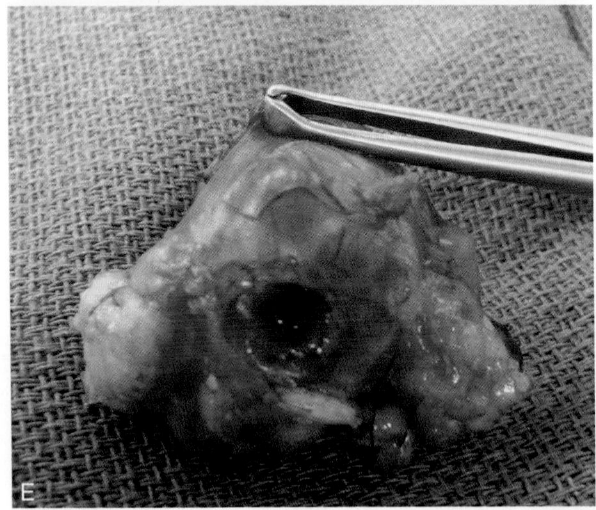

Figure 31.8 Dog with bilateral ureteral obstruction and a urethral obstruction from TCC that had a bladder filled with tumor resulting in the inability to hold urine within the bladder and no room for the pigtails of the ureteral stents to be placed within the bladder. A radical cystectomy was performed with bilateral SUB devices for urinary diversion to the urethra. (A) During surgery the urinary bladder and urethra are isolated. (B) An 18-g IV catheter is advanced into the proximal urethra for guide wire passage. (C) Over the wire the bladder catheter component of the SUB device is advanced down the urethra (D) and the entire bladder and distal ureters are resected en bloc (E).

Notes

1. Percutaneous renal access trocar needle (18 g × 15 cm), Cook Medical, Bloomington, IN.
2. 0.035-inch stiffened hydrophilic Weasel Wire, Infiniti Medical, LLC, Menlo Park, CA.
3. 0.035-inch unstiffened Weasel Wire, Infiniti Medical, LLC, Menlo Park, CA.
4. 5 Fr vascular access sheath, Infiniti Medical, LLC, Menlo Park, CA.
5. 4 Fr 65-cm angiographic Berenstein Catheter, Infiniti Medical, LLC, Menlo Park, CA.
6. 7 Fr Flexor Check-Flo Introducer Sheath, Ansel Modification, Cook Medical, Bloomington, IN.
7. Vet Stent- ureteral cancer stent. Infiniti Medical, LLC, Menlo Park, CA.
8. Vet Stent-Ureter, Double-pigtailed ureteral stents, variable length, Infiniti Medical, LLC, Menlo Park, CA.
9. Marker catheter (5 F, 45 cm), Infiniti Medical, LLC, Menlo Park, CA.
10. Vet Stent Urethra, Infiniti Medical, LLC, Menlo Park, CA.
11. 6 Fr locking-loop nephrostomy tube, Infiniti Medical, LLC, Menlo Park, CA.
12. 7 Fr vascular access sheath, Infiniti Medical, LLC, Menlo Park, CA.

Reference

Berent A, Weisse C, Beal M, et al (2011) Use of indwelling, double-pigtail stents for treatment of malignant ureteral obstruction in dogs: 12 cases (2006–2009). *J Am Vet Med Assoc* 238(8), 1017–25.

Suggested Reading

Berent A (2011) Ureteral obstructions in dogs and cats: a review of traditional and new interventional diagnostic and therapeutic options. *J Vet Emerg Crit Care* 21(2), 86–103.

Carrafiello G, Lagana D, Lumia D, et al (2007) Direct primary or secondary percutaneous ureteral stenting: what is the most compliant options in patients with malignant ureteral obstructions? *Cardiovasc Intervent Radiol* 30, 974–80.

Chitale SV, Scott-Barrett S, Ho ET, et al (2002) The management of ureteric obstruction secondary to malignant pelvic disease. *Clin Radiol* 57, 1118–21.

Henry CJ, Dudley ML, Turnquist SE, et al (2003) Clinical evaluation of mitoxantrone and piroxicam in a canine model of human invasive urinary bladder cancer. *Clin Cancer Res* 9, 906–11.

Rocha TA, Mauldin GN, Patnaik AK (2000) Prognostic factors in dogs with urinary bladder carcinoma. *J Vet Intern Med* 14, 486–90.

Uthappa MC and Cowan NC (2005) Retrograde or antegrade double-pigtail stent placement for malignant ureteric obstruction? *Clin Radiol* 60, 608–12.

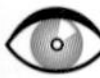

Video clips to accompany this chapter can be found in the online material at **www.wiley.com/go/weisse/vet-image-guided-interventions**

CHAPTER THIRTY-TWO

Cystoscopic-Guided Laser Ablation of Ectopic Ureters

Allyson Berent
The Animal Medical Center, New York, NY

Background / Indications

Ectopic ureters (EU) are the most common cause of urinary incontinence in juvenile female dogs. This is a congenital anomaly of the urinary tract in which the ureteral orifice is inappropriately positioned. It is usually caudal to the urinary bladder (i.e., the bladder neck, urethra, vagina, vestibule, or uterus), but can also be found within the bladder with abnormal ureteral openings or location (termed intravesicularly ectopic ureters). Ectopic ureters are classified anatomically as tunneling either intramurally or extramurally, with over 95% reported to be intramural in dogs. The typical intramural ectopic ureter will enter the distal aspect of the urinary bladder and trigone in a relatively normal position but fail to open into the urinary bladder lumen, tunneling within the submucosa of the urethra. Usually the ectopic orifice is large (1.5–3 times the normal UVJ size) however on occasion it can be small and stenotic (Figure 32.1) resulting in severe hydroureter/hydronephrosis, and potentially a ureterocele. This stenotic opening is most commonly seen in male dogs, particularly Laborador retrievers, and commonly not associated with incontinence. Opening this orifice to improve urine flow and decrease the hydroureter and hydronephrosis is indicated because this is a partial ureteral outflow obstruction.

Concurrent urinary bladder and urethral functional anomalies such as urethral sphincter mechanism incompetence is reported in 75% to 89% of female dogs with EU. Other associated conditions include urinary tract infections (65–85%), persistent paramesonephric septal remnants (~90%), hydroureter (~50%) or hydronephrosis (~25%), short urethras (~20%), vaginal septum/dual vaginas (~10%), renal agenesis (~5%), renal dysplasia (~10%), hormonal imbalances, and ureteroceles (McLoughlin and Chew, 2000, Mayhew et al, 2006, Berent et al, 2012). Hydroureter/hydronephrosis is seen in over 90% of male dogs with EU.

Various methods of surgical correction have been described, requiring a laparotomy, cystotomy, ureterotomy, and/or urethrotomy. The complication rates with surgery vary (16–50%) with 25–50% of dogs receiving ureteral re-implantation developing worsening hydroureter or hydronephrosis and 14% developing uroabdomen (Reichler et al, 2012, McLoughlin amd Chew, 2000). Unfortunately, the postoperative urinary continence rates for female dogs continue to be low regardless of the surgical technique performed varying between 25% and 70% with or without concurrent medical management. The continence rate in male dogs exceeds 70–80% after fixation (Berent et al, 2008, Anders et al, 2012). Many of these dogs are relinquished or euthanized due to persistent urinary incontinence. These disappointing outcomes have encouraged exploration of alternative therapies.

Cystoscopic-guided laser ablation of ectopic ureters (CLA-EU) provides a minimally invasive alternative to surgery in both male and female dogs with intramural EU. This procedure enables simultaneous diagnosis and therapeutic intervention, and may also avoid some of the complications associated with the open surgical techniques. Utilizing cystoscopy and fluoroscopy, the ureteral orifice can be directly visualized, other urinary anomalies can be assessed (vaginal septal remnants, hypoplastic bladder, intrapelvic bladder, hydroureter, and hydronephrosis), and the differentiation of intramural versus extramural tunneling can be made. At the same time, the laser can be used to ablate the medial ectopic ureteral wall to reposition the opening if the EU is intramurally located.

Patient Preparation

All dogs should have a CBC, serum biochemical profile, urinalysis, and urine bacteriologic culture within 2 weeks prior to the procedure. A thorough history and

Veterinary Image-Guided Interventions, First Edition. Edited by Chick Weisse and Allyson Berent.

Companion website: www.wiley.com/go/weisse/vet-image-guided-interventions

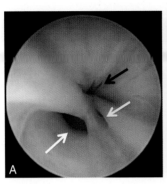

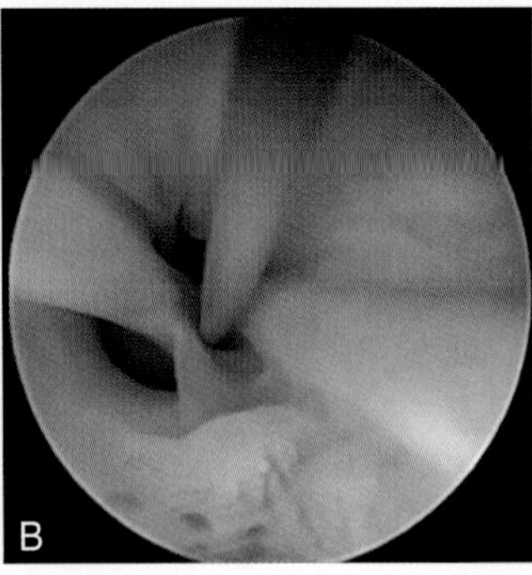

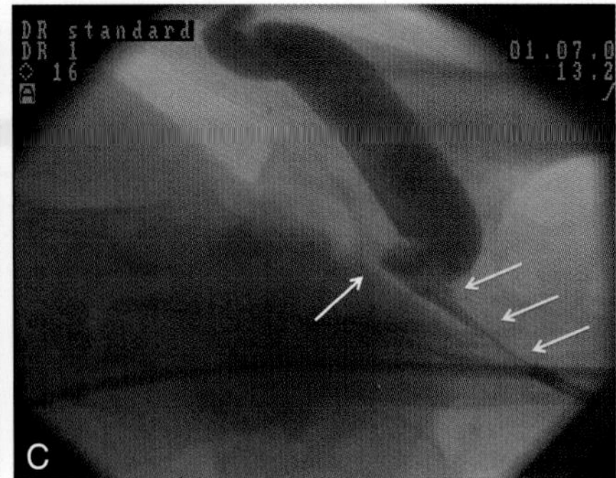

Figure 32.1 (A, B) Female dog with bilateral ectopic ureters during a cystoscopy in dorsal recumbency. In the urethra three openings are identified. The black arrow is the urethral opening at the trigone, the yellow arrow is the small left ectopic ureteral opening and the white arrow is the right ectopic ureteral opening. A guide wire is then advanced into the left ectopic ureteral opening. (C) Fluoroscopy image of a male dog in dorsal recumbency during a retrograde ureteropyelogram and cystourethrogram. Notice the severe hydroureter to the level of the intramural tunnel in the urinary bladder neck (white arrow). The intramural tunnel (yellow arrows) is very narrow, causing a partial outflow obstruction and the severe hydroureter. The ureteral opening is marked by the tip of the flexible cystoscope in the proximal urethra. This is the most common location of ectopic ureteral openings in male dogs.

physical examination should be obtained ensuring there is not a neurologic cause for the urinary incontinence. A urinary tract ultrasonography to assess for any renal pelvic dilation, hydroureter, or renal abnormalities is recommended. Care should be taken when relying on an ultrasonographic interpretation of ectopic ureters as this diagnostic modality is only accurate ~50% of the time. A negative test on ultrasonography should still warrant further investigation through cystoscopy or a computed tomography (CT) scan. The benefit of cystoscopy is that it is 100% accurate for the diagnosis of EU in female dogs when performed by an experienced operator while allowing concurrent treatment with CLA. Performing a CT scan involves greater expense, longer anesthesia times, and is only a diagnostic test. Cystoscopy in male dogs requires more experience for an accurate diagnosis and assessment of the ureterovesicular junction (UVJ).

If a urinary tract infection is present (approximately 65–85% of female dogs) the patient should be treated with appropriate antibiotics and obtain a negative urine culture prior to the procedure when possible.

Potential Risks/ Complications/ Expected Outcomes

An experienced endoscopist comfortable using the laser should perform this procedure. The most substantial risk is performing CLA-EU on an extramural (rather than intramural) ectopic ureter; this is considered a contraindication to the laser procedure. A concurrent ureteropyelogram can confirm the intramural nature of the ureter and is highly recommended by the author but not always performed by others performing the procedure (Figure 32.2). Using rotational fluoroscopy and endoscopy together, the point that the ureter travels extramurally from the urinary bladder can be identified, minimizing the risk of excessive laser ablation (Figure 32.2. Figure 32.3, and Figure 32.4). All operators should be trained in laser safety and appropriate laser goggles should be worn during any laser ablation procedure.

Urethral perforation during cystoscopy is a low risk if the operator is experienced. The urothelial tissue can develop a proliferative reaction along the laser tract that has been termed a "delayed laser reaction" (Figure 32.5). This can ultimately result in a ureteral orifice obstruction and has been seen in approximately 3% of cases in the author's experience (two resulted in obstruction and one was non-clinical). Because of this risk the author recommends a urinary tract ultrasound exam 6 weeks post CLA-EU to confirm there is no development or progression of hydroureter or hydronephrosis.

In a recent study looking at 30 female dogs (48 ectopic ureters) after CLA-EU, 47% were completely continent at a median follow-up of 2.7 years. The addition of medical management (~20% response), transurethral bulking-agent injections (~30% response), and/or the placement of a hydraulic occluder (~80–90% response) improved the overall urinary continence rate to 77% (Berent et al, 2012). Another study reported 18 female dogs evaluated retrospectively using the same technique with similar results (Smith et al, 2011).

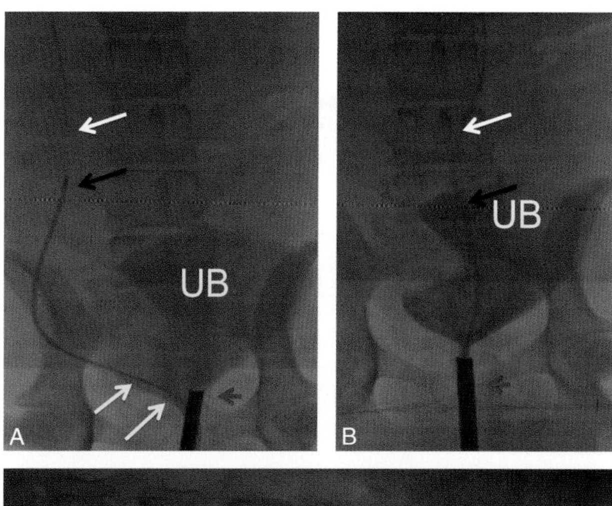

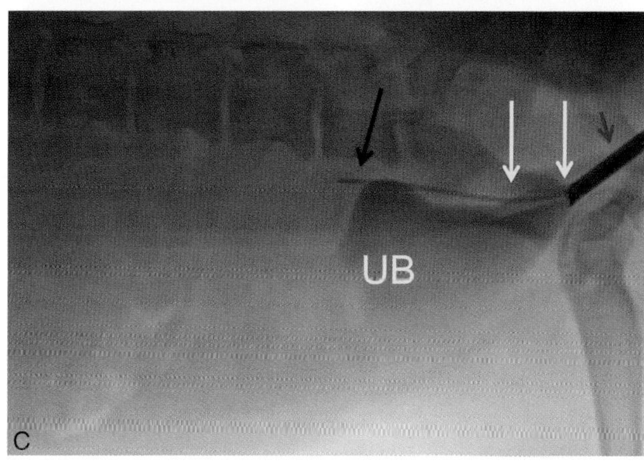

Figure 32.2 Fluoroscopic images of a female dog in dorsal recumbency with bilateral EU documenting the intramural nature of the ureters. (A) VD image with a guide wire (white arrow) and ureteral catheter (black arrow) up the right ureter and contrast within the urinary bladder (UB). The cystoscope (red arrow) is at the trigone. Notice the ureter travelling intramurally (between the yellow arrows) and exiting the bladder wall laterally. (B) A VD image after the left ureter is cannulated with the guide wire (white arrow) and catheter (black arrow). In this image it is hard to tell if this ureter is intramural as the path of the ureter is directly over the bladder (UB). (C) The C-arm is rotated to project a lateral image of the dog (and multiple tangential views as necessary) to confirm the intramural path (between the 2 yellow arrows) of the ureter.

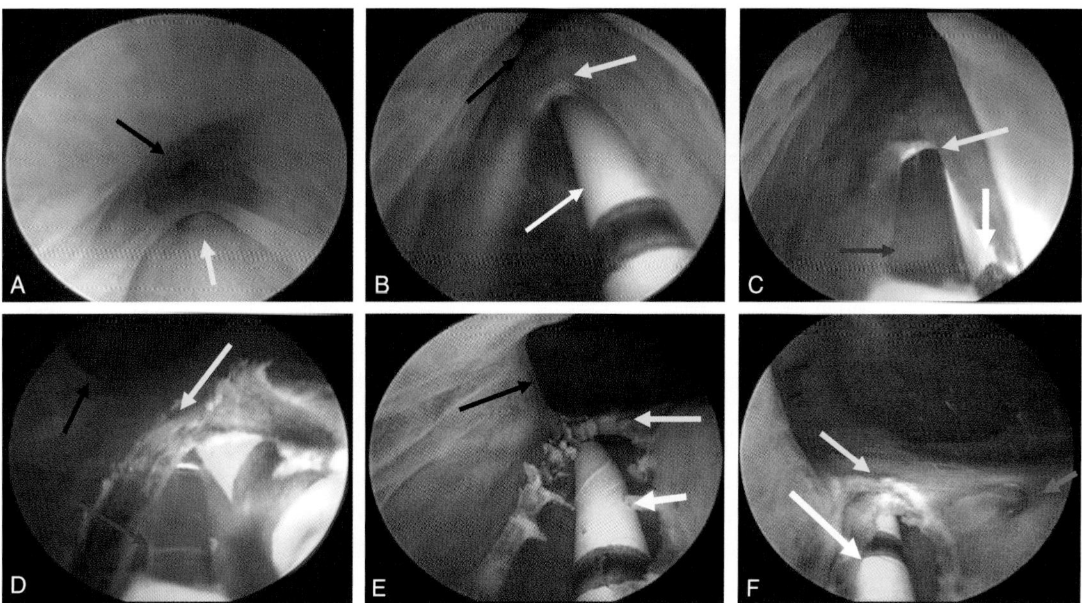

Figure 32.3 Endoscopic images of a female dog with a right ectopic ureter (EU) during a CLA-EU procedure using the diode laser. The dog is in dorsal recumbency. (A) The right ectopic ureteral opening is seen in the dorsal urethral wall (yellow arrow). The urethral lumen is marked with the black arrow. (B) A guide wire/catheter combination (white arrow) advanced into the EU opening (yellow arrow). (C) The diode laser fiber (red arrow) through the working channel of the endoscope as it approaches the EU orifice (yellow arrow). (D) The right ectopic ureteral tunnel as it is advanced to the trigone (black arrow) with the diode laser (red arrow). (E) Opening of the intramural ectopic ureteral tunnel (yellow arrow) to the level of the trigone (black arrow) within the urethra. Notice the ureteral catheter (white arrow) as it aims laterally up the ureter in front of the trigone. (F) The new right ureterovesicular junction (yellow arrow) at the end of the CLA-EU procedure. The opening was advanced into the bladder, in front of the trigone, to the level of the appropriately placed left ureterovesicular junction (blue arrow).

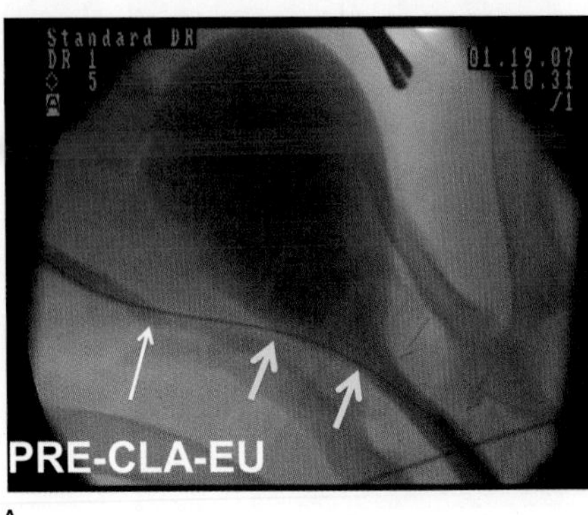

A

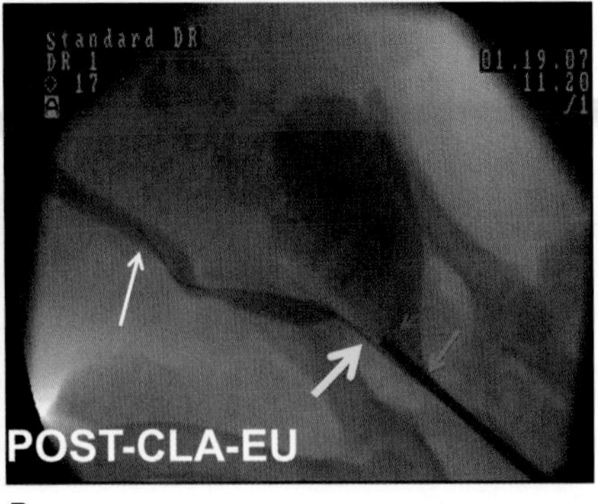

B

Figure 32.4 A female dog in dorsal recumbency during the CLA-EU procedure. Fluoroscopy is used to monitor the intramural and extramural transition. (A) Guide wire (white arrow) is advanced up the right EU and the cystoscope (red arrow) is at the opening of the ectopic orifice. The intramural tunnel within the urinary bladder is documented (between yellow arrows) marking where to stop lasering in front of the trigone (blue arrow). (B) After CLA-EU the endoscope (red arrow) is at the new ureteral opening documenting it is in front of the trigone (blue arrow) with some intramural tunnel remaining (yellow arrow).

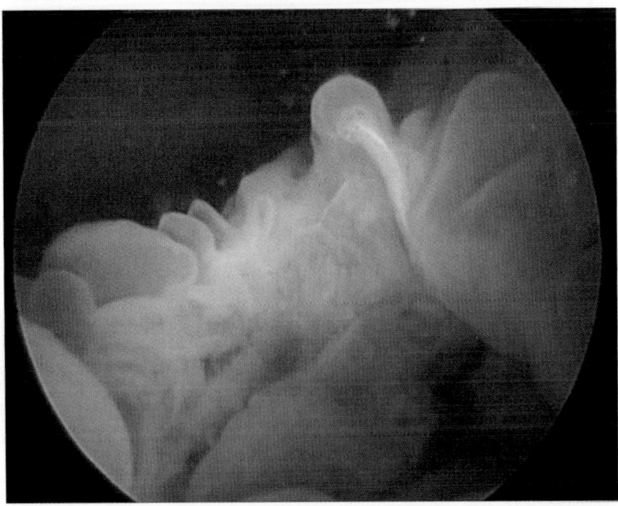

Figure 32.5 Endoscopic image of the left UVJ 1 week after CLA-EU in a female showing a proliferative urethritis/cystitis, likely associated with a reaction to the laser on the tissue.

Four male dogs were previously reported and all were continent after laser ablation (Berent et al, 2008). Nearly 85–90% of male dogs have evidence of hydroureter and/or hydronephrosis on screening ultrasonography and not all male dogs are incontinent, despite the presence of ectopic ureters. Many male dogs present for evaluation of severe "megaureter" and hydronephrosis (Figure 32.1C). Typically, during cystoscopy in these cases, an ectopic ureter is found with a very narrowed intramural tunnel. This has also been seen in a small number of female dogs. Male Labrador retrievers were the most common breed seen in the author's practice with this stenotic condition. Ureterovesicular junction stenosis secondary to ectopic ureters in young male dogs should be a differential for megaureter. To date, approximately 20 male dogs have had CLA-EU performed in the author's practice, and of those that were incontinent to start, 85% were completely continent post-laser ablation; this is consistent with the traditional surgical literature (Anders et al, 2012).

Dogs with a history of EU should have routine urine cultures performed throughout their lives as they are at an increased risk for development of recurrent urinary tract infections, identified in over 80% of female dogs prior to CLA and 35% post-CLA. As these are considered complicated urinary tract infections, treatment is recommended for at least 4 weeks.

Equipment

Endoscopy is typically performed with an appropriate diameter 30 degree rigid cystoscope for female dogs (1.9, 2.7, or 4 mm)[1–3] and 7.5–8.2 Fr flexible ureteroscope[4] for male dogs. Ureteral access is obtained with an appropriately sized angle-tipped hydrophilic guide wire[5] and open-ended ureteral catheter[6] (Table 32.1). A traditional fluoroscopic C-arm is sufficient for visualization during the ureteropyelogram and cystourethrogram to confirm the intramural nature of the EU.

There are two types of lasers that the author has used for this procedure: a diode laser[7,8] and a Holmium:YAG (yttrium, aluminum, garnet) laser.[9] The benefit of the diode laser is that it is a continuous firing laser that has both tissue ablative and coagulative properties. The diode is best used in contact mode resulting in minimal tissue bleeding, edema, or collateral damage, and is very effective for tissue ablation. The diode laser works at 980 nm, which usually provides both coagulation and cutting with essentially no resulting hemorrhage (Figure 32.6E, F). The laser fiber is typically larger for the diode (600 or 1000 μm), making it much harder to

TABLE 32.1
Recommended equipment for female dogs during CLA-EU based on size

Dog size	Guide wire size (inches)	Open-ended ureteral catheter size (French)	Cystoscope size (mm)
Small (<5 kg)	0.018	3 Fr	1.9
Medium (5–20 kg)	0.025	4 Fr	2.7
Large (>20 kg)	0.035	5 Fr	4.0

manipulate during flexible cystoscopy. The Hol:YAG laser works at a wavelength of 2100 nm and can be used for CLA, but has a pulsed activity that results in more of an intermittent surge of pulsing energy resulting in a jumping action during the ablation making treatment less exact. This laser also results in a mild amount of edema, erythema, and hemorrhage (Figure 32.6A–D), which can obscure the cystoscopy image. This is of no clinical consequence for the patient. To avoid excessive bleeding with the Hol:YAG laser, contact mode should be avoided and the laser fiber should be situated 0.1 to 0.5 mm from the desired tissue to be ablated allowing the power to coagulate rather than cut the tissue directly. The laser fibers available for the Hol:YAG are 200, 400, 600, and 1000 µm. Since the advent of laser lithotripsy, more veterinarians have access to a Hol:YAG laser than a diode laser making this a reasonable alternative and more versatile (see Chapter 35). The author prefers the diode laser for CLA-EU as the continuous cutting mode provides an ablation that is fast and exact. The Hol:YAG laser fiber allows more flexibility when performing CLA EU through the male flexible cystoscope when necessary.

Procedure

Dogs are placed in dorsal recumbency and the vulva or prepuce are clipped and aseptically prepared. In male dogs the entire perineum is also clipped and a purse-string suture is placed in the anus. Peri-procedural antimicrobials are given (cefazolin 22 mg/kg [10 mg/lb], IV) in patients that are not currently being treated with an antimicrobial for a previously diagnosed urinary tract infection.

Female Dogs

A rigid cystoscope of an appropriate size (Table 32.1) is advanced into the vestibule and the urethral orifice in a retrograde fashion. Gravity irrigation using sterile saline (0.9% NaCl) solution is typically used. Having a pressure bag for infusion is often helpful though care must be taken to avoid bladder over-distension, as hemorrhage will obscure the image making treatment very difficult. Each UVJ is carefully evaluated paying close attention to the folds of the entire dorsal urethral wall (Figure 32.1). Once an ectopic ureter is identified the cranial EU (if bilateral) should be treated first because the ablation tract can obscure the ectopic opening of the contralateral ureter if any swelling or bleeding occurs. Evaluation of multiple fenestrations, urethral length, and other concurrent bladder, urethral, vaginal, and vestibular defects should be assessed prior to starting laser ablation so the anatomy is not distorted.

Fluoroscopy with retrograde ureteropyelography is then used to confirm the presence of an intramural ectopic tract of the more proximal EU (when bilateral) (Figure 32.2). Using an angle-tipped, hydrophilic guide wire of an appropriate size (Table 32.1) through the working channel of the cystoscope, the EU is cannulated and under fluoroscopic and cystoscopic guidance, the wire is advanced up the ureter (Figure 32.2 and Figure 32.3). An open-ended ureteral catheter is then advanced over the guide wire into the distal portion of the ureter through the ureteral orifice. The guide wire is removed and a retrograde ureteropyelogram is performed with 5 ml of iodinated non-ionic contrast medium (diluted 50:50 with sterile saline solution) through the ureteral catheter (Figure 32.2 and Figure 32.4). The ureter and renal pelvis should be recorded to identify the distal ureteral path within the urethral wall and to determine the anatomic features of the ureter and renal pelvis (if pelvic dilation present). Approximately 2 to 5 ml/kg (2.25 ml/lb) of this mixture is injected into the urethra through the side port of the cystoscope that is within the lumen of the urethra. This allows for a combination retrograde cystourethrogram and ureteropyelogram which together can help identify the path of the EU (Figure 32.2 and Figure 32.4). Evaluation of the urinary bladder trigone in relation to the ureteral orifice and the transition of the ureter from intramural to extramural provides confirmation of its intramural nature. Sometimes the C-arm will need to be rotated to confirm where the ureter exits the bladder wall (Figure 32.2).

Once an intramural ureteral tract is confirmed, the cystoscope is removed over the wire-catheter combination, monitoring under fluoroscopy so catheter access to the ureter is not lost (an assistant can hold the catheter and wire in place). The cystoscope is then reinserted into the urethra, next to the wire-catheter combination, and the laser fiber (600-µm diode or 400-µm Hol:YAG [female], 200-µm Hol:YAG [male]) is inserted into the working channel of the cystoscope

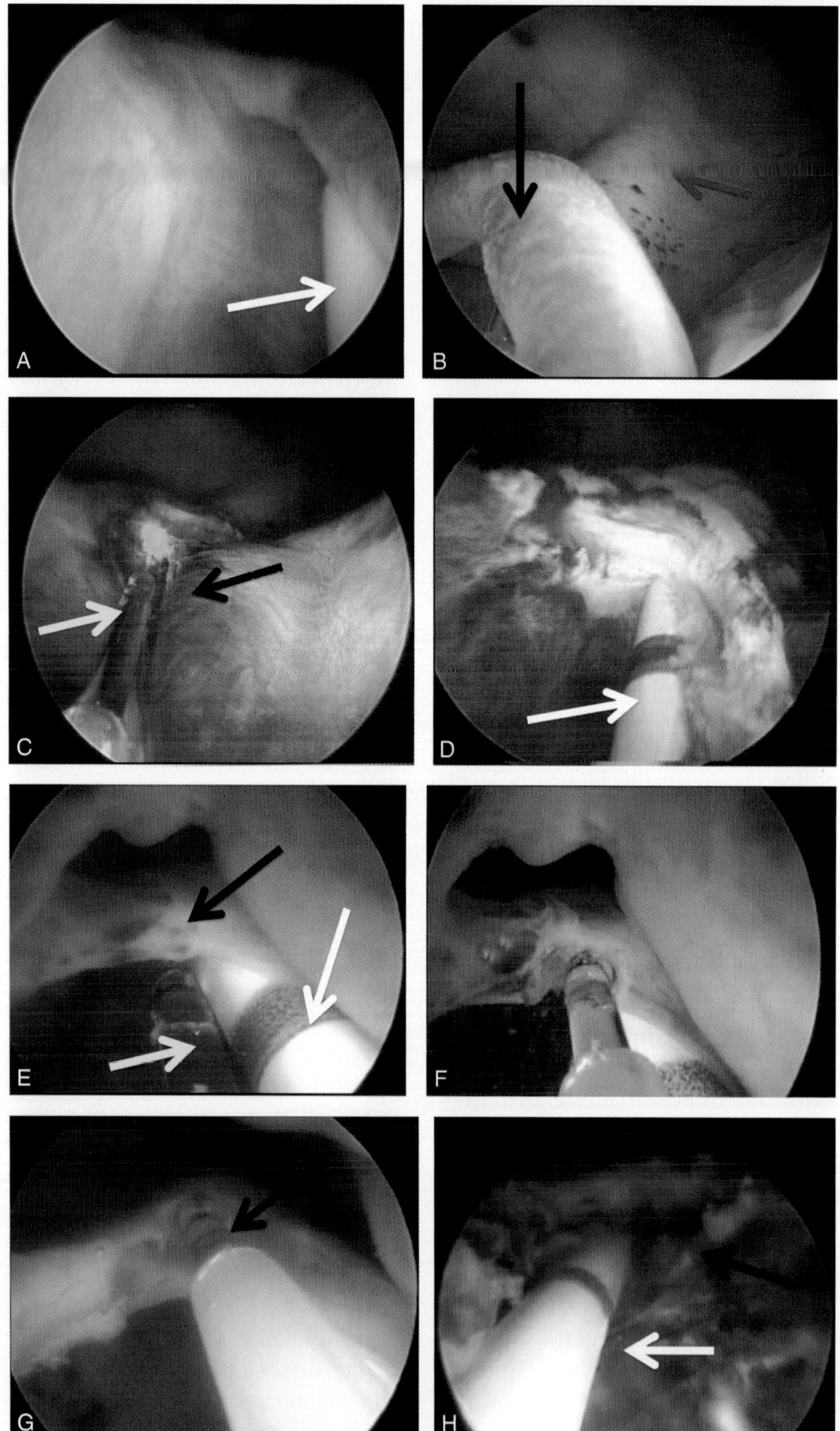

Figure 32.6 Endoscopic images of 2 different female dogs during the CLA-EU procedure of a left EU. The dogs are in dorsal recumbency. A-D is showing the use of a Hol:YAG laser and E-H the diode laser. (A) A ureteral catheter (white arrow) visualized entering the left ectopic ureteral opening in the proximal urethra. (B) The endoscopic view of the intramural tunnel of the ureter within the urinary bladder (red arrow). The catheter bulges the thin intramural tunnel. The ectopic UVJ is pink and smooth (black arrow). (C) The Hol:YAG laser fiber (yellow arrow) advancing the opening of the ectopic UVJ. Notice the tissue is red and edematous (black arrow). (D) The ureteral catheter (white arrow) in the new UVJ after CLA-EU with a Hol:YAG laser. Notice there is some edema and erythema of the tissue. (E) A ureteral catheter (white arrow) within the left ectopic ureteral opening (black arrow) within the mid urethra. The diode laser fiber (yellow arrow) is through the working channel of the cystoscope. (F) The diode fiber is seen cutting the EU opening to advance it cranially. (G) The diode fiber is advancing the EU opening. Notice the lack of erythema, edema, or bleeding. (H) The left EU opening (black arrow) is within the urinary bladder as the catheter (white arrow) remains up the ureter.

and directed onto the ectopic ureteral orifice (Figure 32.3 and Figure 32.6). The cystoscope is deflected toward the urethral lumen to angle the laser fiber tip toward the medial aspect of the ectopic ureteral wall, avoiding the lateral ureteral wall and ureteral catheter; the ureteral catheter helps protect the opposite wall of the ureter. The medial aspect of the ectopic ureteral wall is then carefully cut in a continuous manner by use of the diode laser at 16 to 25 W (Figure 32.6D–F) or a pulsed manner by use of the Hol:YAG laser (10 to 12 Hz and 0.7 to 1.2 J at a pulse width of 700 milliseconds) (Figure 32.6A–C). When the neoureteral orifice is within the urinary bladder lumen, or the ureter appears to be diverging from its path alongside the urethra laterally, suggesting the potential transition from its intramural to extramural course, the lasering is complete and the location is confirmed using fluoroscopy.

A retrograde contrast urethrocystogram and ureteropyelogram are performed in each dog after CLA-EU to ensure there is no extravasation of contrast medium and to document the new location of the ureteral orifice relative to the urinary bladder trigone both cystoscopically and fluoroscopically (Figure 32.4). The operator should be aware that retrograde filling of the vagina and/or uterus in dorsal recumbency during cystourethroscopy will occur and this can mimic peri-urethral contrast. Once the image is seen in lateral (using the C-arm) vaginal filling is confirmed.

This procedure is then repeated on the contralateral side for patients with bilateral ectopic ureters. Once CLA-EU is complete the urethra is again thoroughly scoped to ensure there are no additional fenestrations of the EU.

Finally, since over 90% of patients will have a thick vaginal septal remnant, the vagina is evaluated and laser ablated if indicated. This remnant can result in chronic vaginal pooling and recurrent urinary tract infrctions (UTIs) (see Chapter 42). Due to the non-sterile environment, vaginoscopy should be performed after cystoscopy and CLA.

Male Dogs

Initially all male dogs larger than ~6.0–6.5 kg should have a flexible cystoscopy performed. If EU's are confirmed then the author currently recommends obtaining percutaneous perineal access into the pelvic urethra via the modified Seldinger technique (see Chapter 39) allowing rigid cystoscopy to be performed. This provides superior visibility and facilitates ablation of the EU

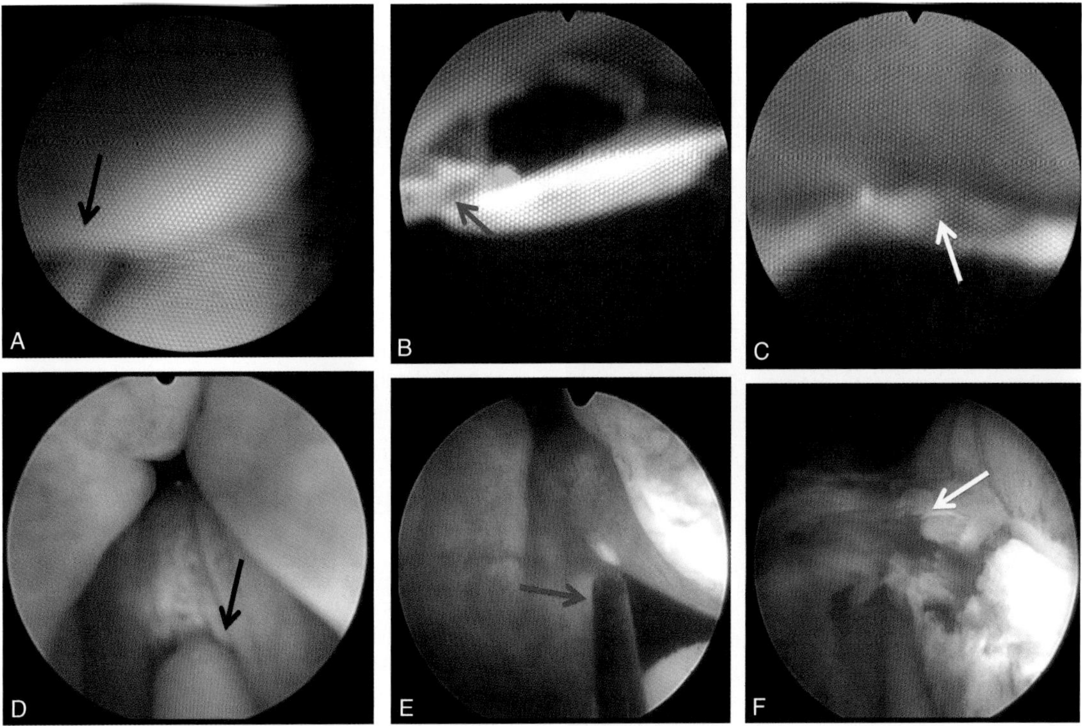

Figure 32.7 Cystoscopic images of two male dogs during CLA-EU. Each patient is in dorsal recumbency. (A–C) CLA-EU is done using the fiberoptic flexible cystoscope; (D–F) the procedure is done with a rigid cystoscope using perineal urethral access. Notice the improved image quality in the latter images. (A and D) The guide wire (black arrow) is in the ectopic ureteral orifice in the proximal urethra. (B and E) The Hol:YAG 200 μm laser fiber (red arrow) is cutting the medial EU wall to advance the orifice. (C and F) The cut tissue of the EU at the new UVJ.

(Figure 32.7). If the EU is minimal and a good angle is obtained using the flexible cystoscope than CLA-EU can be performed using the flexible scope with the 200-µm Hol:YAG laser fiber (Figure 32.7A–C). In male dogs this tissue is typically very thick (Figure 32.7D–F), resulting in a stenotic opening and severe hydroureter. Using the rigid endoscope allows more aggressive ablation to open the tissue maximally without risking extravasation.

Postprocedural and Follow-Up Care

Dogs are given a local urethral infusion of bupivacaine (1 mg/kg [0.5 mg/lb] mixed with saline in a 1:1 solution) for local urethral analgesia after the procedure. Patients also receive a dose of buprenorphine (0.01 mg/kg [0.005 mg/lb]) and are discharged the same day with oral tramadol (2 to 5 mg/kg, [1 to 2.5 mg/lb], PO, q 8 hr) for 3 days and 5 days of a broad-spectrum antibiotic (unless currently being treated for a UTI). Bacteriologic culture of urine samples are performed at 2 to 4 weeks and recommended at 8 weeks, 3 months, 6 months, and then every 6 months thereafter. Repeat urinary tract ultrasonography is recommended at 6 weeks to ensure there is no laser reaction at the UVJ that could result in worsening hydroureter and hydronephrosis. If concerns exist, repeat cystoscopy can be performed; the new EU orifice should heal nicely and nearly resemble a nature UVJ (Figure 32.8).

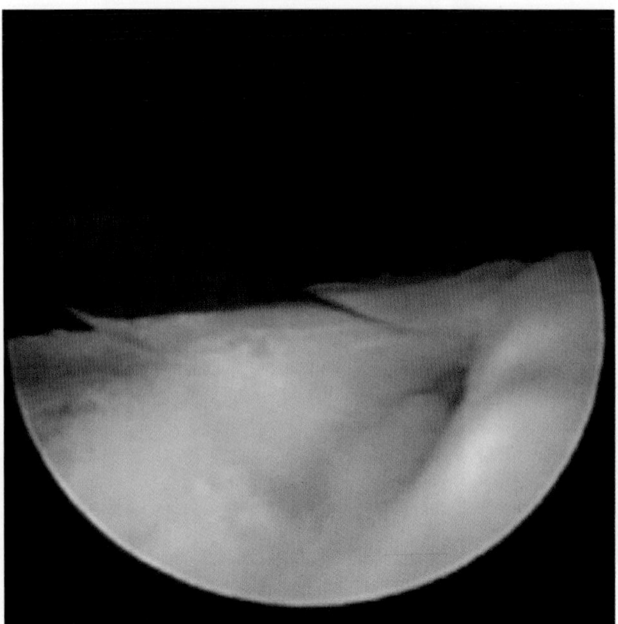

Figure 32.8 Cystoscopic image of a female dog in dorsal recumbency 6 weeks after CLA-EU showing the new left UVJ within the urinary bladder.

Special Considerations/ Alternative Uses/ Complication Examples

The author recommends that patients having ureteral interventions be positioned in dorsal recumbency with the vulva/perineum at the end of the table. Keeping the ureter straight during laser ablation is more problematic if the patient is scoped in lateral recumbency. Cannulating the ureter for other interventions when dogs are in sternal recumbency is also more difficult. The operator should become proficient at dorsal cystoscopy prior to trying any ureteral interventions.

Notes

These are only a few examples of the equipment used for this procedure. There are many variations from different companies available.

1. Rigid endoscope, 1.9-mm 30° lens, Karl Storz Endoscopy, Culver City, CA.
2. Rigid endoscope, 2.7-mm 30° lens, Richard Wolf, Vernon Hills, IL.
3. Rigid endoscope, 4-mm 30° lens, Karl Storz Endoscopy, Culver City, CA.
4. Flex X^2 Flexible ureteroscope, Karl Storz Endoscopy, Culver City, CA.
5. Weasel Wire 0.025- or 0.035-inch hydrophilic angle-tipped guidewire, Infiniti Medical LLC, Menlo Park, CA.
6. 4 or 5 Fr, open-ended ureteral catheter, Cook Medical Inc, Bloomington, IN.
7. 600-µm diode laser fiber and 25-W diode laser, Lumenis Inc, Santa Clara, CA.
8. 600-µm diode laser fiber and 100-W diode Lithotrite, Vectra, Convergent Inc, Alameda, CA.
9. 200 or 400-µm Holmium:YAG laser fiber and 30-W Hol:YAG Lithotrite, Odyssey, Convergent Inc, Alameda, CA.

References

Anders KJ, Samii VF, Chew D, et al. (2012) Ectopic ureters in male dogs: review of 16 clinical cases (1999–2007). *J Am Anim Hosp Assoc* 48, 390–8.

Berent AC, Mayhew PD, and Porat-Mosenco Y. (2008) Use of cystoscopic-guided laser ablation for treatment of intramural ureteral ectopia in male dogs: four cases (2006–2007). *J Am Vet Med Assoc* 232, 1026–34.

Berent A, Weisse C, Mayhew P, and Bagley D. (2012) A prospective study evaluating the cystoscopic guided laser ablation of ureteral ectopia in 30 dogs. *J Am Vet Med Assoc* 240(6), 716–25.

Mayhew PD, Lee KC, Gregory SP, et al. (2006) Comparison of two surgical techniques for management of intramural ureteral ectopia in dogs: 36 cases (1994–2004). *J Am Vet Med Assoc* 229, 389–93.

McLoughlin MA and Chew DJ. (2000) Diagnosis and surgical management of ectopic ureters. *Clin Techn Small Anim Pract* 15, 17–24.

Reichler IM, Specker CE, Hubler M, et al. (2012) Ectopic ureters in dogs: Clinical features, surgical techniques and outcome. *Vet Surg* 41, 515–522.

Smith AL Radlinkay MG, and Rawlings CA. (2010) Cystoscopic diagnosis and treatment of ectopic ureters in female dogs: 16 cases (2005–2008). *J Am Vet Med Assoc* 237, 191–5.

Suggested Reading

McCarthy TC (2006) Transurethral cystoscopy and diode laser incision to correct an ectopic ureter. *Vet Med* 101, 558–9.

CHAPTER THIRTY-THREE

Minimally Invasive Treatment of Bladder and Urethral Stones in Dogs and Cats

Allyson Berent[1] and Larry G. Adams[2]
[1]*The Animal Medical Center, New York, NY*
[2]*Department of Veterinary Clinical Sciences, Purdue University, West Lafayette, IN*

Background/Indications

Lower urinary tract stones, involving the bladder and urethra, can be removed using various minimally-invasive techniques. Removal is typically indicated when the calculi are not amenable to medical dissolution, are causing a urethral obstruction, creating discomfort despite appropriate medical management, or resulting in recurrent infections. Traditional surgical removal of stones via cystotomy or urethrotomy has been the traditional method of choice. Studies have shown that 10–20% of cases have incomplete surgical removal of stones, and this is likely due to poor visualization, hemorrhage, and/or inappropriate technique. Recently, complications associated with traditional surgical cystotomy were reported in 37–50% of cases. In addition, studies have suggested a 40–60% rate of stone recurrence, especially when dealing with calcium oxalate, urate and cystine stones. When sutures are placed in the urinary tract after surgical stone removal the patient can develop suture-induced stones, and this may be associated with even higher stone recurrence rates. In a more recent study looking at the use of laser lithotripsy, stone recurrence rates were 19% over 1–2 years. Ideally, less-invasive and more effective alternatives to traditional surgery for stone removal, with lower stone recurrence rates, should be considered.

The focus of this chapter will be on four procedures: voiding urohydropropulsion, cystoscopic-guided stone basket-retrieval, cystoscopic-guided intracorporeal laser lithotripsy, and a percutaneous cystolithotomy (PCCL) procedure. Each of these procedures has different indications based on species, sex, stone size and stone number (Table 33.1).

VUH

Voiding urohydropropulsion is used for removal of urocystoliths that are smaller than the urethral diameter. The urinary bladder is distended and the small uroliths are flushed through the urethra during manual voiding using gravity with the patient's proximal urethra positioned vertically relative to the effects of gravity.

Basketing

Cystoscopic-guided stone basket-retrieval is also for removal of urocystoliths when the uroliths are smaller than the urethral diameter. This technique allows for removal of slightly larger uroliths than can be removed by VUH by removing them one at a time. Additionally, irregularly shaped uroliths can be repositioned such that the long axis of the urolith is parallel to the urethra permitting passage more easily than if the uroliths moved into the urethra during VUH perpendicular to their long axis.

Laser Lithotripsy

Laser lithotripsy is a minimally invasive technique that fragments uroliths by intracorporeal lithotripsy using a Hol:YAG laser, until the stone fragments are smaller

Veterinary Image-Guided Interventions, First Edition. Edited by Chick Weisse and Allyson Berent.

Companion website: www.wiley.com/go/weisse/vet-image-guided-interventions

TABLE 33.1
Minimally invasive treatment options for the removal of bladder and urethral stones

Procedure	Stone size limit	Patient size limit	Equipment required	Special Indications
VUH	Male dog: 2 mm Female dog: 3–4 mm Female cat: 2–3 mm Male cat: do not perform	Any size patient (not a male cat)	Urinary catheter for male dogs Rigid cystoscope or urinary catheter for female dogs and cats	The author finds it much easier to perform this procedure using a rigid cystoscope to fill the urinary bladder in female dogs and cats rather than repeat blind urethral catheterizations. If cystoscopy is not available, then urethral catheterization is used for bladder filling.
Basketing	Male dog: 2–3 mm Female dog: 4–5 mm Female cat: 2–3 mm Male cat: do not perform	Large enough to accept an appropriately sized cystoscope (not male cats)	Cystoscope and various sized stone baskets	The operator should be prepared for laser lithotripsy in the event the stone gets stuck in the urethra during removal. Do not apply excessive tension on the stone if it is not passively coming through the urethra with irrigation.
Laser lithotripsy	Male dog: 5 mm Female dog: 10 mm Female cat: 5 mm Male cat: no not perform	Must be able to accept the cystoscope comfortably	Various cystoscopes Hol:YAG laser with appropriate fibers FHI	Every operator has their own limits on which patients this is appropriate for. 1. urethral stones 2. no more than 2–4 cystoliths that require fragmentation in female dogs 3. no more than 2 cystoliths that require fragmentation in female cats 4. no more than 2 cystoliths in a male dog.
PCCL	All dogs and cats with any size or number of stones (male or female)	none	Screw trocar (6 mm ± 10 mm for larger stones); 2.7 mm rigid cystoscope; 7.5–8 Fr Flexible cystoscope	Cats are harder to distend and visualize so the author recommends maintaining good apical traction to get the best visualization.

than the urethra. The fragments are then removed by a combination of cystoscopic-guided stone basket-retrieval and VUH. This technique is best suited to female dogs and cats with bladder or urethral uroliths and male dogs with relatively few urethroliths. Animals with larger stone burdens are better suited for PCCL.

PCCL

A newer minimally invasive technique, PCCL, combines cystic and urethral stone retrieval for any size, sex, or species and is easy to perform in both cats and dogs. This technique has been described recently in 27 dogs and cats. In children, when their urethra is too narrow, or the stone burden is too large, PCCL is considered the ideal alternative.

Potential Risks/ Complications/ Expected Outcomes

All of these minimally invasive procedures carry a risk of bladder rupture or perforation, so conversion to a cystotomy should always be possible. Since lavage of the abdomen is not possible with these procedures all patients should have a negative urine culture prior to any procedure and if positive the patient should be treated with an appropriate antibiotic for at least 2–3 days.

VUH

The main risk of this procedure is transient urethral obstruction if the bladder stone is larger in diameter than the urethra or too many bladder stones enter the urethra at once. If forceful bladder expression is continued once the urethra is obstructed, then bladder perforation or rupture may occur. If this occurs, then immediate conversion to open cystotomy and repair of the bladder rupture is required. With proper case selection, VUH is highly successful with all uroliths bring removed in most patients. Active urinary tract hemorrhage may result in blood clots that trap small stones and adhere to the urinary bladder mucosa, thereby preventing their removal by VUH. If this occurs, then waiting 2–5 days until the blood clots resolve and repeating VUH is usually successful. Mild to moderate hematuria is expected post VUH for 8–36 hours.

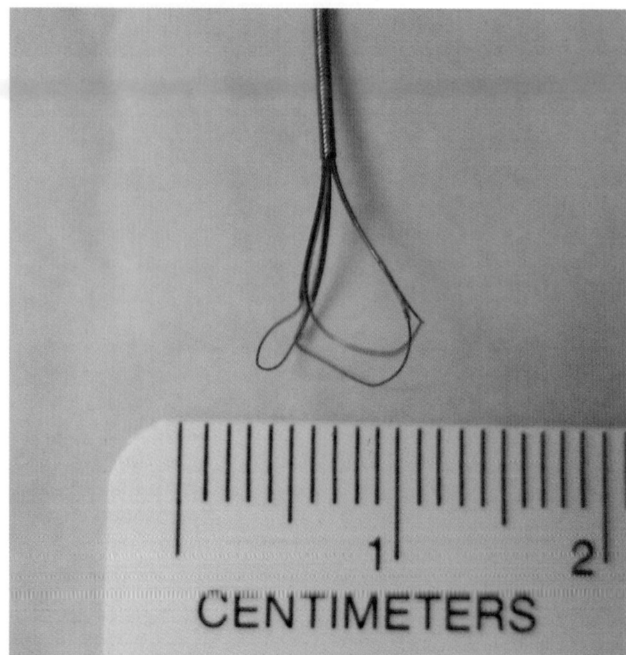

Figure 33.1 Open ended stone basket.

Stone Basketing

In some animals, the stone is too large for voiding urohydropropulsion but small enough to be removed with cystoscopic-guided basket removal, in which case a stone retrieval basket is used to entrap and remove the stone transurethrally. The main risk is wedging of uroliths too large to fit through the urethra during attempts at removal. Avoid firm traction on the stone basket if the urolith does not pass easily. Open-ended baskets (Figure 33.1) allow for easy release of larger uroliths within the urethra to convert to laser lithotripsy if needed. Similar to VUH, basket extraction is highly successful with proper case selection of uroliths smaller than the urethral diameter.

Laser Lithotripsy

Temporary urethral swelling from multiple passes of the endoscope transurethrally is the most common complication, requiring 24 hours of catheterization. This is most common in female dogs and multiple endoscopic passages. Other potential complications include urethral tears, bladder rupture during VUH, urethral strictures, and excessive bleeding. The likelihood of success with laser lithotripsy is directly related to the number and size of uroliths relative to the diameter of the urethra. With proper case selection, all uroliths can be fragmented by laser lithotripsy and removed in 87% of male dogs and 100% of female dogs. See Table 33.1 for guidelines on case selection for laser lithotripsy.

PCCL

There are few risks with this technique other than those that are associated with routine cystotomy. It is very important to be confident of the bladder location on initial digital palpation because of limited visualization. This procedure should never be done in the face of an active urinary tract infection, as the abdomen is not able to be flushed before closure. Urine leakage is kept to a minimum with the use of the Endotip screw trocar with diaphragm (Figure 33.2). If an infection is identified before this procedure, appropriate antibiotic therapy for 3 to 5 days prior to treatment is recommended. The main risk with this procedure is the leakage of urine due to inappropriate incision closure. This is avoided by carefully leak testing the incision after the procedure is complete. A potential complication would be the failure to removal all stone fragments. Because of the excellent visualization before and after the procedure, this risk is far lower than that reported with any other stone removal procedure (<3% versus 10–20%). The main benefit of this procedure is the ability to provide urethroscopy and cystoscopy with improved visualization of the entire lower urinary tract to ensure all stone fragments are removed. The operator should be sure they have appropriate scopes to allow this to occur.

Equipment

Cystoscopes are typically used for all of the minimally invasive stone removal procedures aside from VUH in male dogs. Using the cystoscope to fill the bladder/urethra in female dogs during VUH expedites the procedure. An appropriate diameter 30 degree rigid cystoscope is recommended for female dogs (1.9, 2.7, or 4mm)[1–3] and cats (1.9mm)[1] and 7.5–8.1 Fr flexible ureteroscope[4] for male dogs over 6kg, as previously described in Chapter 2.

Stone retrieval baskets[5–7] come in various shapes and sizes (Figure 33.1 and Chapter 2). An open-ended basket is useful for larger uroliths that will not fit through the urethra.[8] The urolith can easily be entrapped in the urinary bladder and then released within the urethra for laser lithotripsy of the urolith in the urethral lumen. Standard 4-wire stone baskets are more difficult to disengage from the urolith within the urethra than open-ended baskets.

A Holmium:YAG (yttrium, aluminum, garnet) laser is most commonly used for laser lithotripsy.[9] The Hol:YAG laser, as discussed in other chapters, works at a wavelength of 2,100nm, has a pulsed-wave activity resulting in an intermittent surge of pulsing energy. The laser fibers available for the Hol:YAG are 200, 400, 600, and 1000µm.

The PCCL procedure requires the rigid and flexible cystoscopes, as described above, with various stone retrieval baskets, and a 6mm Endotip screw trocar[10] (Figure 33.2). A 10mm trocar can also be helpful for larger stones when necessary.

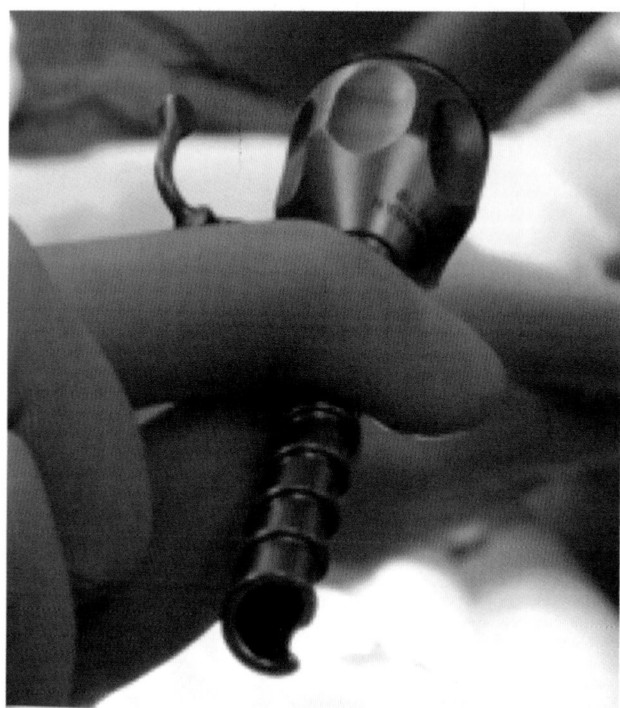

Figure 33.2 Endotip screw trocar that is used during the percutaneous cystolithotomy procedure (PCCL).

Patient Preparation

- Urinalysis and urine culture within 2 weeks
- CBC/serum biochemistry profile preoperatively
- Day of procedure-abdominal radiographs
- Prepuce/vulva flush with chlorhexidine solution.

Procedure

Voiding Urohydropropulsion

The patient is prepped for aseptic catheterization or cystoscopy to fill the urinary bladder. The hair around the vulva or prepucial opening is clipped and cleaned using chlorhexidine scrub and sterile saline rinses similar to surgical preparation. The prepuce or vulva is rinsed two to three times with dilute chlorhexidine solution. Next, the urinary bladder is filled with sterile isotonic crystalloid solution such as 0.9% saline either via cystoscopy or by urinary catheterization. The urinary bladder should be filled until it is moderately turgid. The bladder should not be over-distended to avoid inducing bleeding from damage to the bladder mucosa. The authors prefer to fill the bladder by gravity to less than 80 cmH_2O pressure. It is important to know the bladder filling capacity for the patient, which is typically between 10–20ml/kg. The dog is positioned so that the spine is roughly 25–30 degrees caudal to a line perpendicular to the effects of gravity, such that a line drawn through the proximal urethra into the bladder is vertical (Figure 33.3). The bladder is agitated side to side, and time is allowed for the urocystoliths to settle in the trigone. Intravesicular pressure is gradually increased by manual compression of the bladder to initiate voiding while maintaining forceful urine flow rates to dilate the urethra and flush out the urocystoliths. The bladder is refilled with sterile saline through the cystoscope or a urinary catheter, and the process is repeated until no urocystoliths are passed with the voided fluid. Then post-procedural radiographs or cystoscopy are performed to confirm complete removal of the urocystoliths. If there are a large amount of bladder stones the voiding procedure can be done at a 45 degree angle (Figure 33.3C) so that not all of the stones travel down the urethra simultaneously, which helps to prevent urethral blockage. Then, for the following voids, the patient is placed at a 90 degree angle to the table.

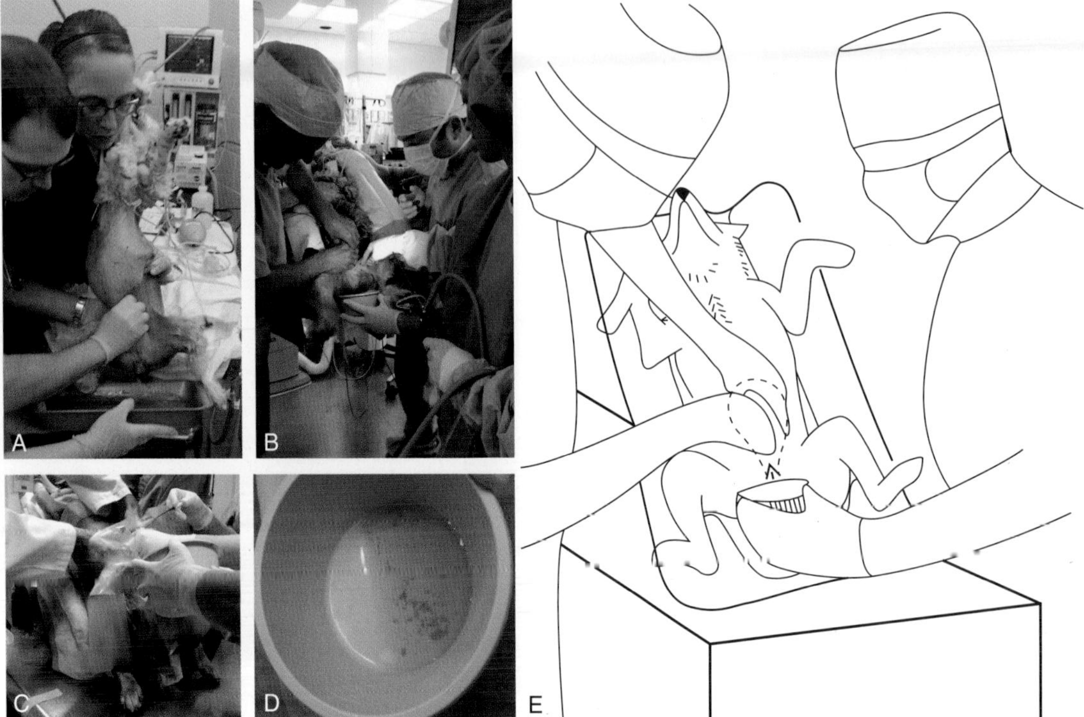

Figure 33.3 Three different dogs positioned for voiding urohydropropulsion. (A) This is a female dog. Note the large urine stream that flushes out the small uroliths along with the fluid as the bladder is expressed. (B) This is a female dog being expressed after filling of the bladder with the aid of a cystoscope. Note this patient is in a small trough, making it easier to lift during the voiding procedure at various different angles. (C) VUH in a male dog, also secured within a trough. (D) Notice the large number of small stones that were voided out during this procedure. (E) Schematic of VUH with a dog in a trough (courtesy of Dr. Alice Defrages).

Cystoscopic-guided Stone Basket Retrieval

Basket retrieval of bladder and urethral stones are routinely performed in both male and female dogs and female cats. This is accomplished by transurethral cystourethroscopy. For female dogs and cats, the dog is positioned in dorsal recumbency with the vulva positioned just beyond the end of the table. For male dogs, the dog is positioned in lateral recumbency. In Chapter 26 diagnostic cystoscopy is described in detail. The prepucial area in male dogs or the perivulvar area in female dogs and cats is clipped and prepped as discussed above for VUH. The prepuce/vulva should be covered with a sterile drape and the operator should wear sterile gloves. For therapeutic cystoscopy the operator should also wear a sterile surgical gown, cap and mask. In females, the cystoscope is positioned in the vaginal vestibule and the vestibule is distended allowing identification of the vaginal cingulum and the urethral orifice (Figure 33.4). In male dogs, the penis is exteriorized and the flexible cystoscope is passed into the penile urethra. For males or females,

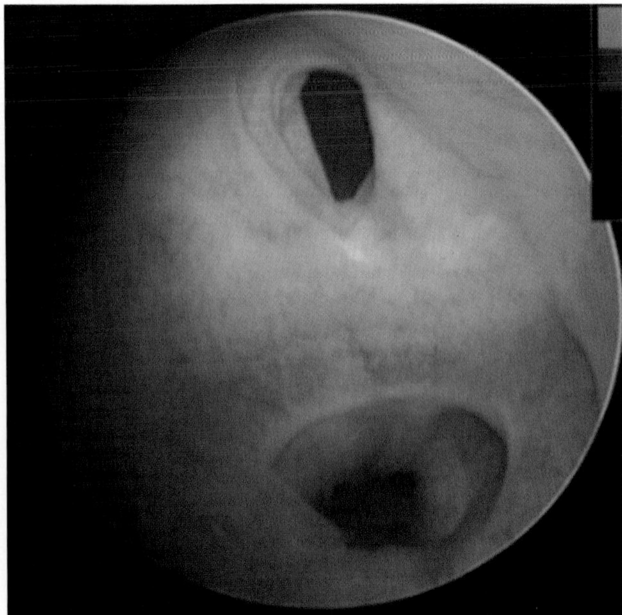

Figure 33.4 Vestibule of female dog distended with fluid as visualized through cystoscope in a dog placed in dorsal recumbency. Note the vaginal cingulum in the lower portion of the image and the urethral orifice above the cingulum.

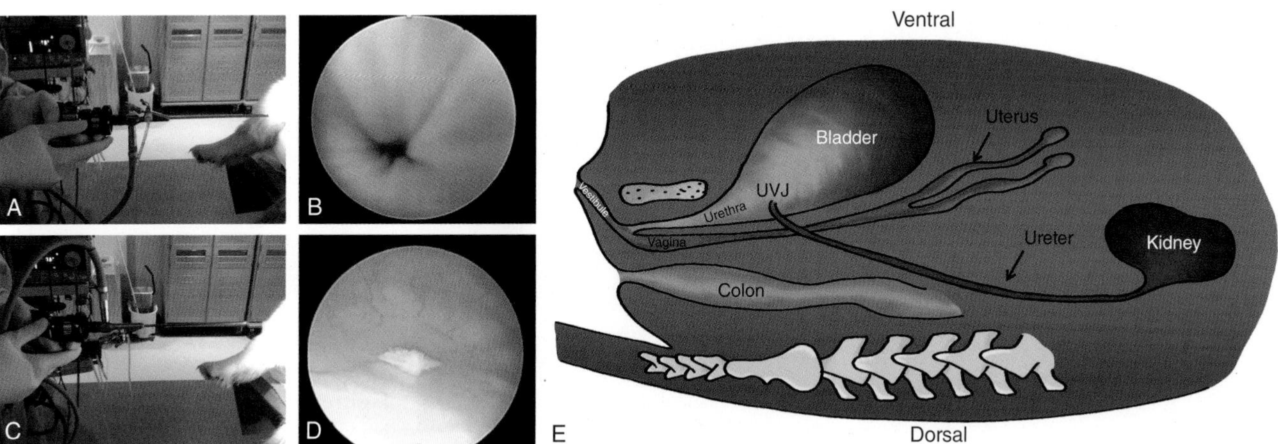

Figure 33.5 Rigid cystoscopy in dorsal recumbency in a female dog using a 30 degree angled cystoscope. (A) Endoscope outside of the patient with the 30 degree angle facing up, and the light cable facing down. (B) Notice the lumen being maintained at the bottom of the screen rather than in the center to prevent trauma to the urethral wall. (C) Endoscope outside of the dog with the 30 degree facing down, and the light cable facing up. This is best to visualize the bottom surface of the urethra or bladder. (D) Visualization of the dependant surface of the bladder wall, where the stone is sitting, facilitated by endoscope position (30 degree down). (E) Schematic of the female dog anatomy when placed in dorsal recumbency (courtesy of Dr. Alice Defarges). UVJ, ureterovesicular junction.

the cystoscope is slowly advanced up the urethra allowing fluid distension and visualization of the urethral lumen during passage of the cystoscope to the urinary bladder. It is important to remember that the female endoscope has a 30 degree angle, making it important to keep the urethral lumen toward the bottom of the image to prevent iatrogenic urethral trauma (see Chapter 26) (Figure 33.5A, B). Next the urinary bladder is drained of urine and refilled with sterile isotonic crystalloid solution such as 0.9% saline. The rigid endoscope should be turned so that the 30 degree angle is facing the dependent portion of the bladder, where the stones are sitting, while keeping the camera in place (Figure 33.5C, D). The largest urocystoliths is visualized and entrapped in the stone basket (Figure 33.6). The urolith is positioned near the end of the cystoscope, then slowly withdrawn through the urethra observing for passage of the urolith through the urethra without the stone engaging the urethral mucosa. If the urolith is too large to pass through the urethra, the urethral mucosa engages then bulges towards the cystoscope and tension is noted on the basket indicating that the urolith is becoming lodged in the urethra. If this occurs, avoid firm traction on the stone basket if the urolith does not pass easily to prevent wedging it in the urethra and causing trauma. Irregular stones may be able to be repositioned with their long axis parallel to the urethral lumen and attempt to basket extract the urolith again. If basket extraction is not possible, the cystoscope should be re-advanced towards the urinary bladder and the urolith released from the basket, then the urolith may be fragmented by laser lithotripsy (see below). If laser lithotripsy is not available, then the urolith should be placed back into the urinary bladder and removed by PCCL or traditional cystotomy. Urocystoliths of less than 4–5 mm in female dogs and less than 2–3 mm in female cats can be routinely retrieved by basket extraction, depending on the size of the patient; in male dogs stones typically need to be less than 2–3 mm to be retrieved, depending on the size of the patient. After the procedure topical bupivacaine (0.3 mg/kg diluted in saline) is usually infused into the urethra for temporary local analgesia.

Laser Lithotripsy

Laser lithotripsy is typically performed by fragmentation of uroliths using a Hol:YAG laser. Cystoscopy is performed and an appropriate diameter laser fiber is advanced through the working channel of the cystoscope until it touches the stone. The recommended sizes are 200 µm for the flexible cystoscope and 1.9 mm rigid cystoscope, 365–400 µm for the 2.7 mm cystoscope and 600–1000 µm for the 4 mm rigid cystoscope. The laser fiber should not be in contact with the bladder or urethral mucosa during laser lithotripsy. Ideally, the laser fiber should be parallel to the mucosa and perpendicular to the stone while targeting the urolith for laser lithotripsy. Continuous irrigation with an isotonic crystalloid helps flush away stone particles and maintain visualization throughout the procedure.

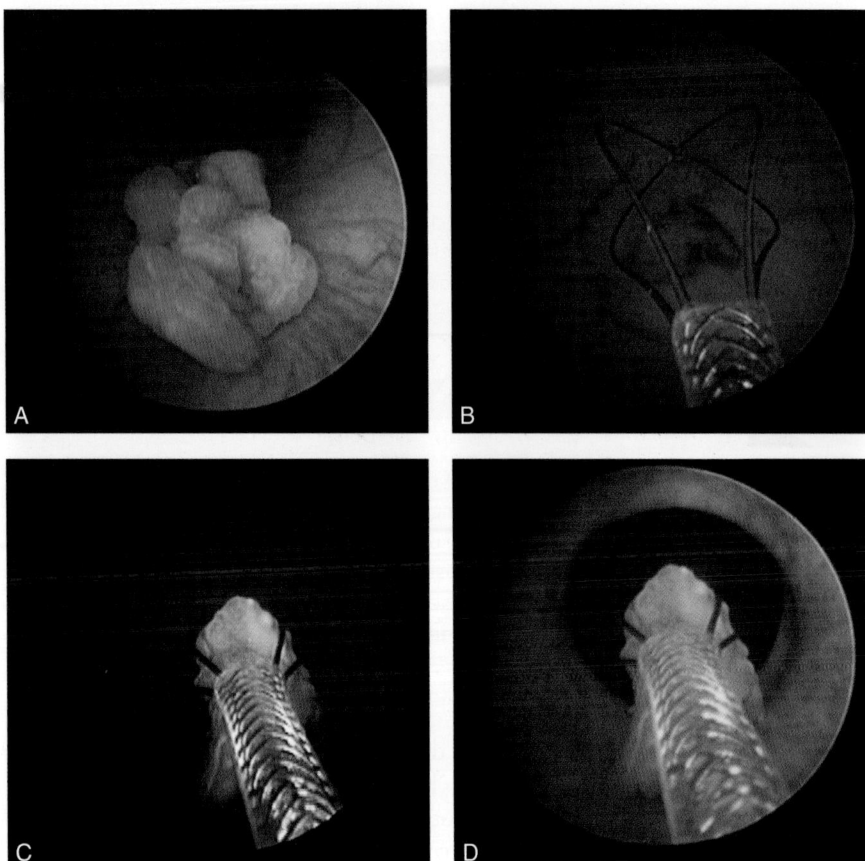

Figure 33.6 Endoscopic images of basket retrieval of a calcium oxalate bladder stone in a female dog that is placed in dorsal recumbency. (A) Cystoscopic image of calcium oxalate urocystolith within urinary bladder. (B) A four-wire stone basket opened above the urocystolith. (C) Urocystolith entrapped in stone basket and positioned near end of cystoscope for basket extraction. (D) The urocystolith in the stone basket being withdrawn into the proximal urethra. Note that the urolith is smaller than the urethral diameter and the urolith is not engaging the urethral mucosa.

If the cystoscope is large enough to occlude the urethra, then care must be taken not to overdistend the bladder and cause injury or rupture of the bladder wall. Monitoring bladder size throughout the procedure is essential. Likewise, bleeding from overdistension or direct laser injury to the mucosa should be avoided because the resultant blot clots tend to trap stone fragments and prevent removal of the fragments by VUH at the end of the procedure. The stone is fragmented until the stone fragments are small enough to be removed normograde through the urethral orifice, by a combination of basket extraction and VUH (Figure 33.7). This process is useful for cystic and urethral calculi in dogs and cats, as well as for renal calculi in dogs (see Chapter 27). Laser lithotripsy and removal of urethral stones is easier than laser fragmentation of urocystoliths, especially in male dogs. Therefore, the authors prefer to move smaller urocystoliths into the urethra, release the stone in the urethra and perform laser lithotripsy within the urethral lumen. Dogs with urethroliths that have been present for weeks or months often have mucosal proliferations (Figure 33.7D and Figure 33.8) or strictures that may make removal of uroliths proximal to the narrowing of the urethra more difficult by these transurethral techniques.

Laser settings vary based on urolith location and hardness of the uroliths. For female animals, initial laser settings for fragmentation of urocystoliths are usually 0.6–0.8 J and 10 Hz. If the urolith is not fragmenting appropriately, then increasing the Hz increases the speed of fragmentation. For very hard calcium oxalate monohydrate uroliths, increasing the power may be required to fragment the uroliths. For urethral stones, the authors prefer to start at 0.6 J and 6–8 Hz and increase frequency as needed to achieve fragmentation of the uroliths. The speed and efficiency of laser lithotripsy increases with increased operator experience.

All canine and feline stone types can be fragmented effectively with laser lithotripsy. Success rates in stone retrieval in female dogs with laser lithotripsy are superior to that of male dogs (100% and 87%, respectively) (Adams et al, 2008).

PCCL

Animals are placed under general anesthesia and positioned in dorsal recumbency. The location of the urinary bladder apex is determined and marked for the appropriate place for the abdominal incision. The patient's abdomen and prepuce/vulva are clipped,

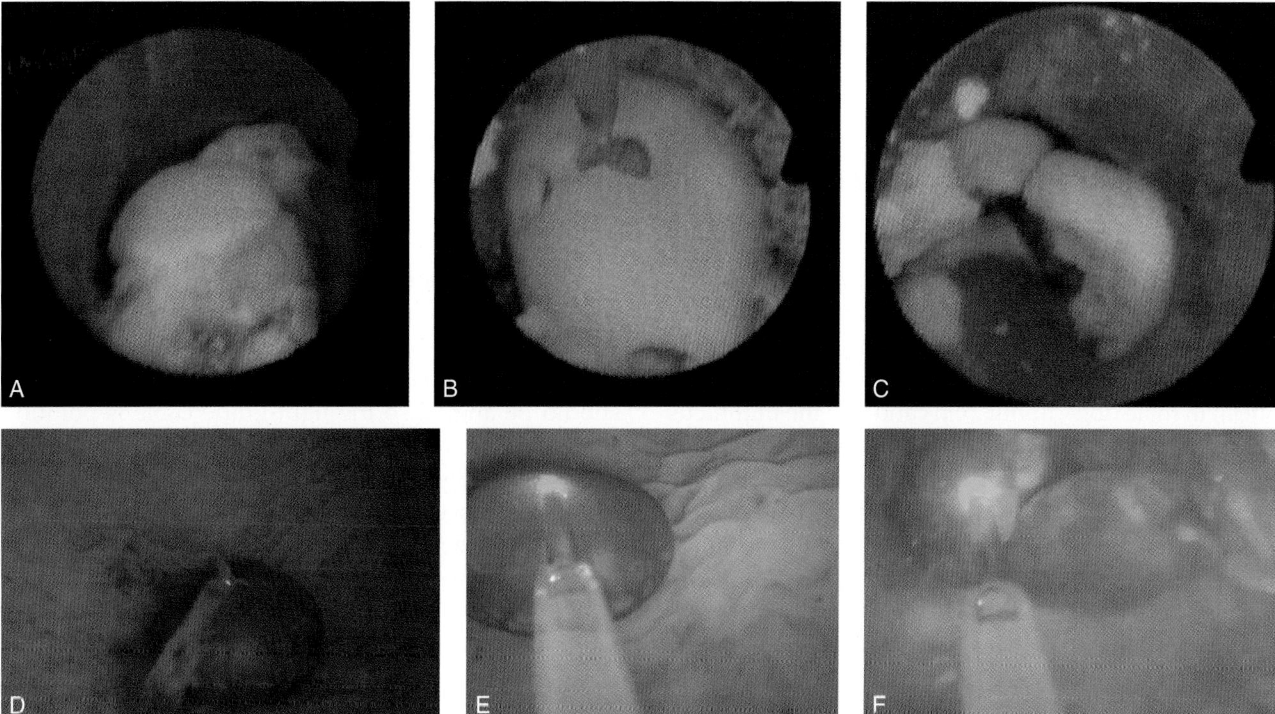

Figure 33.7 Cystoscopic images of stones in two dogs during laser lithotripsy. (A–C) is a urethrolith in a male dog and (D–F) is a urocystolith in a female dog. (A) A partially obstructive urethrolith in male dog. Analysis of the urolith fragments revealed a compound urolith composed of layers of calcium oxalate, struvite and calcium phosphate. (B) Laser lithotripsy of the urethrolith. Note that the laser fiber is in direct contact with the urolith surface and several areas of the urolith had laser damage. Also note small dust like stone fragments coating the urethral wall that have been cleared from stone surface by irrigation. (C) Laser lithotripsy has fragmented the urethrolith into multiple fragments smaller than the urethral diameter. The largest fragment was removed by basket extraction and the smaller fragments were flushed out of the urethra normograde by bladder compression. (D) A bladder stone in the bladder of a small female dog. Notice the polypoid lesion on the bladder wall next to the stone. (E) The laser fiber is in contact with the stone prior to fragmentation. Because the stone is flat the laser fiber is used to place pressure on the surface of the stone during careful fragmentation. (F) The stone fragmented into three parts that could be retrieved through the urethra with a stone basket.

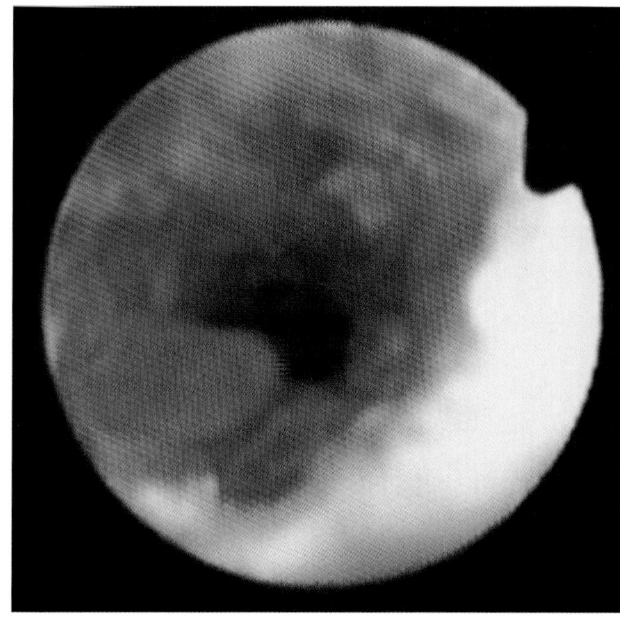

Figure 33.8 Proliferative polyp-like structures in the urethral lumen at the site of prior long-term urethrolith that was removed by laser litiptripsy. Note the narrowing of the urethral lumen at the site of the mucosal proliferation.

asceptically prepared, and draped in, as for routine surgery. A urethral catheter (3.5 to 8 Fr) is placed in male dogs and cats, and sterile saline is infused into the urinary bladder to accurately confirm and palpate the location of the apex. Care should be taken to avoid overdistension of the bladder, as the bladder capacity is typically (10–15 ml/kg). In female dogs and cats this is not typically done and the apex is determined based on previous abdominal radiographs. A small ventral midline skin incision, approximately 1.0 to 2.0 cm in length is made over the bladder apex. This incision is typically just cranial to the prepuce or slightly parapreputial in male dogs, about 2 cm caudal to the umbilicus in female dogs, and just caudal to the umbilicus in male and female cats. A 1–1.5-cm incision is made into the abdominal cavity through the linea alba to accept one finger for digital palpation of the full bladder. A Gelpy forcep is placed in the abdominal incision. Once the bladder is identified, the urinary bladder is emptied through the urethral catheter (in males) so that the vesicle location can be confirmed during digital palpation. The bladder apex is grasped atraumatically with forceps or one finger and brought to the level of the incision. Three stay sutures are placed in a triangle at the apex using 3–0 or 4–0 polydioxanone (one apical and two lateral) (Figure 33.9). The bladder is pulled to the abdominal incision with the stay sutures and the incision is packed with dry gauze reduce urine contamination. Using a #11 scalpel blade, a stab incision is made into the bladder lumen between the stay sutures. A 6-mm metallic Endotip screw trocar,[10] with a diaphragm, is advanced from the stab incision into the bladder lumen angled toward the urethra. The cap is unscrewed from the trocar and the urine is drained with a pool tip suction. The apical stay suture and trocar should be retracted cranially throughout the procedure to keep tension on the bladder. A rigid (2.7-mm, 30-degree lens) cystoscope is advanced through the trocar into the urinary bladder with saline irrigation until the bladder is appropriately distended, aiming caudally toward the trigone/urethral lumen. Care should be taken to avoid over-distention as that will result in hemorrhage and poor visualization. The scope should be angled so the light-guide cable is pointing up to avoid getting caught up on the sternum during cystoscopy (Figure 33.10 and Figure 33.11). The entire mucosal surface of the bladder and proximal urethra can be visualized, and the location and number of uroliths are identified. (Figure 33.10) Slow saline irrigation is used to maintain bladder distension and visibility while tension is maintained on the apex to keep the stone fragments and debris at the trigone for removal.

In female dogs and cats a guidewire can be passed in an antegrade manner, down the urethra and out the vulva so a urinary catheter can then be advanced into the bladder over the wire for irrigation. To aid in passage the tip of the urinary catheter should be cut off so that it is easily passed over the guidewire. The catheter should also be flushed with saline prior to advancing over the wire.

If there are many small fragments the scope is removed and the pool suction is used to suction the

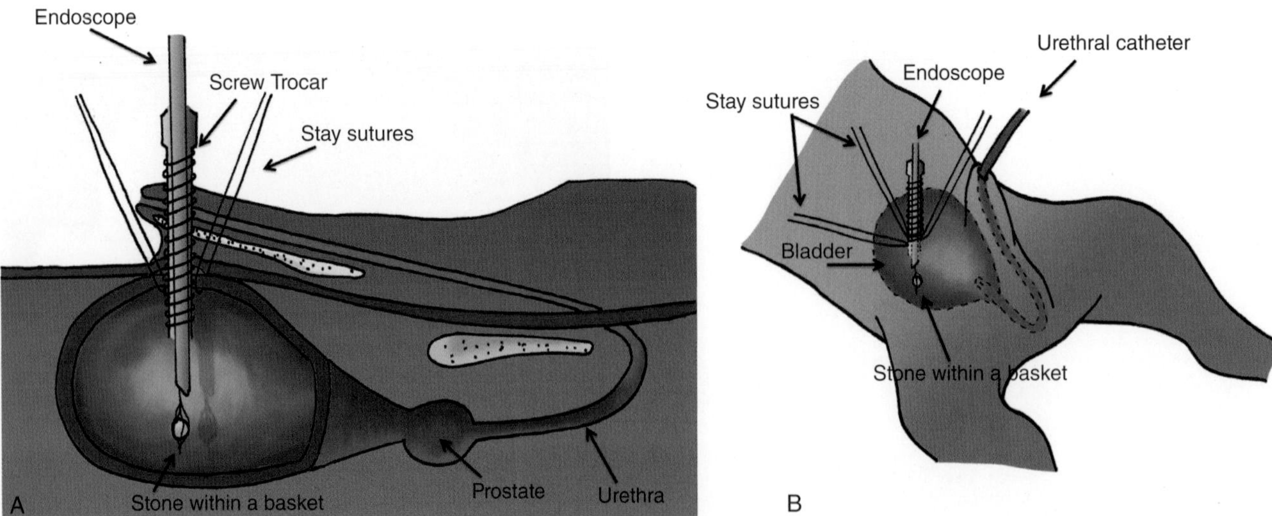

Figure 33.9 Percutaneous cystolithotomy (PCCL). (A) Schematic of this procedure showing the small incision bringing the bladder up to the body wall for insertion of a screw trocar and the endoscope with a basket retrieval of the stone. This approach allows for continual distention and superior visualization (courtesy of Dr. Alice Defarges). (B) Schematic from a ventral projection showing the same as (A) (courtesy of Dr. Alice Defarges).

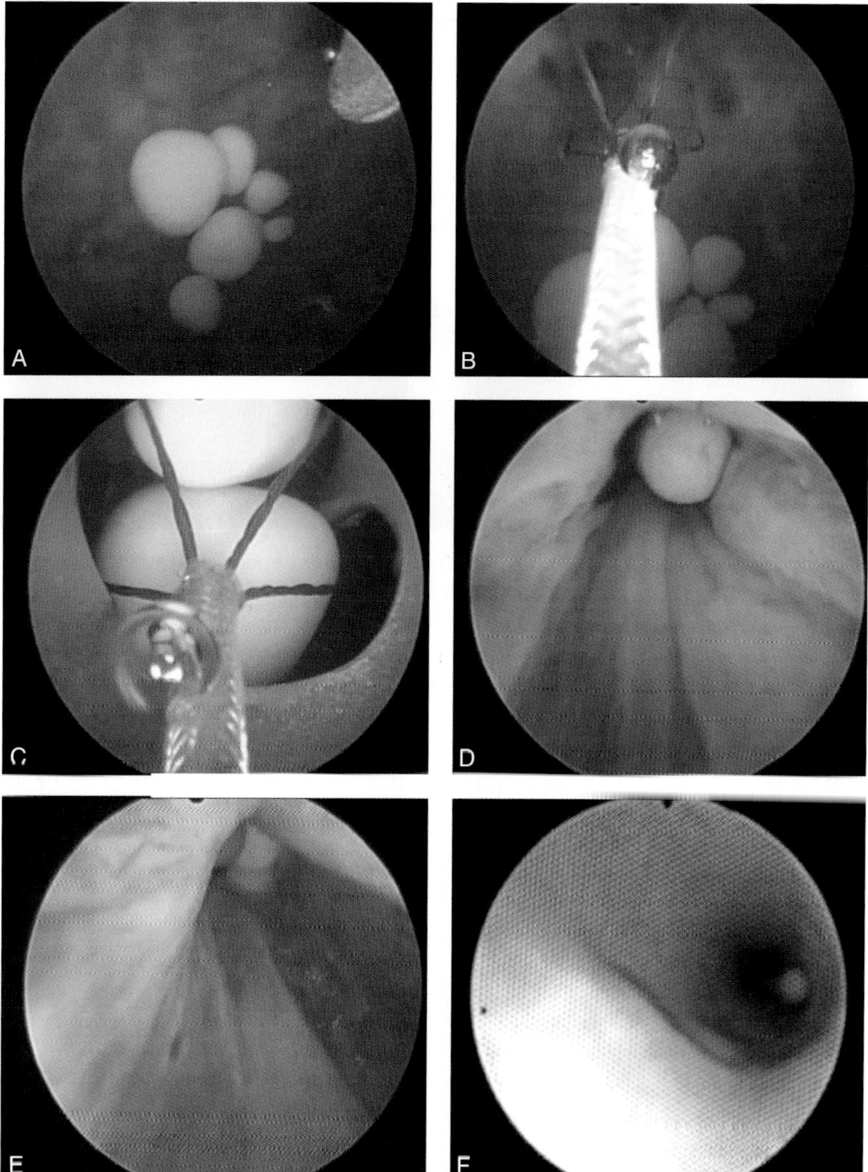

Figure 33.10 Percutaneous cystolithotomy procedure in a dog. (A) Antegrade cystoscopic image through the screw trocar from the apex looking caudal to the trigone, where a pile of calcium oxalate monohydrate stones are sitting. (B) Stone retrieval basket through the working channel of the cystoscope which will entrap the stones and remove them through the trocar, without traumatizing the bladder mucosa. (C) Two stones in the basket as they are pulled through the trocar. (D) Antegrade urethroscopy into the prostatic urethra. Notice the red rubber urinary catheter that is pulled into the urethra to assist in flushing any stones back into the bladder that could be stuck in the urethra. (E) Urethroscopy in the prostatic urethra. Notice the prostatic ductules (small slits) and two stones entrapped between the red rubber catheter and urethral wall. These will be retrieved by the basket. (F) Antegrade urethroscopy using the flexible cystoscope in the penile urethra. Notice the red rubber catheter is pulled back into the distal penile urethra as the flexible endoscopy is advanced down the urethra to confirm all stone fragments have been removed.

saline through the port, while the urinary catheter is used to irrigate the bladder and urethra vigorously. Then the scope is replaced into the bladder, and the remaining larger stones are retrieved with a stone retrieval basket guided through the working channel of the cystoscope (Figure 33.10). For stones larger than the trocar (6 mm), the stone is entrapped into the stone basket and pulled to the end of the trocar. Then, the trocar, scope and basket are all removed from the bladder together, suctioning at the incision to avoid leakage of fluid into the abdomen. Once the stone is at the incision the stone is carefully manipulated through

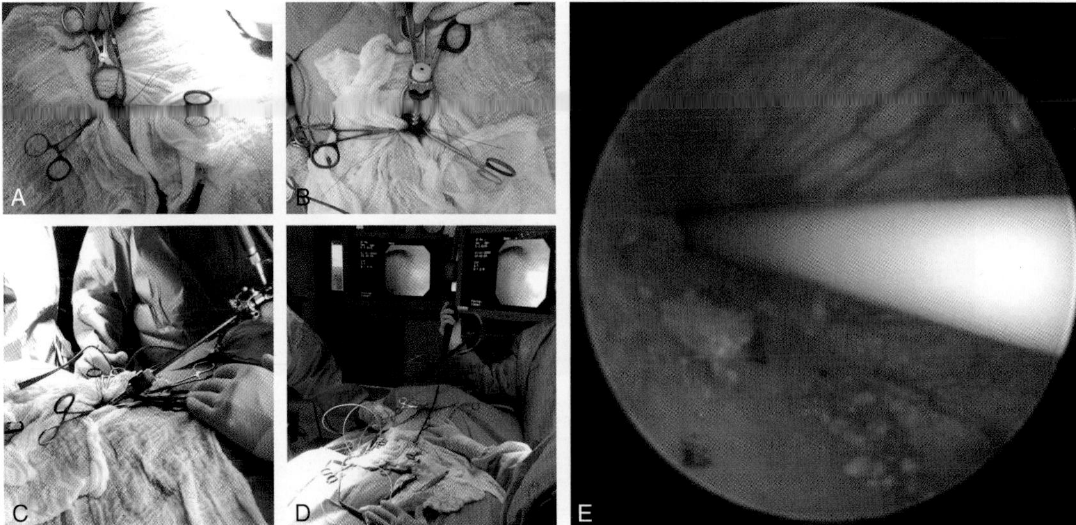

Figure 33.11 PCCL procedure in a dog. (A) Image of the urinary bladder exposed at the ventral abdominal incision being suspended with stay sutures. (B) The PCCL port placed into the bladder lumen at the apex. (C) The rigid cystoscope inserted into the bladder lumen through the port. (D) The flexible endoscope visualizing the flexible urethra in this male dog in an antegrade manner. (E) Antegrade cystoscopic image visualizing the trigone of the bladder with stones in the dependent portion of the bladder. A urethral catheter is seen entering the bladder from the urethra. Notice the left ureteral opening at the trigone.

the incision until retracted. This typically does not extend the incision due to the elasticity of the bladder. The bladder wall stretches while the stone is removed. Once the stone is out the trocar is screwed back into the incision and the scope is replaced.

Finally, after the bladder is free of stone material, the urethra should always be evaluated with the cystoscope (flexible in males and rigid in females). This is done in an antegrade manner using a 1.9 mm scope in female cats, a 2.7 mm scope in female dogs, and a 7.5–8 Fr flexible ureteroscope in male dogs. The endoscope is advanced distally down the length of the urethra to ensure that no stone fragments remain, while the urethra is simultaneously flushed in a retrograde manner through the urinary catheter (Figure 33.10D–F). This in not possible in male cats so the 1.9 mm rigid scope is advanced to the mid/distal urethra and careful flushing is performed distally to ensure no stones are left behind. In male dogs the entire urethra can typically be visualized with the flexible scope, and if <4 kg the scope can usually get to the mid/proximal os penis.

During this procedure the bladder can be explored carefully for polyps or masses, which can be removed with the laser or sampled, if necessary. Once the scope and trocar are removed, the incision is closed with the use of 3–0 or 4–0 poliglecaprone (Monocryl) suture in a simple interrupted or cruciate pattern. The abdominal incision is closed routinely in three layers without skin sutures.

In addition to stone retrieval, this technique can be utilized for evaluation of bladder polyps and tumors, ureteral or renal bleeding, or ureteral access for ureteral stent placement. Patients are typically discharged the same day as this procedure with a 3 day course of antibiotic therapy and tramadol (3–5 mg/kg BID PO).

Prognosis

VUH and Stone Basket Retrieval

The prognosis for complete urolith removal is excellent if the proper size stone(s) and patient are chosen for each procedure.

Laser Lithotripsy

The prognosis for complete urolith removal by laser lithotripsy is excellent in female dogs with 100% of all stone fragments removed in one recent study. In male dogs, complete urolith removal was only possible in 87% of patients. Therefore for male dogs with larger numbers of stones, PCCL is preferred over laser lithotripsy.

PCCL

In a recent study published on this procedure (Runge et al, 2011) less than 3% of patients had a stone fragment found on postoperative radiographs. This is likely because we routinely perform antegrade urethroscopy, allowing confirmation of all stone fragment retrieval

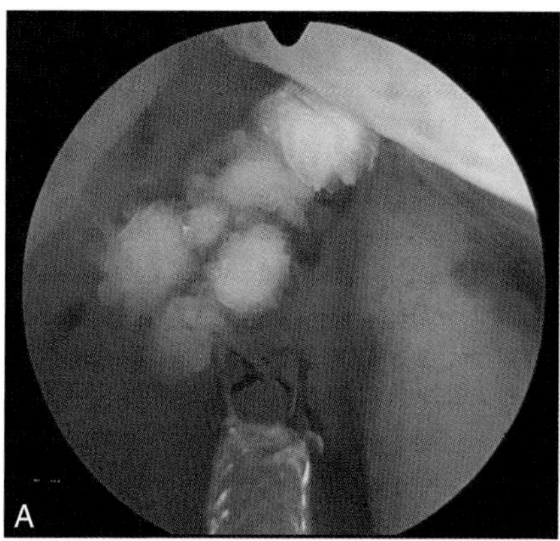

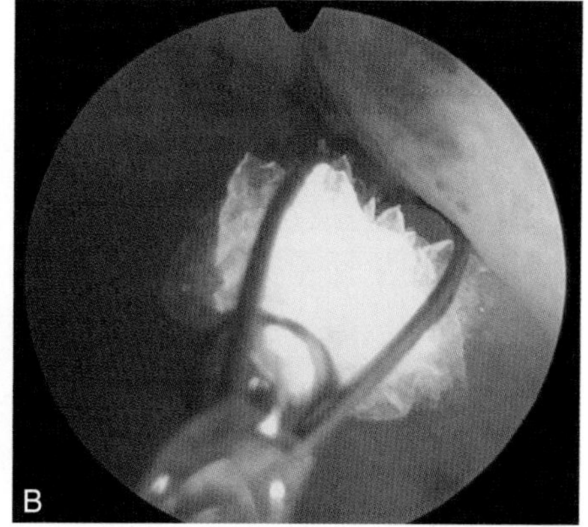

Figure 33.12 PCCL in a male cat. Notice the pile of small, sharp, calcium oxalate dehydrate stones. (A) The stone basket is in the working channel of the endoscope and used to entrap each stone individually. (B) One of the stones in the basket prior to removal through the trocar.

prior to closure. The authors do recommend that if a post-stone removal cystoscopy is not possible due to poor visualization or bladder distension difficulty then a postoperative radiograph should always be taken to ensure appropriate stone retrieval. Otherwise, a radiograph is not routinely performed after PCCL provided complete visualization of the bladder lumen confirms complete urolith removal.

Special Considerations

Minimally invasive management of urolithiasis in veterinary medicine is following the trend seen in human medicine. Over the past 10 years, the veterinary community has made great strides in adapting the technology used for humans to be more applicable to small animal veterinary patients. Conditions that were traditionally considered major therapeutic dilemmas, like stone recurrences and urethral obstructions, now have new, effective, and safe options.

Notes

1. Rigid endoscope, 1.9-mm 30° lens, Karl Storz Endoscopy, Culver City, CA.
2. Rigid endoscope, 2.7-mm 30° lens, Richard Wolf, Vernon Hills, IL.
3. Rigid endoscope, 4-mm 30° lens, Karl Storz Endoscopy, Culver City, CA.
4. Flex X^2 Flexible ureteroscope, Karl Storz Endoscopy, Culver City, CA.
5. Dimension® Basket, 2.4 Fr, Bard Medical, Covington, GA.
6. N-Compass™ stone retrieval basket, Cook Medical, Bloomington, IN.
7. Sur-Catch® NT, No Tip Nitinol Basket, Olympus/Gyrus ACMI, Southborough MA.
8. N Gage, Cook Medical, Bloomington, IN
9. 200 or 400–μm Holmium:YAG laser fiber and 30-W Ho:YAG Lithotrite, Odyssey, Convergent Inc. Alameda, CA.
10. Endotip Trocar, Karl Storz Endoscopy, Culver City, CA.

References

Adams LG, Berent AC, Moore GE, et al (2008) Use of laser lithotripsy for fragmentation of uroliths in dogs: 73 cases (2005–2006). *J Am Vet Med Assoc* 232, 1680–7.

Runge JJ, Berent AC, and Mayhew PD (2011) Transvesicular percutaneous cysotolithotomy for the retrieval of cystic and urethral calculi in dogs and cats: 27 cases (2006–2008). *J Am Vet Med Assoc* 239, 344–9.

Suggested Reading

Bevan JM, and Lulich JP (2009) Comparison of laser lithotripsy and cystotomy for the management of dogs with urolithiasis, *J Am Vet Med Assoc* 234,1286–1294

Grant DC, Harper TA, and Werre SR (2010) Frequency of incomplete urolith removal, complications, and diagnostic imaging following cystotomy for removal of uroliths from the lower urinary tract in dogs: 128 cases (1994–2006). *J Am Vet Med Assoc* 236, 763–766.

Grant DC, Werre SR, and Gevedon ML (2008) Holmium: YAG laser lithotripsy for urolithiasis in dogs. *J Vet Intern Med* 22, 534–539.

Lulich JP, Osborne CA, Albasan H, et al (2009) Efficacy and safety of laser lithotripsy in fragmentation of urocystoliths and urethroliths for removal in dogs, *J Am Vet Med Assoc* 234, 1279–1285.

Lulich JP, Osborne CA, Carlson M, et al. (1993) Nonsurgical removal of urocystoliths in dogs and cats by voiding urohydropropulsion. *J Am Vet Med Assoc* 203, 660–663.

Thieman-Mankin KM, Ellison GW, Jeyapaul CJ, et al. (2012) Comparison of short-term complication rates between dogs and cats undergoing appositional single-layer or inverting double-layer cystotomy closure: 144 cases (1993–2010). *J Am Vet Med Assoc* 240, 65–68.

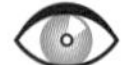

Video clips to accompany this chapter can be found in the online material at **www.wiley.com/go/weisse/vet-image-guided-interventions**

portion of the urethra versus the entire abnormal portion of the urethra; the former resulting in a shorter stent than the latter, but perhaps an increased risk of requiring a repeat stenting in the future as the tumor progresses. Patients with prostatic tumors anecdotally seem to have more aggressive tumors and shorter survival times, and males are significantly more likely to have persistent tenesmus (~47%) following stent placement compared to females (~10%). As these dogs die from systemic disease, survival time likely depends upon the stage and progression of disease at the time of stent placement. Non-steroidal anti-inflammatory drugs (NSAIDs) and chemotherapy are strongly recommended as these medications have a significant effect on median survival times following urethral stent placement (pre-stent NSAIDs and post-stent chemotherapy MST 251 days versus 78 days [range, 7–536] without medications) (Blackburn, 2013).

Equipment

A list of recommended equipment can be found in Figure 34.1. Laser-cut, self-expanding metallic stents are most commonly used for urethral stenting procedures. Balloon-expandable stents are too rigid, risk compression, and are often very short. Mesh self-expanding stents have been used in the urethra but the foreshortening that occurs is unpredictable and could result in excessive lengths of the urethra being stented. Uncovered stents are most commonly used for tumors. Covered stents are more expensive, have larger delivery systems, may be at greater risk of migration, can cover the prostatic ducts in males, and may be associated with increased risk of infection. Covered stents are typically reserved for recurrent urethral strictures.

Urethral stenting is best performed using fluoroscopy. Digital radiography and ultrasound-guided placement have been described but these techniques are less exact and more unpredictable for precise stent placement. Urethral stents are not reconstrainable so only fluoroscopy provides real-time monitoring of both the cranial and caudal edges of the stent during deployment to ensure proper placement. Fluoroscopy entails the risk of radiation exposure so care must be taken to reduce exposure through beam collimation, reducing dose, and wearing standard radiation protection gear.

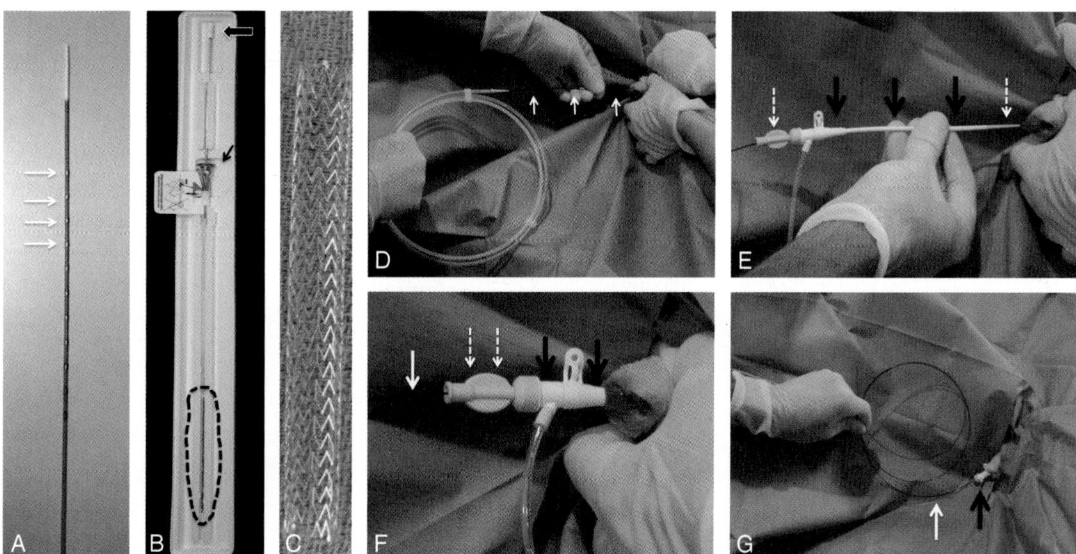

Figure 34.1 Common equipment used for urethral stenting. (A) Straight marker catheter with radiopaque marks (white arrows) 10 mm apart from the beginning of one mark to the beginning of the next mark. This catheter is usually placed within a 14 Fr red rubber catheter that is advanced into the rectum and colon. (B) Stent delivery system with constrained laser-cut, self-expandable metallic (nitinol) stent (SEMS) (black dotted line) inside the delivery sheath with Y-piece (black arrow) containing diaphragm and side-port. The hub (block arrow) is flushed with saline, as is the side-port (black arrow), prior to use in order to flush out any air. (C) A deployed urethral SEMS – these should NOT be deployed outside the patient as they are typically NON-RECONSTRAINABLE stents. (D) 0.035″ angled, hydrophilic guide wire (white arrows) advanced into urethra of a male dog. (E, F) ~7 Fr introducer sheath (black arrows) and dilator (white dotted arrow) advanced over-the-wire up to the penis and sutured to the prepuce. (G) The dilator is removed and the penis released. The sheath (black arrow) provides access throughout the procedure.

Fluoroscopic Procedure

The patient is placed under general anesthesia and positioned in lateral recumbency on a fluoroscopy table. A marker catheter[1] (Figure 34.1A) is placed within a 14 Fr red rubber catheter, introduced per rectum, and gently advanced into the descending colon under fluoroscopic guidance. The patient's prepuce or perineum/vulva are clipped, scrubbed, and draped. Long drapes are recommended to avoid contamination of the relatively long guide wires and stent delivery systems. Perioperative antibiotics are routinely used, unless the patient is already receiving systemic antibiotic therapy. Guide wire and catheter access of the urethra and urinary bladder are obtained using different techniques in male and female dogs.

Male Access

In male dogs, the penis is manually extruded from the prepuce (Figure 34.1). A 0.035″ angled, floppy-tip hydrophilic guide wire[2] is inserted into the urethral orifice and advanced into the urinary bladder under fluoroscopic guidance. A 7 or 8 Fr vascular sheath[3] and dilator are placed over the guide wire and advanced into the penile urethra. The penis is released and allowed to retract into the prepuce. The sheath is sutured to the prepuce and the dilator is removed. A 4 Fr angiographic catheter[4] is advanced over the wire and into the urinary bladder. The guide wire is removed.

Female Access

In female dogs without urethral catheters in place, access is obtained using a speculum, endoscope, or, when necessary, via percutaneous antegrade urethral access (Figure 34.2). When placing a urinary catheter in a female, cut the tip of the urinary catheter off to permit guide wire access if an interventional procedure may be anticipated. This will facilitate guide wire placement in the future. For antegrade catheterization, details are expanded upon in Chapter 40. In brief, a cystocentesis is performed with an 18-gauge over-the-needle catheter advanced trans-abdominally into the urinary bladder using either palpation or ultrasonographic guidance. The stylet is removed and the urinary bladder is partially drained if excessively full and then infused with an iohexol:saline mixture, sufficient to fluoroscopically see the outline of the urinary bladder and proximal urethra. This procedure is easier to perform with a moderate to large bladder, so avoid excessive drainage. A 0.035″ angled, floppy-tip hydrophilic guide wire is advanced through the catheter and into the urinary bladder, and under fluoroscopic guidance directed towards the bladder trigone. The wire is advanced antegrade into the urethra and out the vulva, resulting in "through-and-through" access. Once the wire is in (via either antegrade or retrograde access) a 7 Fr vascular sheath and dilator are advanced retrograde over-the-wire and into the urinary bladder. If a urethral catheter is already in place, a guide wire can be passed through the catheter when possible and coiled into the urinary bladder. The catheter is then removed over-the-wire and the

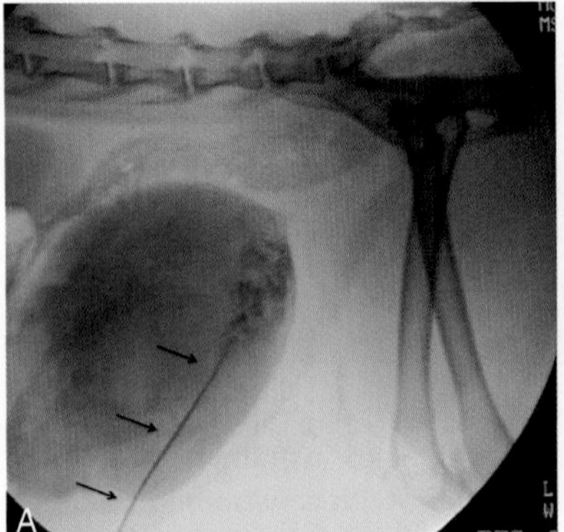

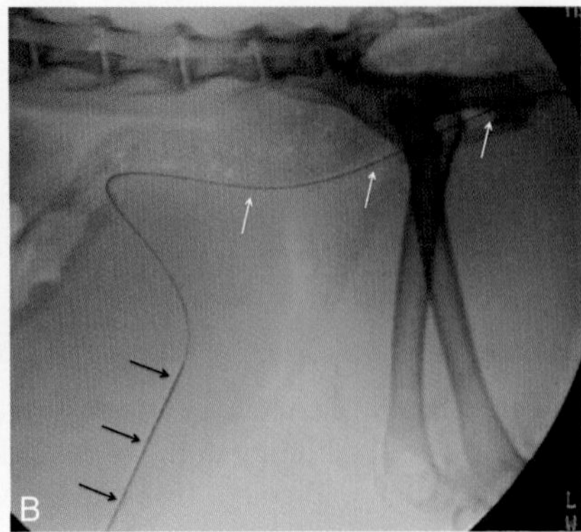

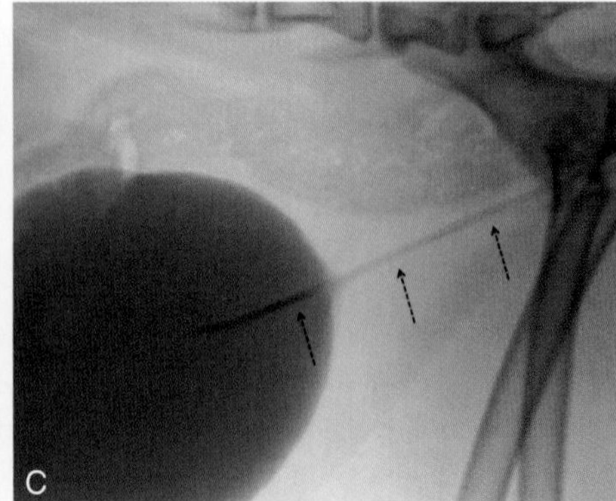

Figure 34.2 Serial lateral fluoroscopic images in a cat during percutaneous antegrade urethral access. The head is to the left in each image. (A) 18-gauge intravenous catheter (black arrows) is used for the cystocentesis to sample urine and instill iodinated contrast (iohexol) until bladder is distended and urethra is visible. (B) 0.035″ angled, hydrophilic guide wire (white arrows) advanced antegrade down the urethra. (C) Following through-and-through access, a 5 Fr catheter with the tip cut off (black dotted arrows) is advanced retrograde over-the-wire, the wire removed, and access is completed. Alternatively, the vascular introducer sheath can be placed over-the-wire and urethrograms performed to determine urethral diameter.

vascular sheath and dilator are advanced over the wire into the bladder. It is a good idea to obtain urine for a urinalysis, culture and sensitivity before adding contrast when possible. Many of these dogs have concurrent urinary tract infections.

Urethrocystogram

After achieving bladder access with the catheter (male) and/or sheath (female), the urinary bladder is distended with an approximately 50:50 mixture of iohexol[5] and sterile saline. Do not use excessive amounts of contrast or you will not be able to visualize the guide wire and stent; Use just enough contrast in your mixture so you can identify the borders of the bladder and urethra and still identify the location of your devices. In addition, it is important to completely fill the urinary bladder so you do not mistake an undistended urinary bladder for the proximal urethra. This is done using the catheter rather than the penile sheath in males as contrast will occasionally extravasate into the tumor making the urethral lumen difficult to visualize (Figure 34.3). In females this should be done using the side-port of the sheath while the wire remains coiled within the urinary bladder.

Following bladder distension, a fluoroscopy run is recorded to determine the stenosis length and normal urethral diameter. To perform this part of the procedure, the catheter (male) or sheath (female) is withdrawn into the distal urethra while continuously injecting contrast under sufficient manual pressure to maximally distend the urethra. In the females, the sheath is injected while withdrawn over-the-wire to avoid losing guide wire access (Figure 34.4) to the bladder. In males, the catheter can simply be withdrawn during the fluoroscopy run, as urethral access in males is typically easy. The length of the urethral obstruction and maximal diameter of the adjacent normal urethral lumen are extrapolated using the colonic marker catheter as a reference to account for magnification (Figure 34.5). In males, using digital subtraction angiography is often useful, as it aids in visualizing the intrapelvic urethra. This is difficult to use in female dogs due to the motion during the urethrogram. An appropriately sized stent is chosen based upon these measurements. The stent diameter is typically chosen by matching the normal urethral diameter caudal to the urethral obstruction (as cranially the urethra is often distended or within the bladder lumen. Matching (or slightly increasing) stent diameter to the urethral diameter ensures adequate mucosal apposition and minimizes chance of migration. The stent length is chosen either (1) to span the narrowed lumen but not to extend further than 1cm cranially and 1cm caudally when possible, or (2) just span the obstructed portion of the urethra. This also depends upon available stent sizes. Balloon-expandable (BEMS) or mesh self-expanding metallic stents (SEMS) can be placed but the author prefers laser-cut SEMS[6] due to ease of use, predictable and precise placement, available lengths, flexibility, biocompatibility, self-expanding nature, and known outcomes.

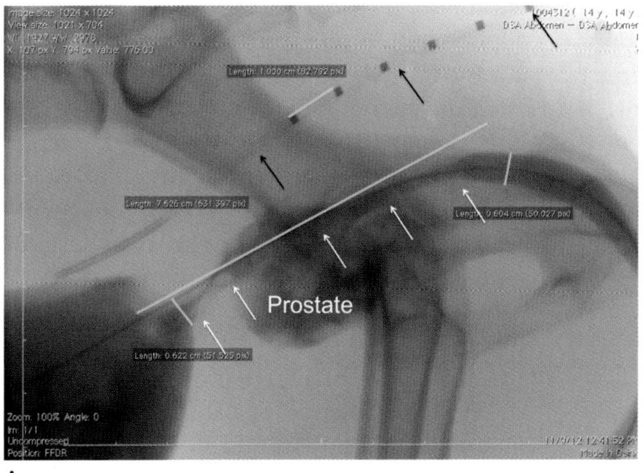

A

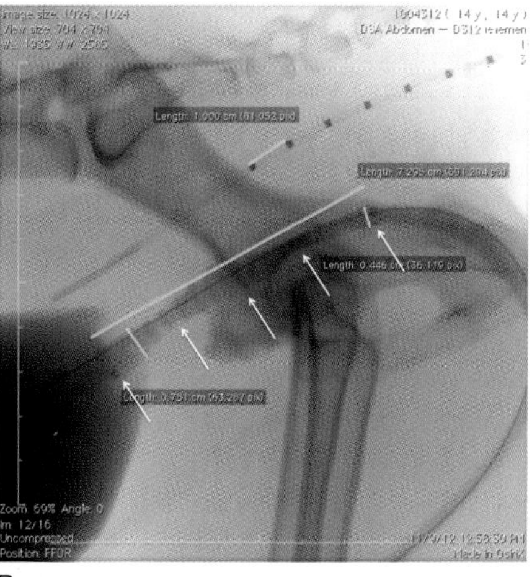

B

Figure 34.3 Lateral caudal abdominal fluoroscopic images of a dog with a prostatic tumor. The dog's head is to the left in each image. (A) The marker catheter (black arrows) is in place in the colon. The 0.035″ angled, hydrophilic guide wire is in the urethra, and the prostatic tumor is narrowing the urethra (white arrows). Notice the extravasated contrast within the prostatic tumor making identification of the urethral dorsal and ventral wall borders difficult to see. The normal urethral wall diameter is 6 mm and the length of stent necessary to extend ~10mm cranial and caudal to the obstruction is approximately 70 mm. (B) After placement of a 8 × 70 mm laser-cut SEMS (white arrows) the urethral lumen in restored.

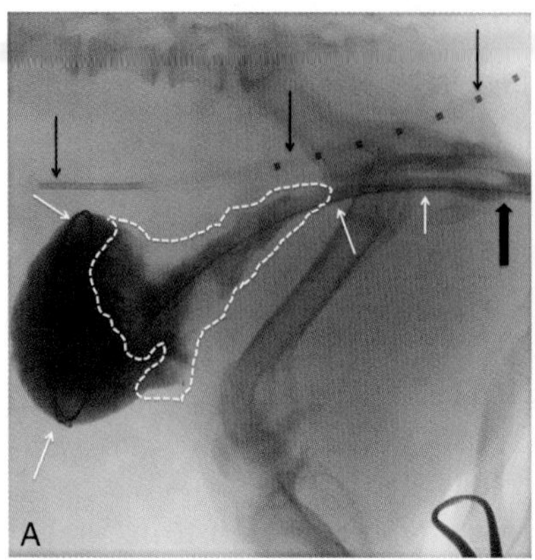

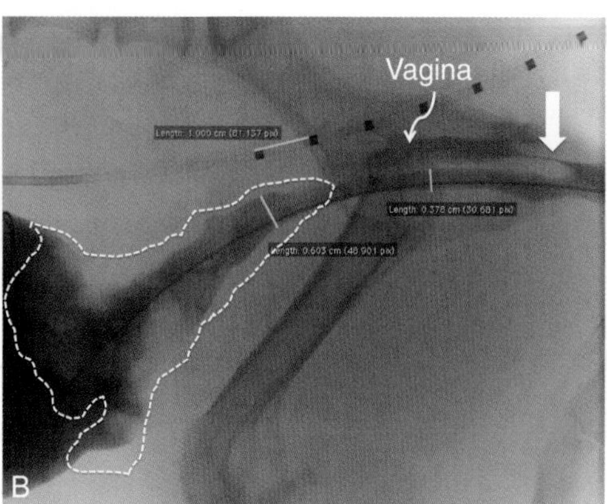

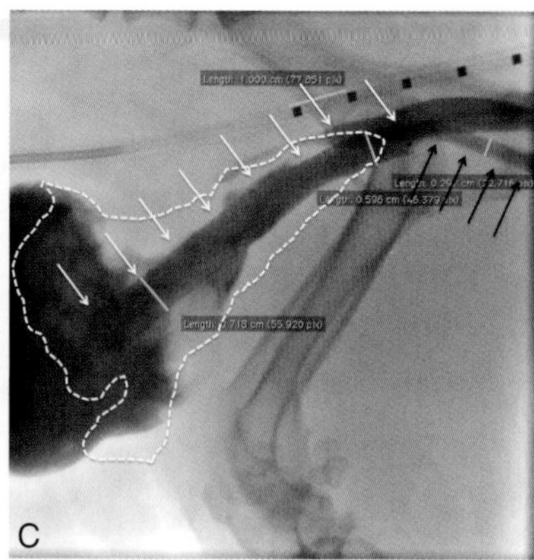

Figure 34.4 Serial lateral caudal abdominal fluoroscopic images of a female dog with urethral and bladder TCC. The dog's head is to the left in each image. (A) A marker catheter (black arrows) has been placed within a 14 Fr red rubber catheter and introduced per rectum in order to calibrate the radiographic images for magnification. A 0.035″ angled hydrophilic guide wire (white arrows) has been advanced through a 7 Fr vascular introducer sheath into the urethra and coiled in the urinary bladder. The bladder has been filled with contrast and saline and a urethrogram (white arrows) is performed as the sheath is withdrawn over the guide wire in order to maintain access to the bladder. The filling defect/obstruction caused by the tumor (white dotted lines) is apparent at the trigone and proximal urethra. The sheath has been withdrawn to the level of the urethral orifice (black block arrow). (B) Following radiographic calibration using the marker catheter the maximal diameter of the distended normal urethra is approximately 6mm. Further caudally the urethra is not sufficiently distended due to leakage of contrast into the vestibule and through the vestibulovaginal junction (white block arrow) and externally. The length of the obstruction is approximately 60–70 mm. (C) Final urethrocystogram after placement of a 8 × 70 mm laser-cut SEMS (white arrows) demonstrating re-established urethral patency. The wire has been removed but the sheath (black arrows) is still seen prior to removal. Notice the overlapping vagina filled with contrast.

SEMS Placement

SEMS are enclosed within a sheath delivery system and are therefore protected from being displaced during positioning across a stenotic lesion. In general, it should be assumed that laser-cut SEMS are *not* reconstrainable unless otherwise specified on the stent packaging. Predilation of the lesion with a PTA balloon is unnecessary. Guide wire access into the urinary bladder is obtained and the catheter (if present) is removed over-the-wire. The stent delivery system is removed from the sterile packaging, examined for any defects, and flushed with sterile saline in both the guide wire hub (proximal end of the delivery system) and the sheath (side port). Saline flushing facilitates advancement over-the-wire, moistens the stent and delivery system, and removes the air which is imperative for vascular procedures.

The stent delivery system is advanced over-the-wire under fluoroscopic guidance and positioned across the malignant obstruction. In order to deploy a laser-cut SEMS, one hand is positioned on the guide wire hub and remains still as the other hand, holding the delivery system sheath, is gently withdrawn. This allows the stent to become unsheathed. When deploying the stent within the bladder, advance the delivery system in slightly farther cranial than necessary, deploy approximately 1 cm of the stent, then withdraw the entire delivery system and stent together caudally to engage the cranial aspect of the stenosis with the open 1 cm of stent. Do *not* try this for intraurethral tumors, as once the stent partially deploys it will engage the urethral wall and it cannot be moved. The stent delivery system is withdrawn and the SEMS deployed. Maintain back tension on the delivery system while completing stent deployment in one smooth step. Make sure you monitor the caudal end of the stent and ensure you are covering the back end of the lesion. In female dogs be sure to back out the sheath prior to stent deployment to avoid opening the stent within the access sheath. Following stent deployment, the delivery system is carefully removed over-the-wire under fluoroscopic visualization to avoid engaging the stent with the delivery system nose-cone. In female dogs, keeping the sheath in the distal urethra while an assistant injects the side-port to maintain a distal urethrogram is very helpful to ensure appropriate distal end placement.

A repeat positive contrast cystourethrogram is performed to document immediate patency of the previously occluded urethra (Figure 34.4C and Figure 34.5D, E). The catheter, and sheath if present, is removed and the animal is recovered from anesthesia without a urinary catheter in place. It is best to leave the bladder slightly distended in order to watch the patient urinate soon after recovering from the procedure. Immediate postoperative radiographs may be obtained to document

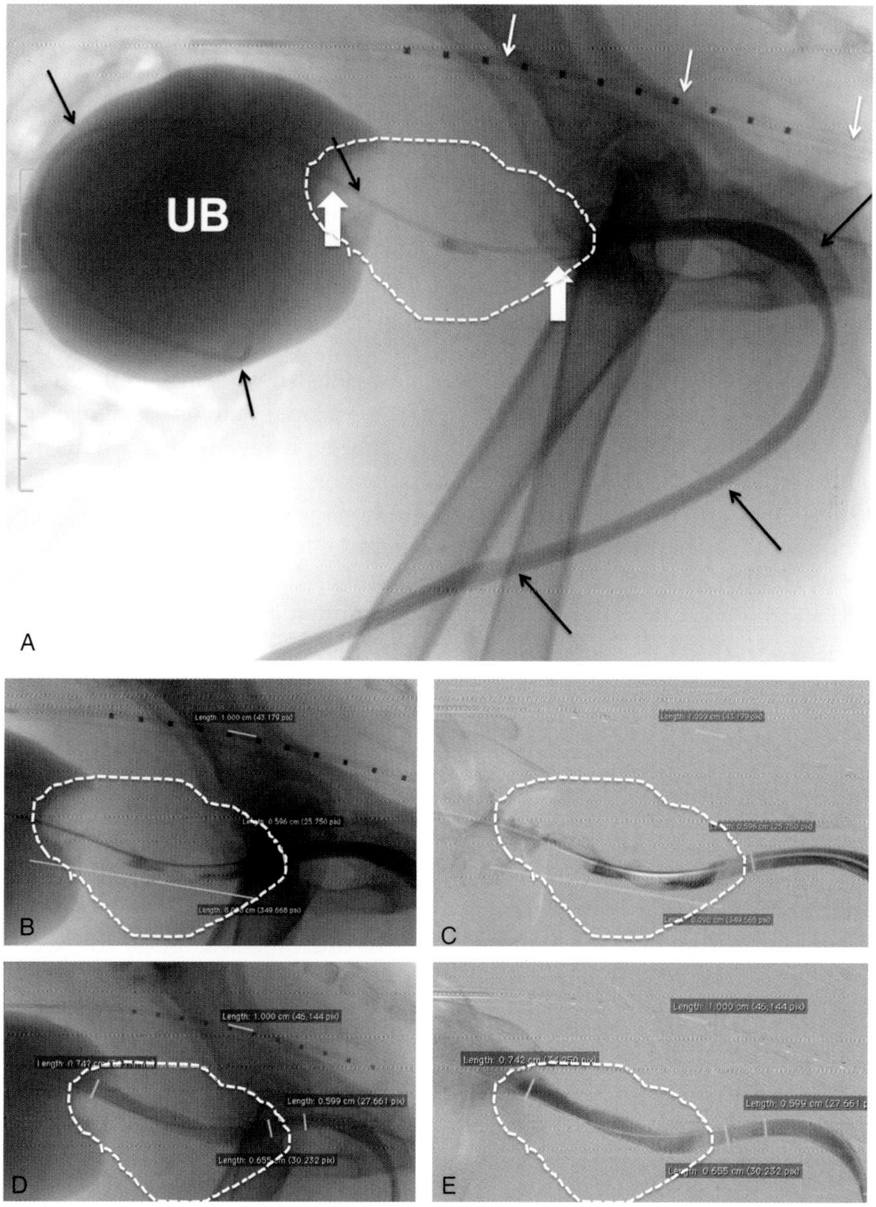

Figure 34.5 Serial lateral caudal abdominal fluoroscopic images of dog with a prostatic urethral tumor extending into the trigone. The dog's head is to the left in each image. (A) A marker catheter (white arrows) has been placed within a 14 Fr red rubber catheter and introduced per rectum in order to calibrate the radiographic images for magnification. A 4 Fr Berenstein catheter (black arrows) has been placed into the bladder over a 0.035″ angled hydrophilic wire that was subsequently removed to fill the bladder with saline and contrast. A urethrogram is performed through the sheath (alternatively the Berenstein catheter can be used) demonstrating a filling defect/obstruction caused by the tumor (white dotted lines) at the level of the trigone and proximal urethra. The urethral narrowing is observed between both white block arrows. Fluoroscopic (B) and subtracted (C) images with maximal urethral measurements showing both views can be helpful in identifying the extent of the obstruction. Maximal urethral diameter of ~6mm and necessary stent length determined to be ~80 mm. Fluoroscopic (D) and subtracted (E) contrast urethrocystogram images following 8 × 80 mm laser-cut SEMS placement demonstrating patency of the urethra through the malignant obstruction has been re-established.

stent location, positioning, and urethral integrity (lack of contrast extravasation). In over 150 procedures, no cases of urethral perforation during urethral stent placement were identified. Occasionally, intravenous fluids can be maintained overnight to maintain urine flow and minimize potential blood clot formation and obstruction though patients are routinely discharged the same day as the procedure after demonstrating the ability to urinate. Patients receive analgesics as necessary (uncommon), antibiotics until urine culture results are available, and are discharged with NSAIDs if not contraindicated.

Follow-Up

Patients are routinely discharged the day of the procedure with antibiotics (pending the culture results) and recheck appointments are generally made for ~1–2 weeks later for oncology consultation if not previously done. It is not uncommon for dogs to demonstrate initial urinary incontinence or persistent low-grade straining post-stenting, which improves over the first week. NSAIDs and chemotherapy are strongly recommended as these have a significant effect on median survival times following urethral stent placement. As urothelial carcinomas rarely have durable remissions following chemotherapy, regular patient evaluations should be recommended in order to identify progressive disease and subsequent ureteral obstructions. Careful history taking will identify problems such as the development of subsequent urethral obstructions, often characterized by incontinence (overflow) or progressive stranguria.

Special Considerations/ Alternative Uses/ Complication Examples

Urethral stenting has also been used for strictures, proliferative urethritis, and reflex dyssynergia in dogs and strictures and tumors in cats (Figure 34.6 and Figure 34.7). The procedure is similar to that described above but there are a few differences. As strictures tend to be more focal, shorter stents can be used. The lesions are spanned by at least 10 mm on each side and care should be taken when using very short stents, as they may have a tendency to "watermelon seed", or slide cranially or caudally when eccentrically placed across a narrowing. In addition, while it is uncommon for tumors to grow through the stent interstices (~2%), strictures have a much greater tendency to do so and clients should be warned about this potential complication. Covered stents, or "stent-grafts", can be used instead of the typical bare stents, however in general, covered stents tend to cost more, exhibit higher migration rates (not in the urethra typically), and require larger profile delivery systems. For these reasons, the author typically uses bare stents initially unless there is only one chance to intervene. Unfortunately, in the author's experience, urethral stenting has not been highly effective in the small number of dogs treated for reflex dyssynergia, in which some dogs remained intermittently obstructed. This could be considered as a salvage procedure in these patients after medical management has failed. Placement of stents for both benign and malignant obstructions in the urinary system is becoming more popular, and is many institutions considered a routine treatment option.

A recent report on cat urethral stenting for benign and malignant obstructions revealed 25% of cats severely incontinent following stent placement (25% mildly incontinent and 50% continent). Long-term outcome was good to excellent in 75% of cats and fair to poor in 25%. Palliative stenting for urethral obstructions in cats can provide a rapid, effective, and safe alternative to more traditional

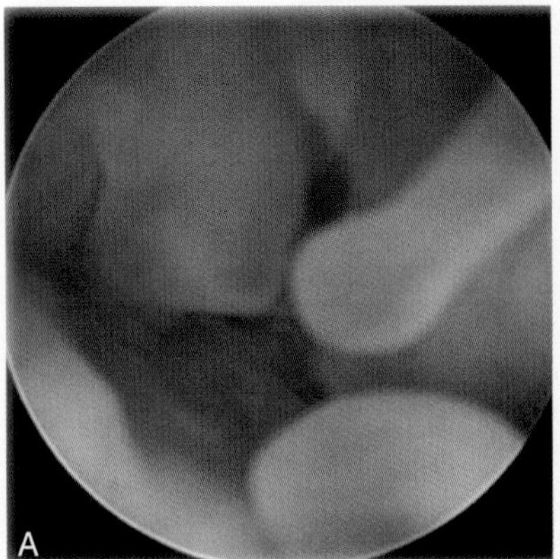

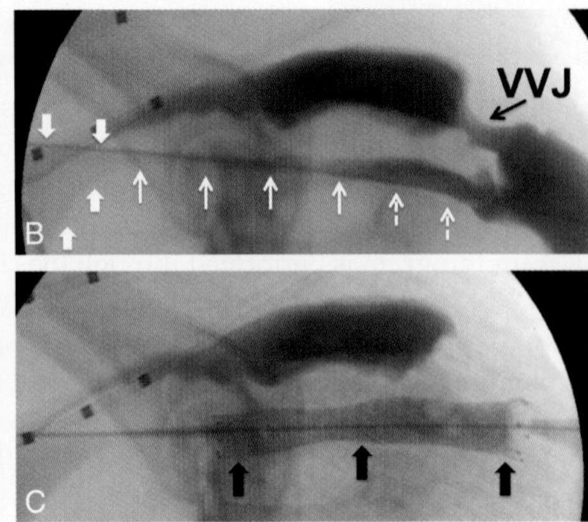

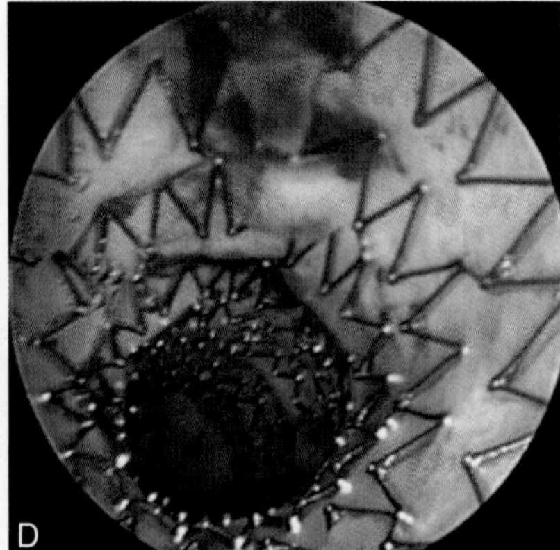

Figure 34.6 Endoscopic (A, D) and fluoroscopic (B, C) images of a female dog with proliferative urethritis causing a distal urethral obstruction. (A) Pre-stent urethroscopy image demonstrating proliferative bands of tissue resulting in urethral obstruction. (B) Contrast vaginourethrocystogram demonstrating a narrowed urethral lumen (white arrows) in the proximal and mid-urethra with filling defects also identified in the distal urethra (white dotted arrows). Note the trigone (white block arrows) is not affected. The vestibulovaginal junction (VVJ) is seen. (C) Contrast urethrogram following urethral stent placement (black block arrows) demonstrating a patent lumen. (D) Post-stent urethroscopy confirming patent urethral lumen. Notice the tight, blanched urethral tissue that is classic for the mucosa associated with proliferative urethritis after stenting.

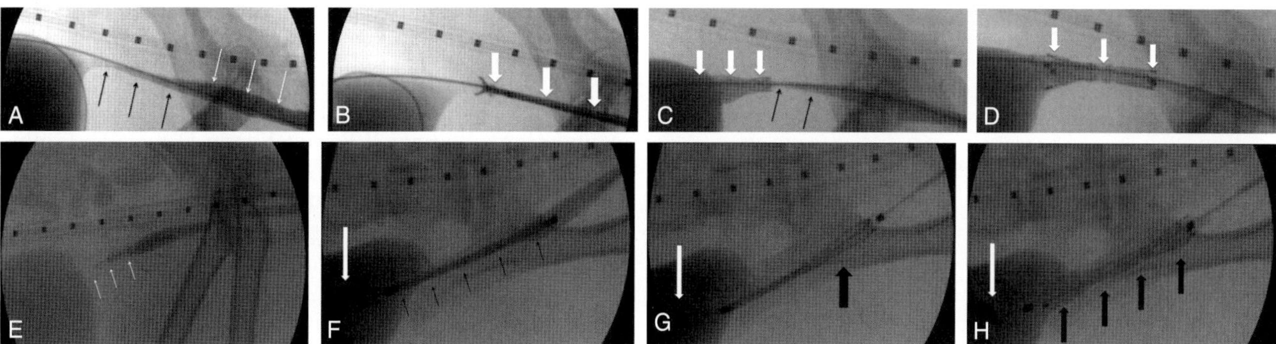

Figure 34.7 Serial fluoroscopic images in two separate cats with urethral obstructions. In all images the head is to the left. (A–D) Female cat with proximal urethral obstruction. A. Retrograde urethral access with a 0.035″ angled, hydrophilic guide wire is obtained and a contrast urethrocystogram is performed through a 5 Fr introducer sheath demonstrating a narrowed proximal urethra (black arrows) and normally dilated distal urethra (white arrows). (B) Retrograde, fluoroscopically-guided 2 mm biopsy device (white block arrows) used to obtain biopsy, directed through the urethral sheath. (C) Retrograde contrast urethrocystogram following SEMS stent placement (white block arrows) and persistently narrowed urethra (black arrows) caudal to stent. (D) Final retrograde contrast urethrocystogram following placement of second overlapping SEMS (white block arrows) demonstrating urethral patency. (E–H) Male cat with a proximal urethral tumor causing obstruction. (E) Retrograde contrast urethrocystogram demonstrating narrowed proximal urethra (white arrows). (F) Screw trocar (white block arrow) placed via mini-cystotomy to allow antegrade 0.035″ angled, hydrophilic guide wire access and stent delivery system (black arrows) across the lesion. The male feline penis is too small to allow passage of the stent delivery system so antegrade access is often needed. (G) The stent is partially deployed (black block arrow). Notice the deployment is from caudal to cranial due to antegrade access of the stent. (H) After final stent deployment (black block arrows), the urethral obstruction has been relieved. Urethral patency is confirmed via urethrogram and/or direct visualization via a scope placed through the screw-trocar (white block arrow).

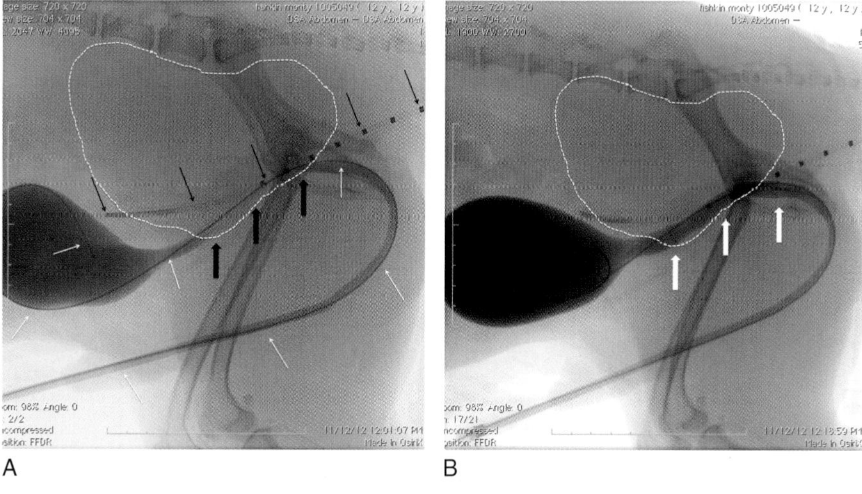

Figure 34.8 Serial lateral caudal abdominal fluoroscopic images of dog with anal sac adenocarcinoma lymph node metastases and subsequent extrinsic urethral compression. The dog's head is to the left in each image. (A) A marker catheter (black arrows) has been placed within a 14 Fr red rubber catheter and introduced per rectum in order to calibrate the radiographic images for magnification. A 0.035″ angled hydrophilic guide wire (white arrows) has been advanced through a 7 Fr vascular introducer sheath into the urethra and coiled in the urinary bladder. The bladder has been filled with contrast and saline and a urethrocystogram performed. The obstruction caused by the extrinsic compression (white dotted lines) is apparent at the level of the prostatic urethra (black block arrows). (B) Urethrocystogram immediately post-stent placement demonstrating patent urethra (white block arrows).

invasive options and long-term survival times in cats with TCC seems to be longer than that seen in dogs (Brace et al, 2012). Urethral stents have also been successfully used for extrinsic (Figure 34.8) malignant urethral obstructions (sublumbar lymph nodes).

Notes

(Examples; Multiple vendors available)

1. Measuring catheter, Infiniti Medical, Menlo Park, CA.
2. Weasel wire, Infiniti Medical, Menlo Park, CA.

3. 7 Fr Vascular introducer sheath, Infiniti Medical, Menlo Park, CA.
4. Cobra head catheter, Infiniti Medical, Menlo Park, CA.
5. Omnipaque (iohexol) injection, Amersham Health Inc., Princeton, NJ.
6. Vet Stent-Urethra, Infiniti Medical, Menlo Park, CA.

References

Bell FW, Klausner JS, Hayden DW, et al (1991) Clinical and pathologic features of prostatic adenocarcinoma in sexually intact and castrated dogs: 31 cases (1970–1987). *J Am Vet Medical Assoc* 199, 1623–30.

Blackburn, A., Berent, A., Weisse, C., et al (2013) Evaluation of outcome following urethral stent placement for the treatment of obstructive carcinoma of the urethra in dogs: 42 cases (2004–2008). *J Am Vet Med Assoc* 242(1), 59–68.

Brace, M., Weisse, C., Berent, A., et al (2012) Evaluation of palliative stenting for management of urethral obstruction in cats. ACVS 2012.

Cerf DJ and Lindquist EC (2012) Palliative ultrasound-guided endoscopic diode laser ablation of transitional cell carcinomas of the lower urinary tract in dogs. *J Am Vet Med Assoc* 240(1), 51–60.

Fries CL, Binnington AG, Valli VE, et al (1991) Enterocystoplasty with cystectomy and subtotal intracapsular prostatectomy in the male dogs. *Vet Surg* 20(2), 104–12.

Goldsmid SE and Bellenger CR (1991) Urinary incontinence after prostatectomy in dogs. *Vet Surg* 20(4), 253–6.

Knapp DW, Glickman NW, DeNicola DB, et al (2000) Naturally occurring canine transitional cell carcinoma of the urinary bladder. A relevant model of human invasive bladder cancer. *Urol Oncol* 5, 47–59.

McMillan SK, Knapp DW, Ramos-Vara JA, et al (2012) Outcome of urethral stent placement for management of urethral obstruction secondary to transitional cell carcinoma in dogs: 19 cases (2007–2010). *J Am Vet Med Assoc* 241(12), 1627–32.

Mutsaers AJ, Widmer WR, and Knapp DW (2003) Canine transitional cell carcinoma. *J Vet Intern Med* 17, 136–44.

Norris AM, Laing AM, Valli VEO, et al (1992) Canine bladder and urethral tumors: a retrospective study of 115 cases (1980–1985). *J Vet Intern Med* 16, 145–53.

Smith JD, Vaden SL, Stone EA, et al (1996) Management and complications following trigonal-colonic anastomosis in a dog: five-year evaluation. *J Am Anim Hosp Assoc* 32, 29–35.

Stone EA, Withrow SJ, Page RL, et al (1988) Ureterocolonic anastomosis in ten dogs with transitional cell carcinoma. *Vete Surg* 17, 147–53.

Upton ML, Tangner CH, and Payton ME (2006) Evaluation of carbon dioxide laser ablation combined with mitoxantrone and piroxicam treatment in dogs with transitional cell carcinoma. *J Am Vet Med Assoc* 228, 549–52.

Weisse C, Berent A, Todd K, et al (2006) Evaluation of palliative stenting for management of malignant urethral obstructions in dogs. *J Am Vet Med Assoc* 229(2), 226–34.

Suggested Reading

Liptak JM, Brutscher SP, Monnet E, et al (2004) Transurethral resection in the management of urethral and prostatic neoplasia in 6 dogs. *Vet Surg* 33, 505–16.

Mann FA, Barrett RJ, and Henderson RA (1992) Use of a retained urethral catheter in three dogs with prostatic neoplasia. *Vet Surg* 21, 342–7.

Stiffler KS, McCrackin MA, Cornell KK, et al (2003) Clinical use of low-profile cystostomy tubes in four dogs and a cat. *J Am Vet Med Assoc* 223(3), 325–9.

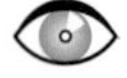

Video clips to accompany this chapter can be found in the online material at **www.wiley.com/go/weisse/vet-image-guided-interventions**

CHAPTER THIRTY-FIVE

Endoscopic Polypectomy and Laser Ablation for Benign Urinary Bladder Lesions

Allyson Berent
The Animal Medical Center, New York, NY

Background/Indications

Urinary bladder polypoid masses can be due to benign or malignant processes, both of which can cause hematuria, chronic urinary tract infections, dysuria and potentially trigonal outflow obstructions. Removal of a polypoid mass can be useful for histopathological analysis and have potential curative results. Masses in the bladder can either be inflammatory polyps, carcinoma *in situ* (CIS), polypoid non-invasive carcinoma, pedunculated invasive carcinoma, or other pedunculated types of masses. Inflammatory polyps are nearly always associated with chronic stone disease or chronic urinary tract infections. Transitional cell carcinoma (TCC) is a likely diagnosis if no infection or stone is documented. Carcinoma *in situ* is rare in animals, and in humans CIS will progress to muscular invasive TCC 83% of the time, with a recurrence rate of 73% after laser ablation. Papillary carcinoma in people can be low or high grade, and high grade is typically invasive beyond the submucosa. This will typically progress to invasive TCC with laser ablation alone, where low grade is reported to have a 39% progression rate in people. This makes ablation alone less than ideal. Since superficial TCC is very common in people (over 75–85%), ablation techniques (like snare polypectomy, electrosurgical ablation, and laser therapy) are routinely performed. Invasive TCC on the other hand, which characterizes over 90% of veterinary TCC, involves the muscular, and often serosal, layers and, as such, for this condition local ablative techniques are not indicated in humans (or animals). Instead, radical surgery with a curative intent, rather than dubulking surgery, is attempted in people when possible. If the tumor is too large than palliation (with stents and catheters or radical cystectomy with urinary diversion) is considered. There has been no survival benefit shown in debulking/local ablation techniques in people for invasive TCC; this is likely the same for invasive TCC in animals. For palliative laser ablation of invasive TCC please refer to Chapter 37.

Polypectomy is rarely necessary in veterinary medicine. If there is a benign polyp than treatment of the urinary tract infection, or removal of the stones, is performed. The polyp should resolve on its own over ~4–6 weeks (depending on the size). If the polyp does not get smaller, or is growing at any point, than biopsy and polypectomy can be considered to attempt to prevent any transformation from polypoid cystitis to carcinoma. If CIS is diagnosed, ablation can be considered but the operator must ablate the base of the mass very well while carefully avoiding perforation (Figure 35.1). Subsequently, serial monitoring with either ultrasonography or cystoscopy should be performed because recurrence is common and progression to invasive TCC may still occur.

The details of electrocautery and laser ablation of respiratory, intestinal, and urogenital lesions are discussed in great detail in other chapters as well (Chapter 10, Chapter 15, Chapter 28, and Chapter 37).

Patient Preparation

A thorough history should be obtained including previous urinary tract infections (number and duration of treatment, time of culture/re-culture, etc.),

Veterinary Image-Guided Interventions, First Edition. Edited by Chick Weisse and Allyson Berent.

Companion website: www.wiley.com/go/weisse/vet-image-guided-interventions

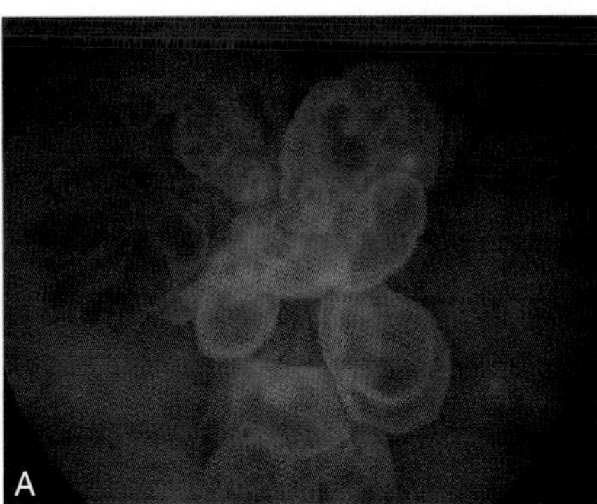

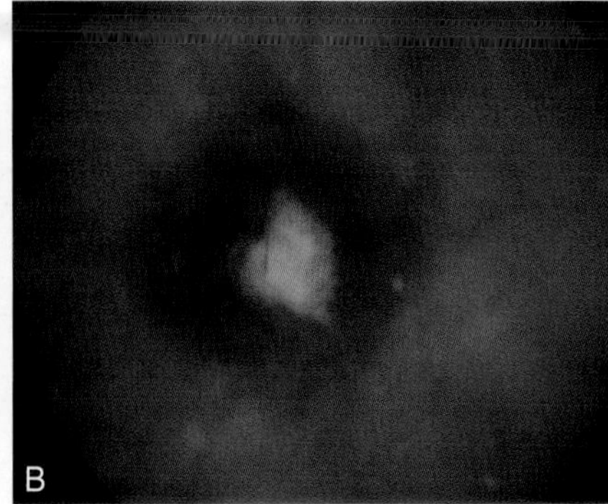

Figure 35.1 Cystoscopic image of a large polypoid mass in the bladder of a female dog before and after endoscopic polypectomy. Notice the base of the mass is white after ablation.

previous urinary tract stones, any previous bladder surgery, and other comorbidities (diabetes mellitus, hyperadrenocorticism, steroid therapy, etc.). An ultrasound exam should be performed evaluating the bladder mass and multiple measurements should be obtained. This is not very accurate for comparison on serial ultrasound exams, but location and size, ideally with a full bladder, are attempted. Local lymph nodes should be evaluated. Thoracic radiography should be performed to assess for any signs of metastatic disease. If an infection is present or uroliths seen, then clearing the infection over 4–6 weeks is necessary while monitoring the size of the mass. If uroliths and an infection are present than this could be associated with struvite urolithiasis, depending on the type of infection (urease-producing bacterial, high pH), and if deemed appropriate dissolution should be attempted over 4–6 weeks. Once the infection is under control and the stones are removed or dissolved then the mass should resolve or get smaller over 4–6 weeks. If it does not resolve, gets progressively bigger, or is found in the face of a negative screen for a UTI or uroliths then a biopsy is recommended. Care should be taken when interpreting an ultrasound exam as an empty bladder can make a mass look polypoid and this can be wrongly interpreted as a benign lesion (and vice-versa).

Prior to considering cystoscopy a patient should have a negative urine culture or be on an appropriate antibiotic for at least 3 days.

Potential Risks/ Complications/ Expected Outcomes

An experienced endoscopist comfortable with cystoscopy, laser surgery, and using ablative devices should perform this procedure. The biggest risks are bladder wall perforation, polyp/tumor regrowth, urethral obstruction, and possible additional tumor seeding. Care should be taken once the stalk is removed, as perforation happens most commonly during ablation of the base. If the masses are removed and too large to then extract from the urinary bladder they can either be ablated to make them smaller for basket retrieval or they can be left in the bladder lumen, in which case they will likely necrose and be urinated out. The author has done this when needed without complication. This could theoretically result in a urethral obstruction. The traditional risks with cystoscopy apply, which include bladder rupture from over-distension, urethral perforation, and a subsequent uroabdomen.

There are no long-term or large studies in veterinary patients looking at any of these techniques for the treatment of either benign or malignant bladder polyps with local ablation techniques. As discussed above, CIS, papillary carcinoma, or invasive TCC are not typically treated with local ablation therapy in human medicine because there has been little to no proven survival benefit. With a histopathological diagnosis the prognosis will vary. If an inflammatory polyp is present this procedure is typically curative. For CIS or non-invasive papillary carcinoma (rare), recurrence rates are high and serial evaluation with repeat ablation and/or intravesicular immunomodulatory infusions, to prevent invasion and spread, should be considered. This is typically an outpatient procedure and patients may have minimal short-lived clinical signs post-cystoscopy such as dysuria, hematuria, and may be considered along with other therapies recommended by an oncologist.

Equipment

Endoscopy is typically performed with an appropriate diameter 30 degree rigid cystoscope for female dogs (1.9, 2.7, or 4 mm)[1–3] or a 7.5–8.2 Fr flexible ureteroscope[4] for male dogs. During cystoscopy the irrigation

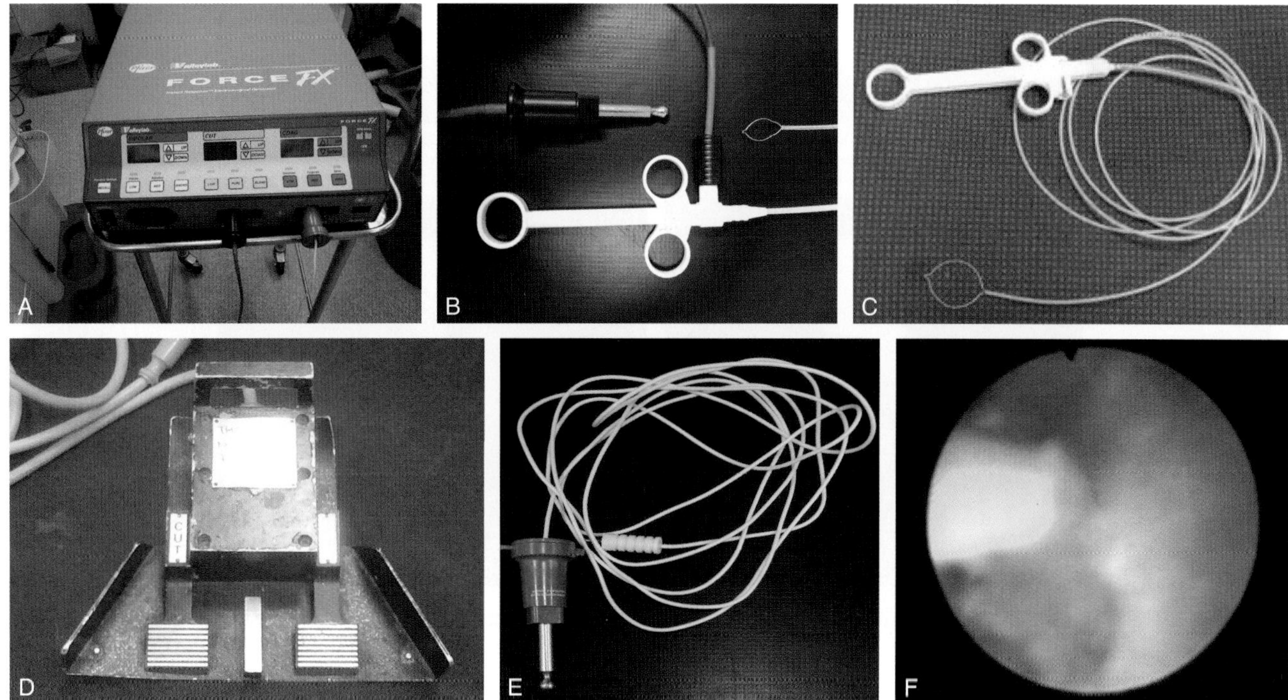

Figure 35.2 Electrocautery unit with various accessories. (A) The electrocautery machine attached to a red and blue/yellow adaptor. (B) The red adaptor connects the electrocautery unit to the snare device. (C) A polypectomy snare device. (D) The foot pedal needed to activate the monopolar devices. (E) The adaptor for the Bugbee cautery probe. (F) The Bugbee cautery probe through the working channel of the flexible cystoscope during mass ablation.

fluid will depend on the modality being chosen for ablation. Electrocautery (snare polypectomy or Bugbee cauterization) requires infusion with sterile water in 5% dextrose (D5W) for conduction and a cautery pad needs to be placed on a patient for grounding. If the diode or Hol:YAG laser are being used than 0.9% sodium chloride infusion is acceptable.

A snare polypectomy device is available in various sizes[5,6] (Figure 35.2 and Figure 35.3), and one should be chosen that is large enough to get around the polypoid mass, but also small enough to fit through the working channel of the endoscope (typically the 2 mm snare catheter fits through the 2.7 and 4.0 mm rigid cystoscope working channel). Retrieval baskets (ranging in basket diameter of 1–3 cm) are needed to remove the mass once it is ablated.[7,8] A Bugbee cautery probe and adaptor[9,10] (Figure 35.2E,F) can be used to ablate small lesions, similar to the lasers (see next paragraph).

There are two types of lasers that the author has used for this procedure: a diode laser[11] and a Holmium: YAG (yttrium, aluminum, garnet) laser[12] (Figure 35.4). The benefit of the diode laser is that it is a continuous firing laser that has both tissue ablative and coagulative properties. The diode is best used in contact mode resulting in minimal tissue bleeding or collateral damage, and is very effective for tissue ablation. The diode laser fibers are available in 600 and 1000 microns and it works at 980 nm that provides both coagulation and cutting with essentially no hemorrhage. The Hol:YAG laser works at a wavelength of 2,100 nm and has a pulsed activity that results in an intermittent surge of pulsing energy that causes a jumping action during the ablation procedure making treatment less precise. This laser also results in a mild amount of hemorrhage that can obscure the cystoscopy image but is of no consequence for the patient post-operatively. For tissue ablation contact mode should be avoided and the laser fiber should be situated 0.1 to 0.5 mm from the desired tissue to be ablated allowing the power to coagulate rather than cut the tissue directly (Figure 35.4). This also results in slightly more tissue edema. The laser fibers available for the Hol:YAG are 200, 400, 600, and 1000 μm. Since the advent of laser lithotripsy more veterinarians have a Hol:YAG laser available than a diode, making this laser a reasonable alternative and more versatile. The smaller Hol:YAG laser fiber allows more flexibility when performing a polypectomy through a male cystoscope.

In small male dogs and cats in which the cystoscope does not fit through the urethral lumen, an antegrade approach as described in Chapter 33 for the percutaneous cystolithotomy procedure can be performed.

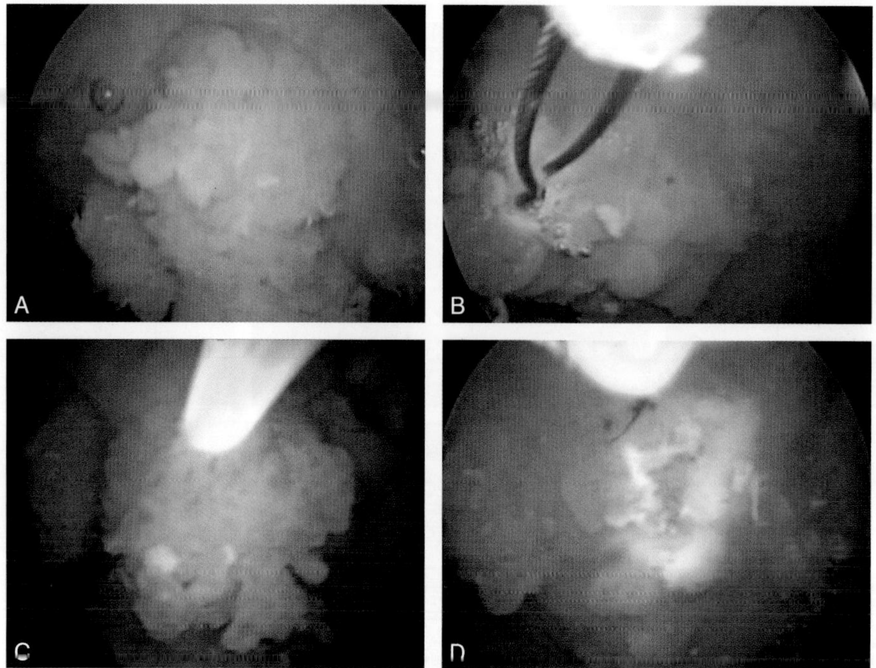

Figure 35.3 Cystoscopic images of a female dog with multiple polypoid masses of the bladder (carcinoma *in situ*). (A) The sessile polypoid mass in the bladder wall. (B) The endoscopic snare device through the working channel of the cystoscope. The tip is extruded to test the power setting on the mass. Notice the bubbles being formed during cautery. (C) The snare is placed around the base of the mass and the entire mass is pulled caudally toward the cystoscope to protect the far wall of the bladder. (D) After the cautery is complete the mass falls off the wall. Notice the lack of bleeding.

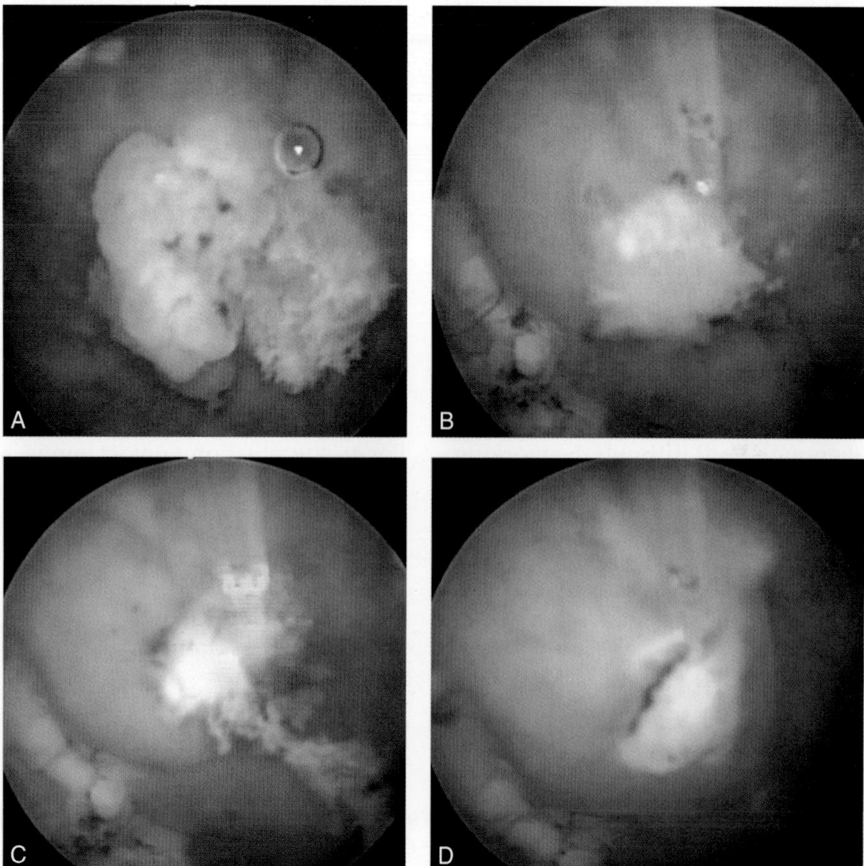

Figure 35.4 Cystoscopic images of a female dog with a small sessile bladder mass. Due to the broad base this mass was laser ablated after biopsy. (A) Mass prior to ablation. (B) Hol:YAG laser being held approximately 0.5–1.0 mm away from the tissue to prevent contact mode and limit bleeding. (C) The mass is being vaporized with the laser energy. (D) The base of the mass after laser ablation. Notice the mass was not removed as with polypectomy but instead vaporized.

This requires the 6 mm screw trocar[13] so rigid cystoscopy can be performed. As this is performed with a small intra-abdominal approach, D5W should not be used (as risk of leakage is higher) so laser ablation is preferred to electrocautery.

Procedure

The patient should be placed in dorsal recumbency and the vulva, prepuce, and ventral abdomen should be clipped and aseptically prepared. Using an appropriately sized endoscope, the urethra and bladder should be evaluated carefully avoiding bladder overdistension. If there is a polypoid mass lesion with a narrow base then starting with the snare polypectomy device is ideal (Figure 35.3). The bladder should be evacuated of 0.9% NaCl irrigation and infused with D5W. The snare can be passed through the working channel of the endoscope. Once it exits the scope it is minimally deployed just so the tip is extracted (Figure 35.3B). The cautery is used on blend or coagulation mode at approximately 15–22 W. The tip is advanced to touch the center of the mass and the cautery is activated with the foot pedal; This allows the operator to adjust the power setting accordingly to see the resultant cauterization that results prior to snare placement. Once an appropriate power setting is chosen the snare is opened and placed around the base of the polypoid mass, gently retracting it to have a relatively tight grip. The device should be pulled toward the scope so the far end of the snare tip is pulled away from the bladder wall (Figure 35.3C). The bladder should be relatively full. The cautery is activated as the snare is slowly tightened to strangulate the blood vessels at the base of the mass while the cautery coagulates the vessels and cuts the tissue. Once the base is completely ablated the polyp will fall to the gravity-dependent portion of the bladder (typically dorsal) (Figure 35.3D). The snare is retracted so that only the tip is exposed and the base can be carefully ablated ensuring to get all the margins and the center (Figure 35.1B). The power should be turned down for this part of the procedure (15–18 W). The author often changes to the diode laser for ablation of the base as it has less thermal damage to normal surrounding tissues and only penetrates 0.1–0.5 mm. To avoid perforation use the laser in non-contact mode by holding the tip of the fiber 0.1–0.5 mm or so from the base and fire the laser so that you see the tissue turn white (Figure 35.4C,D).

For very small polypoid masses, the lasers (diode or Hol:YAG) (Figure 35.4) or the Bugbee cautery (Figure 35.2F) can be used for ablation to the base without snaring them off. This makes biopsy samples difficult to obtain so make certain to biopsy first. The mass will typically vaporize and ablate quickly.

For very large polypoid masses difficult to retract through the urethra after resection, the mass should be ablated and vaporized with a laser or snare tip prior to snaring the base. This will cause the mass to vaporize and shrink in size as the vessels are coagulated. Once it is small enough to pass through the urethra than the snare can be used to resect the mass at the base. In humans, a morcellator can be used, which breaks the mass down into very small pieces that can be voided. The problem is that the smallest morcellator device is 12 mm in diameter that will not fit through the smaller canine urethra. This device can be used through a PCCL approach if necessary. For ablation of larger masses (Figure 35.1), they can be left in the lumen of the urinary bladder in female dogs and will eventually necrose and be passed spontaneously. The risk of urethral obstruction should be considered but has not been experienced in the author's practice.

Once all the masses are ablated, a stone retrieval basket is used to remove them from the bladder floor. They should all be submitted for tissue culture and histopathological evaluation. Ideally each one should be removed individually and a map should be made so that if there are many it is known which are benign and which are malignant. When there are more than three this can be difficult.

Vascular abnormalities have been found in the bladder and urethra in dogs and these too can be ablated with the techniques mentioned above (Figure 35.5).

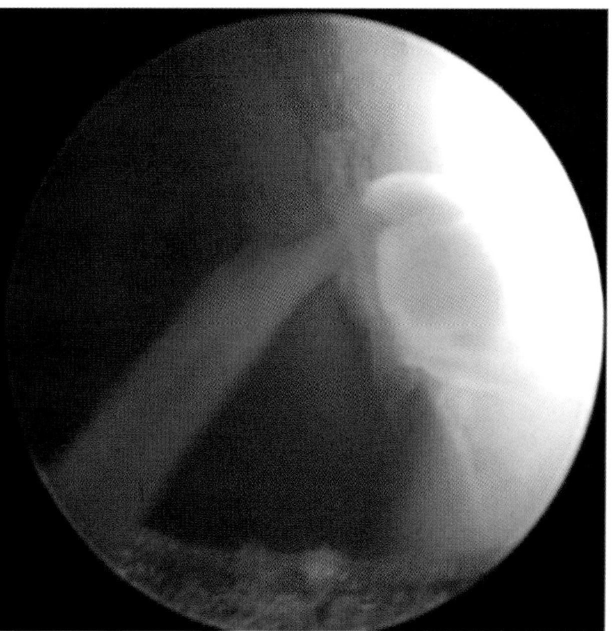

Figure 35.5 Cystoscopic image of a dog with severe hematuria. Notice the small bleeding lesion. This can be laser ablated with either the diode laser (non-contact mode), Hol:YAG laser (non-contact mode), or Bugbee cautery probe (contact mode).

Using the PCCL Approach

This approach is reserved for cats and small male dogs in whom retrograde transurethral cystoscopy is not possible or contraindicated. Please see Chapter 33 for a review on performing this procedure. Once the bladder is accessed with the 2.7 mm rigid cystoscope all of the recommendations made above apply.

Postprocedural and Follow-Up Care

Dogs are given a local urethral infusion of bupivacaine (1 mg/kg [0.5 mg/lb] mixed with saline in a 1:1 solution) for local urethral analgesia. One dose of buprenorphine (0.01 mg/kg [0.005 mg/lb]) is administered and discharge the same day is standard with oral tramadol (2 to 5 mg/kg, [1 to 2.5 mg/lb], PO, q 8 hr) for 3 days and 7–28 days of a broad-spectrum antibiotic pending infection history.

Bacteriologic culture of urine samples are performed at 2 to 4 weeks and recommended at 8 weeks, 3 months, 6 months, and then every 6 months thereafter if the lesion was an infection-induced inflammatory polyp. If CIS or non-invasive papillary TCC is diagnosed a repeat cystoscopy in 4–6 weeks should be considered. If it recurs and partial cystectomy is possible (body or apex) than this is recommended at this time. Consultation with an oncologist should be recommended as well.

Special Considerations/ Alternative Uses/ Complications

This procedure has also been used to ablate bleeding lesions (angioma/hemangioma) in the bladder, urethra, vestibule, and vagina, when needed. The main complication that could be encountered is bladder wall perforation.

Notes

1. Rigid endoscope, 1.9-mm 30° lens, Karl Storz Endoscopy, Culver City, CA.
2. Rigid endoscope, 2.7-mm 30° lens, Richard Wolf, Vernon Hills, IL.
3. Rigid endoscope, 4-mm 30° lens, Karl Storz Endoscopy, Culver City, CA.
4. Flex X^2 Flexible ureteroscope, Karl Storz Endoscopy, Culver City, CA.
5. Polypectomy snare US endoscopy, Mentor, OH.
6. Polypectomy snare, Olympus, Southborough MA.
7. Sur-Catch® NT, No Tip Nitinol Basket, Olympus/Gyrus ACMI, Southborough MA.
8. Dimenstion® Basket, 2.4 Fr, Bard Medical, Covington, GA.
9. Fulgurating electrode Bugbee cautery, 2 Fr, short tip, ACMI-Olympus, Southborough, MA.
10. Cautery machine Valley Lab Force FX, Electrosurgical Generator, Covideien, Boulder, CO.
11. 600-µm diode laser fiber and 100-W diode Lithotrite, Vectra, Convergent Inc, Alameda, CA.
12. 200 or 400-µm Holmium:YAG laser fiber and 30-W Hol:YAG Lithotrite, Odyssey, Convergent Inc, Alameda, CA.
13. Endotip screw trocar, Karl Storz Endoscopy, Culver City, CA.

Suggested Reading

Amling CL (2001) Diagnosis and management of superficial bladder cancer. *Curr Problems Cancer* 25(4), 219–78.

Doloway MS, Bruck DS, Kim SS (2003) Expectant management of small, recurrent, noninvasive papillar bladder tumors. *J Urol* 170(2), 438–41.

Donat SM, North A, Dalbagni G, et al (2004) Efficacy of office fulguration for recurrent low grade papillary bladder tumors less than 0.5 mm. *J Urol* 171(2), 636–9.

Pruthi RS, Bladwin N, Bhalani V, et al (2008). Conservative management of low risk superficial bladder tumors. *J Urol* 179(1), 87–90.

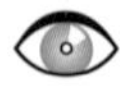
Video clips to accompany this chapter can be found in the online material at **www.wiley.com/go/weisse/vet-image-guided-interventions**

CHAPTER THIRTY-SIX

Intra-arterial Chemotherapy Infusion

Chick Weisse
The Animal Medical Center, New York, NY

Background/Indications

Transitional cell carcinoma (TCC) is the most common tumor of the canine urinary tract. Most dogs with TCC have clinical signs such as hematuria, dysuria, stranguria, and pollakiuria. Dogs with TCC are typically diagnosed with locally advanced tumors involving the trigone of the bladder and are therefore not candidates for complete surgical resection. Furthermore, up to 50% of dogs with bladder tumors have distant metastasis at the time of diagnosis, and aggressive surgical resection is therefore not typically encouraged. However, regardless of stage, most of them die or are euthanized due to signs associated with progressive local disease (Knapp et al, 2000).

Prostatic carcinoma (PCA) is another common malignancy of the male lower urinary tract in which distant metastases are reported in 64–89% of affected animals, and 40% experience dysuria (Bell et al, 1991). In addition, approximately 80% of prostatic tumors are actually TCC. Responses to systemic chemotherapy have been poor, and while early stage prostatic tumors may be amenable to prostatectomy, this often results in incontinence (Goldsmid and Bellenger, 1991) .

Current therapies include chemotherapy, radiation therapy, and surgical debulking, but none are able to consistently produce durable remissions. More effective local tumor control is therefore desirable to improve outcome for TCC and PCA. Current treatments include the use of non-steroidal anti-inflammatory drugs (NSAIDs), with or without chemotherapy. These treatments are directed towards palliating the clinical signs associated with the tumor, but are unlikely to induce complete or durable remissions in the majority of cases. Despite treatment, most dogs die within the first 12 months of diagnosis (Knapp et al, 2000).

Several chemotherapeutic agents, including cisplatin, carboplatin, doxorubicin, and mitoxantrone, have been found to have mild to moderate activity in dogs with TCC, confirming that these tumors are sensitive to chemotherapy. However, all of these agents are associated with systemic toxicity such as myelosuppression, gastrointestinal toxicity and/or renal toxicity. These side effects to normal tissues are dose limiting and significant improvement in outcome through dose escalation is not feasible due to unacceptable toxicity and reduced quality of life. Research suggests that these tumors can respond more favorably to higher concentrations of chemotherapy or non-steroidal anti-inflammatory medications.

Regional dose intensity and efficacy may be increased by targeted delivery of the chemotherapy to the area or region of the tumor. Minimally invasive delivery of systemic doses of chemotherapy directly into the arterial supply of the tumor (called "Intra-arterial [IA] chemotherapy") provides increased intra-tumoral drug concentrations, and may improve the anti-tumor activity. Studies confirm both higher achieved levels of chemotherapy within the targeted tissues as well as improved tumor remissions in laboratory animals.

Research in laboratory rabbits with bladder tumors determined that internal iliac artery infusion of carboplatin and pirarubicin was safely tolerated and resulted in significantly higher chemotherapy levels within the bladder tumor itself (Hoshi et al, 1997). In addition, all tumors receiving intra-arterial therapy reduced in size with 37.5% disappearing compared to those receiving intravenous therapy in which all tumors grew in size. The improved efficacy of the IA drug delivery is thought to result from the initial increased drug concentration in the tumor. Another study in laboratory dogs receiving internal iliac artery

Veterinary Image-Guided Interventions, First Edition. Edited by Chick Weisse and Allyson Berent.

Companion website: www.wiley.com/go/weisse/vet-image-guided-interventions

infusion of pirarubicin demonstrated it was safely tolerated and the bladder mucosa and muscle concentrations of chemotherapy were eight times higher than that of dogs receiving intravenous chemotherapy. In addition, the perivesical adipose tissues, pelvic lymph nodes and prostate all had significantly higher tissue levels when compared with intravenous administration (Sumiyoshi et al, 1991). The increased drug level in the regional tissues and lymph nodes may in fact be an additional advantage with this approach since multifocal vesical implant metastasis, prostatic involvement, and regional lymph node metastasis are common sites of tumor progression in dogs with bladder tumors. These techniques are increasingly being used in human medicine for non-resectable, IV chemotherapy-resistant tumors.

In addition to chemotherapy, NSAIDs have become part of the standard of care for canine TCC and may provide additional benefit if delivered locally. Early reports documented objective tumor regressions in 6 of 34 dogs treated with piroxicam as a single agent, and 2 of these cases demonstrated complete and durable remissions while on therapy. The response to NSAIDs has been confirmed by several follow-up studies (Knapp et al, 1994, Mohammed et al, 2002, Henry, 2003, Henry et al, 2003). As only complete responses are likely to significantly prolong remission and survival in cancer patients, the activity of NSAIDs in canine TCC has received significant attention. Several investigators have attempted to elucidate the mechanisms behind the antitumor activity in canine TCC. It is likely that cyclo-oxygenase inhibitors exert their antitumor activity both via cyclooxygenase dependent and independent pathways. The anti-tumor effects of NSAIDs are likely due to one, or a combination, of various mechanisms including immune-modulatory effects, antiangiogenic effects, antiproliferative, and proapoptotic effects.

Patient Preparation

The patients should receive a complete work-up and tumor staging according to standard practice, including CBC, serum biochemistry profile, urinalysis, urine culture, abdominal ultrasonography, thoracic radiography, and tumor cytology or biopsy. Consultation with an oncologist is critical for developing a treatment plan and ensuring standard-of-care therapies have been discussed. The size of the primary tumor will be measured and the presence of distant metastases will be recorded and documented immediately prior to the first treatment. The presence of metastatic disease should raise the question of the benefit of a regional therapy plan. Lymph node metastases are not life threatening and it is possible that tumor drainage of locally delivered chemotherapy will result in increased lymph node chemotherapy concentrations, however evidence of metastatic disease elsewhere should prompt a discussion about a combination of, or alternating, IA and IV chemotherapy protocol, something the author has been performing more often recently. The clients should provide consent detailing the procedure, risks and benefits associated with this technique, as it remains investigational at this time.

As most dogs with TCC are older, often with a chronic history of urinary tract infections and potentially reduced renal function, a reduced initial dose of chemotherapy should be considered if renal excretion is a concern, in order to avoid serious complications and maintain an acceptable quality of life. Despite this dose reduction, the IA administration will likely provide a significantly higher intratumoral drug concentration than the comparable intravenous full dose.

Premedications include antibiotic coverage for common skin organisms and antinausea medications (Table 36.1).

TABLE 36.1
Procedural and post-procedural medical management

- Antibiotics:
  - Intraoperative: cefazolin (22 mg/kg IV q 2 hr) prn
  - Postoperative: As needed
- Anti-inflammatories:
  - NSAIDs as needed
- Anti-emetics:
  - Perioperative: maropitant (1 mg/kg IV once)
  - Postoperative: ondansetron (0.1–1 mg/kg PO q8–12 hr × 3–7 days)
- Analgesics:
  - Perioperative: opioid premedications
  - Postoperative: tramadol (2–4 mg/kg PO q8–12 hr × 3 days)
  - Postoperative: NSAIDs as needed

Potential Risks/ Complications/Expected Outcomes

Canine patients with severe cardiac, renal, or hepatic comorbidities that would preclude the safe use of general anesthesia or potentially toxic medications such as chemotherapy, NSAIDs, or iodinated contrast agents are not good candidates for intra-arterial therapy, which will require frequent general anesthesia episodes. Many chemotherapeutics will result in bone marrow suppression so patients should be monitored with regular complete blood counts (CBC) and prophylactic antibiotics should be prescribed to dogs with considerably low white blood cell counts. While intra-arterial therapy should result in less systemic exposure to the administered drug, some proportion will still reach the systemic circulation. Dose reductions should be considered in dogs with severely decreased white blood cell counts, and this should be guided by an oncologist. Non-steroidal, anti-inflammatory drugs can cause kidney toxicity, liver toxicity, and gastrointestinal upset/ulceration. Associated clinical signs may be vague or include dullness, depression, anorexia, lethargy, or vomiting, diarrhea, or melena. These signs can be confused with chemotherapy toxicity so any concerns should warrant a veterinary examination.

In the author's experience using IA carboplatin and meloxicam, bloodwork abnormalities were uncommon (<10%) and minor (Weisse et al, 2011). Other complications (~25%) were minor including vomiting/regurgitation and cough for 1 week (4%), gastrointestinal upset (4%), mild hindlimb lameness for a few days (12%), hemorrhagic diarrhea for 1 week (4%), thrombosis of the internal pudendal artery following more distal coil embolization (4%), and vascular access port thrombosis (4%). All treatments were performed safely, rapidly, and without serious adverse side effects. Biological response rates in 17 dogs were 43% in female dogs only 14% in male dogs. Median survival times were 433 days in females and 57 days in males. Additional theoretical complications, not encountered by the author to date, could include more substantial vessel thrombosis and subsequent tissue infarction or non-target delivery of chemotherapy to the rectum (middle rectal artery) with unknown consequences.

The client should also be informed that while IA administration of chemotherapy treatments have been performed in research animals, it has only been performed in a relatively small group of dogs with naturally-occurring tumors.

Equipment

A list of recommended equipment can be found in Figure 36.1. IA chemotherapy procedures require a very little equipment, but the fluoroscopy unit must provide adequate imaging detail to identify very small caliber vessels using digital subtraction angiography (DSA) and road-mapping, as well as the ability to obtain orthogonal imaging when necessary. Failure to identify collateral vessels could lead to non-target delivery and potentially severe consequences.

Fluoroscopic Procedure

The patient is placed under general anesthesia and the groin or neck is clipped and scrubbed (see Chapter 44 for vascular access discussions) for either femoral or carotid arterial access. A surgical cut-down will be made and a 5 Fr introducer sheath[1] will be placed within the femoral or carotid artery. A combination 0.035" angled, hydrophilic guide wire[2] and 4 or 5 Fr reverse-curve catheter[3] (Figure 36.2 and Figure 36.3) (femoral) or 4Fr Berenstein catheter[4] (Figure 36.4) (carotid) is advanced under fluoroscopic guidance to the terminal aorta. A digital subtraction angiogram (DSA) run is performed using 50:50 iohexol[5]:saline to delineate the vascular anatomy and demonstrate the appropriate location for treatment. The 4 or 5 Fr angiographic catheter and guide wire (or more commonly the microcatheter/microwire) combination is advanced into one of the internal iliac arteries. A microcatheter[6,7] and microwire[8,9] combination is then passed coaxially through the Touhy–Borst adapter[10] and Flo-switch[11] (Figure 36.1U) which is attached to the 4 or 5 Fr angiographic catheter. The microcatheter is then advanced over the wire down the internal iliac artery and the c-arm is rotated into a lateral projection. A repeat DSA is performed through the microcatheter, and then the microcather/microwire combination is used to gain superselective access to one of the terminal arteries feeding the tumor (e.g., prostatic artery or vaginal artery) (Figure 36.5). If these vessels are too narrow to accept the microcatheter without being occlusive or causing vessel spasm, the microcatheter is just positioned as distal as possible during treatment within the internal pudendal artery (Figure 36.5C). Standard therapy involves the total systemic chemotherapy dose mixed with an equal volume of iohexol contrast, half of which is injected under fluoroscopic guidance to ensure flow down the target artery without reflux into non-target vessels. The microcatheter is flushed with saline and a repeat angiogram performed to document continued bloodflow

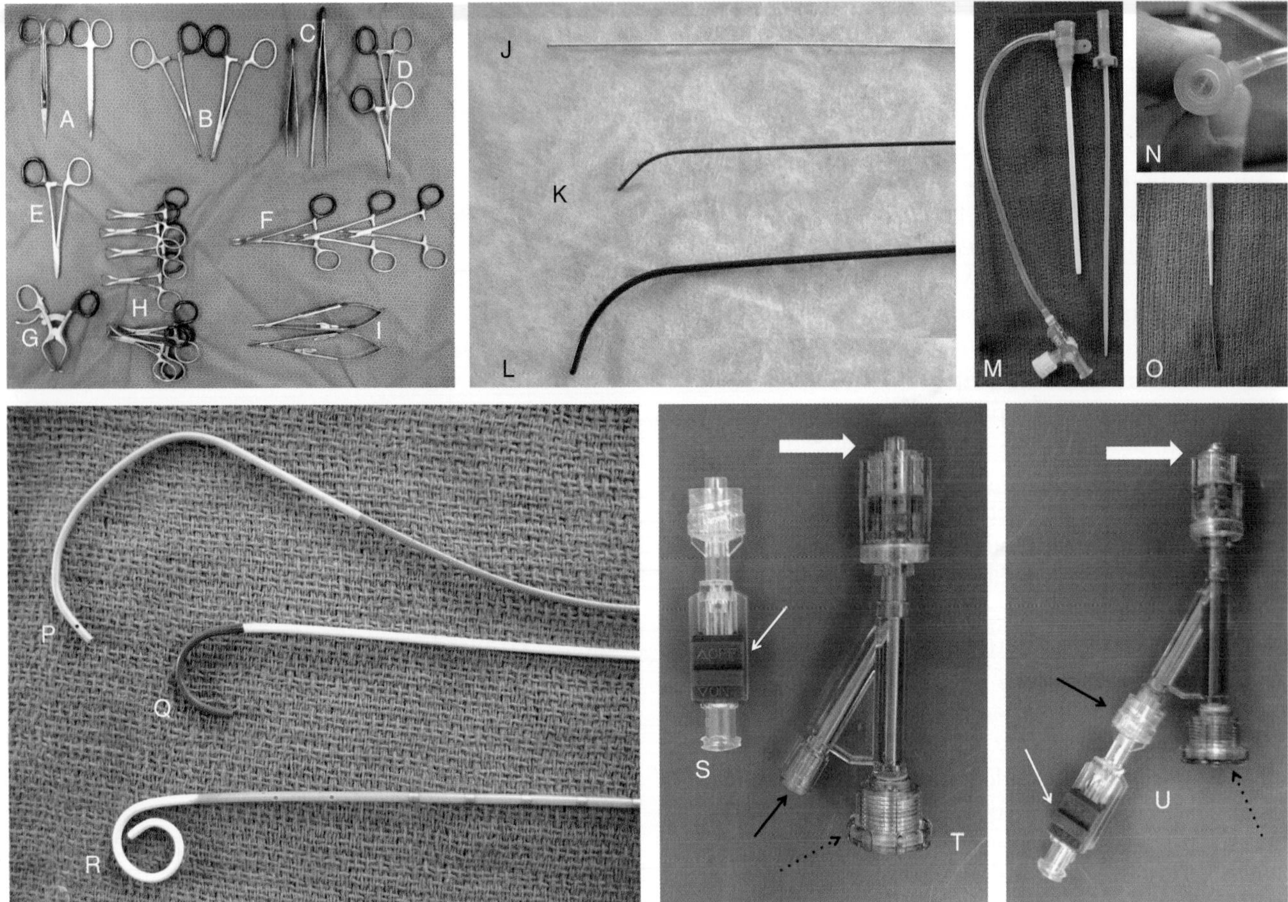

Figure 36.1 (A–I) Sample surgical cut-down set. (A) Sharp-sharps and small Metzenbaum scissors. (B) Right-angled forceps. (C) Brown–Adson and Debakey forceps. (D) Mosquito hemostats. (E) Needle drivers. (F) Kelly hemostats. (G) Small Gelpi retractors. (H) Small Babcock towel clamps. (I) Castroviejo needle drivers for vessel repair. (J–L) Guide wires. (J) 0.018″ microwire. (K) 0.018″ angled, hydrophilic guide wire. (L) 0.035″ angled, hydrophilic guide wire. (M–O) Vascular introducer sheath. 4 Fr vascular introducer sheath made up of shaft (white) with 4 Fr inner diameter, hemostasis valve (N) to prevent bleeding, three-way stop-cock (yellow cap) to flush and/or aspirate, and 4 Fr dilator (blue) to make smooth transition from sheath down to 0.035″ guide wire (O). (P) 4Fr Cobra catheter. (Q) 4 Fr reverse curve RIM catheter. (R) 4 Fr marker pigtail catheter for aortogram and measurements if needed. (S–U) Flo-switch (S) and Touhy–Borst adapter (T), which connect (U) to form a hemostasis valve (dotted black line) and side-port that can be switched on or off (white arrow) for flushing or aspirating. This device is attached to the hub of the 4 Fr catheter (at white block arrow) and allows coaxial passage of a microcatheter/microwire through the 4 Fr catheter.

without vessel spasm or thrombosis. The c-arm is again rotated back into the VD position and the microcatheter/microwire combination is backed up and redirected down the contralateral internal iliac artery. The c-arm is returned into lateral projection and the same process is repeated until superselective access achieved. The remaining half of the chemotherapy and contrast mixture is administered. Alternatively, the total dose can be administered unilaterally to the side with greatest tumor burden, or alternated each treatment to reduce anesthesia times. Upon completion of the repeat angiogram the catheters are removed over-the-guide wire. The catheter and sheath are removed and the femoral or carotid artery ligated. The cut-down site is closed in three layers and the patient recovered.

The dog is monitored during recovery and receives injectable (opiates) and/or oral (Tramadol) analgesia as needed after each treatment and discharged the same day with anti-nausea medications (Table 36.1). Oral NSAIDs are continued the following the day.

Follow-Up

Patients are routinely discharged the same day with a standard protocol to minimize signs associated with adverse chemotherapy side effects (Table 36.1).

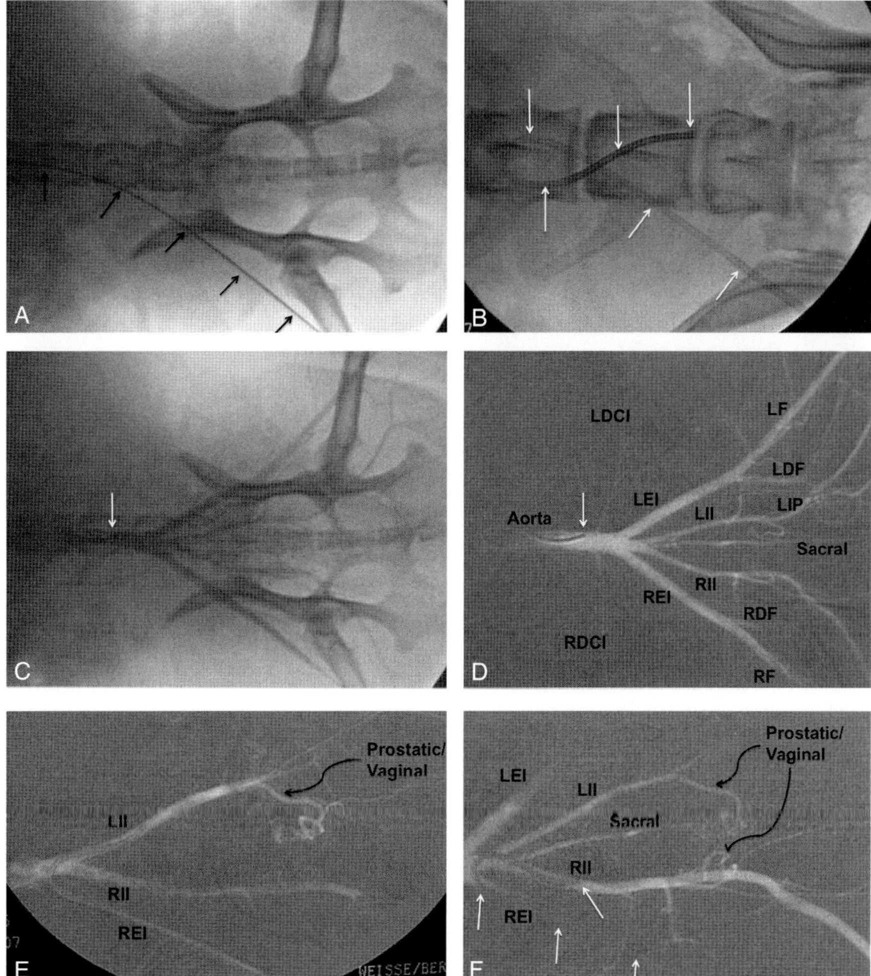

Figure 36.2 Serial VD fluoroscopic images demonstrating use of a 5Fr reverse-curve angiographic catheter to access the ipsilateral and contralateral internal iliac arteries from a femoral artery approach. (A) Right groin vascular access with femoral introducer sheath and 0.035″ angled, hydrophilic guide wire (black arrows) extending from the right femoral artery up the external iliac artery and into the aorta. (B) A 5 Fr reverse-curve angiographic catheter (white arrows) has been advanced over-the-wire and formed into a reverse curve. (C, D) The tip of the catheter (white arrow) is positioned in the terminal aorta and an angiogram (C) and DSA (D) is performed to define the relevant anatomy including left (LDCI) and right (RDCI) deep circumflex iliac, left (LEI) and right (REI) external iliac, left (LDF) and right (RDF) deep femoral, left (LF) and right (RF) femoral, left (LII) and right (RII) internal iliac, left (LIP) and right (RIP) internal pudendal, and sacral arteries. (E, F) The reverse-curve catheter (white arrows) is withdrawn into the LII (E) or RII (F) as needed in order to facilitate subsequent microcatheter super-selective access to each side of the tumor.

Instructions also include limited activity and an Elizabethan collar with regular monitoring of the groin or neck incision for 2 weeks. As with standard chemotherapy treatment, complete blood counts are recommended at 7 and 14 days post-treatment (and prior to subsequent treatment) although systemic levels are expected to be lower following IA versus systemic administration. Toxicity including myelosuppression and gastrointestinal signs should be monitored and recorded. Dose reductions and treatment delay should be instituted and antiemetics and other preventative measures provided as needed according to the standard of care.

Repeat treatments are typically recommended every 3 weeks. Repeat procedures are performed through the same vessel (femoral when possible) by approaching the artery just proximal to the previous ligation. This is standard protocol and the same vessel can be reused in the majority of cases. If thrombosis occurs, the use of both femoral arteries and a single carotid artery can suffice to achieve a minimum of three separate treatments although the author has

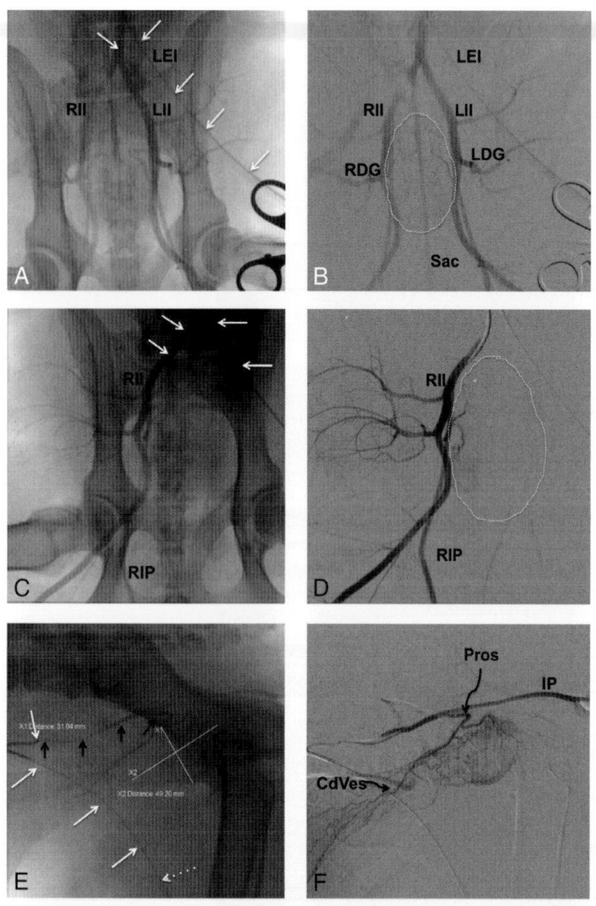

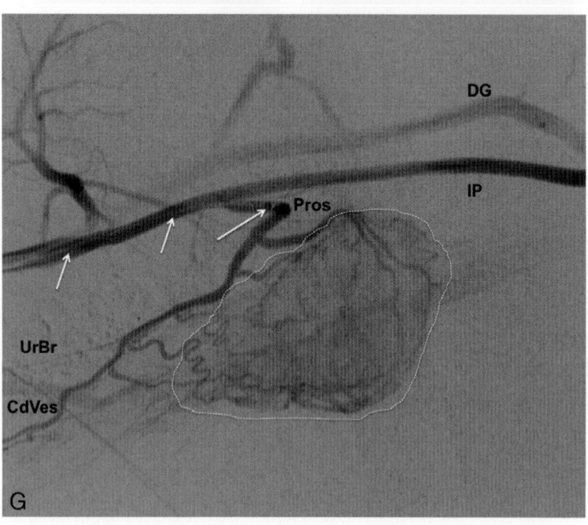

Figure 36.3 Serial fluoroscopic images of a male dog with a prostatic tumor receiving IA chemotherapy via a left femoral artery approach. Angiographic (A) and DSA (B) images showing the reverse-curve catheter (white arrows) extending up the external iliac artery (LEI) and into the orifice of the left internal iliac artery (LII). The right internal iliac artery (RII) can also be seen. Under DSA (B) additional vessels can be seen including the left (LDG) and right (RDG) deep gluteal and sacral (SAC) arteries. The prostatic tumor (white dotted line) can also be seen. Angiographic (C) and DSA (D) images after the reverse-curve catheter has been moved into the contralateral RII. The right internal pudendal artery (RIP) is also identified. (E–G) With the c-arm rotated into lateral positioning, a microcatheter (black arrows) has been passed coaxially through the reverse-curve catheter (white arrows) and a super-selective prostatic (Pros) angiogram (E) and DSA (F, G) performed. The vascular prostatic tumor can be seen as well as the caudal vesical (CdVes) artery going to the urinary bladder. The ureteral artery branch (UrBr) can also be seen.

used a carotid artery twice and an individual femoral artery up to five separate times. It is not recommended to use both carotid arteries if this can be avoided, though this has been done. Response to treatment is assessed by repeat complete staging (CBC, serum chemistry profile, UA, abdominal ultrasonography and chest radiographs) after two (or more) treatment cycles.

Special Considerations/ Alternative Uses/ Complication Examples

Prostatic artery embolization (PAE) is another technique currently being evaluated in research animals and, more recently, humans with intractable

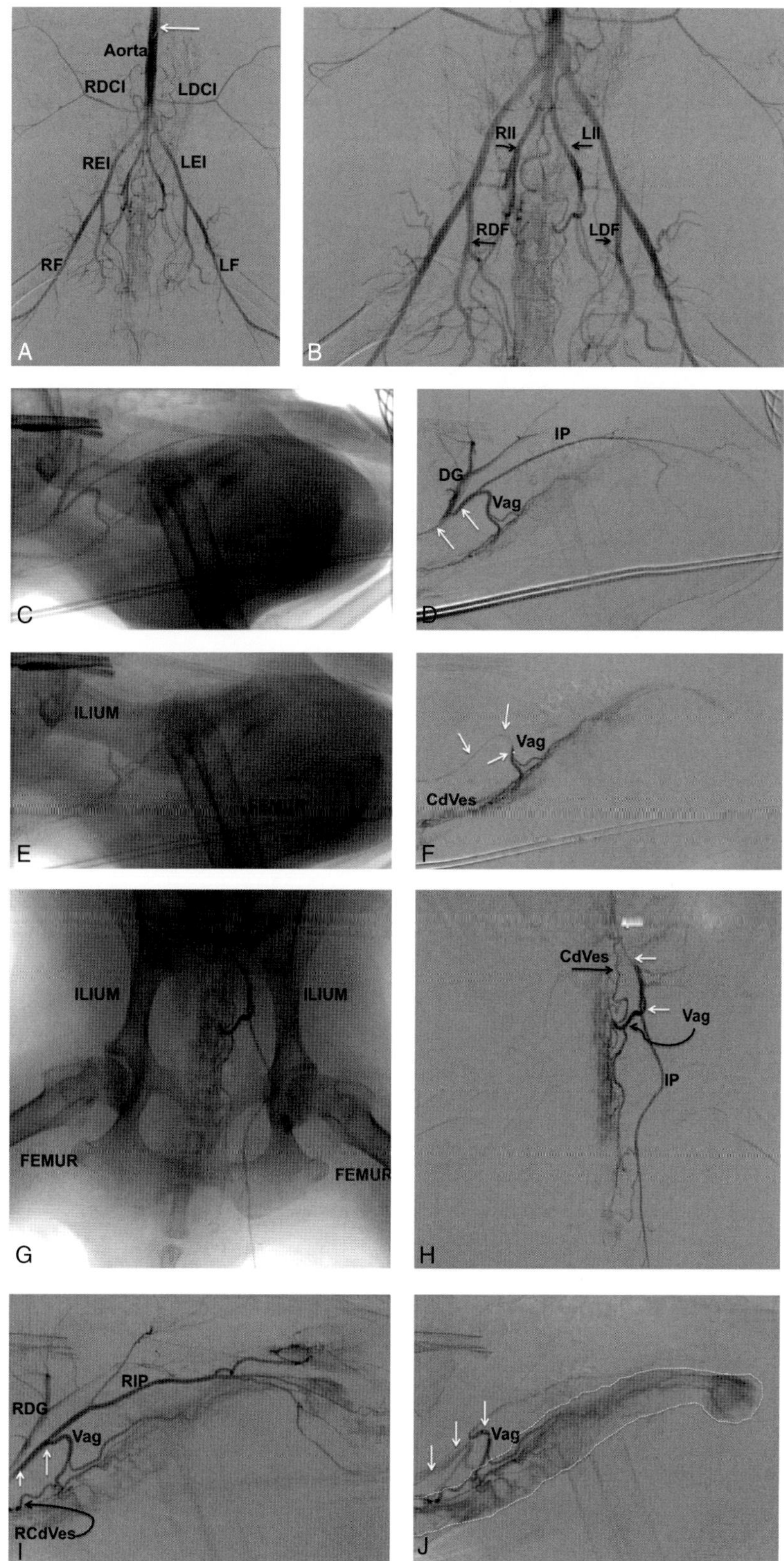

Figure 36.4 Serial fluoroscopic angiograms of a female dog with urethral TCC receiving IA chemotherapy through common carotid artery access. DSA aortogram (A) and close-up (B) through a 4 Fr Berenstein angiographic catheter with the tip (white arrow) in the distal aorta. Relevant vascular anatomy includes the left (LDCI) and right (RDCI) deep circumflex iliac, left (LEI) and right (REI) external iliac, left (LF) and right (RF) femoral, left (LDF) and right (RDF) deep femoral, and left (LII) and right (RII) internal iliac arteries. Lateral super-selective left internal pudendal arteriogram (C) and DSA (D) through a microcatheter (white arrows) demonstrating deep gluteal (DG), internal pudendal (IP), and vaginal (Vag) arteries. Super-selective left vaginal arteriogram (E) and DSA (F) demonstrating vascular urethral tumor and caudal vesical artery (CdVes) going to the urinary bladder. (G, H) Ventrodorsal super-selective vaginal arteriogram (white arrows) demonstrating perfusion only to the left-side and why bilateral treatment is recommended when blood supply evenly distributed. Contralateral (right side) super-selective vaginal arteriogram (I) and DSA (J) demonstrating different perfusion pattern to the urethral tumor (white dotted line) when performed from the right side. In this case, it may be prudent in the future to deliver a higher proportion of chemotherapy via the right side.

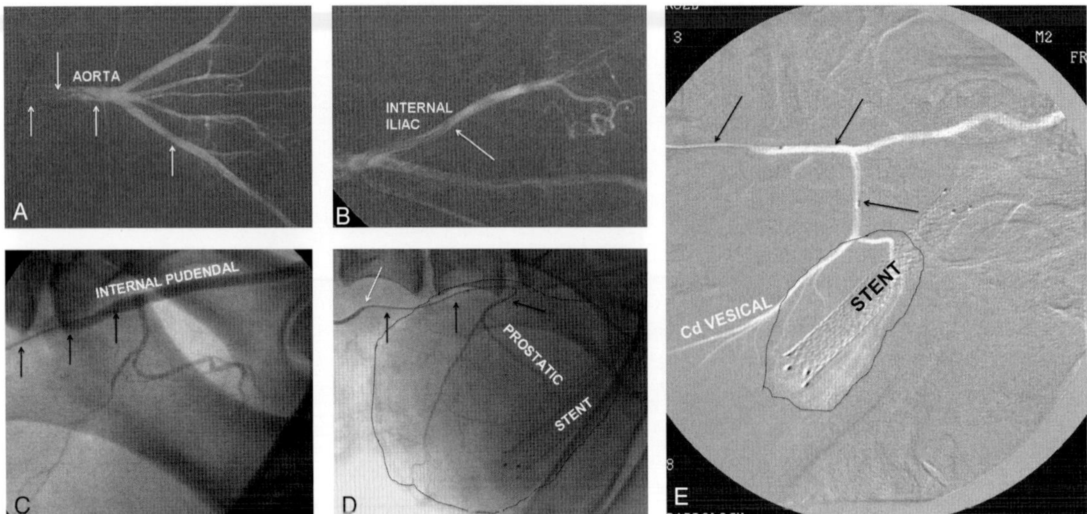

Figure 36.5 Serial fluoroscopic images in a dog with a prostatic tumor receiving serial IA chemotherapy treatments using a femoral artery approach. (A) DSA aortogram via reverse-curve catheter (white arrows) in the terminal aorta. (B) The catheter has been withdrawn down into the left internal iliac artery. (C) Lateral super-selective internal pudendal arteriogram through a microcatheter (black arrows) passed coaxially through the reverse-curve catheter. (D) Further super-selective microcatheterization (black arrows) and prostatic arteriogram demonstrating very large prostate tumor (black dotted line) and urethral stent in place. (E) Follow-up IA chemotherapy ~12 weeks later through microcatheter (black arrows) in the prostatic artery demonstrating substantially smaller prostatic tumor (black dotted line). The caudal vesical artery is visible.

benign prostatic hyperplasia. Although once considered too dangerous to perform due to possibly limited vascularity, PAE has been safely performed in research dogs. The author has performed caudal vesical artery embolization for bladder tumors associated with substantial hemorrhage, and it has been described (along with cranial vesical artery embolization) for hemorrhagic cystitis in humans. This procedure can likely be safely performed in some veterinary patients but too few cases have been performed to recommend it currently. The ideal patients are likely larger dogs in which individual arteries can be identified and super-selectively catheterized to avoid non-target embolization. Figure 36.5 demonstrates IA chemotherapy in a large male dog with a prostatic tumor. The caudal vesical artery can be identified and embolization of this vessel should be avoided when treating a urethral or prostatic tumor with possible embolization. IA chemotherapy delivery to the caudal vesical artery has not been associated with complications in the author's experience to date.

Notes

(Examples; Multiple vendors available)

1. 5 Fr Vascular introducer sheath, Infiniti Medical, Menlo Park, CA.
2. Weasel wire, Infiniti Medical, Menlo Park, CA.
3. Reverse-curve (RIM, Omni or Simmons) catheter, Infiniti Medical, Menlo Park, CA.
4. Berenstein catheter, Infiniti Medical, Menlo Park, CA.
5. Omnipaque (iohexol) injection, Amersham Health Inc., Princeton, NJ.
6. Renegade or Tracker microcatheter, Boston Scientific, Natick, MA.
7. Microcatheter, Infiniti Medical, Menlo Park, CA.
8. 0.018″ Gold-tipped glidewire, Terumo Medical Corp, Somerset, NJ.
9. 0.014 Microwire or 0.018″ Weasel wire, Infiniti Medical, Menlo Park, CA.
10. Touhy–Borst adapter, Cook Medical, Bloomington, IN.
11. Flo-switch, Boston Scientific, Natick, MA.

References

Bell FW, Klausner JS, Hayden DW, et al (1991) Clinical and pathologic features of prostatic adenocarcinoma in sexually intact and castrated dogs: 31 cases (1970–1987). *J Am Vet Medical Assoc* 199, 1623–30.

Goldsmid SE and Bellenger CR (1991) Urinary incontinence after prostatectomy in dogs. *Vet Surg* 20(4), 253–6.

Henry C (2003) Management of transitional cell carcinoma. *Vet Clin N Am Small Anim Pract* 33(3), 597–613.

Henry CJ, McCaw DL, Turnquist SE, et al (2003) Clinical evaluation of mitoxantrone and piroxicam in a canine model of human invasive urinary bladder carcinoma. *Clin Cancer Res* 9, 906–11.

Hoshi S, Mao H, Takhashi T, et al (1997) Internal iliac arterial infusion chemotherapy for rabbit invasive bladder cancer. *Int J Urol* 4(5), 493–9.

Knapp DW, Glickman NW, Denicola DB, et al (2000) Naturally-occurring canine transitional cell carcinoma of the urinary bladder. A relevant model of human invasive bladder cancer. *Urol Oncol*, 5, 47–59.

Knapp DW, Richardson RC, Thomas CK, et al (1994) Piroxicam therapy in 34 dogs with transitional cell carcinoma of the urinary bladder. *J Vet Intern Med* 8, 273–8.

Mohammed SI, Bennett PF, Craig BA, et al (2002) Effects of the cyclo-oxygenase inhibitor, piroxicam, on tumor response, apoptosis, and angiogenesis in a canine model of human invasive urinary bladder cancer. *Cancer Res* 62(2), 356–8.

Sumiyoshi Y, Yokota K, Akiyama M, et al (1991) Tissue levels of pirarubicin (THP) in dogs following intra-arterial infusion. *Gan To Kagaku Ryoho* (Cancer & chemotherapy), 18(10), 1621–6.

Weisse C, Berent AC, Sorenmo K, et al (2011) Response rates following selective and superselective intra-arterial carboplatin +/− meloxicam delivery in a naturally occurring canine model of urothelial cancer. *World Congress on Interventional Oncology*, New York, NY.

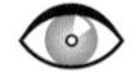 Video clips to accompany this chapter can be found in the online material at **www.wiley.com/go/weisse/vet-image-guided-interventions**

CHAPTER THIRTY-SEVEN

Ultrasound-Guided Endoscopic Laser Ablation for Transitional Cell Carcinoma in Dogs

Dean J. Cerf[1] and Eric C. Lindquist[2]
[1]Ridgewood Veterinary Hospital, Ridgewood, NJ
[2]CEO, SonoPath.com, Sparta, NJ

Background / Indications

Ultrasound-guided endoscopic diode laser ablation (UGELAB) is a palliative procedure used to maintain the flow of urine through the lower urinary tract by decreasing the tumor burden associated with transitional cell carcinoma (TCC). Intuitively, most dogs with obstructive forms of TCC will die of obstruction long before the tumor causes death by metastasis. To this end the elimination of the obstruction may allow additional time for the patient to respond to chemotherapy and provide for a more normal life style. Once luminal patency has been established the chemotherapeutic regimen may be considered, even if it only prevents regrowth in the absence of tumor remission. The UGELAB procedure has been demonstrated to provide a median survival time (MST) equivalent to that of chemotherapy such as mitoxantrone and piroxicam, even in the case of dogs with obstructive lesions in the urethra (Cerf and Lindquist, 2012). In addition, there has been conflicting evidence on whether decreasing the tumor mass prior to initiation of chemotherapy will enhance the effect of the chemotherapeutic agents and overall survival (Upton et al, 2006).

A thorough understanding of laser/tissue interaction is essential to the success of the UGELAB procedure and only those experienced in diode laser surgery, cystoscopy, and ultrasound should attempt this procedure. Ultrasound guidance is essential to the successful laser irradiation of the tumor mass while sparing normal tissues (Cerf and Lindquist, 2012, Moll, 2006, Peavy, 2002, Withrow et al, 1989). Prospective UGELAB operators are encouraged to obtain advanced training and perform less risky laser procedures before attempting this. It is imperative to advise owners that UGELAB does not offer a cure, the tumor will grow back, there is the potential for numerous complications, and chemotherapy is an important component of the overall treatment plan. It is also important to note that these tumors may require numerous UGELAB procedures for maximal effect, which is associated with expense and risk.

Patient Preparation

Prior to performing the UGELAB procedure the patient is staged by performing a thorough physical exam, a CBC and serum biochemical profile, urinalysis, urine culture, blood pressure evaluation, three view thoracic radiographs, abdominal radiographs, and a complete abdominal ultrasound, with special attention to the tumor extent, sublumbar lymph nodes, ureters and renal pelvises. The urine sample for analysis and culture and sensitivity is performed on urine obtained immediately after the endoscope enters the bladder. An extended sensitivity panel is requested to potentially increase the number of antibiotics available for use in the face of multiple drug resistant infections. While most females are treated with UGELAB shortly after diagnosis, surgery in males is sometimes delayed until there is evidence of impending obstruction because the perineal urethrostomy site has resulted in site metastasis.

Veterinary Image-Guided Interventions, First Edition. Edited by Chick Weisse and Allyson Berent.

Companion website: www.wiley.com/go/weisse/vet-image-guided-interventions

Potential Risks/ Complications/Outcomes

The UGELAB procedure can take two to five hours, with the longer surgeries encountered in males, due to the need to perform a perineal urethrostomy for urethral access. Maintenance of core body temperature and blood pressure are necessary through proper use of body warmers and intravenous fluids. Additionally, saline fluids being infused through the endoscope should be warmed prior to and during the application process.

The most immediate and significant risk with the UGELAB procedure is perforation of the urinary tract and resultant leakage of urine into the abdominal cavity. This risk can be reduced by following guidelines below. Experience with UGELAB will decrease the likelihood of perforation. Perforation can be immediate, as the result of extending the activated laser fiber through the urethra or bladder wall, or can be delayed as the result of sloughing of tissue that was devitalized by the laser energy during the procedure. Immediate perforation can be avoided through the skilled use of ultrasound and cautious use of laser energy as the wall of the urethra/bladder is approached. Delayed urine leakage is generally observed within 24 hours but can be seen up to 72 hours after the procedure. Most leakage occurs in the urethra and placement of a urinary catheter for 24–48 hours will typically resolve the leak. In the authors' experience, leakage from tumors treated in the trigone, body and apex is unusual. It is important to remember that canine TCC is typically the invasive type, having invaded the bladder muscle, and often serosal surface. Finding the fine line of depth to remove as much tumor as possible, without perforation of the wall, especially in the thin lining of the urethra, should not be taken lightly.

Infections are a common complication of the UGELAB procedure if a urinary catheter needs to be placed post-operatively. Multiple drug resistant infections are becoming more common with *Enterococcus* spp., *Escherichia coli*, *Klebsiella* spp., and *Pseudomonas* spp. being among the more common nosocomial isolates. Accordingly, urinary catheters are placed only if there is considerable concern for leakage or if an obstruction might occur in the immediate postoperative period because of swelling, inflammation, blood clots, or sloughing of devitalized tumor. Catheters are generally not indicated if the tissue being treated is anterior to the cystourethral junction, unless numerous passes of the endoscope result in urethral swelling. For this reason one should use the narrowest endoscope available with adequate length.

Scar tissue formation within the urethra is an uncommon but frustrating complication of the UGELAB procedure. In the authors experience approximately 6% of dogs experienced the formation of significant scar tissue within the urethra. Early elements of scar tissue formation can develop within a week of the procedure causing complete urethral obstruction shortly thereafter (Figure 37.1A). Stenosis secondary to scar formation is most likely to be encountered when the tumor tissue being treated involves the entire circumference of the lumen, and in most cases are in the proximal one-third of the urethra. Approximately half of these dogs were successfully treated with subsequent laser procedures, and the other half required the placement of a urethral stent (see Chapter 34).

Favorable outcomes for the UGELAB procedure (MST 380 days) without chemotherapy meet or exceed those for other treatments for TCC such as mitoxantrone and piroxicam (MST 350) (Henry et al, 2003). The MST for TCC located in the urethra is also 380 days. If a urethral obstruction exists, the use of mitoxantrone/ piroxicam alone would likely not provide durable relief. Urethral TCC will usually require multiple UGELAB procedures depending on the sensitivity of the neoplasm to chemotherapy, and how aggressive the tumor is, as all TCCs have different biological activity.

Equipment

The essential equipment for the UGELAB procedure consists of a diode laser[1], an ultrasound machine[2], and an endoscope[3] (Figure 37.2A). A 980-nm diode laser is used and should have a range of 0–25 W. Three different laser fibers are used to deliver the laser energy in the following diameters: 400, 600, and 900 μm. It is essential to understand the relationship between the size of the laser fiber and the power density of the laser energy delivered as a decrease in fiber diameter exponentially increases the power density, and therefore has a much more profound effect on the tissue being irradiated. The author commonly uses a 900um laser fiber with wattage of 16–22 W, continuous mode, using both contact and non-contact technique (Moll, 2006, Peavy, 2002). Ultrasound guidance is provided with either a 12 MHz linear or an 8 MHz micro convex ultrasound transducer. When applicable, based on the depth of the tissue being examined with ultrasound, the 12 MHz probe will provide superior detail, which is useful when evaluating the depth of laser energy penetration. The author uses either a 2.7 mm × 18 cm or

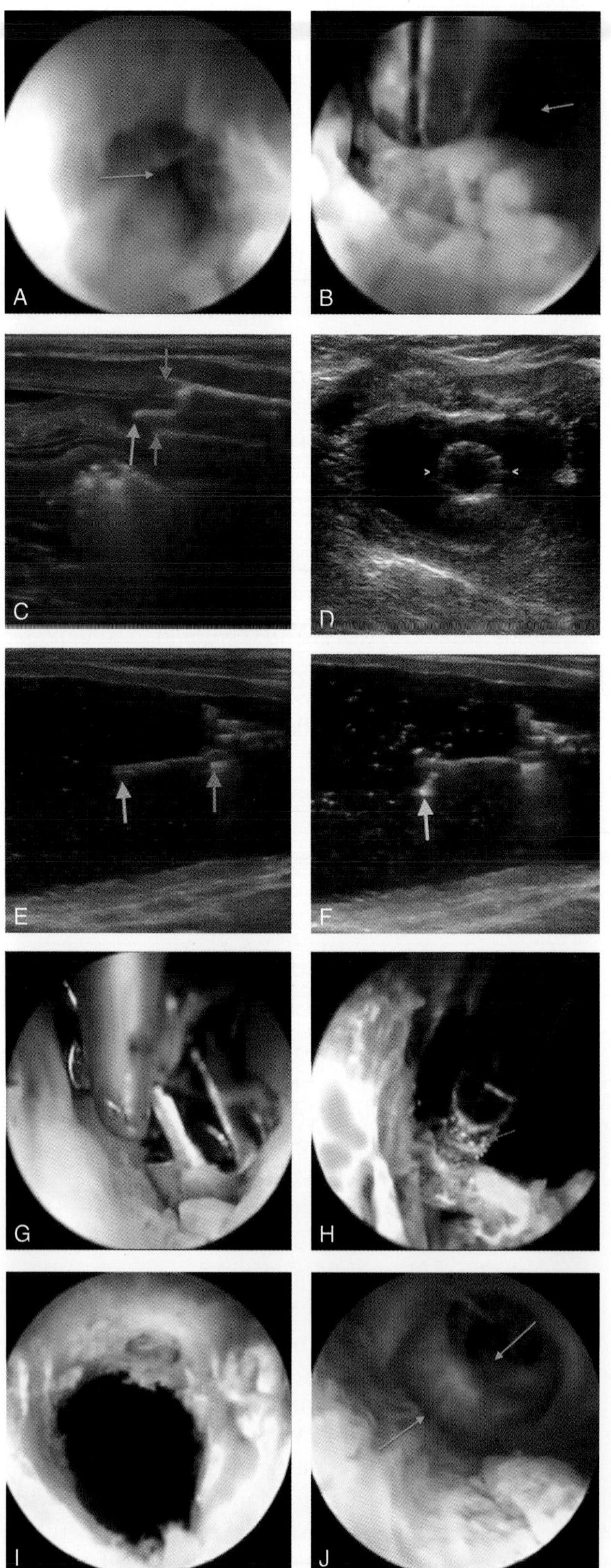

Figure 37.1 (A) Stenosis of the proximal urethra following a UGELAB procedure. The arrow indicates the very small opening in the stenotic lesion. (B) The closed biopsy instrument is positioned at the narrow opening (arrow) in the stenotic lesion. (C) This image demonstrates the placement of a biopsy instrument (blue arrow) though a urethral stent (red arrows) placed for a prior stenosis. The patient developed a subsequent occlusion in front of the stent post-UGELAB that was removed with the UGELAB procedure. This image demonstrates how precisely ultrasound can be used to keep the biopsy instrument and/or laser fiber parallel to the wall of the urethra/bladder wall. (D) Short axis views can be used to further establish the lumen of the bladder, urethra, or a stent (between arrows). (E) The urinary bladder has been distended with saline solution and the closed tip of the instrument (blue arrow) is advanced through the stent (red arrow) into the bladder. (F) The biopsy instrument jaws are opened (arrow) prior to pulling the instrument back out of the bladder. (G) Endoscopic view of biopsy instrument with jaws open as it leaves the stenotic lesion. (H) Laser is used in contact mode to remove the scar tissue which will usually have a pale appearance as compared to normal tissue. (I) Following laser treatment the luminal patency is re-established. (J) In this patient the scar tissue formed again within six weeks. The area between the arrows indicates the extent of new scar formation.

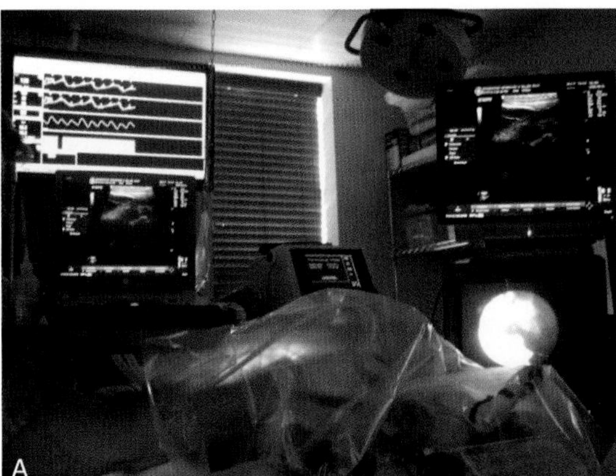

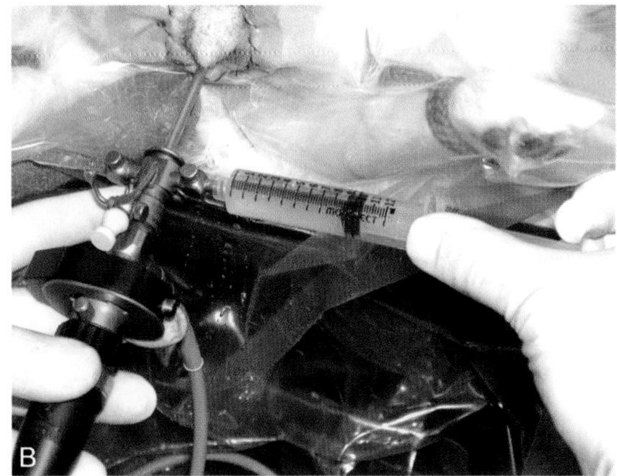

Figure 37.2 (A) Images of a female patient placed in dorsal recumbency with the perineum extending approximately one inch over the end of the table in preparation for a UGELAB procedure. Ultrasound monitors are directed at the ultrasonographer and the laser operator. The laser generator is positioned directly in front of the laser operator (between two ultrasound screens). The endoscope monitor is positioned directly below the ultrasound monitor directed towards the laser operator allowing the operator to quickly view either the ultrasound or the endoscopic view. (B) The three-port sheath allows for ingress of saline from one lateral port, laser application and biopsy from the central port, and egress and sampling from the other lateral port.

a 3.5 mm × 36.5 cm 30° offset rigid endoscope with a three port sheath (Figure 37.2B). The lateral ports provide for saline delivery and fluid drainage. The central port provides the working instrument channel through which the biopsy instrument and laser fiber is placed.

Practical Imaging of the Urinary Tract

With appropriate probe manipulation, the clinical sonographer should attain higher levels of imaging such as evaluation of the deep pelvic urethra, ureteral papillae, ureters, and kidneys. It is important to recognize obstructive or invasive pathology that may be treatable through other interventional radiology techniques concurrently or subsequently (Chapter 31).

The normal urinary bladder wall (Figure 37.3A) thickness changes dependent on the distention of the bladder itself. However, wall thickness must be taken into consideration together with mural contour, transmural deviation of the normal curvilinear appearance, as well as the presence of adhered material or debris (Figure 37.3B). The layers of the urinary bladder represent the hyperechoic outer serosa, three hypoechoic muscularis layers seen on ultrasound as a single hypoechoic line, hyperechoic lamina propria submucosa, and the inner hypoechoic transitional epithelium. Higher resolution is necessary to see all of these layers. Alterations of the natural curvilinear aspects of the wall layers may provide additional information as to the aggressiveness of the lesion (Figure 37.3C).

The deep pelvic urethra can be fully imaged with gentle manual pressure and manipulation of the descending colon with the top of the scanning hand and fingers while angling caudally from the bridge of the pelvic rim into the inguinal area (Figure 37.3D). With practice, using this technique the urethra can be imaged 3–4 cm caudally from the trigone to the level of the cervix in females (Figure 37.3E), and to the point of urethral pelvic curve in male dogs and cats. Deep pelvic urethral imaging is advantageous for pre- and post-UGELAB assessment since tumors (Figure 37.3F) can be located in the distal pelvic urethra as well as within the bladder itself.

The ureteral papillae can be found dorsally and, generally, cranial to the trigone (Figure 37.3G). Ureteral jets may be seen to help identify the ureters (Figure 37.3H). Ureteral dilation (Figure 37.4A) is seen as an anechoic tube dorsal to the urinary bladder and ventral to the colon and may be followed to the corresponding kidney (Figure 37.4B) and ureteral papilla to assess laterality. A dilated ureter will not fill with color flow Doppler (Figure 37.4C). Dilation of the urethra and ureters should be assessed and followed to identify the obstruction. Renal integrity and bladder mass depth should also be assessed (Figure 37.4 and Figure 37.5).

Procedure

The patient is placed in dorsal recumbency on top of a body warming system[4] and a 1.5-inch thick foam pad. The perineum extends over the edge of the table 1–2 inches. The pelvic region and perineum are clipped and aseptically prepared. Tincture of Benzoin is applied to the skin where a fenestrated sterile clear

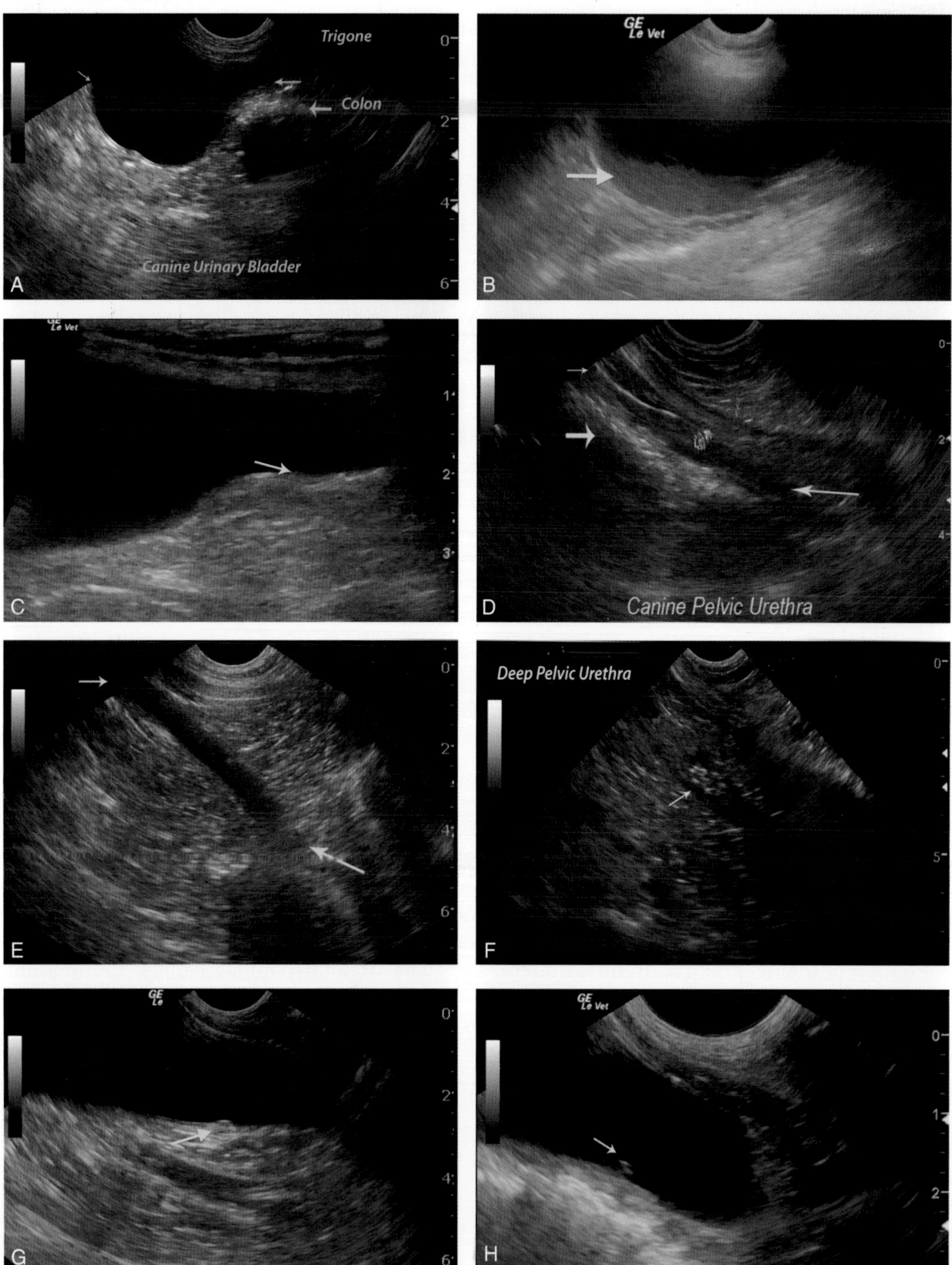

Figure 37.3 (A) Normal 8 MHz global assessment of the urinary bladder in long axis with apex to the left (small arrow) and trigone to the right. The shadow of the colon is positioned dorsal to the bladder. The bladder wall (middle arrow) may be followed separately from the colonic wall (large arrow) to ensure the colonic shadow is not confused with a luminal calculus or mineralized lesion. (B) Dependent bladder debris (arrow) that must not be confused with a bladder mass. Debris will be mobile on ballottment or flushing and will not demonstrate power Doppler color flow. (C) High-resolution (12 MHz) image of the normal urinary bladder demonstrating layer detail (arrow) that is essential to evaluate for transmural penetration of lesions. (D) The pelvic urethra (long arrow) can be imaged 3–4 cm distal from the cystourethral junction (small arrow). The colon (large arrow) may be used as a point of reference to identify the urethra adjacent to it in the near field. (E) 4+ cm of pelvic urethra is imaged in this female geriatric dog. The urethra is excessively dilated in a uniform manner. This is a common finding when distal obstruction is present beyond the sonographic field of view. Small arrow: cystourethral junction, large arrow: caudal extent of pelvic urethra. (F) Pelvic urethral mass (arrow) with multifocal hyperechoic mineralization in a dog that presented with pollakiuria and dysuria. The bladder, cystourethral junction and proximal urethra were normal in this patient. This image evidences the necessity to image the deep pelvic urethra when performing an ultrasound. (G) 8 MHz long axis view of the bladder trigone demonstrating a ureteral papillae (arrow). (H) Global 8 MHz assessment of the urinary bladder in long axis. The ureteral jet (arrow) may be seen at the right ureteral papilla to use as a landmark for resection of mural pathology. Image courtesy of Doug Casey DVM, DABVP, Cert IVUSS.

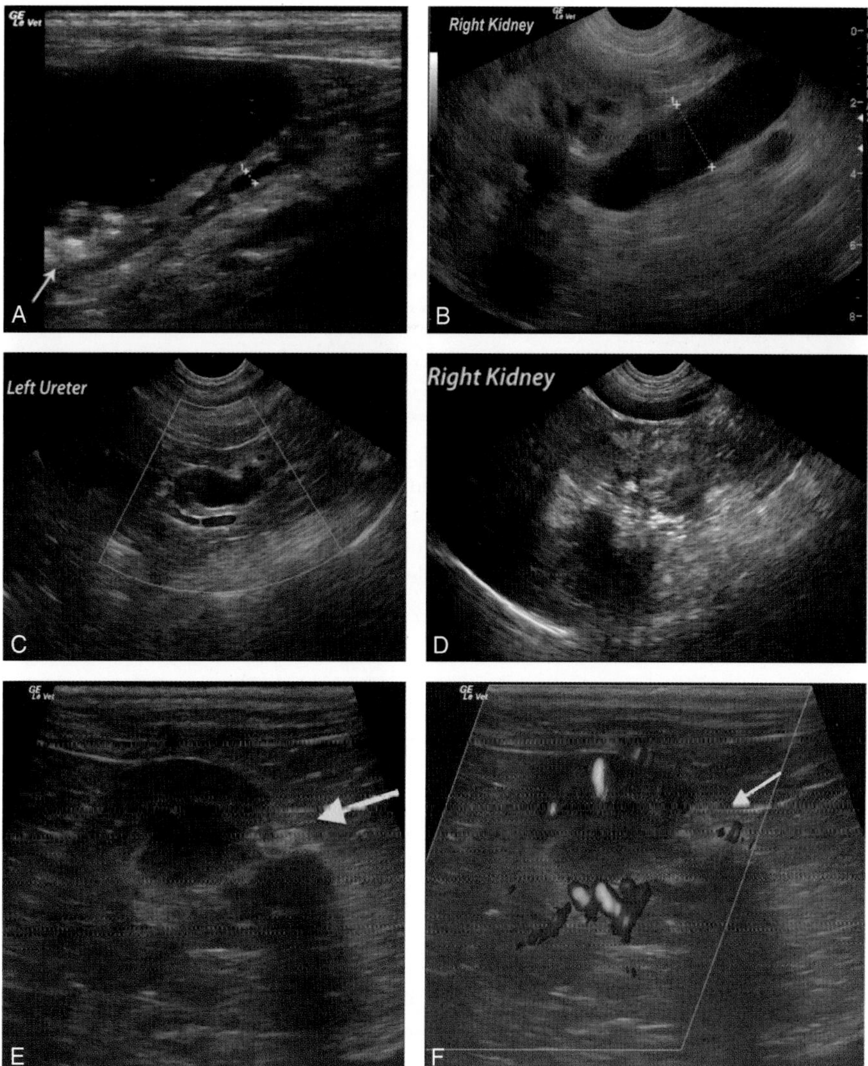

Figure 37.4 (A) Hydroureter seen dorsal to the urinary bladder (0.17 cm) at the end of a UGELAB procedure where a TCC mass was obstructing the ureter. Ureteral decompression was achieved by ablating the mass that enveloped the ureteral papilla. Minimal mass remained (arrow). (B) Severe hydroureter in a dog. Courtesy Andi Parkinson RDMS. (C) Anechoic tubular ureters may be distinguished from blood vessels by means of Color Flow Doppler assessment. A dilated ureter, such as the one in this image, will not demonstrate color flow filling. (D) Incidental finding of renal infarctions in a geriatric MN dog. Note the distinct triangular hyperechoic cortical lesions. (E) Renal infarct (arrow) present in the caudal renal cortex in a dog. Note the focal hyperechoic and mineralized lesion with focal capsular retraction. (F) Power Doppler assessment demonstrating lack of Doppler signals in the infarcted region (arrow) of the kidney but solid signals throughout the remaining cortex which subjectively suggesting blood flow.

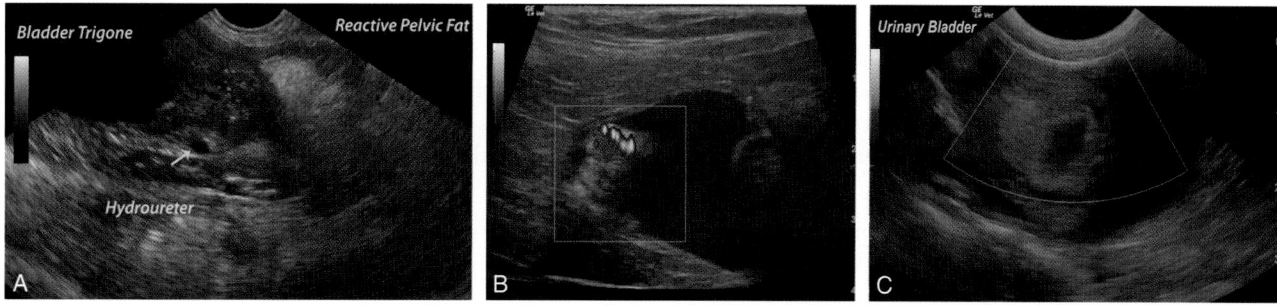

Figure 37.5 (A) Cysto-urethral junction and trigonal mineralizing bladder mass with transmural extension. The ill-defined surrounding echogenic fat in the 2 o'clock position is consistent with regional inflammation typical of transmural disease. Note that the bladder wall layers are indistinguishable and are essentially replaced by the infiltrative mass. Minor hydroureter is noted in mid screen at 3 cm depth (arrow). (B) Mineralizing apical urinary bladder mass (TCC) with strong power Doppler tissue signals that may serve as a target during the UGELAB procedure. (C) Urinary bladder blood clot that resembles a mass. However, power Doppler signals are nonexistent suggesting the presence of blood clot as opposed to tissue mass. This clot resolved 10 days later. Image courtesy of Andi Parkinson RDMS.

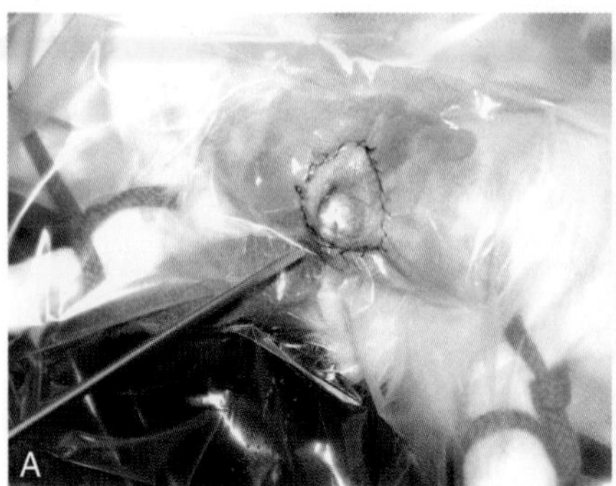

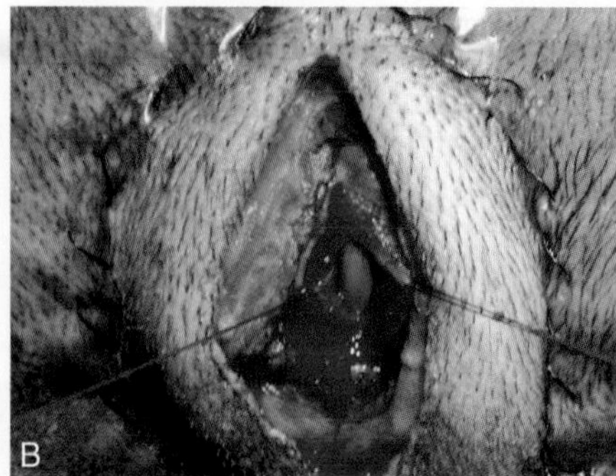

Figure 37.6 (A) A female dog is positioned in dorsal recumbency for a UGELAB procedure. A fenestrated adhesive drape is sutured in place using a nylon suture material. In this photo the endoscope can be seen approaching the vulva. (B) A male dog is positioned in dorsal recumbency. A perineal urethrostomy is used to gain access to the pelvic urethra with the rigid endoscope. Sutures are placed as noted in this photo to aid in placement of the endoscope into the urethra and when closing the urethra at the conclusion of the procedure. Placement of a sterile urinary catheter in the urethra prior to surgery allows the operator to locate the urethra by palpation as well as visualization.

adhesive plastic drape will be placed. A non-fenestrated sterile plastic drape is placed over a tub designed to catch fluids from the endoscopic procedure and both are positioned under the perineum providing a waterproof sterile field. The fenestrated plastic drape with adhesive backing is placed over the vulva/perineal urethrostomy site. The margin of the fenestration is then sutured to the skin using a simple continuous pattern with 2–0 nylon suture (Figure 37.6A). In male dogs a perineal urethrostomy is performed to gain access to the urethra. Polyglactin 910 suture (5–0) material is placed in the margin of the urethral incision at 3 and 9 o'clock to aid in placing the endoscope and in closing the urethra at the completion of the procedure (Figure 37.6B).

The endoscope is introduced into vestibule or the perineal urethrostomy site, with the infusion of sterile saline. In male dogs, the rigid endoscope is directed antegrade, into the penile urethra, to assess for evidence of TCC which, in the authors experience, is an uncommon finding. The endoscope is then directed into the urethra proximal to the urethrostomy site. In female dogs, the vestibule is assessed (Figure 37.7), Understanding the anatomical relationship of the clitoris, vestibule, vagina and urethra is essential to gaining access to the urethra and is further expanded upon in Chapter 26 (urinary imaging) (Figure 37.7).

Once the urethra is entered the operator will encounter either the normal longitudinal pink folds of a collapsed urethra or tumor tissue (Figure 37.8). Allowing saline to fill the bladder will cause the urethra to expand and let the endoscope pass more easily. Care must be taken not to advance the endoscope against significant resistance or the urethra may tear. The bladder should be closely monitored with ultrasound and frequently palpated to avoid over distension and rupture. If the endoscope does not pass freely a closed endoscopic biopsy instrument, or soft hydrophilic guide wire, can be placed into the bladder carefully, using ultrasound to guide it. Care should be taken in doing this blindly, as perforation can occur. The instrument is then opened and gently withdrawn, resulting in creating a small lumen in the center of the urethra. This is repeated until the lumen widens large enough to pass the endoscope (Figure 37.1). If this process is not successful, advanced UGELAB operators may consider performing a similar procedure using the diode laser fiber, activating the laser only as the fiber is withdrawn from the bladder towards the endoscope. This increases the potential for major complication. The laser energy must be turned off before entering the endoscope or the endoscope may get damaged. This should only be done using ultrasound guidance, since the laser fiber is stiff and the end is sharp, so urethral perforation is possible. The safest way to remove tumor within the urethra is to monitor the lumen as the endoscope is withdrawn away from the bladder. Tumor tissue that "falls" into the field of vision is in the middle of the lumen and can safely be vaporized as long as the endoscope remains parallel to the wall of the urethra. Repeating this process many times allows the UGELAB operator to slowly open the urethra, peeling back the layers like an onion. As soon as the endoscope is able to pass into the bladder easily, urine samples are taken as mentioned above. The bladder should be thoroughly examined to map the location of all tumor masses and identify the ureteral papillae. When evaluating the bladder wall the operator should be familiar with using the 30 degree lens of the cystoscope appropriately so that visibility of the

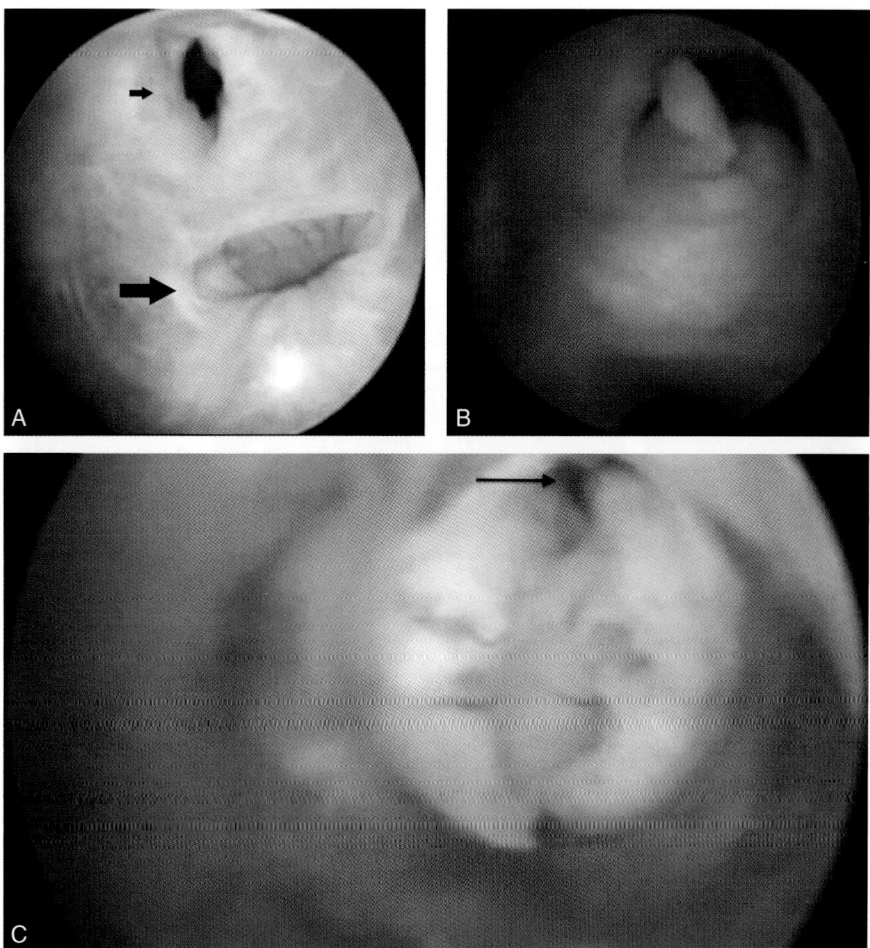

Figure 37.7 (A) endoscope placed in the vestibule of a female dog in dorsal recumbency. The urethral opening is a slit like structure oriented along a ventral-dorsal plane (small arrow). The opening to the vagina is oval, lies dorsal to the urethral opening and will usually display folds in the distal end of the collapsed vagina (large arrow). It is important to understand these anatomical relationships as tumor may distort the normal anatomy making entry into the urethra challenging. (B) A relatively small tumor mass fills the dorsal portion of the urethral orifice. While the mass may need to be removed to gain entry to the urethra the anatomy is normal enough to easily visualize where the endoscope should be placed. (C) The tumor growing in the urethra of this female dog prevents the operator from seeing the urethra and vaginal openings and entry into the urethra is challenging. A very small glimpse of the urethra can be seen ventral to the mass (arrow).

ventral and dorsal bladder wall can be maximized by turning the scope in 180 degrees (Chapter 26).

A similar examination is performed by the ultrasonographer in both short axis and long axis views. The use of the short axis view may better define the site of tumor attachment when the bladder is fully distended (Figure 37.9). At times the tumor may appear, in the ultrasound view, to originate from the ventral or dorsal wall in the long axis view but will be seen to actually originate from the lateral wall in the short axis view. This may allow the experienced UGELAB operator to cut the mass off at the base, which can save considerable time as compared to removing the mass with an ablation technique.

Ablation of tumors isolated to the region of the cystourethral junction is often very rewarding in terms of immediate patient response to treatment and need for limited postoperative care in spite of the life-threatening nature of the obstruction. Tumors of the cystourethral junction often present as complete or nearly complete obstructions (Figure 37.10A). Following the UGELAB procedure many of these patients will have a completely patent urethra (Figure 37.10B). Using the UGELAB procedure dogs with complete obstruction of the trigone and proximal urethra can return to normal urination with one procedure (Figure 37.11); however, it is very likely that the procedure will need to be repeated numerous times to maintain patency as the tumor will continue to regrow. Chemotherapy should also be initiated to attempt to retard growth.

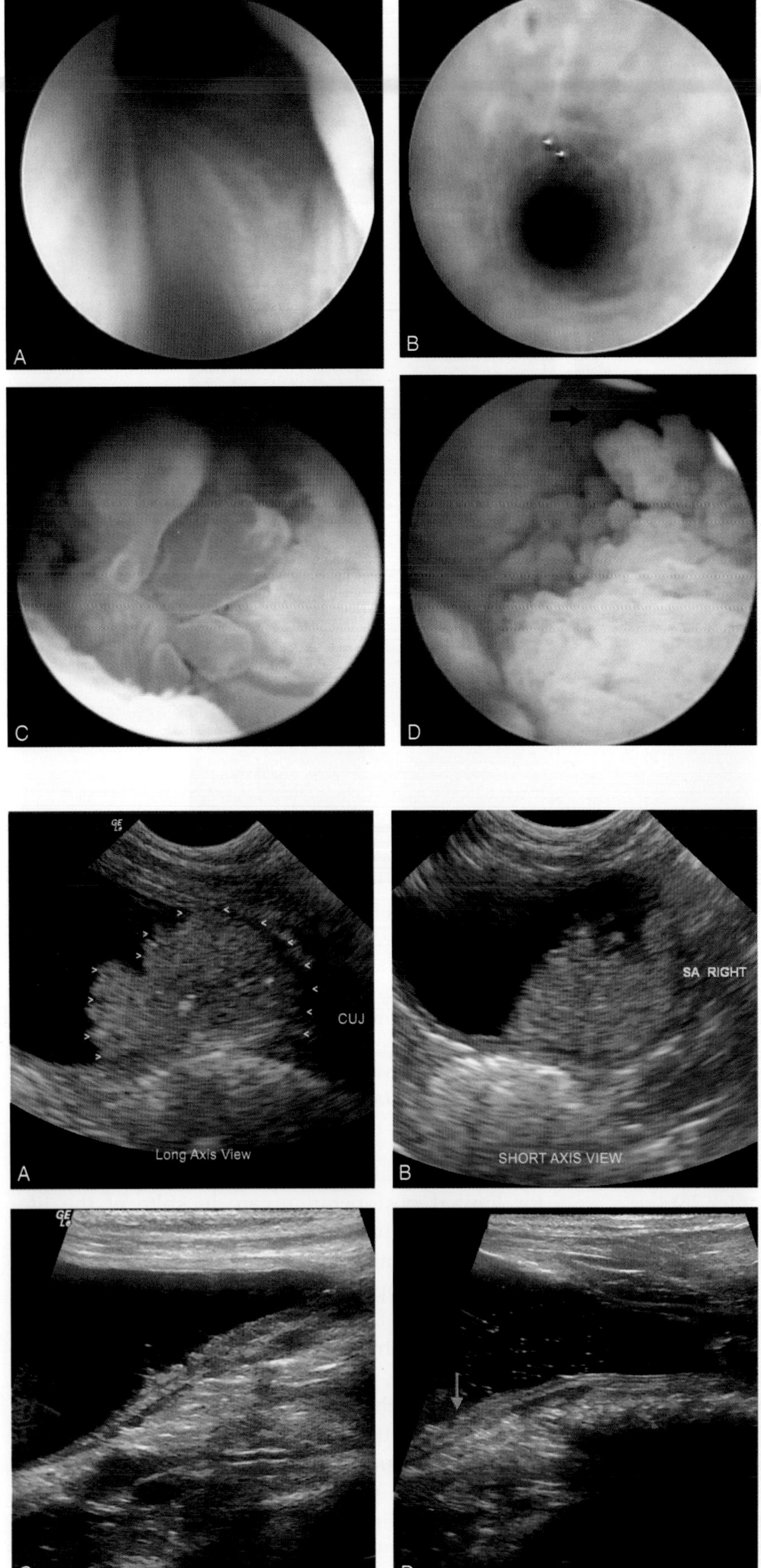

Figure 37.8 (A) Endoscopic view of a female canine urethra. A normal partially inflated urethral has longitudinal folds and has a uniform pale pink color without obvious blood vessels. (B) When fully distended with saline solution the lumen appears very smooth with no projections of tissue into the lumen. In this photo the urethra appears somewhat irritated due to rubbing of the endoscope on the urethra. (C) This image of TCC within a female canine urethra demonstrates the highly vascular nature of TCC. The presence of pigmented hemoglobin enhances the absorption of near infrared diode laser energy and facilitates tumor ablation. (D) Tissue projecting into the lumen of the bladder of a female dog.

Figure 37.9 (A) Long axis view of a TCC appearing to entirely occlude the cystourethral junction (CUJ). (B) Short axis view of the same mass showing attachment to the right dorsal aspect of the CUJ. Using both views as well as the endoscopic view allows the operator to create a mental three dimensional view to allow accurate ablation of the mass. (C) CUJ is entirely patent at the conclusion of the UGELAB procedure. (D) Proximal urethra is entirely patent. Minimal residual tumor is seen (arrow) proximal to the patent urethra.

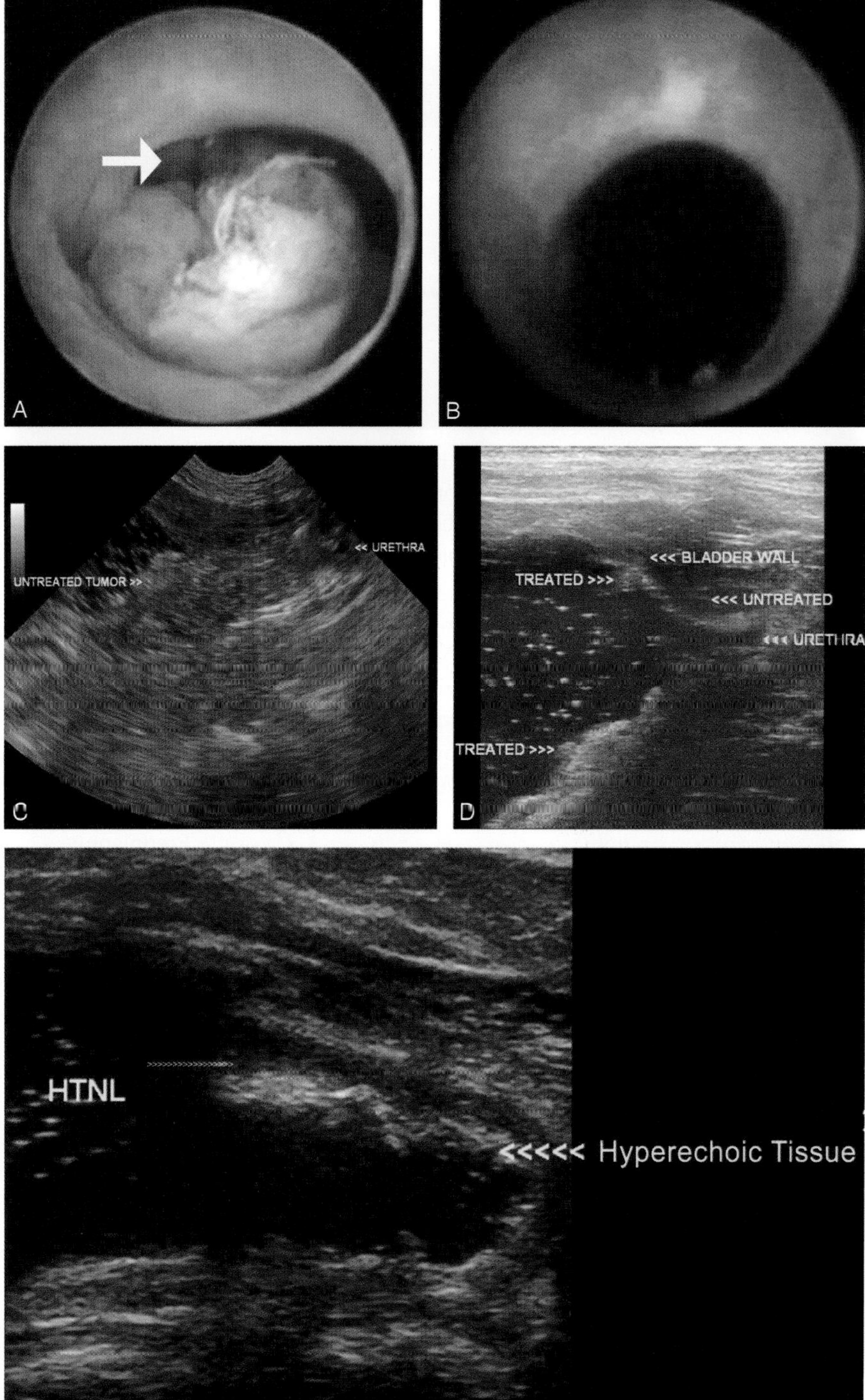

Figure 37.10 (A) Endoscopic view of a TCC occluding nearly the entire cystourethral junction (CUJ) in a female dog in dorsal recunbency. Arrow indicates minimal luminal patency. (B) Following the UGELAB procedure the CUJ is essentially 100% patent. In this individual the lining of the urethra has become irritated by the movement of the endoscope within the lumen. (C) Ultrasound image of the TCC occluding nearly the entire cystourethral junction (CUJ) and proximal urethra prior to the UGELAB procedure. (D) The same patient at the conclusion of the UGELAB procedure. The stippled appearance of the fluid within the bladder/urethra represents tumor debris created by the ablation process. Notice the superior imaging quality of the 12 mHz linear tranducer (D) versus the 8 mHz curved transducer (C).

During the UGELAB procedure ultrasound is used to approach tumor masses, ensure that the laser fiber does not penetrate the bladder or urethral wall, and aid in keeping the endoscope/laser fiber parallel to the bladder wall. In addition, ultrasound is used to monitor the penetration depth of the laser energy, the degree of bladder fullness and monitor for signs of fluid leakage into the peritoneal cavity. As the laser denatures the tumor tissue the devitalized tissue becomes more hyperechoic and appears white compared to non-treated tissue (Figure 37.10D). The demarcation between treated and untreated tissue is referred to as the hyperechoic tissue necrosis line (HTNL) (Figure 37.10E). It is possible that the laser

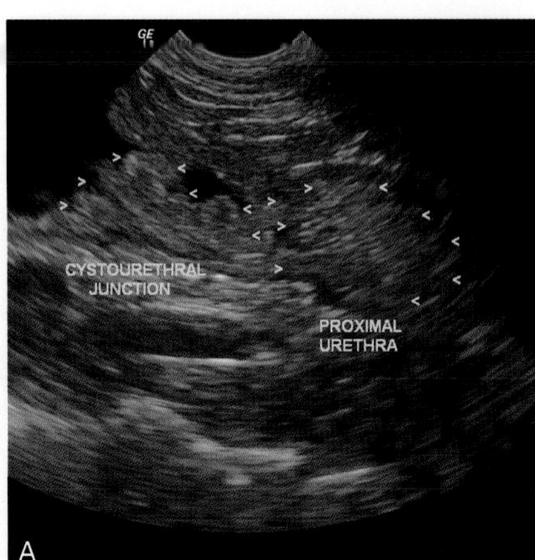

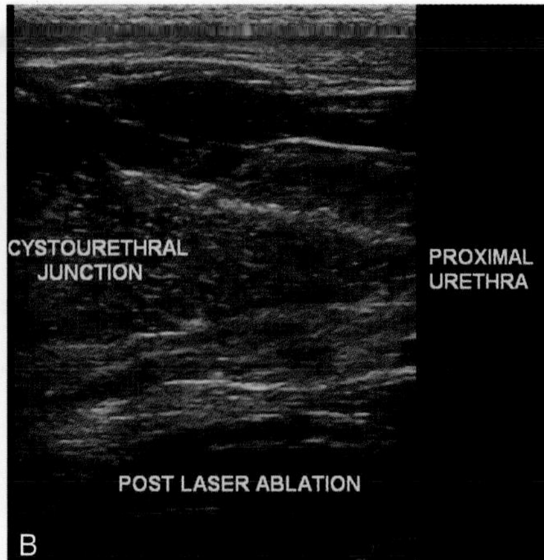

Figure 37.11 (A) ultrasound long axis image image of a female dog with TCC occluding nearly the entire cystourethral junction (CUJ) and proximal urethra prior to the UGELAB procedure. B) The same patient at the conclusion of the UGELAB procedure. The stippled appearance of the fluid within the bladder/urethra represents tumor debris created by the ablation process. Notice the superior imaging quality of the 12 mHz linear tranducer (B) versus the 8 mHz curved transducer (A).

energy could denature tissue below the HTNL and, therefore, it is suggested that the HTNL not be taken to close to the bladder/urethral wall. It is preferable to perform subsequent UGELAB procedures rather than cause a perforation. With greater experience the operator should be able to get the HTNL closer to the wall without adverse consequences. The bladder is intermittently filled and flushed with saline solution during the procedure to better position the mass for laser treatment and to clean debris from the bladder. Likewise, by deflating the bladder, tumor in the apex or body will move caudally and closer to the endoscope and laser fiber which can reduce the need to use a larger/longer endoscope, which could excessively irritate the urethra. It is best not to energize the laser fiber to ablate tumor while deflating the bladder, as this could cause the bladder wall to collapse over the laser fiber resulting in a bladder perforation. At the conclusion of the procedure the bladder is filled and manually expressed repeatedly until ultrasound reveals that all loose debris has been flushed out. Ultrasound evaluation for free fluid in the abdomen should be done at the conclusion of the procedure.

Follow-Up

If significant laser energy is used to treat the urethra, or if the urethral appears swollen, edematous, or overly erythematous, a urinary catheter should be placed for at least 24 hours. The catheter should be removed as early as possible to avoid nosocomial infections. Data would support that with appropriate catheter management like a fully closed, sterile, collection system, cleaning of the urinary catheter with chlorohexidine scrub every 4 hours, and a short indwelling time (ideally <24 hours, but ultimately <48–72 hours), avoidance of nosocomial infections is best (Smarick et al, 2004). When appropriate, patients are placed on antibiotics and these are changed as indicated, based upon the result of the culture and sensitivity testing. As indicated, the operator may consider the use of steroids, bethanechol, phenoxybenzamine, prazosin, diazepam, and/or yunnan paiyou, to facilitate proper urination and to control inflammation, swelling and bleeding, respectively (Table 37.1). Care should be taken in using steroids if there is an active urinary tract infection, and should never be used if the patient is concurrently receiving NSAID therapy.

TABLE 37.1
Commonly used medications - UGELAB

Bethanechol	5–15 mg/dog PO q8h
Diazepam	0.2 mg/kg PO q8h or 2–10 mg (total dose) PO q8h
Phenoxybenzamine	0.25 mg/kg PO q8–12h
Prazosin	1 mg/15 kg PO q8–12h
Prednisone	0.5–1 mg/kg PO per day, reducing dose
Yunnan Paiyou	1 cap sid-tid prn control hematuria

Special Considerations/ Complication Examples

The most immediate and common complication is leakage of urine into the peritoneal cavity. Providing that the laser operator has not used excessive laser energy, this will usually resolve within 24–48 hours after urinary catheter placement. Ultrasound should be used to make sure that the abdominal fluid is resolved before the catheter is removed and the abdomen should then be monitored with ultrasound for an additional 24–48 hours to make sure that there is no subsequent urine leakage. Bladder infections, when encountered, are treated according to standard medical protocols based on the results of culture and sensitivity results. Excessive scar formation within the urethra is an uncommon, but life threatening complication. Tumor regrowth is also common, and repeat UGELAB procedures are often necessary.

Notes

1. CeralasD15, 980 nm Diode Laser, CeramOptec (BioLitec), East Longmeadow, MA.
2. GE Logiq Ultrasound, 12 MHz linear, 8 MHz micro convex ultrasound transducer probe, Milwaukee, WI.
3. HopkinsII 30° rigid telescope, 2.7 mm × 18 cm or 3.5 cm × 36.5 cm and Operating Sheath, Karl Storz Veterinary Endoscopy, Goleta, CA.
4. Bair Hugger, Arizant Healthcare Inc., a 3M company, Eden Prairie, MN 55344.

References

Cerf DJ and Lindquist EC (2012) Palliative ultrasound-guided endoscopic diode laser ablation of transitional cell carcinomas of the lower urinary tract in dogs. *J Am Vet Med Assoc* 240(1), 51–60.

Henry CJ, Dudley ML, Turnquist SE, et al (2003) Clinical evaluation of mitoxantrone and piroxicam in a canine model of human invasive urinary bladder cancer. *ClinCancer Res* 9, 906–11.

Moll JR (2006) Diode lasers in small animal veterinary medicine. In: *Veterinary Laser Surgery* (Berger N and Eeg PH eds.), Blackwell Publishing, Ames IA, pp.111–138.

Peavy GM (2002) Lasers and laser-tissue interaction. In: *The Veterinary Clinics of North America, Small Animal Practice*, Vol. 32, No. 3 (J. Vassallo, ed.), W.B. Saunders, Philadelphia, pp 517–34.

Smarick SD, Haskins SC, Aldrich J, et al (2004) Incidence of catheter-associated urinary tract infection among dogs in a small animal intensive care unit. *J Am Vet Med Assoc* 224(12), 1936–40.

Withrow SJ, Gillette EL, Hoopes PJ, and McChesney SL (1989) Intraoperative irradiation of 16 spontaneously occurring canine neoplasms. *Vet Surg* 18(1), 7–11.

Upton ML, Tangner CH, and Payton ME (2006) Evaluation of carbon dioxide laser ablation combined with mitoxantrone and peroxicam treatment in dogs with transitional cell carcinoma. *J Am Vet Med Assoc* 228(4), 549–52.

Suggested Reading

Benigni L, Lamb CR, Corzo-Menendez N, et al (2006) Lymphoma affecting the urinary bladder in three dogs and a cat. *Vet Radiol Ultrasound* 47(6), 592 – 6.

Blackburn A, Berent A, Weisse C, et al (2013) Evaluation of outcome following urethral stent placement for the treatment of obstructive carcinoma of the urethra in dogs: 42 cases (2004–2008). *Jo Am Vet Med Assoc* 242(1), 59–68.

Cruz-Arámbulo R and Wrigley R (2003) Ultrasonography of the acute abdomen. *Clin TechnSmall Anim Pract* 18(1), 20 31.

Geisse AL, Lowry JE, Schaeffer DJ, et al (1997) Sonographic evaluation of urinary bladder wall thickness in normal dogs. *Vet Radiol Ultrasound* 38(2), 132–7.

Heng HG, Lowry JE, and Boston S (2006) Smooth muscle neoplasia of the urinary bladder wall in three dogs. *Vet Radiol Ultrasound*. 47(1), 83–6.

Holloway A and O'Brien R (2007) Perirenal effusion in dogs and cats with acute renal failure. *Vet Radiol Ultrasound* 48(6), 574–9.

Hylands R (2006) Veterinary diagnostic imaging. Retroperitoneal abscess and regional cellulitis secondary to a pyelonephritis within the left kidney. *Can Vet J* 47(10), 1033–5.

Josel JR, Pagor CA, Glickman MPH, et al (2002). The role of surgical debulkment in dogs with transitional cell carcinoma of the urinary bladder: a retropspective study of 122 dogs. In: *Proceedings of the 22nd Annual Conference of the Veterinary Cancer Society.*, pp 5. Veterinary Cancer Society, New York.

Nyland TG, Mattoon TS, Hergessell ER, et al (2002) Urinary tract. In: *Small Animal Diagnostic Ultrasound*, 2nd edn. Elsevier, Philadelphia, pp 158–95.Nyland TG, Hager DA, and Herring DS (1989) Sonography of the liver, gallbladder and spleen. *Semin Vet Med Surg (Small Anim)* 4, 13–31.

Weisse C, Berent A, Todd K, Clifford C, et al (2006) Evaluation of palliative stenting for management of malignant urethral obstructions in dogs. *J Am Vet Med Assoc* 229(2), 226–34.

CHAPTER THIRTY-EIGHT

Injectable Bulking Agents for Treatment of Urinary Incontinence

Julie K. Byron
Department of Veterinary Clinical Sciences, The Ohio State University, Columbus, OH

Background/Indications

Maintenance of urinary continence relies on many factors. Normally, the major component of urethral tone is comprised of smooth muscle. The mucosal integrity, vasculature, and connective tissue surrounding the urethra also plays an important role in preserving continence. In addition, healthy urothelium, surface tension from glandular secretions, and the pliability of the mucosa contribute significantly to coaptation of the urethral walls, and ultimate continence.

The most common type of urinary incontinence recognized in female dogs is urethral sphincter mechanism incompetence (USMI). Incontinent female dogs have been found to have lower urethral closure pressures than continent dogs, and closure pressure increases in patients successfully managed with medical therapy with either estrogens or α-agonists. The classic signalment is a young-middle-aged spayed female large breed (>20 kg) dog. In the literature large breed dogs (>20 kg) seem to be over-represented compared to smaller breed dogs (<20 kg). There is some evidence that spaying a female dog prior to 3 months of age can increase the risk of urinary incontinence, and there is debate over whether dogs should be spayed prior to the first heat, or after the first heat, in order to further decrease the risk of incontinence.

The best way to obtain a true diagnosis of USMI is based on the results of urethral pressure profilometry. A majority of clinicians don't have access to this equipment, making a diagnosis by exclusion necessary. This is done by using alternative diagnostic imaging (ultrasonography, cystoscopy, CT, contrast urethrocytography, etc.) to rule out other anatomical causes of urinary incontinence. Once the animal is deemed anatomically and neurologically normal than a diagnosis of presumptive USMI can typically be made.

When the disease is localized to USMI alone, complete continence with medical treatment is not guaranteed with medical failures reported in 15–35% of dogs with USMI. Phenylpropanolamine (PPA) is reported to be effective in 74–90% of female dogs and estrogen therapy in 40–85% of dogs, and they are best when used in combination. Other drugs that have been tried, with less success, include GnRH analogues and tricyclic antidepressants (i.e., Imipramine).

Due to the relatively high prevalence of this condition in female dogs, and the overall intolerance by pet owners, a number of procedures, both open and minimally invasive, have been developed to improve continence in dogs failing medical therapy. Many of these have been adapted from human urology, including the use of urethral bulking agents (UBAs).

Injectable UBAs have been used for nearly 80 years in women for treatment of stress and mixed urinary incontinence. During the late 1990s, the use of UBAs was adapted to treat dogs with USMI that failed medical therapy. The principle behind all injectable UBAs is to narrow the diameter of the urethral lumen, thus creating outflow obstruction, increasing the stretch in sphincter muscle fibers, and allowing the urethral muscle to close more effectively. In veterinary medicine injection of UBAs has been performed in selected centers for many years but there is now more widespread application following the introduction of safer and more effective bulking materials.

Veterinary Image-Guided Interventions, First Edition. Edited by Chick Weisse and Allyson Berent.

Companion website: www.wiley.com/go/weisse/vet-image-guided-interventions

Patient Preparation/ Work-Up

Because of the cost, and concerns about the duration of post-procedure urinary continence after the use of UBAs, patient selection for urethral injection is important. The ideal patient has USMI without additional active lower urinary tract disease, including a urinary tract infection. All patients should have a negative urine culture within 2 weeks of injection. Each patient should also have a thorough cystourethroscopy prior to injection to ensure there are not concurrent causes of urinary incontinence, like ectopic ureters. The majority of dogs have failed, or are intolerant of, medical therapy with estrogens or α-agonists. In spite of this, many of these patients have an improved response to medical therapy after injection, unrelated to previous results. Currently, injection therapy is recommended most frequently for those patients with USMI and failure, or declining efficacy, of α-agonist and/or estrogen therapy. As discussed in the following paragraphs, patients with ectopic ureters may benefit from this procedure; however, the location of the ureteral stomata is important.

Potential Risks/ Complications/ Expected Outcomes

The potential risks of using bulking agents for urinary incontinence is material intolerance, abscess formation if concurrent UTI, bleeding during injection, urethral obstruction after injections, and failure of success. Owners should always be aware that there is a chance the injection will not benefit their pet, and that this material is temporary, and will typically require additional injections in the future (within a few months to a few years). With most materials the owners can expect the benefit to last 10–18 months.

Additionally, most of the literature available is on the use of bovine cross-linked collagen, which is no longer on the market. Because of that there are newer materials being used, but the outcomes are unknown at this time.

Equipment

Routine cystoscopy equipment is needed for collagen injections (see Chapter 38). This procedure can not be done through a flexible cystoscope in male dogs and therefore must be approached in an antegrade manner using a rigid cystoscope as descrbied for the PCCL procedure or using retrograde perineal access (see Chapter 33 and Chapter 39).

The different bulking agents reported in the human and veterinary literature include: autologous fat, bovine cross-linked collagen[1], polytetrafluoroethylene (PTFE-Teflon, Polytef) paste[2], polydimethylsiloxane (PDMS-Macroplastique)[3], calcium hydroxylapetite (Coaptite)[4], and carbon-coated zirconium beads[5] (Durasphere). Each dog will need a different volume to be effective and each substance is available in different volumes. Most dogs need between 1.0–2.5 ml to obtain proper coaptation.

An appropriate injection needle will be needed as well, and each brand typically has an appropriate needle to be used. To date the collagen and Teflon are no longer available on the market, and most clinicians are using either PDMS or hydroxyapatite. Some UBAs, like PDMS, must be applied using a specialized injector apparatus due to their viscous nature.

Procedure

The author recommends initially performing a thorough cystourethoscopy to ensure there are no concurrent anatomical anomalies that need to be fixed prior to injection (ectopic ureters, urachal diverticulum, polyps, etc.). Once the anatomy is deemed normal than the cystoscope is removed from the patient and the injection needle should be loaded through the working channel. Care should be taken to avoid trauma to the needle as it will get dull as it is pushed through the port and metal channel, making injections more difficult and leaking of material from the injection site more likely. Using a 4 or 5 Fr open-ended catheter as a sheath the needle can be advanced through the channel while covered by the catheter. Once the needle is pushed out the end of the endoscope the sheathing catheter is then removed and the needle is pulled back into the endoscope.

Prior to entering the urethral lumen the needle should also be primed of bulking agent material to avoid injecting air into the urethral tissue. Once the needle is primed that volume should be recorded so that saline can be used to flush the material from the needle upon completion to avoid wasting material.

Finally, the cystoscope is passed into the external urethral meatus and advanced to the level of the trigone. The scope is then withdrawn to a point just caudal to the bladder neck where the urethra narrows for injection (1–3 cm caudal to the trigone typically). The injection needle is passed and advanced

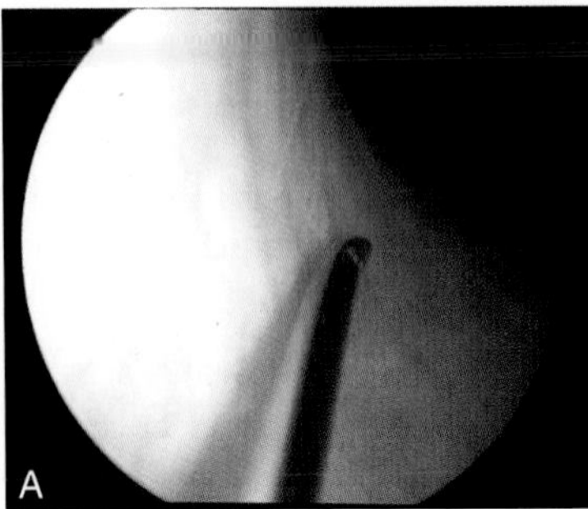

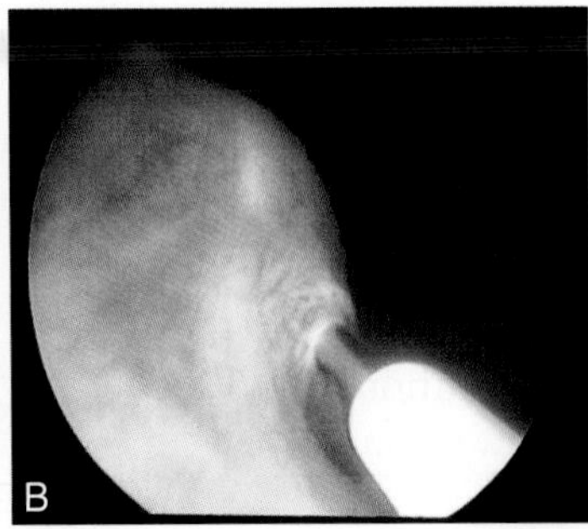

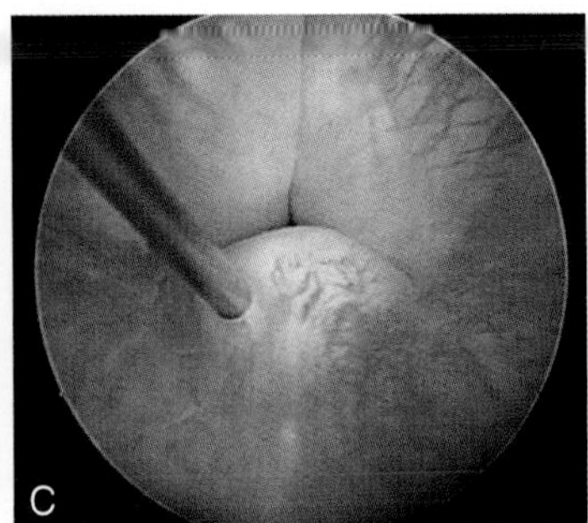

Figure 38.1 Cystoscopic images of the urethra in a female dog. (A) The needle is exiting the working channel of the endoscope within the urethral lumen. Notice that the needle nearly parallel to the urethral mucosa for appropriate depth of penetration. (B) The injection needle is placed through the urethral mucosa, and glutaraldehyde cross-linked bovine (GAX) collagen is being injected under the mucosa creating a "bleb" of material to partially occlude the lumen. (C) Proper placement of submucosal glutaraldehyde cross-linked bovine (GAX) collagen when three "blebs" are made to occlude the urethral mucosa.

submucosally with the bevel pointing toward the mucosa (Figure 38.1). The needle should be nearly parallel to the urethral mucosa, and this is best accomplished by using the 30-degree angle of the cystoscope to line the needle up. Once the bevel is seen to pierce the mucosa, it should not be advanced any deeper (Figure 38.1B). The needle is then rotated 180°, putting the bevel away from the lumen, and the injection is begun, injecting 0.1 ml at a time. The material must be injected slowly with the scope held very still because the urethral mucosa tears easily, leading to loss of the injected material and bleeding. Each bleb is filled with approximately 0.5 to 1 ml of material, or enough material to occlude the urethral lumen by 50–75% per bleb; however, the exact amount needed varies, depending on patient size and conformation, as well as the material injected. Some blebs may be larger than others because the more lateral portions of the wall are easier to fill. It is important that each bleb of material is placed in the same plane to achieve coaptation of the urethral walls (Figure 38.1). The goal is visual occlusion of the urethra (Figure 38.1C). Although there is minimal risk of obstruction, the bladder is manually compressed to verify passage of urine through the urethra. If a concern about obstruction exists, a red rubber catheter can gently be passed into the urethra to flatten the injected material and open the urethra. Typically 3 or 4 blebs are created in the urethral wall at the 2, 6, and 10 o'clock (or 12, 3, 6, and 9 o'clock) positions (Figure 38.1). Some operators will inject two or three rings along the urethral lumen from the proximal to mid-urethra and this too has been effective.

A periurethral approach to injection has also been described in people, has been found to have a slightly higher risk of early postoperative complications. This has not been reported in dogs.

Bulking Agents

The ideal UBA is easily delivered, biocompatible, non-antigenic, non-carcinogenic, stable within tissue, durable, and reasonably cost-effective. Over the past 70 years several different agents have been used as the injected material; however, improvement in continence was rarely achieved without significant scarring or sloughing of the urethra. Development of safer UBAs has improved the outcome of the procedure. The published veterinary literature is limited primarily to bovine cross-linked collagen, however, the use of several other agents has been reported in dogs with USMI including polytetrafluoroethylene (PTFE) paste and polydimethylsiloxane (PDMS). As of June, 2013, only PDMS (Macroplastique), calcium hydroxylapetite (Coaptite), and carbon-coated zirconium beads (Durasphere) are commercially available in the United States.

Polytetrafluoroethylene Paste

Polytetrafluoroethylene (Teflon Polytef Paste) was the first widely used UBA in both humans and dogs. The results of PTFE injection have been reported for 22 dogs that either had failed α-agonist treatment or for which such treatment was unsuitable (Arnold et al 1989). In this group of dogs 36% were continent after one PTFE injection, and an additional 41% were continent after a second injection. The majority of these dogs required adjunct treatment with phenylpropanolamine (PPA) to maintain continence. Fourteen (64%) dogs relapsed after 4 to 17 months. In women, the PTFE particles migrated to other parts of the body, caused a severe inflammatory reaction at the site of injection, and was often extruded, leaving ulcers in the urethral mucosa. With the development of improved injection materials, PTFE has been abandoned as a UBA and is currently unavailable in North America. However, PTFE is still used by some European veterinarians as a more economical alternative to cross-linked collagen, particularly in large breed dogs.

Bovine Cross-linked collagen

Until recently, glutaraldehyde cross-linked bovine (GAX) collagen (Contigen) had been the most widely used UBA in humans and dogs. The collagen is supplied in 2.5-ml syringes and is injected using a 5-Fr transurethral injection needle placed through the instrument port of a rigid cystoscope. Rather than causing an inflammatory reaction, the GAX implant is vascularized and invaded by fibroblasts. Fibroblasts lay down new endogenous collagen, stabilizing the implant. In humans no evidence of migration within the body has been found during 20 years of GAX use. The low morbidity and minimally invasive nature of collagen injection made this UBA attractive for the treatment of refractory incontinence in dogs.

Three reports have described the outcomes of collagen injection in the incontinent female dog. The first report included 32 spayed female dogs refractory to PPA treatment and subsequently treated with periurethral collagen injection (Arnold et al, 1996). Of these dogs, 53% were continent after one or two injections without the addition of PPA. With PPA the success rate increased to 75%. No postoperative complications were observed, and six of these dogs (19%) were observed to be continent longer than 30 months after the first injection. A longer-term follow-up study was performed by the same group of investigators involving 40 dogs over 7 years in which 68% of the dogs were continent for a mean of 17 months (range 1 to 64 months) after collagen injection (Barth et al, 2005). Mild and transient side effects were noted in 15% of treated dogs, including stranguria, hematuria, and vaginitis. A recent retrospective study evaluated the outcome of 36 collagen injections in 31 female dogs (Byron et al, 2011). Ten of these dogs had been diagnosed with ureteral ectopia; 5 had received corrective surgery but had persistent postoperative incontinence. Of the treated dogs with USMI, 66% achieved complete continence immediately after the procedure, and an additional 30% were improved. Of the dogs with improved continence, 46% achieved full continence after the addition of medical therapy. The median duration of complete continence after the procedure was 8 months without additional medical therapy. The majority of dogs had an improved response to medical therapy if added after continence declined. Although little data is available, addressing the success of reinjection following decline in continence after collagen injection in dogs, studies in women have been encouraging. In our experience, repeated injections of collagen, either by "enhancing" the previously placed blebs or by addition of new blebs, has led to improved response and resumption of continence. Reinjection is recommended in patients who do not improve after initial treatment or who experience a decline in continence after a period of time.

Injectable UBAs have been used in a few patients with ectopic ureters. Approximately 50% of these patients continue to have some degree of incontinence after neoureterostomy or laser ablation. Although technically more challenging to implant because of scarring of the urethral mucosa, periurethral injection of collagen appears to improve continence. In addition, injection of collagen distal to the ectopic stoma in patients with proximally placed ureteral ectopia may reduce incontinence without the need for surgical or laser intervention. Unfortunately, the manufacturer of GAX collagen recently removed it from production prompting investigation into alternative bulking agents. At this time there are several on-going studies evaluating the use of these alternatives.

Polydimethylsiloxane (PDMS)

Preliminary results of a study in dogs with urinary incontinence using polydimethylsiloxane (Macroplastique©) revealed that 17/22 (77%) of dogs were continent at 3 months and 16/22 (73%) of treated dogs were continent at 6 months post-injection. An additional 10% of dogs were significantly improved after treatment (Bartges and Callens, 2011). It is important to note that many of these dogs required more than one treatment to achieve continence, and this material is very expensive. This product is of particular interest in that it consists of a silicone elastomer which is suspended in a bioexcretable carrier gel. After implantation using a specialized injector device, the carrier is rapidly absorbed and excreted through the kidneys. The remaining "sponge-like" matrix is quickly encapsulated by fibrin and endogenous collagen which helps to stabilize the implant. This addresses one of the most common reasons for urethral bulking failure, that of implant loss or extrusion. More data is needed on this material to know the true continence rate and duration with each treatment as well as the need for repeat procedures to gain a clinical success.

Newer Agents

Several synthetic and biomaterial agents have been investigated for use as a UBA. These include but are not limited to calcium hydroxylapetite, carbon-coated zirconium beads, autologous cartilage and fat grafts, silicone microimplants, microballoons, and acellular extracellular matrix substances (Kershen et al, 2002; van Kerrebroeck et al, 2003). As tissue engineering advances, more potential materials will be tested. The current limitation of injection therapy is the poor long-term outcome, and this obstacle must be overcome by those working to design new injectable agents. Thus, it is important to educate clients and promote realistic expectations regarding outcomes of canine incontinence therapy with injectable bulking agents.

The use of calcium hydroxyapatite has been effective anecdotally in dogs, with no negative reaction seen in over 10 dogs treated. The major problem with this material is the difficulty in injection since it hardens when it is mixed with saline, requiring very fast injections. Because of this it should not be used unless the operator has a lot of experience with UBAs. This product is more reasonably priced than the PDMS.

Postoperative and Follow-Up Care

After using UBAs in dogs the author recommends 3–7 days of a broad-spectrum antibiotic, in the event bacteria was introduced during cystoscopy. Additionally, 1–3 days of pain medications (non-steroidal anti-inflammatories or tramadol are typically used) are provided. The author requires the patient have one good urination prior to discharge to ensure they are not urethrally obstructed, as this can occur. If the patient is unable to urinate a urinary catheter can be placed for 24 hours. The swelling usually resolves and the obstruction is relieved. This is very rare.

After 2 weeks, if incontinence continues, medical management can be re-instituted. The client should be educated on the fact that UBAs are often used with medical treatment and success will not guarantee that medications will be able to be discontinued. Appropriate expectations on continence rates (50–70% with UBAs and medications) should be set prior to treatment, and the potential need for repeat procedures, as this is a temporary fixation/supplementation, should be clear.

Notes

1. Contigen, Bard, Covington, GA.
2. Teflon paste, Dupont, Fayetteville, NC.
3. Macroplastique, Uroplasty Inc, Minnetonka, MN.
4. Coaptite, Boston Scientfiic, Natick, MA.
5. Durasphere, Coloplast, Minneapolis, MN.

References

Arnold S, Jäger P, DiBartola SP, et al (1989) Treatment of urinary incontinence in dogs by endoscopic injection of Teflon. *J Am Vet Med Assoc* 195, 1369–74.

Arnold S, Hubler M, Lott-Stolz G, et al (1996) Treatment of urinary incontinence in bitches by endoscopic injection of glutaraldehyde cross-linked collagen. *J Small Anim Pract* 37, 163–8.

Bartges JW and Callens A (2011). Polydimethylsiloxane urethral bulking agent (PDMS UBA) injection for treatment of female canine urinary incontinence – preliminary results. *J Vet Intern Med* 25, 748–9.

Barth A, Reichler IM, Hubler M, et al (2005). Evaluation of long-term effects of endoscopic injection of collagen into the urethral submucosa for treatment of urethral sphincter incompetence in female dogs: 40 cases (1993–2000). *J Am Vet Med Assoc* 226, 73–6.

Byron JK, Chew DJ, and McLoughlin ML. (2011) Retrospective evaluation of urethral bovine cross-linked collagen implantation for treatment of urinary incontinence in female dogs. *J Vet Intern Med* 25, 980–4.

Kershen, RT, Dmochowski RR, and Appell RA (2002) Beyond collagen: injectable therapies for the treatment of female stress urinary incontinence in the new millennium. *Urol Clin N Am* 29, 559–74.

van Kerrebroeck P, ter Meulen F, Farrelly E, et al (2003) Treatment of stress urinary incontinence: recent developments in the role of urethral injection. *Urol Res* 30, 356–62.

CHAPTER THIRTY-NINE

Percutaneous Perineal Approach to the Canine Urethra

Chick Weisse
The Animal Medical Center, New York, NY

Background/Indications

Cystourethroscopy has greatly enhanced the diagnosis and treatment of numerous conditions. Rigid telescopes provide well-illuminated highly detailed images using rod lens system technology (Figure 39.1). In addition, the angled lens enables improved field-of-view to facilitate examination of the entire urinary bladder during cystoscopy. Improved suction and irrigation are also provided with the larger accompanying working channel. Retrograde rigid cystoscopy has been limited to female dogs and cats due to the long, narrow, and curved male urethra and narrow feline male urethra and penis. The flexible ureteroscope (2.5–2.8 mm diameter with 1 mm working channel) has been used for male canine urethrocytoscopy but is limited in image quality (Figure 39.1) and procedural abilities due to the fiberoptic system, diminished illumination, difficult deflection, and smaller working channel.

The percutaneous fluoroscopically guided perineal approach using rigid cystoscopy in male dogs is a safe and effective method for facilitating interventional procedures, particularly when obtaining ureteral access for therapeutic endourology.

Patient Preparation

Prior to performing the perineal approach, a complete work-up is required in order to determine that a therapeutic endoscopic procedure is necessary. Dogs should first undergo flexible urethrocystoscopy in order to confirm the distal urethra (penile urethra) is not the source of the problem (obstruction, hematuria, incontinence, etc.). In addition, the pelvic/membranous urethral diameter must be large enough to accommodate a 14 or 16 Fr peel-away sheath (~5–6 mm), which is typically possible in dogs larger than ~8–10 kg.

Potential Risks/Complications/Expected Outcomes

The most concerning potential complications from the percutaneous perineal approach would be hemorrhage from the vascular cavernous tissues of the ischial urethra or stricture formation. Hemorrhage has not been a problem, likely due to the stretching (dilation) of the tissues rather than tearing or cutting that occurs during surgical urethral exposure/access. Strictures are also unlikely to occur with longitudinal incisions, rather than circumferential, and this has been demonstrated experimentally in the urethra. The perineal approach in the male dog is made at the level of the membranous urethra. Longitudinal wounds (including incisions) of the distal membranous urethra do not require urinary diversion and there has been no difference identified in the healing of sutured versus non-sutured prescrotal incisions in experimental dog studies (Weber et al, 1985, Waldron et al, 1985). In one of those studies, primary intention (suturing) healing reduced postoperative hemorrhage but all dogs had mucosal irregularities at 60 days (Waldron et al, 1985). Second intention (non-sutured) healing resulted in increased fibrosis and less inflammation but no strictures were identified (Weber et al, 1985).

Clients should provide consent prior to cystoscopy so this procedure can be performed if necessary. The author has always achieved access using this technique, however sometimes two or three needle sticks are necessary

Veterinary Image-Guided Interventions, First Edition. Edited by Chick Weisse and Allyson Berent.

Companion website: www.wiley.com/go/weisse/vet-image-guided-interventions

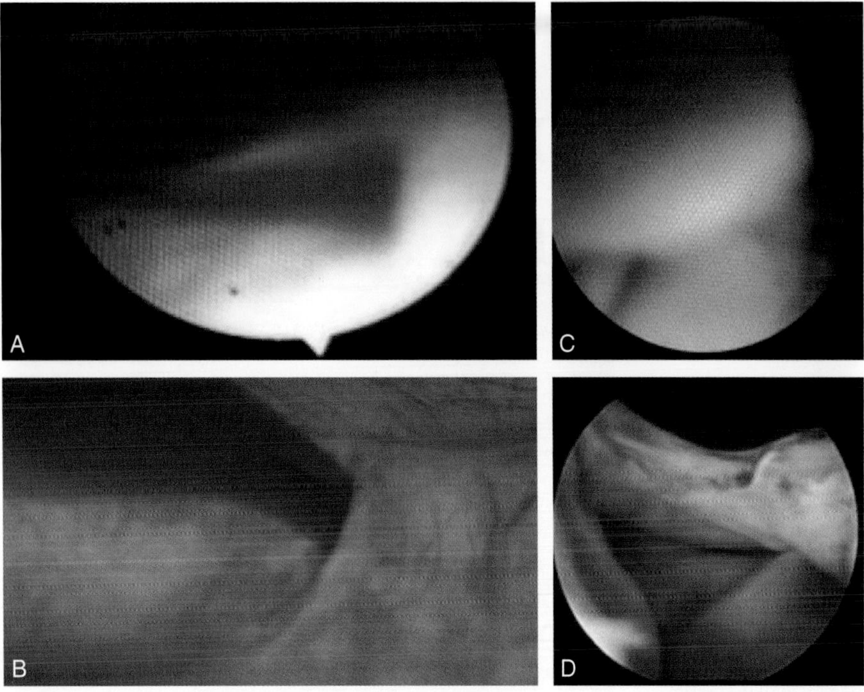

Figure 39.1 Multiple endoscopic images in male dogs. Flexible scope (A) and rigid scope (B) endoscopic images of a male dog with idiopathic renal hematuria demonstrating substantially improved image provided by the rigid scope for hematuria visualization. Flexible scope (C) and rigid scope (D) endoscopic images of a male dog with ectopic ureters. A guide wire is within the ectopic ureteral orifice in image C. The rigid scope provides much better visualization facilitating identification and subsequent laser ablation of the orifice.

to access to the urethral lumen. In a report of 10 dogs (Weisse and Berent, 2012) access time typically took under 30 minutes, half the cases went home the same day of the procedure, and the only complication encountered was one dog leaking urine through the perineal incision 6 hours post-operatively, which did not recur. No long-term complications were identified in any of the dogs with a median follow-up time of ~7 months and some over 3 years. Historical literature describing a similar surgical perineal approach to the urethra also found minimal complications (Brearley et al, 1988).

Equipment

A list of recommended equipment is shown in Figure 39.2. Make certain the rigid cystoscope fits through the peel-away sheath prior to performing this procedure.

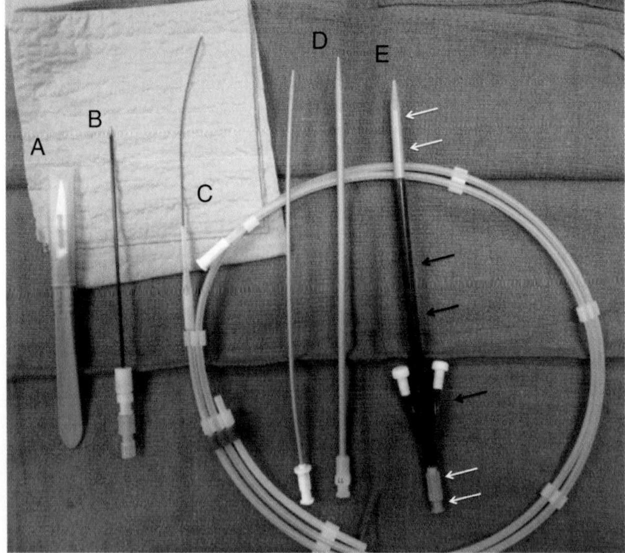

Figure 39.2 Equipment needed for percutaneous perineal approach procedure. (A) Scalpel blade and handle. (B) 18-gauge renal puncture needle. (C) 0.035″ Amplatz super stiff guide wire. (D) dilators between 14 and 16 French. (E) 16 Fr peel-away sheath (black arrows) and dilator (white arrows).

Fluoroscopic Procedure

The perineal approach is performed with the patient placed in dorsal recumbency and the hindlimbs pulled cranially (Figure 39.3). The prepuce and perineal areas are clipped and aseptically prepared. A purse string suture is placed in the anus. This positioning allows access for both retrograde flexible urethroscopy and perineal access. Following flexible urethroscopy, a red rubber catheter is placed and the urinary bladder filled with "diluted iohexol (50% contrast/50% saline). The c-arm fluoroscopy unit is positioned transversely across the dog in order to project a lateral image (Figure 39.4A). The red rubber catheter is pulled into the penile urethra and a strong injection is given to distend the ischial urethra. A 4–5 mm perineal skin incision is made on midline at the level of the ischium. An 18-gauge renal puncture needle[1] is placed under fluoroscopic guidance into the perineum (Figure 39.4A) and advanced parallel and into the pelvic urethra. Ultrasound assistance is often helpful to help line up

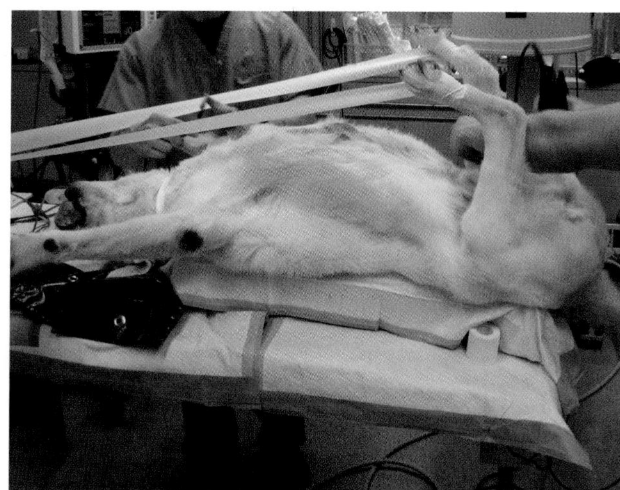

Figure 39.3 Appropriate positioning of a male dog permitting both retrograde flexible urethrocystoscopy as well as the perineal approach if necessary without needing to move the patient.

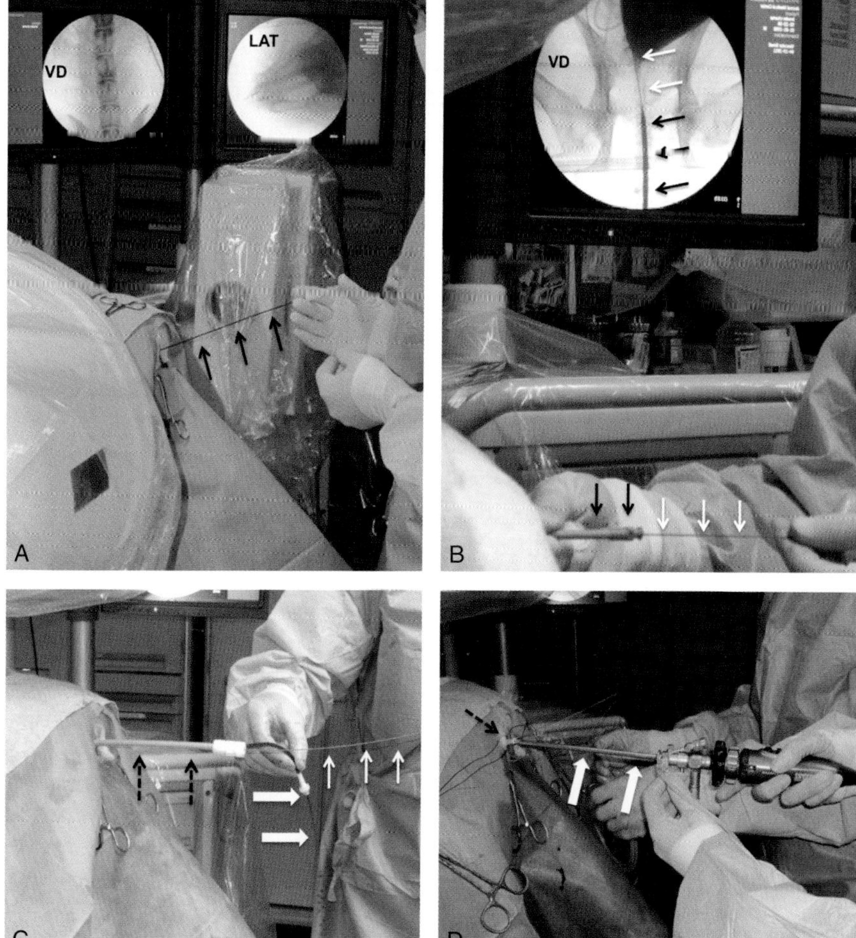

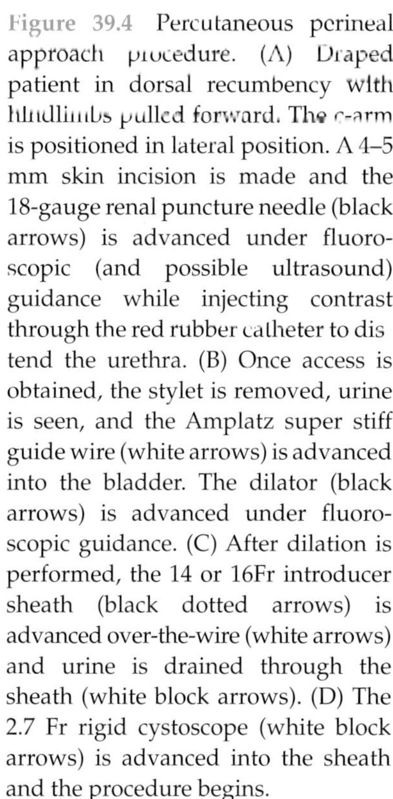

Figure 39.4 Percutaneous perineal approach procedure. (A) Draped patient in dorsal recumbency with hindlimbs pulled forward. The c-arm is positioned in lateral position. A 4–5 mm skin incision is made and the 18-gauge renal puncture needle (black arrows) is advanced under fluoroscopic (and possible ultrasound) guidance while injecting contrast through the red rubber catheter to distend the urethra. (B) Once access is obtained, the stylet is removed, urine is seen, and the Amplatz super stiff guide wire (white arrows) is advanced into the bladder. The dilator (black arrows) is advanced under fluoroscopic guidance. (C) After dilation is performed, the 14 or 16Fr introducer sheath (black dotted arrows) is advanced over-the-wire (white arrows) and urine is drained through the sheath (white block arrows). (D) The 2.7 Fr rigid cystoscope (white block arrows) is advanced into the sheath and the procedure begins.

the needle on the urethral lumen. More commonly a modified technique using a Foley urinary catheter inflated with contrast is used. The Foley balloon is positioned at the desired location for urethral access which distends the urethral lumen facilitating access. Ultrasound and fluoroscopic guidance are used simultaneously to puncture the balloon, indicating urethral lumen access has been achieved. The sharp stylet is removed and urine is identified. Then a 0.035″ angled hydrophilic guide wire[2] is advanced and coiled into the urinary bladder under fluoroscopic guidance. The C-arm is rotated into a dorsoventral projection. The 18-g catheter is then advanced over-the-wire into the prostatic urethra. The hydrophilic wire is exchanged for a 0.035″ amplatz superstiff wire[3] and the 18ga catheter is removed over the wire. Serial dilators[4] (4 Fr, 8 Fr,

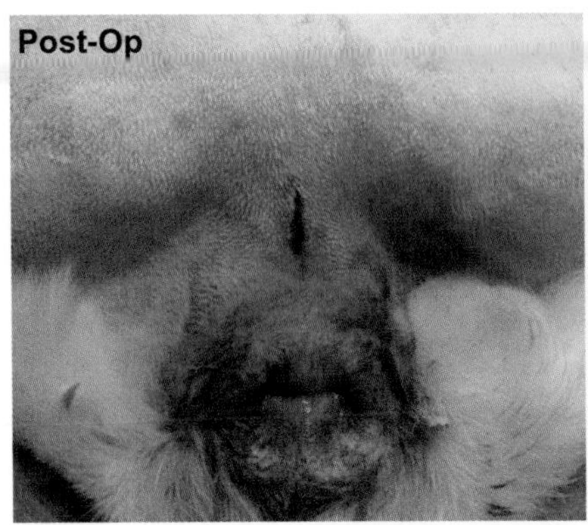

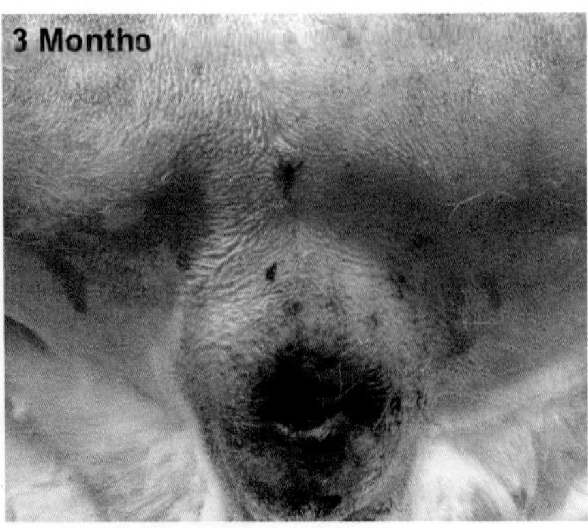

Figure 39.5 Perineal approach site immediately post-operatively (left) and healed site 3 months later (right).

12 Fr, 16 Fr) are used to dilate the tract (Figure 39.4B) to accept a 14 or 16 Fr peel-away sheath[5] (Figure 39.4C). Considerable force is necessary to advance the dilators and stretch the corpus tissues. Once the sheath is within the mid pelvic urethra the dilator is removed and the peel-away sheath is secured to the skin using suture material. A 2.7 mm rigid cystoscope is placed through the sheath and rigid urethrocystoscopy is performed (Figure 39.4D). Upon completion of the intervention, the sheath is removed. A urinary catheter can be placed for a few hours (<12 hours), but this has not been necessary. No sutures are needed to close the perineal incision; a Tega-derm[6] dressing can be placed.

Follow-Up

The patient is recovered with no special treatments for the perineal approach (Figure 39.5); treatments are based upon the underlying condition that was treated. Tramadol (3–4 mg/kg PO BID QID × 3 days) is dispensed to be administered as needed, which is rare. Antibiotic therapy is usually administered for 3–5 days post-procedure, as is typically following cystoscopy.

Special Considerations/ Complication Examples

The increased use of endourologic techniques in male dogs suggests that other potential applications will be utilized with this approach. Some possible procedures include upper urinary tract access, possible bladder stone removal or lithotripsy, and local tumor ablations.

Notes

(Examples, Multiple vendors available)

1. 18gauge Renal puncture needle set, Cook Medical, Bloomington, IN.
2. Weasel wire, Infiniti Medical, Menlo Park, CA.
3. Amplatz Super stiff guide wire, Boston Scientific Corp, Natick, MA.
4. Vessel dilators, Infiniti Medical, Menlo Park, CA.
5. 14 or 16 Fr peel-away introducer sheath, Cook Medical, Bloomington, IN.
6. Tega-derm, 3M, St. Paul, MN.

References

Brearley MJ, Milroy EJ, and Rickards D (1988) A percutaneous perineal approach for cystoscopy in male dogs. *Res Vet Sc* 44(3), 380–2.

Waldron DR, Hedlund CS, Tangner CH, et al (1985) The canine urethra: A comparison of first and second intention healing. *Vet Surg* 14, 213–17.

Weber WJ, Boothe HW, Brassard JA, et al (1985) Comparison of the healing of prescrotal urethrotomy incisions in the dog: Sutured versus nonsutured. *Am J Vet Res* 46, 1309–15.

Weisse C and Berent AC (2012) Percutaneous fluoroscopically-assisted perineal approach for rigid cystoscopy in 9 male dogs. ECVS, Barcelona, Spain.

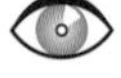
Video clips to accompany this chapter can be found in the online material at **www.wiley.com/go/weisse/vet-image-guided-interventions**

CHAPTER FORTY

Percutaneous Antegrade Urethral Catheterization

Elaine Holmes
Veterinary Specialty Hospital of the Carolinas, Cary, NC

Background

Lower urinary tract diversion is critical for the treatment of patients with various causes of urethral obstructions, trauma, healing after extensive surgery of the urethra, monitoring of urine output, and preventing stagnant urine within the urinary bladder. Retrograde catheterization of the urethra is usually easily achieved, especially in male dogs and cats. However, in certain circumstances, this can be more challenging: female dogs with a urethral obstruction from a space occupying lesion, a distal urethral stricture, a urethral tear, trauma, and small female dogs and cats. In these instances percutaneous antegrade urethral catheterization (PAUC) provides an alternate method to gain access across the urethra, when traditional methods are unsuccessful (Holmes et al, 2012).

Preparation

There are several considerations prior to performing PAUC. The patient must be hemodynamically stable to tolerate general anesthesia. This may require serial decompressive cystocentesis procedures to improve the electrolyte and acid base status. The urinary bladder must be distended and firm for catheter and guide wire placement. If there is concern of bladder necrosis, coagulopathy, or previous abdominal surgery with known adhesions of bowel to the urinary bladder than PAUC should not be performed.

Recommended supplies to perform PAUC:

1. 1½″ 18 gauge over the needle IV catheter (for 0.035″ guide wire; if 5 Fr catheter than need a 0.025″ guide wire and 20 gauge IV catheter; and for a 3.5 Fr catheter than need a 0.018″ guide wire and a 22 gauge IV catheter)
2. Two 20 ml luer lock syringes
3. Two 10 ml syringes containing 100% iodinated contrast agent
4. Sterile saline
5. Three-way stop-cock
6. 0.035″, 0.025″, or 0.018″ angled hydrophilic guide wire[1–3]
   a. If the urethra will not accommodate a 5-Fr drainage catheter, a 0.018″ guide wire should be used
7. Appropriately sized urinary drainage catheter for patient and urethra size.
   a. Large dog: 8–10 Fr and 0.035″ guide wire
   b. Medium dog: 5–8 Fr and 0.035″ guide wire
   c. Small dog: 5 Fr and 0.025″ and/or 0.035″ guide wire
   d. Cat (female): 5 Fr and 0.025″ and/or 0.035″ guide wire
   e. Cat (male): 3.5 Fr and 0.018″ guide wire
8. Sterile drapes
9. Sterile gloves
10. Sterile lubricant
11. Sterile scissors, hemostat, and needle drivers.

The patient must be anesthetized and placed in lateral recumbency. The entire ventrolateral abdomen from cranial to the umbilicus extending to pubis and dorsally to the level of the transverse processes, as well as the perineal region (prepuce, vulva), must be clipped and aseptically prepared. All areas draped routinely with a separate sterile drape covering the surface of the radiology table to maintain sterility during guide wire and catheter passage.

Once the patient is draped the fluoroscopy unit should be set to include imaging of the urinary bladder and entire urethra. Using sterile technique the urinary bladder is palpated and an 18-gauge over-the-needle catheter is inserted transabdominally, along the lateral abdominal wall into the urinary bladder at the level of the cranial bladder body. It should be aimed in the

Veterinary Image-Guided Interventions, First Edition. Edited by Chick Weisse and Allyson Berent.

Companion website: www.wiley.com/go/weisse/vet-image-guided-interventions

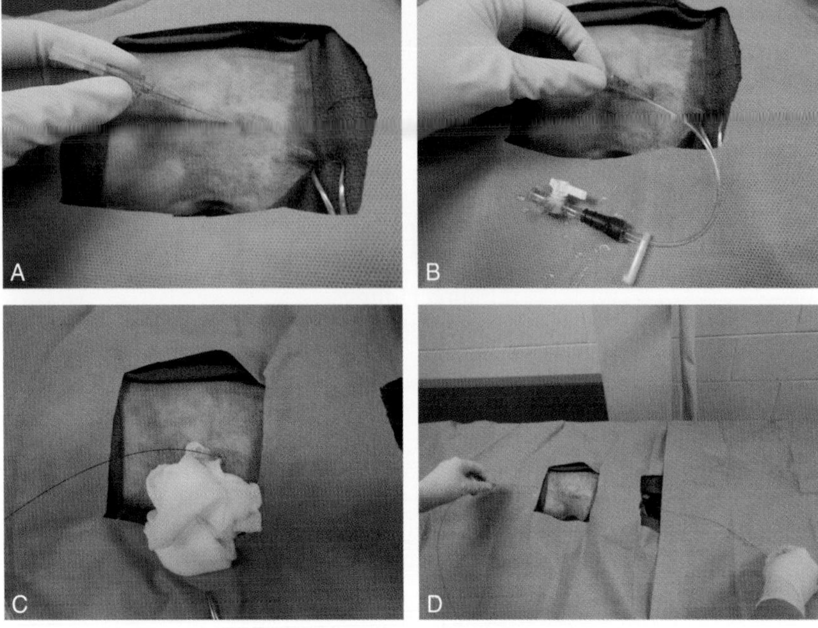

Figure 40.1 (A) Initial urinary bladder puncture. An 18 g over the needle IV catheter is seen puncturing the skin at a 20–30 degree angle. The catheter enters the urinary bladder at the apex and is directed toward the trigone to aid in guide wire manipulations. (B) Complete urinary bladder puncture with contrast to be added. The IV catheter is seated fully within the urinary bladder and a T-port with three-way stop cock is attached. Urine is aspirated and set aside for analysis if needed. The syringe with a 50/50 mixture of contrast and saline and the syringe with 100% contrast will then be attached to the stopcock to perform the cystourethrogram. (C) Guide wire placement. The T-port is detached and the guide wire is placed through the IV catheter under fluoroscopic guidance. A sterile gauze sponge is placed in this patient to collect and urine or contrast that may leak around the guide wire. This is more problematic when a 0.018″ guide wire is used. (D) Fluoroscopic image of a guide wire in the urinary bladder. Access to the bladder has been achieved with a transabdominally placed 18-gauge IV catheter, and a 0.035″ angled hydrophilic guide wire (white arrows), has been inserted and is curled within the urinary bladder.

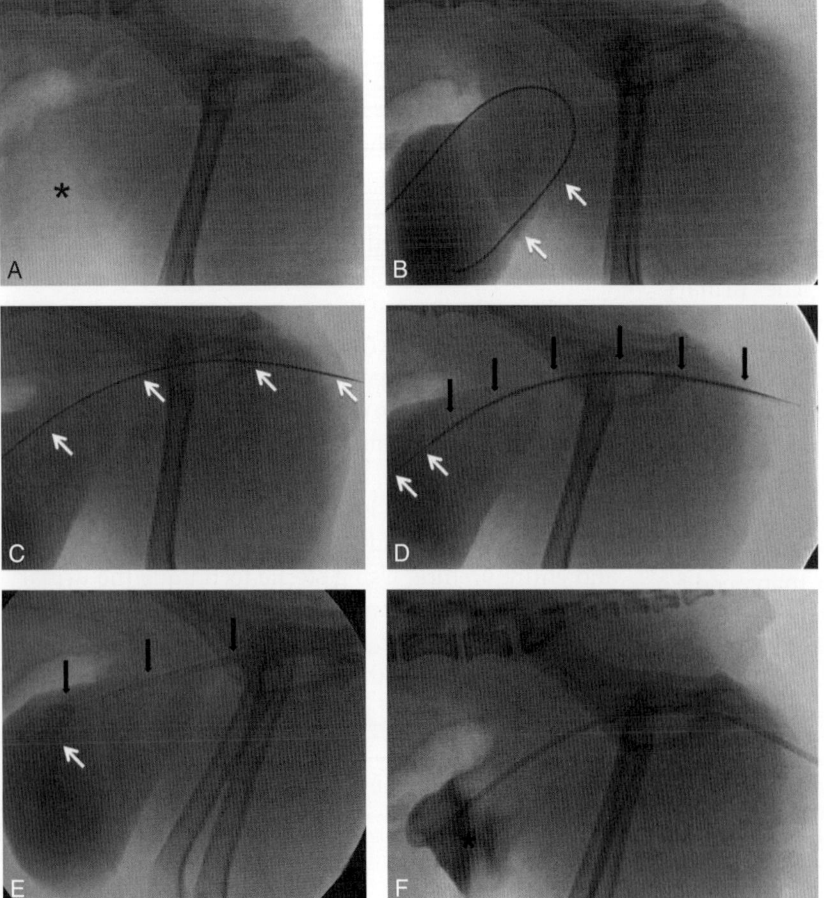

Figure 40.2 Fluoroscopic images during PAUC. (A) Fluoroscopic image of urinary bladder prior to PAUC. (B) Guide wire placement through the over the needle IV catheter into the urinary bladder. The guide wire is seen traversing the urinary bladder (white arrows). (C) Guide wire (white arrows) through-and-through from the urinary bladder, down the urethra and out the prepuce. (D) Urinary catheter placement (black arrows) over the guide wire over being advanced in a retrograde manner. (E) Fluoroscopic image of the urinary catheter (black arrows) after the guide wire is removed. (F) Urinary bladder (black asterisk) drainage after catheter placement.

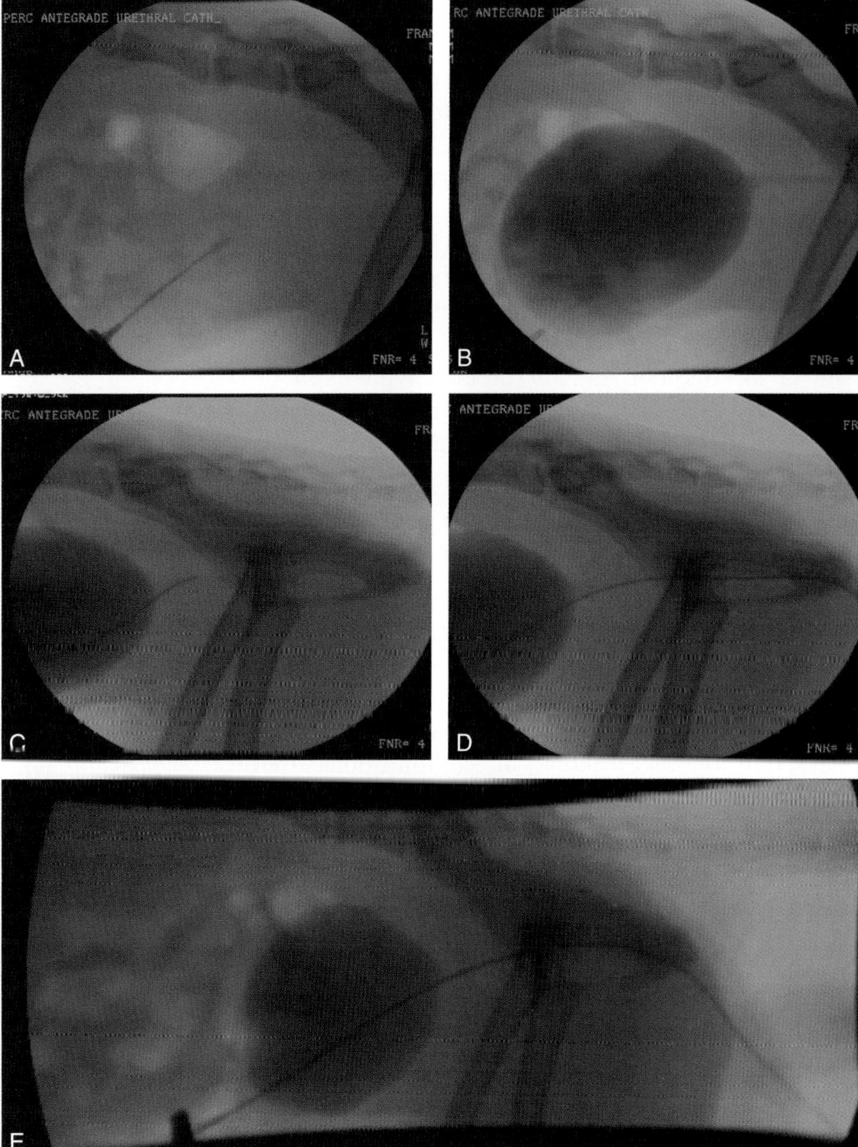

Figure 40.3 Fluoroscopic images during PAUC in a male cat. (A) 18 gauge over-the-needle IV catheter being placed into the urinary bladder aiming toward the urethra. (B) Cystourethrogram using 50% contrast. (C) Guide wire advanced through the guide wire aiming down the urethra in an antegrade manner. (D) Through and through guide wire access. (E) Catheter advanced over the guide wire in a retrograde manner keeping a hemostat on the most cranial aspect of the guide wire to prevent losing access during catheter placement.

direction of the trigone (Figure 40.1). A 2 mm skin incision can be made to facilitate transabdominal puncture. The sharp stylet is removed and an extension set (or T-port) with a three-way stopcock is attached to an empty 10 ml syringe and a 20 ml syringe containing a 50/50 mixture of sterile saline and iodinated contrast. Depending upon urinary bladder size, between 5 and 10 ml of urine is aspirated and submitted for urinalysis and culture. An approximately equal volume of the iodinated contrast mixture is then injected under fluoroscopic guidance until the urinary bladder is moderately distended and the trigone and proximal urethra are clearly visible. A cystourethrogram may be performed at this time if needed, being careful to avoid over distending the bladder. The extension set is removed from the 18-gauge catheter and a 0.035″ hydrophilic angled guide wire is inserted through the catheter (Figure 40.2 and Figure 40.3) and into the urinary bladder, using fluoroscopic guidance. Using a hemostat, the guide wire is manipulated towards the trigone and aimed down the urethra toward the prepuce/vulva. Once it exits "through-and-through" guide wire access is achieved (Figure 40.2 and Figure 40.3). This may require gentle manipulation of the wire within the urethra if there is an obstruction present. For urethral tears that are made in a retrograde manner, the wire usually passes very easily.

Next, an appropriately sized and well-lubricated, open-ended urinary drainage catheter, or red rubber catheter with the tip cut off, is advanced in a retrograde fashion over the guide wire and into the urinary bladder (Figure 40.2 and Figure 40.3). Slight tension on both ends of the guide wire can facilitate catheter passage if necessary. In male cats care should be taken to help the tip of the catheter enter the end of the penis, as it is often swollen. Once the catheter is well placed within the urinary bladder it should be able to drain the urinary bladder readily. The catheter is then sutured securely in place and connected to a sterile urine collection system. The guide wire and over-the needle catheter in the bladder can then be removed. Prior to removing the guide wire, a cystostomy catheter can be placed if deemed appropriate. This is done by using a locking-loop pigtail catheter, which can be placed over this guide wire in an antegrade manner. This is described in more detail in Chapter 41.

Outcome

A case series of nine cats was recently reported (Holmes et al, 2012), in which PAUC was performed for iatrogenic urethral tears and/or strictures. In this series no complications were noted other than the inability to perform the procedure in cats with intraluminal obstructive debris. Theoretical complications that could occur include bladder rupture/tear, infected urine leakage, intestinal contamination, hemorrhage, uroabdomen, etc.

Miscellaneous

Modifications of this catheterization technique include ultrasound-guided percutaneous cystocentesis or visual placement during open abdominal surgery.

Notes

1. 0.035″ Weasel Wire, Infiniti Medical LLC, Menlo Park, CA.
2. 0.025″ Weasel Wire, Infiniti Medical LLC, Menlo Park, CA.
3. 0.018″ Weasel Wire, Infiniti Medical LLC, Menlo Park, CA.

Reference

Holmes ES, Weisse CW, and Berent AC (2012) Use of fluoroscopically guided percutaneous antegrade urethral catheterization for the treatment of urethral obstruction in male cats: 9 cases. *J Am Vet Med Assoc* 241, 603–7.

Suggested Reading

Anderson RB, Aronson LR, Drobatz KJ, and Atilla A. (2006) Prognostic factors for successful outcome following urethral rupture in dogs and cats. *Jl Am Anim Hosp Assoc* 42, 136–46.

Blackburn AL, Berent AC, Weisse CW, and Brown DC (2013) Evaluation of outcome following urethral stent placement for the treatment of obstructive carcinoma of the urethra in dogs: 42 cases (2004–2008). *J Am Vet Med Assoc* 242, 59–68.

Boothe HW (2000) Managing traumatic urethral injuries. *Clin Techn Small Anim Pract* 15, 35–9.

Cooley AJ, Waldron DR, Smith MM, Saunders GK, Troy GC, and Barber DL (1999) The effects of indwelling transurethral catheterization and tube cystostomy on urethral anastomoses in dogs. *J Am Anim Hosp Assoc* 35, 341–7.

Kruger JM, Osborne CA, and Ulrich LK (1996) Cystocentesis: diagnostic and therapeutic considerations. *Vet Clin N Am Small Anim Pract* 26, 353–61.

Meige F, Sarrau S, and Autefage A (2008) Management of traumatic urethral rupture in 11 cats using primary alignment with a urethral catheter. *Vet Comp Orthop Traumatol* 21, 76–84.

Scott RC, Wilkins RJ, and Greene RW (1974) Abdominal paracentesis and cystocentesis. *Vet Clin N Am* 4, 413–17.

Weisse CW, Berent AC, Clifford C, and Solomon J (2006) Evaluation of palliative stenting for management of malignant urethral obstructions in dogs. *Jl Am Vet Med Assoc* 229, 226–34.

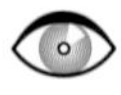

Video clips to accompany this chapter can be found in the online material at **www.wiley.com/go/weisse/vet-image-guided-interventions**

CHAPTER FORTY-ONE

Percutaneous Cystostomy Tube

Elaine Holmes
Veterinary Specialty Hospital of the Carolinas, Cary, NC

Background/Indications

Cystostomy tubes are used to provide temporary or permanent urinary bypass for patients with obstructive, traumatic, motility, or neurologic diseases of the lower urinary tract. Percutaneous cystostomy tube placement can be a rapid and minimally invasive option for patients in which traditional access to the bladder with a urethral catheter is not achievable or desirable. In addition, while fluoroscopy is advantageous in the placement of percutaneous cystostomy tubes, this technique can be accomplished with ultrasound guidance as well. This makes percutaneous cystostomy tubes a widely available option for urinary bypass, both temporarily and permanently. The most common indication for this procedure is for patients with detrusor reflex dyssynergia who have failed medical management, urethral tears, urethral outflow obstructions due to strictures, proliferative tissue, or tumors, and after urethral reconstructive surgery. The cystostomy catheter often allows time for medications to be manipulated while the urethral outflow is assess, as is the case for reflex dyssynergia and proliferative urethritis.

Patient Preparation

There are several relative and absolute preconditions for placement of a percutaneous cystostomy tube. The patient must be hemodynamically stable and able to handle general anesthesia. The urinary bladder must be full to allow accurate placement of the catheter. Any patient with a relative contraindication for cystocentesis, including, but not limited to, severe bladder necrosis, coagulopathy, and previous abdominal surgery with known adhesions of intestinal loops to the urinary bladder, is considered a poor candidate for percutaneous cystostomy tube placement.

Potential Risks/Complications/Expected Outcomes

A retrospective review of surgical cystostomy tube placement reported a 49% complication rate (Beck et al, 2007), and an 85.7% (24 of 28 animals with cultures taken while the tube was in place) urinary tract infection rate. Many of the reported complications were related to tube site irritation and were easily resolved by tube removal. Other complications include persistent straining, premature dislodgement, uroabdomen, ascending infection, tube obstruction, and fistula formation following tube removal (Beck et al, 2007). Gross and microscopic hematuria is expected following percutaneous cystostomy tube placement (Dhein et al, 1989). Some additional complications that could occur include accidental bowl penetration with the needle or catheter, bleeding, splenic puncture if too cranial, bladder wall tearing if the integrity is poor or tissue heath is compromised, and uroabdomen if there is excessive tension or inappropriate puncture.

With a precutaneously placed tube a cystopexy has to form on its own, without surgical assistance. An adhesion between the bladder and the body wall can take 2–4 weeks to form. When using the recommended 5 or 6 Fr in diameter catheter, this stoma will heal quickly once the tube is removed. Premature removal may result in an uroabdomen if an appropriate pexy has not yet been formed.

Equipment

The following is a list of recommended supplies for percutaneous cystostomy tube placement. Please note that different companies and distributors make all of this equipment, so a few recommendations are listed.

Veterinary Image-Guided Interventions, First Edition. Edited by Chick Weisse and Allyson Berent.

Companion website: www.wiley.com/go/weisse/vet-image-guided-interventions

The procedure requires a fluoroscopy unit and/or an ultrasound machine. An 18-gauge access needle[1] or over-the-needle catheter is used for cystocentesis, if the modified-Seldinger technique is being used. In addition a 50% solution of iodinated contrast material[2] will be injected through the catheter attached to an extension set, or T-port adaptor. Then an 0.035″ angle tipped hydrophilic guide wire[3] is used and the locking-loop pigtail catheter[4,5]is placed over the guide wire. For urine drainage a 5 or 6 catheter[4,5] is sufficient. Appropriately sized, non-absorbable monofilament suture is need to secure the catheter once in place and a sterile closed urine collection system will be attached to the catheter upon completion. This procedure is done aseptically, so sterile drapes, gowns and gloves should be used.

Procedure

The patient must be anesthetized and placed in lateral recumbency. The entire ventrolateral abdomen extending from cranial to the umbilicus to pubis and laterally to the level of the transverse processes must be clipped. The area is aseptically prepped and draped routinely. It is often beneficial to initially drape and prep the patient in dorsal recumbency and then roll the patient into lateral recumbency. This can ensure the clinician is able to feel the urinary bladder and stabilize it with one hand during puncture and maintain a sterile field (Figure 41.1).

All manipulations are carried out with fluoroscopic and/or ultrasound guidance. For traditional percutaneous cystostomy tube placement the bladder is palpated and stabilized with one hand or a radiolucent paddle. A 3–4 mm incision is made in the skin and superficial subcutaneous tissues (Figure 41.1) at the level of the mid-bladder body. In particularly over weight patients, it may be useful to bluntly dissect down to the rectus abdominus where the proposed body wall entry point is located. When performing the procedure in lateral recumbency, the preferred location for the body wall entry point is adjacent to the lateral aspect of the rectus abdominus or approximately 2 cm from the linea alba at a level of the body of the urinary bladder, which is typically 2/3 the distance from the umbilicus to the pubis (Cornell, 2000, Diehn et al, 1989). This can change in different patients, so using palpation is very important. This is typically more cranial in cats and more caudal in dogs. The correct orientation of all transabdominal punctures is entering the skin at a 20–30 degree angle from the body wall aiming caudally toward the urethra.

There are two techniques for this procedure: (1) The modified Seldinger technique, which was previously described in detail in Chapter 40 under percutaneous antegrade urethral catheterization (PAUC), and (2) The direct puncture technique where the sharp stylet of the locking-loop pigtail catheter is used to directly puncture the bladder wall, described in Chapter 29 under nephrostomy tube placement using the "one-stab" technique.

1. *Modified Seldinger technique*: After the initial placement of the 18-gauge IV catheter or renal access needle a cystogram is performed using a 50% solution of iodinated contrast material. It is important to remember that, in small patients, the urinary bladder can only hold approximately 5–15 ml/kg of fluid so if the bladder is full an equal amount of urine must be withdrawn prior to infusing contrast (Figure 41.1). Once the bladder is visualized under fluoroscopic guidance a 0.035-inch angle-tipped hydrophilic guide wire advanced through the catheter and coiled within the lumen of the urinary bladder. The stiff part of the shaft of the wire should be within the bladder lumen to provide security during catheter placement. Next, the catheter is removed over the wire, and the wire is left in place within the bladder, being monitored under fluoroscopy. While the wire does not need to exit the urethra, this can be helpful to help give the catheter a stiffer scaffold on which to be placed. Once the IV catheter is removed the locking-loop pigtail catheter is advanced over the guide wire. The sharp stylet is removed and the hollow trocar maintains the stiffness of the catheter. Typically, a #11 scalpel blade is used to provide a stab incision to the abdominal musculature at the wire entry site, as this is where the catheter will often have trouble advancing. The guide wire is held in place and the catheter is advanced over the wire under fluoroscopic guidance, making sure to remain straight on line with the wire under fluoroscopic imaging. Once the catheter punctures through the bladder wall the catheter is advanced off the stiff hollow trocar and onto the guide wire within the urinary bladder. Once the entire pigtail of the catheter and its fenestrations are fully within the urinary bladder the hollow trocar and the guidewire are removed, as the locking string is secured to create the locking loop mechanism. The cystostomy catheter is then withdrawn toward the bladder wall. There should be enough slack to prevent the bladder from being taut against the body wall, whether it is full or empty. This will prevent the catheter from getting pulled out during bladder mobility. Once the

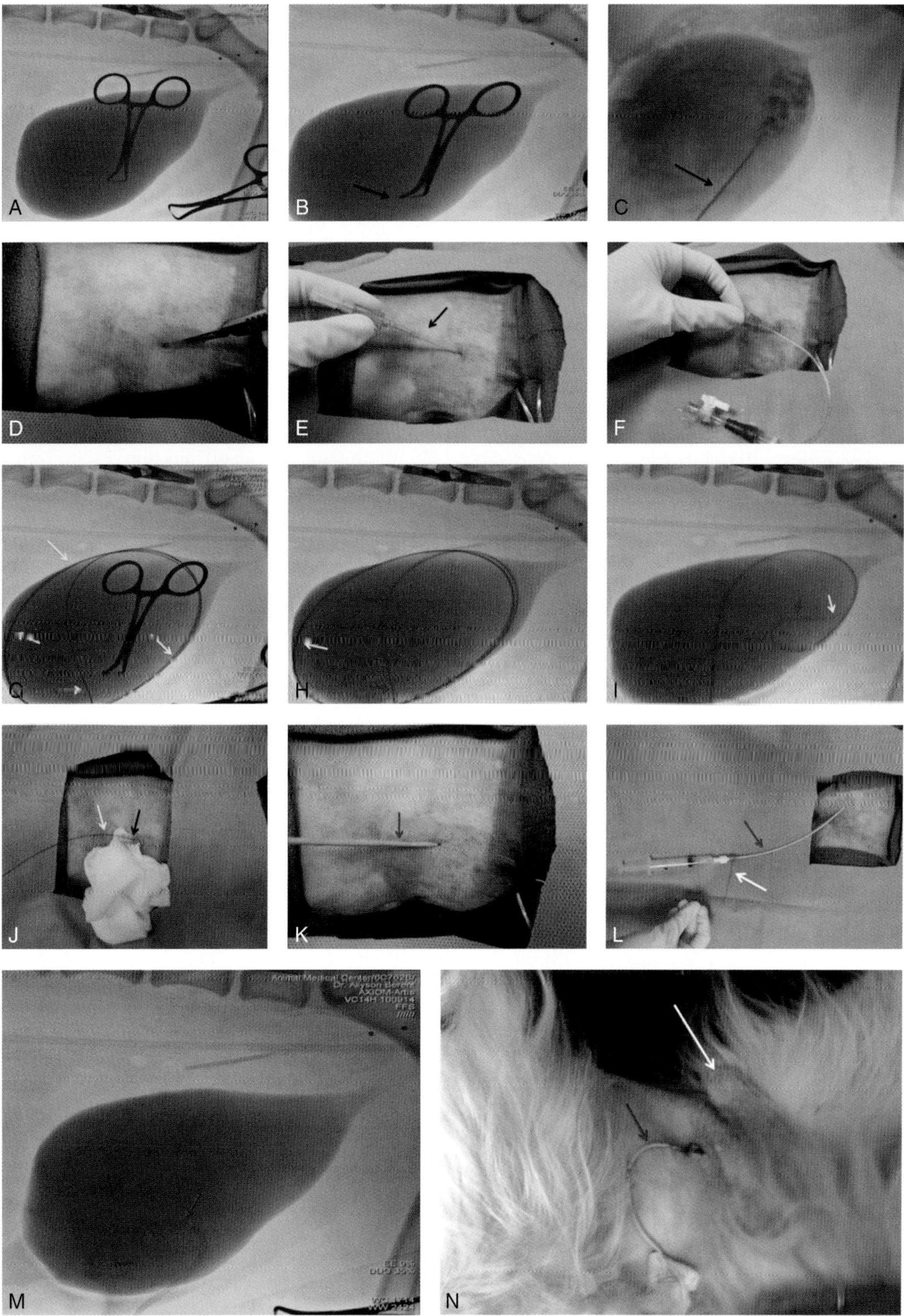

Figure 41.1 Percutaneous modified Seldinger technique for the placement of the locking-loop pigtail cystostomy catheter. (A) Lateral recumbency showing the entire bladder and proximal urethra. (B, C) 18 gauge IV catheter (black arrow) placed within the urinary bladder for a cystogram. (D) Blade used to make a stab incision for placement of the catheter. (E) 18 gauge IV catheter (black arrow) entering the urinary bladder. (F) An extension set on the IV catheter for the cystogram. (G) Guide wire (yellow arrows) coiled in urinary bladder. (H) Cystostomy catheter (red arrows) advanced over the wire (yellow arrows) within the urinary bladder. (I) Locking loop cystostomy catheter (red arrows) making the pigtail curl over the guide wire as the locking string is pulled. (J) Guide wire (yellow arrow) advanced through the IV catheter (black arrow) into the bladder. (K) Locking-loop cystostomy tube (red arrow) being advanced over the guide wire through the body wall. (L) The cystostomy tube (red arrow) exiting the body wall after it is locked in place with the string (white arrow). (M) Fluoroscopy image of the locking loop cystostomy catheter (red arrows) as it is pulled toward the body wall and the wire is removed. (N) Male dog with a cystostomy tube exiting the abdominal wall. This dog is in dorsal recumbency and the cystostomy tube (red arrow) is seen passing lateral to the prepuce (white arrow).

location is satisfactory the bladder is drained and then filled to leak test the fixation. Then the catheter is secured to the body wall using a purse-string suture with a Chinese-finger trap pattern at the incision, and again halfway up the catheter (Figure 41.1 N). The sterile urine collection system is then attached to the catheter for gravity drainage for 24 hours, prior to discharge for intermittent bladder drainage. The patient should have a secure light abdominal wrap to secure the tube and prevent accidental dislodgement.

2. *The "one-stab" technique:* This can be done with fluoroscopic and/or ultrasound guidance. For fluoroscopic guidance, once the stab incision in made at the mid bladder body, the locking-loop pigtail catheter, with the hollow trocar and sharp stylet, are used in combination to enter the bladder wall. The catheter enters the bladder in the lateral bladder wall about midway between the apex and the trigone and is directed caudally toward the trigone. It is often necessary to apply a, firm push to the catheter when entering the bladder, which makes this more difficult than the modified Seldinger technique. Making a skin and muscle incision will aid in passing the catheter into the body wall. Once the catheter within the bladder lumen, the sharp stylet is removed and a urine sample is taken to ensure it is with the lumen. If using fluoroscopy, contrast can then be infused. If using ultrasound this is not needed. Once placement in the bladder is confirmed, the catheter is advanced into the lumen without the sharp stylet. It is then passed off of the hollow trocar so only the soft part of the catheter is advancing within the bladder lumen. Once the entire pigtail and its fenestrations are within the urinary bladder the string on the locking-loop catheter is pulled to lock the loop. This is then secured. The tube is secured to the body wall as described above.

Miscellaneous

This procedure can also be combined with a minimally invasive flank approach, a laparoscopic-assisted approach, or done completely ultrasound-guided (Bray et al, 2009, Zhang et al, 2010, Dhein et al, 1989). A cystopexy is not typically needed for successful tube placement and function so fluoroscopic or ultrasound guidance is typically sufficient.

Percutaneous cystostomy tube can be done using the "one-stab" technique with ultrasound alone, but the bladder must be full. If the urinary bladder is empty, it is recommended to administer a bolus of IV fluids to fill the bladder. If this does not result in sufficient bladder filling ultrasound guidance can be used to perform a cystocentesis for further distension of the urinary bladder. The procedure is typically safer and met with fewer complications when done using a modified Seldinger technique, so this is what is recommended.

Notes

1. TFE-Sheathed Needle with Trochar Stylet, Cook Medical Inc, Bloomington, Indiana
2. Omnipaque (iohexol) injection (240mgI/mL), Amersham Health Inc., Princeton, NJ.
3. 0.035-inch Weasel Wire, Infiniti Medical LLC, Menlo Park, CA.
4. 6.5 French LockingLoop PigTail drainage catheter, Norfolk Vet Products, Skokie, IL.
5. 6 French drainage catheter with locking loop, Infinti Medical LLC, Menlo Park, CA.

References

Beck AL, Grierson JM, Ogden MH, and Lipscomb VJ (2007) Outcome of and complications associated with tube cystostomy in dogs and cats; 76 cases (1995–2006). *J Am Vet Med Assoc* 230, 1184–9.

Bray JP, Doyle RS, and Burton CA (2009) Minimally invasive inguinal approach for tube cystostomy. *Vet Surg* 38, 411–16.

Cornell KK (2000) Cystotomy, partial cystectomy, and tube cystostomy. *Clin Techn Small Anim Pract*15, 11–16.

Dhein CR, Person MW, and Gavin PR (1989) Prepubic (suprapubic) catheterization of the dog. *J Am Anim Hosp Assoc* 25, 261–71

Zhang JT, Wang HB, Shi J, Zhang SX, and Fan HG (2010) Laparoscopy for percutaneous tube cystostomy in dogs. *J Am Vet Med Assoc* 236, 975–77.

Suggested Reading

Hilton P and Stanton SL (1980) Suprapubic catheterization. *Br Med J* 281, 1261–3.

Holmes ES, Weisse CW, and Berent AC (2012) Use of fluoroscopically guided percutaneous antegrade urethral catheterization for the treatment of urethral obstruction in male cats: 9 cases. *J Am Vet Med Assoc* 241, 603–7

Kruger JM, Osborne CA, and Ulrich LK (1996) Cystocentesis: Diagnostic and therapeutic considerations. *Vet Clin N Am Small Anim Pract* 26, 353–61.

Scott RC, Wilkins RJ, and Greene RW (1974) Abdominal paracentesis and cystocentesis. *Vet Clin N Am* 4, 413–17.

CHAPTER FORTY-TWO

ENDOSCOPIC LASER ABLATION OF VESTIBULOVAGINAL REMNANTS (ELA-VR)

Stacy Kathleen Burdick and Allyson Berent
The Animal Medical Center, New York, NY

BACKGROUND / INDICATIONS

Abnormalities in the embryological development of the mullerian ducts and urogenital sinus can lead to various canine urogenital malformations, including an imperforate or persistent hymen, vestibulovaginal stenosis (VVS), vaginal segmental hypoplasia or aplasia, and paramesonephric septal remnants (PPMR). It has been shown in multiple studies that these malformations commonly occur concurrently with other urogenital abnormalities such as a pelvic bladder, recessed vulva, urethral sphincter mechanism incontinence and ureteral ectopia.

Dogs that are clinically affected by these disorders are suggested to display a variety of signs including difficulties during natural breeding, persistent urinary incontinence, vaginal pooling of urine, chronic recurrent urinary tract infections (UTIs), dysuria, infertility, recurrent vaginitis, dystocia, vulvar dermatitis, and ambiguous external genitalia. In a recent study, endoscopic laser ablation of vestibulovaginal septal remnants (ELA-VR) was shown to improve continence scores and decrease urinary tract infections in dogs; however, the small number of dogs without multiple concurrent malformations precluded significance of fixing these lesions (Burdick et al, 2013). As the current implications of these malformations remain unknown, having a non-invasive and effective treatment option such as endoscopic guided laser ablation is ideal.

DEFINITIONS

The definitions of these malformations are not consistent in the literature, making diagnosis, treatment options and outcomes difficult to discuss. The definitions of vestibulovaginal remnants, including PPMR, vaginal septa and dual vagina have been determined by the authors to attempt to clarify this subject (Figure 42.1). They are considered as follows: *vestibulovaginal septal remnant* (VVSR) is used as a general term to describe any dorsoventrally or ventrolaterally directed band or wall of tissue over the vaginal opening that is present between the cervix and vestibule. A *PPMR* is a membrane in which the tissue extends cranially from the vestibulovaginal junction less than 1 cm. A *vaginal septum* is when this tissue extends cranially > 1 cm, stopping prior to the cervix, and a *dual vagina* is when this tissue extends from the vestibulovaginal junction to the cervix, splitting the vagina into two separate compartments. The definition of a *persistent hymen* remains as a thin membrane at the junction of the paramesonephric tubercle and urogenital sinus that is a vertical band over the vaginal opening which can be digital broken down, do not typically require endoscopic- guided laser ablation (ELA). The definition of VVS remains as an annual fibrotic stenosis at the vestibulovaginal junction cranial to the urethral papilla, although at this time, a controversy remains over whether it truly exists as a disease entity and/or is a cause of clinical signs.

PATIENT PREPARATION

Diagnostics utilized to document and characterize vaginal malformations include digital vaginal examination, vaginoscopy, vaginography, and uroendoscopy. Digital vaginal examination and vaginoscopy using a manually held vaginoscope have been performed in awake or sedated animals. These can often give an idea of abnormal vaginal anatomy but are not use in characterizing the extent of the lesion. Positive-contrast

Veterinary Image-Guided Interventions, First Edition. Edited by Chick Weisse and Allyson Berent.

Companion website: www.wiley.com/go/weisse/vet-image-guided-interventions

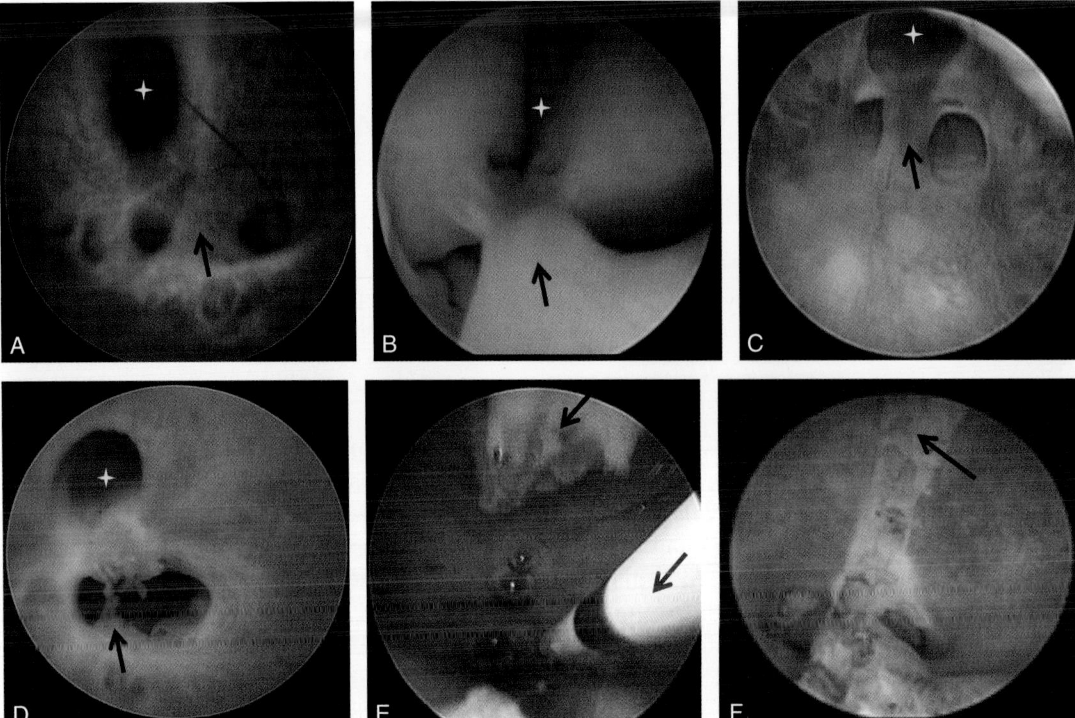

Figure 42.1 Vaginoscopic images of three female dogs in dorsal recumbency with different VVSR after ELA-VR A,D) A dog with a persistent paramesonephric remnant (<1 cm in length) before (A) and after (D) ELA. The urethral meatus is marked by a yellow asterick and the vaginal membrane is marked by a black arrow. (B, E) A dog with a vaginal septum (remnant >1 cm in length) that ends mid vagina (E). The opening to the cervix is seen at the end of the catheter in E. A catheter (red arrow) is seen in the vagina showing the lumen is completely open. The urethral opening is marked by a yellow asterisk and the vaginal membrane by a black arrow. (C, F) A dog with a dual vagina where the remnant (black arrow) at the vaginal opening is seen from the vestibule sitting dorsal to the urethral opening (yellow asterisk). After ELA (F), the entire vaginal membrane is cut with the laser (black arrow) to the level of the cervix

vaginography and computerized tomography (CT) vaginourethrography have also been shown to underestimate the diagnosis of vestibulovaginal septal remnants, likely due to positioning artifact, summation of structures, filling defects, reproductive status and partial volume averaging on CT.

Although, several diagnostic methods to evaluate the urogenital tract have been evaluated, the current gold standard is uroendoscopy, as using other methods may result in a misdiagnosis of the malformation. Uroendoscopy can be utilized to evaluate the vestibule, vagina, urethra, and bladder neck. It has been shown to be superior to CT and conventional vaginography for the diagnosis of vaginal septa and in the diagnosis of concurrent urinary tract anomalies (ureteral ectopia, hypoplastic bladder, intrapelvic bladder and short/wide urethra).

Treatment options for vaginal malformations have traditionally included medical and surgical management, although medical management with antibiotics, steroids and/or hormones has been met with limited to no success. Surgical options are typically invasive and include manual dilation, transection of the vertical septum, T-shaped vaginoplasty, vaginal resection and anastomosis, and vaginectomy with pelvis osteotomy.

Endoscopic guided laser ablation (ELA) of various VVSRs has been recently described as an outpatient procedure, and was shown to be safe and effective with minimal post-operative complications (Burdick et al, 2013). Diagnosis and treatment can be performed concurrently, eliminating the need for two separate anesthetic events. ELA is highly effective for membrane ablation, has been shown to not recur after therapy (Berent et al, 2012), and associated with less morbidity than surgery, especially for a disease process that has unknown implications to the patient.

Prior to performing ELA of any of the various vestibulovaginal remnants, a full work up should be completed. This includes a full physical examination including a digital vaginal exam and evaluation of the vulva. This is to ensure that abnormal anatomy such as a hooded vulva or evidence of vaginitis (erythema, white plaques, mucoid discharge), or urinary incontinence (wet/stained fur or urine scald on the hind limbs, foul odor) is not present. Evaluation for the presence of any comorbidities with baseline diagnostics, such as a complete blood count, serum chemistry, urinalysis, and urine culture should be performed. Specifically, it is vital to ensure the patient does not have an untreated, active urinary tract infection prior to treatment. A negative culture should be obtained within 2 weeks of the procedure if possible. If a positive culture is revealed than an appropriate antibiotic should be used based on sensitivity results for at least 48 hours prior to treatment. Ideally, imaging such as an abdominal ultrasound should be performed to evaluate for concurrent malformations such as ectopic ureters, abnormal urinary bladder positioning and shape, renal or cystic calculi, hydronephrosis, or other abnormalities of the renal anatomy that may have an effect on prognosis or also require treatment.

Potential Risks/Complications/Expected Outcomes

Complications with this procedure are possible and may include urethral tears, vaginal tears, and mucosal trauma. In a recent study evaluating ELA of VVSRs, 5/36 or 14% of the dogs had immediate mild postoperative dysuria that resolved within the first 24–72 hours post-endoscopy (Burdick et al, 2013). Laser perforation of the vaginal wall occurred in one dog. The only effect from this occurrence was that the procedure was discontinued and the remainder of the vaginal tissue had to be re-lasered at the 6–8 week recheck. All dogs that were re-scoped 6 to 8 weeks postoperatively did not have reoccurrence of the malformation.

In this same study, continence scores, vaginitis and urinary tract infections were all improved after endoscopic guided laser ablation. Again, this is difficult to attribute to the fixation of the VVSR, as the majority of dogs in this study had concurrent treatment of other congenital malformations. Future research needs to be performed in order to elucidate the role of vaginal malformations in urinary incontinence, vaginitis and chronic UTIs.

Equipment

Various endoscopes are used for this procedure.[1–3] Typically rigid scopes ranging in size from 1.9–4mm with a 30 degree lens are used. Saline infusion is used to maintain visibility, and this is ideally run on a pressure system to keep the vaginal vault distended. A guide wire[4] and open-ended ureteral catheter[5] is typically used in the authors' practice to evaluate the length and location of the remnant. Finally, the laser that is typically used to ablate the membrane is either a Holmium:YAG laser[6] or a diode laser.[7]

Procedure

The patient is placed in dorsal recumbency and the vulva is clipped and aseptically prepared. Procedural antibiotics are given (cefazolin at 22mg/kg [10mg/lb] IV every 2 hours) in patients that are not being treated with an antibiotic for a previously diagnosed urinary tract infection. A rigid cystoscope with a 30 degree lens and working channel, is advanced into the vestibule using saline irrigation on a pressure irrigation system. The vaginal opening is identified and the urethra is entered in a retrograde manner for a full cystourethroscopy. Following evaluation of the urethra, ureteral openings and urinary bladder, fixation of any anomalies that could be performed endoscopically is conducted (see Chapter 32). The length of the urethra is recorded. The scope is removed from the urethra and the vagina is entered. After each compartment is evaluated with the scope, the guide wire and ureteral catheter are advanced into one of the vaginal compartments. Next, the scope is removed over the wire/catheter combination and re-advanced into the vestibule, using the working channel for the laser fiber (Figure 42.2). The scope can be advanced into the contralateral compartment to evaluate the length of the septum. Each malformation is classified as either a PPMR, vaginal septum or dual vagina based on measurements of the septum with the open ended ureteral catheter (1 cm marks throughout its length).

A laser fiber is then placed inside the working channel of the endoscope (Figure 42.2, Figure 42.3, and Figure 42.3). The laser used is either a diode laser with a 600 μm end-fire laser fiber[6] (at 18–22W) or a Holmium:YAG[8] laser (at 10–12Hz and 0.7 to 1.2J at a pulse width of 700ms) with a 400μm end-fire laser fiber. The malformation is then laser ablated from the caudal aspect to the most cranial aspect. The catheter is used to mark the contralateral vaginal compartment until the vagina is one open tube with one opening (Figure 42.1E, Figure 42.3C, Figure 42.4C).

The patient is administered meloxicam (0.1mg/kg SQ [0.5mg/lb]) upon recovery from the laser procedure if there is no concern of kidney disease, and their urethra, vagina and vestibule is infused topically with a bupivicaine (0.3mg/kg [0.15mg/lb]) and saline mixture (1:1) for local transurethral analgesia.

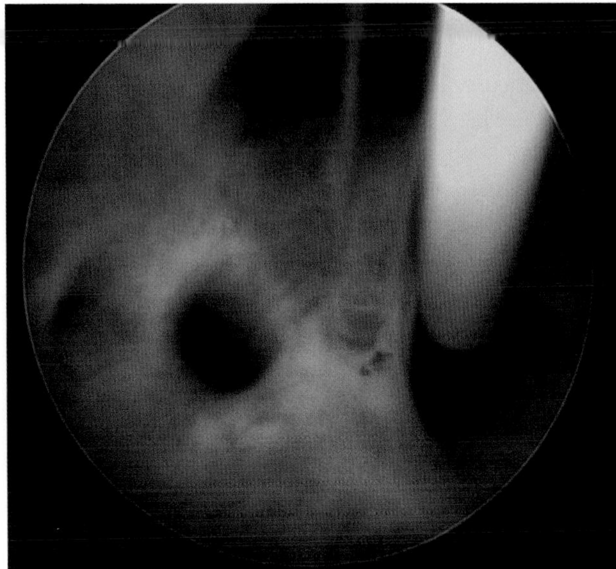

Figure 42.2 Vestibuloscopic image of a female dog in dorsal recumbency with a VVSR. An open-ended ureteral catheter with 1 cm marks on it are advanced within the left side of the vaginal opening, and the laser fiber is advanced through the working channel of the cystoscope and in contact mode with the vaginal membrane prior to ablation.

Follow-Up

The patients are recovered routinely from anesthesia and go home the same day of the procedure. At discharge owners are provided with an analgesic to be administered for signs of discomfort as needed. This is typically a non-steroidal anti-inflammatory drug, meloxicam (0.1 mg/kg PO q 24 h [0.05 mg/lb]), for 1–3 days if there is no concern for kidney disease, or tramadol (2–5 mg/kg PO TID [1–2.5 mg/lb]). Patients are administered amoxicillin-clavulanic acid (15 mg/kg PO BID [7 mg/lb PO BID]) for 3–7 days, depending on underlying disease (PPMR alone versus EU). Bacteriologic culture of urine is performed 2–4 weeks after antibiotic therapy in all patients, and recommended at 8 weeks, 3 months, 6 months, and then every 6 months thereafter if chronic UTIs in in the history. Owners are asked to grade their pets continence level on a scale of 1 through 10 as previously reported (Burdick et al, 2013, Berent et al, 2012), both before and after the procedure is incontinence is the primary concern: 1, minimally continent (leaking all the time), 5, moderately continent

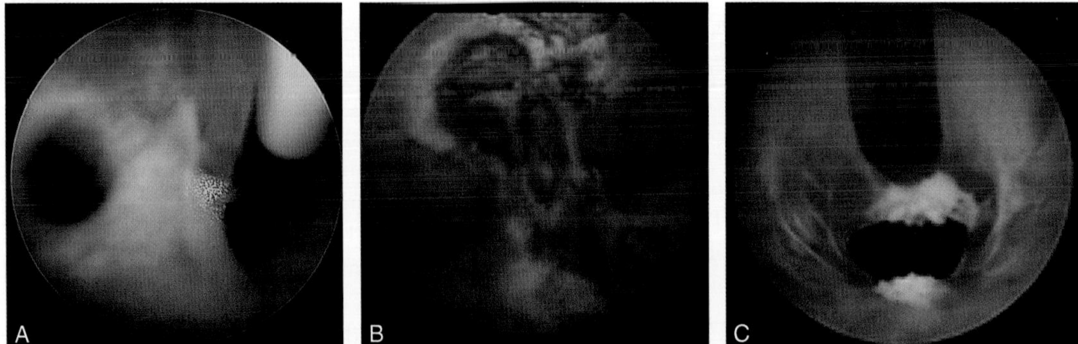

Figure 42.3 Vaginoscopic image of a female dog with a vaginal septum during ELA-VR. Notice the green-light laser beam of the Hol:YAG laser that is being used. (A) The catheter is in the left compartment of the vagina while the laser is in contact mode with the tissue for ablation. (B) As the remnant is being lasered. Notice the charring of the tissue without any hemorrhage. (C) The entire vaginal septum is cut by the laser and the vaginal opening is seen from the vestibulovaginal junction, fully patent.

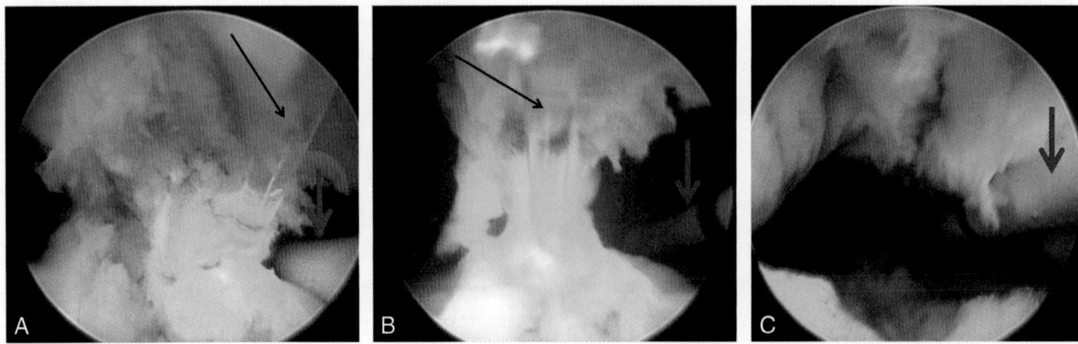

Figure 42.4 Vaginoscopic image of a female dog in dorsal recumbency during ELA-VR using a Holmium:YAG laser. (A) Green light of the laser cutting the tissue at the vaginal opening. Notice the open ended ureteral catheter (red arrow) on the left side of the membrane. (B) The tissue being continuously cut from the right to the left side maintaining catheter visibility. (C) Completion of the ablation, showing one open lumen of the vagina.

(leaking when laying down or when the bladder is full but able to hold urine between urinations and to produce a puddle of urine), and 10, perfectly continent (no leakage at all). Depending on the extent of the lesion, repeat uroendoscopy may be performed 6 weeks after the laser ablation to ensure that regrowth has not occurred. In 30 dogs in which this procedure was performed no dog had re-formation of their VVSR (Berent et al, 2012, Burdick et al, 2013).

Notes

1. Rigid endoscope, 1.9-mm 30° lens, Karl Storz Endoscopy, Culver City, CA.
2. Rigid endoscope, 2.7-mm 30° lens, Richard Wolf, Vernon Hills, IL.
3. Rigid endoscope, 4-mm 30° lens, Karl Storz Endoscopy, Culver City, CA.
4. Weasel Wire 0.025- or 0.035-inch hydrophilic angle-tipped guidewire, Infiniti Medical LLC, Menlo Park, CA.
5. 4–5 Fr open-ended ureteral catheter, Cook Medical Inc, Bloomington, IN
6. 400-μm Hol:YAG laser fiber and 30-W Hol:YAG lithotrite, Convergent Inc, Alameda, CA
7. 600-μm diode laser fiber and 25-W diode laser, Lumenis Inc, Santa Clara, CA.

References

Berent A, Weisse C, Mayhew P, et al (2012) Evaluation of cystoscopic-guided laser ablation of intramural ectopic ureters in female dogs. *J Am Vet Med Assoc* **240**(6), 716–25.

Burdick S, Berent A, Weisse C, et al (2013) Endoscopic-guided laser ablation of vestibulovaginal defects in 36 dogs. *J Am Vet Med Assoc,* **224**(8), 944–9.

Suggested Reading

Cannizzo KL, McLoughlin MA, Mattoon JS, et al. (2003) Evaluation of transurethral cystoscopy and excretory urography for diagnosis of ectopic ureters in female dogs: 25 cases (1992–2000). *J Am Vet Med Assoc* **223** (4), 475–81.

Crawford JT and Adams WM (2002) Influence of vestibulovaginal stenosis, pelvic bladder, and recessed vulva on response to treatment for clinical signs of lower urinary tract disease in dogs: 38 cases (1990–1999). *J Am Vet Med Assoc* **221**, 995–9.

Samii VF, McLoughlin MA, Mattoon JS, et al (2004) Digital fluoroscopic excretory urography, digital fluoroscopic urethrography, helical computed tomography, and cystoscopy in 24 dogs with suspected ureteral ectopia. *J Vet Intern Med* **18**(3), 271–81

Wang KY, Samii VF, Chew DJ, et al (2006). Vestibular, vaginal and urethral relations in spayed dogs with and without lower urinary tract signs. *J Vet Intern Med* **20**(5), 1065–73.

SECTION SIX

Vascular/Lymphatic Systems

Edited by Matthew W. Beal

CHAPTER FORTY-THREE

Lymphangiography

Ameet Singh
Department of Clinical Studies, Ontario Veterinary College, University of Guelph, Guelph, Ontario, Canada

Background and Indications

Imaging of the lymphatic system is recommended when performing surgical treatment of idiopathic chylothorax in dogs and cats. Preoperatively, lymphangiography can provide detailed anatomy of the cisterna chyli and thoracic duct, guiding appropriate selection of a number of available surgical techniques. Intraoperative vital staining of the lymphatic system with methylene blue can aid the surgeon in identification of the cisterna chyli and/or thoracic duct, and postprocedural lymphangiography can determine whether complete occlusion of the thoracic duct has occurred. Incomplete occlusion of all ductal branches has been shown to result in persistent chylous effusion following thoracic duct ligation. If postoperative lymphangiography reveals persistent flow in the thoracic duct, the surgeon should perform complete ductal occlusion.

Lymphatic system imaging can be performed by direct injection of aqueous contrast medium into a lymphatic vessel or lymph node. Radiography, computerized tomography (CT), or intraoperative fluoroscopy can be used to delineate lymphatic anatomy (Figure 43.1).

Minimally invasive techniques for imaging the lymphatic system have been described and are gaining popularity. Percutaneous injection of a popliteal or mesenteric lymph node with iodinated contrast followed by radiography or CT are rapid, minimally invasive techniques that provide adequate delineation of the cisterna chyli and thoracic duct (Figure 43.2).

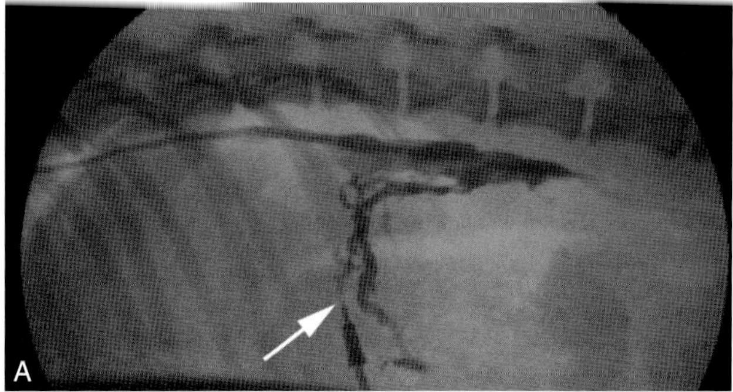

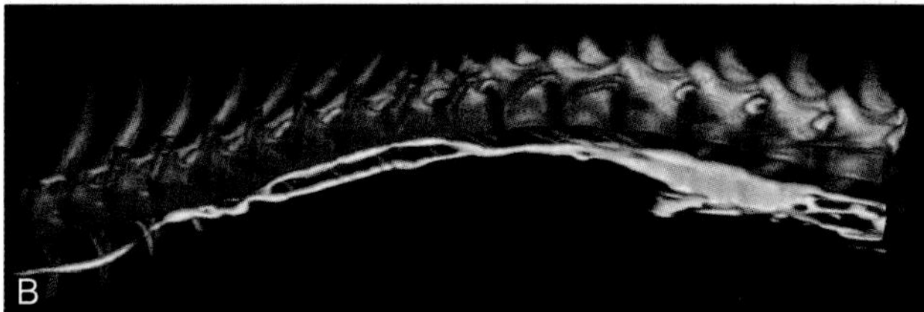

Figure 43.1 Lymphatic system imaging. (A) Fluoroscopic mesenteric lymphangiography is performed by injection of aqueous contrast medium into a catheterized efferent mesenteric lymphatic vessel. The cisterna chyli and its cranial extension, the thoracic duct, are delineated. (B) Three-dimensional CT reconstruction of the cisterna chyli and thoracic duct following popliteal lymphangiography.

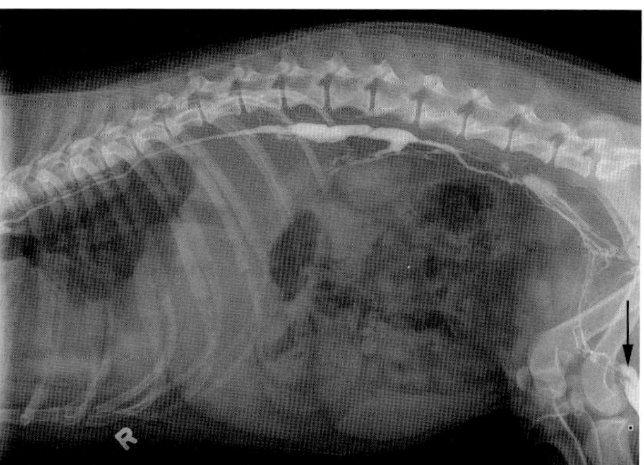

Figure 43.2 Lateral abdominal and thoracic radiograph following popliteal lymphangiography. The popliteal lymph node (arrow), ileolumbar lymphatic centre (ventral to the caudal lumbar vertebrae), cisterna chyli, and thoracic duct are apparent.

Veterinary Image-Guided Interventions, First Edition. Edited by Chick Weisse and Allyson Berent.

Companion website: www.wiley.com/go/weisse/vet-image-guided-interventions

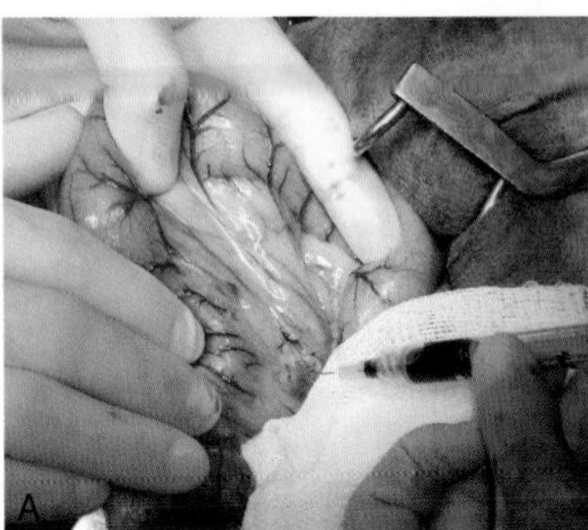

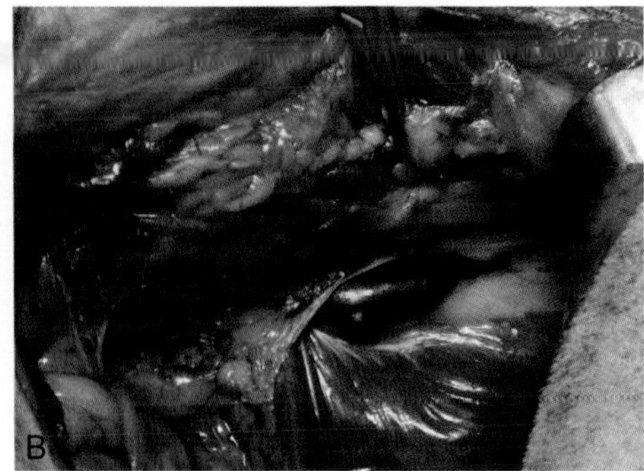

Figure 43.3 Vital staining of the lymphatic system. (A) Intraoperative view following ventral celiotomy and methylene blue injection into a mesenteric lymph node with subsequent delineation of the cisterna chyli and thoracic duct (B). (Image courtesy of Dr. Bryden Stanley.)

Use of minimally invasive techniques for imaging of the lymphatic system negate the need for celiotomy, reducing patient morbidity, anesthesia times, and surgical times; however, they do not aid the surgeon intra operatively. This can be achieved by injection of methylene blue (or contrast) into the mesenteric or popliteal lymph nodes, or directly into a mesenteric lymphatic vessel (Figure 43.3).

Patient Preparation

A complete diagnostic workup focused on identifying any predisposing cause of chylothorax is indicated. A minimum database often includes complete bloodwork (complete blood cell count, serum biochemical profile), urinalysis, thoracic radiography, abdominal ultrasonography, and cytological and biochemical evaluation of pleural fluid.

Potential Risks and Complications

A key factor in the success of percutaneous popliteal lymphangiography is whether the node itself is palpable. If the node is not readily palpable, the author does not recommend blind injection as contrast extravasation and/or through-and-through nodal puncture can occur leading to suboptimal imaging studies. Ultrasound-guidance or an open surgical approach to the node can be used to optimize nodal injection. Clinically significant consequences related to nodal punctures and/or perinodal contrast extravasation have not been found with this technique.

Another potential concern with percutaneous, ultrasound-guided or open popliteal lymphangiography is whether enough pressure can be generated during the injection to open and delineate all thoracic duct branches. Injection into the popliteal lymph node must be performed slowly and the injection pressure is considerably reduced compared with direct mesenteric lymphatic vessel injection. A recent study compared the number of thoracic duct branches delineated using CT following direct mesenteric and popliteal lymphangiography in normal dogs. A significant difference was not found supporting the use of popliteal lymphangiography as a minimally invasive alternative to mesenteric lymphangiography in the perioperative period.

If intraoperative fluoroscopic equipment is not available, the patient will require transfer to the radiology suite multiple times in the perioperative period if pre- and postoperative imaging is performed. Catheter dislodgement from the lymphatic vessel can occur during patient repositioning and transfer to the radiology suite. The catheter in the mesenteric lymphatic vessel must be secured in place with a suture around the lymphatic vessel and an additional suture(s) should be placed between the catheter hub and a segment of bowel.

Toxicities related to administration of methylene blue including Heinz body anemia, pseudocyanosis, and renal failure have been reported with intravenous administration. Using the minimal amount of a 1% methylene blue solution with it diluted 2–5× is recommended (dose is given in the next section). Toxicity in animals undergoing lymphangiography with methylene blue has not been reported.

Equipment List

Minimal equipment is required to perform lymphangiography and/or vital staining of the lymphatic system. Some key equipment includes iodinated, non-ionic, aqueous contrast agent (e.g., Iohexol (350 mg I/ml), GE

Healthcare Canada, Inc., Mississauga, ON, Canada), 1% methylene blue dye, a 25-gauge butterfly catheter, a selection of over-the-needle catheters (22–24 gauge), and a selection of syringes (1–12 ml). Intraoperative fluoroscopy with digital subtraction angiography capabilities can be extremely valuable, and limits patient transfer between the operating room and radiographic suite.

Procedures

Lymphangiography should be performed under general anesthesia. Aseptic technique should be utilized in all of the lymphangiography techniques described below.

In dogs undergoing surgical interventions, in order to dilate and improve direct visualization of mesenteric lymphatic vessels, corn oil or heavy cream (5–10 ml/kg given every hour prior to induction of general anesthesia initiated 3–4 hours preoperatively) can be fed to the patient preoperatively.

Mesenteric Lymphangiography

To perform mesenteric lymphangiography by direct injection of efferent mesenteric lymphatic vessels following standard techniques for celiotomy, see Chapter 50. If the surgeon has elected to perform thoracic duct ligation (± pericardectomy ± cisterna chyli ablation), the patient is positioned in lateral recumbency (left lateral – dogs, right lateral – cats). Lymphangiography or vital dye staining can be performed without patient repositioning by making a standard paracostal approach to the abdomen. Retractors or a reinforced O-ring wound retractor (Applied Medical Corp., Rancho Santo Margarita, CA, USA) can be used to maintain abdominal exposure. A mesenteric lymph node is identified or, alternatively, the cecum is identified and exteriorized allowing for visualization of a colic lymph node. Next, 1 ml/kg of a 1:1 mixture of iohexol:0.9% saline mixture is attached to a three-way-stopcock with extension tubing. This solution is then injected directly into the selected lymph node using a 25-gauge needle (Figure 43.3). Alternatively, a prominent lymphatic vessel can be cannulated using a 25-gauge, ¾ inch over-the-needle catheter and attached to the extension tubing (Figure 43.4). The hub of the catheter can be sutured to a portion of bowel for further stabilization to prevent inadvertent dislodgement. The fluoroscopic equipment is maneuvered into place. Contrast is injected slowly under fluoroscopic guidance. If intraoperative fluoroscopic equipment is not available, the extension tubing attached to the lymphatic catheter is exited from the paracostal incision, which is then closed in a routine fashion followed by patient transfer to the radiology suite. This procedure can be repeated following thoracic duct ligation to confirm complete occlusion of all ductal branches.

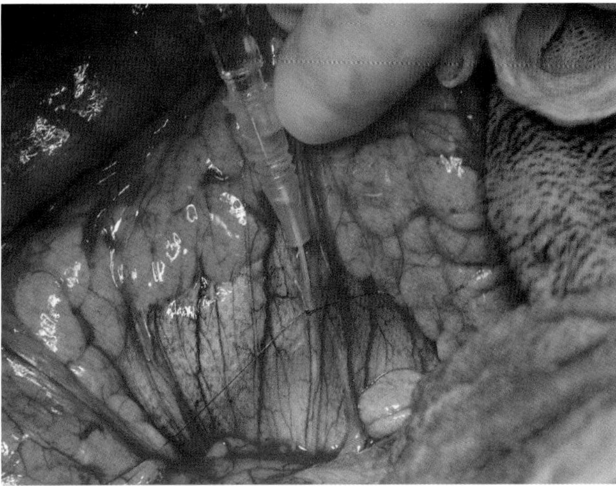

Figure 43.4 Intraoperative view following ventral celiotomy and catheterization of an afferent lymphatic vessel. (Image courtesy of Dr. Bryden Stanley.)

If intraoperative direct visualization of the cisterna chyli and/or thoracic duct is desired at the time of celiotomy, intercostal thoracotomy, thoracoscopy, or a single paracostal approach, methylene blue instead of aqueous iodinated contrast is used. 0.5–1 ml of a 1:1 1% methylene blue:saline mixture is injected into an abdominal lymph node or associated lymphatic vessel (Figure 43.3). The resultant methylene blue:saline solution can be further diluted two- to fivefold. Methylene blue injection can be repeated as required for identification purposes and to confirm complete occlusion of all thoracic duct branches.

Popliteal Lymphangiography

To perform percutaneous popliteal lymphangiography, the patient is routinely anesthetized and placed in lateral recumbency. Injection of left or right popliteal lymph node does not result in variability in number of thoracic duct branches delineated and both can be used. The patient should be positioned on the CT table or in the radiography/fluoroscopy suite depending on imaging modality selected to allow for immediate post-injection imaging without the need for repositioning. Using sterile technique, the non-dominant hand is used to palpate and secure the popliteal lymph node between the thumb and forefinger. A 12 ml syringe

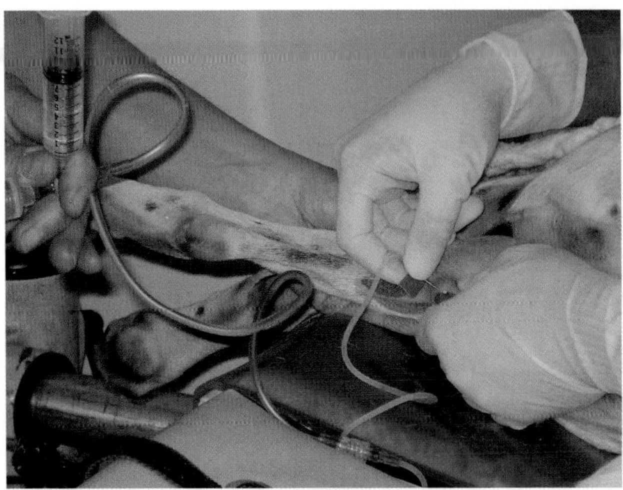

Figure 43.5 Set-up and positioning to perform percutaneous popliteal lymphangiography. The patient is placed in lateral recumbency on the CT radiographic table and using sterile technique, the non-dominant hand is used to secure the popliteal lymph node. The dominant hand is used to puncture the lymph node using a butterfly catheter and a non-sterile assistant performs the injection. (Picture courtesy of Dr. Brigitte Brisson.)

containing 12 ml of diluted aqueous contrast medium is connected to a three-way-stopcock and attached to a 25-gauge butterfly catheter. The syringe is passed to a non-sterile assistant, who performs the injection over 4–5 minutes, following insertion of the butterfly catheter into the popliteal lymph node (Figure 43.5). Radiography or CT is performed immediately following completion of the nodal injection. If thoracic duct ligation is performed following popliteal lymphangiography, percutaneous injection of the contralateral popliteal lymph node can be performed post-thoracic duct ligation to confirm complete ductal occlusion while avoiding multiple injections into the ipsilateral node.

Percutaneous Mesenteric Lymphangiography

Percutaneous injection of a mesenteric lymph node has been shown to adequately delineate the cisterna chyli and thoracic duct anatomy using CT. Ultrasonography is used to visualize a mesenteric lymph node and to guide percutaneous injection. A 27-gauge, 1¼ inch needle is connected to a 3 ml syringe containing aqueous contrast medium (1:1 diluation with 0.9% saline) and extension set with a three-way-stopcock. The node is injected with 1.5–2 ml over the course of 2 minutes immediately followed by radiography, fluoroscopy, or CT. The same procedure can be repeated post-thoracic duct ligation if needed.

Suggested Reading

Birchard SJ, Cantwell HD, and Bright RM (1982) Lymphangiography and ligation of the canine thoracic duct: A study in normal dogs and three dogs with chylothorax. *J Am Anim Hosp Assoc* 18, 769–77.

Enwiller TM, Radlinsky MG, Mason DE, et al (2003) Popliteal and mesenteric lymph node injection with methylene blue for coloration of the thoracic duct in dogs. *Vet Surg*, 32, 359–64.

Fingeroth JM and Smeak DD (1991) Methylene blue infusion. *J Am Anim Hosp Assoc* 27, 259.

Johnson EG, Wisner ER, Kyles A, et al (2009) Computed tomographic lymphography of the thoracic duct by mesenteric lymph node injection. *Vet Surg* 38, 361–7.

Mayhew PD, Culp WT, Mayhew KN, et al (2012) Minimally invasive treatment of idiopathic chylothorax in dogs by thoracoscopic thoracic duct ligation and subphrenic pericardectomy: 6 cases (2007–2010). *J Vet Med Assoc* 241, 904–9.

Millward IR, Kirberger RM, and Thompson PN (2011) Comparative popliteal and mesenteric computed tomographic lymphangiography of the canine thoracic duct. *Vet Radiol Ultrasound* 52, 295–301.

Naganobu K, Ohigashi Y, Akiyoshi T, et al (2006) Lymphography of the thoracic duct by percutaneous injection of iohexol into the popliteal lymph node of dogs: Experimental study and clinical application. *Vet Surg* 35, 377–81.

Osuna DJ, Armstrong PJ, Duncan DE, et al (1990) Acute renal failure after methylene blue infusion in a dog. *J Am Anim Hosp Assoc* 26, 410–12.

Singh A, Brisson BA, Nykamp S, et al (2011) Comparison of computed tomographic and radiographic popliteal lymphanigioraphy in normal dogs. *Vet Surg* 40, 762–7.

Staiger BA, Stanley BJ, and McAnulty JF (2011) Single paracostal approach to the thoracic duct and cisterna chyli: Experimental study and case series. *Vet Surg* 40, 786–94.

CHAPTER FORTY-FOUR

Vascular Access

Chick Weisse
The Animal Medical Center, New York, NY

Background/Indications

In order to perform vascular interventions, access to vascular lumens is necessary and is classified as either arterial or venous. While many different vessels throughout the body may be suitable, the most commonly accessed include the jugular and femoral veins or the common carotid and femoral arteries. Access and potential complications are different between arteries and veins and should be considered separately.

Patient Preparation

Wide clipping and standard surgical scrub should be performed. Whether performing percutaneous or cutdown access, a wide surgical field should be anticipated as patient drape fenestrations are often relatively large, and when used in small veterinary patients, hair contamination can be problematic. For jugular access, extending the neck and placing padding beneath to create an arch, while extending the forelimbs caudally, can help bring the vessel as superficial as possible, flatten excess skin folds and straighten the vessel. For hindlimbs, they should be extended and taped in position to prevent movement in case the anesthetic plane is light and the limb moves with a vascular sheath in place. Antibiotic use is determined by the underlying procedure being performed and whether implants will be placed. Coagulation status evaluation is recommended prior to procedures in those patients at increased risk for hemostatic disorders. The high-pressure arterial system is obviously more likely to result in considerable hemorrhage. The author does not routinely use anticoagulants unless thrombolysis/thrombectomy cases are being performed.

Vessel Selection

Vessel selection should take into account a number of considerations including: vascular anatomy, patient positioning during image acquisition, clinical signs/syndrome, anticipated procedures, and radiation exposure to the operator.

Vascular Anatomy

Knowledge of the "best path" from one location to another is useful when anticipating a procedure. Some anatomical characteristics are uniform among patients and others vary among individuals. For instance, there is a uniformly straight path from the right jugular vein into the vena cava, compared to the more angled path from the left jugular vein, potentially complicating the procedure. The hepatic veins make a gentle angle as they enter the caudal vena cava when approached cranially from the jugular veins. However, the angle is very acute when approached caudally from the femoral veins; this is important if hepatic vein access is anticipated. Other vessels have individual variations, such as the renal artery anatomy leaving the aorta. In some cases the renal artery leaves the aorta in a cranial direction and in others it leaves the aorta in a caudal direction. This can change in the same patient depending upon positioning, stomach filling, the presence of abdominal masses, etc. (Figure 44.1). Knowledge of individual variations using cross sectional imaging prior to a procedure can greatly facilitate access when necessary. Knowing this anatomy helps in the decision making process of which vessel is easiest to access (i.e., carotid versus femoral artery, etc.) to get the best angle, and what shape catheter would aid in cannulating the vessel at that angle (cobra-shape, reverse-curve, etc.).

Veterinary Image-Guided Interventions, First Edition. Edited by Chick Weisse and Allyson Berent.

Companion website: www.wiley.com/go/weisse/vet-image-guided-interventions

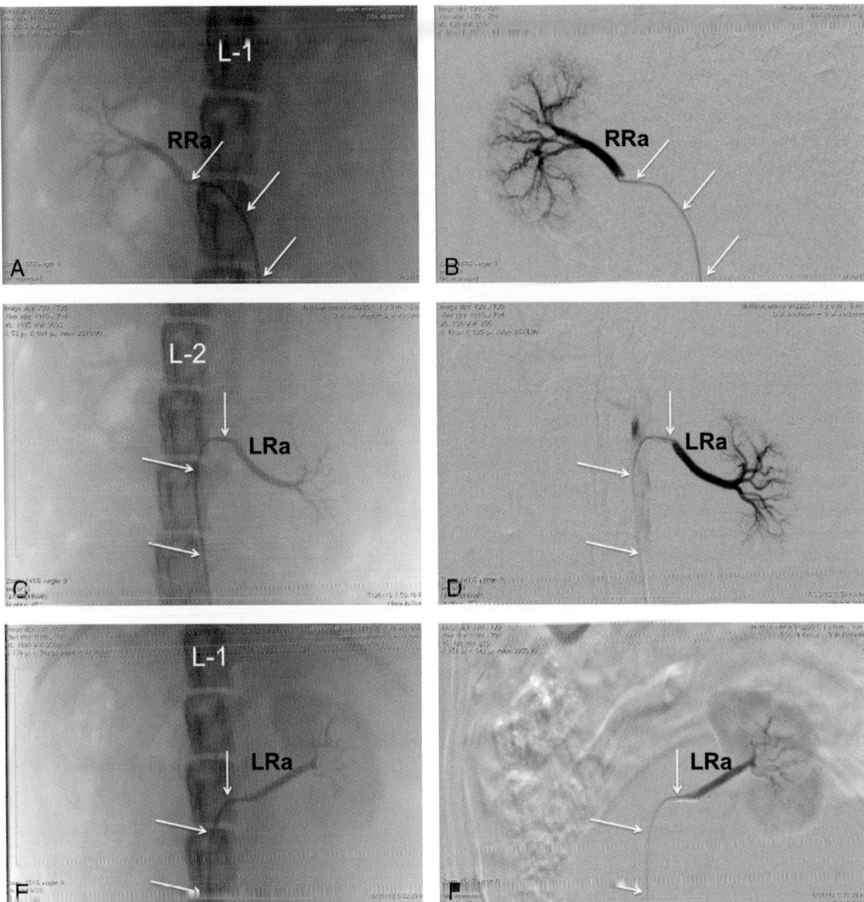

Figure 44.1 Serial renal arteriograms and digital subtraction arteriograms (DSA) in a dog receiving intra-arterial stem cell therapy on different occasions. The patient is in dorsal recumbency with the head at the top of each image and left femoral artery access using a 4 Fr vascular sheath[1] and 4 Fr Cobra catheter[3]. (A) (Non-DSA) and (B) (DSA) right renal arteriograms demonstrating the catheter (white arrows) in the proximal portion of the right renal artery (RRa) extending cranially from the aorta. L-1 is the first lumbar vertebra. (C) (non-DSA) and (D) (DSA) left renal arteriograms with the catheter (white arrows) in the proximal portion of the left renal artery (LRa) extending caudally from the aorta. L-2 is the second lumbar vertebra. (E) (non-DSA) and (F) (DSA) left renal arteriograms in the same dog on a separate occasion demonstrating the same Cobra catheter (white arrows) at the proximal portion of the LRa but now the kidney is extending cranially from the aorta rather than caudally, likely due to patient positioning or reduced stomach contents. Patient positioning may be altered to facilitate catheter placement when necessary.

Patient Positioning

Both the position of the patient during the procedure and the ability to move/rotate the fluoroscopy unit for orthogonal views can be important when considering access sites. For instance, if the procedure will be best imaged with the patient in lateral recumbency and dual access (from above and below) may be indicated, consider contralateral jugular (or carotid) and femoral vein (artery) access. For example, a patient placed in left lateral recumbency will have the right jugular up and the left femoral vein down. It is preferable to have the groin sheath in the down leg to facilitate catheter manipulations however the jugular sheath should be in the face up right jugular vein in this example.

Anticipated Procedure

When treating a lesion in the hind limb, contralateral groin access can be achieved and a reverse-curve catheter used to access the other limb; however, catheter manipulations may be more difficult due to the often tight bend involved when crossing from one external iliac to the other external or internal iliac artery or vein. For instance, carotid (or jugular) access may be preferred when addressing lesions in the caudal abdomen or hindlimbs. Bilateral jugular involvement may be better accessed from below (via a femoral vein approach) in order to access both jugular veins separately. Another important consideration about the procedure is the anticipated use of different devices.

For instance, larger devices require larger access lumens. The venous system is considerably larger diameter than the arterial system. When larger veins are required, the jugular vein may be preferred to the often smaller femoral vein. When larger arteries are required, the carotid artery is considered over the smaller femoral artery. Additionally, when dual lumen access is needed, (i.e., aortic "kissing stents" for a saddle thrombus), two arterial vessels may be needed to have enough room for two delivery systems. If both external carotid arteries are used than both carotid arteries will then need to be ligated, which could result in complications (see below), so in this case using one large sheath in one carotid artery or one carotid artery and one femoral artery might be considered.

Clinical Signs/Syndrome

Often the clinical syndrome will necessitate certain access sites while on other occasions comorbidities will be important. For instance, consider potential thrombolysis of a cranial vena cava clot with subsequent caval syndrome. Swelling of the head and forelimbs may make jugular access more difficult. On the other hand, severe pelvic limb osteoarthritis may prevent extension of the hindlimbs without excessive pain so a jugular approach may be preferred.

Distance from the Radiation Beam

When possible, vascular access at a distance from the treatment area of concern helps keep the operator protected from exposure to radiation. As an example, when the region of interest is in the hindlimbs, access can be obtained from a cervical or contralateral groin approach. The cervical (carotid artery) approach may be preferred to distance oneself from the beam (as well as to have straight access into either limb).

Potential Risks/ Complications

There are generally very few complications associated with vascular access; however, risks include hemorrhage, thrombosis/emboli (with possible sequelae), and vessel wall dissection/damage. Additionally, during carotid arterial access, the vasosympathetic trunk is manipulated and this can rarely result in Horner's syndrome. If this occurs, it is typically temporary and resolves within a few weeks.

Hemorrhage

The most substantial risk during (and following) vascular access is hemorrhage. While most IR procedures in humans are performed using percutaneous access, the inability to limit veterinary patient activity post-operatively has led to the author preferring surgical cut-down and artery ligation or repair (extremely rarely indicated) post-procedure. Venous catheterization is still performed percutaneously in the majority of cases. When large access sheaths (10 Fr or larger) are commonly used in veins, smaller access devices (multilumen catheters or smaller sheath introducers) are often left in place after the procedure to permit the vascular access site to close down partially over the next day before complete removal. Hemorrhage can also be minimized during access by using a modified Seldinger approach (single-wall puncture technique) as opposed to the double-wall (Seldinger) technique (Seldinger, 1953). Single wall puncture is the author's preferred technique for both arterial and venous access. This involves placing the access needle into the lumen of the vessel until a "flash" is identified and then advancing the guide wire into the vessel through that catheter. The double-wall approach involves passing the needle through-and-through both walls of the vessel with a Seldinger needle, removing the inner cannula, and withdrawing the needle until a "flash" is identified. This is often performed percutaneously using anatomical landmarks. The former technique is preferred in patients with bleeding disorders, to avoid the increased risk of hemorrhage associated with the creation of two vessel defects.

Dogs can tolerate ligation of the femoral artery without consequence assuming a patent internal iliac artery and its tributaries. In addition, simultaneous ligation of the femoral artery and vein are typically tolerated although some swelling, edema, and possible pain may be expected temporarily, possibly with fewer clinical signs than if the vein is ligated alone (Butkovic et al, 1996, Perkins and Edmark, 1971). The author has used the femoral artery multiple times in the same patient following ligation. It seems the multiple branches leaving the femoral artery maintain bloodflow proximal to the ligation site, and limit thrombosis, enabling future access (Figure 44.2).

Dogs have also been demonstrated to safely tolerate acute ligation of one or both carotid arteries (in most cases) due to a well-developed vertebral basilar arterial system (Clendenin and Conrad, 1979a, b). While acute occlusion of both carotids may temporarily reduce bloodflow there does not appear to be any deleterious sequelae (Hedlund et al, 1983).

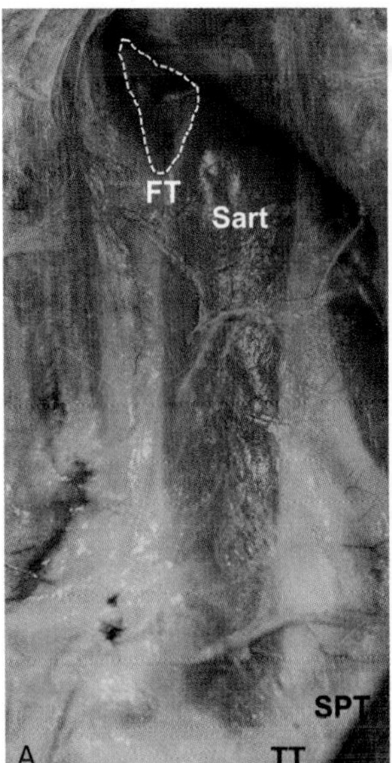

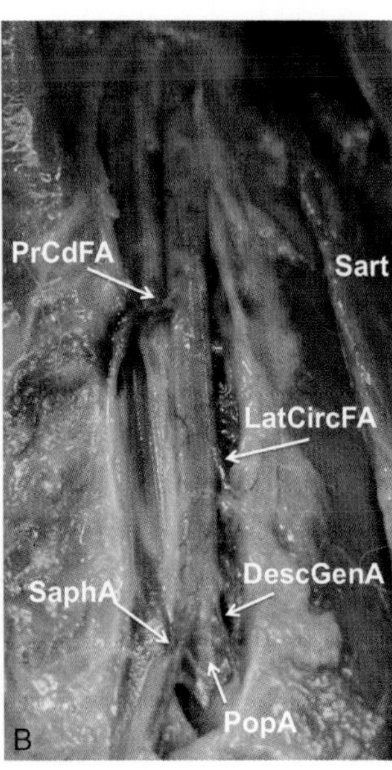

Figure 44.2 Canine cadaveric left hindlimb with skin and subcutaneous tissues removed. The patient is facing to the right. (A) Proximal limb exposure demonstrating femoral triangle (FT) and Sartorius m. (Sart) overlying much of the femoral artery. When vascular access is made more distally, this muscle belly needs to be reflected cranially or divided longitudinally to access the vessels situated more deeply as they extend distally. This is appreciated with digital palpation of the femoral pulse. The tibial tuberosity (TT) and straight patellar tendon (SPT) are seen distally. (B) Sartorius muscle (Sart) reflected cranially to expose the femoral artery between the femoral nerve cranially and the femoral vein caudally. Branches including the proximal caudal femoral (PrCdFA), lateral circumflex femoral (LatCircFA), descending genicular (DescGenA), popliteal (PopA), and saphenous (SaphA) arteries can be identified and accessed if necessary. Alternatively, the femoral can be ligated anywhere along this path safely.

Following experimental chronic unilateral occlusion of the carotid artery, extensive collateralization develops via the ipsilateral cranial thyroid and vertebral artery and contralateral vertebral artery to the caudal auricular and occipital arteries. Blood supply to the terminal branches of the external carotid artery is believed to develop via retrograde flow from the proximal caudal auricular artery. Following experimental chronic bilateral carotid ligation, anastomotic connections from the internal carotid artery to the maxillary ascending pharyngeal arteries develop bilaterally (Clendenin and Conrad, 1979a, b). In the clinical setting, the author avoids ligation of the carotid artery if the contralateral carotid is occluded or has already been ligated as a few patients have recovered from the procedure with transient neurological sequelae or blindness. In such circumstances, vessel repair may be preferred, though if anticoagulants are to be used (i.e., cases of "saddle thrombi") this should be carefully considered.

Although not routinely used, the canine brachial artery can also be safely ligated without apparent lameness, edema or gangrene (Butkovic et al, 1996).

Ligation of the femoral vein acutely is safely tolerated when performed distal to the deep femoral vein, and can likely be tolerated proximal to this, although some edema or lameness may occur temporarily (Perkins and Edmark, 1971). The author avoids ligation of the jugular vein when possible. This low-pressure system rarely results in substantial hemorrhage and bilateral jugular thrombosis does not appear to be well tolerated in the dog acutely.

Thrombosis

Thrombosis may occur more commonly than identified in veterinary patients, but due to the very active fibrinolytic system and rich collateral networks of the vascular system, it does not appear to be a common problem. The sequelae of thrombosis are more concerning in human patients with the considerably reduced ability to tolerate vascular occlusion.

Vessel Wall Dissection/Damage

During vascular isolation the operator should take the time to appreciate the anatomy of each vessel and their associated branches in the region, as the vein, artery and nerves are usually closely associated. Some small-caliber vessels, or branches to the vessel, can be dissected or torn, either during the cut down process, or during the puncture, and this could result in severe hemorrhage, or the inability to salvage the vessel for use. During vessel isolation after the perivascular tissue is dissected off the vessel, a suture (3–0 PDS) is typically placed around the vessel proximal and distal to the point of access. This is typically done by ligating the vessel distal to the access point and having a loop around the vessel proximal to the access point (Figure 44.3). Placing a stay suture on the distal ligature aids in maintaining a hold on the vessel as well as keeping it taught and straight during puncture. In animals, due to the small caliber vessels compared to people, care should be taken to avoid performing puncturing through and though both walls of the vessel, and instead entering the lumen with one wall puncture, using the modified Seldinger technique. This will help to prevent further hemorrhage.

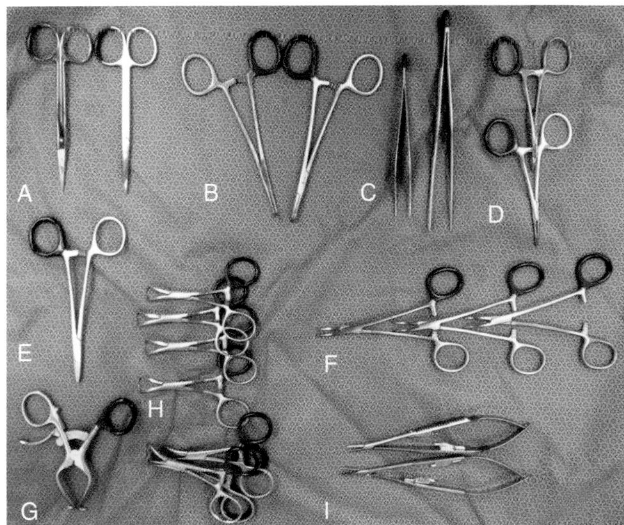

Figure 44.3 Sample surgical cut-down set. (A) Sharp-sharps and small Metzenbaum scissors. (B) Right-angled forceps. (C) Brown–Adson and Debakey forceps. (D) Mosquito hemostats. (E) Needle drivers. (F) Kelly hemostats. (G) Small Gelpi retractors. (H) Small Babcock towel clamps. (I) Castroviejo needle drivers for vessel repair.

Equipment

Arterial access obtained via cut-down requires a few important instruments as well as a scalpel blade and small surgical set (Figure 44.4). Regardless of percutaneous or surgical vessel access, the author uses a single-wall puncture technique using an intravenous catheter for initial access. Venous vascular sheath[1] size (Figure 44.5) is often not limited by the size of the vessel, due to the relatively large diameter of the jugular vein (expect for particularly small patients requiring very large delivery systems. Arterial access is often more difficult in smaller patients due to the relatively narrow arterial diameters. In these patients, a microintroducer set[2] is often preferred for initial access with a smaller gauge needle prior to placing the larger sheath (Figure 44.6) in order to make as few small holes in the vessel wall as possible (if repeated attempts are necessary).

Arterial Vascular Access Procedures

While arterial wall repair can be performed following removal of the sheath at completion of the procedure, the vessel is typically ligated to avoid hemorrhagic complications during recovery. This may be particularly important during carotid artery access to avoid air or thromboemboli to the brain that could occur during the repair of the vessel. The author typically begins with vessel ligation distal to the access point before needle access is made to prevent this potential risk (Figure 44.3D, Figure 44.7D, and Figure 44.8C).

Femoral Artery (Figure 44.3)

In small patients in whom multiple procedures are unlikely to be necessary, a larger femoral artery will be available more proximally on the limb. If relatively larger devices (such as stent delivery systems) may be utilized during the procedure, a more proximal approach may also be necessary. In those patients anticipated to receive multiple procedures in the future, a more distal approach on the limb may be preferred to allow future access to the same artery. More distal limb dissections will find the femoral artery less superficial. In addition, when smaller sheaths and catheters can be used, accessing the perforating branches off the femoral artery will help maintain femoral artery patency in the future.

Common Carotid Artery

While the common carotid artery is positioned deeper than the femoral artery, access is relatively easy and provides a substantially larger lumen. The cut-down can be performed on midline but the author prefers an incision beginning caudal to the larynx and equidistant between the trachea (midline) and the ipsilateral external jugular vein. Both common carotid arteries are equally accessible but care should be taken when dissecting the artery out of the carotid sheath to avoid damage (or incorporation within the ligature) to the vagosympathetic trunk. Both dog (Figure 44.7) and cat (Figure 44.8) common carotid artery access can be easily performed.

Venous Access Procedures

Following appropriate patient positioning, clipping, scrub and draping, percutaneous access is typically made to the jugular vein and cut-down or percutaneous access to the femoral vein if necessary.

External Jugular Vein

Following a 3–5 mm scalpel incision, an over-the-needle catheter is used to gain jugular vein access (Figure 44.9). The guide wires included with the vascular sheaths often have a J-tip or a straight tip. The author prefers using the straight tip as the J-tip is often too large for use

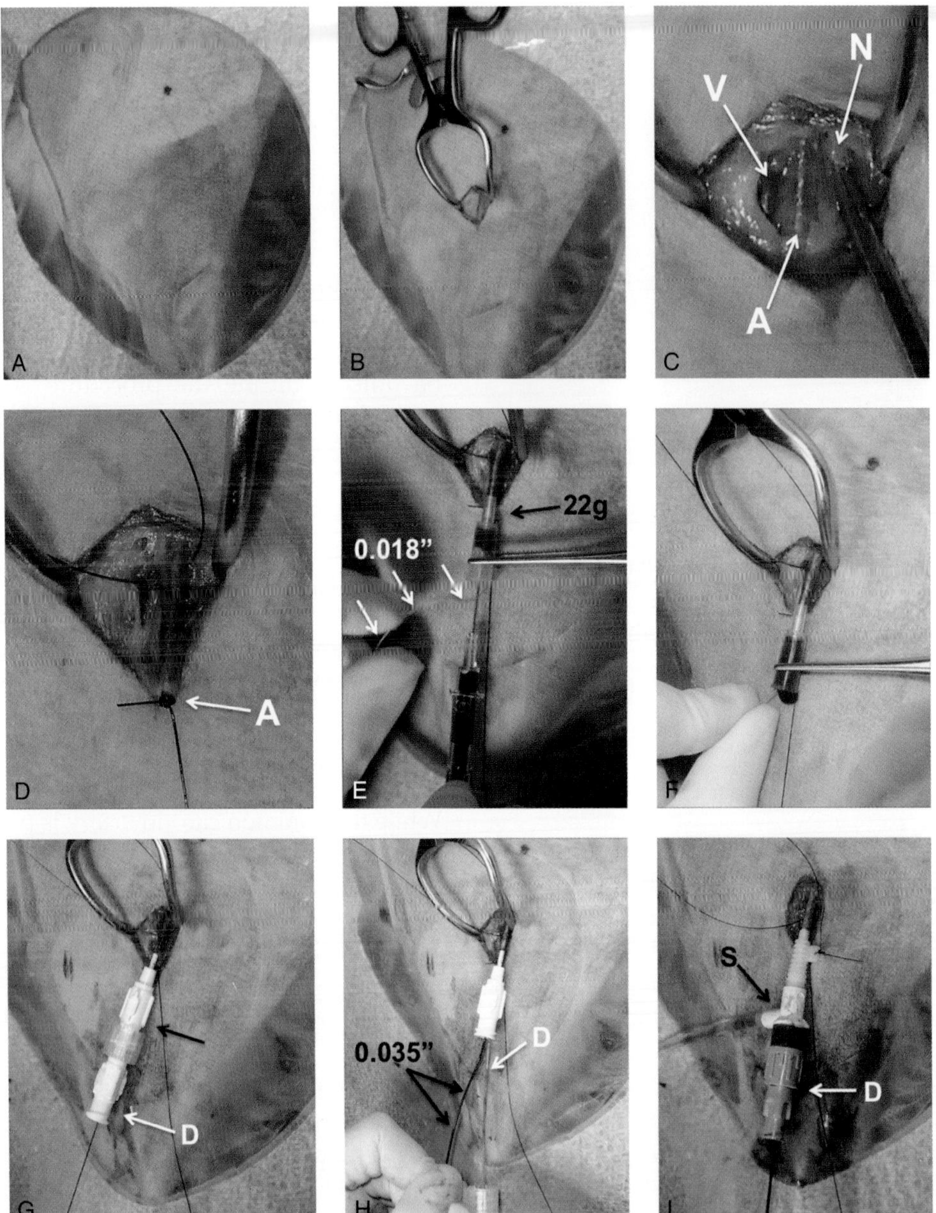

Figure 44.4 Feline left femoral artery access via cut-down and micropuncture[2] introducer. The cat is in dorsal recumbency with the head to the top of each image. The left hindlimb is extended. (A) A wide clip permits a large fenestrated drape to be placed. (B) A 1–2 cm incision is made over the proximal femoral artery and Gelpi retractors placed. (C) Gentle sharp and blunt dissection permits identification of the femoral artery (A), nerve (N) and vein (V). Careful dissection will avoid traumatizing small femoral perforating branches during arterial isolation. These can bleed substantially. (D) Once isolated, the femoral artery is ligated distally and a proximal suture placed for retraction. Ligation prevents back bleeding and introduction of air or emboli distally. (E) For particularly small vessels, a micropuncture set permits vessel access with a 22 g catheter and 0.018″ guide wire. (F) The 0.018″ guide wire is advanced into the aorta under fluoroscopic guidance. (G) The catheter is removed over-the-wire and exchanged for the microintroducer sheath (black arrow) and dilator (D) placed over-the-wire. (H) The 0.018″ guide wire and dilator (D) are removed in unison leaving the sheath (black arrow) in place to accept the 0.035″ guide wire. Substantial bleeding can occur when the dilator is removed, so this is performed quickly. (I) The microintroducer sheath is removed over-the-wire and exchanged for the introducer sheath (S) and dilator (D) that are sutured in place. (J) The dilator is removed over-the-wire and the procedure can commence. (K) Upon completion of the procedure, the wire is removed, the sheath is withdrawn, and the proximal suture is used to ligate the artery (white arrow) proximally before the sheath is completely removed. The puncture site is investigated to make sure there is no bleeding and the ligatures are placed appropriately above and below with no perforating branches between. (L) The incision is closed routinely.

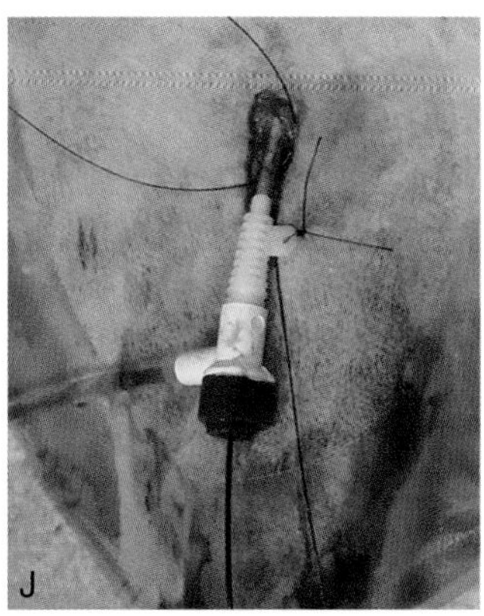

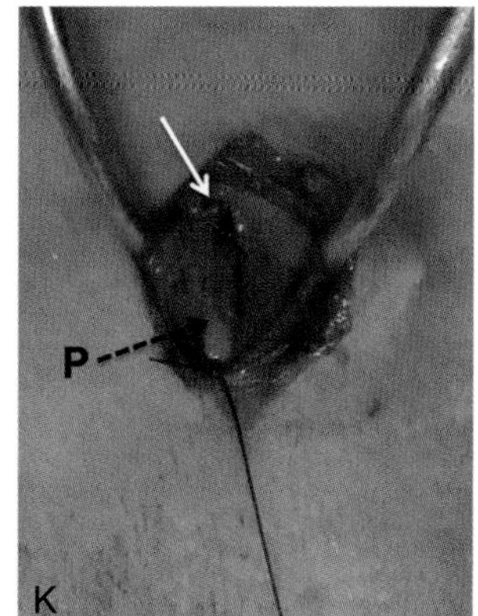

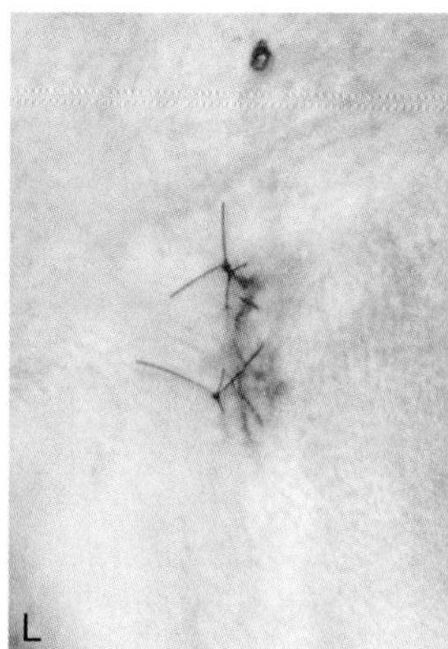

Figure 44.4 (*Continued*)

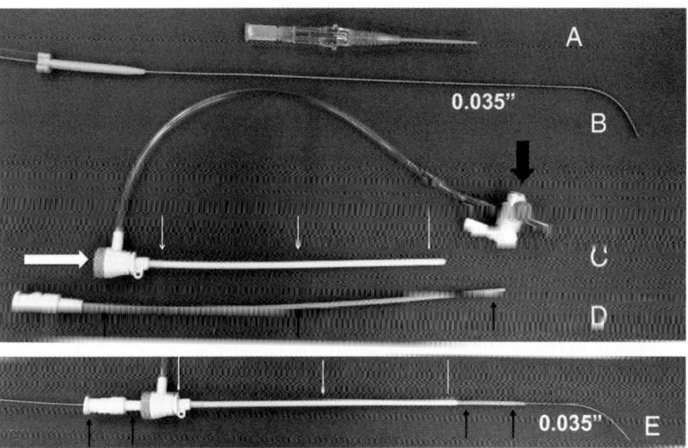

Figure 44.5 Equipment for standard (larger) vessel access. (A) 18-gauge over-the-needle catheter. (B) 0.035″ guide wire with gentle bend manual performed on shapeable tip. The bend permits operator to turn the wire during introduction if it does not pass easily. A straight wire will not change course. (C) 5 Fr vascular introducer sheath[1] made up of shaft (white arrows) with 5 Fr inner diameter, hemostasis valve (white block arrow) to prevent bleeding, and three-way stop-cock (black block arrow) to flush and/or aspirate. (D) 5 Fr Dilator with 5 Fr outer diameter shaft (black arrows). (E) Combination 5 Fr vascular introducer sheath (white arrows) and dilator (black arrows) making smooth transition down to the 0.035″ guide wire.

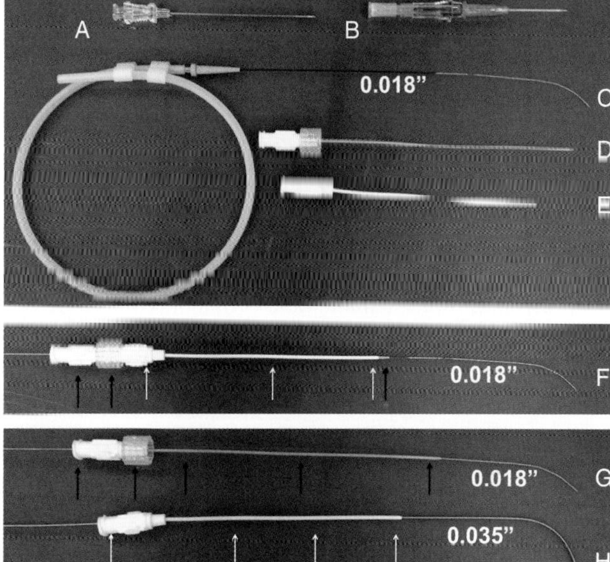

Figure 44.6 Micropuncture set[2] and equipment for smaller vessel access. (A) 22-gauge introducer needle or (B) 22-gauge over-the-needle catheter used for initial vessel access. (C) 0.018″ mandrel wire with shapeable tip and gentle curve manually formed to help direct wire if it does not advance. (D) Microintroducer dilator and (E) Microintroducer sheath. (F) The combination microintroducer dilator (black arrows) and sheath (white arrows) fit snugly and taper down over the 0.018″ guide wire for vessel introduction. (G) Once in place, the combination dilator and 0.018″ guide wire are removed leaving the microintroducer sheath (H) in place to accept a 0.035″ guide wire. Now a standard (larger) vascular introducer sheath can be placed over the 0.035″ guide wire.

in many of animal veins routinely accessed. In addition, the straight-tip wire is typically "shapeable" so a gentle 45-degree curve is manually created prior to access. During wire placement, if an obstruction is encountered with a straight wire tip, turning the wire will have no effect. An angled tip will permit the operator to gently rotate the wire and facilitate selection of the appropriate path down the vessel lumen. If access remains difficult with this wire than a hydrophilic angled guide wire is often very helpful. On rare occasions the author has found very small external jugular veins but hypertrophied internal jugular veins (within the carotid sheath). The internal jugular veins can be used for access instead if necessary but the typical internal jugular vein is substantially smaller than the normal external jugular vein. When large sheaths are removed from the jugular vein (10–12 Fr), a smaller, multilumen catheter (5–7 Fr) is often left in place 24–48 hours to allow the percutaneous access hole to close down slightly before removal of vascular access (Figure 44.10).

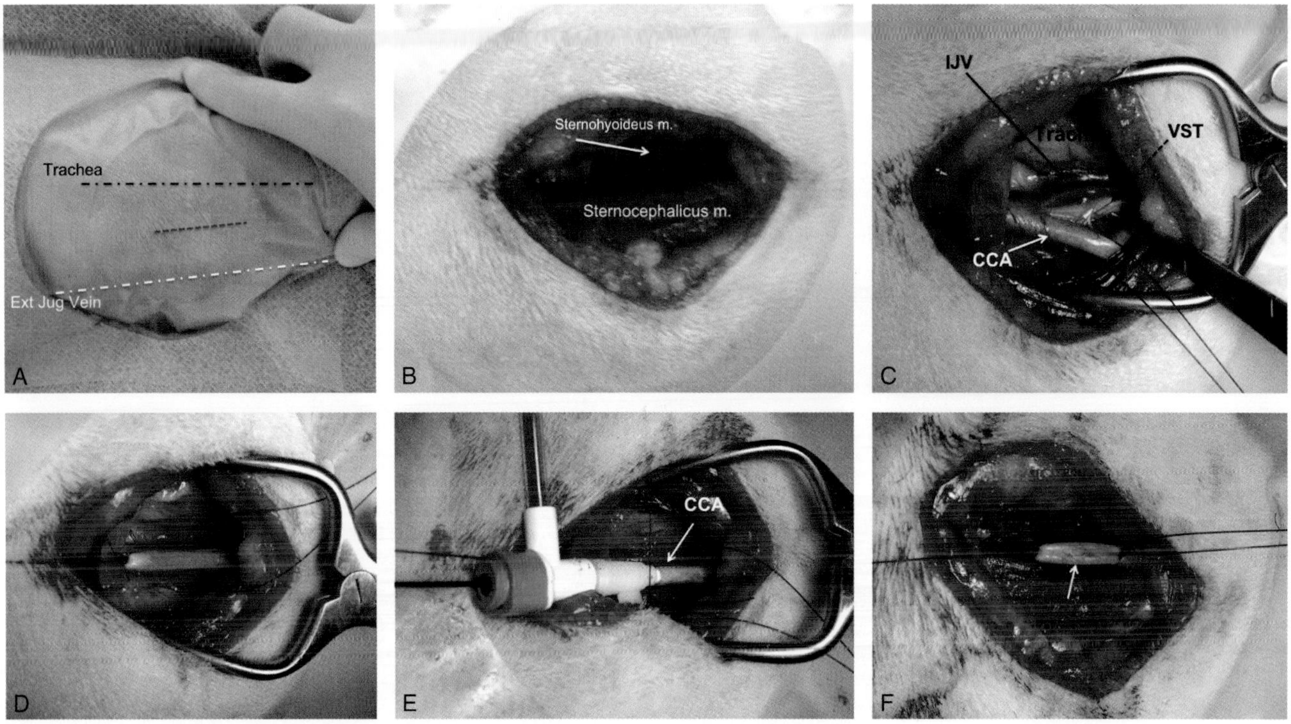

Figure 44.7 Canine carotid cut-down with dog in dorsal recumbency and head to the left in each image. (A) The trachea, larynx, and external jugular vein are identified. The incision (red dotted line) is made between the two and midway between the larynx and thoracic inlet. More cranial incisions may be made if future attempts to re-access the same carotid artery more caudally are anticipated. (B) Sharp and blunt dissection is used to identify and split the often thin connection between the sternohyoideus and sternocephalicus muscles. (C) The carotid sheath is located just dorsal and lateral to the trachea and includes the common carotid artery (CCA), vagosympathetic trunk (VST), and internal jugular vein (IJV). In animals with occluded, small, or absent external jugular veins, the IJV can sometimes be used for venous access. (D) The CCA is ligated cranially and a suture placed caudally for retraction. The ligation prevents back bleeding during the procedure and air and other emboli into the brain. Careful dissection of the CCA is necessary to avoid entrapment of the VST during ligation. (E) Standard single-wall puncture is used to obtain vascular access and an introducer sheath is placed and secured with a suture. (F) Upon completion of the procedure, the sheath is withdrawn as the caudal suture is used for ligation of the CCA prior to sheath removal. The puncture site (white arrow) is then investigated to make certain there is no bleeding prior to releasing the ligatures.

Femoral Vein

This vessel is uncommonly accessed solely but more often used for dual access with the jugular vein or when cardiac procedures are being performed during simultaneous femoral artery access. A cut-down is typically used to access this vessel but sheath introduction is otherwise the same as for jugular access.

Follow-Up

Standard discharge instructions following femoral artery access involve E-collar use as needed and limited activity until suture removal (or recheck if no skin sutures placed) at 10–14 days post-procedure. For carotid access and jugular access sites, no neck leads are used for 10–14 days. The author has accessed a single femoral artery up to five times, but carotid re-access is less commonly achievable more than once or twice, due to thrombosis that occurs; The limited number of perforating arteries leaving the common carotid limit bloodflow and promote vascular stasis with subsequent thrombosis compared to the femoral artery which has multiple branches providing brisk bloodflow at multiple levels.

Special Considerations/ Complication Examples

Dialysis catheter placement is uncommonly performed but more often is used in the temporary dialysis setting so placement is similar to jugular vein access with the use of a peel-away sheath. When using peel-away sheaths, remember to ask the anesthetist for positive-pressure ventilation when feeding

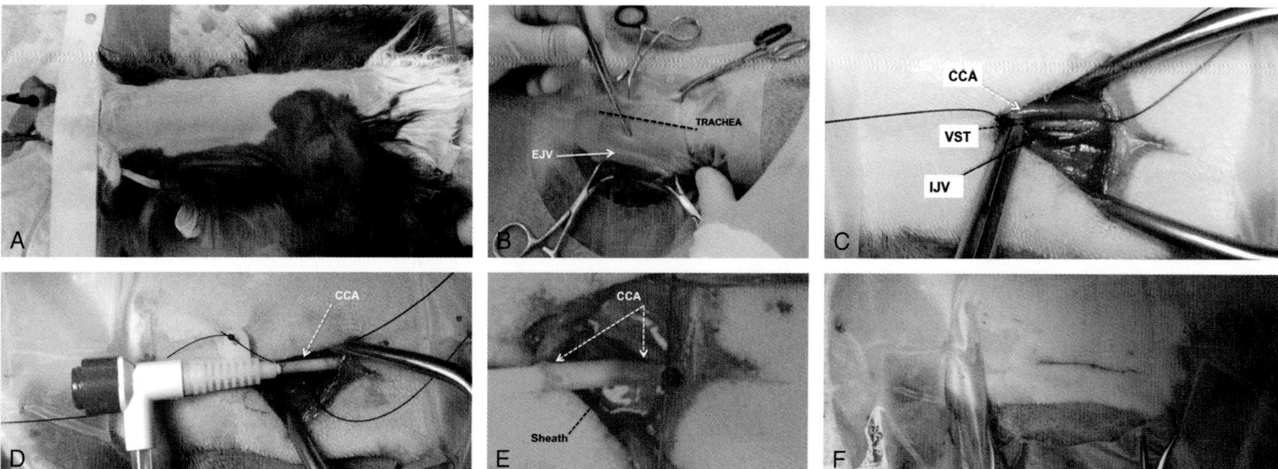

Figure 44.8 Feline carotid cut-down with cat in dorsal recumbency and head to the left in each image. A. The head is extended and forelimbs pulled caudally. A cushion is placed underneath the neck for support and to permit further neck extension in order to place the vessels in a more superficial position. (B) The trachea, larynx, and external jugular vein are identified. The incision is made between the two and midway between the larynx and thoracic inlet. More cranial incisions may be made if future attempts to re-access the same carotid artery more caudally are anticipated. (C) Sharp and blunt dissection is used to identify and split the often thin connection between the sternohyoideus and sternocephalicus muscles. The carotid sheath is located just dorsal and lateral to the trachea and includes the common carotid artery (CCA), vagosympathetic trunk (VST), and internal jugular vein (IJV). The CCA is ligated cranially and a suture placed caudally for retraction. The ligation prevents back bleeding during the procedure and air and other emboli into the brain. Careful dissection of the CCA is necessary to avoid entrapment of the VST during ligation. (D) Standard single-wall puncture is used to obtain vascular access and an introducer sheath is placed and secured with a suture. (E) Upon completion of the procedure, the sheath is withdrawn as the caudal suture is used for ligation of the CCA prior to sheath removal. The puncture site is then investigated to make certain there is no bleeding prior to releasing the ligatures. (F) The incision is closed routinely.

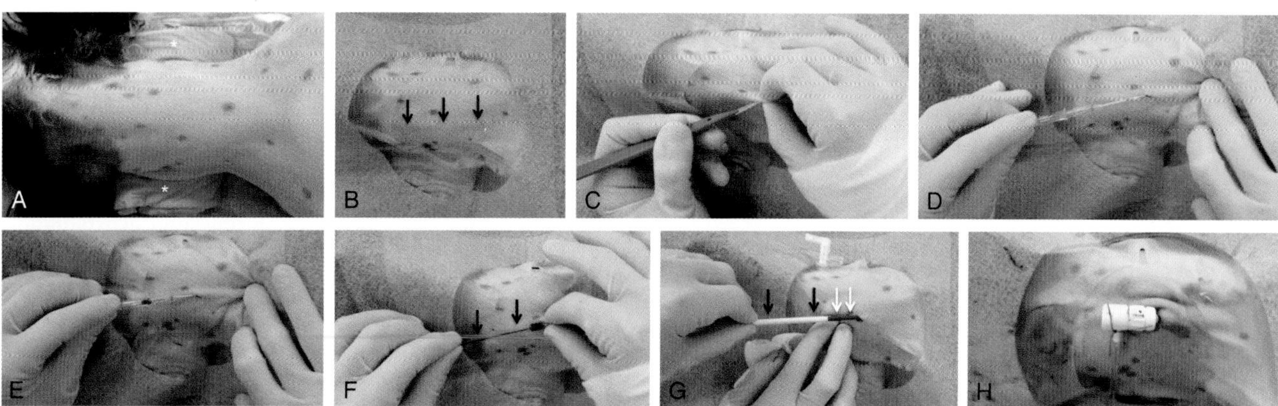

Figure 44.9 External jugular vein access in a dog in dorsal recumbency with the head to the left in each image. (A) The neck is extended with a rolled towel (*) beneath and the forelimbs pulled caudally. (B) Following draping, the right external jugular can be easily identified (black arrows). (C) The skin is tented and a scalpel blade is used make a skin incision slightly larger than the sheath planned for placement. (D) An 18 g catheter is used to gain vascular access. Note the placement of the hand far back on the catheter in order to identify the "flash" of blood. (E) Once the flash is identified, the catheter is advanced. (F) The stylette is removed and a 0.035" guide wire (black arrows) is advanced down the jugular vein. (G) The catheter is removed and the sheath (black arrows) and dilator (white arrows) combination is advanced over the wire into the jugular vein. (H) The sheath is sutured in place and the dilator and wire are removed.

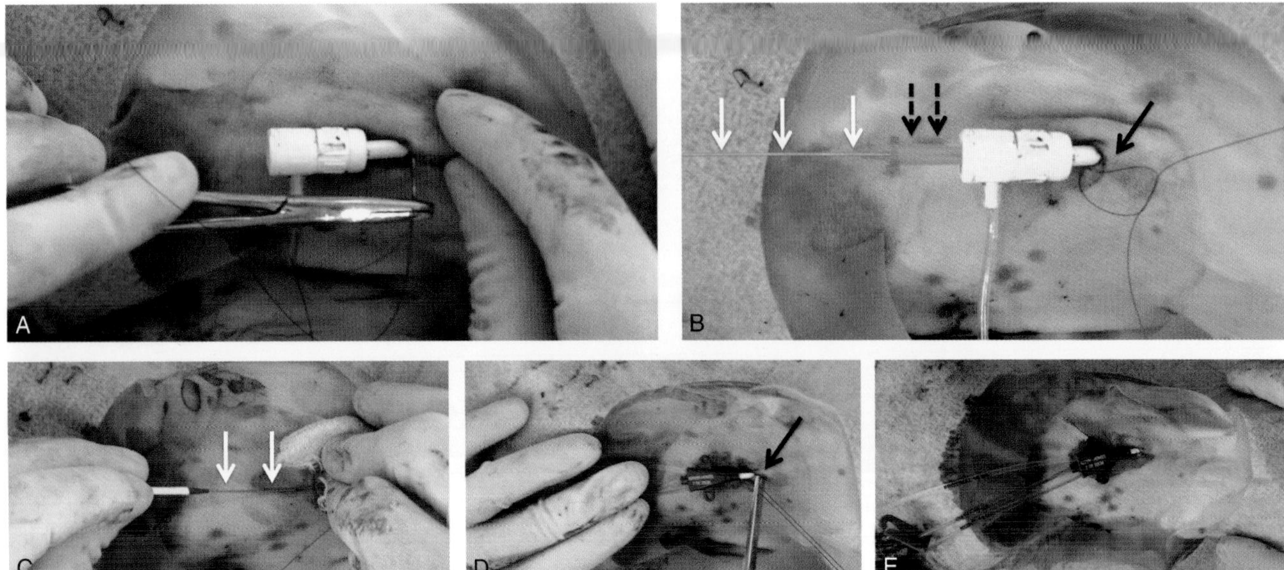

Figure 44.10 External jugular vein large sheath removal and replacement with a smaller multi-lumen catheter. (A) A 3–0 monofilament absorbable purse-string suture is placed around the puncture site. (B) Prior to sheath removal and tying of the purse-string suture (black arrow), an introducer (black dotted arrow) is used to place a guide wire (white arrows) through the sheath. (C) Pressure is placed on the puncture site as the sheath is removed over-the-wire and the smaller multi-lumen catheter is placed over the wire (white arrows). (D) The purse-string suture is gently tightened (black arrow) and cut. (E) The multilumen catheter is secured in place with simple interrupted sutures.

the catheter down the open peel-away sheath as the large lumen can allow an air embolus if the patient takes a large breath simultaneously. Chronic dialysis catheters are rarely used but placement requires tunneling, not unlike vascular access port placement. The author suspects the placement of dialysis catheter tips in the intrahepatic caudal vena cava may allow higher achievable flow rates; this is an area of current investigation.

Notes

(Multiple vendors available)

1. Vascular introducer sheath, Infiniti Medical, Menlo Park, CA.
2. Micropuncture set, Infiniti Medical, Menlo Park, CA.
3. Cobra head catheter, Infiniti Medical, Menlo Park, CA.

References

Butkovic V, Capak D, Stanin, D, et al (1996) Arteriography after ligation of the brachial and femoral artery in the dog. *Vet Med (Praha)* 41(10), 319–22.

Clendenin MA and Conrad MC (1979a) Collateral vessel development, following unilateral chronic carotid occlusion in the dog. *Am J Vet Res* 40, 84–8.

Clendenin MA and Conrad MC (1979b) Collateral vessel development after chronic bilateral common carotid artery occlusion in the dog. *Am J Vet Res* 40, 1244–8.

Hedlund CS, Tanger CH, Elkins AD, et al (1983) Temporary bilateral carotid artery occlusion during surgical exploration of the nasal cavity of the dog. *Vet Surg* 12, 83–5.

Perkins RL and Edmark KW (1971) Ligation of femoral vessels and azygous vein in the dog. *J Am Vet Med Assoc* 159(8), 993–4.

Seldinger SI (1953) Catheter replacement of the needle in percutaneous arteriography; a new technique. *Acta Radiol* 39(5), 368–76.

CHAPTER FORTY-FIVE

Foreign Body Retrieval

William T.N. Culp
School of Veterinary Medicine, University of California – Davis, Davis, CA

Background and Indications

Intravascular foreign bodies, while uncommon, present a unique clinical scenario that may require prompt attention. The majority of intravascular foreign bodies occur iatrogenically as a result of dislodgement of intravascular catheters, or other instrumentation that has been introduced into the vasculature during the performance of a particular intervention. As vascular-based procedures have increased in human patients over the last 20 years, so has the incidence of intravascular foreign bodies (Schechter et al, 2012, Woodhouse and Uberoi, 2012), with the increased performance of vascular interventional procedures in companion animals, a similar scenario is likely to occur.

When foreign bodies are left intravascularly in humans, the reported overall major complication rate ranges from 21–71% (Fisher and Ferreyro, 1978, Gabelmann et al, 2001, Richardson et al, 1974). Major complications (including causes of mortality) identified in humans include arrhythmias, sepsis, catheter-associated thrombosis, pulmonary emboli, endocarditis, ventricular perforation, adrenal infarction, and caval syndrome (Fisher and Ferreyro, 1978, Gabelmann et al, 2001, Richardson et al, 1974). Human studies have shown that clinical signs may be delayed by up to 1 year following embolization (Fisher and Ferreyro, 1978). In all cases, the potential benefits of removing an intravascular foreign body (via open surgical or endovascular techniques) need to be weighed against the potential risks involved with the retrieval procedures.

Patient Preparation

Removal of intravascular foreign bodies by any method in companion animals requires general anesthesia and evaluation of clinical laboratory tests such as complete blood count, biochemistry panel, and urinalysis is indicated prior to initiation of removal. Intravascular foreign bodies that occur during an endovascular procedure are often radio-opaque and clearly visible with radiography and fluoroscopy. Peripheral and central intravenous catheters are often radio-opaque as well (Figure 45.1), but the size and materials of these catheters tend to make visualization less ideal with these imaging modalities. Ultrasonography can be successfully utilized to identify some intravascular

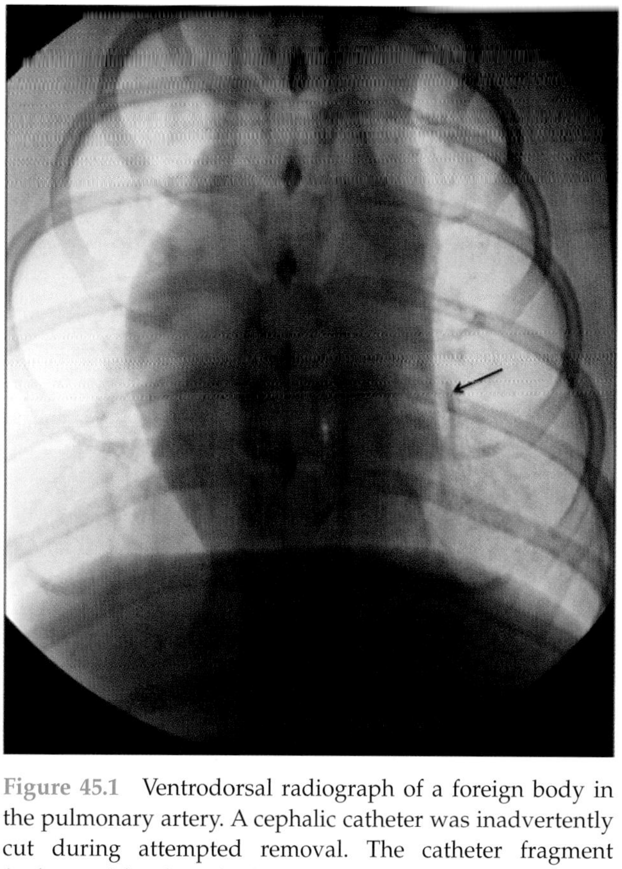

Figure 45.1 Ventrodorsal radiograph of a foreign body in the pulmonary artery. A cephalic catheter was inadvertently cut during attempted removal. The catheter fragment (red arrow) has launched to the pulmonary artery.

Veterinary Image-Guided Interventions, First Edition. Edited by Chick Weisse and Allyson Berent.

Companion website: www.wiley.com/go/weisse/vet-image-guided-interventions

foreign bodies that are peripherally located or located in the cervical region (jugular vein). Computerized tomography and magnetic resonance imaging (MRI) are regularly used diagnostic tests to identify intravascular foreign bodies in humans (Woodhouse and Uberoi, 2012). Ultimately, however, without being able to see the foreign body fluoroscopically, the operator has limited ability to achieve removal of most of these devices.

Potential Risks/Complications/Expected Outcomes

The presence of most intravascular foreign bodies is known immediately, as these tend to occur from accidental catheter dislodgement during removal of peripheral or central intravenous catheters or during endovascular procedures. Historically, removal of intravascular foreign bodies in veterinary patients had been performed via surgical extraction. These procedures may involve considerable morbidity and potential complications associated with the extraction procedure should be considered.

The use of a minimally invasive endovascular technique for foreign body removal is an attractive alternative to historical surgical options. Percutaneous intravascular foreign body removal in humans has a success rate of 90–100% (Dondelinger et al, 1991, Uflacker et al, 1986, Yang et al, 1994). A recent veterinary report documented the percutaneous removal of intravascular foreign bodies in five dogs, a goat, and a horse. All devices were successfully removed with the use of a snare that was controlled with fluoroscopic-guidance (Culp et al, 2008).

It should be noted that not all patients are good candidates for intravascular foreign body retrieval due to comorbidities that may put them at greater anesthetic risk. Additionally, certain foreign bodies are more difficult to remove due to their composition, size, and/or location; the amount of time that a foreign body has been present may also play a role in the decision-making process. Stents that are not easily compressible can be difficult to collapse when snared, and some devices have sharp edges that can traumatize the blood vessel during removal. Additionally, some instrumentation is too large to be removed through a vascular access sheath. Foreign bodies that are located in a region where a free end of the foreign body is not accessible present a particularly difficult scenario as snaring and grasping techniques are often utilized to remove the foreign bodies. Foreign bodies are more likely to become embedded in a vascular wall as time progresses; however, several human studies have described the retrieval of foreign bodies that have been present for extended periods of time (Chu et al, 2007, Savage et al, 2003, Thanigaraj et al, 2000). The complication rate associated with intravascular foreign body retrieval tends to be low with lack of retrieval and temporary arrhythmias (if accessing a foreign body in the heart or pulmonary arteries) predominating (Culp et al, 2008, Dondelinger et al, 1991). Surgical removal or the decision to leave a foreign body in situ likely carries much higher risks in some of these cases.

Equipment

Some examples of recommended equipment can be found in Figure 45.2, Figure 45.3, Figure 45.4 and Figure 45.5, and the use of this equipment is described next. Fluoroscopy is most commonly the imaging modality of choice for retrieving foreign bodies; however, this requires the foreign body to be radio-opaque in most situations. Occasionally, fluoroscopy can be utilized for foreign bodies that are not radio-opaque or minimally radio-opaque if a filling defect can be clearly identified. In those situations where this is not the case, the treating clinician can decide if guidance with ultrasonography or MRI is more suitable; this has been rarely attempted in veterinary medicine.

Fluoroscopic Procedure

Most intravascular foreign bodies are peripheral or central intravascular catheters that have migrated to the great veins, heart, or pulmonary arteries. However, foreign bodies that occur in the arterial system secondary to an arterial intervention can also dislodge and typically migrate to a vascular bifurcation. The approach for the particular intravascular foreign body depends on the location of the foreign body and the vascular access that already exists.

If the foreign body is secondary to a procedure that is currently underway, the vascular access that has already been established can be utilized to introduce the instrumentation (e.g., catheters and snares) that would be used to remove the foreign body. For cases of peripheral and central venous catheters that have become intravascular foreign bodies, vascular access for removal may need to be obtained. Many of these foreign bodies can be removed via access to the jugular vein; jugular vein vascular access is discussed in detail in Chapter 51.

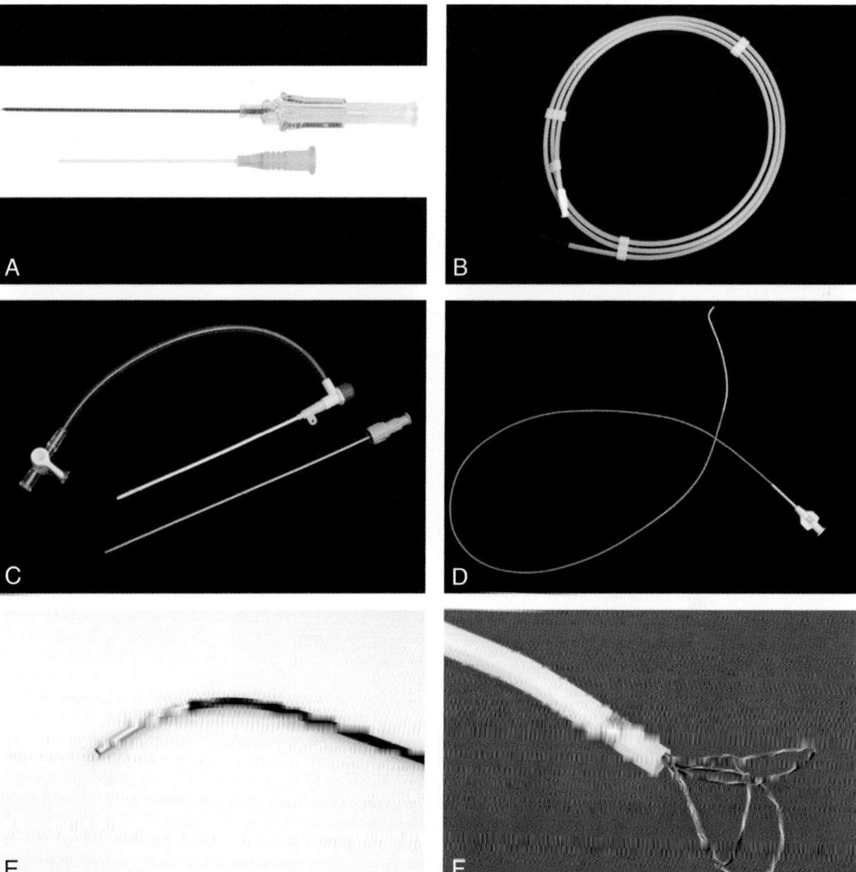

Figure 45.2 Equipment utilized during vascular foreign body retrieval procedures (A) 18 gauge over the needle catheter. (B) 0.035-inch angled, hydrophilic guide wire. (C) Vascular introducer sheath (white) and dilator (blue). (D) 4 Fr angled selective catheter (Berenstein). (E) 6 Fr guiding sheath. (F) Endovascular snare with multiple loops.

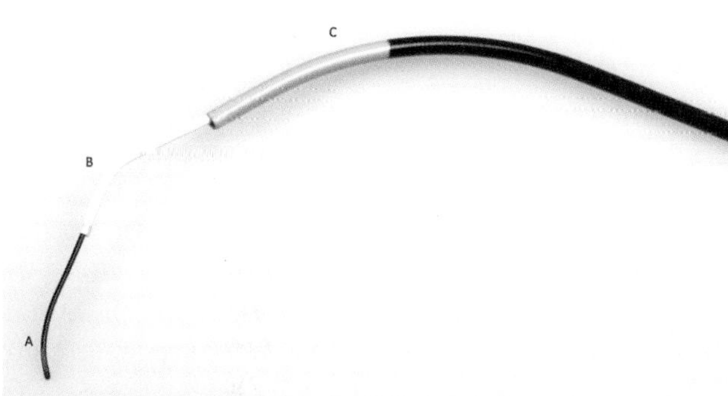

Figure 45.3 Image demonstrating the interaction between multiple instruments that may be utilized during intravascular foreign body retrieval. (A) 0.035-inch angled, hydrophilic guide wire. (B) 4 Fr angled selective catheter (Berenstein). (C) 6 Fr guiding sheath.

A large introducer sheath[1] (generally 10–12 Fr or larger) is recommended for the retrieval of intravascular foreign bodies as this will allow for the removal of the foreign body with the least chance of complication. When an introducer sheath has been placed in the jugular vein for retrieval of a foreign body in the great veins, heart or pulmonary arteries, a 0.035-inch hydrophilic angled guide wire[2] is passed through the sheath into the jugular vein and further into the right atrium. The guide wire can be further passed into the right ventricle and into the pulmonary artery of interest (depending on the location of the foreign body) or the guide wire can be placed in the jugular vein and a selective or guiding catheter introduced over the guide wire and used to direct the guide wire to the desired location. The catheters recommended by the author for guidance through the vascular system include either a Berenstein (4 or 5 Fr angled catheter)[3] or a Cobra (4 or 5 Fr hook catheter)[4]. In some cases, a guiding sheath[5] may be needed for increased stiffness; a catheter and guide wire combination may be more easily passed and maintained in a particular location if placed through a guiding sheath (Figure 45.3). Additionally, for intravascular foreign bodies located in smaller vessels, some retrieval devices have been designed that are passed through a microcatheter (3 Fr)[6] (Schechter et al, 2012).

When the catheter has been placed in the vessel containing the foreign body (Figure 45.4), the guide wire can be removed. If the vascular anatomy is not obvious during passage of the guide wire, an angiogram (utilizing a contrast[7]/saline mixture; generally 50%/50%) can be performed at any point, through the catheter, to determine location. In complex anatomy (such as the pulmonary vasculature), using the

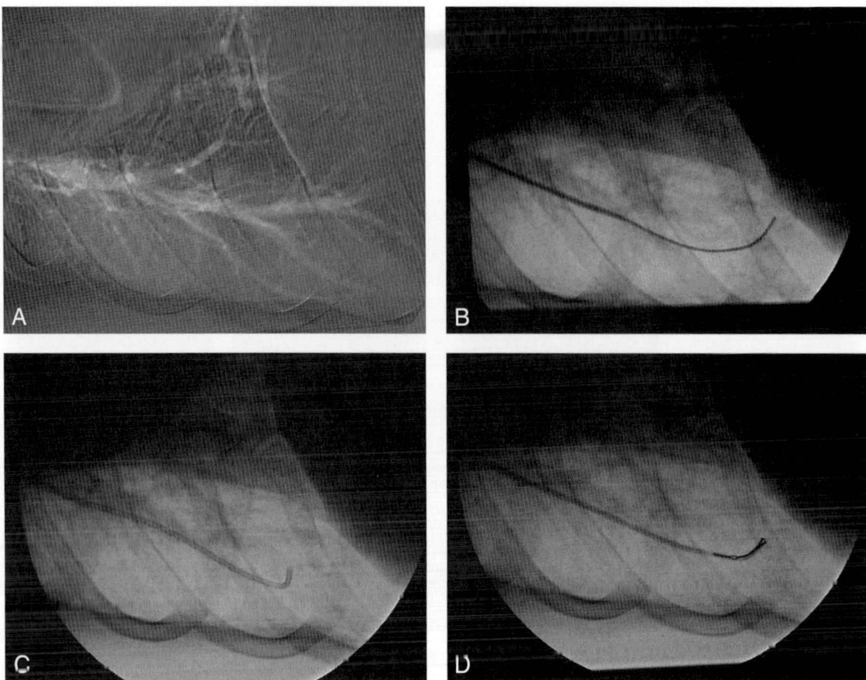

Figure 45.4 Fluoroscopic image series of the procedure of intravascular foreign body retrieval. A pulmonary angiogram has been performed to identify the pulmonary vasculature where the intravascular foreign body is located (A). The 0.035-inch hydrophilic guide wire is passed into the pulmonary artery branch that has been identified to contain the intravascular foreign body; an angled catheter is placed over the guide wire and is being advanced simultaneously (B). After the angled catheter is placed into the appropriate vessel, the guide wire is removed (C). A goose-neck snare has been introduced through the angled catheter, passed beyond the intravascular foreign body, engaged the catheter fragment and has then been withdrawn to engage the foreign body against the catheter tip (D).

"roadmapping" function of the fluoroscopy system can be useful in gaining access to the target vessel. Alternatively, rotating the c-arm can help identify a preferred projection. When the clinician is satisfied with catheter position, a device utilized for foreign body retrieval can be inserted through the catheter to the point of the foreign body.

The techniques most commonly employed to grasp an intravascular foreign body include the snare loop technique, the use of helical baskets and the use of intravascular forceps/graspers (Dondelinger et al, 1991, Gabelmann et al, 2001, Woodhouse and Uberoi, 2012). For cases where a free end of the foreign body exists, the snare technique is likely the easiest and most reliable technique (Cahill et al, 2012, Culp et al, 2008, Savage et al, 2003, Wolf et al, 2008). A 90-degree snare[8] (the snare loop, when exposed, is positioned perpendicular to the catheter used to introduce the snare) can be utilized in the majority of cases (Figure 45.5). Many of these snares are currently made from nitinol wire that expands to the width of the blood vessel (the chosen snare diameter should equal the target vessel size); this allows the snare to loop around the free end of the foreign body making grasping of the foreign body significantly easier (Gabelmann et al, 2001, Savage et al, 2003, Woodhouse and Uberoi, 2012). Currently, several versions of multiloop snares exist, and these have the potential to increase a clinician's chance to grasp a foreign body.

To snare a foreign body, several techniques can be employed. The snare is passed through the guiding catheter to the foreign body. The combination of instruments are then advanced into the blood vessel beyond the foreign body. The guiding catheter is retracted to allow the snare to become exposed; the snare is then retracted to loop the foreign body. The guiding catheter is advanced over the snare, which closes the snare down and locks the foreign body inside the snare and up against the guiding catheter (Figure 45.5). It is preferable to snare just the free end as grasping the foreign body in a central location will cause it to be positioned perpendicular to the catheter once the snare has been withdrawn into the catheter.

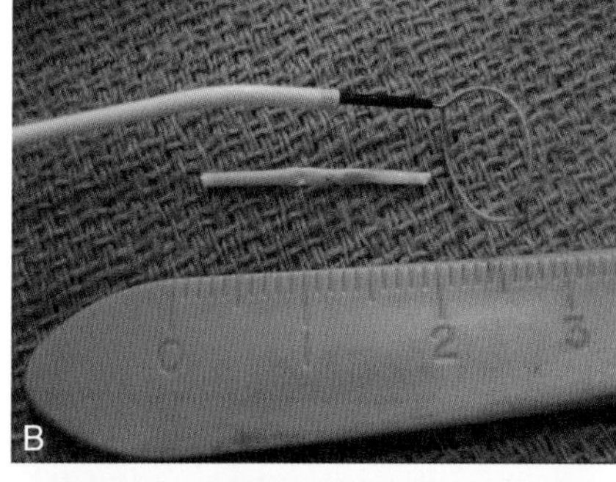

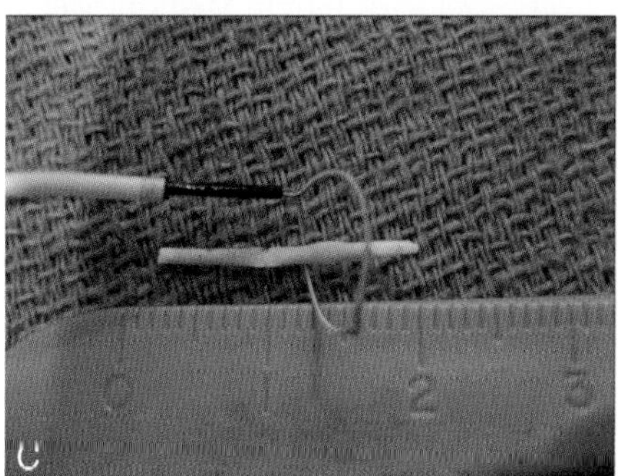

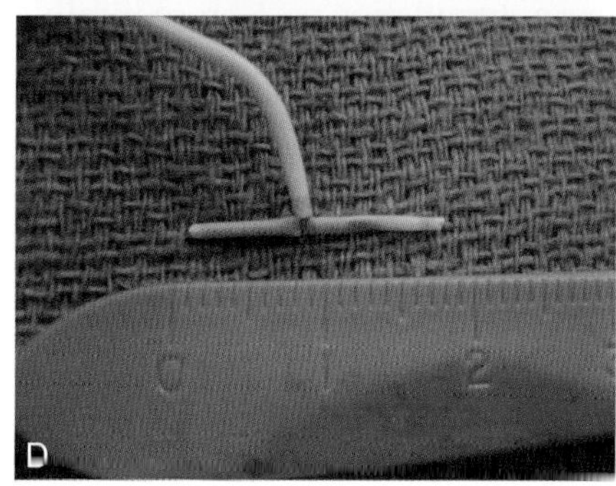

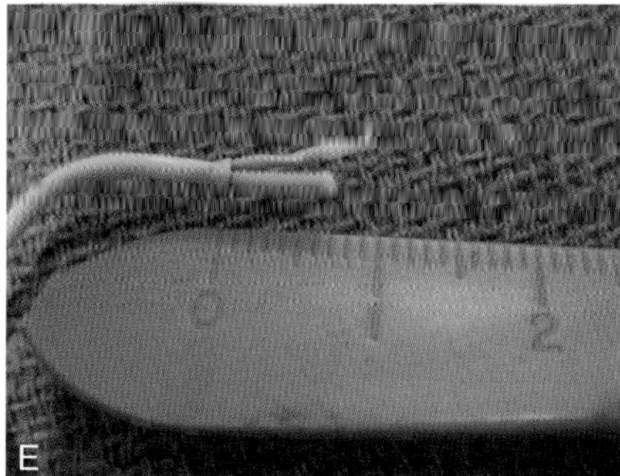

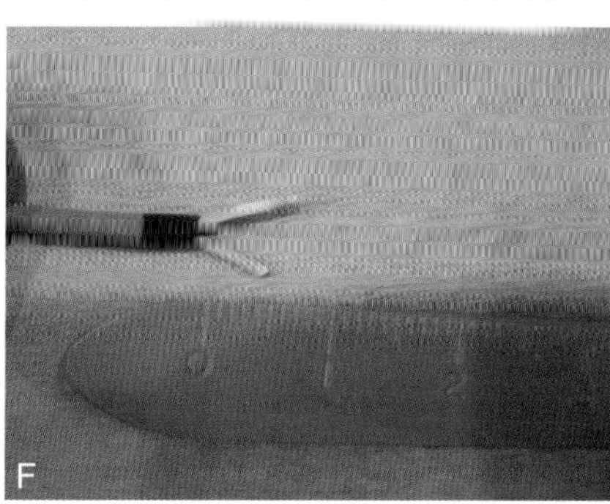

Figure 45.5 Ex vivo example of intravascular foreign body retrieval. The catheter pictured here is an actual intravascular foreign body, a cephalic catheter that was inadvertently cut during catheter removal (A). A snare is advanced out of the angled catheter past the foreign body and opened to fill the lumen of the vessel containing the foreign body (B). The snare is positioned around the foreign body (C) and then the snare is pulled back into the angled catheter (D). As the snare is pulled further into the angled catheter, the foreign body collapses which allows safer removal (E). The snare and angled catheter combination are pulled into a guiding sheath for removal out of the blood vessel (F).

When a foreign body has been firmly grasped with a snare, it should be retracted gently and pulled into the large introducer sheath and removed. The removal process should be monitored with fluoroscopic-guidance to prevent inadvertent dislodgement of the foreign body and re-introduction into the vascular system.

The use of helical baskets may be considered in certain situations. Helical baskets are useful in the retrieval of spherical or ovoid objects. Most vascular helical baskets are large, requiring a guiding sheath with an increased diameter; however, ureteral stone baskets could be considered if a smaller device is needed (Schechter et al, 2012). While forceps and graspers were utilized in many of the early intravascular foreign body retrieval cases, the indication for these devices is currently rare as the risk of damaging the vascular wall or perforating a blood vessel exists (Schechter et al, 2012). Other snares also exist that have multiple loops[9] that increases the ability to capture a foreign body (Figure 45.2).

Follow-Up

After removal of the foreign body, a contrast angiogram should be performed to document there has been no damage or perforation of the target vessel resulting in hemorrhage. The vascular introducer sheath can then be removed. If the sheath was present in a vein, then compression of the vessel for 5–10 minutes should be sufficient for hemostasis. If the sheath was present in an artery, vascular repair or ligation (depending on the artery) may need to be considered.

Postoperative complications are uncommon with intravascular foreign body removal if the procedure was performed uneventfully and no anesthetic complications develop. Surgical sites should be monitored for bleeding or seroma accumulation post-procedurally and patients can generally be discharged on the same or following day. Discharge from the hospital would also be dependent on whether the foreign body was introduced as part of another procedure or whether it was associated with an intravenous catheter removal.

Special Considerations

A few unique situations should be discussed. When foreign bodies do not have free ends, other devices can be introduced into the blood vessel to attempt to move the foreign body into a more favorable position or expose a free end. Examples of these devices may include guide wires with hooked tips, pigtail catheters (which can be spun), and deflecting wires (guide wire introduced into a catheter to alter the position of the catheter tip).

When a stent has been deployed into an incorrect position and retrieval is not possible due to the stent size, composition or position, a balloon catheter may be utilized to reposition some stents into a more favorable position. As an example, if a stent migrates into the heart, a balloon catheter can be placed into the lumen of the stent, gently inflated and utilized to reposition the stent into a vessel where it will likely not cause further trauma or migrate (e.g., iliac veins) (Schechter et al, 2012, Woodhouse and Uberoi, 2012). When a stent is placed in a vessel and appears to be poorly sized or migration is noted, a second larger stent can be placed within the first stent to essentially "lock" the first stent into place (Gabelmann et al, 2001). When performing this procedure, the second stent should be oversized to the diameter of the blood vessel (generally 10–20%) within which the migrating stent will be positioned. Lastly, an endovascular procedure can sometimes reposition an intravascular foreign body into a location that is more favorable for extraction (by surgery or an endovascular technique); a foreign body in the heart could be repositioned into the jugular vein or femoral vein allowing for easier exposure and extraction as well as less potential procedural morbidity.

Notes

1. Vascular introducer sheath, Infiniti Medical, Menlo Park, CA.
2. Weasel wire, Infiniti Medical, Menlo Park, CA.
3. Berenstein catheter, Infiniti Medical, Menlo Park, CA.
4. Cobra catheter, Infiniti Medical, Menlo Park, CA.
5. Flexor® Check-Flo® introducer sheath, Cook Medical, Bloomington, IN.
6. Microcatheter, Infiniti Medical, Menlo Park, CA.
7. Omnipaque (iohexol) injection, Amersham Health Inc., Princeton, NJ.
8. Amplatz GooseNeck snare, Covidien, Dublin, Ireland.
9. EN Snare® endovascular snare system, Merit Medical Systems, Inc., South Jordan, UT.

References

Cahill AM, Ballah D, Hernandez P, and Fontalvo L (2012) Percutaneous retrieval of intravascular venous foreign bodies in children. *Pediatr Radiol* 42, 24–31.

Chu TS, Tso WK, and Lie AK (2007) Percutaneous retrieval of a chronic foreign body with both intravascular and extravascular components. *Australas Radiol* 51, 179–81.

Culp WT, Weisse C, Berent AC, Getman LM, Schaer TP, and Solomon JA (2008) Percutaneous endovascular retrieval of an intravascular foreign body in five dogs, a goat, and a horse. *J Am Vet Med Assoc* 232, 1850–6.

Dondelinger RF, Lepoutre B, and Kurdziel JC (1991) Percutaneous vascular foreign body retrieval: experience of an 11-year period. *Eur J Radiol* 12, 4–10.

Fisher RG and Ferreyro R (1978) Evaluation of current techniques for nonsurgical removal of intravascular iatrogenic foreign bodies. *AJR Am J Roentgenol* 130, 541–8.

Gabelmann A, Kramer S, and Gorich J (2001) Percutaneous retrieval of lost or misplaced intravascular objects. *AJR Am J Roentgenol* 176, 1509–13.

Richardson JD, Grover FL, and Trinkle JK (1974) Intravenous catheter emboli. Experience with twenty cases and collective review. *Am J Surg* 128, 722–7.

Savage C, Ozkan OS, Walser EM, Wang D, and Zwischenberger JB (2003) Percutaneous retrieval of chronic intravascular foreign bodies. *Cardiovasc Intervent Radiol* 26, 440–2.

Schechter MA, O'Brien PJ, and Cox MW (2012) Retrieval of iatrogenic intravascular foreign bodies. *J Vasc Surg* 57, 276–81.

Thanigaraj S, Panneerselvam A, and Yanos J (2000) Retrieval of an IV catheter fragment from the pulmonary artery 11 years after embolization. *Chest* 117, 1209–11.

Uflacker R, Lima S, and Melichar AC (1986) Intravascular foreign bodies: percutaneous retrieval. *Radiology* 160, 731–5.

Wolf F, Schernthaner RE, Dirisamer A, et al (2008) Endovascular management of lost or misplaced intravascular objects: experiences of 12 years. *Cardiovasc Intervent Radiol* 31, 563–8.

Woodhouse JB and Uberoi R (2012) Techniques for intravascular foreign body retrieval. *Cardiovasc Intervent Radiol* 36, 888–97.

Yang FS, Ohta I, Chiang HJ, Lin JC, Shih SL, and Ma YC (1994) Non-surgical retrieval of intravascular foreign body: experience of 12 cases. *Eur J Radiol* 18, 1–5.

CHAPTER FORTY-SIX

Hemorrhage Embolization

Chick Weisse
The Animal Medical Center, New York, NY

Background/Indications

Life-threatening hemorrhage in veterinary patients is typically identified secondary to vascular tumor rupture (e.g., splenic hemangiosarcoma, hepatic or adrenal tumors), trauma (e.g., during or immediately following surgery from dehiscence or bleeding vascular pedicle, or fracture-associated hemorrhage), or severe coagulopathy (e.g., rodenticide ingestion, disseminated intravascular coagulation, etc.). Occasionally, other conditions including intractable epistaxis, idiopathic renal hematuria, severe gastrointestinal ulceration/hemorrhage, or tumor surface or intraparenchymal bleeding, can lead to chronic blood loss with intermittent large hemorrhagic episodes, resulting in the need for red blood cell transfusions and/or additional therapies. In most circumstances, treatment of the underlying condition, with or without surgery, is successful in preventing further bleeding, at least temporarily. In other cases, continued hemorrhage is not amenable to traditional therapies and interventional radiology techniques may be able to offer suitable alternatives in some circumstances.

Transarterial embolization (TAE) for life-threatening hemorrhage has been performed in humans since the 1970s and has evolved to successfully control hemorrhage for many of the above conditions, and many more. The benefits of TAE for life-threatening hemorrhage are numerous. First, the procedure can be performed in unstable, critical patients (conscious sedation rather than general anesthesia). Angiographically identified hemorrhage is sometimes easier to confirm than surgical exploratory in the head, blood-filled abdomen (or gastrointestinal tract), or thorax. In humans, in whom ligation of larger arteries is not tolerated without severe complications (such as the carotid and femoral arteries), TAE provides superselective control without the risk of damage to nearby tissues through dissection. While surgical exploration can allow evacuation of the hematoma, it will also result in loss of tamponade and may result in more severe massive hemorrhage. Once embolized, the intact hematoma can actually act to continue to tamponade venous bleeding (Chen et al, 2009). Lastly, TAE can often provide better control than surgical ligation or clipping as embolization obstructs bloodflow at the level of the actual bleeding; The level of occlusion can be much further distal with TAE than that achieved during an open surgical procedure. Super-selective, distal embolization reduces the development of substantial collateralization compared with proximal ligation so that if bleeding recurs, repeated embolization can be performed because larger, more proximal vessels remain patent. Intractable epistaxis is an excellent example of this point (see Chapter 4 for additional information). TAE is also used for gastrointestinal bleeding not identified or amenable to endoscopic control, pelvic fractures in which very large blood volumes can be lost, and a variety of tumors known to bleed excessively during surgical dissection (renal, brain, bone, hepatic, etc.). Hepatic and splenic trauma, as well as excessive urogenital bleeding (uterine, bladder, renal pelvis, etc.) has also been successfully treated with TAE.

In veterinary patients, the non-emergent use of TAE is growing and has been performed to reduce blood supply to primary tumors and metastases, to reduce bleeding associated with intractable epistaxis, tumors, renal hematuria, and vascular anomalies (see Chapters 4, 5, 22, 28, 46, and 48). In the emergent setting, TAE has been performed successfully to stop severe intractable epistaxis in dogs (Weisse et al, 2004) and guttural pouch hemorrhage in horses (Leveille et al, 2000). The author has also performed TAE to reduce hemorrhage

Veterinary Image-Guided Interventions, First Edition. Edited by Chick Weisse and Allyson Berent.

Companion website: www.wiley.com/go/weisse/vet-image-guided-interventions

associated with a large pelvic tumor, hemorrhagic cystitis, transvaginal uterine fibroid hemorrhage (Weisse et al, 2002), and metastatic liver tumors. The author has also attempted this technique for intractable intestinal bleeding but a lesion could not be identified to embolize so the procedure was aborted. TAE for control of life-threatening arterial hemorrhage in veterinary patients is possible but the indications and ideal circumstances have not yet been elucidated.

Patient Preparation

As a variety of cases may benefit from TAE to control hemorrhage, each must be taken individually in regards to appropriate work-up. Important preoperative information includes the underlying primary condition (if known) such as cancer, coagulopathy, trauma, etc., as well transfusion history and previous other treatments and medications administered. Minimal diagnostic testing should include complete blood work (CBC and chemistry panel), urinalysis, blood pressure, and coagulation screen with platelet count and possible function testing, blood type, red blood cell crossmatch (if transfusion history). Diagnostic imaging might include radiography and/or ultrasonography; however, computerized tomography (CT) or magnetic resonance imaging (MRI) should probably be avoided unless the patient is systemically stable and can tolerate multiple anesthetic episodes with the procedure delayed. Both CT and MR studies would require prolonging anesthetic times as well as additional exposure to potentially nephrotoxic contrast agents (iohexol more so than gadolinium). In debilitated patients this would necessitate diuresis overnight followed by the therapeutic procedure the following day. The additional risk might not be necessary in many patients for whom the TAE procedure might be considered on an emergency basis. For those patients receiving preoperative imaging, arterial phase CTA or MRA is recommended as those lesions with little arterial supply are perhaps less likely to respond to arterial embolization. In certain circumstances, endoscopy might provide useful information without the risk of substantially prolonging anesthesia (can be performed simultaneously) or additional exposure to contrast agents (Figure 46.1). This has been performed for gastrointestinal bleeding, bladder bleeding, and upper urinary tract bleeding (see Chapter 28). Should neoplasia be involved, consultation with an oncologist is critical for developing a treatment plan and ensuring standard-of-care therapies have been discussed. Embolization can be performed with chemotherapy (see Chapters 5, 23, and 65). If a tumor is the underlying source of hemorrhage, the operator should evaluate for the (rare) potential of associated arteriovenous communications within the mass that could results in distal embolization to the venous circulation (e.g., lungs).

Premedications include typically broad-spectrum antibiotic coverage, anti-inflammatories (corticosteroids or non-steroidal anti-inflammatory drugs (NSAIDs), if not contraindicated and post-embolization syndrome is a possibility), and analgesics (Table 46.1).

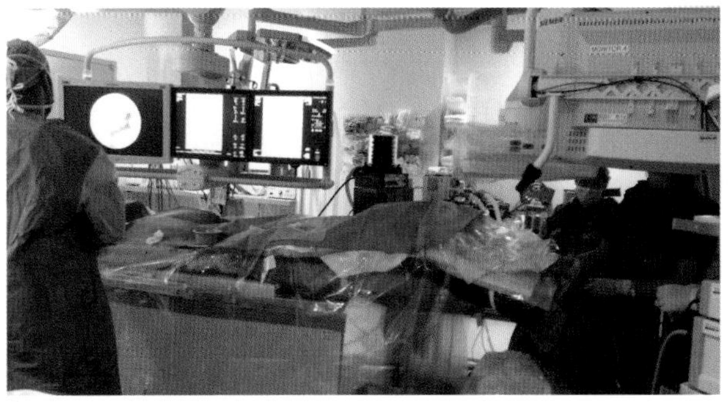

A

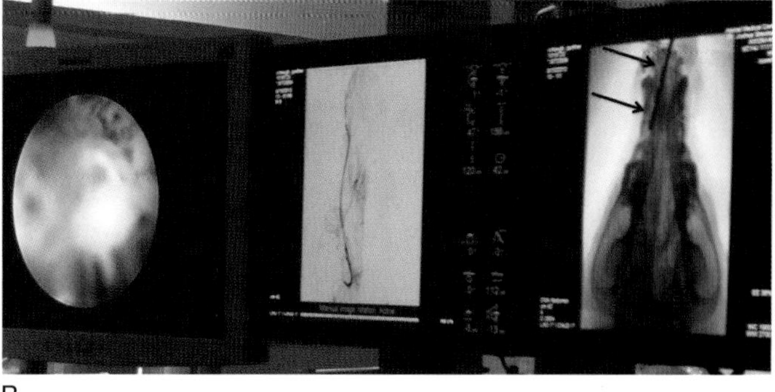

B

Figure 46.1 Combined IR and rhinoscopic biopsy procedure in a dog with severe life-threatening epistaxis. (A) The patient is draped in the angiography suite. The operator on the left side of the image has performed a nasal embolization procedure via a femoral artery approach. On the right hand side, at the head of the patient, the endoscopist is performing the rhinoscopy and biopsy. The angiographic catheter remains in place during the procedure in case excessive hemorrhage occurs following the diagnostics biopsies. (B) Close-up view of the three monitors used during the procedure. On the left is the rhinoscopy image during the biopsy. In the center is the carotid angiogram performed immediately post-embolization of the right sphenopalatine artery. On the right monitor is the fluoroscopic image of the head during the biopsy documenting the location of the endoscope (black arrows) in the right nasal cavity. The previous angiograms performed can help guide the endoscopist as to where a more vascularized biopsy specimen may be found (as opposed to necrotic tissues).

Table 46.1
Procedural and post-procedural medical management

- Antibiotics:
  - Intraoperative: cefoxitin (30 mg/kg IV once, then 20 mg/kg IV q2 hr)
  - Postoperative: clavamox (13.75 mg/kg PO BID × 14 days)
- Anti-inflammatories (if indicated):
  - Intraoperative: dexamethasone SP (0.1 mg/kg IV once at induction)
  - Postoperative: prednisone if indicated (1 mg/kg/day PO × 3 days, then 0.5 mg/kg/day PO × 3 days, then 0.5 mg/kg/q2 days PO)
- Analgesics:
  - Perioperative: opioid premedications
  - Postoperative: tramadol (2–4 mg/kg PO q8–12 hr × 3–5 days)

Blood transfusions and intravenous fluids should be provided to help restore hypovolemia prior to anesthesia if possible. Although potentially increasing the risk of general anesthesia, the ideal time for the procedure is during the hemorrhagic episode as angiographic contrast extravasation will be most readily identifiable at this time; once hemorrhage has ceased the procedure may be more difficult if the source of the bleed is not already known.

Potential Risks/ Complications/ Expected Outcomes

Anticipated complications would most likely be those related to placing unstable patients under general anesthesia, continued hemorrhage, and signs associated with non-target embolization and tissue necrosis that can occur if embolization is performed too distally or within adjacent normal tissues; complications would then be associated with those organs that are damaged. During hypovolemic shock, arterial and venous vasoconstriction can led to vessel spasm, prevent identification of hemorrhage sites, and therefore prevent safe and effective treatment to be delivered. Other standard complications associated with interventional radiology procedures include guide wire- and catheter-induced trauma, and pericatheter thrombosis. An absolute contraindication to arteriography is a known severe allergy to contrast media. Patients suffering from life-threatening hemorrhage are likely at increased risk for contrast nephropathy as the incidence of this complication is highest in volume-depleted animals. Complications associated with neuroembolization procedures (those performed cranial to the aortic arch) include stroke, blindness, neurological deficits, etc. (refer to Chapter 4 for more information); similarly for renal embolization, complete renal infarction is possible resulting in complete loss of renal function on that side (see Chapter 28). These procedures should be attempted only by individuals with experience in embolization procedures and superselective catheterizations.

The durability of embolization likely depends upon the disease process, target vessels, and degree of embolization performed. Bleeding can occur from the arterial supply, the venous drainage, or both. Discussions with the client should explain the difference and, as only arterial embolization is possible, venous bleeding will continue. Arterial embolization of venous bleeding may reduce the significance of the bleeding (common example of "stepping on a garden hose"); however, continued minor bleeding may continue and hopefully this will no longer be life threatening. In addition, these procedures can be repeated as necessary as the feeding target vessel typically remains patent if not "over-embolized".

Equipment

A list of recommended equipment is shown in Figure 46.2 and Figure 46.3. Transarterial embolization procedures require very little equipment but the fluoroscopy unit must provide adequate imaging detail to identify very small caliber vessels using digital subtraction angiography (DSA) and the ability to obtain orthogonal imaging when necessary. Failure to identify collateral vessels could lead to non-target embolization and severe consequences.

Fluoroscopic Procedure

Prior to the procedure, the operator should review the relevant anatomy. When performing TAE in uncommon locations it is often prudent to have anatomical drawings, photocopies, or textbooks in the angiography suite for review during the procedure if necessary. General anesthesia protocols should take into consideration the debilitated state of these patients and emergency drugs should be calculated preoperatively. Blood products and colloid fluid therapy should be available and the

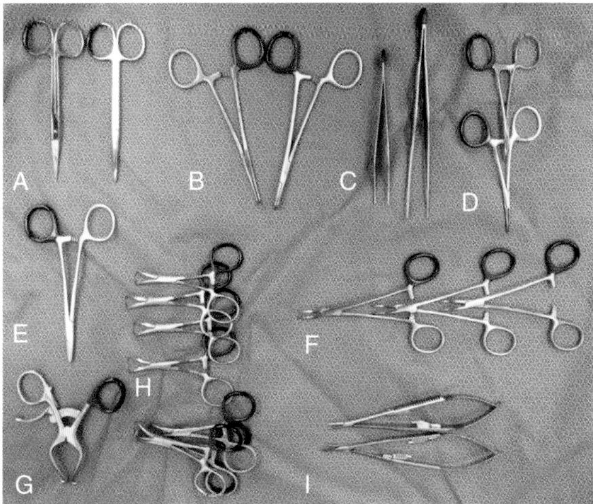

Figure 46.2 Sample surgical cut-down set. (A) Sharp-sharps and small Metzenbaum scissors. (B) Right-angled forceps. C. Brown–Adson and Debakey forceps. (D) Mosquito hemostats. (E) Needle drivers. (F) Kelly hemostats. (G) Small Gelpi retractors. (H) Small Babcock towel clamps. (I) Castroviejo needle drivers for vessel repair if necessary.

anesthetist should serially monitor the packed cell volume throughout the procedure. Neuromuscular blockade may be considered in order to minimize patient movement during fluoroscopic imaging, reduce contrast load delivered, and prevent treatment/procedural delays (avoid longer anesthesia times).

Depending upon region targeted, the standard femoral artery or carotid approach is used, hair clipping and sterile preparation is performed accordingly, and arterial access is obtained routinely using a 4 or 5 Fr vascular introducer sheath[1] (see Chapter 44 for more information). A 4 Fr angled catheter[2,3] and 0.035-inch hydrophilic angled guide wire[4] combination are passed through the sheath, into the aorta, and advanced to the targeted region (Figure 46.4). A digital subtraction angiogram is performed to define the anatomic features; it is imperative that the patient be positioned as evenly as possible and motionless prior to the DSA. A Touhy–Borst adapter[5] and Flo-switch[6] are attached to the 4 Fr catheter. With the tip of the 4 Fr catheter securely

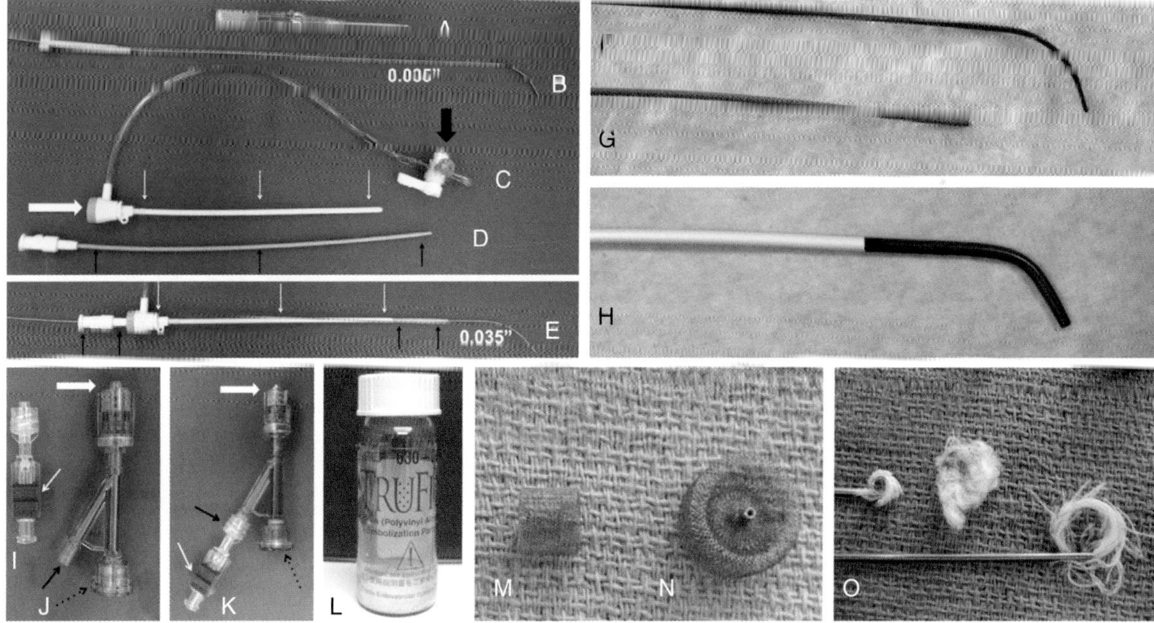

Figure 46.3 Equipment for standard hemorrhage embolization procedure. (A) 18-gauge over-the-needle catheter. (B) 0.035″ guide wire with gentle bend manually formed on shapeable tip. The bend permits operator to turn the wire during introduction if it does not pass easily. A straight wire will not change course. (C) 5 Fr vascular introducer sheath made up of shaft (white arrows) with 5Fr inner diameter, hemostasis valve (white block arrow) to prevent bleeding, and three-way stop-cock (black block arrow) to flush and/or aspirate. (D) 5 Fr Dilator with 5 Fr outer diameter shaft (black arrows). (E) Combination 5 Fr vascular introducer sheath (white arrows) and dilator (black arrows) making smooth transition down to the 0.035″ guide wire. F. 0.035″ angled, hydrophilic guide wire. (G) Standard soft-tipped 0.035″ Teflon guide wire for pushing coils. (H) 4 Fr Berenstein (hockey stick) angiographic catheter. Flo-switch (I) and Touhy–Borst adapter (J), which connect (K) to form a hemostasis valve (dotted black line) and side-port that can be switched on or off (white arrow) for flushing or aspirating. This device is attached to the hub of the 4 Fr catheter (at white block arrow) and allows coaxial passage of a microcatheter/microwire through the 4Fr catheter. (D) Polyvinyl alcohol particles (or PVA hydrogel microspheres can be used instead). (M, N) Vascular plugs in orthogonal views. The receptacle for the specialized delivery wire to screw in can be seen in (N). (O) Variety of thrombogenic coils with Dacron fibers. These coils are advanced through the angiography catheter once in position within the target vessel.

positioned in the proximal artery, a microcatheter[7,8] and compatible angled microwire[9,10] are used to select the smaller feeding arterial branch using the fluoroscopy roadmap setting. Care must be taken when selecting this vessel as it is often small and can spasm easily or the catheter can be occlusive preventing embolization. If spasm occurs, it may relax after 5 or 10 minutes. Alternatively, some have recommended infusion of lidocaine to minimize vessel spasm. If both strategies fail, one may have to treat the contralateral side first (if a bilateral case), wait longer, or return at a later date.

Arterial hemorrhage can only be identified when active (>0.5 ml/min) (Baum et al, 1973). Occasionally, the author has placed radio-opaque markers around the tumor to help identify the mass angiographically (Figure 46.4) when superficially located, or endoscopic clips can be placed if and when accessible. If bleeding has ceased and the origin is no longer apparent, "provocative testing" has been performed in humans. This involves injecting heparin or tPA into the region of interest in hopes of restimulating the bleed while immediate treatment (TAE) is possible. Of course, the danger in performing this procedure in a patient with recent life-threatening hemorrhage cannot be overstated and this is not routinely recommended. When the origin of hemorrhage is unclear but the area (around tumor or hematoma) is identified, gelfoam embolization can be used in larger feeding vessels (unilateral or bilateral internal iliac artery embolization for instance for pelvic hemorrhage) (Figure 46.5).

After proper location of the microcatheter is confirmed angiographically, embolization can be safely performed with an embolic and iohexol[11] slurry until flow through the vessels is substantially diminished angiographically (Figure 46.4). The appropriate size of polyvinyl alcohol (PVA)[12] or other embolization particles[13], gelfoam[14], or devices[15,16] (see Chapter 1) are chosen on the basis of vascular architecture and operator comfort. Use of undersized particles carries the risk of extreme distal vascular occlusion and increases the risk of necrosis and

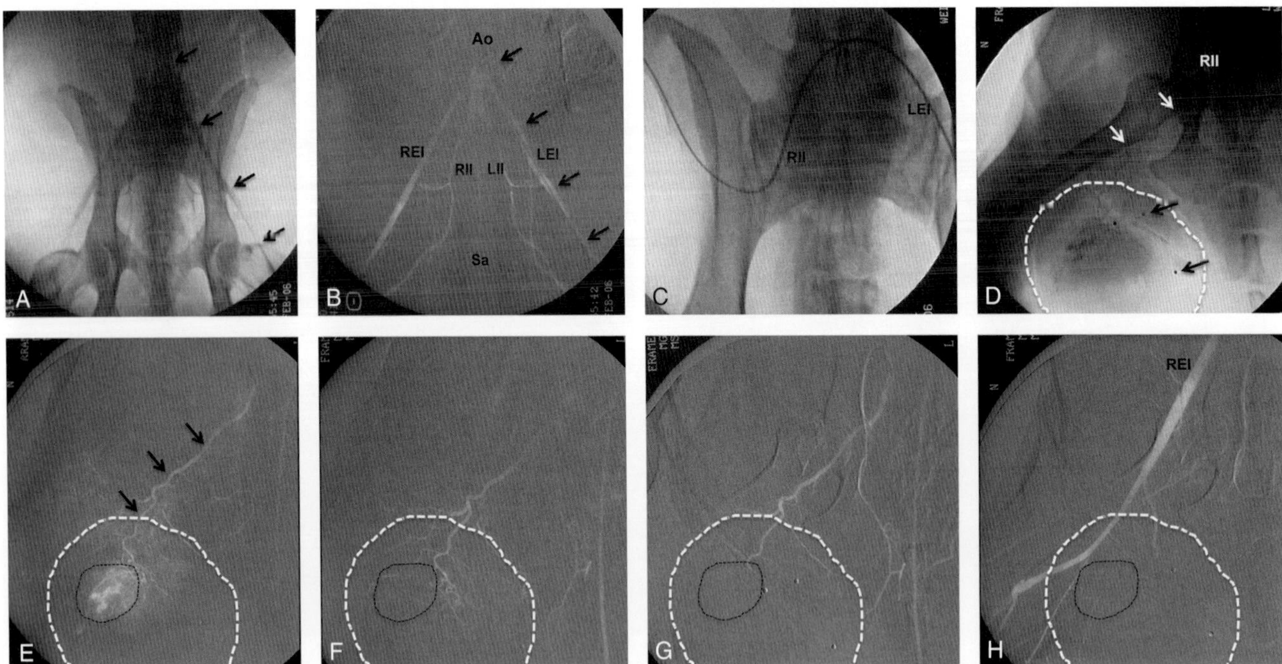

Figure 46.4 Serial ventrodorsal angiograms of a dog with intractable life threatening hemorrhage from a right-sided pelvic liposarcoma. Repeated attempts at manual surgical ligation in the emergency room were unable to stop the hemorrhage. Aortogram (A) and digital subtraction aortogram (B) via left femoral artery access and catheterization (black arrows) of the terminal aorta (Ao) demonstrating the left and right external iliac arteries (LEI, REI), the left and right internal iliac arteries (LII, RII), and the sacral artery (Sa). (C) Up-and-over catheterization from the LEI to the RII with the guide wire advanced into a distal branch. (D) Superselective catheterization and angiography of a distal internal iliac branch (white arrows) showing the tumor blush (white dotted lines) and radio-opaque markers (black arrows) placed on the tumor surface to help identify the mass during angiography. (E) Superselective DSA of distal internal iliac branch (black arrows) with target vessel showing tumor blush (white dotted lines) and contrast extravasation (black dotted lines) indicating ongoing hemorrhage. (F) Same DSA study after initial embolization with PVA particles showing reduced tumor blush and reduce ongoing contrast extravasation. (G) Final superselective DSA study showing lack of tumor blush and contrast extravasation confirming successful TAE of hemorrhage. (H) DSA of REI to confirm no contributing arterial supply to the tumor hemorrhage. Lack of tumor blush confirms there is no contribution.

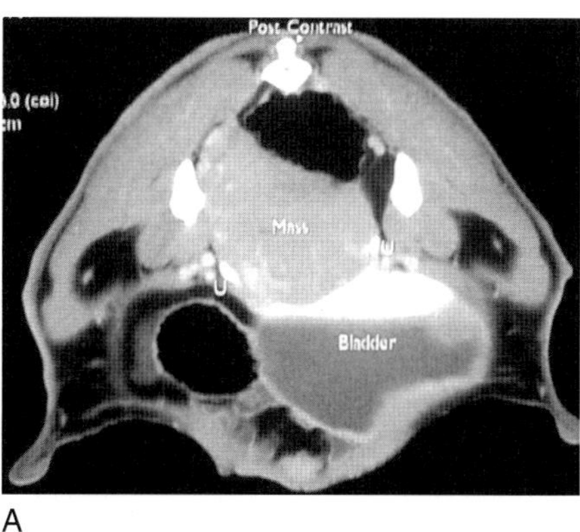

A

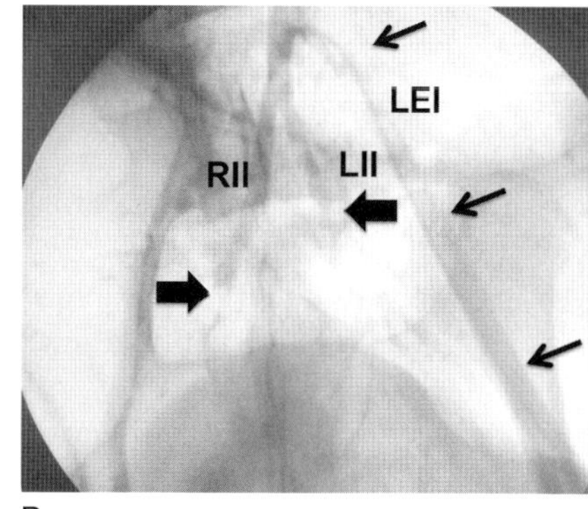

B

Figure 46.5 CT (A) and angiographic (B) images of a goat with a large, bleeding intrapelvic uterine leiomyoma (fibroid). (A) Axial contrast CT image demonstrating the intrapelvic mass (mass) compressing the bladder and colon with ureters (U) adjacent to the mass. (B) Angiographic images following bilateral internal iliac gelfoam embolization performed due to severe, life-threatening transvaginal hemorrhage. A sheath in the left femoral artery was placed and a catheter (black arrows) advanced into the terminal aorta. The angiogram demonstrates the left external iliac artery (LEI) and both right and left internal iliac arteries (RII, LII). A 4 Fr catheter was advanced into both the LII and RII and gelfoam torpedoes injected until stasis of bloodflow was confirmed angiographically. This is demonstrated by the abrupt attenuation of the contrast within the internal iliac arteries (black block arrows). Gelfoam is temporary and the proximal delivery and collateral bloodflow prevents ischemic complications. The hemorrhage was successful controlled with this procedure.

tissue sloughing. On the other hand, use of inappropriately large particles gelfoam thrombogenic coils or plugs carries the risk of proximal vessel thrombosis that may allow for development of collateral vessels that bypass the proximal occlusion and re establish perfusion over time. The author has used PVA-200 particles[12] (180–300 μm) or 300–500 μm PVA hydrogel microspheres[13] for nasal embolization; these sizes should also be effective elsewhere. Alternatively, gelfoam[14] torpedoes or slurry can be used for more temporary bleeding when recanalization of the embolized tissue is desirable (after the process has been effectively treated for instance). Gelfoam resorption following intravascular use is reported to recur within 7–21 days (Van Allen and Pentecost, 1992). Larger embolics such as gelfoam pledgets and coils may be preferred for organs with rich collateral supply (stomach, etc.) without the risk of ischemia. In humans with peptic gastrointestinal bleeding, if bleedings is not confirmed with angiography (or no aneurysm is identified), stomach bleeding is typically managed with left gastric artery embolization and duodenal bleeding with gastroduodenal artery embolization (using thrombogenic coils for example).

The chosen embolic (if particles or microspheres) is primed for delivery by preparing it as a slurry with iodinated contrast material. To do so using PVA, the embolic is loaded into a syringe, the plunger replaced, and all of the air evacuated to densely compact the material. This syringe is connected with a three-way stopcock to a second syringe filled with contrast material, and the contents are vigorously mixed to form the slurry. The viscosity is adjusted by additional dilution of the PVA with sterile saline as necessary to match the caliber of the delivery catheter and the flow in the vessel to be embolized. Relatively dilute concentrations are required to prevent occlusion of microcatheters or clumping within the small caliber vessels and subsequent proximal embolization. Microspheres can just be gently mixed with a contrast/saline mixture (~1:1 or 2:1) to keep them evenly suspended; Vigorous mixing is not typically necessary.

Embolization is performed by injecting the slurry via a 1 ml luer-lock polycarbonate syringe[17] through a selectively placed microcatheter under fluoroscopic visualization using digital roadmapping software. The slurry is radio-opaque due to the contrast mixture and can thus be seen perfusing the target region. Care is taken to prevent reflux of particles into non-target vessels. As embolization proceeds, flow decreases. Embolization is performed subjectively to near-stasis of blood flow; complete stasis is avoided to permit future embolization if hemorrhage recurs, reduce the risk of tissue necrosis, and reduce the risk of embolic material reflux and non-target embolization. Prior to complete blood flow stasis (and periodically during the embolization procedure), the catheter is flushed of slurry by injecting saline solution gently. A gentle injection avoids flushing particles into non-target vessels. Selective arteriography is performed to evaluate the success of the procedure. If embolization is successful, slow to no blood flow is seen in the target vessels. When performing bilateral embolization, the author prefers to embolize until reduced flow is present rather than complete bloodflow stasis as bilateral embolization carries a higher risk of ischemic consequences; alternatively, larger particles could be used. The microcatheter is withdrawn and repeat angiography is performed through the 4 Fr catheter to identify persistent perfusion through other vessels or decreased perfusion elsewhere due to non-target embolization. This procedure can be repeated on the contralateral side if necessary for midline targets (urinary bladder for instance) by selecting the contralateral artery. The procedure is then repeated, as above.

When using larger devices such as coils for more proximal, larger vessel embolization it is important to treat both sides of the bleeding artery when possible to avoid the "backdoor" effect of reverse bleeding. For instance, if a vessel is transected in surgery, both sides need to be ligated to arrest hemorrhage from both sides; the same technical consideration is required for TAE.

Following embolization, the catheter and sheath are removed. Hemostasis of the arterial access site is typically achieved with artery ligation. The patient is recovered in the intensive care unit for monitoring overnight. Treatment instructions include intravenous fluids at maintenance rates (unless contraindicated) or higher rates if excessive (>3ml/kg) volumes of iodinated contrast were necessary. Analgesics are typically recommended but often not necessary; NSAIDs seem to provide sufficient palliation for any discomfort from the surgical cut-down site (unless corticosteroids have been administered prior); NSAIDs should be avoided in hypovolemic patients or those with other comorbidities (renal or hepatic dysfunction). Blood products may be needed so monitoring of PCV and coagulation status should be performed when indicated.

Follow-Up

Postoperative patient care is typically dependent on underlying conditions; however, the TAE procedure should add little morbidity, and stable patients can typically be discharged the following day. "Postembolization syndrome", a series of clinical signs, including general malaise, fever, nausea, and pain, is not normally associated with these types of TAE procedures (compared to those involving chemotherapy, or certain viscera including the liver, kidneys, uterus, etc.).

Typically, analgesics and antibiotics should be considered due to diminished bloodflow and possible ischemic consequences. Activity is limited for 2 weeks while the groin or neck incision heals until suture removal 10–14 days later.

Special Considerations/ Alternative Uses/ Complication Examples

The author has successfully performed TAE for hemorrhage associated with intractable epistaxis, urinary bladder hemorrhage, prostatic hemorrhage, a bleeding hindlimb/pelvic tumor, vaginal bleeding associated with a large uterine fibroid, and metastatic liver disease

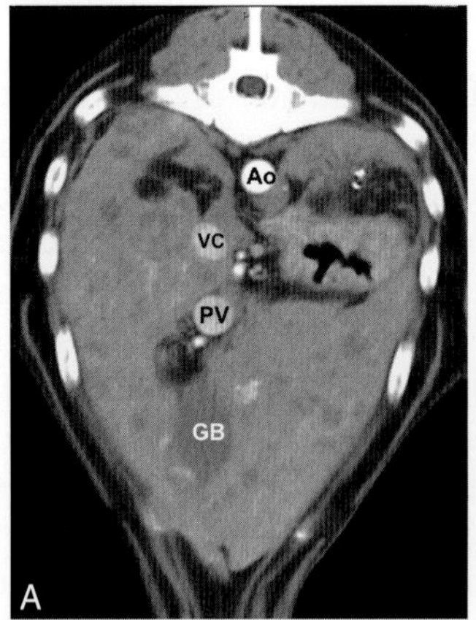

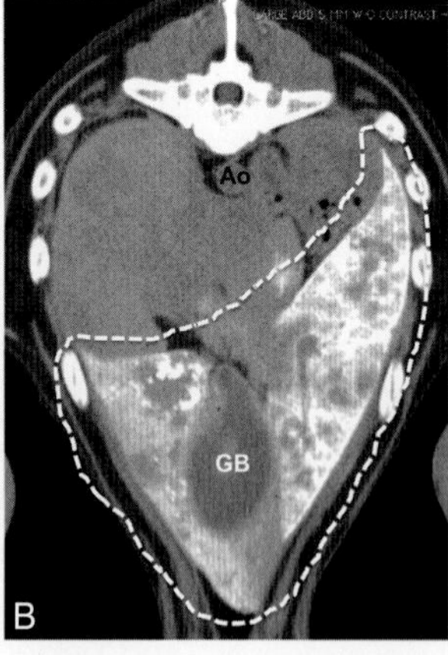

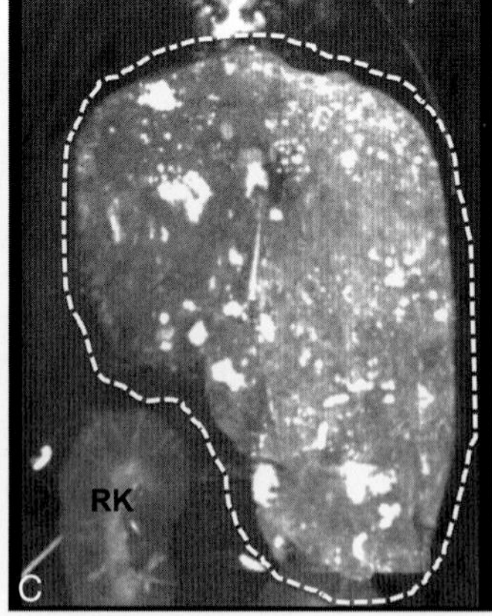

Figure 46.6 Serial images in a dog with splenic hemangiosarcoma that received splenectomy and subsequent systemic chemotherapy. This dog developed recurrent hemoabdomen from diffuse metastatic liver hemangiosarcoma bleeds treated with repeated red blood cell transfusions. (A) Contrast axial CT angiogram demonstrating the aorta (Ao), caudal vena cava (VC), portal vein (PV) and gall bladder (GB) as well as a diffusely mottled liver with numerous hypoattenuating lesions consistent with hepatic hemangiosarcoma metastases. (B) Repeat CT without contrast immediately following hepatic artery TAE of approximately 2/3 of the liver (white dotted line) to decrease the bleeding. (C) Coronal reconstruction of the liver demonstrating the contrast uptake (white dotted lines) within the portion of the liver receiving the TAE. Note the focal areas of increased contrast uptake consistent with more vascularized tumors within the liver parenchyma. The right kidney (RK) can also be seen in this image. This procedure was successfully performed multiple times to reduce the tumor-associated bleeding.

(Figure 46.6). Embolization was successful at subjectively reducing hemorrhage or improving visual evaluation at the time of surgery.

Notes

(Examples; Multiple vendors available)

1. 4 Fr or 5 Fr vascular introducer sheath, Infiniti Medical, Menlo Park, CA.
2. Berenstein catheter, Infiniti Medical, Menlo Park, CA.
3. Cobra catheter, Infiniti Medical, Menlo Park, CA.
4. Weasel wire, Infiniti Medical, Menlo Park, CA.
5. Touhy–Borst adapter, Cook Medical, Bloomington, IN.
6. Flo-switch, Boston Scientific, Natick, MA.
7. Renegade or Tracker microcatheter, Boston Scientific, Natick, MA.
8. Microcatheter, Infiniti Medical, Menlo Park, CA.
9. 0.018 Transend or V-18 microwire, Boston Scientific, Natick, MA.
10. 0.014 Microwire or 0.018 Weasel wire, Infiniti Medical, Menlo Park, CA.
11. Omnipaque (iohexol) injection, Amersham Health Inc., Princeton, NJ.
12. PVA-200 particles, Cook Medical Inc., Bloomington, IN.
13. Beadblock 300–500 μm PVA hydrogel microspheres, Biocompatibles UK Limited, Farnham, UK.
14. Gelfoam absorbable gelatin, Pharmacia and Upjohn Company, Kalamzoo, MI.
15. Cook embolization coils, Cook Medical Inc., Bloomingdale, IN.
16. Amplatzer vascular plug, AGA Medical Corp, Golden Valley, MN.
17. 1 ml polycarbonate syringes, Merit Medical, South Jordan, UT.

References

Baum S, Athanasoulis CA, Waltman AC, et al (1973) Gastrointestinal hemorrhage: angiographic diagnosis and control. *Adv Surg* 7, 149–98.

Chen, H., Chen, J., Chen, Y, et al (2009) Arterial embolization for controlling life-threatening traumatic pelvic hemorrhage. *Mid Taiwan J Med* 14, 16–26.

Leveille R, Hardy J, Roberston JT, et al (2000) Transarterial coil embolization of the internal and external carotid and maxillary arteries for prevention of hemorrhage from guttural pouch mycosis in horses. *Vet Surg* 29(5), 389–97.

Van Allen RJ and Pentecost MJ (1992) Transcatheter control of hemorrhage in cancer patients. *Semin Intervent Radiol* 9, 38–44.

Weisse C, Clifford C, Nicholson M, et al (2002) Percutaneous bland arterial embolization and chemoembolization for the treatment of benign and malignant diseases. *J Am Vet Med Assoc* 221, 1430–6.

Weisse C, Nicholson ME, Rollings C, et al (2004) Use of percutaneous arterial embolization for treatment of intractable epistaxis in three dogs. *J Am Vet Med Assoc* 224(8), 1307–11.

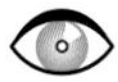 Video clips to accompany this chapter can be found in the online material at **www.wiley.com/go/weisse/vet-image-guided-interventions**

CHAPTER FORTY-SEVEN

Thrombectomy and Thrombolysis: The Interventional Radiology Approach

Marilyn E. Dunn[1] and Chick Weisse[2]
[1]*Department of Clinical Sciences, Faculty of Veterinary Medicine, University of Montreal, Quebec, Canada*
[2]*The Animal Medical Center, New York, NY*

Background

Thrombosis is recognized as a common complication of many acquired diseases, including cardiovascular (left atrial thrombosis, aortic thrombosis), endocrine (aortic thrombosis), inflammatory, hepatic (portal vein thrombosis), renal (aortic thrombosis), and neoplastic disorders (Table 47.1). The authors suspect that due to the difficulty of identifying thrombosis in veterinary medicine many patients with thrombosis go undiagnosed, making the true prevalence difficult to estimate. Limited therapeutic options and confusion regarding medical management often leads to a decision not to treat these patients. This chapter will describe minimally invasive treatments for thrombosis including a multimodality approach centered on interventional radiology, antiplatelet and anticoagulant therapy, and thrombolytics. Little information is published in veterinary medicine and therefore many of these recommendations are based on the authors' experiences.

Suspecting and Finding the Thrombus

Clinical signs resulting from compromised blood flow to an organ can be variable and depend on the affected organ. Actual detection of thromboemboli can be challenging. A combination of Doppler ultrasonography, angiography, venography, ventilation-perfusion scans, and contrast enhanced computerized tomography (CT) and/or magnetic resonance imaging (MRI) imaging can aid in identification; however many cases likely go undiagnosed.

Venous Versus Arterial

Normal hemostasis is maintained through a delicate balance between endogenous anticoagulants and procoagulants. The net effect is preservation of blood flow in the systemic vasculature with localized coagulation at sites of vessel injury. Changes in this balance can tip the scales to either excessive bleeding or thrombus formation. The primary disorder influences the site of thrombus formation (arterial or venous vasculature), the composition of the occluding thrombus, and the approach to antithrombotic therapy. The relative proportions of platelets and fibrin in the clot depend on the shear forces within the injured vessel. Arterial thrombi form under high shear forces and therefore tend to contain a large number of platelets held together by fibrin strands. Venous thrombi form under low shear forces and consist primarily of fibrin and red blood cells. Mixed thrombi are an intermediate form and occur in the pulmonary vasculature. Strategies to inhibit arterial thrombogenesis typically include the use of antiplatelet drugs, whereas anticoagulants are the mainstay of venous thromboprophylaxis.

An important consideration in the decision making process in a thrombotic patient is the site of the clot. An arterial thrombus is often considered an emergency and time to intervention is critical unless collateral circulation is present (or has developed), in which case

Veterinary Image-Guided Interventions, First Edition. Edited by Chick Weisse and Allyson Berent.

Companion website: www.wiley.com/go/weisse/vet-image-guided-interventions

TABLE 47.1
Commonly associated conditions with venous and arterial thrombosis in dogs

	Dog	Cat
Arterial	Protein losing nepropathy Hyperadrenocorticism Neoplasia Glucocorticoid therapy	Left-sided cardiovascular disease
Venous	Adrenal neoplasia Liver disease (inflammatory, neoplastic, other)	Adrenal neoplasia Liver disease (inflammatory, neoplastic, other)
Mixed (including pulmonary thromboembolism	Sepsis Pancreatitis	Sepsis Pancreatitis

the condition is less emergent (e.g., aortoiliac occlusive disease). Venous thrombosis tends to present less acutely and the decision to intervene may be more difficult to make. For instance, if a patient presents with a partially obstructive vena caval thrombus, and the underlying hypercoagulability can be managed, the patient's fibrinolytic system may slowly eliminate the clot. Subsequent migration or embolism of the clot must be considered and monitored for.

Anticoagulation of the Thrombotic Patient

Once the patient is confirmed to have a thrombus, a number of factors will affect the decision whether to anticoagulate the patient and which agent(s) should be used. Some of these factors include venous versus arterial thrombus, coagulation status of the patient, the patient's cardiovascular stability, previous or impending surgery, the presence of hemorrhage, whether the patient will undergo an intervention, financial concerns, and of course the underlying disease and associated prognosis.

Antiplatelets

Aspirin

Aspirin is the most common antiplatelet drug used in veterinary medicine. It acts through irreversible acetylation of the platelet cyclooxygenase active site leading to decreased thromboxane A_2 synthesis. The effects of aspirin are permanent and last for the lifespan of the platelet (7–10 days). It is estimated that 70% of dogs may be resistant to the antiplatelet effects of aspirin due to a mutation in the G-coupled-protein receptor. This may explain the variable responses to aspirin noted in platelet aggregation studies. Identifying which patients may possess this mutation is not practical. This is an important consideration when deciding to treat a patient with aspirin alone. Recommended doses and monitoring are given in Table 47.2.

Clopidogrel

Clopidogrel irreversibly inhibits the binding of ADP to specific platelet ADP receptors (P2Y12). ADP receptor blockade impairs platelet release, reaction, and ADP-mediated activation of GPIIb/IIIa, thereby reducing the primary and secondary aggregation response. It is metabolized by hepatic cytochrome p450, with significant platelet inhibition occurring within 3 hours after initiation of therapy in healthy Beagles. The concurrent use of aspirin and clopidogrel appears well tolerated and has been reported in the human literature to maximize platelet inhibition. Concurrent use of clopidogrel with proton pump inhibitors should be avoided as the latter may inhibit its metabolism thus rendering it inactive. Resistance has not been reported in cats and dogs. Recommended doses and monitoring are referred to in Table 47.2.

Anticoagulants

Warfarin

Warfarin is a vitamin-K antagonist that alters the synthesis of vitamin-K dependent clotting proteins (Factors II, VII, IX, X) and the anticoagulant proteins C and S. Warfarin interferes with hepatic reductase activity leading to impaired post-translational carboxylation. Warfarin's anticoagulant activity is delayed (4–5 days) as the newly synthesized inactive clotting proteins gradually replace their functional counterparts. Its narrow therapeutic range has resulted in a high rate of bleeding complications in cats (20%). Warfarin has been used safely in both healthy dogs and those with aortic thrombosis. Recommended doses and monitoring are given in Table 47.2.

Heparin

Heparin is a heterogeneous mixture with 1/3 of molecules possessing a pentasaccharide sequence that binds to antithrombin (AT). Heparin has been the anticoagulant of choice in acute settings as its short half-life allows rapid dose adjustments and it can be antagonized

TABLE 47.2
Anticoagulant, antiplatelet and thrombolytic (fibrinolytic) drugs commonly used in clinical patients and the recommended doses and frequency of administration

Drug	Dog	Cat	Monitoring
Anticoagulants			
Unfractionated heparin	150–300 units/kg SC q8 hr CRI 25–50 units/kg/hr*	250–300 units/kg SC q8 hr CRI 25–50 units/kg/hr*	adjust to achieve 1.5–2 times baseline PTT values
Low molecular weight heparin			
Dalteparin	150 units/kg SC SID–TID**	150 units/kg SC BID–QID**	Anti-Xa activity 2–3 hr (dog) or 90 min (feline) post dose 0.4–1.0 U/ml TEG: normocoagulable tracing
Enoxaparin	0.8 mg/kg SC QID*	1.5 mg/kg SC QID*	Anti-Xa activity 2 hr (dog) or 60 min (feline) post dose 0.4-1.0 U/ml
Rivaroxaban	2 mg/kg PO BID*	unknown	unknown
Warfarin	0.2 mg/kg PO BID	0.5 mg/cat PO SID	adjust to achieve 1.5-2 times baseline PT values INR 2–3**
Antiplatelets			
Acetylsalicylic acid	0.5 mg/kg PO BID	5 mg/cat PO q72 hrs	Platelet aggregation/PFA-100
Clopidogrel	0.5–1 mg/kg PO SID	18.75 mg/cat PO SID	Platelet aggregation/PFA-100
Thrombolytics			
IV dose can be given directly at the site of the clot			
Tissue plasminogen activator	0.5 mg/kg IV over 30–60 minutes Can be repeated up to 3 times within 24 hours***	0.5 mg/kg IV over 30–60 minutes Can be repeated up to 3 times within 24 hours	
Streptokinase	90 000 units IV over 30 minutes followed by CRI 45 000 units/hr IV 6–12 hr	90 000 units IV over 30 minutes followed by CRI 45 000 units/hr IV 6–12 hr	

SC: subcutaneous
CRI: constant rate infusion
*Please note that these doses have been taken from abstracts and personal data and are unpublished.
**INR, International Normalized Ratio (INR). This ratio is calculated from the patient prothrombin time ($PT_{patient}$), the laboratory reference mean prothrombin time ($PT_{reference}$), and the International Sensitivity Index (ISI) of the thromboplastin reagent which is calculated by the reference laboratory: $INR = [PT_{patient}/PT_{reference}]^{ISI}$.
***The author has never used greater than 9 mg of TPA systemically per dog at one time.

by the administration of protamine. Despite its widespread use, heparin has a complex pharmacokinetic profile that produces an unpredictable anticoagulant effect. Due to its extensive binding to macrophages and endothelial cells, low-dose subcutaneous heparin has poor bioavailability. Recommended doses and monitoring are given in Table 47.2.

Low molecular weight heparins (LMWH)

LMWH are produced by depolymerization of heparin and bind to AT and accelerate its inhibition of Factor Xa. LMWHs bind poorly to plasma proteins and cells and undergo first order renal clearance resulting in a more predictable pharmacokinetic profile. In humans, peak anti-Xa (measured 3–4 hours following the dose) activity appears to correlate more closely to efficacy, however the relationship between target anti-Xa activity and clinical outcome remains to be defined. Dalteparin (Fragmin) and enoxaparin (Lovenox) have been used in small animals. Dalteparin has been evaluated more extensively in small animals and is currently the author's personal preference. Recommended doses and monitoring are given in Table 47.2.

Direct Xa inhibitor

Rivaroxaban is a direct factor Xa inhibitor used in humans for the prevention and treatment of thromboembolic disorders at a fixed-dose without the need for laboratory monitoring. Its *per os* administration makes it an attractive anticoagulant for clinical use. It has been shown to exert Xa inhibition and decreased thrombin generation in healthy dogs. Clinical experience with this drug is very limited. Recommended doses and monitoring are given in Table 47.2.

Thrombolytic Drugs

Thrombolytic drugs target the clot directly by accelerating fibrinolysis. Side effects reported with these agents are bleeding tendencies, pulmonary embolism (when treating venous thromboembolism) and reperfusion injury. Tissue plasminogen activator (tPA), streptokinase, and urokinase have been administered intravenously in cats and dogs with thrombosis with variable success. TPA has been considered a superior thrombolytic agent as it directly binds and activates plasminogen at the site of the clot thus resulting in less systemic side effects associated with excessive fibrinolysis. Administering tPA directly at the site of the clot (catheter directed thrombolysis) may theoretically be more efficacious, but this has not been routinely substantiated. The authors have used tPA in both dogs and cats with variable efficacy and very few complications.

Thrombolytic drugs are reported to be most efficacious in the 60 minutes to 6 hours following an embolic event. This does not preclude its use later in the disease process; however, the sooner it can be administered the greater the potential benefit. Recommended doses and monitoring are given in Table 47.2.

Central Venous Thrombosis

Clinical Signs

Clinical signs depend upon the site of the thrombus, the completeness of occlusion, and the collateral circulation present. Obstruction of the cranial vena cava may result in edema of the head and neck and/or forelimbs and may be associated with pleural effusion, obstruction of the portal vein may result in ascites, and caudal vena caval thrombosis can result in edema of the hindlimbs. Collateral circulation may alleviate venous congestion and therefore many patients may have few to no clinical signs related to their central venous thrombosis.

Diagnostics

Underlying disease and predisposing factors to consider in patients with central venous thrombosis are hyperadrenocorticism, protein losing nephropathy, protein losing enteropathy, neoplasia (including adrenal), sepsis, glucocorticoid therapy, pancreatitis, and complications of a central venous catheter placement or previous surgery. Portal vein thrombosis has been reported following inflammatory, infectious, and neoplastic liver disease. Diagnostic testing can include a complete blood count, biochemistry panel, urinalysis, urine protein to creatinine ratio, and abdominal and chest imaging (radiography and ultrasonography plus or minus CT or MRI). Endocrine and liver function testing is performed as indicated. Clotting times (PT and PTT) may be useful to detect hypocoagulability, but are not useful in the detection of hypercoagulability. FDPs and D-dimers would be expected to be elevated. TEG would be expected to indicate a hypercoagulable state.

Intervention

Treatment of venous thrombi must be based upon consideration of the overall clot burden and extent, the resulting clinical signs associated with the venous obstruction, and the ability to control the underlying cause of the clot if it is identified. In addition, one of the most problematic complications in humans with venous obstruction is "post thrombotic syndrome (PTS)", a group of conditions including swelling, pain, skin ulceration, and discoloration resulting from chronic untreated deep vein thrombosis (DVT). The cause is unclear but likely associated with chronic inflammation and damaged venous valves. It is unclear if this occurs in animals. The major goals of venous thromboembolism (VTE) treatment includes resolution of clinical signs, avoidance of PTS, and reduction in the risk of pulmonary thromboembolism (PTE). While anticoagulation and systemic thrombolysis continues to play a predominant role in VTE, catheter-based techniques may help improve outcomes when considering the goals stated above. These techniques are generally divided into three categories, including : (1) Passive infusion of thrombolytics into the clot through infusion catheters called "catheter directed thrombolysis (CDT); (2) "percutaneous mechanical thrombectomy (PMT)" involving mechanisms of clot aspiration and maceration ; and (3) lytic-assisted devices providing pharmacomechanical and sonically enhanced thrombolysis techniques. Most techniques do not require extensive equipment (Figure 47.1). The chosen vessel for access is often based upon avoiding the affected area (see Chapter 44). For instance, femoral vein access may be used for cranial cava thrombosis to avoid further damage to the potentially thrombosed jugular veins. Alternatively, if a jugular catheter is already in place, access is already present and this vessel may be used for tPA infusions and subsequent interventions. For further information on the venous techniques, see Chapter 49.

CDT is technically easy and relatively inexpensive to perform (Figure 47.2); however, improved outcomes

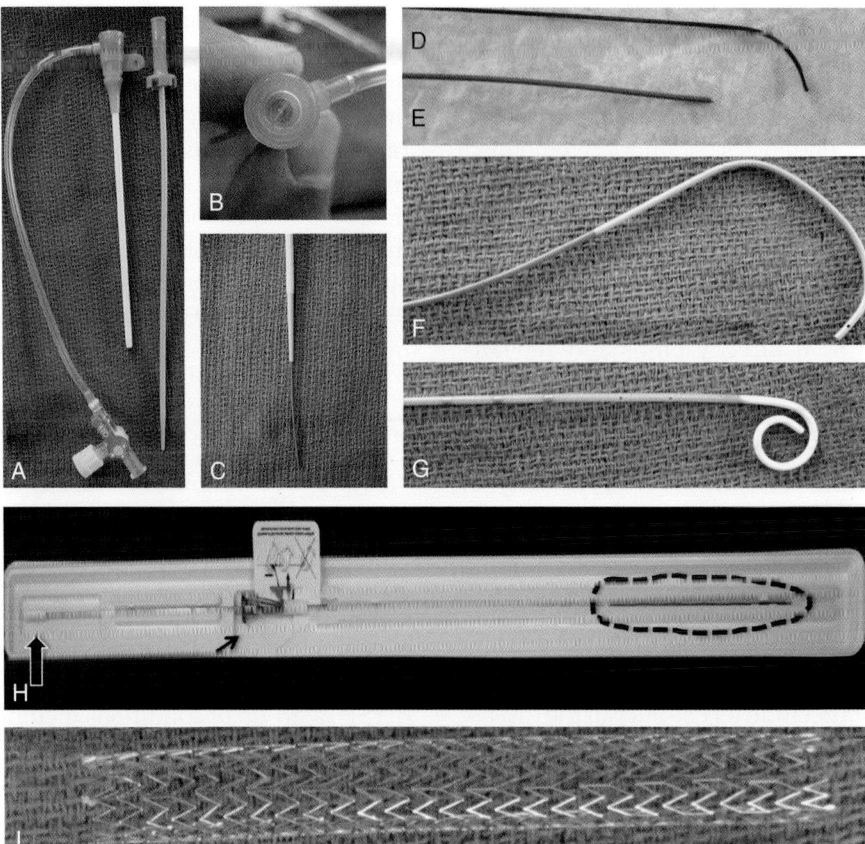

Figure 47.1 Common equipment used for thrombolysis/thrombectomy/vascular stenting procedures. 5–8Fr vascular introducer sheath[1] and dilator (A) with hemostasis valve (B) and smooth transition from sheath to dilator to 0.035" guide wire (C). (D) 0.035" angled hydrophilic guide wire[2], typically 150 or 180 cm in length. (E) Floppy tip PTFE guide wire[3], typically 150–260 cm long. (F) 4Fr Cobra catheter[4] (Alternatively a Berenstein catheter[5] can be used) to select appropriate vessels for catheter-directed thrombolysis, fragmentation, or stent placement. (G) Pigtail marker catheter[6]. The radio-opaque marks are 10 mm from the beginning of one mark to the beginning of the next. Spinning this catheter alone or over a guide wire exiting one of the proximal holes can be used for percutaneous mechanical thrombectomy via fragmentation. (H) Stent delivery system with constrained laser-cut, self-expandable metallic (nitinol) stent[7] (SEMS) (black dotted line) inside the delivery sheath with Y-piece (black arrow) containing diaphragm and side-port. The hub (block arrow) is flushed with saline, as is the side-port (black arrow), prior to use in order to flush out any air. Other types of SEMS can be used as well[8,9]. (I) A deployed laser-cut SEMS[7] – these should NOT be deployed outside the patient as they are typically non-reconstrainable stents.

have not yet been documented and prolonged infusion times and increased risk of bleeding are the potential problems. PMT provides an elegant approach and has been demonstrated to work well with hyperacute thrombi ; however, they tend to fall short in more chronic thrombi that are 2–3 weeks old, which is commonly seen in veterinary patients. The lytic-assisted devices are the new frontier and work well in smaller vessels; however, larger vessels may also require adjunctive CDT or vascular stenting. Venous stenting is often employed where large veins may be externally compressed leading to recurrent thrombosis ; however, stents are often avoided at the confluence of veins or in the limbs where stent fracture and other complications can occur. Stenting has been used more often at the author's institution due to the relative ease and rapidity of placement, immediate resolution of clinical signs, and general chronicity of most of the clots encountered in our patients.

Portal vein thrombosis is generally treated with systemic lytic agents along with anticoagulants. Unless a portosystemic shunt is present, it is not easily accessed using CDT through a minimally invasive approach.

Embolic trapping devices range from baskets to "spider-like"' endovascular implants to trap emboli and prevent them from reaching the lungs. Once trapped, emboli can undergo fibrinolysis. The most commonly used embolic trapping devices are vena cava filters placed in humans with DVTs. Filters are

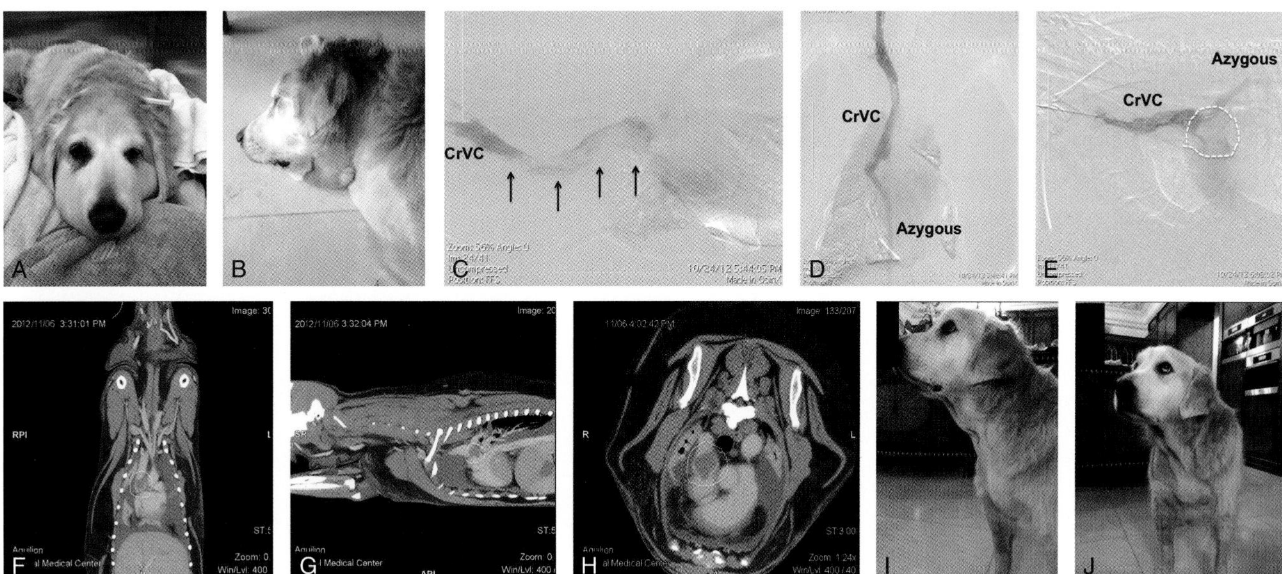

Figure 47.2 Catheter-directed thrombolysis (CDT) in a dog with cranial vena cava (CrVC) syndrome following thrombosus secondary to central line placement. (A, B) Dog with swollen head and neck due to CrVC thrombosus. This patient also had respiratory difficulty secondary to pleural effusion. Lateral (C) and ventrodorsal (D) DSA CrVC venogram via jugular sheath placement demonstrating contrast pooling in CrVC and filling defect (black arrows) due to large clot burden. The azygous vein is retrograde filling and demonstrates reversal of bloodflow to decompress the CrVC via the caudal vena cava (CaVC). (E) Lateral DSA CrVC venogram through jugular sheath following ~24 hr tPA CDT via infusion catheter[10]. There is some retrograde filling of azygous vein but normograde emptying has resumed. A smaller remnant thrombus (white dotted line) remains between the azygous vein and right atrium. [illegible] CT angiogram one week later demonstrating thrombolysis but persistence of small thrombus (white dotted line). (I, J) Images 2 weeks later with resolution of swelling and pleural effusion.

indicated in patients with a high risk of pulmonary embolism. Filters can be inserted fluoroscopically into the vena cava using jugular or femoral vein access, depending on the ease of vessel access and the size of the patient. Filters must be placed downstream from the clot. Filters are made of nitinol or stainless steel and are biocompatible and non-thrombogenic. Some complications reported with filters include migration and tearing, or perforation, of the vena cava. To the author's knowledge, these devices are not routinely used in clinical veterinary patients for venous thrombosis.

Long-Term Therapy/Follow-up

As long as the thrombus is visible, it may be advisable to maintain anticoagulant therapy with the intent of continuous Xa inhibition. For example, if the patient is receiving dalteparin, TID administration would be recommended. Once the thrombus is no longer visible, if the underlying disease predisposing to thrombosis has been stabilized and/or the thrombus has been stable over a period of weeks, a decrease to SID administration in dogs could be considered. Following the patient's coagulation status (TEG, D-dimer) may also help in the decision process. As it is believed that platelets play a minor role in the pathogenesis of venous thrombosis, long-term antiplatelet therapy is unlikely necessary. See Box 47.1 for an algorithm for the treatment of venous thrombosis.

Arterial Thrombosis

Clinical Signs

The most common sites of arterial thrombosis in dogs and cats are the distal aorta, iliac arteries, and brachiocephalic arteries. Arterial obstructions often present with more severe clinical signs, depending upon the amount of tissue risking devitalization. Severe pain, muscular rigidity, paresis, and paralysis are most commonly observed; however, the author has observed chronic presentations. Peripheral arterial thrombi are less commonly diagnosed in veterinary patients, likely due to the vast and abundant collateral perfusion throughout much of the body. The classic arterial thromboembolism scenario in veterinary medicine is the saddle thrombus occluding unilaterally or bilaterally the pelvic limbs. In severely affected animals the attending clinician often does not have the luxury of time to determine if systemic anticoagulation

BOX 47.1

Algorithm for the treatment of central venous thrombus

CENTRAL VENOUS THROMBUS
Fortuitous finding
Mild/moderate clinical signs

Stabilize patient as needed
Complimentary diagnostic tests as needed
Goal: identify and treat cause of hypercoagulability
Decision to intervene based on clinical condition and risk assessment

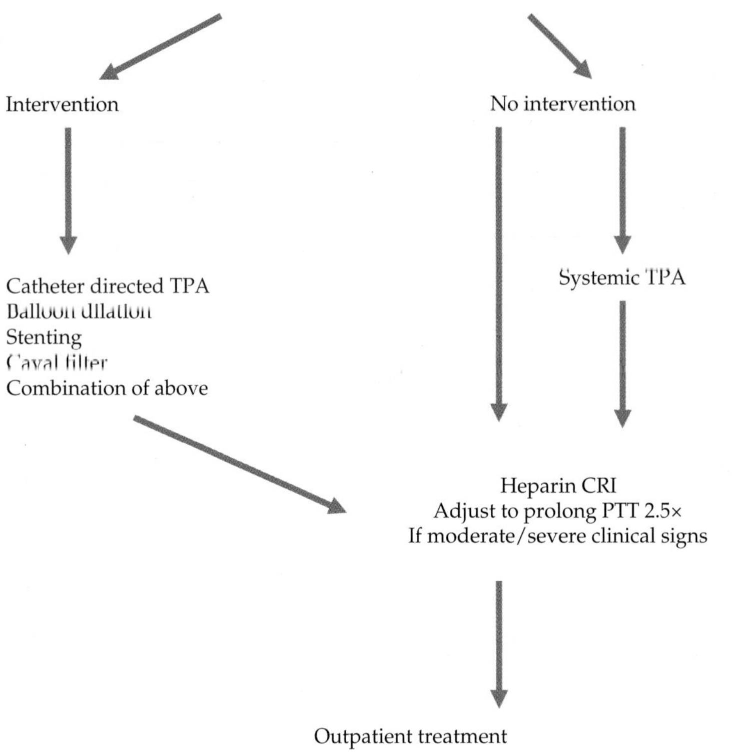

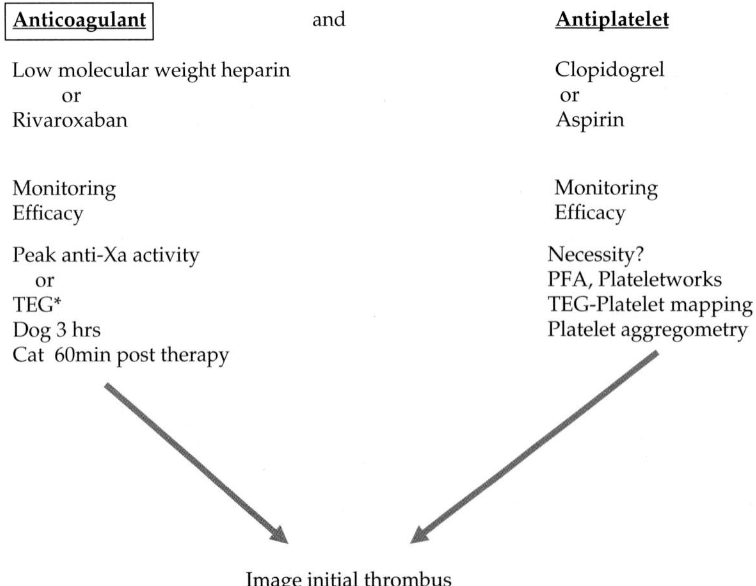

*In order to observe patient's coagulation status without the effect of heparin and without stopping heparin therapy, TEG run with a heparinase cup

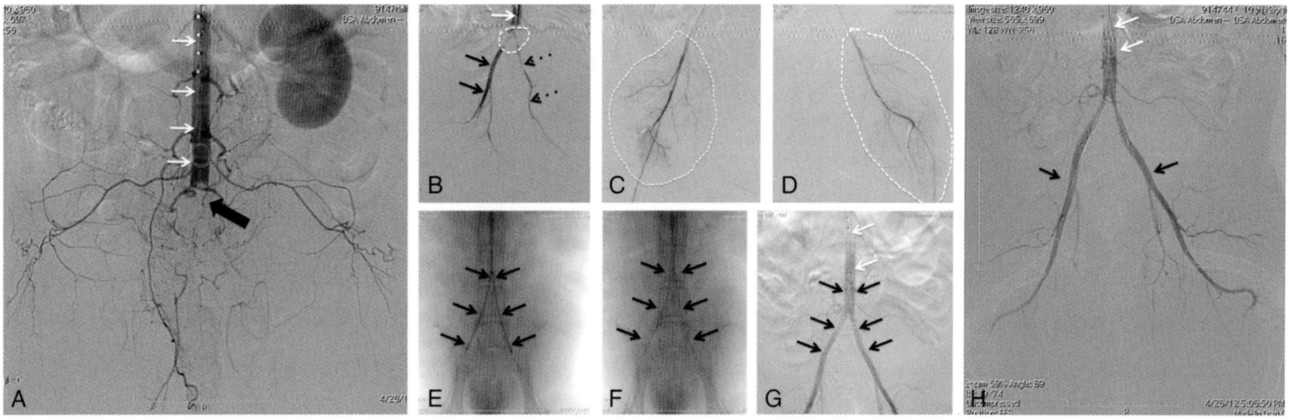

Figure 47.3 Serial angiograms of a dog with an aortic saddle thrombus receiving catheter-directed thrombolysis (CDT) and vascular stenting. (A) Initial DSA aortogram via pigtail marker catheter (white arrows) placed through carotid artery. Complete aortic attenuation is identified (block arrow). (B) DSA arteriogram through Berenstein catheter (white arrow) demonstrating patent right external iliac (REI) artery (black arrows) and faintly patent left internal iliac (LII) artery (black dotted arrows) with clot present at aortic trifurcation (white dotted line). (C) Close up REI artery DSA showing perfusion to muscles (white dotted line) so not completely thrombosed. (D) Close up LII artery DSA showing perfusion to muscles (white dotted line) so not completely thrombosed). (E–G) Serial images showing bilaterally placed « kissing » external iliac artery stents[7] (black arrows) prior to deployment (E), immediatley following deployment (F), and after DSA aortogram (G) via marker pigtail catheter (white arrows) showing re-established bloodflow through both external iliac arteries. (H) Final DSA aortogram via marker pigtail catheter (white arrows) showing extensive bloodflow through both external iliac arteries (black arrows).

and/or lytic therapy will be effective. Historically, surgical thrombectomy has been performed and rheolytic thrombectomy has been described. Both techniques are effective, but unfortunately the underlying cardiac disease and fragile systemic condition of the patient often results in poor longer-term outcomes in approximately 50% of the patients. In addition, acute reperfusion of both pelvic limbs would be associated with malpractice litigation if performed in humans, due to the anticipated risk of death from reperfusion injury. Before performing such a procedure the attending clinician should have a long conversation with the pet owner about this sequela.

Diagnostics

Underlying disease and predisposing factors to consider in patients with arterial thrombosis are similar to that described above for venous thrombosis. These include, but are not limited to, left-sided heart disease (cats), hyperadrenocorticism, protein losing nephropathy (most common cause in the authors' experience), protein-losing enteropathy, neoplasia (including adrenal), sepsis, and glucocorticoid therapy. Diagnostic testing should include a complete blood count, biochemistry panel, urinalysis, urine protein to creatinine ratio, abdominal and chest imaging (radiography and ultrasound) and more detailed imaging, like constrast CT or MIR. Clotting times (PT and PTT) are not useful in the detection of hypercoagulability, but can detect hypocoagulability and/or disseminated intravascular coagulation. FDPs and D-dimers would be expected to be elevated. TEG would be expected to indicate a hypercoagulable state.

Intervention

It has been the authors' experience that dogs (and likely cats) can likely tolerate occlusion of both the internal iliac arteries without clinical signs. Once the thrombus grows and extends beyond this bifurcation, clot begins travelling down the external iliac arteries and into the femoral arteries. This is the point of clinical presentation. As long as both external iliac arteries can remain patent the animal can recover. The use of infusion thrombolysis with vascular stenting has been successful in a small number of these patients treated by the author (Figure 47.3). This technique appears to provide a more delayed reperfusion than the hyperacute reperfusion encountered during complete clot removal (Figure 47.4). Vascular access (see Chapter 44) is chosen based upon avoiding affected vessels. For instance carotid artery access is chosen for saddle thrombi to avoid further damage to distal limb perfusion following therapy. Recently, Winter et al (2012) described improved clinical signs and no side effects in a small number of dogs with aortic thrombi using a systemic warfarin based therapy.

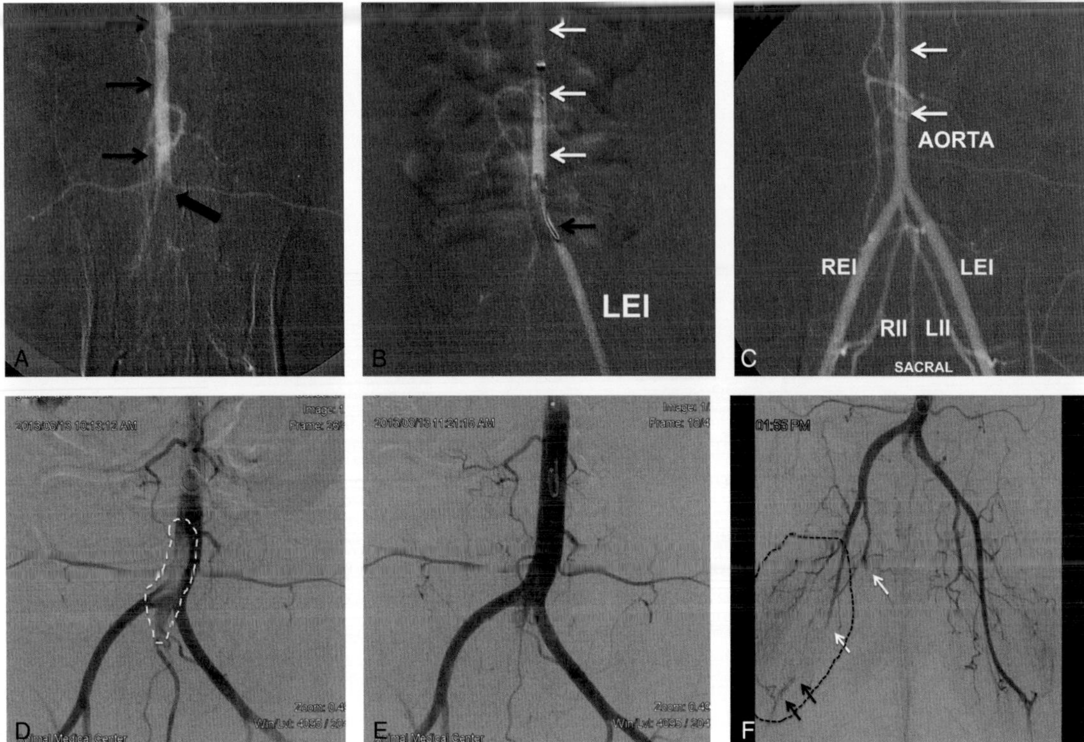

Figure 47.4 Serial DSA aortograms in a cat (A–C) and dog (D–F) with a saddle thrombus receiving rheolytic thrombectomy. (A) Cat aortgram through pigtail catheter (black arrows) placed via carotid artery demonstrating complete attenuation of contrast (block arrow). (B) Rheolytic thrombectomy catheter[11] (white arrows) in aorta over guide wire (black arrow) and aortogram showing left external iliac artery (LEI) patency. (C) Final aortogram through sheath (white arrows) following complete rheolytic thrombectomy and now complete filling of left and right external iliac (REI,LEI), left and right internal iliac (RII,LII), and sacral arteries. This cat would be at high risk for reperfusion injury. (D) Dog distal aortogram through pigtail catheter placed via common carotid cutdown demonstrating thrombus filling defect (white dotted line) occluding both internal iliac arteries and partial obstruction of right external iliac artery. (E) Following rheolytic thrombectomy, repeat aortogram demonstrates no filling defect but internal iliacs still occluded due to chronicity of thrombus. Better filling of local small vessels also apparent. (F) Repeat proximal hindlimb angiography post-thrombectomy demonstrates additional obstructions of femoral artery and branches (white arrows). Collateral blood vessels are apparent (black dotted line) reconstituting the distal femoral artery (black arrows) suggesting chronicity to this obstruction. tPA was adminstered into these obstructed vessels prior to removing the catheters. Because of the patent external iliac arteries and collateral recanalization of the distal hindlimb arteries, reperfusion injury would be low risk in this patient.

Interestingly, the author has recognized more chronic distal aortic occlusions in dogs (atherosclerotic in humans) between the renal and external iliac arteries (Aortoiliac Occlusive Disease); the chronicity is identified by collateral circulation and the clinical signs associated with claudication rather than acute hindlimb ischemia (Figure 47.5). These patients should not be "lumped in" with saddle thrombi patients. These patients can respond to vascular therapy very well as the risk of acute reperfusion injury is not expected. Aggressive and early physical therapy should be performed as the author has seen muscle contracture following arterial ischemia of the pelvic limb in a dog. See Box 47.2 for an algorithm for the treatment of arterial thrombosis.

Ischemia–Reperfusion Injury

Ischemia-reperfusion is a cascade of events leading to cell damage, cell death, increased vascular permeability, tissue necrosis and multi-organ dysfunction. The acute absence of perfusion creates an environment that, upon return of blood flow, results in injury primarily by oxidative damage. Reperfusion injury is a major concern in patients suffering from arterial thromboembolism and is believed to create more injury than the ischemia. Routine laboratory results associated with ischemia–reperfusion injury are metabolic acidosis, hyperkalemia, and hyperphosphatemia.

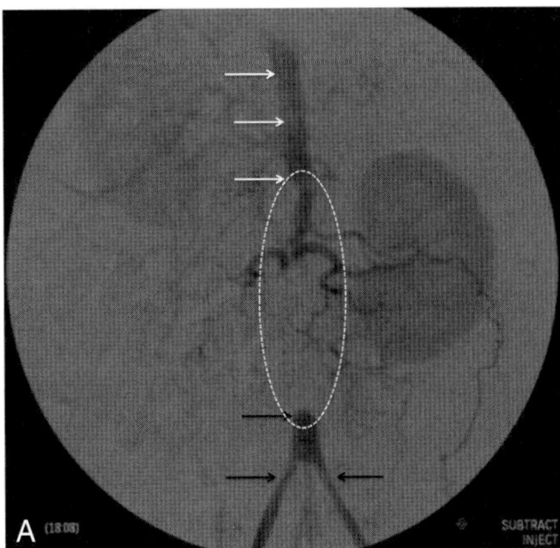

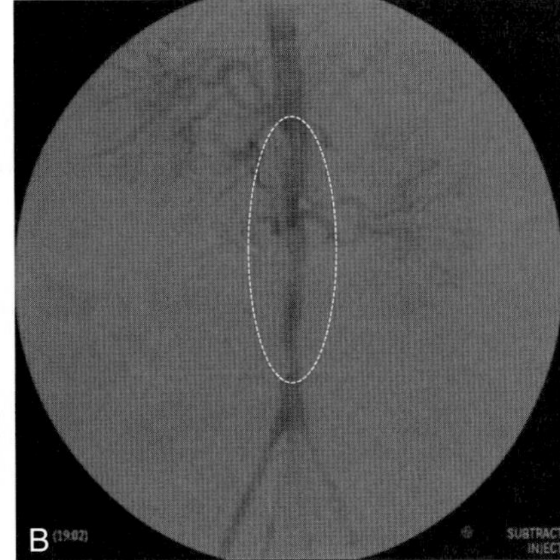

Figure 47.5 Pre (A) and Post (B) DSA aortograms in a dog with aortoiliac occlusive disease demonstrating claudication (hindlimb weakness/pain) after short walks. (A) Initial aortogram shows proximal aorta contrast filling (white arrows), large segmental defect at level of thrombus obstruction (white dotted line), and reconstitution of terminal aorta and iliac arteries (black arrows) due to collateral circulation. (B) Aortogram following aortic stent[7] placement with now patent aorta and lack of collateral filling. This dog is unlikely to develop any reperfusion injury due to the collateral circulation that was present.

Numerous treatment strategies have been investigated both prior to and following reperfusion. Given the lack of markers of injury and variable treatment results, it has been difficult to conclude on the effectiveness of the agents used.

Treatment

To decrease oxidative damage *N*-acetylcysteine, mannitol, vitamin E, vitamin C, calcium channel blockers, and allopurinol have been investigated, but appear to exert the best effect when given experimentally prior to the ischemic event. Free radical scavengers: Deferoxamine, dimethylsulfoxide (DMSO), 21-aminosteroids (lazaroids), and nitric oxide (NO) have also been investigated. Hyperbaric oxygen therapy has also been suggested as a means to improve tissue perfusion during an ischemic event and may help alleviate reperfusion injury. Treatment for hyperkalemia should be initiated and monitored for immediately after re-establishing perfusion as this can be abruptly life-threatening and medically controlled.

Author's Recommendations

Given the lack of clinically relevant data and therefore lack of veterinary guidelines the approach used in a few clinical patients now follows. See Table 47.3 for dosing guidelines. Please note that many of the abovementioned agents have not been investigated in cats and dogs and therefore no dose can be recommended at this time).

Upon presentation following an acute ischemic event.

1. Perform baseline blood gas along with electrolytes and phosphorus. Correct abnormalities with supportive therapy as required.
2. Administer mannitol as long as the patient is not anuric nor in heart failure. Ensure hydration is appropriate prior to general anesthesia for the procedure given the diuretic effects of mannitol.
3. Procedure aimed at restoring blood flow.
4. Monitor blood gas, electrolytes, phosphorus for signs of electrolyte disturbances, and administer allopurinol if the patient is able to take oral medications for 72 hours.

Long-Term Therapy/Follow-up

Platelets are considered to be the major players in the pathogenesis of arterial thrombosis and therefore antiplatelet therapy is recommended long term/lifelong in these patients. As long as the thrombus is visible, it may also be advisable to maintain anticoagulant therapy with the intent of continuous Xa inhibition. For example, if the patient is receiving dalteparin, TID administration would be recommended. Once the thrombus is no longer visible, if the underlying disease predisposing to thrombosis has been stabilized and/or the thrombus has been stable over a period of weeks, a decrease to SID administration could be considered. Following the patient's coagulation status, (TEG, D-dimer) may also help in the decision process. Following 1–2 months without signs of thrombosis, the anticoagulant could be stopped while maintaining antiplatelet therapy.

BOX 47.2

Algorithm for the treatment of arterial thrombus

ARTERIAL THROMBUS
Treated as an emergency

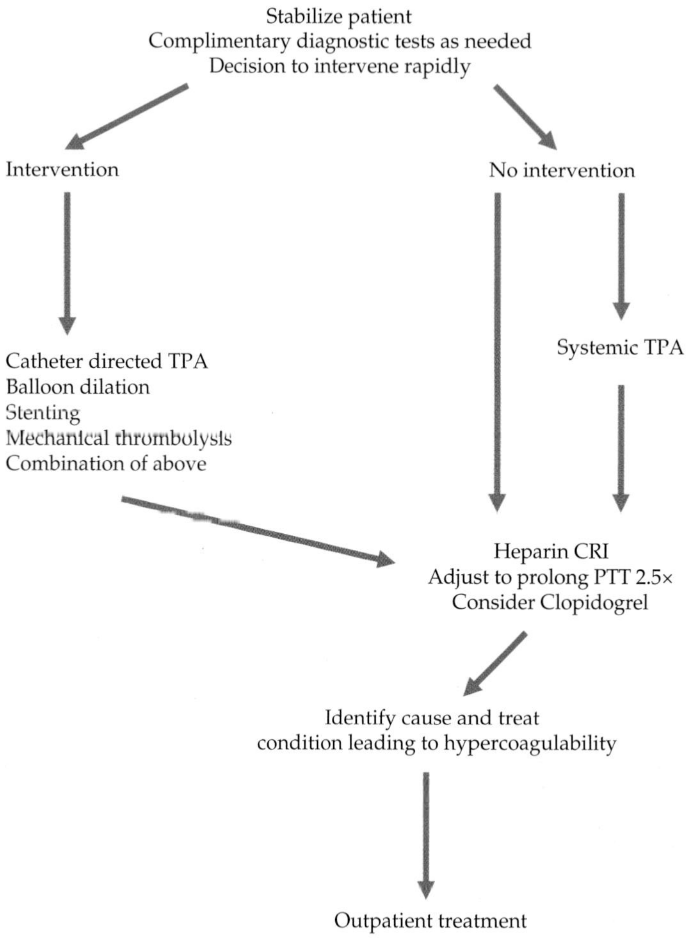

Antipatelet and **Anticoagulant**

Antipatelet	**Anticoagulant**
Clopidogrel or Aspirin	Low molecular weight heparin or Rivaroxaban
Monitoring Efficacy	Monitoring Efficacy
Necessity? PFA, Platelet works TEG-Platelet mapping Platelet aggregometry	Peak anti-Xa activity or TEG* Dog 3 hrs Cat 60min

Imaging initial thrombus
Adjust therapy

* In order to observe patient's coagulation status without the effect of heparin and without stopping heparin therapy, TEG run with a heparinase cup.

TABLE 47.3
Agents used in the prevention and treatment of schema-reperfusion injury in dogs and cats

Drug	Dog	Cat
Allopurinol	20–50 mg/kg PO BID for 2 days	None reported 9 mg/kg PO SID (for urate urolithiasis)*
N-acetylcysteine	140 mg/kg PO or slow IV once then 70 mg/kg slow IV QID for 8 doses (acetaminophen toxicity dose)	100 mg/kg PO BID
Deferoxamine	15 mg/kg/hr IV CRI (iron toxicosis)*	None reported
Vitamin C	None reported	250 mg/cat PO BID
Vitamin E	300 UI/dog PO BID*	50 mg/kg PO SID
Mannitol	0.5–1 g/kg IV over 10–15 minutes (single dose)*	0.5–1 g/kg IV administer over 20 minutes (2 doses)*
DMSO	82 mg/kg SC 3 times/week (dose for systemic amyloidosis*)	None reported

SC: subcutaneous
CRI: constant rate infusion
*Please note that these doses have been taken from experimental studies or have been indicated to treat other conditions.

Pulmonary Thromboembolism (PTE)

Clinical Signs

The cause of PTE in veterinary patients is likely different from those in humans who often suffer from migration of DVT; as such the treatments are likely to be different. In humans, PTE carries an approximate 30% mortality rate if left untreated compared to ~8% when treated. Not all PTEs are the same, however, so careful risk stratification must be pursued in order to determine which patients will benefit from intervention and which patients may be harmed. As such, the terms "massive pulmonary embolism (PE)" and "submassive PE" have been used. In massive PE, hemodynamic instability (systemic hypotension and circulatory collapse) is likely an absolute indication for intervention (thrombolysis for instance). In submassive PE, right ventricular dysfunction (RV:LV ratio greater than or equal to 1 in humans), high clot burden, or concomitant DVTs may raise the consideration for intervention.

Clinical signs related to obstructive/massive PTE include signs related to congestive heart failure and decreased cardiac output: severe weakness, dyspnea, cough, and hemoptysis. Pleural and abdominal effusion, hepatic congestion, and distended jugular veins can be observed.

Diagnostics

Underlying disease and predisposing factors to consider in patients with in situ obstructive PTE include heartworm disease and neoplasia. Central venous clots can detach from their primary site and result in obstructive PTE. In these cases, underlying diseases that predispose to central venous thrombosis should be investigated (Table 47.1). Arterial blood gas analysis or pulse oximetry will reveal hypoxemia. Thoracic radiography may reveal an enlarged right heart, increased or decreased pulmonary artery size and decreased visibility of the pulmonary vasculature, pleural effusion, and an enlarged vena cava. Echocardiography is an easily accessible modality useful in confirming a thrombus in the proximal pulmonary artery. Angiography, contrast-enhanced CT and MRI are also useful modalities in confirming and locating the PTE.

Intervention

The absence of DVTs (highly uncommon in veterinary patients) makes the use of vena cava filters a rare consideration in our patients while it is a very common, rapid, minimally-invasive and safe procedure in humans. These implantable basket-like devices allow bloodflow to persist through the vena cava but catch any blood clots launching up the vena cava, preventing further PTE. In addition, the clot is trapped in an area of high bloodflow, facilitating lysis.

Systemically administered thrombolysis is contraindicated in patients with recent surgery, known or recent hemorrhage, intracranial disease (bleeding, tumor, trauma, or stroke). While this treatment is appealing, in humans there has been statistically significant clinical evidence that systemic thrombolysis is associated with improved mortality over anticoagulation therapy alone. There is growing evidence that shorter infusion times (<2 hr) may be preferred over the historically longer infusion times (~12 hr for

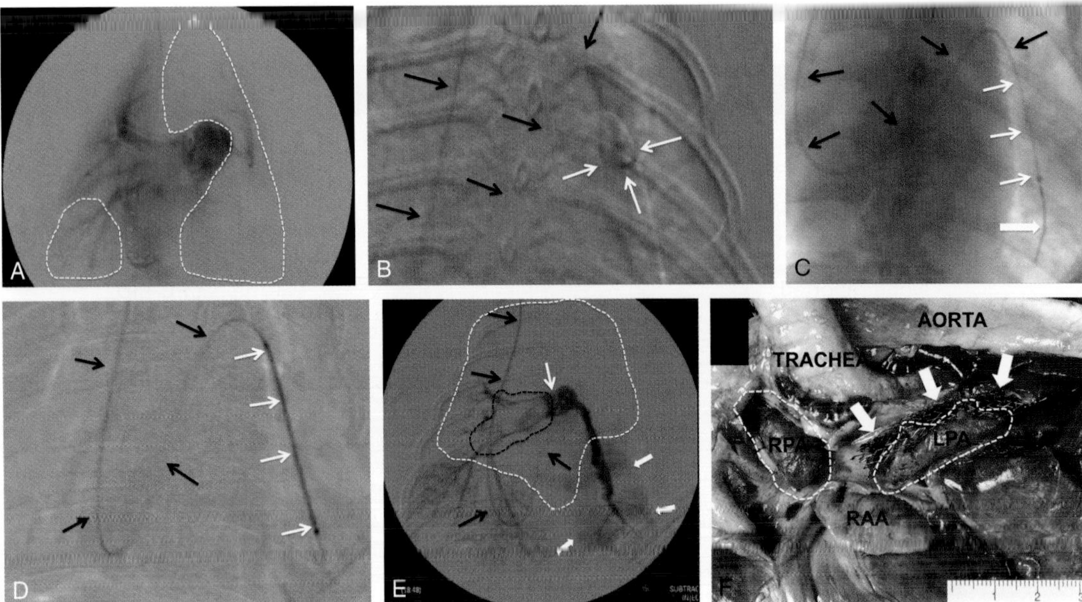

Figure 47.6 Serial images of a dog with a massive PTE receiving CDT, fragmentation and stenting. (A) DSA pulmonary arteriogram via catheter placed in the right jugular vein demonstrating lack of perfusion to the entire left lung and diminshed perfusion to the right caudal lung (white dotted lines). (B) Pigtail catheter (black arrows) with tip (white arrows) in left main pulmonary artery. The catheter is spun to fragment the thrombus. (C) Infusion catheter (black arrows) with multi-fenestrated tip (white arrows) placed over a guide wire (white block arrow) in the left main pulmonary artery. The catheter is infused with tPA. (D) Continued obstruction treated with stent delivery system (black arrows) placed over a guide wire. The constrained stent (white arrows) is evident. (E) Following stent[7] placement within the left main pulmonary artery, repeat DSA arteriogram through the pigtail catheter (white arrow) demonstrates improved perfusion to the left caudal lung lobe (white block arrows). The right main pulmonary artery thrombus (black dotted line) remains and has migrated during manipulations to obstruct perfusion to the right cranial lung lobe. There is still diminished perfusion to the left cranial lung (white dotted line). The dog died at this point during the procedure. (F) Post-mortem image of this patient with both the left (LPA) and right (RPA) pulmonary artery thrombi in situ. The LPA stent (white block arrows) can be identified bypassing the thrombus. The aorta, trachea, and right atrial appendage (RAA) can be seen as well.

instance) in terms of more rapid clot lysis and fewer bleeding sequelae. For PTEs, there is evidence that systemic thrombolysis does not provide sufficient clot exposure to the compound and more localized therapy is therefore warranted (consider an open bottle of wine "breathing" without a decanter).

Surgical embolectomy is associated with high morbidity and mortality in human hospitals without substantial experience and multidisciplinary approaches. As such, the risks associated with the procedures performed in veterinary patients is likely to be at least as high but may be considered in those patients with massive PE and contraindications to thrombolysis. Catheter-based techniques delivering localized tPA through infusion catheters, pigtail fragmentation catheters, thrombectomy devices, etc., offer a more elegant and theoretically improved clot removal approach (Figure 47.6). Until recently little evidence existed supporting an advantage; however, more recently, evidence supporting catheter-based techniques is growing for massive PTE. Access is typically acheived via the external jugular vein (see Chapter 44).

Long-Term Therapy/Follow-up

Anticoagulants are the mainstay of therapy in humans with PTE, given the frequent venous origin of the thrombus. Recommendations are therefore similar as to those in the central venous section. As long as the thrombus is visible or believed to be present, it may be advisable to maintain anticoagulant therapy with the intent of continuous Xa inhibition. For example, if the patient is receiving dalteparin, TID administration would be recommended. Once the thrombus is no longer visible or suspected to have resolved and if the underlying disease predisposing to thrombosis has been stabilized, a decrease to SID administration could be considered. Following the patient's coagulation status, (TEG, D-dimer) may also help in the decision process. As it is believed that platelets play a minor role in the pathogenesis of venous thrombosis, long-term antiplatelet therapy is unlikely to be necessary.

Preoperative and Postoperative Anticoagulant/Antiplatelet Considerations

Prior to, during, and following thrombosis intervention, the question of medical anticoagulation becomes important. If the underlying disease that predisposed to hypercoagulability and thrombus formation is not addressed, the patient will likely thrombose other sites or have recurrence at the same treated site. Another consideration is handling patients already receiving anticoagulant therapy that must undergo intervention for thrombosis. As bleeding from catheter sites, peri- and postoperatively is a concern, it is generally recommended to discontinue anticoagulant and antiplatelet therapy prior to the procedure, unless very minimal vascular access is anticipated. The length of time to discontinue therapy is variable and dependent on the half-life of the agent being used. Given the short half-life of standard heparin it can be stopped 2–5 hours before a procedure. Given the longer half-life of LMWH, these should be stopped 8 hours prior to a procedure. Despite aspirin's antiplatelet properties, clinical bleeding with aspirin therapy appears to be uncommon. Clopidogrel is a potent antiplatelet medication and complications in humans undergoing interventional procedures have been reported. It may therefore be prudent to discontinue clopidogel at least 7 days prior to a procedure.

Despite these recommendations, in an emergency situation, an intervention can be performed despite anticoagulant/antiplatelet therapy. The clinician must be prepared for bleeding complications and if needed, may be able to reverse the effects of heparin with the use of protamine or by transfusion of activated clotting factors in the case of LMWH.

There is very little information in the veterinary literature on whether to continue anticoagulant and/or antiplatelet medication postoperatively. According to human recommendations, the presence of a vascular stent does not augment thrombogenesis. Anticoagulant/antiplatelet medication should be continued as long as the underlying disease that led to thrombosis is present.

Notes

(Examples; Multiple vendors available)

1. 5–8 Fr vascular introducer sheath, Infiniti Medical, Menlo Park, CA.
2. Weasel wire, Infiniti Medical, Menlo Park, CA.
3. Basset (or Bentson) wire, Infiniti Medical, Menlo Park, CA.
4. Cobra head catheter, Infiniti Medical, Menlo Park, CA.
5. Berenstein catheter, Infiniti Medical, Menlo Park, CA.
6. Marker Pigtail catheter, Infiniti Medical, Menlo Park, CA.
7. Vet Stent-Urethra or Vet Stent-Trachea, Infiniti Medical, Menlo Park, CA.
8. Vet Stent Trachea, Infiniti Medical, Menlo Park, CA.
9. Wallstent, Boston Scientific, Natick, MA.
10. Uni-Fuse Infusion catheter, AngioDynamics, Latham, NY.
11. Rheolytic thrombectomy catheter, Possis Medical, Minneapolis, MN

Reference

Winter RL, Sedacca CD Adams A, et al (2012) Aortic thrombosis in dogs : presentation, therapy and outcome in 26 cases. *J Vet Cardiol* 14, 333–42.

Suggested Reading

Arellano MP and Tapson VF (2012) Pulmonary embolism treatment strategies. *Endovasc Today* 11, 74–8.

Cunningham SM, Ames MK, Rush JE, et al (2009) Successful treatment of pacemaker-induced stricture and thrombosis of the cranial vena cava in two dogs by use of anticoagulants and balloon venoplasty. *J Am Vet Med Assoc* 235, 1467–73.

Dunn M and Brooks MB (2009) *Kirk's Current Veterinary Therapy XIV*. Philadelphia, Saunders, pp 24–28.

Kitrell D and Berkwitt L (2012) Hypercoagulability in dogs : Treatment. *Compendium on Continuing Education Practice* 34, 1–5.

McMichael M and Rustin MM (2004) Ischemia-reperfusion injury : pathophysiology Part I. *J Vet Emerg Crit Care* 14, 231–42.

McMichael M and Rustin MM (2004) Ischemia–reperfusion injury : assessment and treatment Part II. *J Vet Emerg Criti Care* 14, 242–52.

Razavi MK (2011) Catheter-based therapies for DVT. *Endovasc Today* 10, 45–8.

Reimer SB, Kittleson MD, and Kyles AE (2006) Use of rheolytic thrombectomy in the treatment of distal aortic thromboembolism. *J Vet Intern Med* 20, 290–6.

Schlicksup MD, Weisse CW, Berent AC, et al (2009) Use of endovascular stents in three dogs with Budd-Chiari syndrome. *J Am Vet Med Assoc* 35, 544–50.

Vajdovich P (2008) Free radicals and antioxidants in inflammatory processes and ischemia-reperfusion injury. *Vet Clin Small Anim* 38, 31–123.

Welch KM, Rozanski EA, Freeman LM, et al (2010) Prospective evaluation of tissue plasminogen activator in 11 cats with arterial thromboembolism. *J Feline Med Surg* 12, 122–8.

Whelan MF and O'Toole T (2007) The use of thrombolytic agents. *Compendium: Continuing Education for Veterinarians* 29, 476–82.

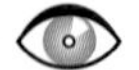

Video clips to accompany this chapter can be found in the online material at **www.wiley.com/go/weisse/vet-image-guided-interventions**

CHAPTER FORTY-EIGHT

Peripheral Arteriovenous Fistulas and Vascular Malformations

Chick Weisse
The Animal Medical Center, New York, NY

Background/Indications

Vascular anomalies have not been completely classified in the veterinary literature; however, it is likely that many of the same types of lesions identified in humans occur in animals. In addition, appropriate classification based upon histology and biological behavior is likely important as misdiagnosis (wrong classification) in humans is not uncommon and subsequently leads to inappropriate treatments or recommendations (Vaidya et al, 2008). The same situation occurs in veterinary medicine. For example, hepatic arteriovenous malformations (AVMs) were historically (and continue to be) inappropriately classified as hepatic arteriovenous fistulas (AVFs), although both may exist. These two lesions may be difficult to distinguish; however, the biological behaviors, and therefore the treatments, are very different. Classification of vascular anomalies is beyond the scope of this chapter; however, for ease of discussion, these lesions can be divided into "high-flow" and "low-flow" groups. The "high-flow" group includes AVMs and AVFs, differentiated by the presence of a "nidus" or "nest" of feeding vessels in the AVM. The AVF is identified by the lack of an intervening nidus and consists of a direct arteriovenous communication. Multiple AVFs are possible. Both of these high-flow lesions can be congenital but the AVFs can also be acquired secondary to vascular trauma (ligation of artery to vein, bite wound, biopsy site, catheter placement, etc.) or tumors. Identification of a pulsatile, blood-filled structure on the distal limb (site of previous catheter placement) or over a previous surgery site should alert the clinician to the possibility of an AVF. True AVMs are congenital and grow at the same rate as the individual; this often leaves time for conservative management in many cases with more invasive treatments reserved for those lesions resulting in unacceptable clinical signs. Reported absolute indications for treatment of AVMs in humans include hemorrhage, worsening high output cardiac failure, complications associated with venous hypertension, lesions in a limb-threatening location, or lesions threatening vital functions (Lee, 2005, Legiehn and Heran, 2010). The most common locations of human AVMs are the central nervous system, the pelvis, and distal extremities; in dogs the liver seems to be the most common site in the author's experience, but they have also been identified in the peripheral limbs, head, and pelvis. Low-flow lesions involving the veins or lymphatics are exceedingly rare (or rarely diagnosed) in veterinary patients. The author has identified and treated only one venous malformation in the distal hindlimb of a cat. Venous malformations have not been characterized in veterinary patients.

Clinical signs associated with AVFs/AVMs are typically associated with the nearby structures. Elevated venous pressures can result in edema, thickened veins, thickened skin, hyperpigmentation, and even ulceration. Importantly, most of the clinical lesions are located downstream from the actual lesion instead of directly over it. Distal limb lesions that might otherwise be subclinical are at greater risk to be repeatedly traumatized resulting in potential for substantial hemorrhage. Bloodflow shunted through the vascular anomaly can result in a "steal" phenomenon resulting in diminished perfusion through the native arteries. This is readily apparent angiographically but has yet to be demonstrated to cause clinical sequelae in animals, aside from arguably reduce hepatic function in those patients with HAVM. Theoretically, high-output

Veterinary Image-Guided Interventions, First Edition. Edited by Chick Weisse and Allyson Berent.

Companion website: www.wiley.com/go/weisse/vet-image-guided-interventions

cardiac failure can result as the blood shunting continues to expand over time. This is a rare sequela in humans as well. Venous malformations may only appear as distended vascular structures.

Ultrasonography and cross-sectional imaging can be helpful in confirming the often palpable pulsatility associated with high-flow malformations and identifying the abnormal bloodflow directionality and velocities. In the author's experience, however, a combination of cross-section imaging and direct angiography provide for optimal characterization of these complex lesions. For example, large arterial vessels may feed the AVM; however, the smaller vessels that are also contributing may be unapparent on cross sectional imaging. Selective arteriography of the surrounding vascular beds will often identify these vessels, particularly once the major feeders have been embolized.

Therapy for AVFs involves ligation or embolization of the abnormal arteriovenous communication, such as is achieved during treatment of a patent ductus arteriosus (see Chapter 58). Acute occlusion of an AVF is well tolerated and typically provides a "cure". Alternatively, treatment of an AVM is performed by targeting the nidus rather than the feeder vessels. Inappropriate treatment such as proximal occlusion (surgically or interventionally) will exacerbate the lesion by stimulating growth and making future treatments more difficult. Understanding the difference between AVFs and AVMs is important in order to recommend the appropriate therapy, relay a realistic prognosis, and provide reasonable expectations for the pet owners. Treatment of AVMs is often considered more palliation than cure as repeat treatments can be anticipated in the human experience. In rare cases, small AVMs may be resectable and that may be the best chance for a true "cure", however "skeletonization", or ligation of feeding vessels, virtually always fails in human patients (Rosen and Blei, 2006).

Transcatheter therapies for AVFs include coils, plugs, or stent-grafts while treatments for AVMs typically involve cyanoacrylate glue (*n*-BCA), or more recently "Onyx" (ethylene-co-vinyl alcohol [EVOH] in dimethyl sulfoxide [DMSO]), a slower polymerizing agent. Particles such as PVA have been described but these are less commonly used for high-flow lesions because of problems with recanalization; newer microspheres may reduce the risk of recanalization. Sclerosants such as 95% ethanol have also been used but can cause substantial toxicity to local tissues, particularly skin and mucosal surfaces and neural structures. The inability to opacify the ethanol without reducing its sclerosant ability is also problematic. Venous malformations have been traditionally treated with percutaneous sclerosants like ethanol or more recently three percent sodium tetradecyl sulfate (STS) foam, again more likely for palliation of clinical signs rather than a cure.

Patient Preparation

Preoperative medical management is based upon individual patient comorbidities or associated clinical signs. A cardiac evaluation is recommended prior to the procedure as high-output cardiac failure is a perceived sequela of AVMs/AVFs (although the author has only seen this in one cat with a chronic (>10 years) peripheral hindlimb AVM). Routine laboratory workup (complete blood count, serum biochemical profile, and urinalysis) is performed prior to the procedure, as is additional screening to ensure the vascular anomaly is not associated with a tumor (three view thoracic radiographs, regional lymph node evaluation, and possible cross-sectional imaging when indicated). Coagulation assessment may be indicated in select patients.

Cross-sectional imaging such as dual-phase computerized tomography angiography (CTA) has greatly enhanced pre-surgical planning for hepatic AVMs (HAVM) and is highly recommended whether surgical or interventional treatment is pursued. This imaging may also help in planning for peripheral AVFs/AVMs. As HAVMs likely change over time, the imaging should be performed as close to the procedure as possible. Embolization is typically performed under a separate anesthetic event as the contrast load (total iodinated contrast volume administered to the patient) will be reached when performing the CTA. This delay also provides additional time to review the images and develop a plan of approach. While human interventionalists often prefer magnetic resonance imaging (MRI) due to the reduced radiation exposure and improved soft-tissue detail, CTA is the author's diagnostic cross-sectional imaging of choice with the arterial phase being the most important for identification of feeders. When an AVM/AVF is suspected, rapid acquisition of images is necessary to differentiate arteries from veins if possible. Even when cross-sectional imaging is acquired appropriately, multiple treatment plans should be prepared in the event that one treatment plan is aborted during the actual therapeutic procedure. In the author's experience, the CTA will often underestimate the degree of vessel contributions that will become more evident during embolization of the major feeding branches and subsequent angiography. However in humans, CT and MRI may demonstrate the full extent of the lesions, perhaps even better than angiography (Rosen and Blei, 2006).

It is the responsibility of the individual performing the procedure to have an extensive knowledge of the local vascular anatomy and become comfortable reading cross-sectional imaging on such cases. Understanding the anatomy will hopefully prevent embolization of a necessary vessel, particularly of concern in the distal limbs (where limited tissue exists and overlying skin and neural structures are often adjacent to the lesion), the pelvis (where essential organs may be adjacent or involved), or the head.

Prior to performing AVF/AVM embolization, discussions about surgical resection (historical standard-of-care) should occur and owner consent obtained. Pre-medications may include broad-spectrum antibiotic coverage. Some may recommend pre-operative corticosteroids to help mitigate the anticipated ensuing inflammatory response associated with the embolization procedure. Post-embolization syndrome can occur and should be treated symptomatically (see Chapter 23).

Potential Risks/ Complications/Expected Outcomes

The major complications associated with AVF/AVM embolization is non-target embolization of: (1) important arterial branches resulting in critical ischemia to limb, adjacent organs/structures and/or overlying skin, and (2) distal migration of embolics into the venous/pulmonary circulation. Identifying normal arterial anatomy in these cases is often difficult as chronicity leads to vascular hypertrophy of both arterial feeders and venous drainage. Development of collateral venous vessels secondary to the high venous pressures complicates identification of the more normal native arteries that are typically under-perfused, smaller caliber, and otherwise difficult to discern. High-flow lesions can permit migration of glue or other embolics through the AVM/AVF and into the pulmonary circulation. Small amounts of migrated embolics are likely insignificant but larger volumes or bigger devices could occlude progressively larger vessels and result in higher risk of substantial morbidity and/or mortality.

Local sclerotherapy treatments such as 95% ethanol and STS foam have additional potential complications such as pain, thrombosis, pulmonary hypertension, hematoma, ulceration, cellulitis, infection, and anaphylaxis.

Historical complications associated with general anesthesia, arterial access site hemorrhage/infection, and contrast allergies/nephropathy must be discussed as well.

Depending upon the lesion type, the risk of recurrence is currently unknown. For patients with AVMs and venous malformations, the owners should anticipate the potential need for multiple procedures. In a recent human publication reporting on patient satisfaction following percutaneous treatment for AVMs, complete or partial symptomatic relief was initially achieved in 58% of patients, which declined to ~40% after 3 to 5 years (van der Linden et al, 2009).

Patient neutering should be discussed but perhaps performed under a separate anesthetic episode or when imaging is obtained. Many of these lesions are congenital in nature but a genetic component may exist (as it does in humans). In addition, acute progression or expansion of an AVM is associated with hormonal stimulation and/or during pregnancy; the author has witnessed exacerbation of an HAVM during estrus in a dog (Rosen and Blei, 2006).

Human interventionalists typically undergo special training in the use of embolic agents such as n-BCA and/or Onyx prior to performing these procedures. It is recommended by the author to have someone with such training present when performing these procedures for the first time, as the potential for causing irreversible harm to the patient is real and cannot be overstated.

Equipment

Recommended equipment can be found in Figure 48.1. Glue embolization procedures require very little equipment but do need a separate embolization area to avoid ionic contents from contacting the glue. 5% dextrose in water is needed for preparation of the glue. The details are further described below. The fluoroscopy unit must provide adequate imaging detail to identify very small caliber vessels using digital subtraction angiography and the ability to obtain orthogonal imaging when necessary. Failure to identify collateral vessels could lead to non-target embolization and severe consequences or continued AVF/AVM flow. A cut-down set is required for non-percutaneous vascular access. All staff in the room MUST wear eye protection during handling of liquid embolics to prevent contact with the cornea. Onyx use requires the use of DMSO-compatible catheters and other specialized equipment.

Fluoroscopic Procedure

High-flow Lesions

General considerations

Patient positioning depends upon femoral versus common carotid access; see Chapter 44 for further clarification. For a forelimb lesion the femoral artery is typically used for access and for a hindlimb lesion the

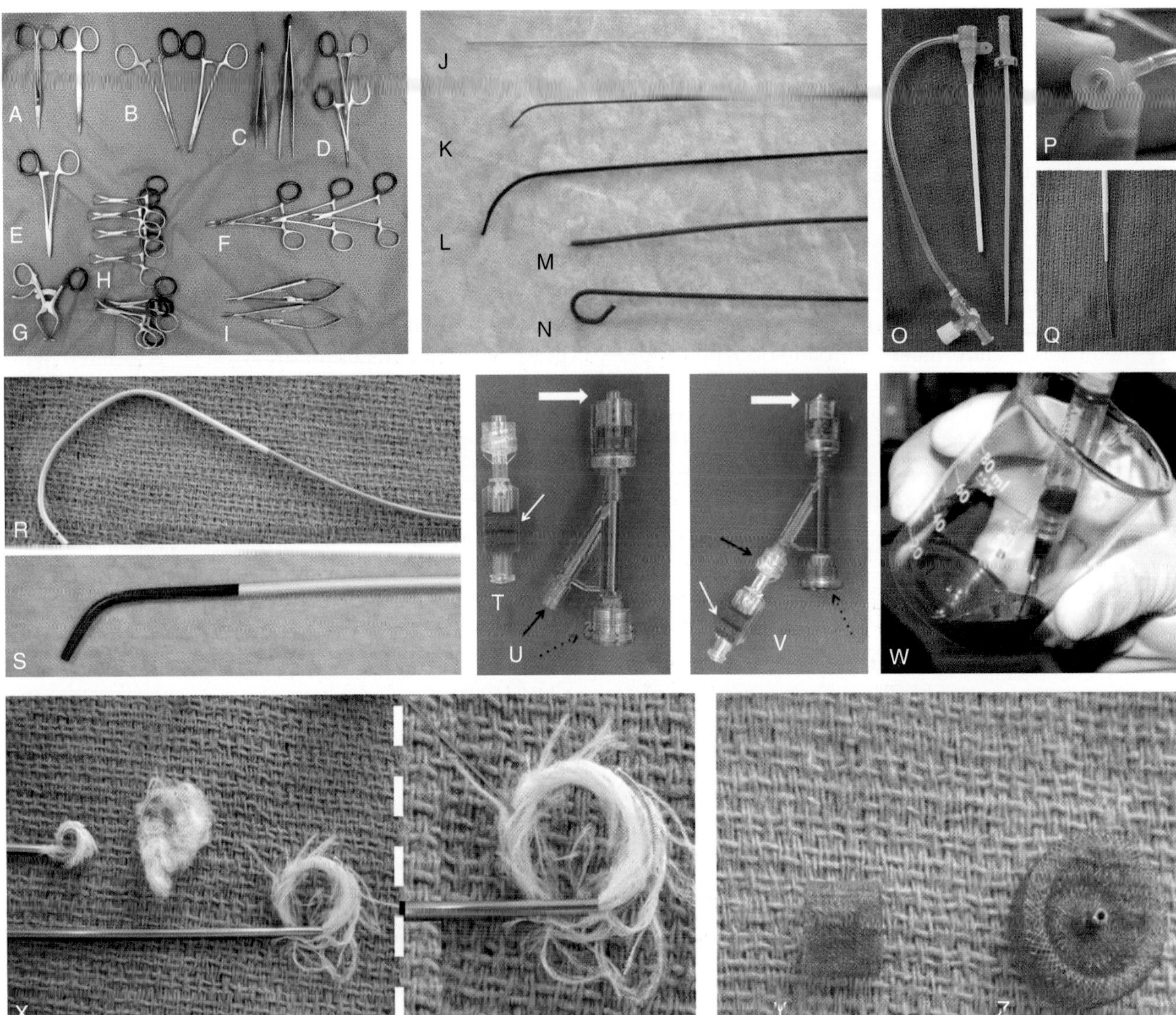

Figure 48.1 (A–I) Sample surgical cut-down set. (A) Sharp-sharps and small Metzenbaum scissors. (B) Right-angled forceps. (C) Brown–Adson and Debakey forceps. (D) Mosquito hemostats. (E) Needle drivers. (F) Kelly hemostats. (G) Gelpi retractors. (H) Small Babcock towel clamps. (I) Castroviejo needle drivers for vessel repair. (J–N) Guide wires: (J) 0.018″ microwire, (K) 0.018″ angled, hydrophilic guide wire, (L) 0.035″ angled, hydrophilic guide wire, 0.035″ straight PTFE wire (M) and 0.035″ Rosen PTFE wire (N), both of which are uncommonly used for this procedure. (O–Q) Vascular introducer sheath. 4 Fr vascular introducer sheath made up of shaft (white) with 4 Fr inner diameter, hemostasis valve (P) to prevent bleeding, three-way stopcock (yellow cap) to flush and/or aspirate, and 4 Fr dilator (blue) to make smooth transition from sheath down to 0.035″ guide wire (Q). (R) 4 Fr Cobra catheter. (S) 4 Fr Berenstein catheter. Flo-switch (T) and Touhy–Borst adapter (U), which connects (V) to form a hemostasis valve (dotted black line) and side-port that can be switched on or off (white arrow) for flushing or aspirating. This device is attached to the hub of the 4 Fr catheter (at white block arrow) and allows coaxial passage of a microcatheter/microwire through the 4 Fr catheter. (W) Glue (cyanoacrylate), iodinated poppy-seed oil, and tantalum mixture prepared prior to injection. (X) Three thrombogenic coils (left) and one close-up view (right) demonstrating Dacron fibers to increase thrombogenicity. Side view (Y) and front view (Z) of an Amplatz vascular plug.

carotid artery or opposite hindlimb femoral artery is used. When small caliber femoral arteries are encountered, micropuncture sets[1] are used for initial access. A sheath no larger than the catheter used is selected. Typically a 4 Fr Berenstein[2] catheter, 4 Fr Cobra catheter[3], or 5 Fr reverse-curve catheter[4,5] is used in combination with a 0.035″ angled hydrophilic guide wire[6] to select the major vessel feeding the limb or region. A diagnostic arteriogram is performed using 50:50 iohexol[7]:saline mixture. For hindlimb lesions, it is

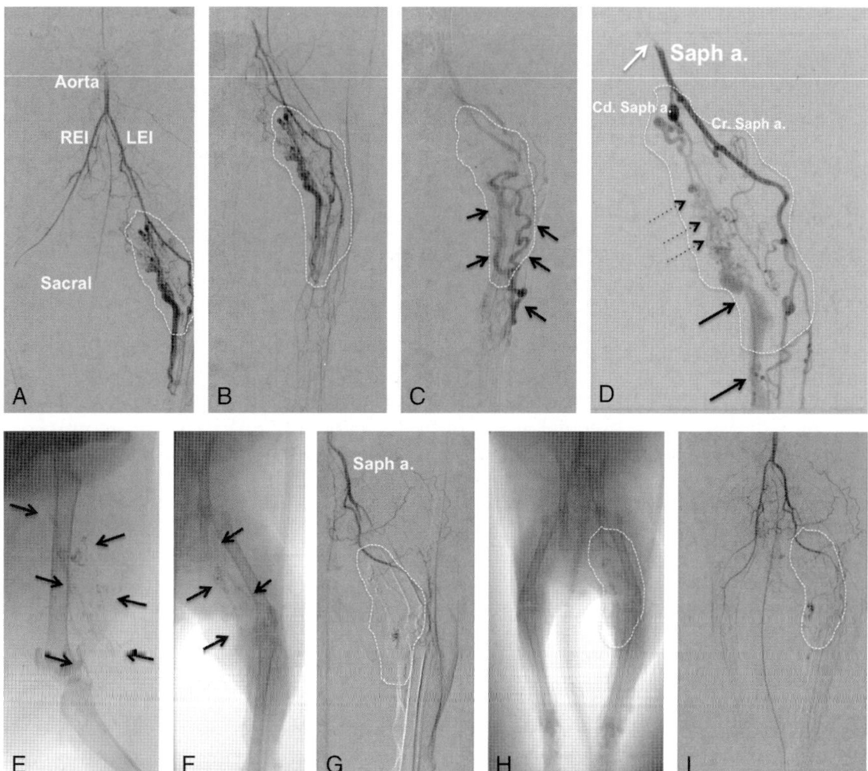

Figure 48.2 Serial fluoroscopic images of a cat with a left hindlimb AVM receiving glue embolization via a common carotid approach. Early arterial (A), later arterial (B) and early venous phases (C) of a distal DSA aortogram performed through a Berenstein catheter in the distal aorta demonstrating the right (REI) and left (LEI) external iliac and sacral arteries. The left hindlimb AVM is identified (white dotted line) with the draining veins (black arrows). (D) Saphenous DSA arteriogram with catheter tip (white arrow) in saphenous artery demonstrating the origin of the AVM (white dotted line) off the caudal ramus of the saphenous artery with contribution from the cranial ramus of the saphenous artery. The AVM nidus (black dotted arrows) is apparent draining into the medial saphenous vein (black arrows). Following glue embolization through a coaxially placed microcatheter, the radio-opaque glue (black arrows) can be seen in the lateral (E) and ventrodorsal (F) views. (G) Repeat saphenous DSA arteriogram showing very little filling of AVM (white dotted line). Final aortogram (H) and DSA aortogram (I) showing persistent perfusion of aorta, iliacs and sacral arteries with mostly embolized LHAVM (white dotted line). A pedal pulse was still present. While complete occlusion was the goal, additional embolization was deemed too dangerous in this setting and the owner warned of potential recurrence of the AVM.

best to include both limbs in the field for this first arteriogram to compare the normal and abnormal limbs (Figure 48.2). This would make using carotid arterial access more ideal. All contrast studies should be performed under digital subtraction angiography (DSA) in order to identify small caliber vessels. In addition, for very high-flow lesions, using higher frame rates (~15 fps or higher) will permit improved identification of vessels and differentiation of arterial and venous filling but will also result in higher radiation exposure. All non-critical personnel should leave the room during the acquisition of these runs. The use of a tourniquet may be helpful in reducing the rate of bloodflow through the lesion temporarily and improve visualization of other branches. The author tries to limit total iohexol administration to 3 ml/kg for the entire procedure when possible (however "safe" and "unsafe" contrast doses have not been clearly determined for veterinary patients). As these patients may have received diuretic therapy, intra-procedural and post-procedural care to avoid contrast-induced nephropathy must be taken.

AVF

For AVFs receiving coil embolization, the treatment can often be performed using larger catheters as the feeding vessel is often substantially hypertrophied in high-flow lesions (Figure 48.3), even in small patients. Options typically include standard thrombogenic coils[8,9], detachable coils[10], or vascular plugs[11]. Alternatively a stent-graft can be placed across the artery (or vein) for

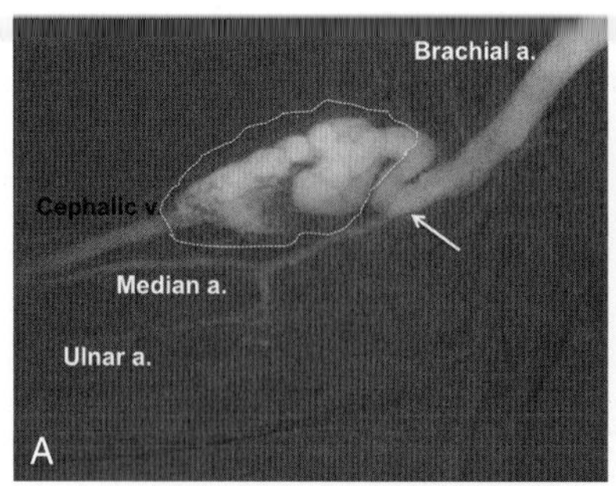

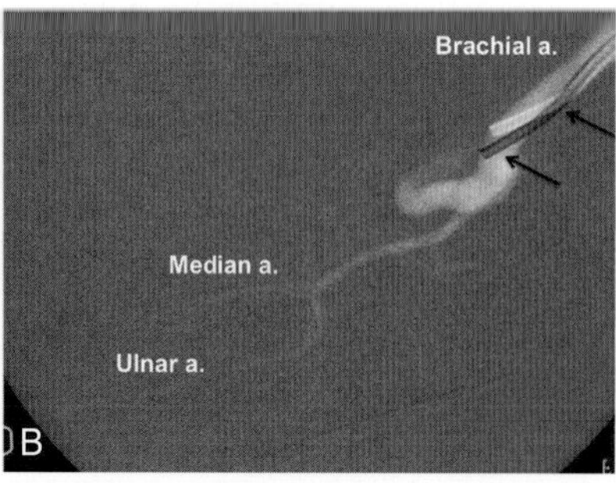

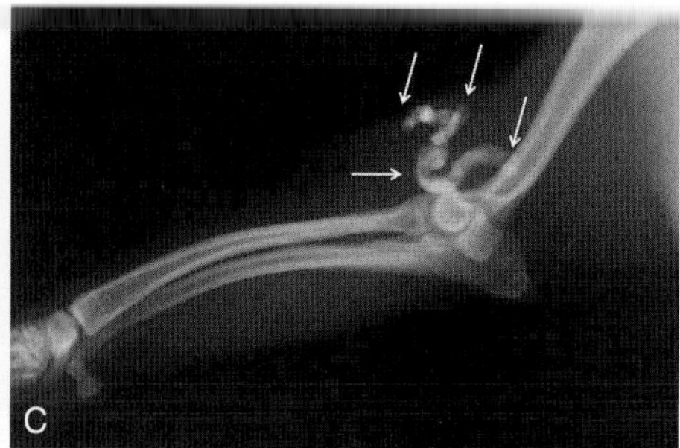

Figure 48.3 Serial images of a dog with a forelimb AVF receiving glue embolization. Pre- (A) and post- (B) brachial DSA arteriogram through a Berenstein catheter (black arrows) demonstrating large AVF (white dotted line) likely arising from the superficial brachial artery and entering the cephalic vein with retrograde bloodflow. Small median and ulnar arterial flow can be seen as well dramatic hypertrophy of the brachial artery until the level of the AVF (white arrow). Following embolization, the AVF is completely occluded but the median and ulnar arteries are still patent. (C) Postoperative radiograph demonstrating the radio-opaque glue embolus (white arrows) in the AVF.

"window"-type communications but this should be avoided in areas of high motion.

AVM

For AVMs, the larger 4 Fr or 5 Fr catheter remains in position or can be advanced distally but proximal to the lesion of interest. A Touhy–Borst adapter[12] and Flo-switch[13] are attached to permit a 1.9 to 3 Fr microcatheter[14,15] to be coaxially introduced. The microcatheter/microwire[16,17] combination are used to superselect the particular vessel supplying the AVM (Figure 48.2). The primary vessels are substantially hypertrophied so access is typically straightforward as it is the preferential path the microcatheter will take. Due to the vascular "steal" of the AVM, the standard tributaries of the neighboring arteries may not be visible making identifying the catheter location more difficult for those not well versed in the regional vascular anatomy. Repeat DSA is performed through the microcatheter using 100% iohexol via a 1 ml luer-lock polycarbonate syringe[18] as needed to identify the AVM anatomy and target the nidus if possible. Once the proper location is identified, the microcather is flushed and liquid embolic preparation can begin.

The following is a description of *n*-BCA embolization (as the author has not used Onyx clinically at the time of this manuscript). A dry, unused section of the surgical table is isolated and surgical gloves are changed. Any moisture (ionic liquid) will cause premature glue polymerization. Separate syringes are used. Five percent dextrose in water (D5W) is poured into a basin; this will be used for catheter flushing as this non-ionic liquid will not lead to glue polymerization in the catheter but saline or contrast will. One ml of *n*-butyl-cyanoacrylate glue[19] (nbca) is mixed with iodized poppy seed oil[20] (Ethiodol or Lipiodol) in a 1:1 to 1:3 mixture of glue to oil inside a sterile shot glass (round-bottom and convenient, easily cleaned glass container). If necessary, a small amount of tantalum powder[21] can be added to the mixture to lend radio-opacity to the mixture (not often necessary as the oil is radio-opaque). The oil slows polymerization time and the tantalum delays the start of polymerization. The ratio of the mixture is based upon personal experience and adjusted with the rate of flow through the AVM. Once mixed, approximately 0.1 to 0.5 ml of the glue mixture is drawn up into two or three different 1 ml polycarbonate syringes, and two or three 1 ml polycarbonate syringes are filled with D5W as well. Time is now important as the longer the glue is exposed to the environment the more likely polymerization will begin. While one person is preparing this glue mixture, an assistant is washing the hub of the microcatheter with sterile D5W to remove any saline and contrast. The assistant then flushes the microcatheter with a 1cc syringe of D5W to clear out the lumen to prevent glue polymerization within the microcatheter from the contrast and saline that was previously injected. The anesthetist is asked to hyperventilate to avoid breathing during the glue delivery (avoid motion artifact during fluoroscopy). This is usually not necessary for peripheral AVMs. The glue mixture syringe is attached to the microcatheter and under fluoroscopic guidance the mixture is injected into the catheter. The empty syringe is removed and the full 1 ml syringe with D5W is attached and injected slowly while watching under fluoroscopy. During the slow D5W injection, the small volume of glue will begin to be visualized exiting the microcatheter. The rate of injection is commensurate with the flow through the AVM in order to fill the nidus if possible. Once injected, the microcatheter is removed as an assistant is holding the 4Fr catheter to prevent it from moving during microcatheter removal. Care must be taken to avoid injecting the D5W as the

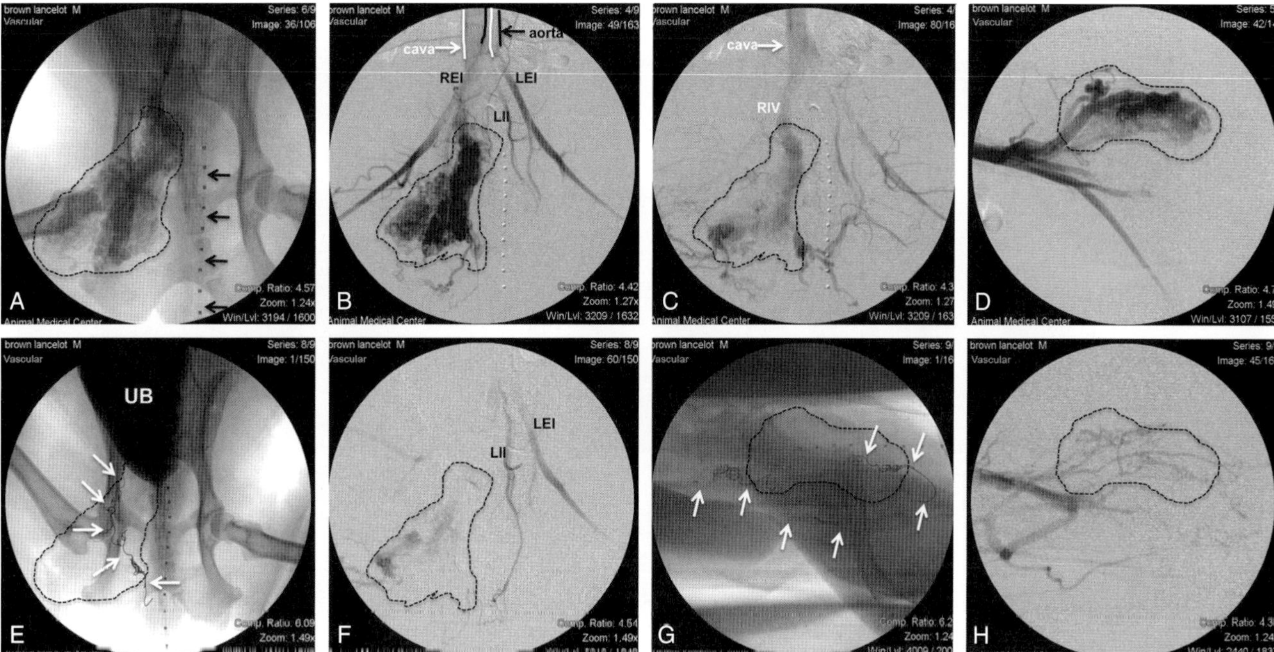

Figure 48.4 Serial fluoroscopic images of a dog with a right pelvic AVM receiving coil embolization. Ventrodorsal early right internal iliac arteriogram (A), DSA arteriogram (B), and delayed DSA arteriogram demonstrating the large AVM originating off the right internal iliac artery. A marker catheter is in the rectum (black arrows). (B) The right external (REI), left external (LEI), and left internal (LII) iliac arteries are evident as is the aorta (black lines) and early filling of the vena cava (white lines) in the arterial phase suggesting a vascular anomaly. (C) The right iliac vein (RIV) is draining the AVM (black dotted line). (D) Lateral aortogram demonstrating the AVM (black dotted line) in the region of the pelvis. (E) Ventrodorsal image showing the placement of thrombogenic coils (white arrows) chosen over glue due to the potential risk of non-target glue embolization off adjacent viscera in the pelvic canal. The urinary bladder (UB) is filled with contrast draining from the kidneys. (F) Late arterial DSA aortogram demonstrating diminished perfusion of the HAVM. The left internal (LII) and left external (LEI) iliac arteries are identified. (G) Lateral image showing the presence of the multiple thrombogenic coils (white arrows). (H) Lateral DSA aortogram showing diminished HAVM perfusion.

microcatheter is being removed. Now a repeat DSA run can be performed through the 4 Fr or 5 Fr catheter to identify the remaining perfusion to the AVM. Sometimes the microcatheter can be reused before removal but this adds the risk of potentially gluing the catheter in place or the glue polymerizing within the catheter and losing a substantial amount of expensive glue mixture. The procedure is repeated as necessary with subsequent selective and super-selective arteriograms using a new microcatheter to evaluate the success of the procedure. The author has used as many as eight separate microcatheters for a single glue embolization procedure when many vessels were involved. Alternatively, "Onyx"[22] can be used to embolize the AVM; see package insert for special handling and instructions for use.

Ideally, the procedure is completed when there is no longer any flow identified to the AVM; Multiple vessels should be interrogated to make sure embolization is complete. It is not uncommon to identify more and more feedings vessels as previous vessels are occluded. Complete/absolute AVM occlusion may not be achieved (Figure 48.4). A post-procedure radiograph is recommend to document the embolic location. Chest radiographs are also recommended to document whether distal pulmonary circulation embolization (with glue) occurred.

Following embolization, all catheters and sheaths are removed. Hemostasis is typically achieved with artery ligation. All animals recover from anesthesia in an intensive care unit for monitoring.

Low-Flow (Venous) Malformations

The author recommends having an experienced interventionalist available during sclerotherapy of these lesions when possible. Even in experienced hands, 95% ethanol can be very dangerous and result in skin sloughing and severe necrosis needing amputation. These procedures are typically performed percutaneously with direct injection into the abnormal vascular structure (Figure 48.5); reflux or extravasation can

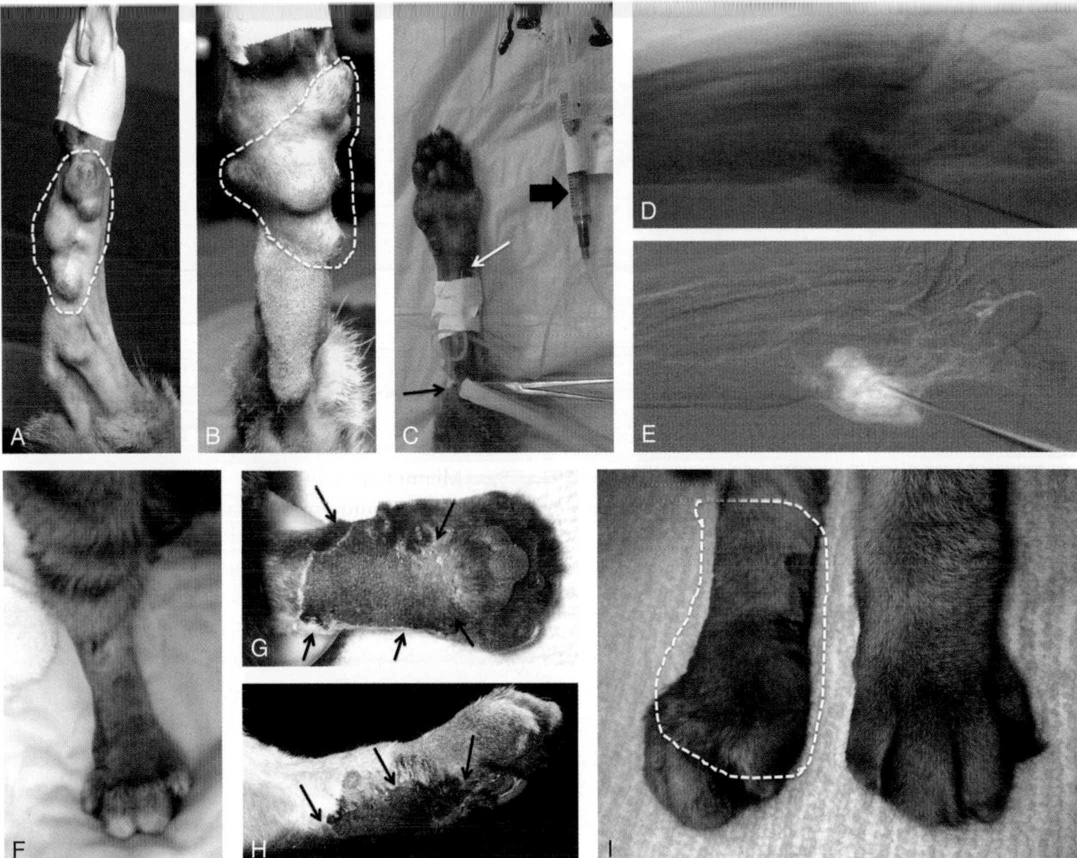

Figure 48.5 Serial images of cat with hindlimb venous malformation receiving percutaneous ethanol sclerotherapy. (A, B) Preoperative images at time of biopsy demonstrating multiple large dilated vascular structures on ventral and medial surfaces (white dotted line) of the hindlimb. (C) Percutaneous ethanol sclerotherapy procedure with tourniquet (black arrow) to reduce reflux of ethanol, injection needle taped in place (white arrow), and syringe with ethanol (black block arrow). Fluoroscopic images of one of three contrast injections performed. The fluoroscopic image (D) is inferior to the DSA image (E) below, which better demonstrates collateral vessels. (F) Immediately post-sclerotherapy demonstrating hyperemia and swelling. (G, H) Short-term follow-up images showing superficial skin necrosis (black arrows) but otherwise no major limb complications. (I) Long-term follow-up demonstrating partial hair regrowth and diminished vascular dilations (white dotted line) compared to the initial images (A, B).

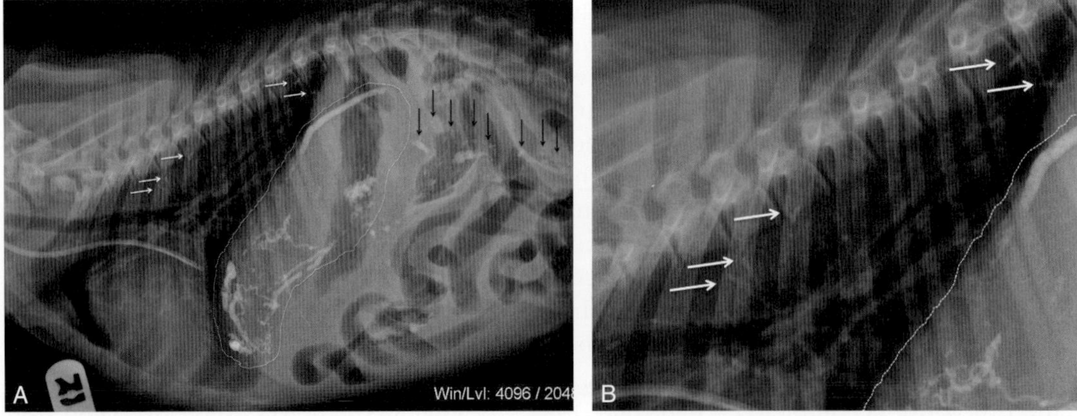

Figure 48.6 Potential complication following HAVM glue embolization in one dog. (A) Lateral radiograph following HAVM (white dotted line) glue embolization demonstrating non-target embolization of small pieces of glue within pulmonary circulation (white arrows) and within multiple acquired extrahepatic portosystemic shunts (black arrows). (B) Close-up view of pulmonary vasculature non-target embolization (white arrows).

result in severe morbidity. The use of STS foam[23] or other sclerosants is beyond the scope of this chapter.

Follow-Up

Postoperatively, periodic assessments for ischemic skin and neurological changes in the affected limb are performed. The patient is typically discharged the following day assuming there is no evidence of substantial skin or adjacent tissue necrosis. Instructions also include limited activity and an Elizabethan collar with regular monitoring of the groin/neck incision for two weeks. Repeat treatments are typically recommended if perfusion persists or clinical signs are worsening.

Special Considerations/ Alternative Uses/ Complication Examples

Examples of potential non-target embolization (Figure 48.6) and tissue ischemia (Figure 48.5G, H); Each of these complications was inconsequential in these patients but substantial morbidity could result in other patients.

Notes

(Examples; Multiple vendors available)

1. Micropuncture set, Infiniti Medical, Menlo Park, CA.
2. Berenstein catheter, Infiniti Medical, Menlo Park, CA.
3. Cobra head catheter, Infiniti Medical, Menlo Park, CA.
4. Rim catheter, Merit Medical Systems, South Jordan, UT.
5. Modified hook catheter Merit Medical Systems, South Jordan, UT.
6. Weasel wire, Infiniti Medical, Menlo Park, CA.
7. Omnipaque (iohexol) injection, Amersham Health Inc., Princeton, NJ.
8. MREye thrombogenic coils, Cook Medical, Bloomington, IN.
9. Nester thrombogenic coils, Cook Medical, Bloomington, IN.
10. Flipper detachable coils, Cook Medical, Bloomington, IN.
11. Amplatz vascular plugs, Infiniti Medical, Menlo Park, CA.
12. Touhy–Borst adapter, Cook Medical, Bloomington, IN.
13. Flo-switch, Boston Scientific, Natick, MA.
14. Renegade or Tracker microcatheter, Boston Scientific, Natick, MA.
15. Microcatheter, Infiniti Medical, Menlo Park, CA.
16. 0.018″ Gold-tipped glidewire, Terumo Medical Corp, Somerset, NJ.
17. 0.014 Microwire or 0.018 Weasel wire, Infiniti Medical, Menlo Park, CA.
18. 1 ml polycarbonate syringes, Merit Medical Systems, South Jordan, UT.
19. TRUFILL *n*-BCA liquid embolic system, Cordis Neurovascular, Miami Lakes, FL.
20. Lipiodol/Ethiodol, Guerbet LLC, Bloomington, IN.
21. TRUFILL tantalum powder, Cordis Neurovascular, Miami Lakes, FL.
22. Onyx liquid embolic system, Micro Therapeutics, Inc., Irvine, CA.
23. Sotradecol (Sodium tetradecly sulfate injection, 3%), Mylan Institutional, Morgantown, WV.

References

Vaidya S, Cooke D, Kogut M, et al (2008) Imaging and percutaneous treatment of vascular anomalies. *Semin Intervent Radiol* 25(3), 216–33.

Lee BB (2005). New approaches to the treatment of congenital vascular malformations (CVMs)—a single centre experience. *Eur J Vasc Endovasc Surg* 30, 184–97.

Legiehn GM and Heran MKS (2010) A step-by-step practical approach to imaging diagnosis and interventional radiologic therapy in vascular malformations. *Semin Intervent Radiol* 27(2), 209–31.

Rosen RJ and Blei F (2006) Hemangiomas and vascular malformations. In *Abrams' Angiography* (Baum S and Pentecost MJ, eds). Lippincott Williams & Wilkins, Philadelphia, pp 1180–212.

Van Der Linden E, Pattynama PM, Heere BC, et al (2009) Long-term patient satisfaction after percutaneous treatment of peripheral vascular malformations. *Radiology* 251, 926–32.

Suggested Reading

Takasawa C, Seiji K, Matsunaga K, et al (2012) Properties of n-butyl cyanoacrylate-iodized oil mixtures for arterial embolization: In vitro and in vivo experiments. *J Vasc Intervent Radiol* 23(9), 1215–21.

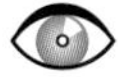
Video clips to accompany this chapter can be found in the online material at **www.wiley.com/go/weisse/vet-image-guided-interventions**

CHAPTER FORTY-NINE

Central Venous Vascular Obstruction

Michael David Schlicksup[1] and Matthew W. Beal[2]
[1] *Veterinary Specialty Care, Mount Pleasant, SC*
[2] *College of Veterinary Medicine, Michigan State University, East Lansing, MI*

Background/Indications

Although rare, venous vascular obstruction is a condition that, if necessary, is amenable to image-guided endovascular intervention. Generally, peripheral venous obstruction rarely causes clinical signs due to effective collateral venous and lymphatic drainage. However, central venous obstruction is more likely to manifest with clinical signs. Some of the most well-documented of these conditions include Budd–Chiari syndrome, Budd–Chiari-like syndrome, cranial vena cava syndrome, and acute caudal vena cava obstruction (caudal to the liver). Budd–Chiari syndrome is an obstruction of blood flow between the liver and the junction of the caudal vena cava and right atrium (Schlicksup et al 2009). Budd–Chiari-like syndrome involves intrahepatic obstruction of hepatic venous drainage (Schlicksup et al 2009). Significant debate exists regarding classification of these syndromes. These conditions result in the accumulation of ascites due to obstruction of hepatic venous drainage with or without hindlimb edema. Hindlimb edema occurs due to acute caudal vena cava obstruction. Cranial vena cava syndrome, or cranial cava obstruction (Palmer et al 1998), results in edema of the head and forelimb(s). Concurrent pleural effusion and/or chylothorax may also result due to obstruction of lymphatic drainage from the thoracic duct. Venous vascular obstruction resulting in these conditions may occur due to congenital, traumatic, thrombotic, neoplastic, infectious, or a combination of these conditions (Cunningham et al, 2009, Fine et al, 1998, Haskal et al, 1999, Miller et al, 1989, Rollois et al, 2003, Schlicksup et al, 2009, Whelan et al, 2007).

The goal of endovascular therapy is the return of laminar blood flow to a previously obstructed vessel. In the central circulation, stent placement is often the principle technique for accomplishing this goal. Catheter-directed thrombolysis, thrombectomy, and the use of inhibitors of hemostasis may also play a role when stents are not indicated, or are contraindicated. While stent placement can be a primary treatment modality, it is more often used to provide palliation of clinical signs. For a summary of interventions for thrombus-induced vascular obstruction, please see Chapter 47.

Patient Preparation

Animals should undergo a thorough diagnostic workup in order to elucidate the cause and exact location of the vascular obstruction as well as co-morbid conditions. To determine location, Doppler ultrasonography in the hands of an experienced ultrasonographer can provide valuable information. Helical dual-phase computerized tomographic angiography (CTA), magnetic resonance angiography, or selective angiography are essential to determine location, severity, and length of the obstruction as well as adjacent normal vessel size (Figure 49.1).

Additional diagnostic testing prior to intervention is appropriate. In addition to assessment of overall health and major body system function (complete blood count (CBC), serum biochemical profile, and urinalysis), assessment of primary hemostasis (platelet count from CBC) and secondary hemostasis (prothrombin time (PT) and activated partial thromboplastin time (aPTT) at minimum; with TEG recommended) are indicated prior to any vascular intervention. In dogs with known or breed specific platelet function abnormalities, buccal mucosal bleeding time assessment is also indicated. Management of primary and secondary hemostatic abnormalities prior to vascular intervention is indicated to minimize the chance of hemorrhage. In animals with renal dysfunction, minimizing iodinated contrast load (during CTA and selective

Veterinary Image-Guided Interventions, First Edition. Edited by Chick Weisse and Allyson Berent.

Companion website: www.wiley.com/go/weisse/vet-image-guided-interventions

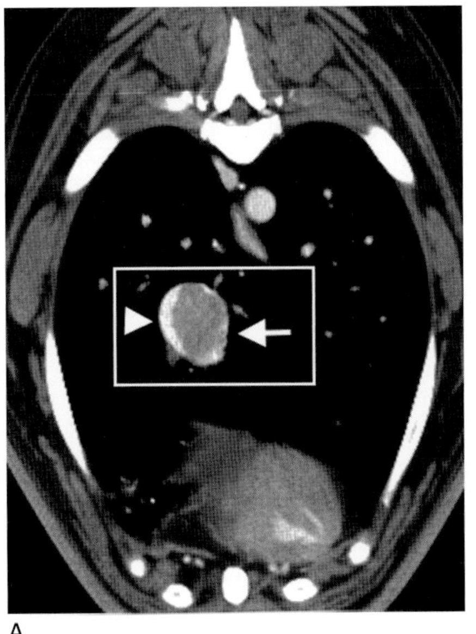

A

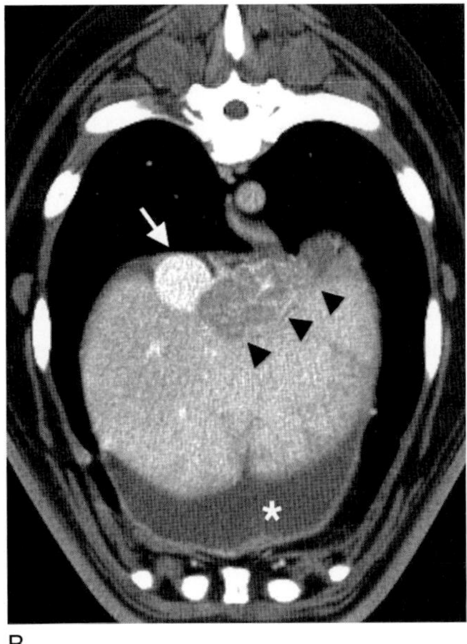

B

Figure 49.1 CTA study of a dog with a suspected neoplastic obstruction of the left hepatic vein and thoracic caudal vena cava in sternal recumbency. Dorsal is to the top of the images. (A) Delayed phase axial image of the caudal thorax. Within the white box is the caudal vena cava. The white arrow represents a partial vascular obstruction occluding approximately 90% of the vessel's diameter. The white arrowhead demonstrates a rim of contrast material passing around the obstruction. (B) Identical study and positioning to (A). Image of the cranial liver. The white arrow represents normal contrast material filling the intrahepatic vena cava. The black arrowheads represent the suspected neoplastic tissue occluding the left hepatic vein. Note the ascites present surrounding the liver (asterisk).

angiography) is important to help minimize the likelihood of contrast-induced-nephropathy. In animals with vascular obstruction associated with neoplasia, appropriate staging is indicated prior to therapeutic intervention. Appropriate premedication for potential neuroendocrine tumors is indicated in those patients to reduce the risk of tachyarrhythmias and hypertension.

Potential Risks/ Complications/ Expected Outcomes

Complications associated with the endovascular management of venous obstruction may include hemorrhage at vascular access sites, hemorrhage due to vascular perforation, arrhythmias during catheter and wire manipulations or misplaced stents, embolization of tumor or thrombus (pulmonary thromboembolism), and acute rethrombosis after restoration of flow. Hemorrhage can be prevented by identifying and managing hemostatic abnormalities prior to intervention, careful attention to properly securing the vascular introducer sheath(s) to the skin, ensuring that endovascular manipulations of catheters and other devices are always performed over a guide wire, ligation or repair of the access vessel (if vascular access is performed via cutdown), and via placement of a light pressure bandage at the access site after the procedure. Guide wire manipulations within the heart may cause arrhythmias. These may be identified via ECG and are optimally managed by avoidance if possible. Pharmacologic management of arrhythmias may be necessary. If pheochromocytoma (or other neuroendocrine tumors) with caval invasion is the cause of vascular obstruction, manipulations of guide wires, catheters, and stents in contact with the tumor may result in arrhythmias with or without hypertension. Temporary cessation of vascular manipulations or, in cases of severe hypertension, the administration of peripheral vasodilators or selective beta-blockers may be necessary. Appropriate preoperative medical management of these types of tumors is always recommended, if possible, prior to therapeutic intervention. Careful guide-wire-directed manipulations of endovascular devices will help minimize the risk of thrombus or tumor thrombus embolization. The most important strategy for preventing acute rethrombosis after restoration of flow is to ensure that flow is maintained. The role of antihemostatic agents in the perioperative and postoperative period requires further investigation in veterinary medicine (see Chapter 47 for more information).

Stent related complications may include malpositioning, migration, and fracture. Stent malpositioning is minimized by using laser-cut stents because they do not foreshorten and can be deployed precisely. Use of a stent guide to serve as an anatomical reference during stent deployment is an inexpensive yet valuable tool. Appropriate stent sizing to provide adequate outward radial force will help minimize the chance of stent migration. Most endovascular stents are oversized by 10–20% beyond the maximum adjacent normal vessel dimension. Fracture of centrally located endovascular stents is rare due to the lack of motion in these vessels. In addition, advances in stent design and manufacturing also help make stent fracture less likely. Stents placed peripherally across joints should be avoided when possible as they are still at significant risk of fracture due to the motion in these areas.

If successful, endovascular management of venous obstruction should result in restoration of laminar flow and rapid relief of clinical signs. The primary benefit of these techniques lies in their minimally invasive nature and the expected rapid resolution of clinical signs. In cases of vascular obstruction where surgical resection includes significant risk of both morbidity and mortality, endovascular techniques can palliate clinical signs, with little risk to the animal, for extended periods.

TABLE 49.1
Instrumentation for endovascular stent placement

Instrumentation
18 ga 1.5″ over the needle IV catheter[1]
Hydrophilic guide wire (0.035″ 150–260 cm standard stiffness, hydrophilic angled guide wire)[2]
8–14 Fr Vascular introduction sheath[3]
4 Fr Berenstein catheter[4]
5 Fr Marker catheter[5]
Floppy-tip PTFE (polytetrafluoroethylene) 0.035″ × 260 cm guide wire[6]
Rosen Wire (polytetrafluoroethylene) 0.035″ × 260 cm guide wire[7]
Omnipaque (iodinated contrast material)[8]
5 Fr Pigtail angiographic catheter[9]
Endovascular stent(s)

Equipment

Endovascular interventions require a thorough knowledge of vascular anatomy and are performed under fluoroscopic guidance. Commonly utilized equipment is illustrated in Table 49.1 and Figure 49.2. Stents are a critical device for the management of venous obstruction. Numerous human and veterinary stents are available. Deployment characteristics such as the ability to reconstrain stents during deployment and foreshortening should be verified with manufacturer instructions prior to placement. In general, laser-cut stents are desirable in the vascular space because they do not foreshorten. This allows for precise stent deployment. On the other hand, mesh stents tend to be available in a wider variety of sizes, including larger diameters. A variety of stent sizes should be on hand during the procedure to ensure correct sizing. Stent diameter is chosen to be 10–20% larger than the diameter of the "normal" portion of the vessel adjacent to the obstructive lesion and should, at absolute minimum, span the entire length of the obstruction. Both covered and bare (uncovered) stents are available. Covered stents prevent tissue ingrowth, especially in neoplastic obstruction, but may occlude the

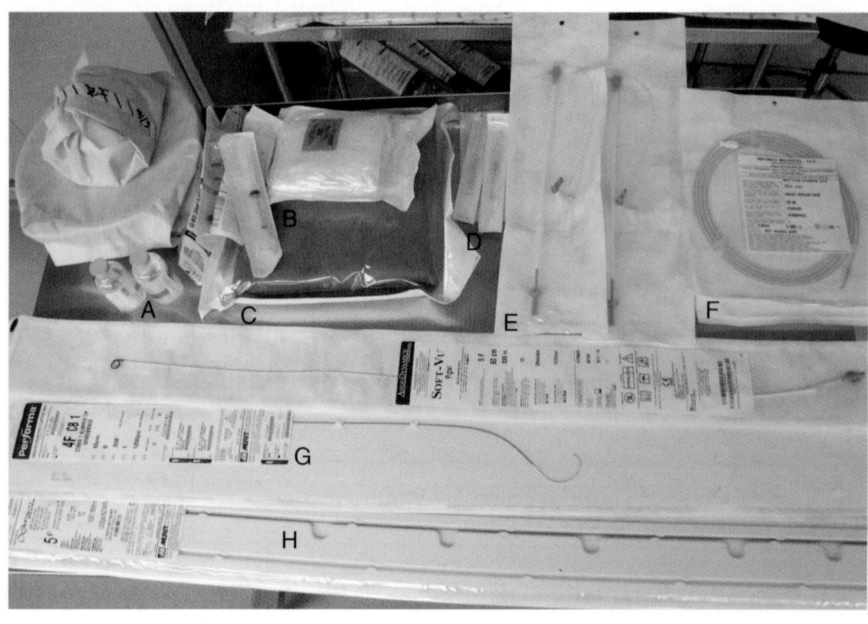

Figure 49.2 Material required for endovascular stent placement. (A) Iodinated contrast material. (B) Sterile dome covers for fluoroscopy unit. (C) Water impermeable sterile drapes. (D) 18 g intravenous over-the-needle catheters. (E) Vascular sheath introducers of a size appropriate for the procedure and stent delivery system. (F) 0.035″ angled hydrophilic guide wires. (G) Angiographic catheters: Pigtail catheter (above) and Cobra catheter (below). (H) 5Fr marker catheter. Not pictured: Berenstein catheter.

ostia of draining vessels. In the authors' experience, placement of bare stents across the ostia of draining vessels has not been associated with complications. Bare stents also have a high success rate at palliating clinical manifestations of vascular obstruction. Placement of a stent-guide under the patient and parallel to the occluded vessel will provide radiographic reference points for stent deployment; however, these marks should not be used for calibration of measurement tools due to the distance between the table top and the target vessel. Marker catheters placed within the lumen of the target vessel will provide more accurate calibration measurements.

Procedure

Positioning and preparation of access sites will vary depending on the location of the vascular obstruction to be relieved. Animals are placed under general anesthesia and ECG, respiratory rate, oxygen saturation, end-tidal CO_2, and blood pressure are ideally monitored. Use of neuromuscular blocking agents to eliminate respiratory motion artifact during angiography is desirable. Because most interventions involve the central venous system, positioning is most often dorsal recumbency. The following is a description of the procedures for stent placement in the central venous circulation for the relief of Budd–Chiari syndrome and cranial vena cava syndrome.

Budd Chiari Syndrome

Avoid the use of hindlimb peripheral catheters for anesthesia in these patients as venous return is impaired. The ventral cervical and the medial aspect of both thighs are clipped and aseptically prepared to allow access to both external jugular veins and both femoral veins. The right (and occasionally left) jugular vein are most commonly utilized due to favorable anatomy that facilitates ease of access to the thoracic caudal vena cava and left hepatic vein. Relief of Budd–Chiari syndrome via decompression of the left hepatic vein is typically preferred due to its large size, substantial hepatic drainage, gentle curve off the caudal vena cava, and general ease of access; however, other hepatic veins have been used. Occasionally, achieving access across the obstruction from one side (cranial or caudal access) may be more difficult than the other so planning possible access from both locations concurrently is best. Draping should be performed to permit aseptic access to all locations and should provide ample aseptic area for the manipulation of guide wires (Figure 49.3):

1. The modified Seldinger technique is used to gain access to the right external jugular vein. An 18ga over the needle IV catheter[1] is introduced into the right jugular vein, the needle is removed, and a 0.035″ 150–260 cm standard stiffness, hydrophilic angled guide wire[2] is introduced and manipulated, using fluoroscopic guidance, into the cranial vena cava, through the right atrium and into the caudal vena cava to the level of the obstruction. The IV catheter is exchanged for an appropriate sized vascular introducer sheath[3] (most often 8–14 Fr depending on stent delivery system diameter), which is sutured in place to the adjacent skin (Figure 49.4). In suitably sized patients, a large enough sheath may be placed to permit side-by-side stent delivery systems in one jugular vein.
2. The guide wire[2] is manipulated through or around the obstruction and positioned distal to the obstruction into the abdominal caudal vena cava. Use of a Berenstein catheter[4] may be necessary to direct the guide wire past the obstruction. The Berenstein catheter is exchanged for a marker catheter and the guide wire is removed. Caval angiography is used to

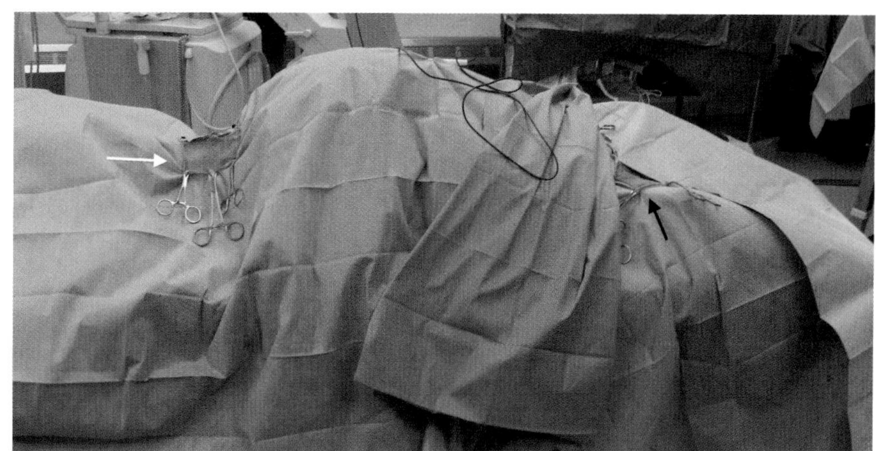

Figure 49.3 Animal positioned for endovascular stent placement in dorsal recumbency with the head to the left. The right external jugular vein (white arrow) and right femoral vein (black arrow) have been aseptically prepared and draped. Note that ample drape material is placed both cranially and caudally for aseptic guide wire manipulations.

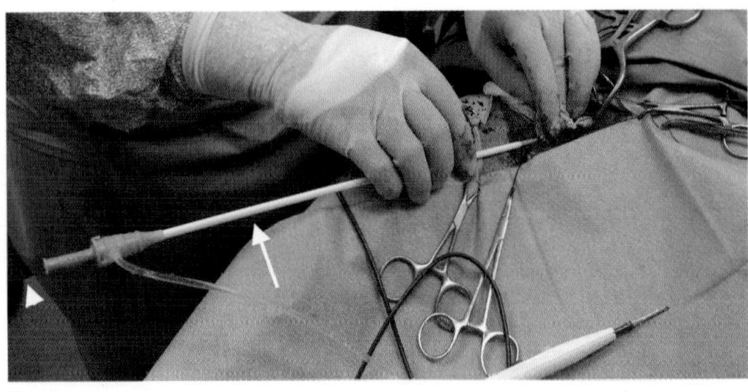

A

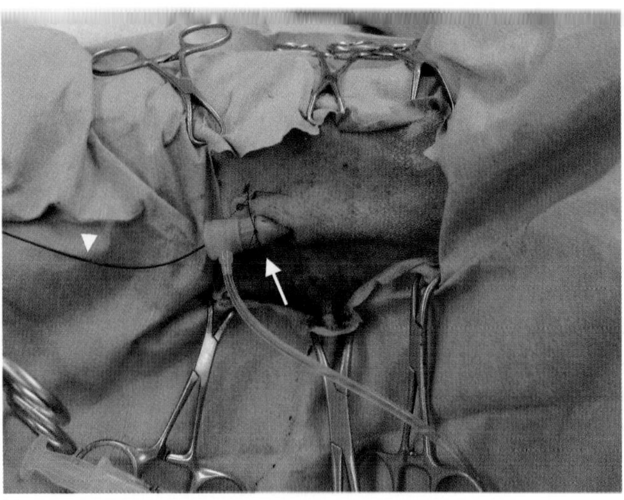

B

Figure 49.4 (A) Following removal of the 18 g over the needle IV catheter a 12 Fr vascular introduction sheath (white arrow) is placed over the 0.035″ angled hydrophilic guide wire (white arrowhead) and inserted into the right jugular vein. (B) Vascular introduction sheath (white arrow), placed via the modified Seldinger technique, over a 0.035″ hydrophilic guide wire (white arrowhead) in place within the right external jugular vein.

illustrate the caudal most aspect of the obstruction and pressure measurements are performed at this time through the marker catheter[5]. An angiographic determination can be made as to whether the caudal vena cava is being decompressed via the vertebral venous plexus and azygous vein. Digital subtraction angiography will aid in making these determinations. A measurement of the caudal vena cava caudal to the obstruction may be made at this time. Caudal vena cava pressure measurements caudal to the obstruction are recommended and compared to right atrial pressure for additional information concerning starting pressure gradients across the obstruction. If no gradient exists, stenting is unlikely to improve the situation. Marker catheters typically have multiple side holes so catheter placement is important when measuring pressures to ensure the side holes are not spanning the entire obstruction.

3. With this access, endovascular biopsy forceps could be used to acquire samples for histopathology if the obstruction is believed to be endovascular and of neoplastic origin.
4. A second 0.035″ 150–260 cm standard stiffness hydrophilic guide wire[2] is introduced into the cranial vena cava via the introducer in the right jugular or via a separate introducer in the left jugular vein or femoral vein. Dual jugular sheaths may be avoided if hypercoagulability is a concern in this patient. If a second sheath is necessary, the caudal sheath is used for caval access and the cranial sheath for hepatic vein access. A 4–5 Fr Berenstein[4] catheter can be used to help direct the guide wire into the left (preferred) or other hepatic vein and the Berenstein catheter is then advanced over it. Pressure measurements and angiography are performed at this time and the diameter of the hepatic vein is determined. Left hepatic vein pressure is compared to right atrial pressure to help support the diagnosis of obstruction. The marker catheter in the vena cava can be used for calibration of measurement instruments (Figure 49.5A).
5. Concurrent angiograms of both the caudal vena cava caudal to the obstruction and the left hepatic vein will illustrate the exact anatomy and length of the obstruction. Simultaneous injection through the jugular sheath can often help delineate the cranial aspect of the obstruction.
6. In cases of Budd–Chiari syndrome, multiple hepatic veins and the caudal vena cava are commonly obstructed. If there is no clinical evidence of caudal vena cava obstruction (swollen hindlimbs) because it is being successfully decompressed via the vertebral venous plexus to the azygous vein, it is likely only necessary to restore patency to a single hepatic vein to provide resolution of clinical signs. A stent is ideally placed in the left hepatic vein, which is the largest hepatic vein and has a gentle curve where it enters the caudal vena cava, thus preventing stent kinking. If there is clinical evidence of both caval and hepatic venous obstruction, then restoration of patency to a hepatic vein and the caudal vena cava is indicated. Concurrent deployment of both

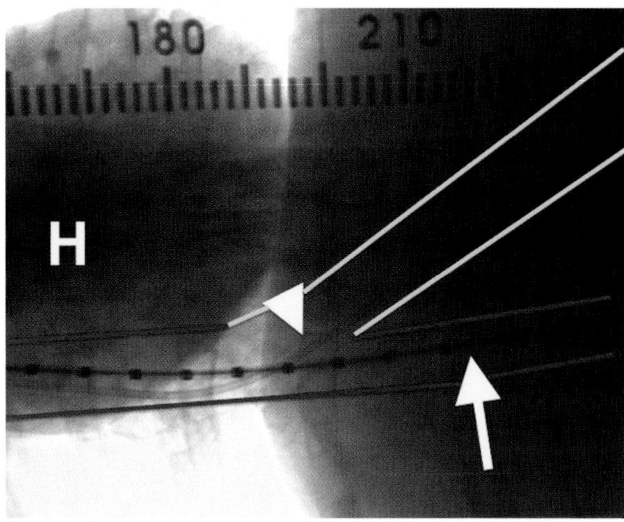

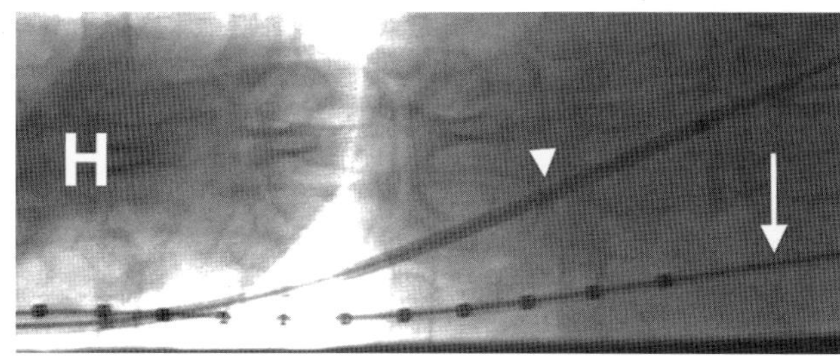

Figure 49.5 Fluoroscopic images during endovascular stent placement with the dog placed in dorsal recumbency. Cranial is to the left and caudal to the right. (A) The caudal vena cava is highlighted in red and the left hepatic vein in yellow. A marker catheter is present within the caudal vena cava (white arrow) and a Berenstein catheter has been advanced from the caudal vena cava into the left hepatic vein (white arrowhead). The heart is labeled H. (B) The marker catheter remains in place within the caudal vena cava (white arrow). A 0.035″ × 260 cm floppy-tip PTFE guide wire has been advanced through the Berenstein catheter into the left hepatic vein and the Berenstein catheter has been removed and exchanged for a stent delivery system (white arrowhead).

stents is necessary in this "kissing stent" scenario and stent diameter should be chosen anticipating two stents sharing a single lumen (caudal vena cava in this case).

7. Stent deployment is usually performed over 0.035″ × 260 cm floppy-tip polytetrafluoroethylene (PTFE) guide wires[6] to provide stability and enough length for the delivery system to fit over it. Sometimes a Rosen wire[7] (short tight curled end) is preferred for the hepatic vein due to the limited "running room" beyond the obstruction; this wire provides stiffness up to the tight curl which prevents distal damage/penetration into the liver parenchyma. The Berenstein catheter in the left hepatic vein is removed over the PTFE guide wire and is exchanged for a stent delivery system (Figure 49.5B). If caval patency is also needed, the same can be performed in the vena cava.
8. Positioning of the delivery system(s) is confirmed by repeat venography prior to deployment. This can be performed through the delivery system(s).
9. The stent(s) are then deployed under fluoroscopic guidance (Figure 49.6 and Figure 49.7). If two stents are being used they are deployed simultaneously and allowed to engage at the vascular confluence thus providing patency of both vessels. The delivery system(s) are then removed over the guide wires.

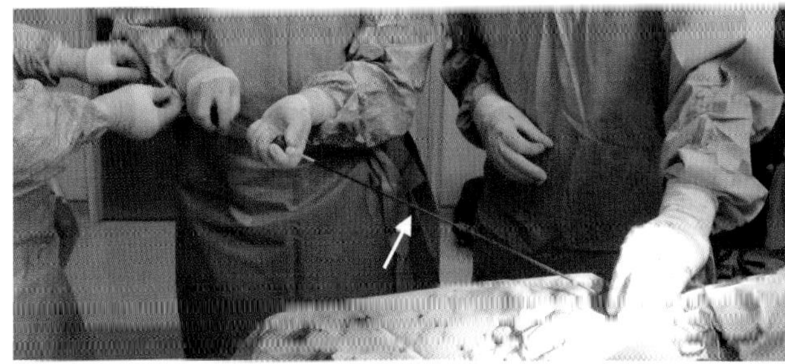

Figure 49.6 Endovascular stent deployment. The stent delivery system (white arrow) is placed over a 0.035″ PTFE guide wire.

10. Catheters for angiography (Berenstein[4], marker[5]) are then advanced over the guide wires to perform caudal vena cava and hepatic venous angiography to illustrate resolution of the obstruction, measure post-stent deployment pressures, and to allow the placement of an angioplasty balloon if additional stent expansion is desired (uncommon).
11. The jugular introducer sheath(s) are removed or exchanged for smaller standard venous access catheters. When large vascular sheaths are utilized, exchanging for a smaller device that may be removed 12 hours later may minimize the chance for hemorrhage. Placement of a purse-string suture at the insertion site and use of a light wrap over the neck will also help minimize the likelihood of hemorrhage.

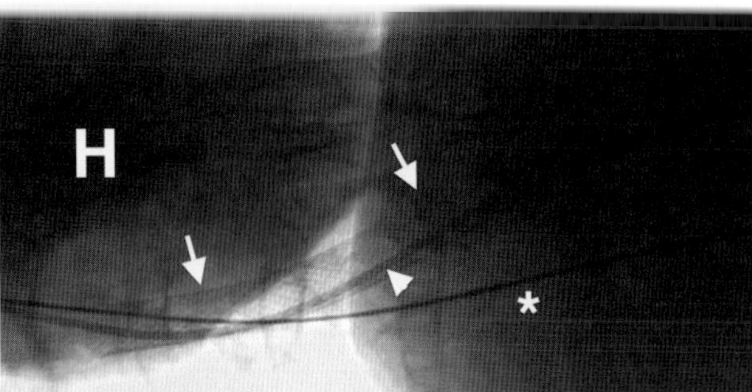

Figure 49.7 Identical positioning to Figure 49.5. An endovascular stent (white arrow) has been deployed within the left hepatic vein extending into the caudal vena cava. The stent delivery system remains in place within the vessel (white arrowhead) and a 0.035″ angled hydrophilic guide wire (asterisk) remains in place within the caudal vena cava.

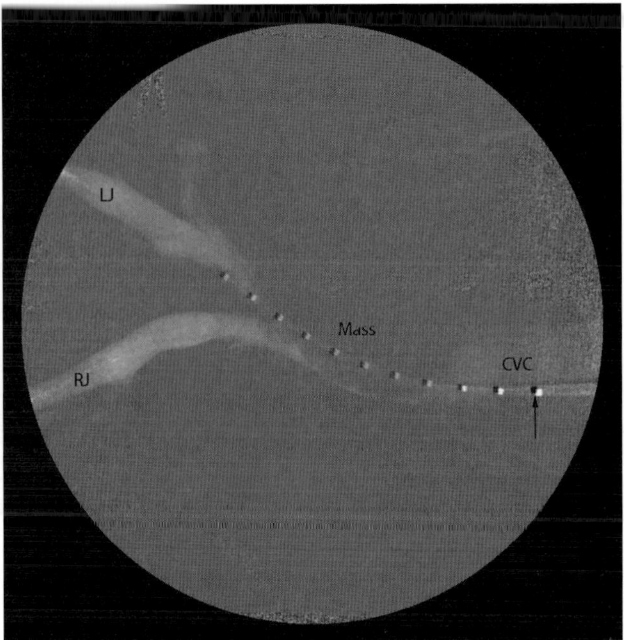

Figure 49.8 Ventrodorsal image from digital subtraction angiogram of a dog with cranial vena cava syndrome due to a large mass (Mass) located at the confluence of the jugular veins. Cranial is to the left of the image and caudal is to the right. Angiography was performed via bilateral femoral vein access and a marker catheter (arrow) has been advanced into the left jugular vein (LJ) while a Berenstein catheter is advanced into the right jugular vein (RJ). The cranial vena cava (CVC) is patent beyond the mass.

Cranial Vena Cava Syndrome

Avoid the use of forelimb peripheral catheters for anesthesia in these patients as venous return is impaired. Draping and preparation should be performed to permit aseptic access to all locations (bilateral jugular veins and bilateral femoral veins). In contrast to endovascular management of Budd–Chiari syndrome, the femoral vein(s) are the logical access sites for the endovascular management of cranial vena cava syndrome. Jugular venous access may be undesirable for multiple reasons. Cervical edema may make jugular venous access challenging although these obstacles may be mitigated via ultrasound guided vascular access. High jugular venous pressures may potentiate hemorrhage. The potential involvement of the external jugular veins in the underling pathologic process coupled with the proximity of the access site to the pathology in the cranial vena cava will create additional challenges. Additionally, femoral venous access allows the operator to distance him or herself from the source of the ionizing radiation (fluoroscope).

If cross-sectional imaging (CTA) suggests there is a distance of 1–2 cm between the confluence of the jugular veins and the obstructive lesion, unilateral femoral venous access may be all that is required as only a cranial vena cava stent will be required. The 1–2 cm between the confluence of the jugular veins and the obstructive lesion will serve as the "landing zone" for the cranial aspect of the stent. However, if the obstruction extends to, or into the jugular veins (Figure 49.8), then bilateral access will most likely be required to allow for concurrent angiography of both jugular veins and concurrent deployment of stents extending from both jugular veins to a location caudal to the obstruction. Alternatively, introduction of one large, or two smaller introducers into a single femoral vein may also accomplish this goal. A description of the technique for concurrent deployment of two stents that extend from the jugular veins to span the obstruction and terminate just outside the right atrium is detailed below.

1. Femoral vein access may be performed either percutaneously (using the modified Seldinger technique as described above) or via surgical cutdown (preferred) for the placement of vascular sheath introducers. See Chapter 44.
2. 0.035″ standard stiffness, angled tip, hydrophilic guide wires are introduced up the femoral veins, into the caudal vena cava, through the right atrium, and negotiated past the obstruction. Use of exchange length guide wires (260 cm) may be necessary in a large-breed dog. Use of a Berenstein catheter may help direct the guide wires beyond the obstruction. This maneuver will result in guide wire access to both jugular veins.

3. The Berenstein catheter is advanced into one jugular vein for angiography and jugular vein pressure determination.
4. A marker catheter is advanced over the other guide wire into the opposite jugular vein. The marker catheter will be used for calibration of measurement instruments and will facilitate angiography of one jugular vein and the cranial vena cava. It will also allow for jugular vein pressure determination (Figure 49.8). Marker catheters typically have multiple side holes so catheter placement is important when measuring pressures to ensure the side holes are not spanning the entire obstruction.
5. The guide wires are removed and angiography is performed through both catheters to illustrate the exact location of the obstruction. Digital subtraction angiography is used to illustrate the obstruction with greater detail (Figure 49.8). Bilateral jugular vein pressures are determined and compared to right atrial pressure.
6. The diameter of the normal jugular vein adjacent to the obstruction is determined bilaterally and stents are chosen that are 10–20% greater than this diameter. The distance from a point approximately 1–2 cm cranial to the obstruction to a point 1–2 cm caudal to the obstruction is determined in order to choose an appropriate stent length. Laser-cut stents can be precisely deployed as they do not foreshorten, and are strongly recommended for this type of intervention.
7. 0.035″ floppy-tip PTFE wires (180–260 cm) are advanced through the catheters utilized for angiography as described in point (5) and the catheters are removed.
8. The stent delivery systems are advanced over the PTFE wires into each jugular vein and are deployed concurrently across the obstruction (Figure 49.9).
9. Repeat angiography and jugular vein pressure measurement may be performed via the stent delivery systems. Alternatively, the stent delivery systems may be removed over the PTFE guide wires and exchanged for the aforementioned Berenstein catheter and marker catheter as described in point (5). Angiography and pressure measurement will demonstrate resolution of cranial vena cava obstruction (Figure 49.10).
10. If percutaneous access was performed, the femoral vein introducer sheaths are removed and direct pressure is applied to the insertion sites for 15–20 min. If access was performed via cutdown, repair or sacrifice of the vessel is performed and the cutdown site is closed routinely. Post-procedural radiographs are performed (Figure 49.11).

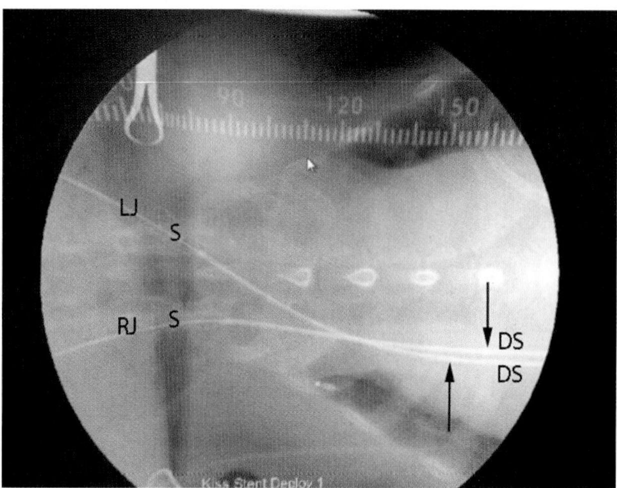

Figure 49.9 Ventrodorsal image illustrating stent deployment in the dog from Image 8. Note that the stent delivery (DS) systems and partially deployed stents (S) extend from positions in the jugular veins (RJ and LJ) cranial to the obstructing mass to one 1–2 cm caudal to it. Arrows illustrate the caudal margin of the laser-cut-stent still within the delivery system (DS).

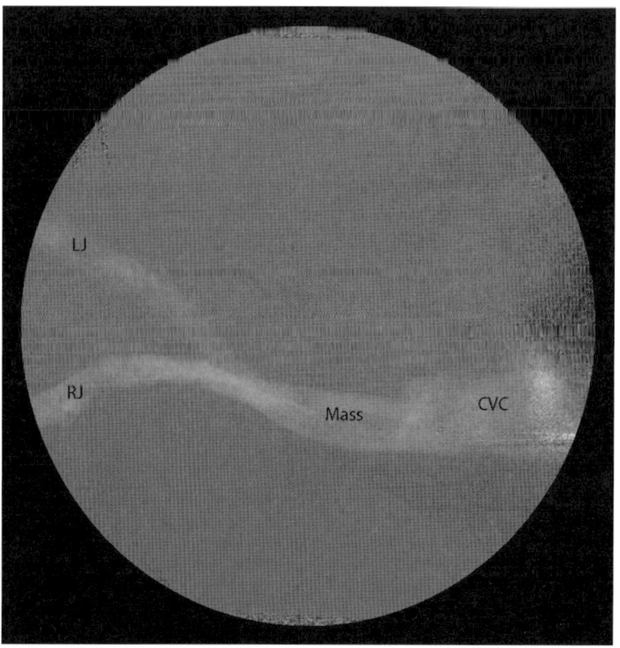

Figure 49.10 Ventrodorsal image from digital subtraction angiogram of a dog with cranial vena cava syndrome due to a large mass (Mass) located at the confluence of the jugular veins. Cranial is to the left of the image and caudal is to the right. Stents have been deployed to span the length of the mass and thus decompress the cranial venous drainage.

Follow-Up

Orthogonal radiographs are performed immediately following the procedure to provide simple, repeatable monitoring of stent location. Animals usually remain

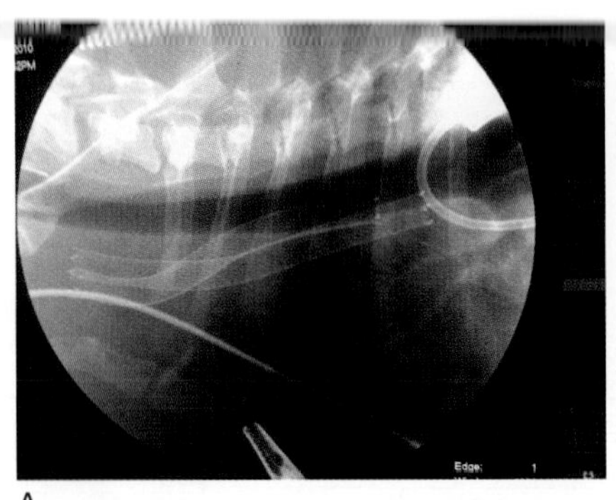
A

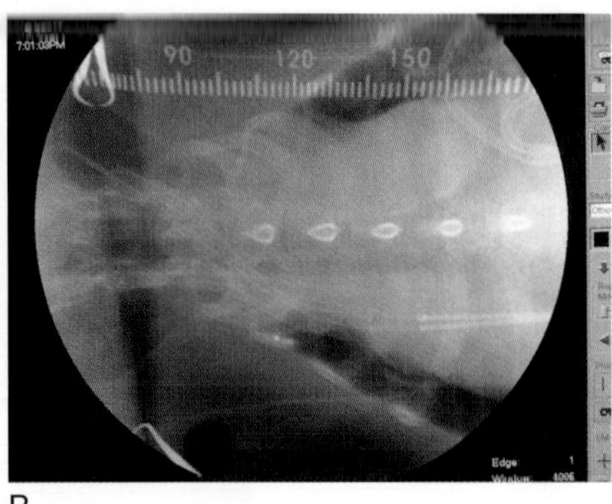
B

Figure 49.11 (A, B) Lateral and ventrodorsal radiographs of the dog in Figure 49.8–Figure 49.10, illustrating stents spanning a mass located at the confluence of the jugular veins.

hospitalized for approximately 24 hours. Follow-up therapy is dictated by the health of the animal and the underlying disease process. If clinical signs of vascular obstruction recur, radiographs, CT angiography, or selective angiography may be needed to determine the reason. Most endovascular stents remain in place for the lifetime of the animal. Inhibitors of hemostasis are often indicated to minimize the chance of thrombosis of the stent(s). Treatment with these medications is dependent on the underlying cause of the venous obstruction.

Notes

1. Braun Medical, Bethlehem, PA.
2. Infiniti Medical LLC, Menlo Park, CA.
3. Infiniti Medical LLC, Menlo Park, CA.
4. Infiniti Medical LLC, Menlo Park, CA.
5. Infiniti Medical LLC, Menlo Park, CA.
6. Infiniti Medical LLC, Menlo Park, CA.
7. Infiniti Medical LLC, Menlo Park, CA.
8. GE Healthcare, Milwaukee, WI.
9. Cook Medical, Bloomington, IN.

References

Cunningham SM, Ames MK, Rush JE, et al (2009) Successful treatment of pacemaker-induced stricture and thrombosis of the cranial vena cava in two dogs by use of anticoagulants and balloon venoplasty. *J Am Vet Med Assoc* 235, 1467–73.

Fine DM, Olivier NE, Walshaw R, et al (1998) Surgical correction of a late-onset Budd-Chiari like syndrome in a dog. *J Am Vet Med Assoc* 212, 835–7.

Haskal ZJ, Dumbleton SA, and Holt DE (1999) Percutaenous treatment of caval obstruction and Budd-Chiari syndrome in a cat. *J Vasc Intervent Radiol* 10, 487–9.

Miller MW, Bonagura JD, DiBartola SP, et al (1989) Budd–Chiari like syndrome in two dogs. *J Am Anim Hosp* 25, 277–83.

Palmer KG, King LG, and Van Winkle TJ (1998) Clinical manifestations and associated disease syndromes in dogs with cranial vena cava thrombosis: 17 cases (1989–1996). *J Am Vet Med Assoc* 231, 200–24.

Rollois M, Ruel Y, and Besso JG (2003) Passive liver congestion associated with caudal vena cava compression due to oesophageal leiomyoma. *J Small Anim Pract* 44, 460–3.

Schlicksup M, Weisse C, Berent A, et al (2009) Use of endovascular stents in three dogs with Budd–Chiari syndrome. *J Am Vet Med Assoc* 235, 544–50.

Whelan, MF, O'Toole TE, Carlson KR, et al (2007) Budd–Chiari like syndrome in a dog with a chondrosarcoma of the thoracic wall. *J Vet Emerg Crit Care* 17, 175–8.

Suggested Reading

Phillips H and Aronosn L (2012) Vascular surgery. In: *Veterinary Surgery Small Animal* (Tobias KM and Johnston SA, eds). Elsevier Saunders, St. Louis, MO, pp 1854–70.

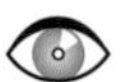
Video clips to accompany this chapter can be found in the online material at **www.wiley.com/go/weisse/vet-image-guided-interventions**

CHAPTER FIFTY

Cisterna Chyli and Thoracic Duct Glue Embolization

Ameet Singh

Department of Clinical Studies, Ontario Veterinary College, University of Guelph, Guelph, Ontario, Canada

Background

A variety of treatments for naturally occurring, idiopathic chylothorax in animals have been reported, yet evidenced-based recommendations are lacking in the veterinary literature. Specific treatment is oriented towards an underlying cause if one is discovered. Conservative therapy in cases of idiopathic chylothorax, consisting of intermittent pleural evacuation, ± low fat diet, and neutraceutical therapy, is unlikely to resolve this condition. Thoracic duct ligation, pericardectomy, ± cisterna chyli ablation are the procedures most frequently performed for the management of idiopathic chylothorax, often requiring one or two intercostal thoracotomy approaches and a celiotomy. Thoracoscopic thoracic duct ligation and pericardectomy with cisterna chyli ablation have been recently described as minimally invasive alternatives to open surgical procedures.

Glue embolization of the cisterna chyli and thoracic duct via percutaneous puncture using fluoroscopic guidance has been described for treatment of traumatic and non-traumatic chylothorax in humans, and has gained popularity over thoracic duct ligation because of its minimally invasive approach. A similar percutaneous technique has been described in dogs in an experimental study. Glue embolization of the cisterna chyli and thoracic duct via mesenteric lymphatic injection at the time of celiotomy has also been performed in dogs and cats with idiopathic chylothorax. Advantages of cisterna chyli and thoracic duct glue embolization via mesenteric lymphatic injection compared with traditional open surgical techniques are numerous. They include shorter anesthesia and surgery times, technical ease and single cavitary approach potentially resulting in shorter postoperative hospitalization. Furthermore, glue embolization allows for the ability to occlude smaller tributary branches of the thoracic duct that cannot not be easily visualized otherwise. Depending upon visual observation may contribute to persistent or recurrent postoperative chylothorax.

Pericardectomy is currently accepted by most veterinary surgeons as a routine adjunctive procedure to thoracic duct ligation for the treatment of idiopathic chylothorax. Transdiaphragmatic pericardectomy can be performed at the time of celiotomy for cisterna chyli and thoracic duct glue embolization, if desired.

Previous reports of cisterna chyli and thoracic duct embolization in dogs have used cyanoacrylate glue as an embolic agent. Limitations with this agent include rapid, unpredictable polymerization time and an exothermic polymerization reaction. Addition of a specific radiopaque contrast medium delays cyanoacrylate polymerization time in blood and polymerization ceases in the presence of 5% dextrose. A non-adhesive, liquid embolic agent (Onyx™, ev3 Endovascular Co., Irvine, CA, USA) has been used successfully in humans and dogs for cisterna chyli and thoracic duct embolization. An advantageous feature of this novel agent is its cohesive property, which prevents rapid polymerization. This allows for physical manipulation of the embolus under fluoroscopic guidance by controlled injection and reduces the risk of the catheter being glued within the lymphatic vessel.

Patient Preparation

Both dogs and cats presenting with idiopathic chylothorax are candidates for cisterna chyli and thoracic duct glue embolization. This technique may be used as

Veterinary Image-Guided Interventions, First Edition. Edited by Chick Weisse and Allyson Berent.

Companion website: www.wiley.com/go/weisse/vet-image-guided-interventions

the initial surgical procedure or in patients in which other techniques (e.g., thoracic duct ligation and pericardectomy) have failed to resolve chylothorax. Chronic cases of chylothorax can have severe metabolic and nutritional derangements that should be corrected prior to undertaking general anesthesia.

Lymphangiography is a helpful step prior to performing cisterna chyli and thoracic duct glue embolization as it provides the surgeon with relevant lymphatic anatomy (see Chapter 43 for further details). In order to dilate and improve visualization of mesenteric lymphatic vessels, corn oil or heavy cream (5–10 ml/kg) (given every hour prior to induction of general anesthesia initiated 3–4 hours preoperatively) can be fed to the patient preoperatively.

Potential Risks/Complications/Expected Outcomes

Technical challenges can occur relating to the ability to visualize and/or catheterize efferent mesenteric lymphatic vessels and catheter dislodgement. With experience, identification of efferent lymphatics in the mesoduodenum will become routine as they are a predictable anatomical finding in the cranial abdomen. Feeding patients triglyceride-laden meals preoperatively will result in lymphatic vessel dilation and improved visualization.

The risk of greatest concern when performing cisterna chyli and thoracic duct glue embolization is inadvertent flow of the glue embolus into the venous system at the lymphaticovenous anastomosis in the cranial thorax (Figure 50.1). If this occurs intraoperatively, the anesthetist should be notified immediately, as deleterious consequences can occur. The glue embolus can remain within the central venous system and remain inconsequential to the patient or travel to the pulmonary circulation. Should the embolus lodge within the pulmonary arterial system, depending on its extent and location, life-threatening decompensation under general anesthesia may occur requiring advanced cardiovascular support. However, many pulmonary thromboemboli in dogs are subclinical in nature. Patients in which inadvertent cranial flow of the glue embolus into the venous/pulmonary system occurs should be recovered in the intensive care unit

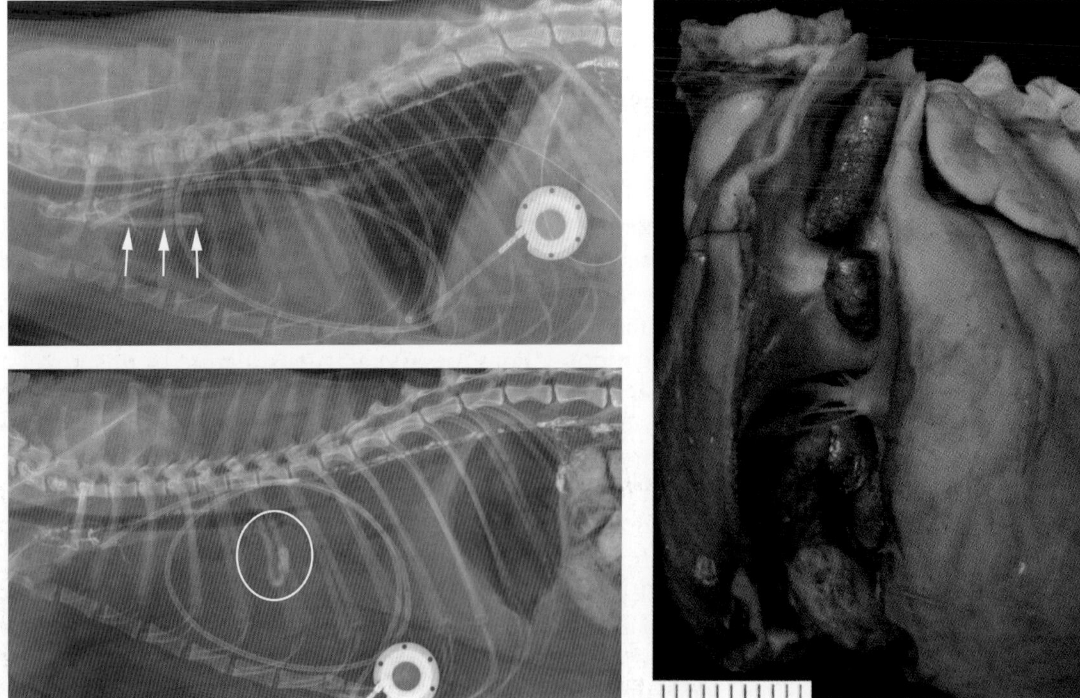

Figure 50.1 Thoracic radiographs in a cat post-cisterna chyli and thoracic duct glue embolization. (A) Immediate postoperative view demonstrating inadvertent migration of the embolic mixture of cyanoacrylate glue and aqueous contrast medium into the cranial vena cava (arrows). (B) 20 days postoperatively. The embolic mixture has migrated into the pulmonary arterial system leading to acute death. (C) Post-mortem image of the cat in A and B demonstrating presence of the embolus in the main pulmonary artery, right atrium and ventricle. Images courtesy of Dr. Chick Weisse.

with appropriate cardiovascular monitoring. Postoperative radiographic evaluation should be performed to determine the location of the radiopaque glue embolus within the central venous or pulmonary circulation. Frequent reevaluation of the patient in the postoperative period is recommended, and the owners should be warned of potential respiratory signs associated with a pulmonary thromboembolic event.

Chyloperitoneum was reported to occur 3 days postoperatively in 1/8 dogs in an experimental study in which cisterna chyli and thoracic duct glue embolization was performed. This complication can occur as a result of abdominal lymphatic vessel obstruction, concurrent abdominal lymphangiectasia, or from chyle leak at the site of mesenteric lymphatic vessel catheterization. Spontaneous resolution of chyloperitoneum commonly occurs as chyle can be reabsorbed through the large surface area of the peritoneum during the time that new lymphaticovenous anastomoses are forming. Histopathological evaluation of the jejunum at 6 weeks and 6 months post cisterna chyli and thoracic duct embolization in normal dogs revealed only mild dilation of lacteals. This finding indicates cisterna chyli and thoracic duct embolization in normal dogs does not lead to severe intestinal abnormalities in the post-operative period. Delayed complications in humans undergoing cisterna chyli and thoracic duct embolization have been reported and are non-specific in nature including lower limb edema and diarrhea.

As with other surgical techniques for chylothorax, persistent (chylous or non-chylous) effusion is a potential occurrence postoperatively. Appropriate owner education should be performed prior to undertaking surgical intervention. It has been suggested that persistent chylothorax following thoracic duct ligation is as result of incomplete occlusion of all thoracic duct branches, allowing chyle to flow into the thoracic cavity and subsequently leak into the pleural space. Delayed recurrence of chylothorax can occur >1 year postoperatively and a common finding at time of lymphangiography is collateral lymphatic vessel development around the thoracic duct ligation site, which allows for recurrent chyle leak into the pleural space. It has been suggested that collateral vessel development is a result of lymphatic hypertension within the cisterna chyli. Based on these findings, preventing chyle flow into the thoracic cavity by occluding the cisterna chyli, through embolization or ablation techniques, should theoretically result in improved success for resolution of idiopathic chylothorax. Prospective data from a large number of patients undergoing cisterna chyli and thoracic duct glue embolization for the treatment of naturally occurring, idiopathic chylothorax in veterinary medicine is required to make additional evidence-based recommendations.

Equipment List

- Selection of over-the-needle vascular catheters (22–24 gauge)
- Extension set connected to a three-way stopcock
- Cyanoacrylate glue (Vetbond Tissue Adhesive, n-butyl cyanoacrylate, 3M Health Care, St. Paul, MN, USA)
- Lipiodol (480 mg I/ml, Guerbet, Bloomington, IN, USA)
- Iodinated, nonionic, aqueous contrast agent (e.g. Iohexol (350mgI/ml), GE Healthcare Canada, Inc., Mississauga, ON, Canada)
- Sterile saline
- 5% dextrose in water solution
- Intraoperative fluoroscopy with digital subtraction capabilities.

Procedure

Routine techniques are used to perform an exploratory celiotomy and all abdominal structures are thoroughly examined. The mesoduodenum and duodenum are retracted medially and the caudate process of the caudate live lobe retracted cranio-laterally to expose efferent mesenteric lymphatic vessels (Figure 50.2). The efferent lymphatics are larger than the afferents, and do not have lymph nodes preventing glue flow to the cisterna chyli. Depending on whether preoperative oil or heavy cream feeding was used, the lymphatic vessels will appear clear (Figure 50.2A) or milky white (Figure 50.2B). Manual retraction is then optimized to allow for unobstructed and direct catheterization of the efferent lymphatic vessel using an over-the-needle catheter (24 gauge, ¾ inch most often). The catheter is sutured in place and an extension set primed with iodinated contrast medium attached (Figure 50.3). Intraoperative fluoroscopic equipment is maneuvered into place and mesenteric lymphangiography performed (Figure 50.4). The volume injected to fill the cisterna chyli and thoracic duct should be recorded to prevent overfilling when using the glue mixture.

Once cisterna chyli and thoracic duct anatomy have been verified, the embolization procedure can be performed. A three-way-stopcock is connected to the extension set. A syringe containing 5% dextrose is attached to one port and a 6 ml syringe containing 6 ml of a 1:2.5 ratio of cyanoacrylate:lipiodol mixture

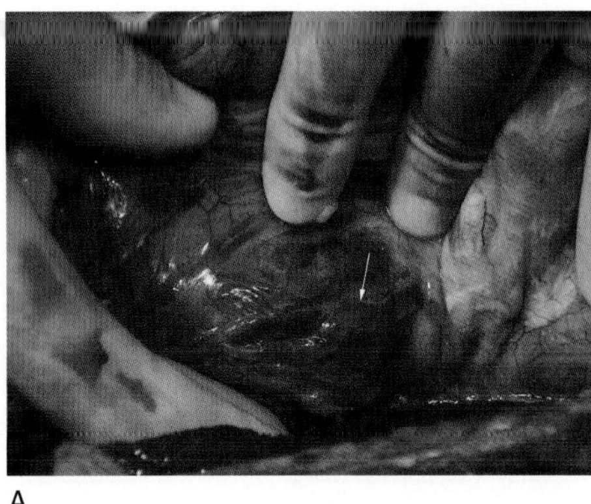

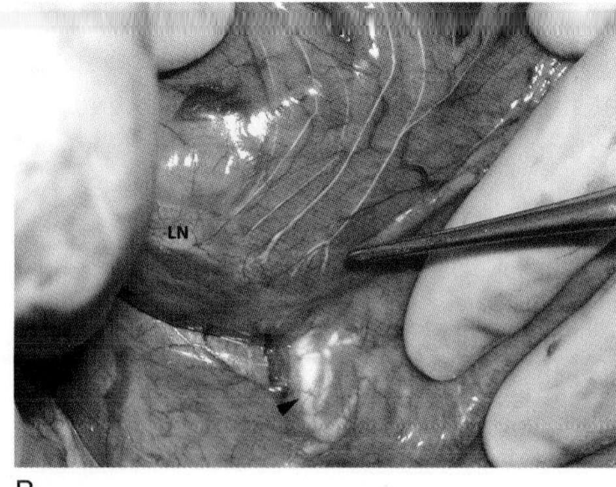

Figure 50.2 Intraoperative view of mesenteric lymphatic vessels in the mesoduodenum readily apparent with the duodenum retracted medially. (cranial aspect to the left, caudal to the right). (A) Large, efferent lymphatic vessel suitable for catheterization is apparent (arrow). (B) Following preoperative feeding of a triglyceride laden meal, small, milky white, multiple afferent lymphatics are seen coursing towards a lymph node (LN) along with larger, dilated efferent lymphatics (arrowhead). Images courtesy of Dr. Chick Weisse.

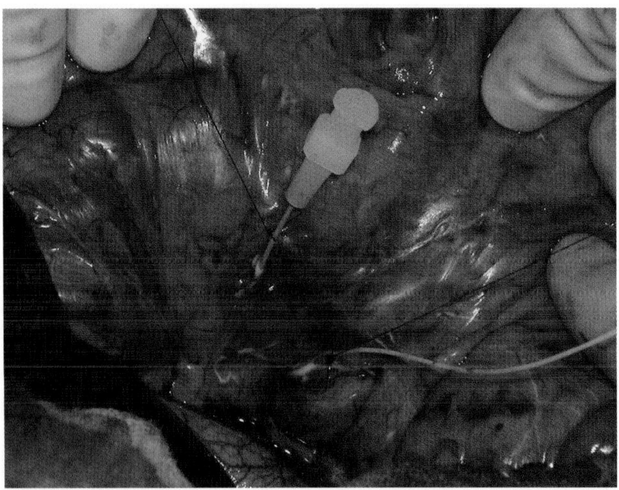

Figure 50.3 Intra-operative view of two separate catheterized efferent mesenteric lymphatic vessels. Image courtesy of Dr. Chick Weisse.

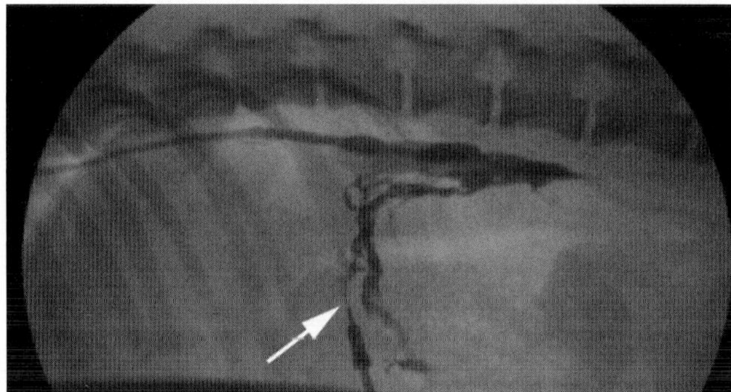

Figure 50.4 Fluoroscopic mesenteric lymphangiography delineating the cisterna chyli and thoracic duct. Aqueous contrast medium is injected into a catheterized efferent mesenteric lymphatic vessel (arrow).

connected to the second port. The catheter is flushed with 5% dextrose in water to remove any remaining contrast form the cisterna chyli and thoracic duct, which could lead to premature glue polymerization. Prior to injection of the embolic mixture, confirm the anesthetist is maintaining a positive pressure breath hold to reduce forward flow in the thoracic duct. With fluoroscopic guidance, 2–4 ml (or a similar volume to previously injected during the lymphangiogram) of the solution is injected over the course of 3–5 seconds. Fluoroscopic guidance is pivotal in determining the volume required as embolus location within the cisterna chyli and thoracic duct can be directly visualized. Care must be taken to prevent rapid craniad movement of the glue embolus. In an experimental study in dogs (mean weight 29.75 kg), a mean volume of 2.8 ml was required in order to embolize the cisterna chyli and thoracic duct approximately to the level of the mid-thoracic vertebrae. This volume is only to be used as a guide, since large variability exists in the amount of embolic agent required among patients. Maintaining breath hold during positive pressure ventilation for 2–3 seconds following injection can be used to prevent further cranial flow of the glue mixture and allow polymerization time to occur.

Following fluoroscopic confirmation of appropriate embolus location within the cisterna chyli and thoracic duct, the catheter is flushed with 0.25–0.5 ml 5% dextrose in water. A repeat lymphangiogram is performed to document complete occlusion. Repeat glue embolization can be performed if forward flow is identified. Otherwise, the catheter is removed from the efferent lymphatic vessel that is ligated both proximal and distal to the puncture site (Figure 50.5). These steps must be performed in an efficient and organized manner as timely removal of the catheter is necessary otherwise it can become glued into the lymphatic vessel.

The celiotomy incision is closed in routine fashion and a method for pleural evacuation (if not already in place) is typically inserted. This author prefers the use of a small-bore, wire-guided chest drain (MILA International Inc, Erlanger, KY, USA) that can be placed using the modified Seldinger technique prior to recovery from anesthesia. A PleuralPort (Norfolk Medical Inc., Skokie, IL, USA) can also be placed either via image guidance or a minimal surgical approach to the thorax. This device has a fenestrated silicone drain that is inserted into the pleural space and is connected to a titanium port that is placed in the subcutaneous tissues, which can be aspirated with a non-coring Huber needle. Placement of a PleuralPort may allow for faster discharge from hospital as owners can be instructed how to use the port for evacuation of the pleural space at home.

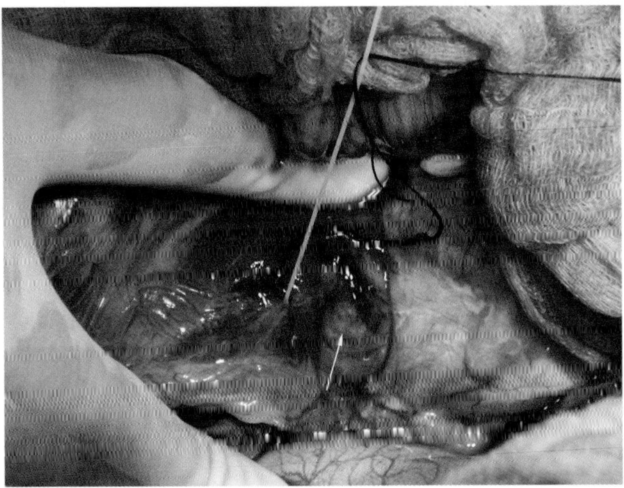

Figure 50.5 Intraoperative view following glue embolization of the cisterna chyli and thoracic duct. The catheter is being pulled from the efferent lymphatic vessel. Cyanoacrylate glue is apparent within the cisterna chyli (arrow). Image courtesy of Dr. Chick Weisse.

Orthogonal postoperative thoracic and abdominal radiographs are performed (Figure 50.6) and the patient recovered in the intensive care unit. Following successful embolization of the cisterna chyli and thoracic duct, chylous effusion typically resolves in <7 days, but serosanguinous effusions can persist longer. Careful monitoring of pleural fluid amounts and consistency should be performed. Hypoproteinemia and fibrosing pleuritis may have developed in cases with persistent, chronic chylothorax. The time to patient discharge depends on the volume and clinical signs related to post-operative chylous effusion. Orthogonal thoracic radiographs are obtained at time of discharge and then at 1, 3, and 6 months postoperatively, and every 6 months thereafter to monitor for pleural effusion. Owners are educated on clinical signs associated with recurrence of pleural effusion.

Suggested Reading

Allman DA, Radlinsky MG, Ralph AG, et al (2010) Thoracoscopic thoracic duct ligation and thoracoscopic pericardectomy for treatment of chylothorax in dogs. *Vet Surg* 39, 21–7

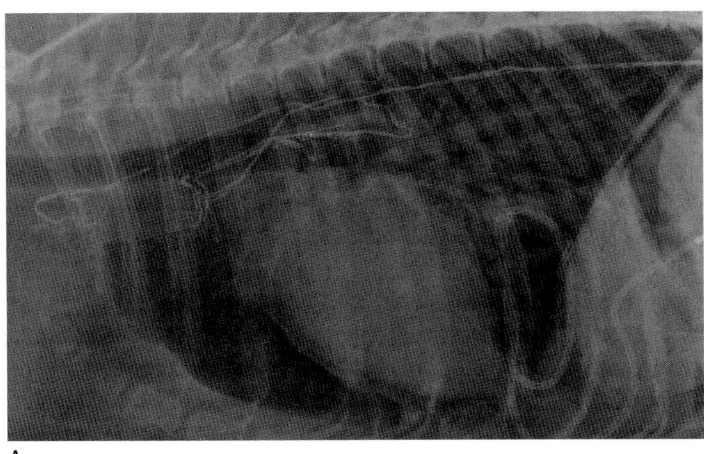

A

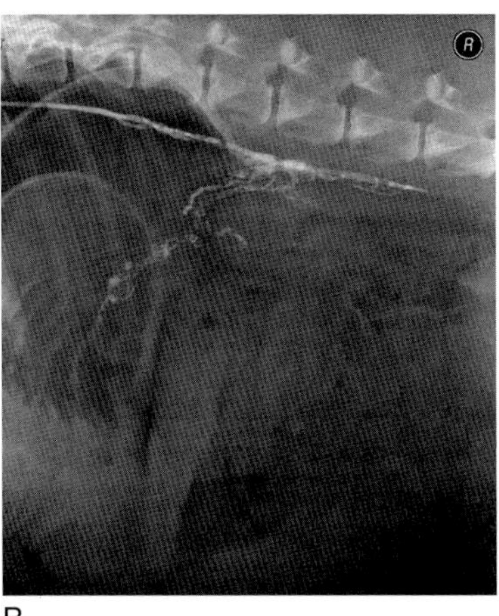

B

Figure 50.6 Lateral thoracic (A) and abdominal (B) radiograph in a dog post-cisterna chyli and thoracic duct glue embolization. The mixture of cyanoacrylate glue and oily contrast medium (Lipiodol) is apparent within the thoracic duct and branches (A) and efferent mesenteric lymphatic vessels and cisterna chyli (B). Images courtesy of Dr. Chick Weisse.

Birchard SJ, Smeak DD, and McLoughlin MA (1998) Treatment of idiopathic chylothorax in dogs and cats. *J Am Vet Med Assoc* 212, 652–657.

Cope C (2004) Management of chylothorax via percutaneous embolization. *Curr Opin Pulm Med* 10, 311–14.

Cromwell LD and Kerber CW (1979) Modification of cyanoacrylate for therapeutic embolization. *Am J Roentgenol* 132, 799–801.

Fossum TW, Jacobs RM, and Birchard SJ (1986) Evaluation of cholesterol and triglyceride concentrations in differentiating chylous and nonchylous pleural effusions in dogs and cats. *J Am Vet Med Assoc* 188, 49–51.

Itkin M, Kucharzcuk JC, Kwak A, et al (2010) Nonoperative thoracic duct embolization for traumatic thoracic duct leak: experience in 109 patients. *J Thorac Cardiovasc Surg* 139, 584–9.

Kunstlinger F, Brunelle F, Chaumont P, et al (1981) Vascular occlusive agents. *Am J Roentgenol* 136, 151–6.

Laslett D, Trerotola SO, and Itkin M (2012) Delayed complications following technical successful thoracic duct embolization. *J Thorac Cardiovasc Surg* 23, 76–9.

Mayhew PD, Culp WT, Mayhew KN, et al (2012) Minimally invasive treatment of idiopathic chylothorax in dogs by thoracoscopic thoracic duct ligation and subphrenic pericardiectomy: 6 cases (2007–2010). *J Am Vet Med Assoc* 241, 904–9.

Nadolski GJ and Itkin M (2012) Thoracic duct embolization for non-traumatic chylous effusion: experience in 34 patients. *Chest* 143, 158–163.

Pardo AD, Bright RM, Walker MA, et al (1989) Transcatheter thoracic duct embolization in the dog. An experimental study. *Vet Surg* 18, 279–85.

Sakals S, Schmiedt CW, and Radlinsky MG (2011) Comparison and description of transdiaphragmatic and abdominal minimally invasive cisterna chyli ablation in dogs. *Vet Surg* 40, 795–801.

Sicard GK, Waller KR, and McAnulty JF (2005) The effect of cisterna chyli ablation combined with thoracic duct ligation on abdominal lymphatic drainage. *Vet Surg* 34, 64–70.

Singh A, Brisson BA, O'Sullivan ML, et al (2012) Feasibility of percutaneous catheterization and embolization of the thoracic duct in dogs. *Am J Vet Res* 72, 1527–34.

Weisse CW, Berent AC, Todd KL, et al (2008) Potential applications of interventional radiology in veterinary medicine. *J Am Vet Med Assoc* 233, 1564–74.

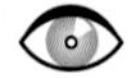

Video clips to accompany this chapter can be found in the online material at **www.wiley.com/go/weisse/vet-image-guided-interventions**

SECTION SEVEN

Cardiac System

Edited by Brian A. Scansen

CHAPTER FIFTY-ONE

Radiographic Cardiac Anatomy

Brian A. Scansen
Department of Veterinary Clinical Sciences, The Ohio State University, Columbus, OH

Introduction

Performing image-guided interventions within the heart and great vessels requires detailed knowledge of thoracic and cardiovascular anatomy. An understanding of thoracic anatomy and image interpretation is important prior to intervention for appropriate diagnosis, planning and equipment selection, as well as during catheterization to verify the intervention is being performed at the correct site and to troubleshoot unexpected findings or complications. This chapter serves as a review of cardiovascular anatomy and provides a framework for the subsequent chapters on specific cardiac pathologies that may require intervention.

Equipment

The basic requirements of an interventional lab have been discussed previously in Chapter 1. However, a few comments regarding fluoroscopic imaging of the heart are pertinent. The thorax is a complex three-dimensional shape with a wide variation in the radiographic opacity of thoracic structures (e.g., air opacity of the lung vs. mineral opacity of the rib cage vs. soft tissue opacity of the heart and vessels). Capturing this complex structure onto a two-dimensional radiograph or live fluoroscopic image leads to superposition of structures and variable attenuation of the radiographic beam. In addition, the heart is a rapidly moving organ with a complex spatial relationship, having chambers that twist around one another. Delineation of cardiovascular anatomy by injection of iodinated contrast can help to visualize specific chambers, but the high rate of blood flow within the beating heart minimizes the time available for contrast visualization and quickly leads to dilution of delivered contrast agents.

The difficulty in evaluating cardiovascular anatomy due to the complex structure of the thorax can be mitigated by review of multiple image planes, selective injection of iodinated contrast material, use of a power injector, and by digital-subtraction angiography (DSA). Many human catheterization laboratories, particularly those that treat congenital heart disease, now employ bi-plane fluoroscopic systems that provide real-time imaging of two orthogonal views to improve anatomic guidance. There is also a new generation of fluoroscopic systems that perform rotational angiography to circumferentially record a single injection from all angles and create a three-dimensional reconstruction of the anatomy. Alternatively, some systems have the capability of importing anatomic landmarks from cross-sectional imaging studies (computed tomography (CT) or magnetic resonance imaging (MRI)) onto the two-dimensional fluoroscopic image to improve guidance during the intervention. Few veterinary catheterization facilities have these capabilities, but most current veterinary interventions can be performed using a portable C-arm fluoroscope that easily rotates the field of view around the thorax to numerous projection angles. The fluoroscopic system chosen should provide high resolution (at least 512 × 512 and optimally a 1024 × 1024 matrix), generate sufficient energy to penetrate the thorax of a large dog, and be capable of displaying and recording fast frame rates (25–30 fps or higher). It is imperative that fast frame rates be employed when cardiac imaging is recorded. The rapid heart rates of dogs and cats, often 50 to 120 bpm or more under general anesthesia, cause contrast filling of the structure of interest to be temporally brief and a frame-by-frame review of a recorded angiographic run is often needed to visualize the anatomy and perform measurements. Fast frame rates prevent the operator from "missing" the lesion during contrast injection into a high-flow organ such as the heart.

Veterinary Image-Guided Interventions, First Edition. Edited by Chick Weisse and Allyson Berent.

Companion website: www.wiley.com/go/weisse/vet-image-guided-interventions

It is generally not possible by hand injection to achieve a sufficiently tight bolus of contrast to optimally opacify a chamber of the heart in medium-sized and larger dogs. Automated power injectors are therefore used that allow the operator to program the volume, flow rate, and pressure of an injection to maximize opacification of the heart or great vessels within one to two cardiac cycles. Importantly, angiographic catheters and high-pressure tubing should be in place if a power injector is used. An end-hole catheter is a poor choice for recording an angiographic study, particularly within the heart, as the full force of the injection is directed through the single end hole and catheter recoil is likely. Additionally, if the end hole is against a vessel wall or the endocardium, a high-pressure injection may damage the vessel or endocardium. The preferred angiographic catheter is the largest diameter possible for the task, of the shortest length possible, and with multiple side holes and a closed or tapered tip – all to maximize flow and minimize vessel trauma. Figure 51.1 shows a selection of angiographic catheters that fulfill these criteria; for intracardiac injections and angiographic studies in large vessels, the author prefers the Berman or pigtail catheter. See Table 51.1 for general guidelines on power injector settings for ventricular injections, noting that whichever catheter is chosen will have unique settings for maximal flow rate and pressure that must be reviewed and not exceeded.

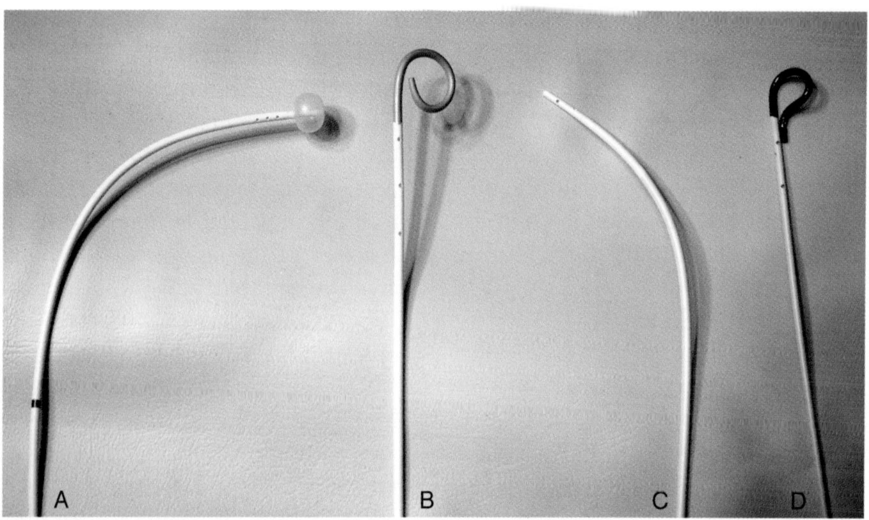

Figure 51.1 Catheters for angiographic injection. In order to maximize flow rate, angiographic catheters should be chosen to have the largest diameter and shortest length for the task. Additionally, catheters with multiple side holes are preferred to a single end hole in order to avoid catheter recoil and minimize endothelial trauma. The Berman catheter (A) is a closed-tip, flow-directed catheter; the pigtail catheter (B) has multiple side holes as well as an end hole allowing it to be delivered over a wire; variations of the pigtail catheter with different configuration of the loop are available, with the Omni catheter (D) shown here; the NIH or Gensini (C) catheter has a tapered distal tip with multiple side holes.

TABLE 51.1

General guidelines for power injector settings during ventriculography in dogs

Parameter	Typical setting
Injection volume	Dependent on anatomic site of injection. For most RV or LV studies, a volume of 1–2 ml/kg is chosen
Flow rate	Varies by catheter chosen; in general, a flow rate is chosen to provide an injection duration comprising 1–2 cardiac cycles (~2 s)
Injection pressure	Varies by catheter chosen, usually between 100 and 1200 PSI for angiographic catheters; in general, choose the lowest pressure that will deliver the desired volume within the desired time
Rate of rise	0.5 to 1 s is generally chosen to prevent recoil of the catheter and to move the tip of the catheter away from the endocardium prior to maximal injection

Note, that maximal injection volumes, flow rates, and pressure settings are specific to the catheter being used and MUST BE VERIFIED prior to each individual injection.

Normal Thoracic Anatomy

Lateral Perspective

Many interventions for cardiovascular disease are performed with the animal positioned in right or left lateral recumbency. Lateral positioning allows the operator to monitor dorsal-ventral and cranial-caudal motion of catheters and wires as they are advanced into the thorax. Right-to-left lateral deflection, however, is less clearly visualized. Figure 51.2 is a representation of the normal cardiac structures superimposed over a lateral thoracic radiograph to indicate their relative position in this projection. Figure 51.3 shows a series of images following injection of iodinated contrast into the cranial vena cava of a normal dog, with the catheter placed at the entrance of the right atrium.

Ventrodorsal Perspective

Although less common than lateral imaging for cardiac intervention, the ventrodorsal projection allows visualization of left-to-right laterality and the cranial-caudal position of catheters introduced into the thorax. The location of catheters or wires in the dorsal-ventral plane, however, is challenging in the ventrodorsal perspective. Figure 51.4 is a representation of the normal cardiac structures superimposed over a ventrodorsal thoracic radiograph to indicate their relative position in this projection. Figure 51.5 shows a series of images following injection of iodinated contrast into the cranial vena cava of a normal dog, highlighting the path of blood flow through right heart and outflow tract, to the pulmonary arteries and lungs, followed by pulmonary venous return to the left atrium and

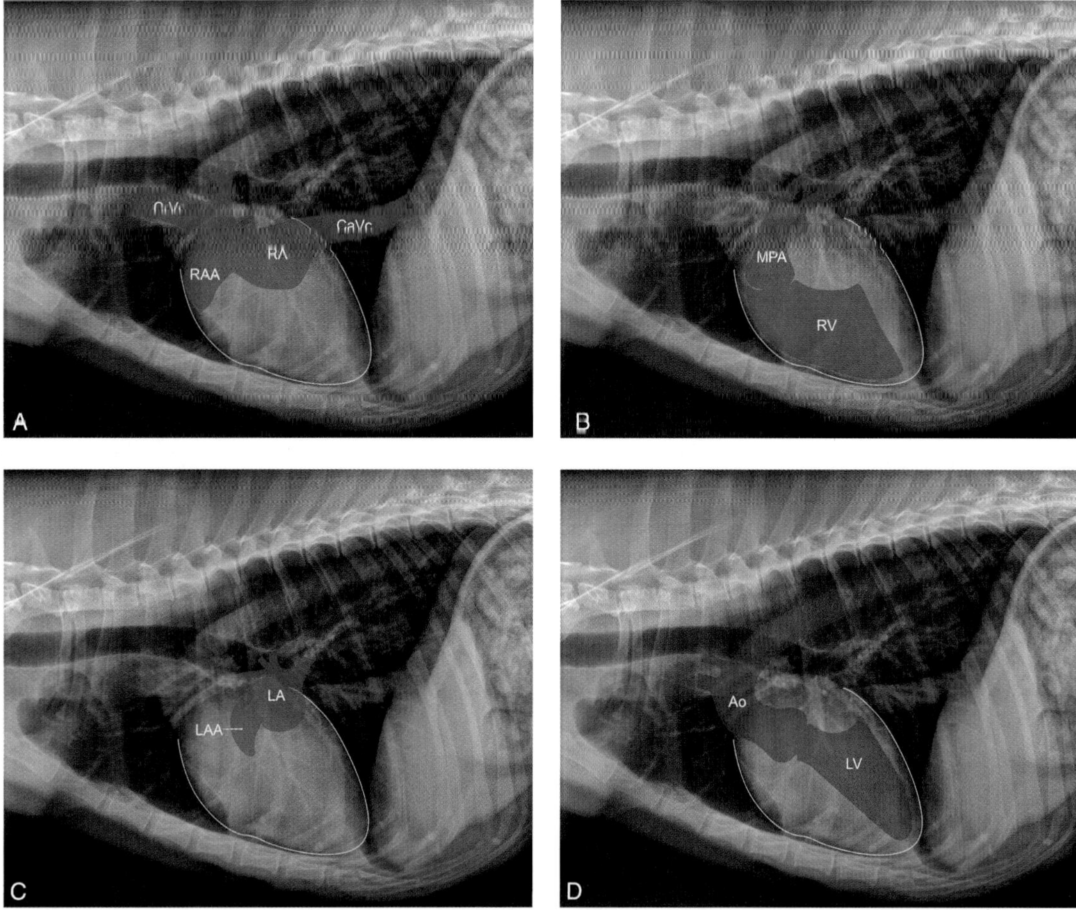

Figure 51.2 A schematic representation of the anatomical relationship between cardiovascular structures on a radiograph as viewed from the lateral perspective. The cardiac silhouette is outlined in yellow and the approximate position of the four cardiac chambers are individually highlighted in each panel. Panel A highlights the relative position of the cranial vena cava (CrVc), caudal vena cava (CaVc), right atrium (RA), and right auricular appendage (RAA). Panel B highlights the right ventricle (RV) and main pulmonary artery (MPA). Panel C highlights the left atrium (LA) and left auricular appendage (LAA). Panel D highlights the left ventricle (LV) and aortic arch (Ao). (Copyright by The Ohio State University.)

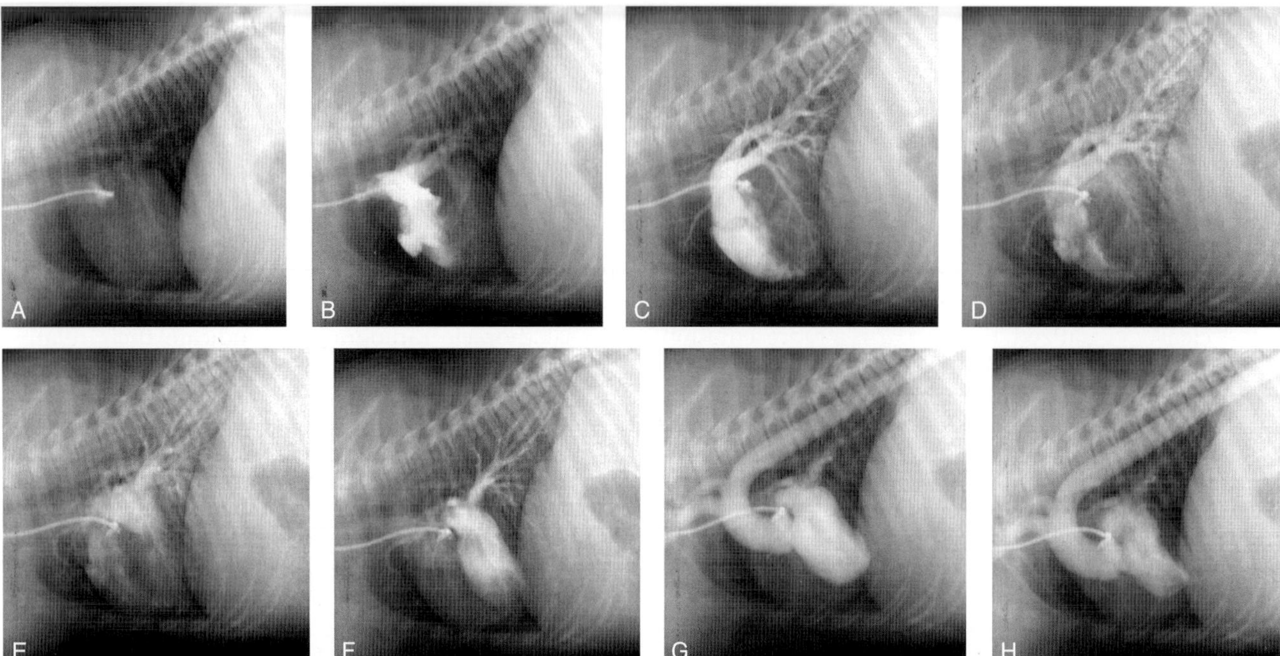

Figure 51.3 Sequential passage of iodinated contrast through the heart and great vessels in a normal dog as viewed from the lateral perspective. The catheter in (A) is positioned at the junction of the cranial vena cava and right atrium and contrast can be visualized entering the right atrium and ventricle (B), the right ventricular outflow tract and pulmonary arterial system (C), the distal pulmonary arteries and lungs (D), before returning in the pulmonary veins to the left atrium (E), and left ventricle (F), and finally being ejected into the aorta and systemic arterial system (G & H). (Courtesy of JW Buchanan.)

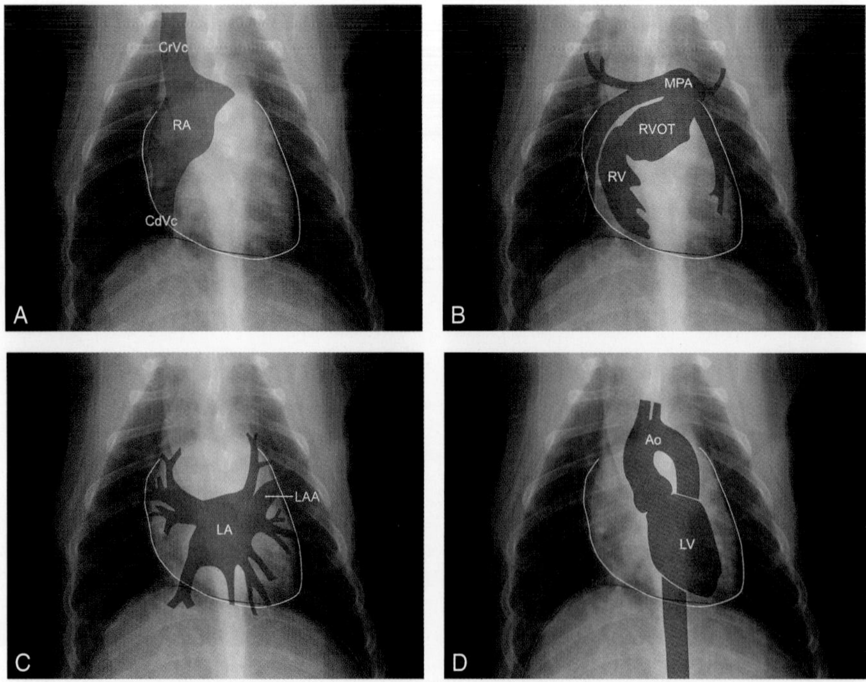

Figure 51.4 A schematic representation of the anatomical relationship between cardiovascular structures on a radiograph as viewed from the ventrodorsal perspective. The cardiac silhouette is outlined in yellow, the diaphragm in orange, and the approximate position of the four cardiac chambers are individually highlighted in each panel. Panel A highlights the relative position of the cranial vena cava (CrVc), caudal vena cava (CaVc), and right atrium (RA). Panel B highlights the right ventricle (RV), right ventricular outflow tract (RVOT), and main pulmonary artery (MPA). Panel C highlights the left atrium (LA) and left atrial appendage (LAA). Panel D highlights the left ventricle (LV) and aorta (Ao). (Copyright by The Ohio State University.)

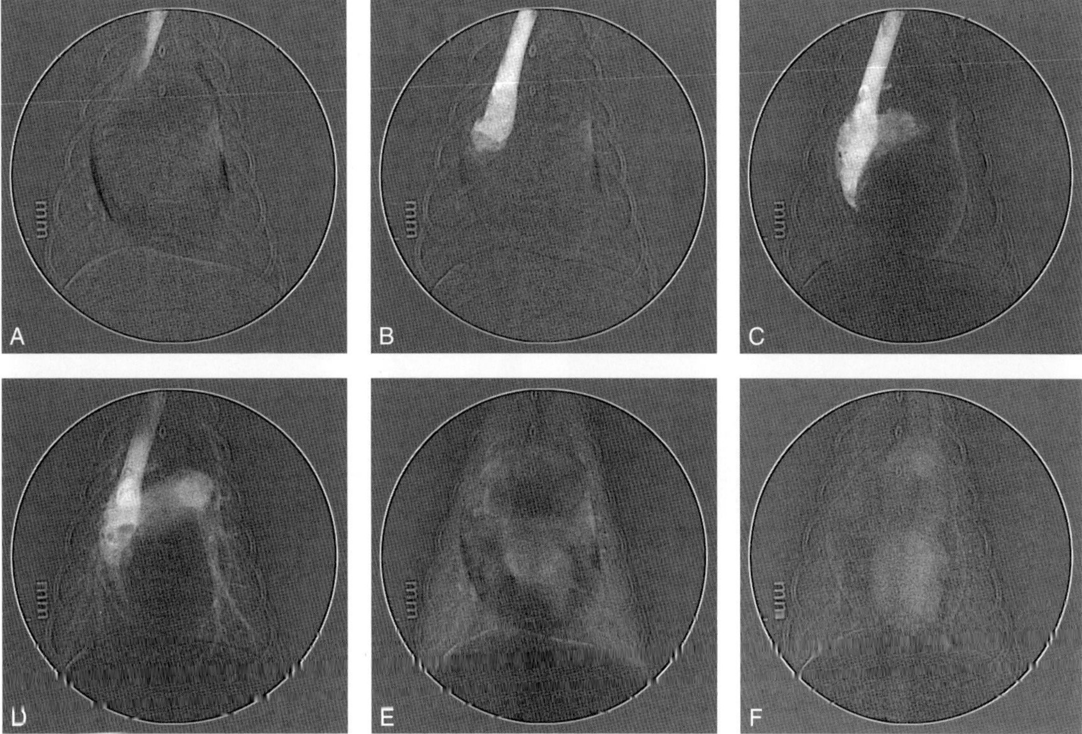

Figure 51.5 Sequential passage of iodinated contrast through the heart and great vessels in a normal dog as viewed from the ventrodorsal perspective and under digital subtraction angiography. The catheter is within the cranial vena cava and the injection of contrast first highlights the cranial vena cava (A); then the right atrium (B); the right ventricle and right ventricular outflow tract (C); followed by the main pulmonary artery and distal pulmonary arterial system (D); the lungs, pulmonary venous system, and left atrium (E); and finally the left ventricle and aorta (F).

ventricle, and finally ejection of the contrast bolus from the left ventricle with opacification of the aorta and cranial branch vessels.

Oblique Perspectives

Several additional imaging planes are used in human medicine to highlight and optimize imaging of cardiac structures. Variations from the traditional lateral or ventrodorsal projection are typically given by an angle, which refers to the position of the image intensifier in relation to the animal's thorax in a ventrodorsal position. Commonly used angulations in human medicine include the right and left anterior obliques (RAO and LAO, respectively) with variable cranial or caudal angulation. Typically, the image intensifier is rotated 30° to the animal's right (RAO) or left (LAO) and a variable 10° to 30° of cranial or caudal angulation may also be employed. Altering the angle of the C-arm can elongate structures (e.g., the left ventricular outflow tract in subaortic stenosis) or provide a more directly perpendicular visualization plane during device deployment (e.g. the atrial septum). These viewing angles have not been standardized in veterinary medicine and are largely operator and case-dependent. In practice, adjusting the angle of the C-arm is most useful to optimize an angiogram for measurement, such as improving visualization of the minimal ductal diameter of a patent ductus arteriosus, or to compensate for suboptimal positioning of the animal while on the table.

Variations From Normal

While an understanding of normal angiographic anatomy is critical to guide intervention, most interventions are undertaken in animals with cardiovascular pathology. As such, structural malformations and chamber remodeling are common and may markedly deviate the expected position of normal structures. Figure 51.6 shows an angiogram from a Chihuahua dog with pulmonary valve stenosis and patent ductus arteriosus; note that the position of the pulmonary valve in this dog is ventrally displaced (adjacent to the sternum) and directed more in a craniocaudal position than the expected dorsoventral position seen in the normal dog of Figure 51.3. Rotation and altered orientation of cardiac structures in this dog were a

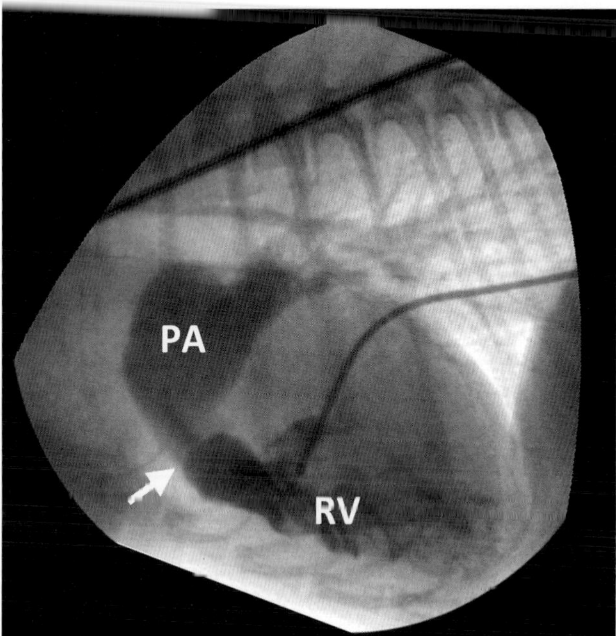

Figure 51.6 Lateral thoracic angiogram from a young Chihuahua dog with both pulmonary valve stenosis and a patent ductus arteriosus, which demonstrates the altered position of normal cardiac structures in the setting of cardiovascular pathology. The pulmonary valve (arrow) is displaced cranially and ventrally in this image (adjacent to the sternum) due to severe dilation of the main pulmonary artery as well as left and right ventricular hypertrophy. PA = main pulmonary artery; RV = right ventricle.

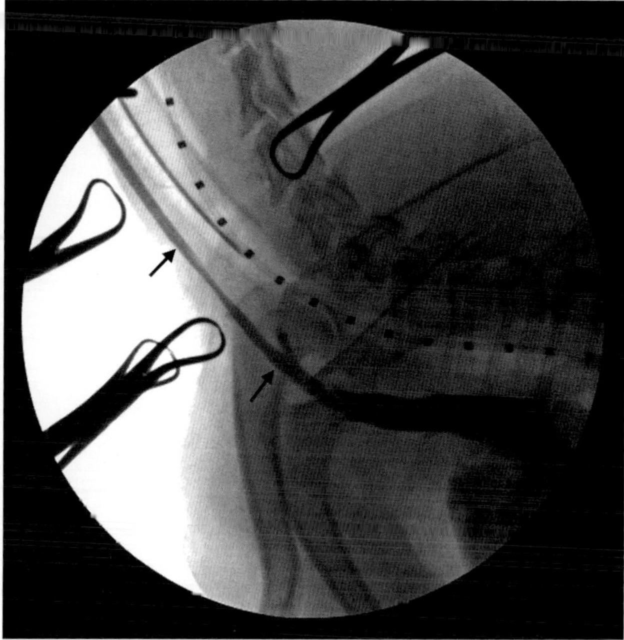

Figure 51.7 Lateral thoracic angiogram of the right external jugular vein and cranial vena cava from a Jack Russell Terrier that had undergone percutaneous catheterization of the same vein 2 months previously. Note the narrowing of the jugular vein throughout the neck (arrows) secondary to prior vascular access, which prevented passage of an appropriately-sized introducer at the time of reintervention.

result of severe dilation of the main pulmonary artery and hypertrophy of the right and left ventricles due to the congenital heart defects.

Just as cardiac pathology can distort the expected position and appearance of cardiovascular structures, prior intervention may also distort normal anatomy. Figure 51.7 provides an example of a dog with narrowing of the right external jugular vein due to percutaneous venous access with a large introducer into that vein 2 months prior. Note that the jugular vein is of much small diameter in this dog than would be expected given the diameter of the cranial vena cava. The venous stenosis in this dog's right jugular vein necessitated that repeat access be obtained in the left external jugular vein to introduce a sheath of sufficient size for further intervention.

In addition to cardiac pathology and prior intervention distorting normal angiographic anatomy, clinically silent anatomic variants may also complicate cardiac intervention. The most commonly encountered anatomic variant relevant to cardiac intervention is the persistent left cranial vena cava. Dogs and cats normally have only a right-sided cranial vena cava. However, when the left anterior cardinal vein fails to regress in these species, a persistent left cranial vena cava is present that is of no clinical consequence. The left cranial vena cava may occur singularly or, more often, both left and right cranial cava are present (Figure 51.8). Buchanan described two types of persistent left cranial vena cava in the dog – complete and incomplete – and the size of a persistent left cranial vena cava is inversely proportional to the size of any co-existent right cranial vena cava. It is important to remember that the left cranial vena cava enters the caudal aspect of the right atrium at the coronary sinus, due to this structure's embryologic origin. The persistent left cranial vena cava generally poses no clinical problem for the animal, although a case report of an incomplete persistent left cranial vena cava in a Brittany spaniel did suggest the possibility of this structure causing megaesophagus if partially atretic. Transpositional venous anomalies, such as the persistent left cranial vena cava, are common in animals with transpositional arterial anomalies such as persistent right aortic arch. A persistent left cranial vena cava carries importance for the interventionalist as left jugular venous access results in an unexpected catheter path. As such, most venous interventions performed

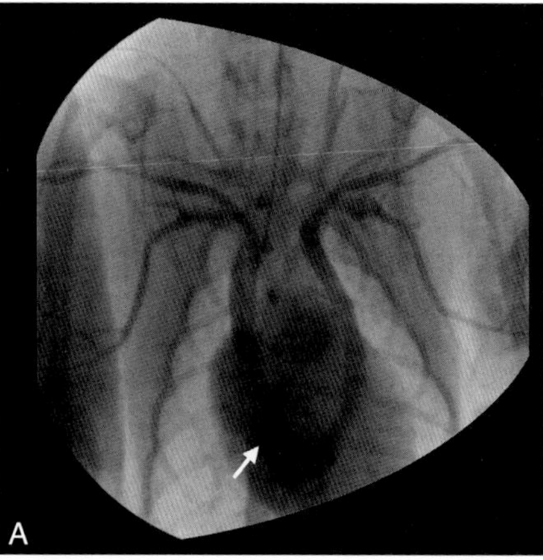

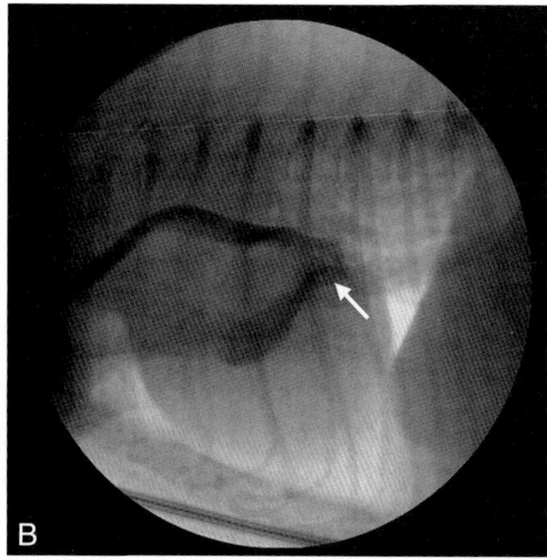

Figure 51.8 Images of persistent left cranial vena cava in the dog. The ventrodorsal projection (A) was made by simultaneous injection of iodinated contrast into both left and right cephalic veins and highlights the separate and comparably sized right and left cranial vena cava. The lateral projection (B) shows selective injection into the left external jugular vein and highlights the caudal communication between the left cranial vena cava and the coronary sinus. In both, note that the entrance of the persistent left cranial vena cava is at the dorsocaudal aspect of the cardiac silhouette at the location of the coronary sinus (arrows).

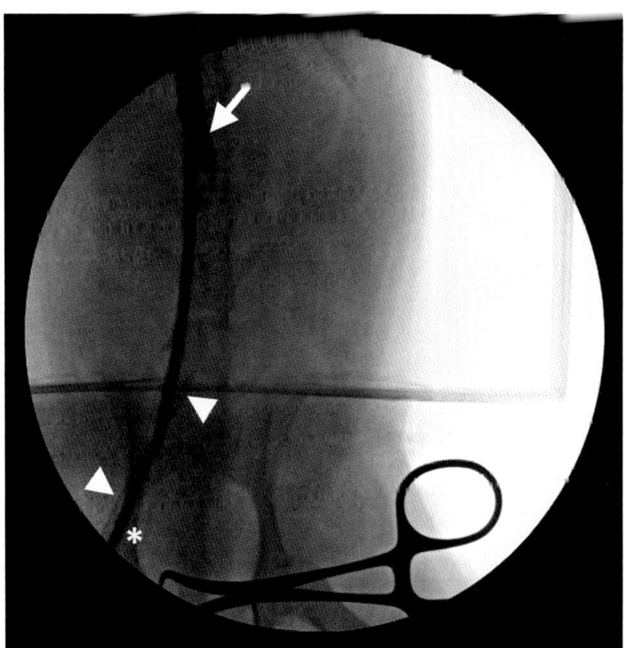

Figure 51.9 Femoral venous injection in a Cavalier King Charles spaniel showing a narrowed right caudal vena cava with reflux (arrow) back into the duplicated left caudal vena cava at the level of the renal veins. A vascular sheath is present in the right femoral vein (*) through which the injection is made, adjacent to a second vascular sheath in the right femoral artery (arrowheads).

from the cranial half of the body should be undertaken through the right external jugular vein or normal cranial vena cava anatomy should be confirmed prior to intervention. Reports of pacemaker implantation and heartworm extraction through a persistent left cranial vena cava exist in the literature and the author has performed balloon pulmonary valvuloplasty through a persistent left cranial vena cava, although these procedures are technically more challenging than the standard route.

Numerous abnormalities of the caudal vena cava have also been reported in humans and animals. The caudal vena cava may display duplication, leftward transposition, or interruption (often with azygous continuation), and these malformations may also be associated with portosystemic shunts. Most caudal caval anomalies are asymptomatic (unless concurrent with portocaval shunting), but may affect venous approaches from the femoral vein during cardiac intervention and should therefore be considered. Figure 51.9 is taken from a Cavalier King Charles spaniel with duplication of the caudal vena cava incidentally detected during femoral venous catheterization for pulmonary valve stenosis. Note that the right femoral vein in this dog does not increase in diameter as the contrast enters the external iliac vein and caudal vena cava as would be expected. Rather, this dog has a small right caudal vena cava as well as a duplicated left caudal vena cava, the cranial aspect of which can be seen by the reflux of contrast at the level of the renal veins.

Suggested Reading

Buchanan JW (1963) Persistent left cranial vena cava in dogs: angiocardiography, significance and coexisting anomalies. *J Am Vet Radiol Soc* 4, 1–8.

Buchanan JW and Patterson DF (1965) Selective angiography and angiocardiography in dogs with congenital cardiovascular disease. *J Am Vet Radiol Soc* 6, 21–39.

Hamlin RL (1959) Angiocardiography for the clinical diagnosis of congenital heart disease in small animals. *J Am Vet Med Assoc* 135, 112–16.

Mullins CE (2006) *Cardiac Catheterization in Congenital Heart Disease: Pediatric and Adult*. Blackwell Publishing, Malden, MA.

Schwarz T, Rossi F, Wray JD, et al (2009) Computed tomographic and magnetic resonance imaging features of canine segmental caudal vena cava aplasia. *J Small Anim Pract* 50, 341–9.

Tashjian RJ and Albanese NM (1960) A technique of canine angiocardiography with the interpretation of a normal left lateral angiocardiogram. *J Am Vet Med Assoc* 136, 359–65.

CHAPTER FIFTY-TWO

Pericardial Disease

Steven G. Cole
Los Angeles, CA

Background/Indications

Symptomatic pericardial disease is relatively common in dogs and quite rare in cats. While constrictive pericardial disease and infiltrative pericardial neoplasia can be encountered, pericardial effusion and subsequent cardiac tamponade is most commonly seen, and this is the condition in which image-guided intervention has its role.

Pericardial effusion in dogs occurs as a result of pericardial or, more commonly, cardiac-associated masses, and these include hemangiosarcoma, heart base masses (e.g., chemodectoma/paraganglioma), mesothelioma, carcinoma, and lymphoma, among other less common tumor types. Other causes of pericardial effusion in dogs include inflammatory disease (e.g., idiopathic pericarditis), infectious disease (with bacterial and fungal disease recognized most commonly), congestive heart failure, coagulopathy, and trauma. Pericardial effusion in cats is generally the result of congestive heart failure, infectious disease (e.g., FIP), or neoplasia (e.g., lymphoma).

The signs resulting from pericardial effusion are related to the degree of cardiac tamponade present, and this is dependent upon the volume of effusion, the rate at which the pericardial fluid has accumulated, and the compliance of the pericardium. As such, patients with rapidly accumulating fluid (e.g., secondary to a ruptured hemangiosarcoma) may present with signs of acute collapse and cardiogenic shock, whereas patients with slowly accumulating fluid and a compliant pericardium commonly present for abdominal distension and ascites secondary to right-sided congestive heart failure.

Pericardiocentesis is the initial treatment of choice for patients with symptomatic pericardial effusion/cardiac tamponade, and this may be life-saving in dogs with severe cardiac tamponade/cardiogenic shock. This procedure has been described in detail previously. Surgical options are also well established to address both the underlying cause of pericardial effusion (e.g., right atrial mass excision), as well as recurrent fluid accumulation (e.g., subtotal pericardiectomy). Minimally invasive techniques (e.g., thoracoscopic pericardial window, thoracoscopic subtotal pericardiectomy) have also been developed to address chronic/recurrent pericardial effusion with less morbidity than is seen with thoracotomy, with success rates equivalent to open techniques in many cases.

Balloon pericardiotomy is an alternative, image-guided technique to prevent cardiac tamponade in patients with chronic/recurrent pericardial effusion. This procedure is minimally invasive (equivalent to pericardiocentesis), does not require thoracoscopic equipment (and thus is often cost effective), and may be performed relatively easily by those skilled in cardiovascular intervention. Limitations of the technique stem from the fact that a portion of the pericardium is not removed. This has two implications, as no sample is obtained for histopathology, and it is also possible for the dilation site to seal and result in eventual failure of the procedure. Despite this, balloon pericardiotomy remains a viable option, especially in patients with advanced/multicentric disease that would otherwise make them poor surgical candidates.

Patient Preparation

Prior to balloon pericardiotomy, patients should have a complete cardiac workup, including chest radiographs, ECG, and echocardiogram. Baseline bloodwork and a coagulation profile are recommended, with additional screening (e.g., abdominal ultrasonography), depending upon the clinical situation. In contrast to thoracotomy and thoracoscopy, which can be

Veterinary Image-Guided Interventions, First Edition. Edited by Chick Weisse and Allyson Berent.

Companion website: www.wiley.com/go/weisse/vet-image-guided-interventions

performed with minimal pericardial effusion, balloon pericardiotomy requires at least a moderate volume of pericardial fluid to be performed safely. As such, the procedure is most often performed at some point following the initial diagnosis of pericardial effusion, and it is important to monitor for the redevelopment of clinical signs and to screen for recurrent effusion if balloon pericardiotomy is planned.

Potential Risks/ Complications/ Expected Outcomes

Risks associated with balloon pericardiotomy are related to both the anesthetic procedure, as well as to the balloon technique itself. Because the presence of pericardial effusion is required to allow initial access to the pericardium, there is a risk of decompensation at the time of anesthetic induction. Adequate periprocedural volume expansion with IV crystalloids and/or colloids is very important, and the operator should be ready to obtain pericardial access immediately following sedation/anesthetic induction. This is generally best achieved by using ultrasonography to identify an appropriate window, and then marking the skin prior to beginning the procedure.

Complications related to the balloon procedure itself can occur both acutely and chronically. Acute complications include hemorrhage (from the pericardium, inadvertent cardiac puncture, or from trauma to or rupture of a cardiac-associated mass) and pneumothorax (generally due to air ingress around the dilators/balloon catheters at the access site). While serious hemorrhage is relatively rare, some degree of pneumothorax is common, although easily managed. Chronic complications associated with the procedure include closure of the dilation site and recurrent pericardial effusion (although this does not preclude additional intervention), the development of constrictive pericardial disease, as well as seeding of the thoracic cavity and subcutis with tumor cells in patients with pericardial neoplasia (similar to that described with thoracoscopic techniques).

While large-scale studies of balloon pericardiotomy have not been performed in veterinary patients, a pilot study describing a single balloon technique demonstrated initial procedural success in six of six patients with no recurrence of effusion in four of six dogs over an extended time frame (5–32 months). The author has employed the double-balloon technique, described below, which has been adapted from human medicine. This allows for a larger, eccentric dilation of the pericardium and has produced similar results, with no recurrence of effusion over an extended time frame (6–12 months or greater) in the majority of cases.

Equipment

Balloon pericardiotomy requires materials to obtain initial access to the pericardium, as well as to perform the procedure itself. Initial access is generally obtained with a 14 or 16 gauge over-the-needle catheter, although a smaller catheter may be used initially, and a microintroducer may be employed to allow passage of a larger guide wire for subsequent introducer placement. Two vascular introducers (generally 10–12 Fr, 11 cm) are needed, as are two PTFE guide wires (generally 0.035″ dia., 150–180 cm, 1.5 mm J-tip). Finally, two balloon valvuloplasty catheters (generally 16–25 mm dia., 4–5 cm balloon length) are required. The diameter of the balloon catheters used (and the introducers required) is dependent upon the size of the patient and the desired rent in the pericardium. A single balloon technique may also be employed in smaller patients, or if the double balloon technique is technically challenging.

It is noted that balloon pericardiotomy can be technically challenging, and this may result in protracted procedure times and subsequent exposure to ionizing radiation. It is imperative to take all steps to minimize fluoroscopy times, as well as to use proper protective gear at all times.

Fluoroscopic Procedure

Initial Access

Following sedation/anesthetic induction, the patient is placed in lateral recumbency (right lateral recumbency is most often employed), and the lateral thorax is aseptically prepared and draped. The side of the thorax that is accessed is dictated by the clearest window for pericardial access as assessed by transthoracic ultrasound. Accessing the pericardium from the right ventral thoracic wall provides the benefit of the cardiac notch, which is a natural separation between the right cranial lung lobe and the right middle lung lobe in dogs. Additionally, the right ventricle is of lower pressure if inadvertent cardiac puncture occurs and there are fewer major coronary arteries at risk of laceration. The alternative arguments in favor of accessing the pericardium from the left thoracic wall are the greater thickness of the left ventricular wall as compared to the right, which is less likely to be perforated and also more likely to seal if intracardiac puncture is mistakenly performed. Initial access to the pericardium is obtained through a stab skin incision with a 14–16 g. over the needle catheter (or a smaller catheter followed by a microintroducer), and the pericardium is partially decompressed by withdrawing pericardial fluid if cardiac tamponade is present prior to the procedure, or if the patient is hypotensive and/or tachycardic following induction. A sample of the pericardial fluid may be retained for analysis if not performed previously.

Introducer Placement

After initial access to the pericardium is achieved, a small volume of a non-ionized contrast medium is instilled to verify proper placement of the over the needle catheter within the pericardial space (Figure 52.1A). The following technique is then employed to allow two introducers to be placed through the same hole in the pericardium. First, the initial catheter is exchanged for a 10 to 12 Fr, 11 cm vascular introducer using the modified Seldinger technique. The short, access guide wire used for the placement of the introducer is left in place, and a 150 or 180 cm, 0.035″, J-tip, PTFE guidewire is inserted into the introducer alongside the access guide wire and then advanced into the pericardium, with its position confirmed via fluoroscopy (Figure 52.1B).

The introducer is then withdrawn along the long PTFE guide wire until the short, access guidewire is no longer within the introducer. At this point, the access guide wire and the long guide wire will traverse the chest wall and pericardium at the same points. A second 10 to 12 Fr, 11 cm vascular introducer is then placed via the short, access wire and is advanced into the pericardium. The original introducer may then be advanced over the long guide wire and into the pericardium. Finally, the short, access guide wire is removed and replaced with a second 150 to 180 cm, 0.035″, J-Tip, PTFE guide wire, and the position of this wire within the pericardium is confirmed with fluoroscopy.

Balloon Placement

Following placement of the introducer sheaths, the guide wires are advanced into the pericardium. It is noted that the guide wires will generally travel along the pericardium and will not contact the heart as they are advanced. It is important that the guide wires be well within the pericardium, so that access is not lost during subsequent manipulation of the catheters (Figure 52.1C). The balloon valvuloplasty catheters are then advanced over the guide wires and into the pericardial space, and the radiopaque markers may be used to determine the position of the balloons. Once the valvuloplasty catheters are in place, the introducers are withdrawn from the chest cavity, as the balloon inflation must take place just inside the chest wall.

Balloon Dilation

The ability to perform this technique is dependent upon balloon inflation on either side of the pericardium, and this can be challenging in some cases. From a patient positioning standpoint, this may be facilitated by placing the forelimbs in sternal recumbency after introducer/guidewire placement, as this allows the pericardium to fall away from chest wall. One catheter is slowly withdrawn until the proximal marker is at the level of the chest wall, and this generally ensures that the balloon is positioned across the pericardium (Figure 52.2A). Visualization of the

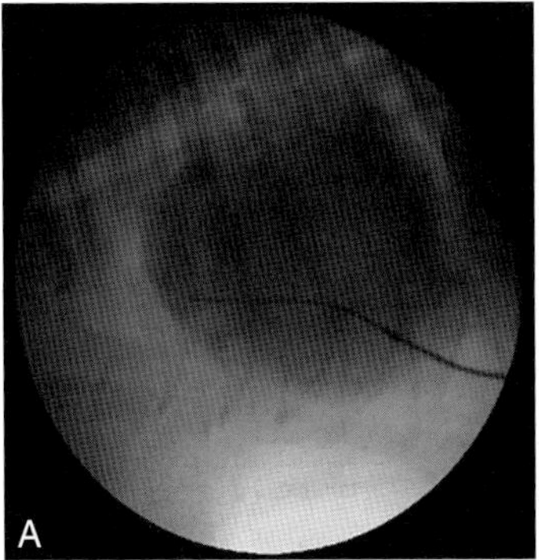

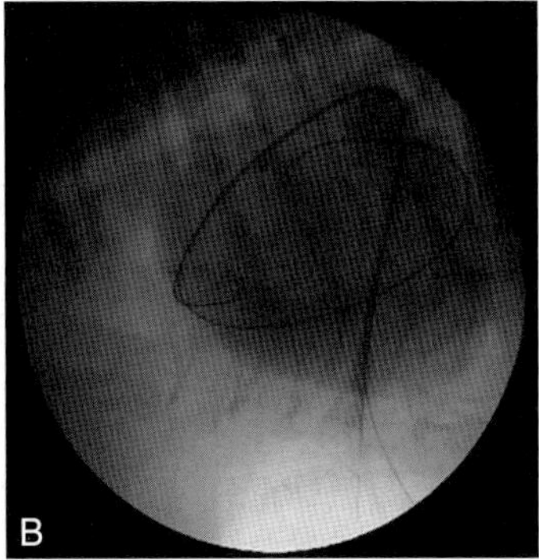

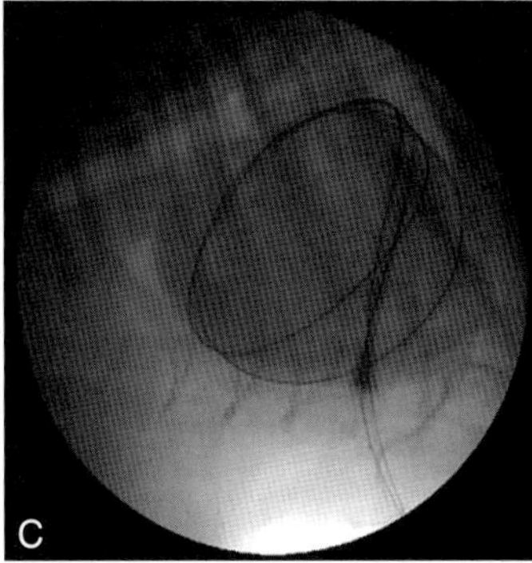

Figure 52.1 (A) Over the needle catheter placement within the pericardial space. Iodinated contrast medium has been instilled into the pericardial space to verify catheter placement. (B) A vascular introducer with both the initial short access guide wire and long J-tip guide wire in place through the same introducer. (C) Both vascular introducers and long PTFE guide wires in place. Note the point at which the dilators cross is the location of the pericardium. The guide wires lie along the inner aspect of the pericardium and do not contact the heart.

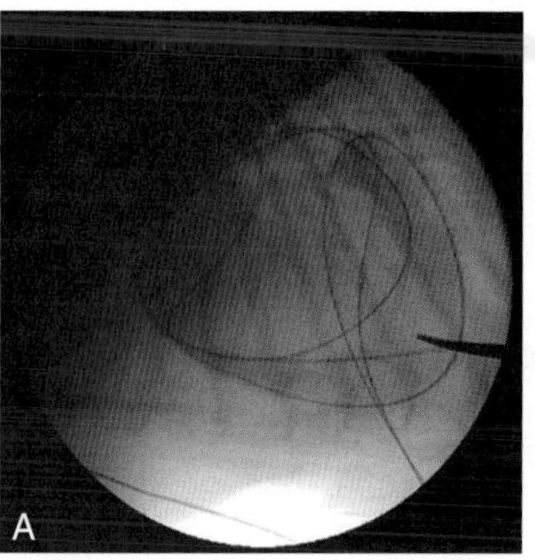

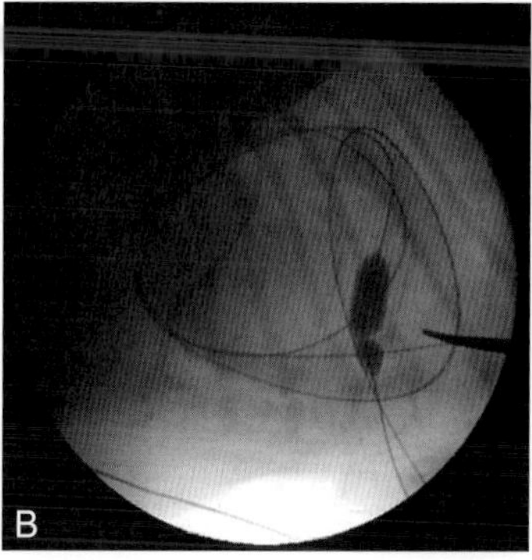

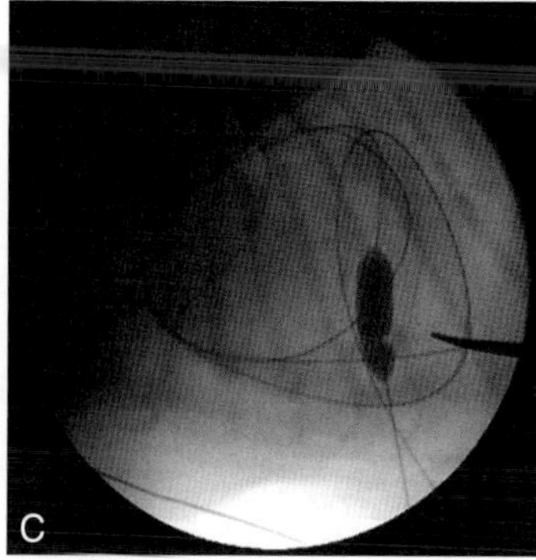

Figure 52.2 (A) Positioning of a single balloon (note the radiopaque marker bands along the more caudal guide wire) across the pericardium prior to inflation. (B) Partial inflation of the initial balloon. The "waist" seen in the balloon is created by the pericardial constriction at this site. (C) Further inflation of the initial balloon results in a partial disappearance of the 'waist' during dilation of the pericardium.

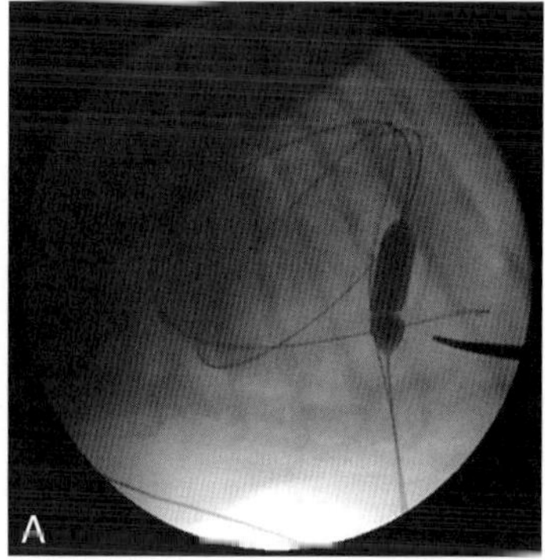

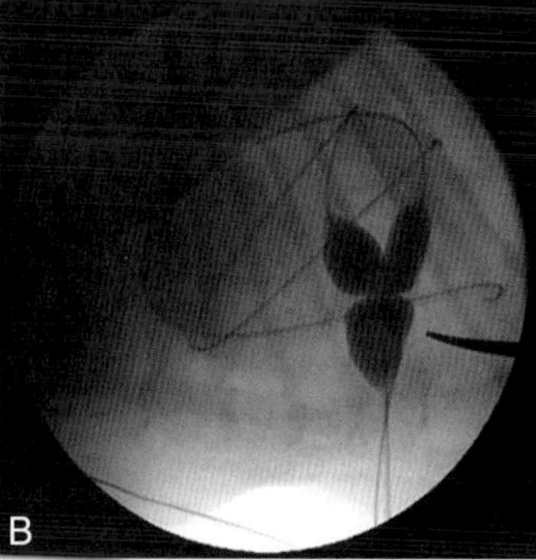

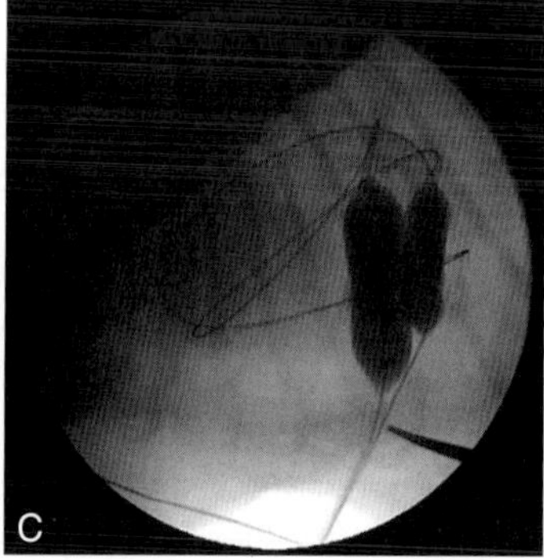

Figure 52.3 (A) Positioning of the second balloon across the pericardium has now been performed (note the radiopaque marker bands along the more cranial guide wire). The first balloon should remain inflated during positioning of the second balloon to localize the pericardium. (B) Partial inflation of the second balloon catheter. As before, the "waist" seen in the balloons is created by the pericardium. (C) Complete inflation of both balloons. The balloon diameters in this case were 16 mm and 25 mm, respectively. Note that contrast within the pericardium has disappeared as the pericardial effusion has drained through the dilation site and into the pleural space.

balloon can be improved if a very small amount of contrast is instilled during positioning. Once positioned, the balloon is inflated, and the presence of a 'waist' indicates proper placement (Figure 52.2B, C). The second catheter is then withdrawn until the balloon is positioned across the pericardium and is inflated alongside the first balloon (Figure 52.3A–C). The balloons are typically left inflated for 5 minutes, and the dilation may be repeated for a total of three inflations. Following the dilation procedure, the valvuloplasty balloons and guide wires are removed. The small skin incision can then be closed with a single suture.

Follow-Up

In addition to standard postoperative care, it is recommended that chest radiographs be obtained following the procedure. Additional monitoring for the development of pleural effusion and/or signs of hemorrhage (tachycardia, hypotension, pallor, anemia, hypoproteinemia) is also important during the perioperative period. Serial echocardiography is also recommended, with recheck imaging at 2 weeks, 6 weeks, 12 weeks, and then at 3-month intervals.

Special Considerations/ Complication Examples

One potential difficulty that may arise during the procedure is prolapse of the balloon into the pleural space, and advancing the valvuloplasty catheter into the pericardium may be difficult if this occurs. As long as the PTFE guide wire remains within the pericardial space, this may be remedied by removing the balloon catheter and reinserting the vascular introducer. The balloon catheter may then be advanced over the guidewire and through the introducer into the pericardium.

As already noted, some degree of pneumothorax is not uncommon in patients following balloon pericardiotomy, as it is difficult to eliminate ingress of air around the balloon catheters during the procedure. Additionally, pleural effusion (generally a small volume) is invariably present following drainage of the pericardial fluid into the chest cavity following balloon dilation. This can be addressed at the time of the procedure by replacing an introducer into the chest cavity and draining any air and/or fluid through the infusion port. Alternatively, a chest tube may be placed, or most commonly, thoracocentesis may be performed as necessary following the procedure.

Suggested Reading

Cobb MA, Boswood A, Griffin GM, and McEvoy FJ (1996) Percutaneous balloon pericardiotomy for the management of malignant pericardial effusion in two dogs. *J Small Anim Pract* 37(11), 549–51.

Iaffaldano RA, Jones P, Lewis BE, et al (1995) Percutaneous balloon pericardiotomy: a double-balloon technique. *Catheter Cardiovasc Diagn* 36(1), 79–81.

Sidley JA, Atkins CE, Keene BW, and DeFrancesco TC (2002) Percutaneous balloon pericardiotomy as a treatment for recurrent pericardial effusion in 6 dogs. *Journal of Veterinary Internal Medicine* 16(5), 541–6.

Wang HJ, Hsu KL, Chiang FT, et al (2002) Technical and prognostic outcomes of double-balloon pericardiotomy for large malignancy-related pericardial effusions. *Chest* 122(3), 893–9.

CHAPTER FIFTY-THREE

Cardiac Pacing

Amara H. Estrada
College of Veterinary Medicine, University of Florida, Gainesville, FL

Backgroung/Indications

Symptomatic bradycardia remains the most compelling indication for pacemaker therapy in dogs and cats. Pacemaker therapy is the treatment of choice for certain bradyarrhythmias such as third degree or complete atrioventricular (AV) block, high grade second degree AV block, sick sinus syndrome/sinus node dysfunction (SSS/SND), or persistent atrial standstill (not associated with hyperkalemia). Syncope is not, however, the only symptom which might be associated with a bradyarrhythmia. Patients may also show signs of exercise intolerance, near-syncope or presyncope, weakness, ataxia, generalized muscle weakness, or even development of congestive heart failure. Many factors determine whether a bradyarrhythmia will cause clinical signs including rate of escape rhythms, length of sinus pauses, presence and extent of any underlying cardiac disease process such as myocardial failure or valvular degeneration, and overall health of the patient. Pacing therapy is not a "one size fits all" practice and some options and considerations for pacemaker type, lead location, and programming are important for patients with different types of bradyarrhythmias that require artificial pacing.

Atrioventricular (AV) Block

Dogs versus cats

AV block is the most common indication for permanent pacemaker implantation. Dogs and cats differ in the rate of their intrinsic escape rhythms, with cats typically having a faster ventricular escape rhythm (90–120 bpm) such that they do not frequently require artificial cardiac pacing. Occasionally, cats with cardiomyopathy will develop bradyarrhythmias concurrent with a slow escape rhythm, and pacemaker therapy is required to either keep them out of congestive heart failure or improve quality of life if the rate is slow enough to affect their activity. There have been reports of cranial vena caval obstruction and resultant development of chylothorax in cats with transvenous pacing, and thus most cardiologists choose to place an epicardial lead on the left ventricular apex through an abdominal/diaphragmatic approach in cats if pacing is required. There are, however, small diameter leads (4.1 Fr) that may be suitable to use in cats, but thus far the experience with this is minimal.

Single- versus dual-chamber pacing

Most dogs affected by AV block (whether second degree or complete) have been treated by single-chamber ventricular-based pacemaker (VVI; see Table 53.1) implantation. These systems consist of one right ventricular apical lead and therefore do not maintain AV synchrony or the normal ventricular activation sequence. Numerous studies in humans and animals have shown negative consequences of such non-physiologic pacing. The term pacemaker syndrome is used in human medicine to describe adverse clinical and hemodynamic consequences of non-physiologic pacing. Dual-chamber pacing systems, particularly those with two leads, are more time consuming to place in dogs because of smaller vessels and the requirement for two leads. Additionally, dual-chamber pacemakers require slightly more complex programming. Thus, it has been assumed that implantation of dual-chamber pacemakers would have higher complication rates both initially and in the long-term. Recent studies, however, show that while dual-chamber pacing and the implantation of multiple leads do prolong anesthesia and procedural time, dogs do not have any increased incidence of either short-term or long-term complications associated with multiple leads or longer anesthesia/procedural time. Another

Veterinary Image-Guided Interventions, First Edition. Edited by Chick Weisse and Allyson Berent.

Companion website: www.wiley.com/go/weisse/vet-image-guided-interventions

TABLE 53.1
North American Society of Pacing and Electrophysiology/British Pacing and Electrophysiology Group generic code (NBG Code) for pacing system nomenclature

Position	I	II	III	IV	V
Category	Chamber(s) paced **O**=None **A**=Atrium **V**=Ventricle **D**=Dual (A+V)	Chamber(s) sensed **O**=None **A**=Atrium **V**=Ventricle **D**=Dual (A+V)	Response to sensing **O**=None **T**=Triggered **I**=Inhibited **D**=Dual (T+I)	Rate modulation **O**=None **R**=Rate modulation	Multisite Pacing **O**=None **A**=Atrium **V**=Ventricle **D**=Dual (A+V)

The NBG Code is used in veterinary medicine and comprises five positions to describe antibradycardia pacing.
From Bernstein AD et al (2002) PACE 25, 260–4.

type of pacing, atrial synchronous pacing (via VDD implantation), allows for dual-chamber pacing with only a single lead. For atrial synchronous pacing, 1 lead is implanted in the right ventricle, but unlike standard VVI systems, this lead has a floating electrode in the right atrium that is capable of sensing inherent atrial electrical activity and stimulating ventricular contraction after an appropriate delay, therefore allowing for AV synchrony. Although atrial synchronous pacing has been reported in veterinary medicine, the set distance between the floating atrial electrode and ventricular pacing tip often prevents its use in small dogs.

Right ventricular apex vs. right ventricular septum vs. left ventricular free wall vs. biventricular pacing

As early as 1925 Wiggers demonstrated that pacing at the right ventricular apex (RVA) leads to asynchronous ventricular contraction and reduced cardiac function. In the last decade there has been a surge of interest in the human pacing arena in the sequence of ventricular activation and the search for more optimal ventricular pacing sites. In adults with chronic RVA pacing, there is a higher risk of development of left ventricular systolic dysfunction, heart failure, and atrial fibrillation. The author's team has investigated both biventricular pacing as well as left ventricular free wall pacing via a coronary sinus/vein lead implantation, and in dogs with appropriate anatomy, leads can be placed and remain stable in this location. However, the time, cost and experience required for left ventricular lead placement, and the high failure rates we have experienced due to absent, unsuitable, unusable, or unattainable venous anatomy, argue that at the moment RV septal lead placement may be technically and financially the best alternative to RVA pacing. Within this chapter, the author describes the placement of leads within these locations but also offers pros and cons to each location.

Sinus Node Dysfunction/Sick Sinus Syndrome

Atrial pacing vs. dual-chamber pacing vs. ventricular back up pacing

The majority of dogs with SND retain the ability to conduct through the AV node. This is important, not only because this may be used for conduction of antegrade pacing from the atrial myocardium during atrial-based pacing, but also because retrograde conduction of impulses through the AV node may occur with ventricular-based pacing systems. It is therefore important that if using VVI pacing in dogs with SND, it is used only as 'back up' for periods of bradycardia in order to retain as much AV nodal conduction as possible. Another important consideration for dogs with SND is the concurrent high incidence of degenerative valve disease in this patient population. New or worsened mitral regurgitation has been documented in humans both acutely and with chronic RVA pacing as a direct result of the abnormal activation sequence of the ventricles. Thus, the ideal pacemaker for these dogs would be one that alleviates their symptoms associated with bradycardia, but also maintains AV synchrony and normal ventricular activation; atrial-based pacing (AAI) accomplishes these goals but methods for achieving this in small breed dogs have not yet been optimized. Conventionally, the atria have been paced from the right atrial appendage, however several complications have been reported when this site was attempted in small breed dogs with naturally occurring SND, including partial and complete lead dislodgement, pneumothorax and lead perforation. While atrial-based pacing is preferable in such patients, the right auricular appendage does not appear to be an ideal site for these small dogs. Alternative atrial pacing sites such as the interatrial septum appear possible, but there is a learning curve for placement of leads in this location.

Atrial Standstill

Atrial standstill is an uncommon arrhythmia, which is usually found to be associated with an atrial myocarditis whereby the atrial myocardium is replaced by fibrous connective tissue. Atrial standstill occurs when the atria fail to depolarize from a sinus initiated impulse. Junctional or ventricular escape rhythms are usually present. Pacemaker implantation is indicated in this disease as increasing the heart rate will not only improve any clinical signs of exercise intolerance or syncope but will assist in the management of congestive heart failure if present. Because of the inability of the atria to depolarize, single-chamber ventricular pacing (VVI) is the only option.

Preoperative Patient Preparation

Prior to permanent pacemaker implantation, a full diagnostic work up is recommended, if this is possible. Patients with very low escape rates are the exception to this as there may not be time to fully evaluate a patient prior to permanent pacing. An echocardiogram to evaluate underlying cardiac structure and function is always performed. When time does permit, bloodwork consisting of a serum chemistry panel, complete blood cell count with manual differential and possibly a troponin I level should be assessed. While myocarditis is an uncommon cause of bradyarrhythmias, these patients can be especially arrhythmogenic when placing temporary or permanent pacing leads. If there is reason to suspect myocarditis (evidence of systemic inflammation on bloodwork, fever, ventricular ectopy), troponin I may be helpful in making treatment decisions (i.e., delaying the procedure if possible). A urinalysis along with a thorough skin and ear exam is also recommended in attempt to avoid implanting a patient who may subsequently infect their pacing system. If urinary tract infections, pyoderma, or serious ear infections are present, and the procedure can be safely delayed to allow for appropriate therapy, this is preferable.

Potential Risks/Complications/Expected Outcomes

Complications following pacemaker implantation have been shown to be directly related to the experience of the implanter in both veterinary and human medicine. Development of a seroma (nearly always sterile) is a fairly common occurrence but can be easily managed with wrapping of the neck with gentle pressure. The author therefore prefers to keep the patient's neck and surgical site wrapped with clean bandages allowing for slight pressure on the implantation site for 2 weeks postoperatively. It is important to note that if seroma formation does occur, drainage of fluid surrounding the generator should not be performed because of the risk of introduction of bacteria to the site and also for concern of damage to the leads and generator within the pocket. Rebandaging with slight pressure is instead used as long as there are no signs of infection (heat, swelling, discharge, etc.).

The incidence of infection following pacemaker implantation is reported to be anywhere from 5 to 10%, which is much higher than the author's experience and reports in human medicine with an incidence of less than 2%. Should infection occur, the optimal treatment of an infected pacemaker is removal of the entire system (lead and generator) if possible, appropriate long-term antibiotic therapy (via culture and sensitivity), and replacement of the pacing system on the opposite side of the neck if delay is not feasible. Treatment with antibiotic therapy alone is rarely associated with eradication of the infection.

Partial or silent venous thrombosis of the jugular vein is likely common following transvenous lead placement, but does not typically cause clinical signs. Thrombus adherence/formation on the lead is also sometimes visualized on recheck echocardiograms without clinical signs noted by owner. In the author's experience, these types of thrombi do not typically dislodge or grow bigger over time. It is advisable however, to treat patients with antithrombotic agents such as low-dose aspirin or clopidogrel if a thrombus is recognized.

Lead perforation of the myocardium is a possible, and likely an under-recognized occurrence, but can cause pericardial effusion and pneumothorax. In fact, the only signs of perforation may be a rising stimulation threshold, a change in the ventricular depolarization pattern on surface electrocardiogram or diaphragmatic contraction with each output stimulus.

The most common complication, especially in the immediate postoperative period, is lead dislodgment. While "macro"-dislodgement of a lead away from the myocardial surface can be easily recognized on thoracic radiographs, smaller movements associated with "micro"-dislodgement will not be seen. Small amounts of motion at the lead tip can lead to re-initiation of the inflammatory cycle and acute rises in pacing threshold. In patients with suspected lead dislodgment, strict limitation of patient activity is important to allow for lead tip stabilization.

Sometimes, dogs will have contraction of their neck or diaphragm with each pacing stimulus. This is usually due to either high voltage output or phrenic nerve stimulation and can be avoided by lowering the voltage output. Pacemakers that are donated from pacing manufacturers will often have etching on the back to indicate they are not for use in people. This can sometimes lead to voltage leak around the generator and it should be implanted with the etched side down in attempt to avoid contraction of the overlying musculature.

Pulse generators have a typical life span ranging from 10 to 12 years when manufactured. Most generators implanted in veterinary medicine today have not been used previously but remaining battery life at implant is variable and can be assessed prior to implantation using a programmer. With development of more sophisticated pacing algorithms, pacing modes, tracking of rhythm abnormalities, performing of daily threshold testing, ability to assess for intrinsic conduction, pacing mode switching, and multiple other functions now incorporated within newer generators, knowledge of basic programming or collaboration with a local pacing company technical consultant can be invaluable in maximizing the function and lifespan of a pulse generator. There are many functions, which may automatically be turned on when manufactured, that can drain battery life. In contrast, there may also be functions that can be utilized to help sustain pacing systems for the duration of an animal's life if utilized correctly. When a generator is close to battery depletion, an *end of life* or *elective replacement indicator* is turned on. Most commonly, this is signaled by a gradual decrease in pacing rate, thus giving ample time to replace the generator prior to complete failure of the generator.

Fluoroscopic Procedure

The patient's fur is clipped prior to entering the catheterization lab. A large area around the neck and jugular veins is clipped as well as any sites that may be used for temporary pacing. Antibiotics are typically administered (cefazolin, 22 mg/kg, IV) at the start of the procedure before a skin incision is made and then repeated every 2 hours after the first dose.

Temporary Pacing

For patients with bradyarrhythmias, the safest way to implant a permanent pacemaker is after some method of temporary pacing has been employed. There are various ways that this can be accomplished with pros and cons for each technique.

Transvenous temporary pacing

Temporary transvenous pacing is accomplished using no or mild sedation. If sedation is necessary, a strong pure mu opiod such as hydromorphone is given along with atropine to avoid an increase in vagal tone, which may reduce escape rates. The equipment typically used for transvenous pacing is shown in Figure 53.1. A lateral saphenous or jugular vein is clipped and sterilely prepped for catheter placement. A 22-gauge catheter is placed within the vein and an appropriately sized guide wire is advanced. Once the guide wire is in place, a 5 or 6 Fr introducer is placed within the vein to allow for catheter placement and hemostasis, a small nick in the skin with a #11 blade may be necessary to advance the introducer. At this point, a temporary pacing lead is placed, either blindly or with fluoroscopic guidance and patient restraint, into the apex of the right ventricle. Temporary pacing leads are available with balloon tips to facilitate placement in a critical setting without fluoroscopic guidance. The balloon is inflated after the lead is past the tip of the introducer and advanced, with the help of normal blood flow, into the right ventricle. Once appropriately positioned in the right ventricular apex, the temporary pacing lead is attached to a temporary pulse generator (Figure 53.2). The ECG is monitored until consistent pacing and capture of ventricular depolarization is accomplished. Temporary transvenous pacing does require considerable training and skill as well as fluoroscopic guidance in most cases. This can sometimes lead to a delay in achieving a stable rhythm and can also add time to the length of the overall procedure.

Transthoracic temporary pacing

Transthoracic temporary pacing of the dog ventricle has been shown to be successful using commercially available transthoracic pacing systems with adhesive patches applied to the right and left hemithoraces directly over the heart. While transthoracic pacing is safe and effective, it is not without complications and must be performed after the patient is under general anesthesia. It produces mild to severe muscle movement in most dogs, sometimes requiring neuromuscular blockade to allow surgical procedures to continue. Additionally, it is a painful procedure often times necessitating a deeper plane of anesthesia.

Transesophageal temporary pacing

Transesophageal pacing is accomplished using a commercially available system for children and can readily achieve atrial pacing in dogs. Transesophageal pacing also requires general anesthesia and elicits considerable patient movement similar to transthoracic

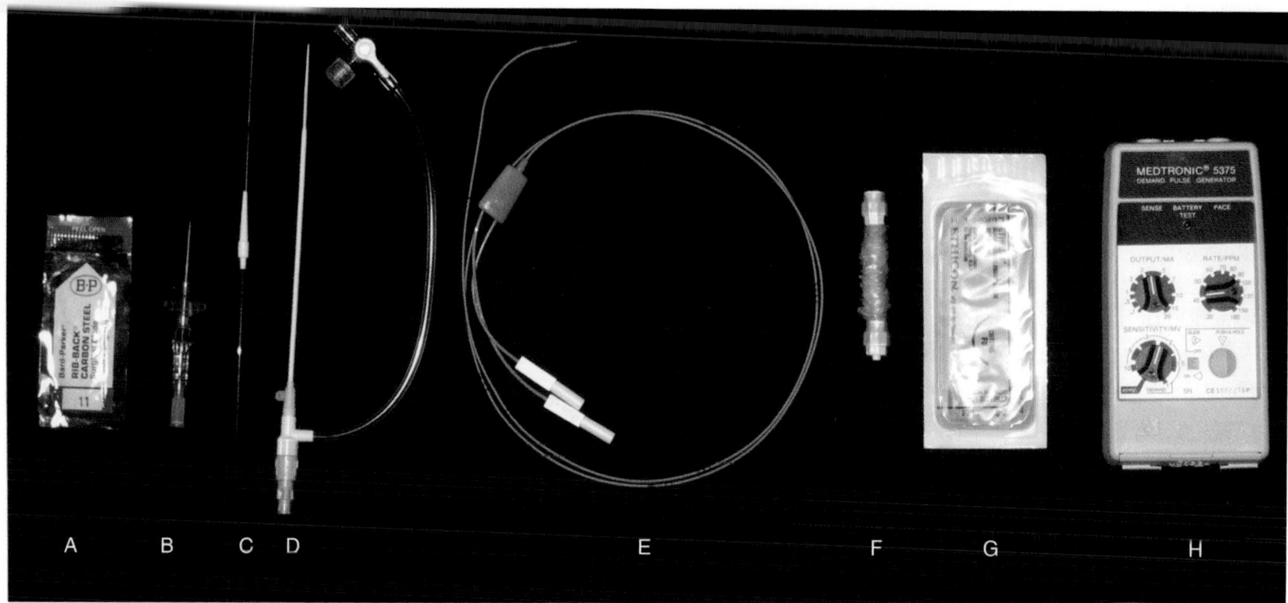

Figure 53.1 Supplies used for temporary transvenous pacing include an #11 blade (A) to create a small skin incision over the vein, a 22-gauge over-the-needle catheter (B) for initial venous access, an 0.018″ guide wire (C) and microintroducer sheath (D) for vascular access, the pacing lead (E), optional sterile sleeve (F) to cover the pacing lead that is external to the introducer, nylon suture (G) to suture the introducer to the skin, and a external pulse generator (H) to provide the pacing stimuli.

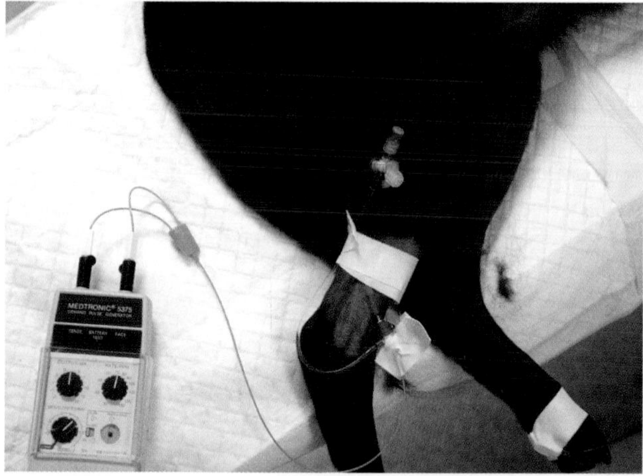

Figure 53.2 The lateral saphenous or contralateral jugular vein is typically used for temporary pacing. In this dog, the microintroducer sheath has been placed in the right lateral saphenous vein, the pacing lead advanced to the right ventricle, and the lead then connected to the external pulse generator.

pacing, but does not appear to be as painful and does not appear to cause esophageal irritation with short-term pacing. It is not possible, however, to pace the ventricles as the lead system is too far away from the ventricular myocardium to achieve ventricular capture. Thus, transesophageal temporary pacing systems might be a realistic option for short-term pacing in patients with SND, but not for dogs requiring pacing of the ventricular myocardium.

Lead Placement

In veterinary medicine, the majority of permanent pacemakers are placed transvenously through a jugular vein approach under general anesthesia. At the author's practice, once the rhythm is controlled with temporary pacing, anesthesia is induced with etomidate and anesthesia is maintained with inhalant anesthesia. Animals are typically also maintained on lidocaine and fentanyl infusions in order to reduce anesthetic requirements. Once the patient is anesthetized and a stable rhythm is achieved via temporary pacing as described above, a 3 to 4 cm vascular cut-down over the jugular vein, as low as possible – essentially at the thoracic inlet, is made. Placing leads in this location leads to far less motion of the lead body and tip (and therefore decreased likelihood of dislodgement) once the patient is awake. The jugular vein is isolated and stabilized with stay sutures and the cranial aspect is ligated. The cranial suture around the jugular is secured but not cut so that the suture can assist in manipulating the jugular vein. A small venotomy incision is made with use of small thumb forceps and iris scissors for insertion of the permanent pacing leads. Leads are passed from the jugular vein and into the chamber and location that has been selected for permanent pacing (right ventricular apex, right ventricular septum, left ventricular free wall via coronary sinus, right auricular appendage or right atrial septum; methods for locations described in subsequent sections) via fluoroscopic guidance. The choice of lead type is based largely on availability of leads, clinician preference, and patient size (with concern for multiple leads leading to cranial caval syndrome in smaller patients). Other factors, however, that should be taken into consideration include the desired chamber(s) for pacing, the underlying rhythm disorder in the patient, and underlying myocardial and valvular function.

Right ventricular apical lead

Placement of a pacing lead within the right ventricular apex is generally very straightforward and is currently the most common location for permanent artificial cardiac pacing. Pacing leads are typically packaged together with multiple stylets that are either curved or straight at the tip; such stylets can also be purchased separately. These stylets are long thin wires that can be shaped to the operator's preference and placed within the pacing lead to improve lead stiffness/stability during advancement into the animal's vein and also allow the operator to create a shape in the lead that facilitates intracardiac placement. The author uses only a straight stylet when implanting right ventricular apical leads but prefers the 14 gauge guide wire as these are more flexible at the tapered end. These also have a ball at the tip of the stylet, which assists in locking them into the lead better; the author feels this allows for more control for lead guidance. A small 60 to 80 degree curve is shaped into the straight stylet via fingers or a hemostat, roughly 10 to 15 cm from the stylet tip, which will create a ventrally directed bend that will help the lead cross the tricuspid valve. This stylet is then inserted into the lead and the lead advanced into the venotomy site and directed with fluoroscopic guidance into the caudoventral aspect of the cardiac silhouette. Once across the tricuspid valve with the pacing lead, as determined by presumed position of the valve on the cardiac silhouette and/or development of ventricular arrhythmias, the curved stylet is removed and exchanged for a straight stylet in order to guide the lead into the RV apex. Orthogonal views can be helpful to confirm placement of the lead tip in the RV apex; the lead is appropriately at the RV apex when the tip is seen to be at the caudoventral aspect of the cardiac silhouette on a lateral view (Figure 53.3A), and deviates slightly toward midline on the ventrodorsal projection (Figure 53.3B). If the lead is active fixation, then it is secured appropriately (4–5 clockwise rotations of the lead). Passive fixation leads (e.g., plastic tines on the lead tip) will secure by entrapment in the trabeculations of the RV and do not require rotation. To determine whether the location of the pacing lead is adequate, several measurements are now made using an external pacing system analyzer. With a ventricular lead, the R wave height is measured to ensure that the pacing lead can 'see' complexes well enough. Generally, an appropriately placed pacing lead will measure/sense an R wave that is at least 10 mV (and usually higher). Next, the impedance is determined. Impedance is the total resistance to current flow and gives information regarding the integrity of the pacing system. Impedance should generally be between 500 and 1000 Ω at time of implantation. Lastly, and most importantly, the threshold for pacing is determined.

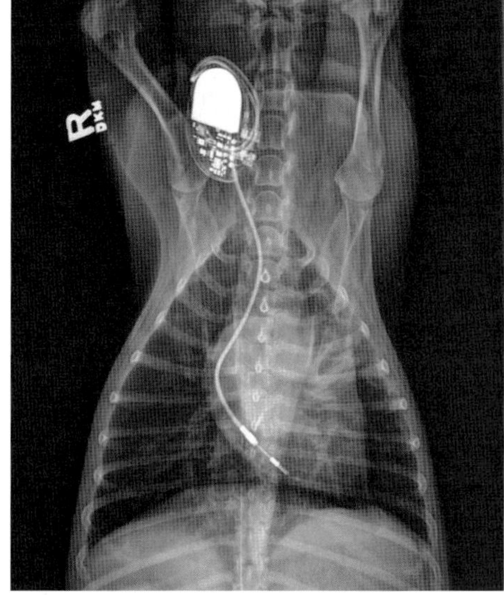

A

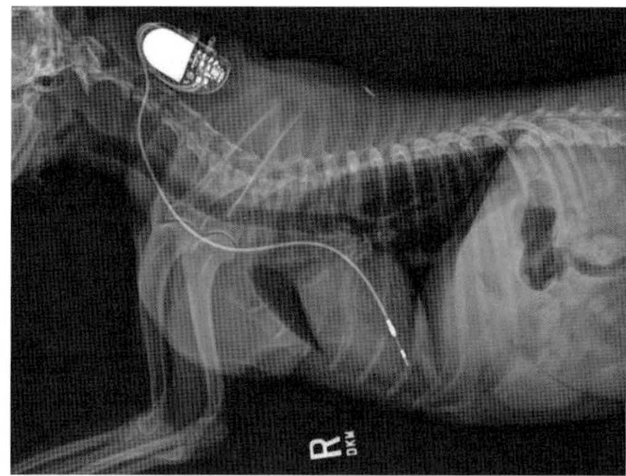

B

Figure 53.3 Orthogonal view thoracic radiographs showing lead position in the right ventricular apex (RVA). The lead tip is seen to be at the caudoventral aspect of the cardiac silhouette on a lateral view (A), and deviates slightly toward midline on the ventrodorsal projection (B).

Right ventricular septal lead

The author has recently begun to try and implant leads within the right ventricular septum from a jugular vein approach. For this location, an active fixation lead with an extendable helix is necessary. To implant in this region, the patient is positioned in left lateral recumbency and the technique is similar for RVA leads as described above. The stylet used, however, is customized at the surgical table to have a smaller curve at the end such that the guide wire and lead can be rotated together in a counter-clockwise manner and directed towards the septum and not the free wall. Use of a rotational fluoroscopic or a biplane unit is preferable in order to visualize the correct orientation towards the septum versus the free wall of the RV. The appearance of this lead tip location is slightly more cranial within the RV (Figure 53.4A) and directed more medially (Figure 53.4B) than an RVA lead position. Once the lead has been placed in this location, the tip should be stable such that it cannot be directed either towards the free wall or septum, because it has settled into this orientation. With RV septal placement of leads, the R wave amplitude will be much smaller than with RVA leads. Acceptable R wave amplitude in these locations is 4–5 mV because of the perpendicular alignment of the dipoles and also because there is less muscle and vector in this plane.

Left ventricular free wall lead (LVF) via coronary sinus

To place a Medtronic® LVF lead, first the coronary sinus is cannulated with a steerable electrophysiology catheter such as a 5 Fr RF Mariner SCXL steerable electrophysiology catheter (Figure 53.5). This catheter is then used to position a 9 Fr Attain 6218 guide catheter into the coronary sinus. Next, a retrograde venogram is done through the guide catheter with a balloon-tipped end-hole catheter to obtain a map of the coronary venous system and select the appropriate coronary vein for lead placement. A uni- or bipolar over-the-wire LVF lead is then placed in the selected coronary vein through the guide catheter with the use of a 180 cm 0.014″ guidewire. The guide catheter is then simultaneously removed and cut from the LVF lead with the supplied cutting device. When using the cutting device for LV leads, the hand that holds the cutting device (usually the right hand) is completely frozen and still on the animal, positioned directly on the animal's neck. The other hand (usually the left) pulls the guiding catheter very steadily and slowly to cut the lead off. It is very important that the slitter/cutting device is lined up in the groove before the sheath of the guiding catheter is pulled or the lead will dislodge. The difficulty with using this lead has been the variability of coronary venous anatomy in dogs and the inability to effectively position leads over the left ventricular free wall as intended.

Right auricular appendage lead

An active or passive fixation lead can be placed within the right auricular appendage (Figure 53.6) but care should be taken in selecting an appropriate lead as these are manufactured for adult human-sized atria. The author prefers to use a lead that has a tip surface area that is greater than 4 mm^2. Small electrode tips have been theorized to place an increased force per

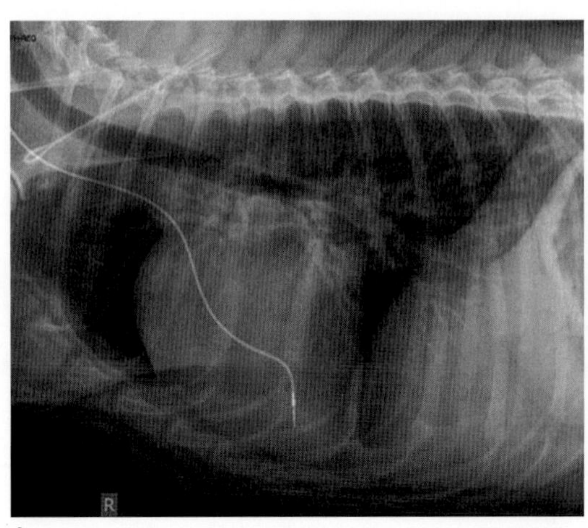

A

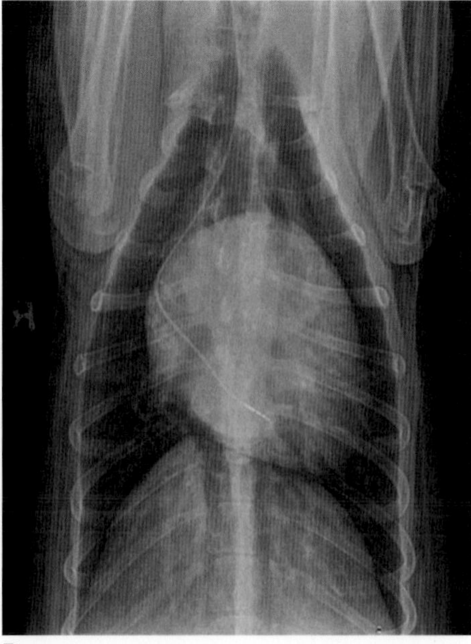

B

Figure 53.4 Orthogonal view thoracic radiographs showing lead position in the right ventricular septum (RVS). The appearance of this lead tip location is slightly more cranial within the RV (A) and directed more medially (B) than an RVA lead position. Images courtesy of Dr. N. Sydney Moise, DVM, DACVIM (Cardiology and Internal Medicine).

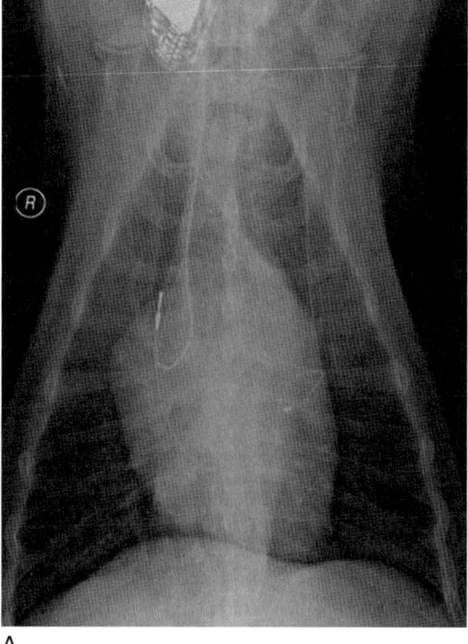

A

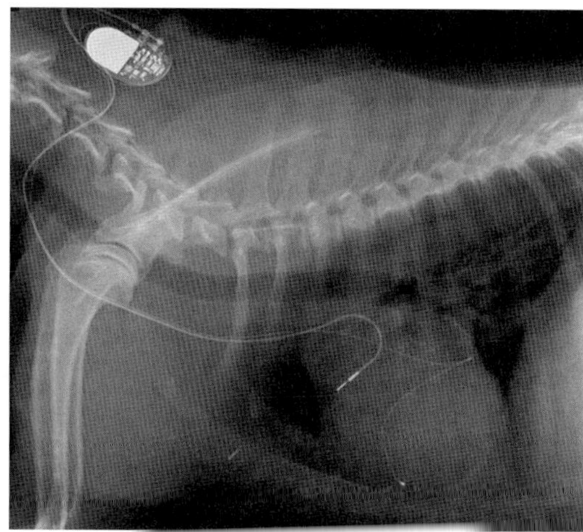

B

Figure 53.5 Orthogonal view thoracic radiographs showing a dual-chamber pacing system utilizing a left ventricular lead placed via the coronary sinus. There are passive fixation leads in both the right auricular appendage and within a cardiac vein overlying the interventricular septum.

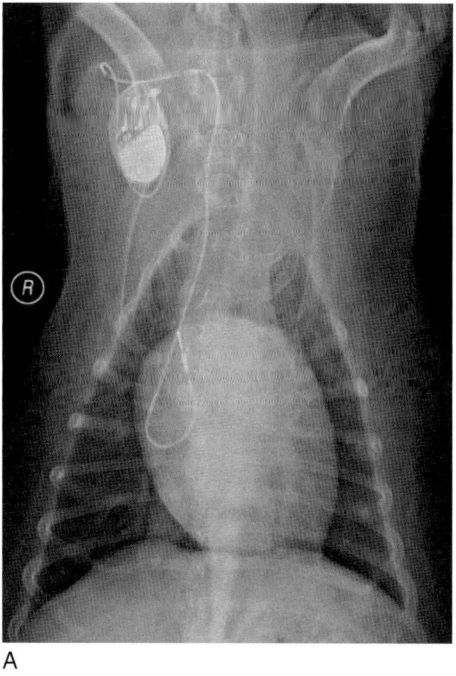

A

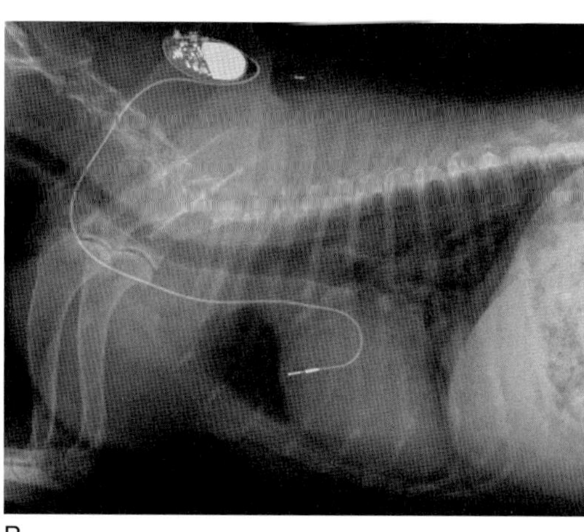

B

Figure 53.6 Orthogonal view thoracic radiographs showing a single-chamber right auricular pacing system. There is a passive fixation lead within the right inter-atrial septum.

unit area on the thin atrial myocardium, making it more likely for perforation to occur. Use of a straight stylet within the right atrial body to straighten the lead during initial passage is first used. Once the lead tip is at the edge of the caudal vena cava (but still within the body of the right atrium), either a preformed J-shaped stylet or a straight stylet customized at the surgical table with a J-shaped curve is used to direct the lead into the right auricular appendage. The author then watches the lead tip for a 'wind shield wiper' motion during atrial contraction, suggesting that the tip is appropriately implanted within the auricular appendage.

Right atrial septal lead

The author has some experience with placing leads within the right atrial septum from a jugular venous approach (Figure 53.7). For this location, a thin (4.1 Fr)

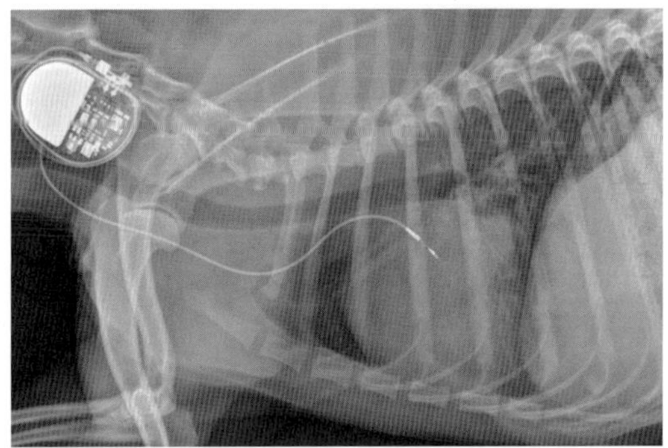

A

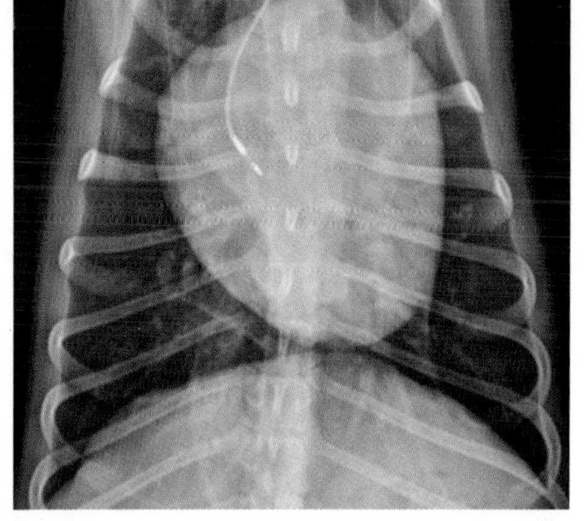

B

Figure 53.7 Orthogonal view thoracic radiographs showing a single-chamber right atrial septal pacing system. There is an active fixation lead placed within the right auricular appendage.

lumenless fixed screw-in lead (Select Secure 3830 from Medtronic) is used, which is passed through a steerable catheter delivery system (Select Site, Medtronic Inc.). We have found that there is a significant learning curve to using this lead. The advantages of the 3830 leads include: (1) smaller lead body which is more flexible and may fit into small dog atria easier, and (2) smaller lead French size, which may reduce the likelihood of cranial caval syndrome in small dogs. Because it is not an extendable helix, a disadvantage is there is no set number of turns to make or any visual aid on fluoroscopy to help you know when it has been effectively implanted. It is a matter of "feel" to know how much resistance is present in order to not over-drive through the myocardium. The optimal placement is typically four to five rotations of the lead. In small dogs, the guiding catheter which comes with the 3830 leads is far too large. Thus, we use the LV delivery system guiding catheter which has a very small bend at the tip allowing us to place the 3830 in the RA septum while using the cutting technique described above with a modified 'handle'. The guiding catheter and lead are placed together with the lead fully inside of the guiding catheter and the bend pointed down towards the RV/floor of the RA. The guiding catheter is then rotated counterclockwise and directed toward the right atrial septum with the operator's left hand on the guiding catheter. Next, the 3830 lead is advanced out of the guiding catheter with the right hand and rotated once clockwise and then stabilized with the left hand after the full rotation. This is repeated four to five times, until the resistance grows. The lead is then released, at which point the slack of the lead should spin within the fingers if it has been driven into the atrial myocardium. In this location, P waves of at least 2 mV should be seen if the lead is appropriately placed. Optimal lead impedance for this lead in this location is 900–1200 Ω. The guiding catheter is then cut off as previously described above for LV free wall leads.

Dual-chamber pacing systems

The lead positions described above may be combined to allow for dual-chamber sequential pacing (right atrium and right or left ventricle; Figure 53.8), dual-chamber sensing with a single pacing lead (Figure 53.9), or biventricular pacing (right atrium, right ventricle, and left ventricle; Figure 53.10).

Lead Testing

Once a lead is placed, it is important to determine whether the location of the pacing lead is adequate. Several measurements are now made using an external

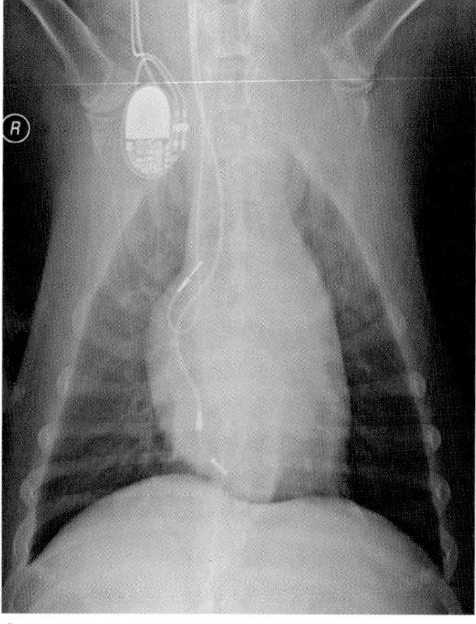

A

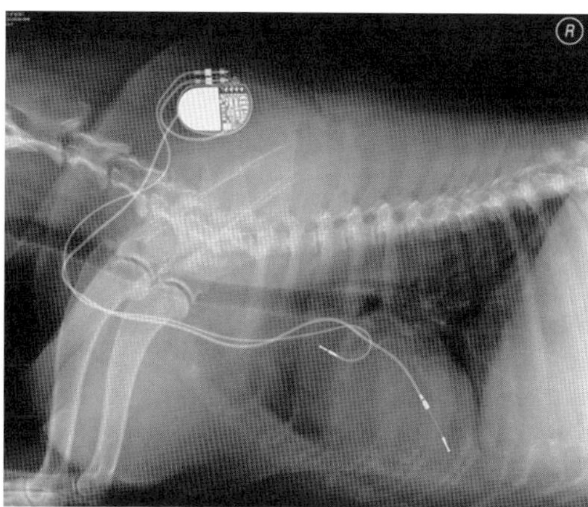

B

Figure 53.8 Orthogonal view thoracic radiographs showing a dual-chamber pacing system. There are passive fixation leads in both the right auricular appendage and right ventricular apex.

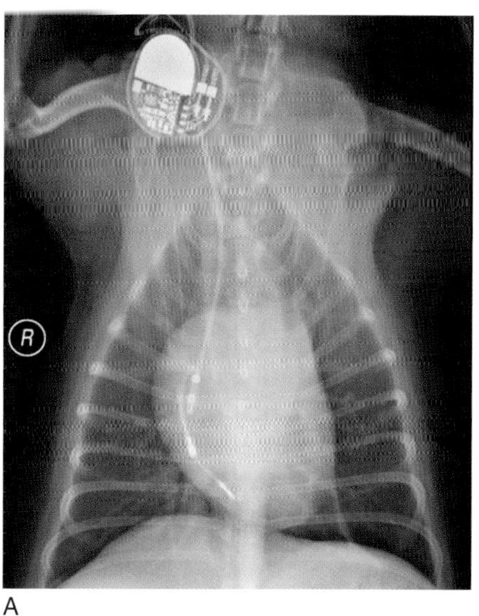

A

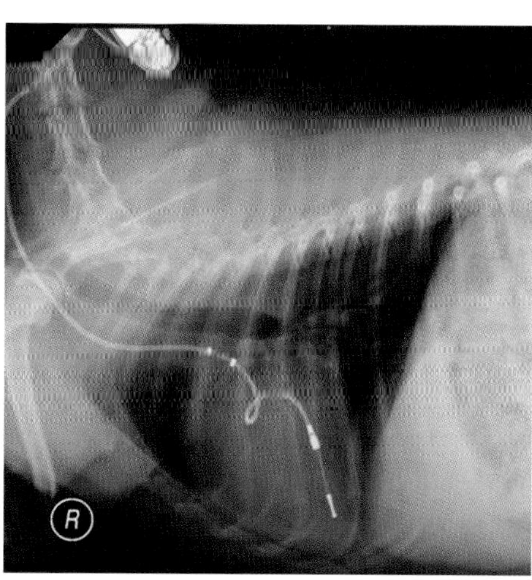

B

Figure 53.9 Orthogonal view thoracic radiographs showing a dual-chamber pacing system utilizing a sensing only floating atrial electrode. There is passive fixation of the lead in the right ventricular apex and a loop created in the right atrium such that the floating atrial electrode is within the cranial portion of the right atrium.

pacing system analyzer. With a ventricular lead, the R wave height is measured to ensure that the pacing lead can 'see' complexes well enough using the guidelines given above for each lead.

Next, the *impedance* is determined. Impedance is the total resistance to current flow and gives information regarding the integrity of the pacing system. Impedance should generally be between 500 and 1000 Ω at time of implantation. Lastly, and most importantly, the *threshold* for pacing is determined. The threshold for cardiac pacing is the minimal electric stimulus required to cause cardiac muscle contraction. For safety reasons, a margin of two to three times this minimal value is programmed to ensure that capture/contraction will occur. Once the pacing leads are in place and determined to be functioning appropriately, they are secured within the jugular vein by encircling ligatures. The author uses 2–0 braided polyester for securing the lead and ties it tight (nearly to the point of breaking). With this type of suture material, it is not necessary to be concerned about causing damage to the lead insulation. The first ligature is placed around the lead and jugular vein. Next, in order to simulate neck and head motion when the patient is awake, the cranial suture that is tied off on the jugular vein is gently pulled while watching the lead body and tip on fluoroscopy to

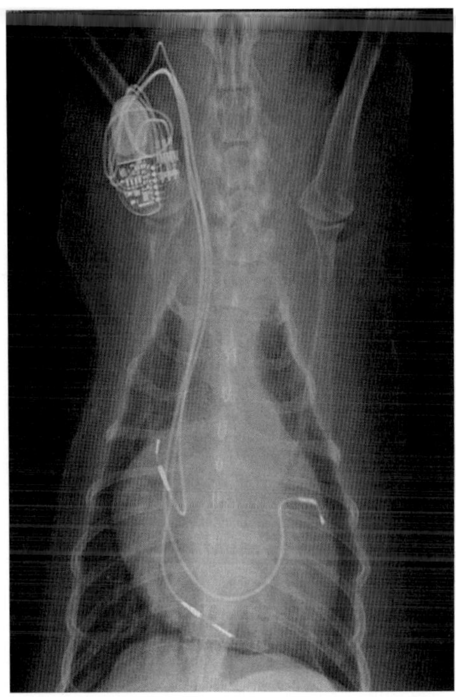

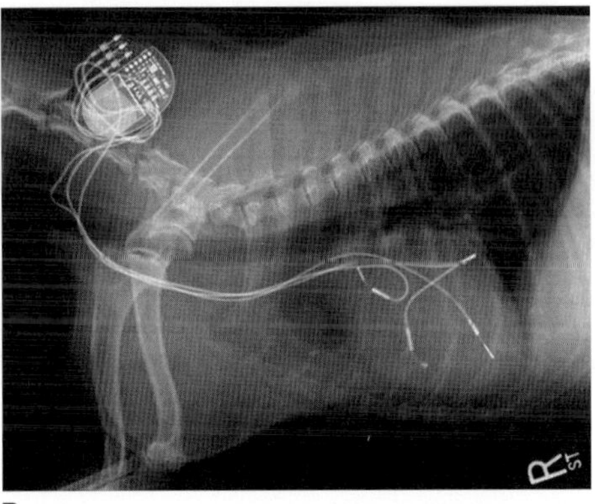

Figure 53.10 Orthogonal view thoracic radiographs showing a dual-chamber biventricular pacing system. There are passive fixation leads in the right auricular appendage, the right ventricular apex and within a cardiac vein overlying the interventricular septum via the coronary sinus.

ensure that there is enough slack within the lead such that it does not move from the desired position during motion. When a single lead is used, the anchoring sleeve is placed into the jugular vein and two to three additional ligatures are placed encircling the jugular vein, lead and anchoring sleeve. When multiple leads are placed, the anchoring sleeve is cut off with iris scissors and leads are individually secured to the jugular vein by encircling ligatures. The author currently uses 2–0 braided polyester suture, as this type of suture material can be tied very tightly without causing lead damage, even when secured directly onto the lead, in order to avoid lead migration.

Generator

Once the leads have been secured and tested, a subcutaneous pocket is dissected either dorsal to the jugular vein in the neck or a second incision is made above the first incision and a subcutaneous pocket is bluntly dissected with the fingers (Figure 53.11A). If a second incision is made (this is the author's preference) the leads are then tunneled up to the second incision with hemostats (Figure 53.11B). The leads are then connected to the appropriate port(s) of a pulse generator (Figure 53.11C). The lead must be firmly advanced into the pulse generator to ensure the lead electrodes fully engage the electrodes of the generator (see inset in Figure 53.11C). A wrench, supplied by the pacemaker manufacturer, is then inserted into the screwhole(s) on top of the generator and turned clockwise until a clicking sound is heard, confirming the lead is tightly screwed into the generator. The remaining lead lengths and the generator are placed in the subcutaneous pocket and the incision is closed routinely (Figure 53.11D). The neck is wrapped with a sterile bandage, which is left in place for 2 weeks, and changed when necessary. Basic programming is performed at this time but further fine tuning and adjustment of pacing parameters are typically performed the following day.

Pacemaker Programming

All contemporary pacemakers have many programmable parameters that can be altered to optimize and troubleshoot pacemaker function. Pacemakers can be programmed and evaluated non-invasively to adjust and fine-tune the pacing parameters. Programming and interrogation of pacemakers typically occur in the immediate (24 hour) post-operative period, at a 4–6-week recheck, at 3 and 6 months and then yearly to assess not only function but also battery life. All manufacturers of pacemakers also make programmers. These are not, however, interchangeable and a specific device will require a certain programmer. A detailed description of pacemaker programming is

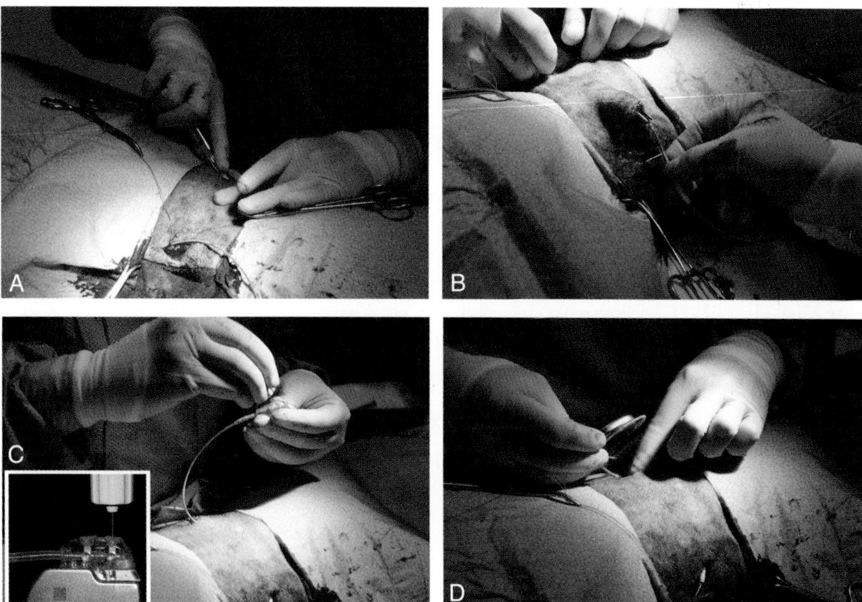

Figure 53.11 Images during permanent pacemaker implantation. (A) The second incision created above the initial lead placement site for insertion of the pulse generator. (B) The lead(s) is (are) then tunneled under the skin up to this location. (C) The attachment of the pacing lead to the pulse generator. Note that the lead must be firmly advanced into the generator and fully seated to engage the electrodes (inset). The lead is then screwed into the generator tightly by clockwise rotation of the wrench into the small screwhole(s) on top of the generator until a clicking sound is heard. (D) The subcutaneous pocket that is created dorsal to this incision using blunt dissection with the fingers where the leads and pulse generator are then buried.

beyond the scope of this text. A few of the most critical parameters merit mention here.

Pulse Width and Voltage Amplitude Programmability

Output programming is probably the most important aspect of programming that should be performed routinely. There are two aspects of voltage output that can be programmed: the *voltage*, or amplitude of the impulse; and the *pulse width*, or how long this voltage is applied to the myocardium. The combination of these make up the output delivered to the myocardium. The output must be high enough to allow an adequate pacing margin of safety but should also be programmed with the intent of maximizing pacemaker longevity. There is no consensus of the best way to program output parameters, but values are usually set at either twice the voltage amplitude at threshold or three times the pulse width at threshold. The less output used, the longer the battery will last. A pacing lead usually has its lowest threshold at the time of implantation. Over a period of 2 to 6 weeks, the threshold rises to its highest level at approximately three to four times the acute level and then falls to a chronic threshold that is usually stable at approximately two or three times the acute level.

Follow-Up

Threshold testing is performed the day following implantation and voltage amplitude and pulse width are left at three times the threshold settings in anticipation of the rise that occurs and peaks at approximately 4–6 weeks postimplantation. The implant incision sites are checked for any signs of inflammation or infection and bandages are changed. This is typically done with the owner of the patient so that they can see what the surgical site looks like at time of discharge from hospital and so that they can be shown how to correctly bandage the neck. Owners are sent home with two to three sets of rebandaging material and instructed to keep the bandages clean and dry. Suture removal is scheduled for 3–4 weeks (typically with the family veterinarian).

In the 4–6 week postoperative period, there should be strict exercise restriction with leash walks only. A harness, instead of a neck collar, is used from now on and typically is purchased by the owner prior to hospital discharge such that the pet can be sent home using this. The owners should be counseled to have the pet avoid any jumping and running in order for the lead to become stable within the implanted location. Owners are also taught how to take the pet's heart rate either via auscultation with a stethoscope or palpation of the femoral pulse and given instructions if and when to call with reports of abnormal heart rates. Patients are continued on antibiotics (cephalexin 22 mg/kg PO, BID) for 2 weeks.

Recheck evaluation for pacemaker programming and threshold testing is performed at 6 weeks post-implantation. At this point in time, output settings can be lowered to twice the threshold as maximal inflammation and highest threshold will have occurred by this point. The pet can also start to resume normal activity at this time. The patient is then rechecked again at 6 months postimplantation for an electrocardiogram, threshold testing, and echocardiogram (basic echocardiographic evaluation, assessment of lead for clot or thrombus, etc.). Recheck evaluations are then scheduled on a yearly basis. Heart rate trends are continued at home by the owner once per week as initial depletions of battery will typically lower the output rate in order to provide an early indication of need for replacement.

Suggested Reading

Adachi M, Igawa O, Yano A, et al. (2008) Long-term reliability of AAI mode pacing in patients with sinus node dysfunction and low Wenckebach block rate. *Europace* 10, 134–7.

Hillock RJ and Mond HG (2012) Pacing the right ventricular outflow tract septum: time to embrace the future. *Europace* 14(1), 28–35.

Khan MN, Joseph G, Khaykin Y, et al (2005) Delayed lead perforation: a disturbing trend. *Pacing Clin Electrophysiol* 28, 251–3.

Kikuchi K, Abe H, Nagamoto T, et al (2003) Microdislodgment: a likely mechanism of pacing failure with high impedance small area electrodes. *Pacing Clin Electrophysiol* 26, 1541–3.

Mahapatra S, Bybee KA, Bunch TJ, et al (2005) Incidence and predictors of cardiac perforation after permanent pacemaker placement. *Heart Rhythm* 2, 907–11.

Masumoto H, Ueda Y, Kato R, et al (2004) Long-term clinical performance of AAI pacing in patients with sick sinus syndrome: a comparison with dual-chamber pacing. *Europace* 6, 444–50.

Pioger G, Leny G, Nitzsche R, and Ripart A. (2007) AAIsafeR limits ventricular pacing in unselected patients. *Pacing Clin Electrophysiol* 30, S66–S70.

Sharma AD, Rizo-Patron C, Hallstrom AP, et al; DAVID Investigators. (2005) Percent right ventricular pacing predicts outcome in the DAVID trial. *Heart Rhythm* 2 (Suppl 2), S75–76.

Van De Wiele CM, Hogan DF, et al (2008) Cranial vena cava syndrome secondary to transvenous pacemaker implantation in two dogs. *J Vet Cardiol* 10, 155–61.

Wess G, Thomas WP, Berger DM, et al (2006) Applications, complications, and outcomes of transvenous pacemaker implantation in 105 dogs (1997–2002). *J Vet Intern Med* 20, 877–84.

CHAPTER FIFTY-FOUR

Arrhythmia Ablation

Roberto A. Santilli and Manuela Perego
Clinica Veterinaria Malpensa, Samarate Varese, Italy

Introduction

Radiofrequency energy is a sinusoidal current with a band of 0.3 to 30 MHz used in medicine for ablating, coagulating, and cauterizing tissues. For catheter ablation, radiofrequency is delivered to the cardiac tissue through a small endocardial or epicardial electrode to provide effective tissue heating. The range of tip temperatures used during radiofrequency catheter ablation is 50 °C to 90 °C, although temperatures ranging between 60 °C and 70 °C are the target for many temperature-controlled catheters. These temperatures induce a rise of electrode–tissue interface temperature that provokes myocardial damage through resistive heating of the superficial layers and through a conductive heating of the deeper layers. Thermal injuries vary according to the temperature reached: abnormal automaticity has been observed at temperature >45 °C, while conduction block develops at temperatures between 51.7 °C and 54.4 °C. Temperatures above 50 °C induce an irreversible loss of cellular excitability.

Four to 5 days after catheter ablation, well-circumscribed areas of coagulation necrosis, surrounded by a peripheral zone of hemorrhage, and mononuclear cell and neutrophil infiltration appear. In 2 months, areas of fibrosis, granulation tissue, fat cell deposition, cartilage formation, and chronic inflammatory cell infiltration develop.

Indications

Radiofrequency catheter ablation is the first line treatment for most common supraventricular arrhythmias reported in the dog, such as focal atrial tachycardia, atrial flutter, and bypass-tract mediated tachycardia as well as for ventricular tachycardia refractory to medical treatment. Radiofrequency catheter ablation can also be used to modulate the ventricular rate in cases of tachycardia-induced cardiomyopathy caused by incessant supraventricular arrhythmias through ablation of the His bundle followed by permanent ventricular pacing.

Potential Risks, Complications and Follow Up

In human medicine radiofrequency catheter ablation of cardiac arrhythmias has a global success rate of 97.4% and a significant complication rate of 0.14%. The success rate of radiofrequency catheter ablation of atrioventricular nodal reciprocating tachycardia is reported as 96.1% with a 1% risk of iatrogenic atrioventricular block occurrence, while ablation of accessory pathways is reported successful in 94% of cases with a complication rate of 1.83%. The acute success rate of radiofrequency catheter ablation of atrial flutter is 86% with a complication rate of 1.3%, while radiofrequency catheter ablation of atrial tachycardia is associated with 80% success for a right atrial focus, 72% for left atrial foci, and 52% for septal foci. The success rate of radiofrequency catheter ablation for ventricular tachycardia is higher for humans with idiopathic ventricular tachycardia compared to those with ventricular tachycardia due to ischemic heart diseases or cardiomyopathy. Iatrogenic atrioventricular block was the most common complication derived from radiofrequency catheter ablation (5.1%), while procedure-related death ranged between 0.08 and 0.13%. Recurrence rates reported after radiofrequency catheter ablation of accessory pathways, focal atrial tachycardia and atrial flutter were respectively 5.5%, 8%, and 7%.

In the author's electrophysiology laboratory, overall success rate has been 92.3% (100% for cavotricuspid isthmus (CTI)-dependent atrial flutter; 98% for

Veterinary Image-Guided Interventions, First Edition. Edited by Chick Weisse and Allyson Berent.

Companion website: www.wiley.com/go/weisse/vet-image-guided-interventions

accessory pathways; 79% for focal atrial tachycardia). Recurrence rates of 7.2% have been observed (15% CTI-dependent atrial flutter; 4.5% accessory pathways; 2% focal atrial tachycardia) with a complication rate of 6.2% (2% accessory pathways; 5.2% focal atrial tachycardia).

Equipment

Radiofrequency catheter ablation is preceded by a detailed endocardial or epicardial mapping study under electro-anatomic guidance. The equipment needed to perform catheter ablation includes:

1. A C-arm fluoroscopic unit that allows positioning of catheters within the cardiac chambers and vascular tributaries using two views: right lateral and 30 degree dorsoventral oblique (Figure 54.1).
2. An electrophysiologic system, which displays 12 surface and 10–12 endocavitary electrographic leads and permits the mapping of endocavitary potentials to analyze the sequence of activation and to perform atrial and ventricular stimulations.
3. Several different electrode catheters, introduced with the modified Seldinger technique, which differ depending on the area of interest: quadripolar, to map the His potentials; decapolar, to map the coronary sinus and the right atrial wall potentials; and a Lasso catheter, to map the pulmonary venous ostia (Figure 54.2).
4. A transseptal puncture kit to obtain left atrial access. It is composed of a specially designed needle, a long

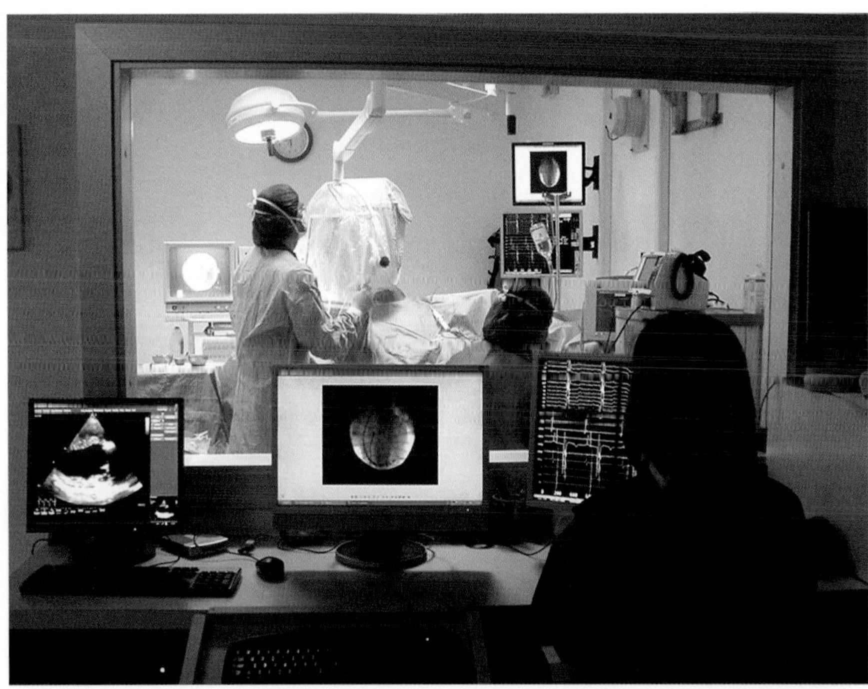

Figure 54.1 Electrophysiologic laboratory including an external workstation where one operator analyzes intracardiac and surface electrograms, performs mapping and pacing and activates radiofrequency energy; and a surgery room, equipped with a C-arm fluoroscopic unit, cardioverter defibrillator and multiple screens. Here a second operator places the electrocatheters with fluoroscopic and intracardiac electrographic guidance.

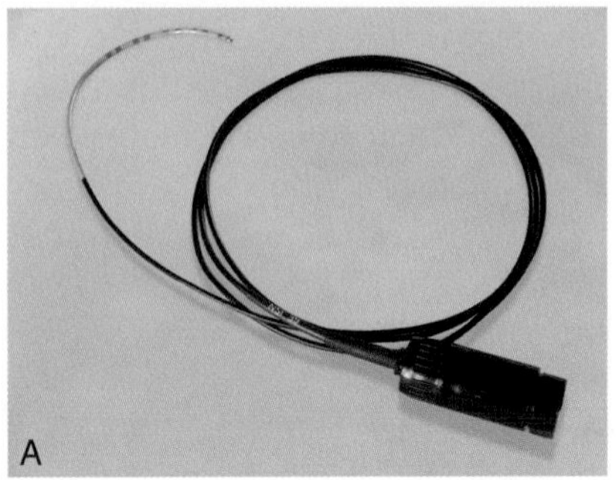

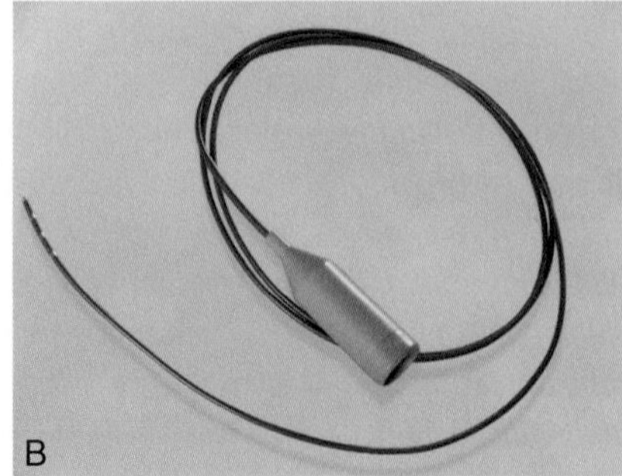

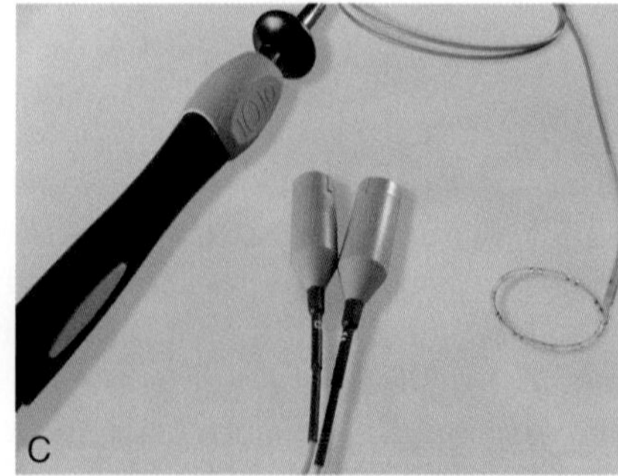

Figure 54.2 Electrodes used for endocardial mapping: (A) decapolar electrode used to map coronary sinus potentials and right atrial potentials; (B) quadripolar electrode used to map His potentials; (C) lasso catheter used to map pulmonary vein potentials.

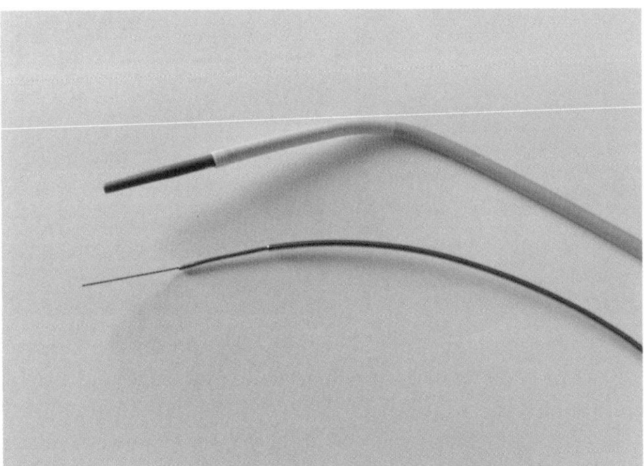

Figure 54.3 Transseptal puncture kit, including a 100 cm introducer set and a specially designed transseptal needle.

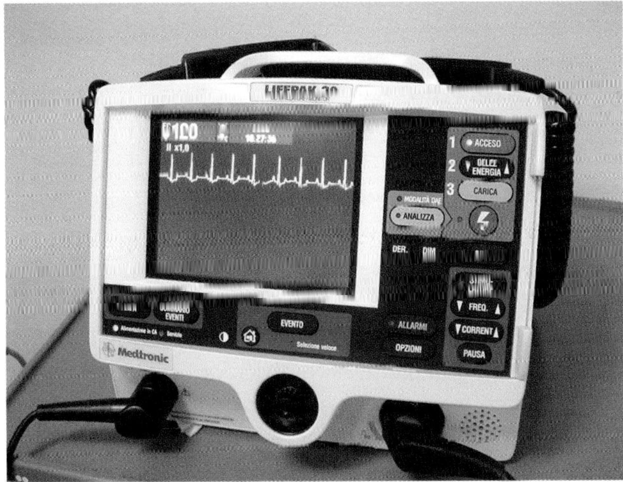

Figure 54.4 Biphasic cardioverter defibrillator with external pacing used to perform cardioversion of atrial fibrillation or asynchronous defibrillation of malignant ventricular arrhythmias.

introducer set to reach the fossa ovalis from a caudal approach and a 0.018″ wire (Figure 54.3).

5. A specially designed needle for pericardiocentesis and transpericardic epicardial approach in cases of epicardial ventricular tachycardia.
6. A biphasic cardioverter/defibrillator to perform electrical cardioversion and defibrillation (Figure 54.4).
7. A temperature-controlled ablation system and, in the case of low blood flow target sites such as the coronary body ostium or the pulmonary vein ostium, a thermocool irrigated ablation system.
8. A 7 Fr steerable ablation catheter with a tip diameter of 4–8 mm to deliver radiofrequency energy (Figure 54.5).

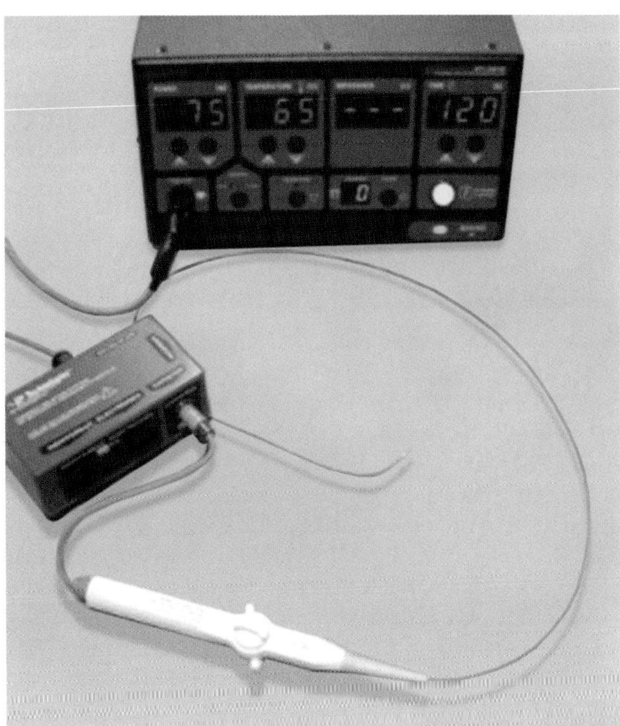

Figure 54.5 Ablation system with controlled temperature and the possibility to monitor power, impedence and time of radiofrequency erogation, as well as 7 Fr, 4 mm thermocoupled-tipped steerable catheter to perform radiofrequency catheter ablation.

Mapping Procedure

To perform radiofrequency catheter ablation the arrhythmic substrate and the target site should be established through a detailed electrophysiological study. The procedure is conducted under general anesthesia induced with propofol 4 mg/kg IV bolus, after pre-anesthetic medication with midazolam 0.2 mg/kg IM, and maintained with a mixture of isoflurane (1–2%) and oxygen (100%). Antiarrhythmic drugs should be discontinued for at least five half-lives before the procedure. Dogs are placed in dorsal recumbence and venous accesses for endocardial mapping are obtained using a modified Seldinger technique (see Chapter 44). Under fluoroscopic and intracardiac ECG guidance one decapolar and one quadripolar electrode catheter are placed respectively through the right external jugular vein into the coronary sinus (CS), and through the right femoral vein to the tricuspid valve annulus to record His bundle potentials. An ablation catheter with a deflectable curve is then positioned through the right or left femoral vein into the high right atrium, right ventricular apex, or tricuspid annulus to perform atrial or

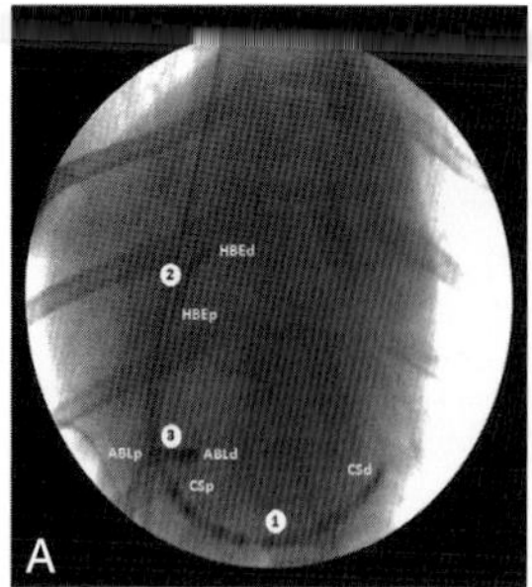

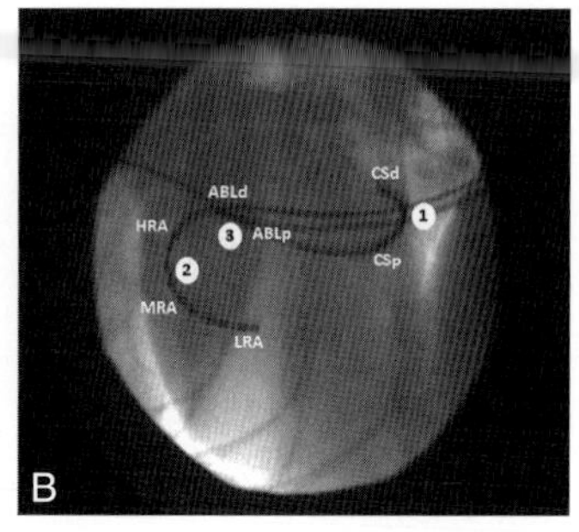

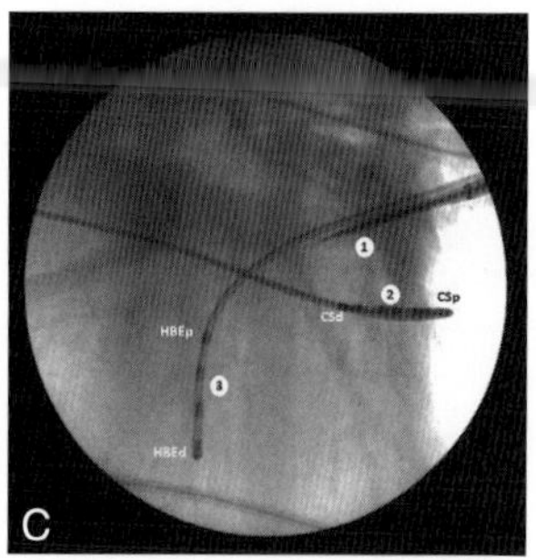

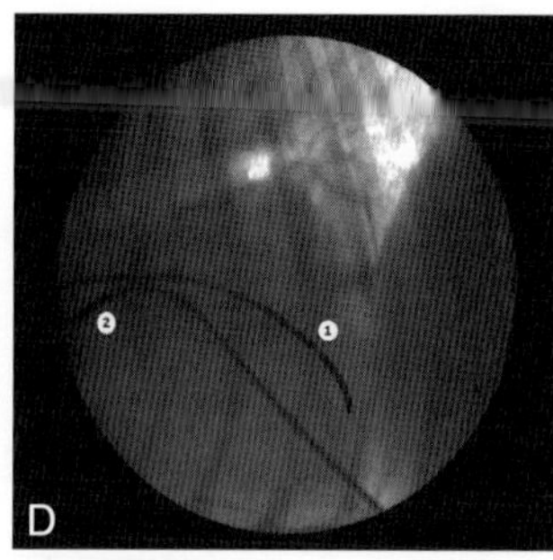

Figure 54.6 (A) Left-anterior 30° oblique fluoroscopic view with standard positioning of the electrodes for endocardial mapping of accessory pathways: (1) decapolar electrode placed into the coronary sinus body to map left atrial potentials (CSd) and the right atrial posterior wall (CSp); (2) quadripolar electrode placed at the His bundle (HBEp, HBEd); (3) 7 Fr, 4 mm thermocoupled-tipped steerable catheter placed in the mid-septal area to perform radiofrequency catheter ablation of an accessory pathway (ABLp, ABLd). (B) Right lateral fluoroscopic view with standard positioning of electrodes for endocardial mapping of right atrial flutter or right atrial focal tachycardia: (1) decapolar electrode placed into the coronary sinus body to map left atrial potentials (CSd) and the right atrial posterior wall (CSp); (2) decapolar electrode placed along the right atrial free wall recording the right atrial roof (HRA), crista terminalis (MRA) and low posterior right atrium (LRA); (3) 7 Fr, 4 mm thermo-coupled-tipped steerable catheter placed at the right atrial roof to perform radiofrequency catheter ablation of an atrial ectopic focus. (C) Right lateral fluoroscopic view used to guide transseptal needle (1) at the fossa ovalis; (2) decapolar electrode placed into the coronary sinus body to map left atrial potentials (CSd) and right atrial posterior wall (CSp); (3) quadripolar electrode placed at the His bundle (HBEp, HBEd). (D) Right lateral fluoroscopic view after transpericardic placement of an introducer into the pericardial sac to map the epicardial surface of the right ventricular outflow tract: (1) decapolar electrode placed at the right ventricular apex; (2) 7 Fr, 4 mm thermo-coupled-tipped steerable catheter placed at the epicardial surface of the right ventricular outflow tract to perform radiofrequency catheter ablation of an epicardial circuit.

ventricular programmed electrical stimulation, unipolar, and bipolar endocardial mapping, respectively (Figure 54.6A). In case of suspected focal atrial tachycardia or atrial flutter, a second decapolar electrode catheter is inserted through the right femoral vein and placed in the right atrium to record the anterolateral aspect of the crista terminalis (HRA) potentials with the proximal electrodes pairs, the middle lateral right atrium (MRA) potentials with the middle pairs and the low posterolateral right atrium (LRA) potentials with the distal pairs (Figure 54.6B). To map left atrial wall or pulmonary vein ectopic foci a transseptal puncture should be performed. Under fluoroscopic guidance a specially designed guide wire, inserted into a transseptal needle, is placed at the fossa ovalis through the femoral veins and pushed into the left atrium. The technique relies on fluoroscopic landmarks to identify anatomical boundaries. The movement of the tip of the needle, which resembles a "jump" from the thicker muscular septum to the thin wall of the fossa ovalis, is an indirect radiological sign of the position of the fossa that can be detected by experts without the need for adjunctive imaging modalities (Figure 54.6C). Once the wire is in the left atrium the dedicated needle is pushed across the interatrial septum to produce a larger hole and an introducer set is left in place and used to guide the Lasso catheter or the ablation catheter. The Lasso catheter is used to map pulmonary venous ostia while the ablation catheter is used to map ectopic foci at the left atrial wall, the pulmonary veins and the left appendage. Rarely, in cases of epicardial ventricular tachycardia in dogs with arrhythmogenic right ventricular cardiomyopathy, a detailed epicardial mapping study can be conducted with a retro-xyphoid transpericardic approach. A special designed needle is advanced in the pericardial sac with an ultrasound-guided technique. Once the tip of the needle is in the pericardial cavity, contrast medium is injected to assess the proper position, then a guide wire is positioned and over the wire an introducer placed to permit the insertion of an electrode catheter (Figure 54.6D).

Twelve-lead ECG and intracardiac signals are displayed and analyzed with an electrophysiologic recorder at paper speed of 100 or 300 mm/second. The intracardiac electrograms are recorded at a filter setting of 50–500 Hz. Pacing is performed using stimuli that are twice the diastolic threshold and 2 ms in duration.

During basal electrophysiologic study, conduction times (AH and HV) and refractoriness of the atrioventricular node and the eventual accessory atrioventricular connections are assessed with incremental and programmed atrial and ventricular pacing protocols. Incremental atrial and ventricular stimulation are performed by the coronary sinus and right ventricular apex with a progressively shorter cycle length to evaluate the antegrade and retrograde Wenckebach point of the atrioventricular node and of the accessory pathway, respectively. In some cases, rapid atrial pacing can induce focal atrial tachycardia caused by enhanced abnormal automaticity. Programmed atrial and ventricular stimulation is used to assess the antegrade and retrograde effective refractory period of the atrioventricular node and the accessory pathways and to induce re-entrant tachycardia, such as atrioventricular reciprocating tachycardia, micro-re-entrant atrial tachycardia, typical and atypical atrial flutter, and re-entrant ventricular tachycardia. Programmed atrial and ventricular pacing is performed using a protocol of a train of eight paced beats with a cycle length shorter than the intrinsic rhythm cycle length followed by an extrastimulus with a progressively shorter coupling interval. Antegrade conduction along an accessory pathway is considered present in the case of ventricular pre-excitation (either abnormally short or negative His to ventricular interval) during normal sinus rhythm or during atrial pacing at progressively shorter cycle lengths. The occurrence of retrograde conduction along an accessory pathway is demonstrated by the evidence of eccentric ventriculoatrial activation during ventricular programmed pacing or reciprocating tachycardia.

To determine the electrogenic mechanism of different supraventricular tachycardias, definitive electrophysiologic tests are performed. Orthodromic atrioventricular reciprocating tachycardia and permanent junctional reciprocating tachycardia are diagnosed in the case of eccentric ventriculoatrial activation when a single ventricular extrastimulus, which is introduced during tachycardia while the His bundle is refractory, pre-excites the atrium with an identical activation sequence. Termination of the tachycardia without atrial activation by a ventricular extrastimulus when the His bundle is refractory has also been considered diagnostic for bypass-tract mediated tachycardia. Resetting of the tachycardia circuit is used to differentiate a reciprocating tachycardia from a focal atrial tachycardia. After overdrive atrial pacing from the coronary sinus area during tachycardia, the presence of a variable first beat (more than 10 ms from baseline) ventriculoatrial interval after pacing is considered diagnostic for focal atrial tachycardia. Macro re-entrant atrial tachycardia, such as typical and atypical atrial flutter, are defined by entrainment with concealed fusion in the isthmus area. Pacing 10–20 ms faster than the atrial tachycardia cycle length at a site with presystolic activity or mid-diastolic potential can entrain a re-entrant tachycardia to the pacing rate without changing the morphology of F waves or the intracardiac electrogram sequence. As soon as the isthmus pacing is terminated, tachycardia should return to the initial cycle length including the first post-pacing interval.

For focal atrial tachycardia characterization, programmed atrial and ventricular stimulation, burst atrial pacing and a isoproterenol hydrochloride 0.04–0.1 μg/kg/min IV constant rate infusion are used to verify the electrogenic mechanism. Automatic focal atrial tachycardias are characterized by initiation only under isoproterenol infusion, while no effect of programmed stimulation on the initiation nor on termination should be observed, and the tachycardia can be transiently suppressed with overdrive pacing. Non-automatic focal atrial tachycardias are defined when the underlying mechanism is micro-reentry or delayed and triggered activity is reproducible during initiation of the tachycardia with incremental atrial pacing, programmed atrial pacing or burst atrial pacing.

Radiofrequency Catheter Ablation

Radiofrequency catheter ablation is performed with controlled temperature via a thermocouple-tipped steerable 7 Fr catheter. Radiofrequency current is generated by a conventional generator that monitors catheter tip temperature, power output, and impedance. Radiofrequency current is delivered at the atrial or ventricular endocardium or epicardium target area depending on the technique used with controlled temperature of a maximum of 65 °C and 75 W for 60 s. In cases of ablation of the isthmus area of atrial flutter, 65 °C and 100 W for at least 45 s are used. The erogation of current is terminated immediately in case of an increase in impedance or displacement of the catheter. Energy is usually applied during tachycardia to evaluate the interruption of the arrhythmia with no recurrence for at least 45 minutes post-ablation.

Accessory Atrioventricular Pathways

Accessory pathways are muscular connections between the atrial and ventricular myocardium (Kent fibers) or the atrioventricular node and the ventricle or the right bundle (Mahaim fibers). The anatomical distribution and electrophysiologic properties of Kent fibers have been reported in the dog. In most cases accessory pathways are right-sided, located in the posteroseptal and right posterior area, display non-decremental conduction, and 70% of them are concealed and mediate orthodromic atrioventricular reciprocating tachycardia.

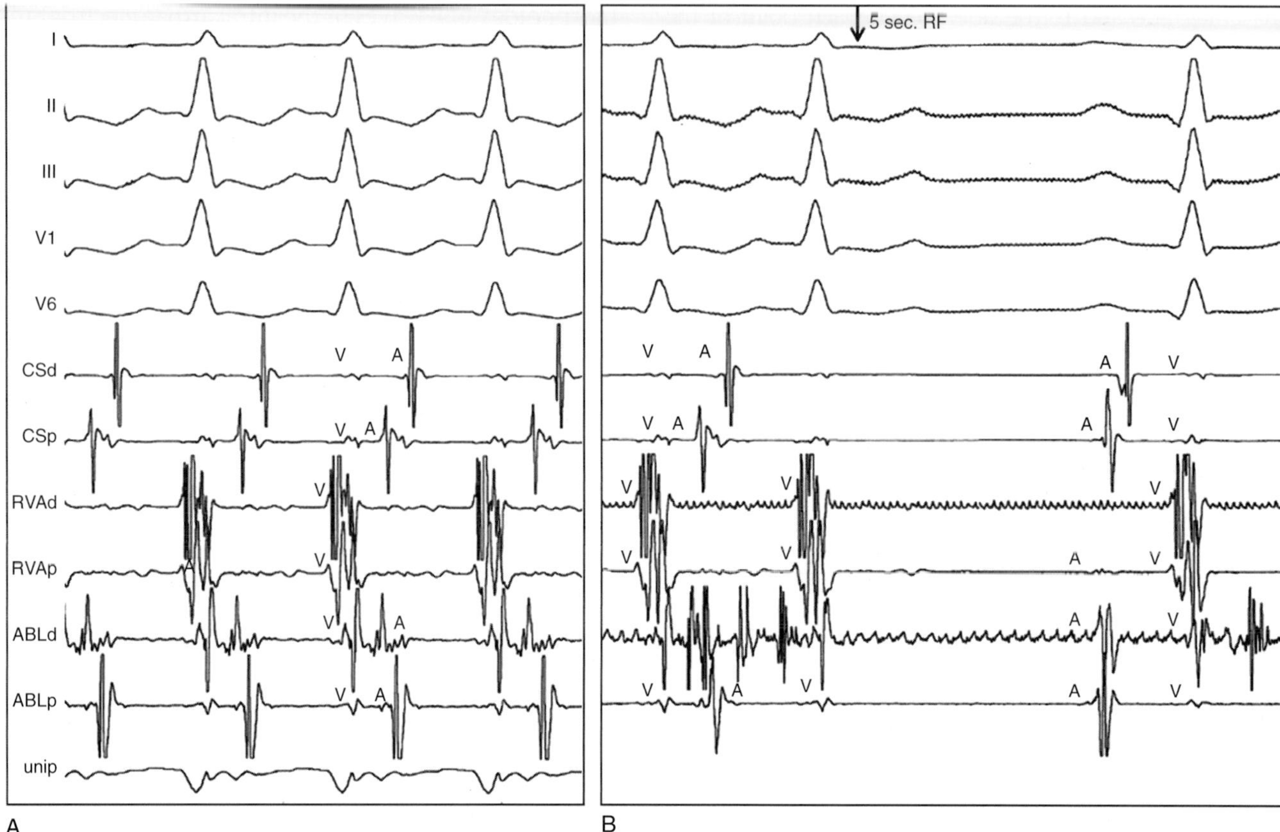

Figure 54.7 Surface and intracardiac electrograms obtained during endocardial mapping (A) and radiofrequency (RF) catheter ablation (B) of a midseptal accessory pathway in a dog with paroxysmal supraventricular tachycardia. Recordings displayed include: leads I, II, III, V1, and V6 of surface electrocardiogram and intracardiac atrial (A) and ventricular (V) potentials from the distal to the proximal portion of the coronary sinus (CSd, CSp), from the distal to the proximal portion of the right ventricular apex (RVAd, RVAp), from the distal to the proximal portion of the ablation catheter (ABLd, ABLp) and from the unipolar electrode (unip) placed on the distal dipole of the ablation catheter. In (A) notice the sequence of atrial and ventricular activation during orthodromic atrioventricular reciprocating tachycardia with a cycle length of 220 ms with a shorter V-A interval at the level of the ABLd located in the mid-septal area with sharp and negative unipolar recording. In (B) notice retrograde block of the macro-reentrant atrioventricular tachycardia along the accessory pathway (before the tachycardia termination in CSd, CSp, ABLp is visible V not followed by A) after 5 seconds of radiofrequency energy delivery with restoration of a normal sinus rhythm.

To map the tricuspid annulus area and to find the target of ablation, an adapted left anterior 30 degree oblique fluoroscopic view and intracardiac electrogram guidance should be used. The insertion of an accessory pathway is established by recording the earliest site of ventricular activation during antegrade conduction in the case of ventricular pre-excitation (during sinus rhythm or atrial pacing) and the site of earliest atrial activation during a reciprocating tachycardia or ventricular pacing in the case of a concealed accessory pathway. Sharp and negative unipolar waveforms are also used to localize the pole closest to the bypass tract (Figure 54.7). Left-sided accessory pathways are isolated with epicardial mapping through the coronary sinus multipolar catheter, while the right free wall and septal accessory pathways are mapped from the endocardium with a deflectable ablation catheter. Disappearance of accessory pathway conduction after successful radiofrequency catheter ablation of a particular target is also used as further proof of the bypass tract's anatomical site.

Focal Atrial Tachycardia

Focal atrial tachycardia is defined as an atrial activation starting rhythmically in a small area (focus) from which it spreads out centrifugally. Focal atrial tachycardia can be caused by enhanced abnormal automatism (automatic) as well as by either micro-re-entry or delayed triggered activities (non-automatic).

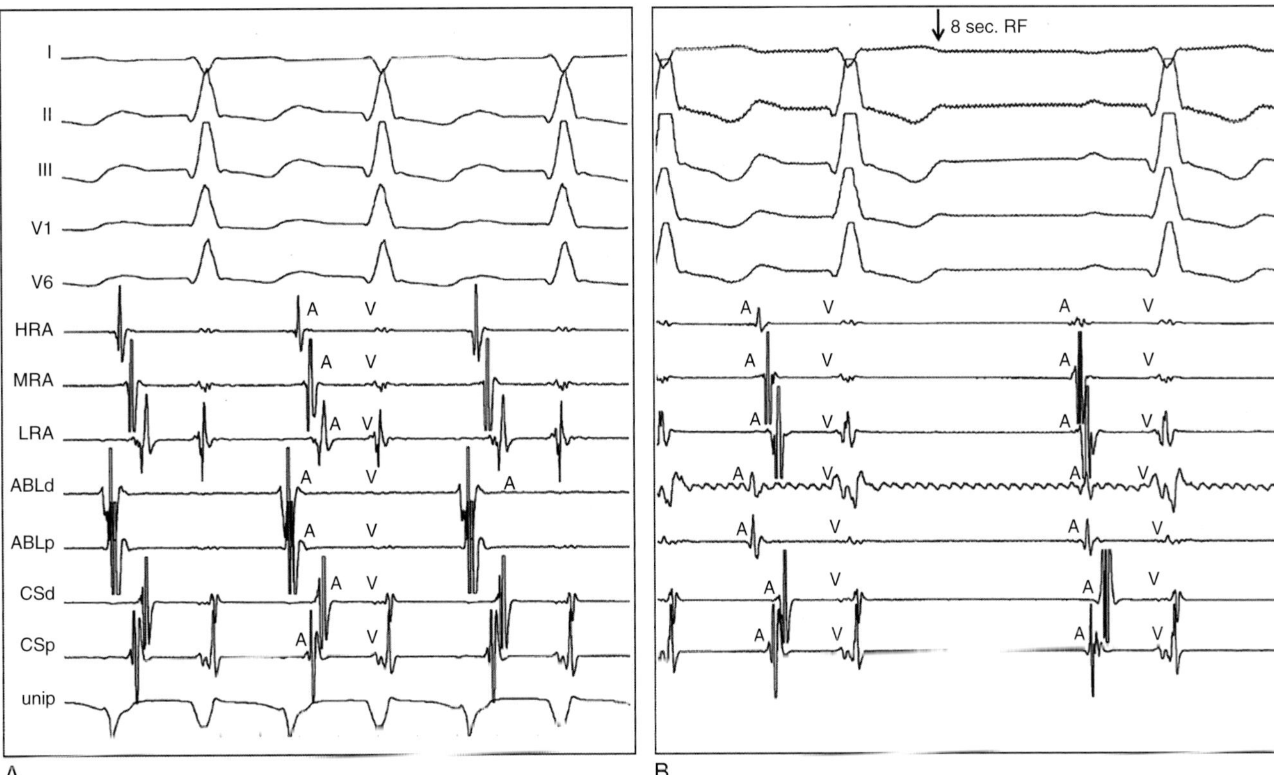

Figure 54.8 Surface and intracardiac electrograms obtained during endocardial mapping (A) and radiofrequency (RF) catheter ablation (B) of a focal atrial tachycardia in a dog with incessant supraventricular tachycardia and tachycardia-induced cardiomyopathy. Recordings displayed include leads I, II, III, V1, and V6 of surface electrocardiogram and intracardiac atrial (A) and ventricular (V) potentials from the antero-lateral aspect of the crista terminalis (HRA), middle lateral right atrium (MRA) and low postero-lateral right atrium (LRA), from the distal to the proximal portion of the ablation catheter (ABLd, ABLp), from the distal to the proximal portion of the coronary sinus (CSd, CSp), and from the unipolar electrode (unip) placed on the distal dipole of the ablation catheter. In (A) notice the sequence of atrial and ventricular activation during focal atrial tachycardia arising from the crista terminalis with a cycle length of 300 ms and the earlier site of atrial activation at the level of the ABLd located at the crista terminalis with sharp and negative unipolar recording. In (B) notice the termination of the automatic tachycardia after 8 seconds of radiofrequency energy delivery with restoration of a normal sinus rhythm.

In dogs, the majority of focal atrial tachycardias reported are automatic and the ectopic foci are usually right-sided (63%) located particularly near the crista terminalis and coronary sinus ostium. In about one third of dogs the atrial ectopic foci are left-sided and located in the pulmonary venous ostia. The atrial ectopic foci are localized at the site of the earliest presystolic activity relative to the onset of the P wave during tachycardia (–39.9 + 17.7 ms) where the sharp and negative unipolar recording, with QS pattern, appears. To determine the site of origin of focal atrial tachycardia, mechanical interruption caused by application of pressure to the focus and the presence of fragmented, long duration, low amplitude electrograms are considered diagnostic for the ablation target area. Fractioned potentials consist of three or more consecutive negative deflections with low peak-to-peak amplitude (Figure 54.8).

Atrial Flutter

Atrial flutter is a macro-re-entrant atrial tachycardia characterized by an anatomical circuit that includes an area of slow conduction called an isthmus. According to the location of the isthmus area, atrial flutter is usually divided into typical and atypical subtypes. In typical atrial flutter, the isthmus involved is the CTI, an area of the low posterior right atrium bounded by the inferior (caudal) vena cava and the Eustachian ridge posteriorly and the tricuspid valve annulus anteriorly. According to their rotation pattern around the tricuspid valve annulus, two form of CTI-dependent atrial flutter have been identified, both in humans and in dogs: typical (counterclockwise) and reverse typical (clockwise). The activation sequence of the right atrium and tricuspid valve annulus during clockwise atrial flutter presents a superior-to-inferior activation of the

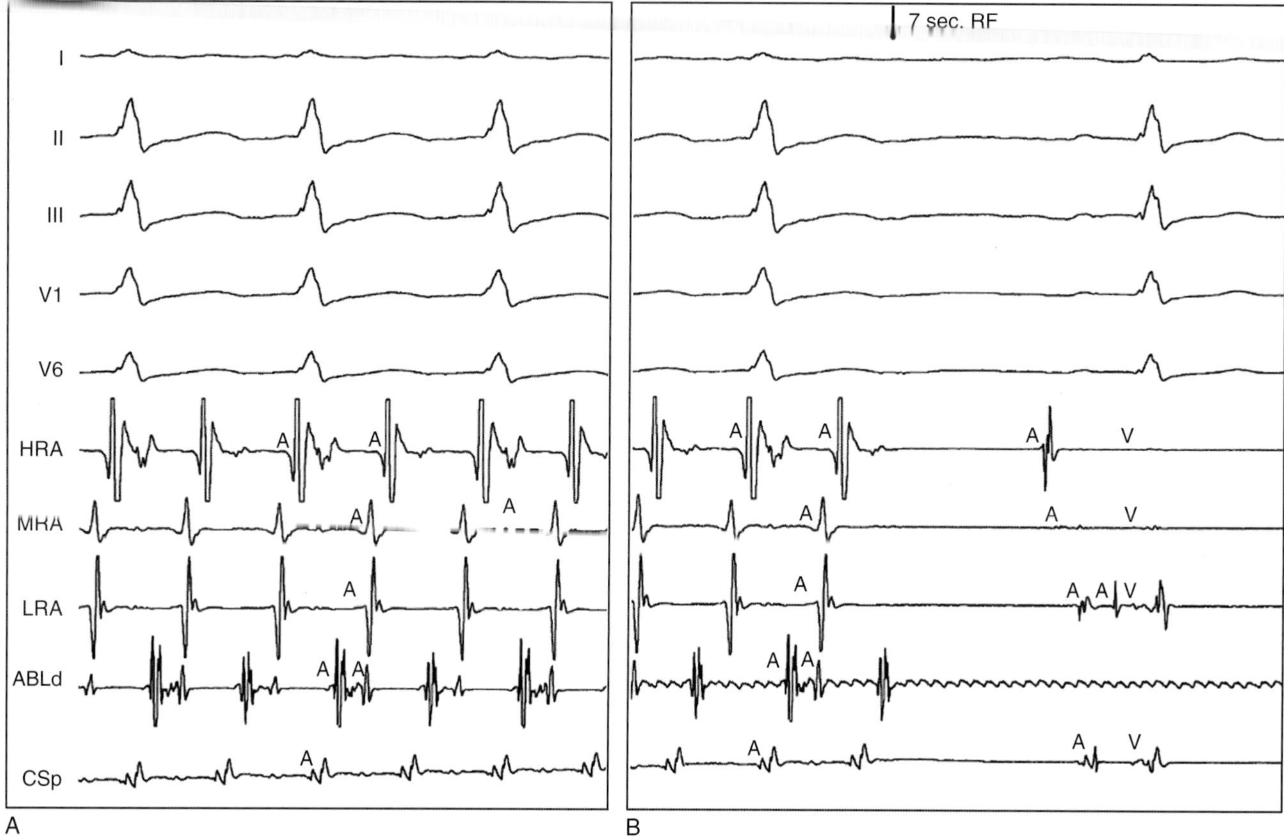

Figure 54.9 Surface and intracardiac electrograms obtained during endocardial mapping (A) and radiofrequency (RF) catheter ablation (B) of a reverse typical cavotricuspid isthmus dependent atrial flutter with 2:1 atrioventricular conduction ratio in a dog with incessant supraventricular tachycardia. Recordings displayed include: leads I, II, III, V1, and V6 of surface electrocardiogram and intracardiac atrial (A) and ventricular (V) potentials from high right atrium (HRA), middle right atrium (MRA) and low right atrium (LRA), from the distal portion of the ablation catheter (ABLd) and from the proximal portion of the coronary sinus (CSp). In (A) notice the sequence of atrial and ventricular activation during atrial flutter with an atrial cycle length of 140 ms and a ventricular cycle lengh to 280 ms and with a clockwise rotation around the tricuspid valve annulus from CSp, to ABLd, to LRA, to MRA, to HRA and back to CSp. A double potential suggesting a line of block is present at the ABLd site. In (B) notice the termination of the macroreentrant right atrial circuit after 7 seconds of radiofrequency energy delivery with restoration of a normal sinus rhythm. A double potential suggestive of a line of block is present at the LRA site.

interatrial septum and inferior-to-superior activation of the right atrial free wall. The atrial wavefront proceeds from the His area timed with the beginning of the suspected F wave, to the CS ostium, the LRA, the MRA, the HRA, to reach the His bundle again. During counterclockwise atrial flutter, the activation pattern of right atrium and tricuspid valve annulus presents an inferior-to-superior activation of the interatrial septum and superior-to-inferior activation of the right atrial free wall. Once the diagnosis of CTI-dependent AFL is made, the CTI conduction time should be assessed by measuring the activation time from the LRA to the CS ostium or from the CS ostium to the LRA during pacing from the controlateral site (Figure 54.9).

To interrupt atrial flutter a bidirectional conduction block should be achieved at the isthmus area using radiofrequency energy. The ablation of the CTI is performed using both an anatomical and electrophysiological approach guided, respectively, by the right lateral fluoroscopic view and the presence of concealed entrainment at the target site. Radiofrequency application is performed during tachycardia by positioning the catheter in the mid-portion of the CTI starting from the tricuspid valve annulus. The catheter is then gradually withdrawn toward the caudal vena cava to produce a linear lesion. The endpoint of the procedure is the termination of the macro-reentrant atrial tachycardia, the impossibility of re-induction of the arrhythmia with programmed atrial stimulation both from the CS ostium and the LRA, and the presence of a CTI bidirectional block lesion. The presence of CTI bidirectional block is assessed by alternatively pacing the CS ostium and LRA searching for a prolongation of CTI conduction time, the presence of double potentials at the site of ablation, and

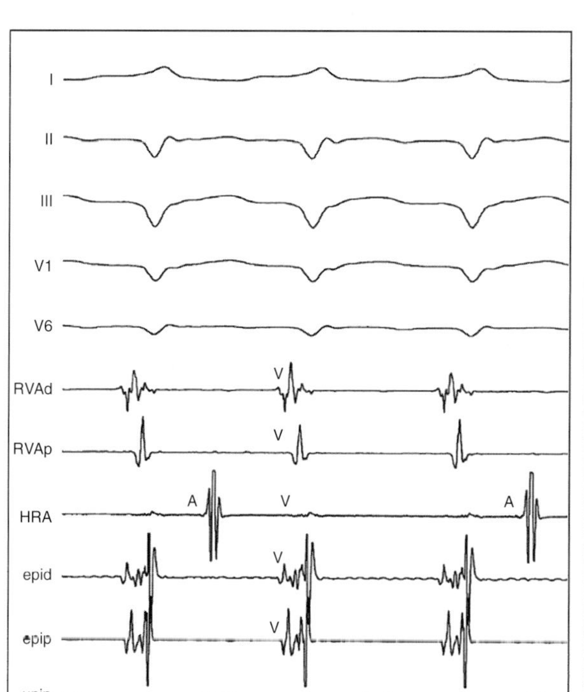

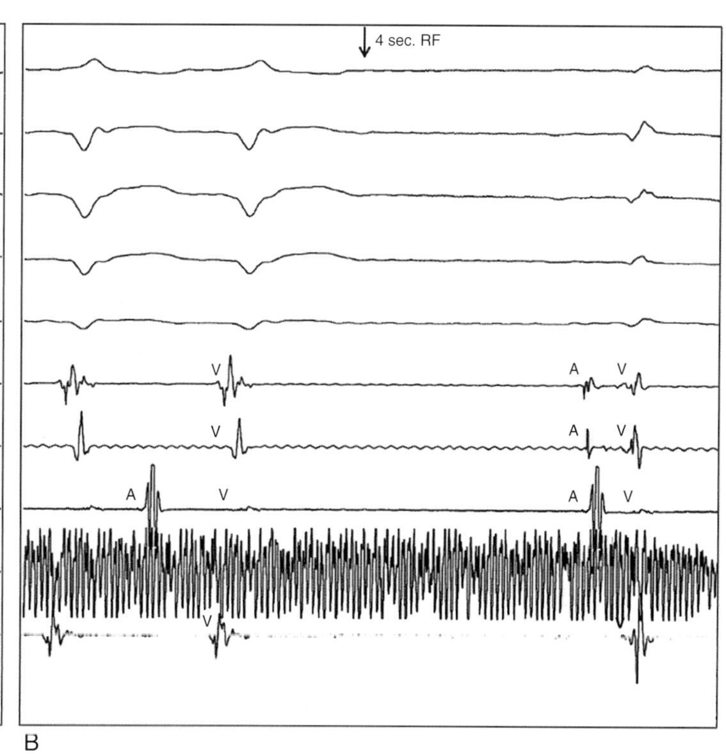

Figure 54.10 Surface and intracardiac electrograms obtained during simultaneous endocardial and epicardial mapping (A) and radiofrequency (RF) catheter ablation (B) of a reentrant ventricular tachycardia in a English Bulldog with segmental arrhythmogenic right ventricular tachycardia. Recordings displayed include: leads I, II, III, V1, and V6 of surface electrocardiogram and intracardiac and epicardial atrial (A) and ventricular (V) potentials from distal to proximal right ventricular apex (RVAd, RVAp), from high right atrium (HRA), from the distal to the proximal portion of the ablation catheter placed after a transpericardic approach at the level of the epicardial surface of the right ventricular outflow tract (epid, epip), and from the unipolar electrode (unip) placed on the distal dipole of the ablation catheter. In (A) notice the sequence of atrial and ventricular activation during ventricular tachycardia with a cycle length to 270 ms and the earlier site of ventricular activation at the epicardial level where a sharp and negative unipolar recording appears. In (B) notice the termination of the reentrant right ventricular circuit after 4 seconds of radiofrequency energy delivery with restoration of a normal sinus rhythm.

the presence of a change from a bidirectional activation pattern of the right free wall with a collision site at the right atrial free wall or inter-atrial septum to a superior-to-inferior activation post-ablation.

Ventricular Tachycardia

Radiofrequency catheter ablation is also indicated in patients with ventricular tachycardia associated with the segmental form of arrhythmogenic right ventricular cardiomyopathy. This type of myocardial disorder has been reported in the English bulldog and it is characterized by the presence of a segmental dilatation of the right ventricular outflow tract. Dogs affected present with incessant ventricular tachycardia having a left bundle block appearance that induces cardiogenic shock. The anatomical circuit can be either endocardial or epicardial. In the former, ablation can be performed with an ablation catheter introduced into the pulmonary artery to map the aneurysmatic area; in the latter case, a transpericardic approach is needed and the ablation catheter is introduced into the pericardial sac (Figure 54.10). In these cases the ventricular tachycardia is usually very rapid and the ablation site can be identified during sinus rhythm by searching for fragmented diastolic potentials that suggest inhomogeneous and slow conduction within the circuit.

Suggested Reading

Atkins CE, Kanter R, Wright K et al (1995) Orthodromic reciprocating tachycardia and heart failure in a dog with a concealed postero-septal accessory pathway. *J Vet Intern Med* 9(1), 43–9.

Foster SF, Hunt GB, Thomas SP, et al (2006) Tachycardia-induced cardiomyopathy in a young Boxer dog with supraventricular tachycardia due to an accessory pathway. *Aust Vet J* 84(9), 326–31.

Santilli RA, Bontempi LV, and Perego M (2011) Ventricular tachycardia in English bulldogs with localized right ventricular outflow tract enlargement. *J Small Anim Pract* 52(11), 574–80.

Santilli RA, Critelli M, and Baron Toaldo M (2010) ECG of the month. Pre-excited atrial fibrillation in a dog with an atrioventricular accessory pathway. *J Am Vet Med Assoc* 237(10), 1142–4.

Santilli RA, Diana A, and Baron Toaldo M (2012) Orthodromic atrioventricular reciprocating tachycardia conducted with intraventricular conduction disturbance mimicking ventricular tachycardia in an English Bulldog. *J Vet Cardiol* 14(2), 363–70.

Santilli RA, Perego M, Crosara S, et al (2008) Utility of 12-lead electrocardiogram in differentiating paroxysmal supraventricular tachycardias in the dog. *J Vet Intern* 2(4), 915–23.

Santilli RA, Perego M, Perini A, et al (2010) Electrophysiologic characteristics and topographic distribution of focal atrial tachycardias in dogs. *J Vet Intern Med* 24(3), 539–45.

Santilli RA, Perego M, Perini A, et al (2010) Radiofrequency catheter ablation of cavo-tricuspid isthmus as treatment of atrial flutter in two dogs. *J Vet Cardiol* 12(1), 59–66.

Santilli RA, Ramera M, Perego M, et al. (2014) Radiofrequency catheter ablation of atypical atrial flutter in five dogs. *J Vet Cardiol* 16(1): 9–17.

Santilli RA, Spadacini GM, Moretti P, et al (2006) Radiofrequency catheter ablation of concealed accessory pathways in two dogs with symptomatic atrioventricular reciprocating tachycardia. *J Vet Cardiol* 8(2), 157.

Santilli RA, Spadacini GM, Moretti P, et al (2007) Anatomic distribution and electrophysiologic properties of accessory atrioventricular pathways in dogs. *J Am Vet Med Assoc* 231(3), 393–8.

Sherlag BJ, Wang X, Nakagawa H, et al (1993) Radiofrequency ablation of a concealed accessory pathway as treatment for incessant supraventricular tachycardia in a dog. *J Am Vet Med Assoc* 203(8), 1147–52.

Wright KN, Bright JM, Cox JW Jr, et al (1996) Transcatheter modification of the atrioventricular node in dogs, using radiofrequency energy. *Am J Vet Res* 57(2), 229–35.

Wright KN, Hines DA, and Bright JM (1996) Cardiac electrophysiologic measurements in dogs before and after administration of atropine and propranolol. *Am J Vet Res* 57(12), 1695–701.

Wright KN, Mehdirad AA, Giacobbe P, et al (1999) Radiofrequency catheter ablation of atrioventricular accessory pathways in 3 dogs with subsequent resolution of tachycardia-induced cardiomyopathy. *J Vet Intern Med* 13(4), 361–71.

CHAPTER FIFTY-FIVE

Heartworm Extraction

Ashley B. Saunders
Department of Small Animal Clinical Sciences, College of Veterinary Medicine and Biomedical Sciences, Texas A&M University, College Station, TX

Background

In animals with heartworm disease, a life-threatening condition (caval syndrome) can occur when heartworms move from the pulmonary arteries back into the right atrium, venae cavae and across the tricuspid valve into the right ventricle. In dogs, it is typically but not always associated with a larger number of heartworms, while only a few heartworms can result in caval syndrome in cats and ferrets. A combination of red blood cell lysis, partial obstruction of inflow into the right heart, reduced cardiac output, and pulmonary hypertension manifests clinically as weakness, collapse, cough, dyspnea, and hemoglobinuria. A right sided systolic heart murmur correlates with tricuspid regurgitation secondary to the physical presence of the worms or elevated right heart pressures. Jugular venous distension and ascites occur with elevated right heart pressures and right-sided heart failure. Physical removal of heartworms is typically recommended to alleviate caval syndrome and may be beneficial in animals with large heartworm burdens and/or hemodynamic compromise. Without heartworm removal, hemolytic anemia, disseminated intravascular coagulation, hepatorenal dysfunction, and heart failure result, at which point prognosis is considered guarded to poor, often resulting in death within a few days.

Diagnosis and Patient Evaluation

Presenting complaints are typically related to acute signs of hemolysis, shock, or right-sided heart failure. The most common presenting clinical signs in dogs are hemoglobinuria, characterized as dark red or port wine colored urine, dyspnea, exercise intolerance, ascites, and cough. Cats with caval syndrome have been described with dyspnea secondary to chylous effusion or abdominal distension related to pulmonary hypertension. The ferret in one report presented for acute lethargy and collapse and had pulmonary artery enlargement on radiographs that led to the diagnosis.

A complete diagnostic work-up is recommended to assess clinical status, determine anesthetic risk, be able to appropriately advise owners, and create a treatment plan. Evaluation includes but may not be limited to a complete blood count, biochemistries, coagulation testing, heartworm testing, urinalysis, blood pressure, thoracic radiography, and echocardiography. If heartworm extraction is being considered, it is prudent to avoid acquiring blood samples from the right jugular vein to prevent hematoma formation or damage to the vessel prior to the procedure. The most common laboratory abnormalities are anemia, thrombocytopenia or other evidence of coagulopathy, elevations in alanine transferase, azotemia, proteinuria, and hemoglobinuria. Thoracic radiographs provide information regarding disease severity related to heart size, the pulmonary vasculature, and pulmonary parenchymal abnormalities. Echocardiography is used to assess heart size and function, determine the presence and severity of pulmonary hypertension, and to confirm the location of the heartworms that appear as hyperechoic, parallel lines (Figure 55.1 and Figure 55.2). Additional diagnostic tests may be indicated depending on clinical status or presenting signs.

Pulmonary hypertension is a common complicating factor, occurring in 65% of dogs with caval syndrome in one study. Dogs with significant pulmonary hypertension and signs of right heart failure with few heartworms apparent by echocardiography and without signs of hemolysis are not typically considered for heartworm extraction. Removing the heartworms will most likely not contribute to a clinical improvement in these patients.

Veterinary Image-Guided Interventions, First Edition. Edited by Chick Weisse and Allyson Berent.

Companion website: www.wiley.com/go/weisse/vet-image-guided-interventions

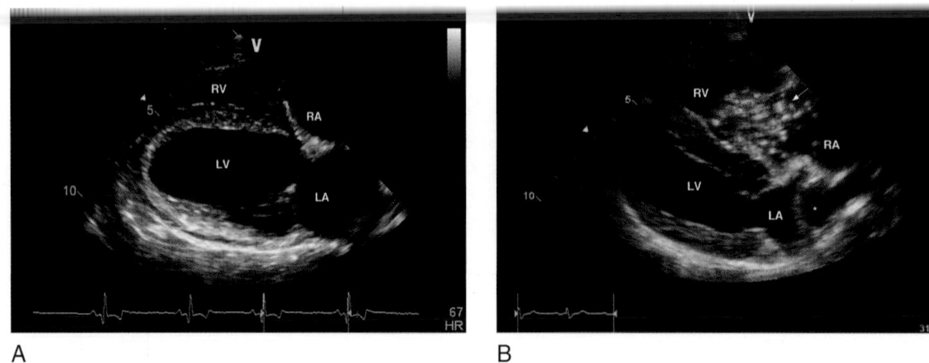

Figure 55.1 Transthoracic echocardiographic images taken in a right parasternal long axis view in two dogs. (A) Images from a normal dog with the left atrium (LA), left ventricle (LV), right atrium (RA) and right ventricle (RV) labeled for comparison purposes. (B) A dog with heartworms in the RA and RV. Heartworms were visualized echocardiographically as parallel white lines (arrow). The right pulmonary artery (*) is enlarged secondary to pulmonary hypertension.

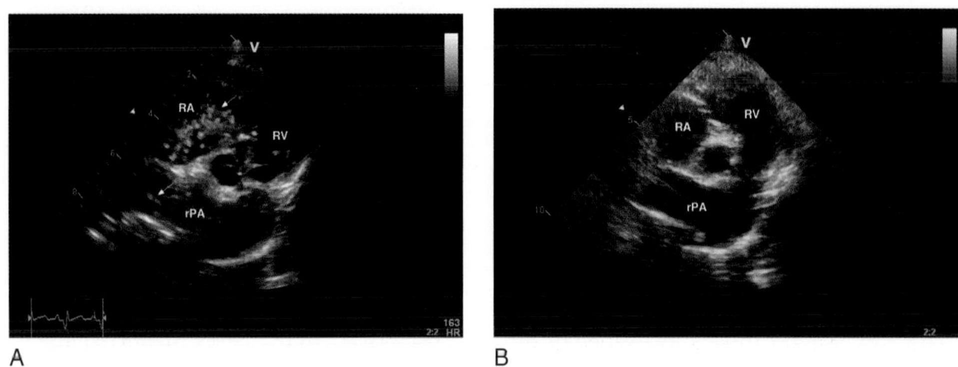

Figure 55.2 Transthoracic echocardiographic images from a right parasternal short axis view in a dog with caval syndrome and pulmonary artery enlargement. (A) Preoperative images documenting heartworms (arrows) in the right atrium (RA), right ventricle (RV), and right pulmonary artery (rPA). (B) Images obtained in the same dog 24 hours following heartworm extraction. Heartworms were no longer visualized.

Patients can present at various stages of caval syndrome from developing hemoglobinuria with no other overt clinical signs to those that are severely compromised. The urgency of performing the procedure depends on the clinical status at the time of evaluation. Patient stabilization, in preparation for the procedure, may require oxygen supplementation, thoracocentesis or abdominocentesis, vasopressors, and intravenous fluid therapy or blood products to address dyspnea and to improve cardiac output and tissue perfusion. Life-threatening arrhythmias should be addressed when present. In each case, the administration of medications prior to the procedure is considered and may include corticosteroids, diphenhydramine, low-molecular weight heparin, clopidogrel, bronchodilators, and antibiotics. Prior to therapy it is important to take into account any use of corticosteroids, doxycycline, non-steroidal anti-inflammatory medication and aspirin prior to presentation. Medications are selected to address airway inflammation, thromboembolism, and an increased risk of antigen release and acute circulatory collapse associated with possible damage to the heartworms during the removal process.

Potential Risks/ Complications/ Expected Outcomes

Patients that are clinically affected and have hemolytic, metabolic, and pulmonary aberrations are generally considered high risk for anesthesia. In order to perform the procedure, local anesthesia, sedation or general anesthesia is selected, based on clinical status in each case. When general anesthesia is required, a balanced protocol that minimizes systemic hypotension is recommended.

Complications that can occur during heartworm extraction include thromboembolism, hemorrhage, arrhythmias, and death. Damage to heartworms during extraction can result in acute circulatory collapse, especially in cats.

Physical removal of intact heartworms provides an immediate benefit compared to natural causes of heartworm death or death following the administration of an adulticide. However, it is not always possible to remove every heartworm during the procedure, particularly those present in the distal pulmonary arteries. Migration of heartworms from the right atrium and ventricle back out into the pulmonary arteries has been reported following general anesthesia due to changes in right heart hemodynamics. Additionally, heartworms can be adhered to valve tissue, most likely related to thrombus formation, preventing their removal.

In a recent retrospective analysis of dogs with caval syndrome, 14 of 21 that had heartworm extraction performed were discharged from the hospital. Six dogs died intraoperatively or in the immediate postoperative period. Elevations in alanine transferase and the presence of heartworms in the pulmonary arteries on echocardiography were associated with a poor prognosis. The most common reasons for euthanasia in the study were poor prognosis and financial constraints. The authors concluded that dogs that have heartworm extraction performed and survive to discharge have a good long-term prognosis.

Equipment

Various devices have been utilized for heartworm extraction including rigid, flexible or three-pronged tripod forceps, endoscopic baskets, snare catheters, and horse hair brushes (Figure 55.3). Ideally, a device should be able to remove heartworms without causing damage to the worms or to the patient's vascular structures or valve tissue. Additionally, device selection is influenced by the size of the patient and the location of heartworms in the right heart and pulmonary arteries.

Rigid forceps provide a direct means of accessing the cranial vena cava and right atrium, but do not provide access to the right ventricle or pulmonary arteries, are generally too large to be introduced into the jugular vein of small dogs, cats, or ferrets, and allow for only a few heartworms to be removed at a time. Blind introduction of forceps can result in inadvertent damage to the tricuspid valve and right atrium. Variation in the jaws of these types of forceps can cause unintended damage to heartworms or in some cases make them difficult to grasp and remove. Flexible alligator forceps introduced in the 1980s provide access to more distal structures, including the pulmonary arteries using fluoroscopic guidance, but are no longer readily available.

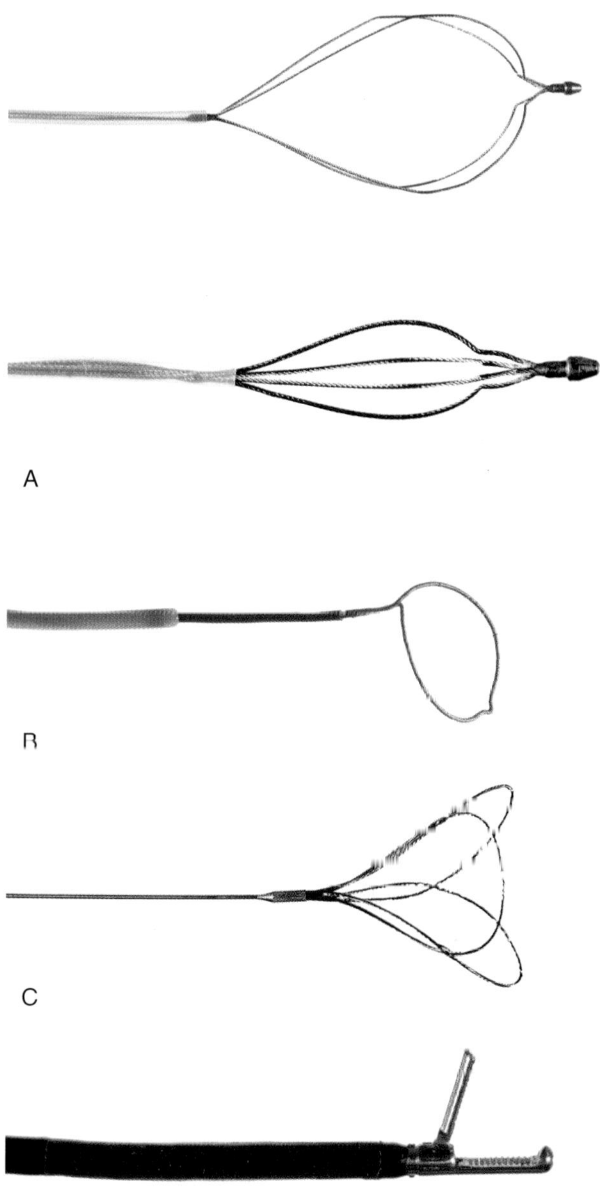

Figure 55.3 Devices used for heartworm extraction. (A) Endoscopic basket retrieval device (Olympus, San Jose, CA) with four wires shown fully open and partially closed. (B) Single loop Amplatz Goose Neck™ Snare with the cable advanced out the end of the snare catheter. (C) Three interlaced loop EN Snare®. (D) Flexible alligator forceps.

Endoscopic baskets, designed for intraluminal use, are made up of multiple wires housed in a sheath. They are flexible and come in various sizes and shapes (flat wire, helical) that can be employed in a wide range of patient sizes. The basket is advanced or retracted from the sheath using a handle. Snares are made to capture objects using a radiopaque cable with a single loop (Amplatz Goose Neck™ Snare, Covidien, Plymouth, MN) or three interlaced loops (EN Snare®, Merit Medical, South Jordan, UT) when combined with a snare catheter.

Both the basket and snare cable are housed in a sheath or catheter, respectively, making them less likely to cause damage during positioning for heartworm extraction. The flexibility of the snare can help when obtaining access to more distal structures by advancing the snare catheter over a guide wire positioned in a pulmonary artery. Pulmonary artery access with a basket retrieval device has been described with the use of a long flexible introducer positioned over a preplaced guide wire. The author and colleagues prefer to use a snare device for heartworm retrieval in ferrets and cats, while an endoscopic basket device is preferred for dogs.

Imaging During the Procedure

Fluoroscopy does not provide direct visualization of heartworms; however, real-time imaging allows the operator to follow the location of the retrieval device within the cardiac and vascular structures as well as to observe device manipulation, including monitoring the opening and partial closure of the basket retrieval device (Figure 55.4). Echocardiography provides direct visualization of the heartworms, is helpful when assessing heartworm retrieval success, and can assist with locating and positioning the device. Transthoracic echocardiographic imaging may require interruption of the procedure when using fluoroscopy and requires a non-sterile member of the team to acquire the images. In dogs and cats of adequate size, transesophageal echocardiography can provide valuable information during the extraction procedure, but requires general anesthesia. The author prefers to use a combination of fluoroscopy and echocardiography for real-time imaging during the procedure, when possible (Figure 55.5).

Procedure

When using a basket retrieval device or snare catheter, one operator is typically in charge of the jugular vein and hemostasis control while the second operator manipulates the device. Both right and left jugular venous approaches have been described with the right being used most often. Left jugular venous access to the right atrium does not follow a straight course and can be problematic if a persistent left caudal vena cava is present. The author and colleagues have encountered a rare case of a congenital absence of the right jugular vein in a dog.

For the procedure, the patient is positioned in left lateral recumbency with the neck extended to fully visualize the right jugular furrow. Tightly rolled surgical towels can be placed under the neck for additional support. An area over the right jugular vein is clipped from the point of the mandible to the thoracic inlet and approaching midline both in a ventral and dorsal direction. This can also be performed prior to placing the patient in lateral recumbency. Following sterile preparation of the surgical site, an appropriately sized incision is made to expose the jugular vein. Once the jugular vein is identified and dissected from the surrounding soft tissues, circumferential suture or umbilical tape is placed loosely around the vessel proximal and distal to the intended venotomy site for hemostasis control (Figure 55.6). If the vein will ultimately be sacrificed at the end of the procedure, the suture cranial to the venotomy can be used to ligate the vessel. Intravascular access is achieved by making a

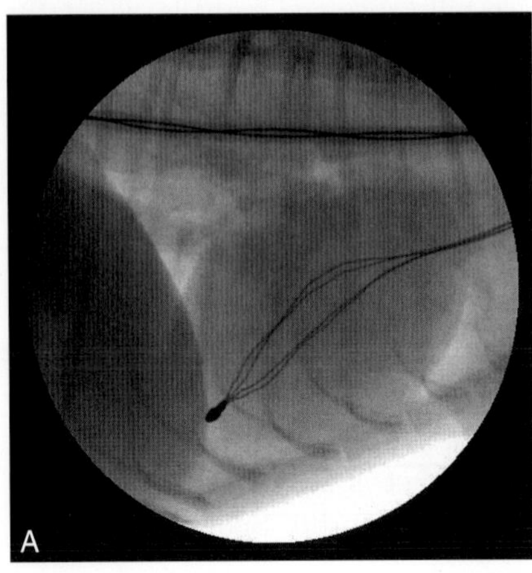

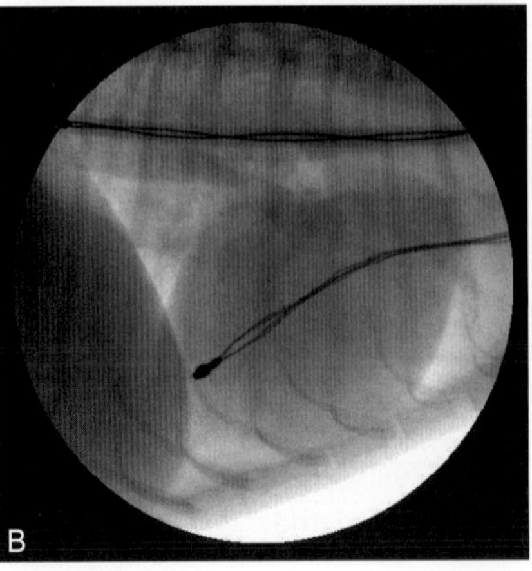

Figure 55.4 Fluoroscopic image from a dog with caval syndrome demonstrating the basket retrieval device in the right atrium and crossing the tricuspid valve into the right ventricle. (A) The basket retrieval device is shown fully open. (B) To avoid transecting the heartworms prior to removal, the device is only partially closed. Where the wires come together represents the end of the radiolucent sheath.

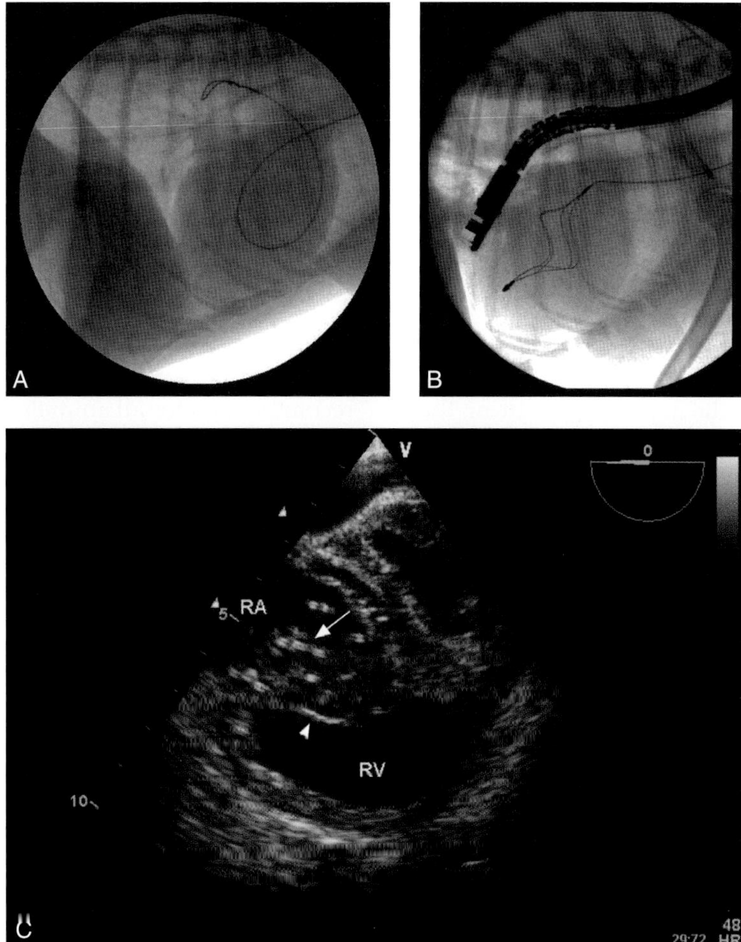

Figure 55.5 Imaging during the heartworm extraction procedure. (A) Fluoroscopic image depicting a snare in the pulmonary artery of a dog. (B) Fluoroscopic image of a basket retrieval device in a dog. The transesophageal echocardiography probe was used to provide real-time visualization of the heartworms. (C) Transesophageal echocardiographic image, from the same dog as B, documented heartworms (arrow) in the right atrium (RA) and crossing the tricuspid valve (arrow head) into the right ventricle (RV).

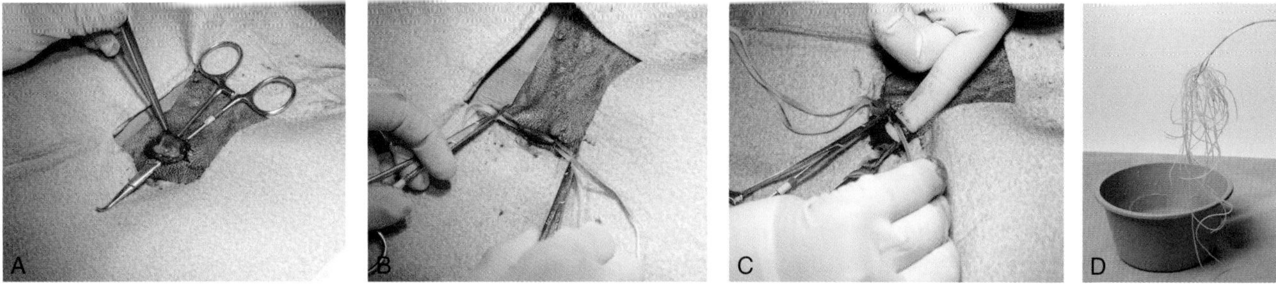

Figure 55.6 Intraoperative images during heartworm extraction in a dog with caval syndrome. After making a surgical incision in the jugular furrow, the jugular vein was identified. (A) A hemostat can be placed behind the jugular vein to maintain visibility while dissecting the vessel free from surrounding tissues. (B) The jugular vein was isolated and encircled loosely with umbilical tape prior to performing the venotomy. (C) Once the venotomy was made, the basket retrieval device was introduced into the vessel and advanced into the cranial vena cava and right atrium. (D) Multiple heartworms were extracted with the basket retrieval device.

small venotomy with tenotomy scissors or a number 11 scalpel blade, being careful to not transect the vessel. The selected retrieval device is inserted through the venotomy in the jugular vein and advanced into the cranial vena cava and right atrium. Rigid forceps should not be advanced past this point. A snare or endoscopic basket device is advanced out of the catheter/sheath by the operator and passed into the vena cava, right atrium and across the tricuspid valve using fluoroscopic guidance. Gentle advancement and rotation of the device is used to capture heartworms, followed by partial closure of the device prior to gentle withdrawal out of the jugular vein. Complete closure of the endoscopic basket device or tightening of the snare must be avoided to prevent partial or complete transection of the heartworms. When a large amount of heartworms are located in the pulmonary arteries, a snare catheter can be advanced into a pulmonary artery over a guide wire that is exchanged for a snare cable. It is possible for heartworms to become lodged at the thoracic inlet or in the jugular vein during their removal, particularly if a large amount of heartworms become incorporated into the device or in patients with small jugular veins. If the operator senses that the device is becoming difficult to retract into the jugular vein, the device is returned to the right atrium and fully opened to release some of the worms. After multiple passes of the retrieval device without removing heartworms, echocardiography is utilized to document the location of remaining heartworms. The jugular vein is ligated proximal and distal to the venotomy or the venotomy site is repaired, depending on the preference and expertise of the operator. The subcutaneous tissues and skin are closed in a routine manner.

The use of a vascular introducer sheath large enough to accept a retrieval device has been reported to support access to more distal structures, in dogs of adequate size. With the use of an introducer, damage to the heartworms could occur during removal and may require removal of the retrieval device and introducer simultaneously.

Follow-Up

Following the procedure, the right-sided heart murmur may resolve if it was related to the physical presence of heartworms across the tricuspid valve, while a murmur can persist in dogs with tricuspid regurgitation secondary to pulmonary hypertension. Hemoglobinuria typically resolves quickly within a few days. Reassessing the patient for resolution of anemia and hepatic and renal function is recommended within 1–4 weeks and especially prior to adulticide therapy. Patients with symptomatic pulmonary hypertension or congestive right heart failure typically require continued medical management that is often long-term or lifelong. This is particularly important to communicate to owners in order to provide them with realistic expectations following the procedure.

Advantages of heartworm extraction include a rapid improvement in clinical status and reduction in the heartworm burden; however, the procedure does not typically result in all heartworms being removed. In dogs, additional adulticide therapy with the "split-dose" or "three dose" protocol of melarsomine dihydrochloride (Immiticide®, Merial, Duluth, GA) is recommended in the weeks to months following extraction, to eliminate remaining heartworms. Adulticide therapy with melarsomine dihydrochol-oride is not recommended for cats and ferrets. The administration of a macrocyclic lactone preventative is recommended for all animals. Please see the American Heartworm Society's website (www.heartwormsociety.org) for the most up-to-date guidelines.

Suggested Reading

Atkins CE (1987) Caval syndrome in the dog. *Semin Vet Med Surg Small Anim* 2(1), 64–72.

Bove C, Gordon SG, Saunders AB, et al (2010) Outcome of minimally invasive surgical treatment of heartworm caval syndrome in dogs: 42 cases (1999–2007). *J Am Vet Med Assoc* 236(2), 187–92.

Bowman DD and Atkins CE (2009) Heartworm biology, treatment, and control. *Vet Clin N Am: Small Anim Pract* 39(6), 1127–58.

Bradbury C, Saunders AB, Heatley JJ, et al (2010) Transvenous heartworm extraction in a ferret with caval syndrome. *J Am Anim Hosp Assoc* 46(1), 31–5.

Howard PE and Pitts RP (1986) Use of a fiberoptic accessory for retrieval of adult heartworms in a dog with postcaval syndrome. *J Am Vet Med Assoc* 189(10), 1343–4.

Jackson RF, Seymour WG, Growney PJ, and Otto GF (1977) Surgical treatment of the caval syndrome of canine heartworm disease. *J Am Vet Med Assoc* 171(10), 1065–9.

Morini S, Venco L, Fagiolo P, et al (1998) Surgical removal of heartworms versus melarsomine treatment of naturally-infected dogs with high risk of thromboembolism. In: *Recent Advances in Heartworm Disease: Symposium '98* (Seward LE and Knight DH, eds). American Heartworm Society, Batavia, IL, pp. 235–40.

Small MT, Atkins CE, Gordon SG, et al (2008) Use of a nitinol gooseneck snare catheter for removal of adult *Dirofilaria immitis* in two cats. *J Am Vet Med Associ* 233(9), 1441–5.

Venco L, Borgarelli M, Ferrari E, et al (1998) Surgical removal of heartworms from naturally-infected cats In: *Recent Advances in Heartworm Disease: Symposium '98* (Seward LE and Knight DH, eds). American Heartworm Society, Batavia, IL, pp. 241–6.

Yoon WK, Han D, and Hyun C (2011) Catheter-guided percutaneous heartworm removal using a nitinol basket in dogs with caval syndrome. *J Vet Sci* 12(2), 199–201.

CHAPTER FIFTY-SIX

Transcatheter Mitral Valve Therapies

E. Christopher Orton
Department of Clinical Sciences, College of Veterinary Medicine and Biomedical Sciences, Colorado State University, Fort Collins, CO

Background

Mitral regurgitation (MR) occurs in humans and most domestic animal species due to a variety of etiologies. Degenerative MR is widely regarded as the most important acquired heart disease in dogs. The overall prevalence of degenerative MR in dogs is estimated to be as high as 7% of the canine population (Atkins et al, 2009). The prevalence is highest in small and toy breeds of dog and increases with age. A significant portion of dogs with degenerative MR will progress to develop clinical signs of heart failure (Stage C disease). Once dogs become symptomatic for heart failure secondary to severe MR, the condition will be fatal without an interventional therapy. Open surgical mitral valve repair is the current standard of care for humans with uncomplicated severe degenerative MR (Bonow et al, 2008). While successful open mitral valve repair has been reported in dogs (Griffiths et al, 2004, Uechi et al, 2012), cost and availability severely limit open mitral repair as a practical intervention for dogs. Several transcatheter approaches are under development for treatment of severe MR. Some of these approaches hold promise as an interventional therapy for dogs with severe MR.

Classification of Mitral Regurgitation

MR is classified according to its underlying etiology (Box 56.1). These etiologies are considered primary if the underlying pathology directly involves the mitral leaflets. Secondary MR, also referred to as functional MR, results from remodeling of the left ventricle secondary to myocardial disease (e.g., dilated cardiomyopathy). MR is also classified according to the underlying functional derangement of the valve apparatus causing regurgitation (de Marchena et al, 2011). Any of these functional derangements, alone or in combination, will result in MR. Functional classification of MR is important because interventional therapies to correct MR are directed at one or more of these underlying functional causes. Degenerative MR, the most common etiology in humans and dogs, results from leaflet prolapse (type II defect) and secondary annular dilation (type I defect). An intervention intended to correct or palliate degenerative MR must therefore address one or both of these derangements. Functional MR secondary to dilated cardiomyopathy results from dilation of the mitral annulus (type I defect) and papillary muscle displacement during systole (type IIIb defect). Interventions directed at palliation of functional MR must address at least one of these functional derangements.

Indirect Transcatheter Mitral Annuloplasty

Several devices are under development for indirect transcatheter mitral annuloplasty. All exploit the proximity of the coronary sinus and great cardiac vein to the mitral annulus and are designed to apply circumferential traction on the mitral annulus via the great cardiac vein. These devices are intended to reduce the size of the mitral annulus and thereby decrease MR by correcting the annular dilation (type I) component. The MONARC device consists of a springlike cord between two self-expanding anchors (Figure 56.1). It is deployed transvenously via a jugular vein and directed into the great cardiac vein via the coronary sinus. The distal anchor is placed at the transition between the anterior interventricular vein and the great cardiac vein. The proximal anchor is positioned in the coronary sinus ostium. A biodegradable component is incorporated

Veterinary Image-Guided Interventions, First Edition. Edited by Chick Weisse and Allyson Berent.

Companion website: www.wiley.com/go/weisse/vet-image-guided-interventions

BOX [illegible]
Classification of mitral regurgitation (MR)

Etiologic classification

Congenital MR
- leaflet defect (cleft or perforation)
- valve dysplasia (leaflet fusion & thickening, chordae fusion and shortening, aberrant chordae)

Degenerative MR
- idiopathic (myxomatous) degeneration
- connective tissue disorders (e.g., Marfan syndrome)
- drug-induced (serotoninergic drugs)
- carcinoid syndrome

Inflammatory MR
- endocarditis
- rheumatic heart disease

Traumatic MR
- papillary or chordae rupture
- leaflet perforation

Infiltrative MR
- neoplasia
- amyloidosis

Functional MR
- dilated cardiomyopathy
- ischemic cardiomyopathy
- hypertrophic cardiomyopathy

Functional classification

Type I:	Normal leaflet motion	Leaflet perforation
		Annular dilation
Type II:	Increased leaflet motion	Leaflet prolapse
		Chordae rupture or elongation
		Papillary rupture
Type IIIa:	Restricted leaflet motion during diastole (and systole)	Chordae fusion and shortening
		Aberrant chordae
		Leaflet thickening or fusion
Type IIIb:	Restricted leaflet motion during systole	Papillary muscle displacement due to cardiac remodeling

into the springlike connecting cord and maintains it in an elongated state at implantation. After implantation, the biodegradable component absorbs over approximately 1 month, allowing the spring to apply active tension between the anchors. This active tension places a circumferential traction force on the mitral annulus reducing its circumference.

The MONARC device has been evaluated in a phase I clinical trial of 72 human patients with functional MR (Harnek et al, 2011). The device was successfully deployed in 59 patients (82%). MR was reduced by ≥1 grade in 50% of patients. This study identified an important anatomic variation in 55% of patients where branches of the circumflex coronary artery pass between the great cardiac vein and mitral annulus and are susceptible to compression when the device engages. Compression was documented in 15 patients and infarction in 2 patients. An indirect transcatheter annuloplasty device is currently not available for dogs. There are several reasons why this strategy will not likely to be the best for dogs. The device only addresses annular dilation (type I) and not the leaflet prolapse (type II) mechanism of MR. As such, the device appears to be better suited for functional MR rather than degenerative MR. The problem of coronary artery compression may limit application of the device in humans. The importance of this anatomic variation in dogs is unknown.

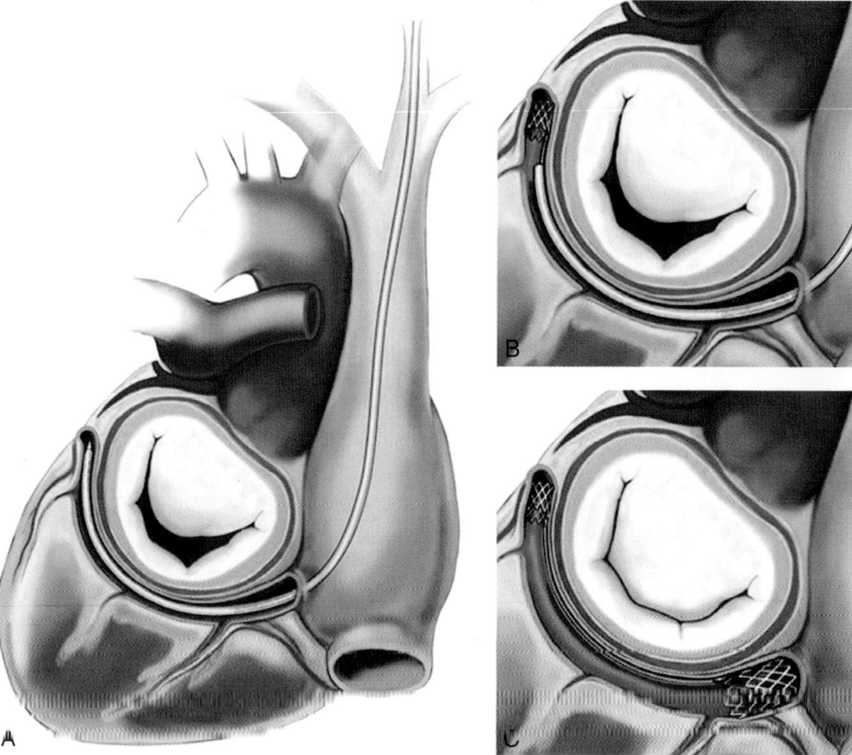

Figure 56.1 Indirect transcatheter mitral annuloplasty with MONARC device. Indirect mitral annuloplasty exploits the proximity of the great cardiac vein to the mitral annulus. The MONARC device consists of a springlike cord between two self-expanding anchors. It is deployed transvenously via the jugular vein and directed into the great cardiac vein via the coronary sinus (A). The distal anchor is placed at the transition between the anterior interventricular vein and the great cardiac vein (B). The proximal anchor is positioned in the coronary sinus ostium (C). A biodegradable component is incorporated into the springlike connecting cord and maintains it in an elongated state at implantation. After implantation, the biodegradable component absorbs resulting in the application of active tension to the mitral annulus. (Used with permission from Harnek J, Webb JG, Kuck KH, et al 2011. Transcatheter implantation of the MONARC coronary sinus device for mitral regurgitation: 1-year results from the EVOLUTION phase I study (Clinical Evaluation of the Edwards Lifesciences Percutaneous Mitral Annuloplasty System for the Treatment of Mitral Regurgitation). J Am Coll Cardiol: Cardiovasc Interv 4, 115–22, Elsevier.)

Transcatheter Mitral (Edge-to-Edge) Repair

Transcatheter mitral repair is based on the edge-to-edge (Alfieri) technique for open mitral valve repair (Alfieri et al, 2004). The MitraClip (Abbott) clip device is approved for use in humans (Feldman et al, 2009). Deployment of the device utilizes a caudal transvenous (percutaneous) approach with a high transseptal puncture to gain access to the left atrium (Figure 56.2). The opposing mitral leaflets are grasped under transesophageal echocardiography (TEE) guidance and a clip is deployed to permanently fix the opposing mitral leaflets together at the point of greatest regurgitation/prolapse. Patients must have favorable anatomy based on coaptation depth and length as well as flail gap and width to be eligible for the procedure (Figure 56.3). These eligibility criteria make it necessary to intervene at an earlier stage of the disease and before the onset of significant secondary dilation of the mitral valve annulus.

The MitraClip device has undergone a pivotal phase II clinical trial (EVEREST II) in humans. Human patients ($n = 279$) with severe degenerative or functional MR were randomized to MitraClip or open mitral valve repair (Feldman et al, 2011). The primary efficiency endpoint of freedom from death, reoperation, or severe MR at 1 year was significantly better for open surgery (73% vs. 55%). However the primary safety endpoint of freedom from an adverse event at 30 days was better for the MitraClip (15% vs. 48%). Thus MitraClip is considered less effective than surgery, but safer in patients with severe degenerative or functional MR. Currently, there is no device for transcatheter mitral repair in dogs. The MitraClip device is too large to be deployed in dogs. However, the concept would likely be applicable to dogs if the technology could be downsized. Eligibility

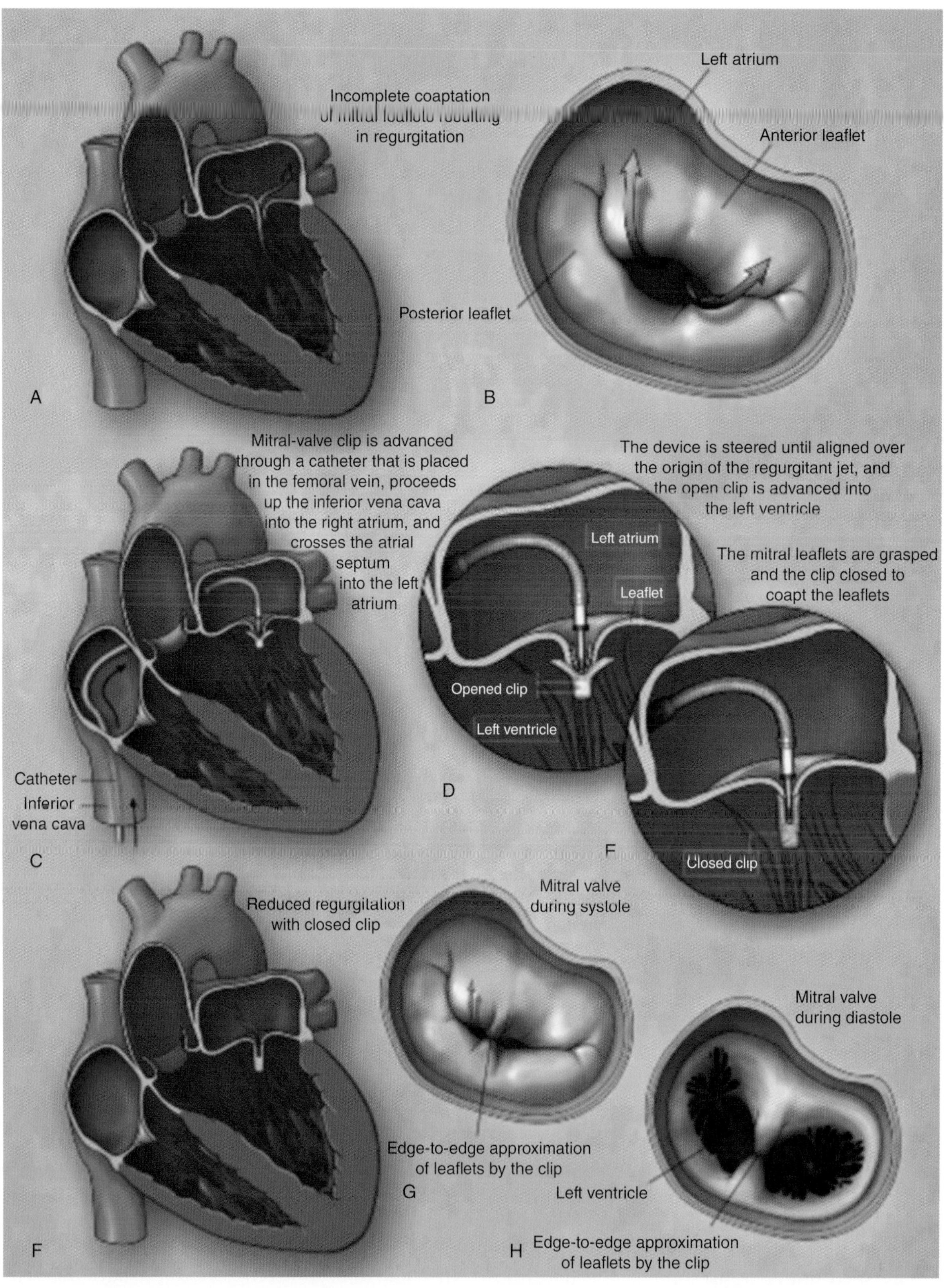

Figure 56.2 Transcatheter mitral repair with MitraClip device. The MitraClip device is designed to correct mitral regurgitation caused by leaflet prolapse (A & B) based on the edge-to-edge mitral repair technique. Deployment of the device utilizes a transvenous approach with high transseptal puncture to gain access to the left atrium (C). The device is steered through the mitral valve at the origin of the regurgitant jet and opposing mitral leaflets are grasped under transesophageal echocardiography guidance (D). The clip is deployed to permanently fix the opposing mitral leaflets together at the point of greatest regurgitation/prolapse (E & F). The clip prevents leaflet prolapse during systole (G) and results in a double office opening during diastole (H). (Used with permission from Feldman T, Kar S, Rinaldi M, et al 2009. Percutaneous mitral repair with the MitraClip system: safety and midterm durability in the initial EVEREST (Endovascular Valve Edge-to-Edge REpair Study) cohort. J Am Coll Cardiol 54, 686–94, Elsevier.)

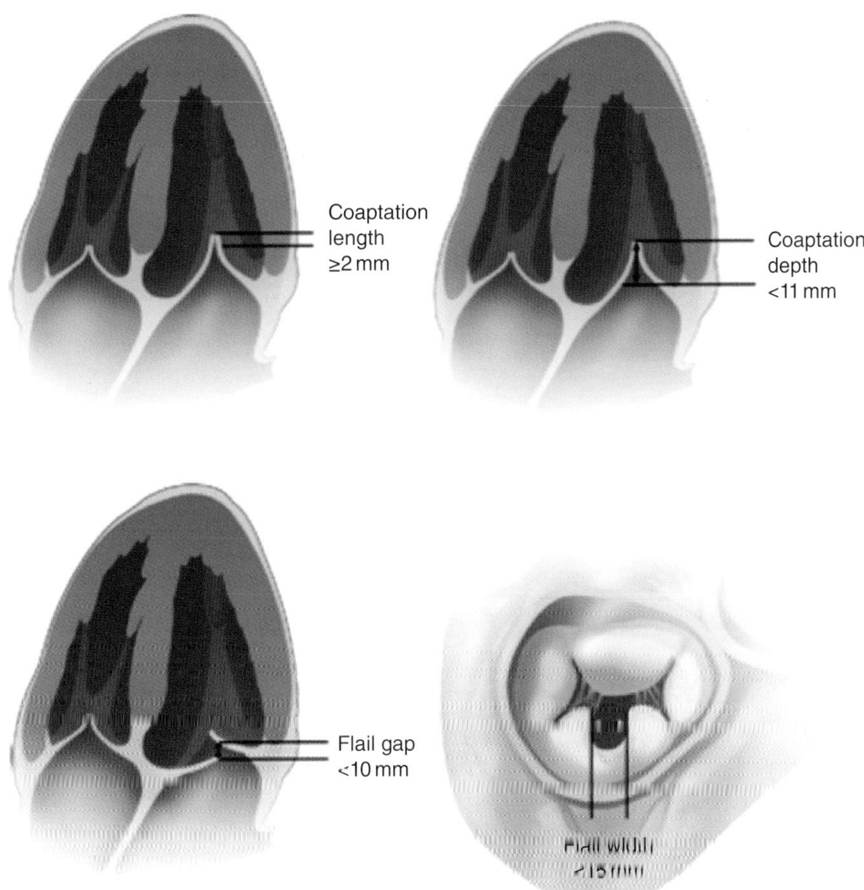

Figure 56.3 Eligibility criteria for transcatheter mitral edge-to-edge repair in human patients. (Used with permission from Feldman T, Kar S, Rinaldi M, et al 2009. Percutaneous mitral repair with the MitraClip system: safety and midterm durability in the initial EVEREST (Endovascular Valve Edge-to-Edge REpair Study) cohort. J Am Coll Cardiol 54, 686–94, Elsevier.)

criteria would likely require early intervention before significant secondary annular dilation occurred. Percutaneous transcatheter delivery could prove challenging in small dogs. A hybrid transcatheter approach where delivery is performed through the left ventricular apex (transapical) might be adaptable to dogs.

Transcatheter Mitral Valve Implantation

Development of transcatheter mitral valve implantation (TMVI) is based upon the success the Sapien device (Edwards Lifesciences), which is approved for transcatheter aortic valve implantation (TAVI) in humans. The Sapien device employs a bioprosthetic valve in a ductal stent that can be deployed into a calcified stenotic aortic valve. The device is anchored by radial traction against the calcified aortic annulus. Because the mitral annulus is distensible, a similar approach cannot be used to anchor a prosthetic device in the mitral position. Several prosthetic devices are in development for TMVI; each exploring different mechanisms to overcome the challenge of anchoring a prosthesis in the mitral position. The MitralSeal device (Avalon Medical) is being developed specifically for TMVI in dogs. The device is a bioprosthetic valve mounted within a self-expanding Nitinol stent (Figure 56.4). The stent consists of a Dacron covered cuff that prevents displacement of the device into the ventricle and a cylindrical portion that houses the valve leaflets. The device has three tethers on its ventral aspect that aid with manipulation of the device during deployment and anchor the device to prevent dislodgement into the atrium. The prosthesis is compressed into a delivery loading tube for transcatheter deployment (Figure 56.5). The delivery system consists of a 0.032″ guidewire, delivery catheter with introducer, a loading tube, and a delivery obturator (Figure 56.6). The MitralSeal device is deployed using a hybrid surgical-transcatheter approach through the left ventricular apex

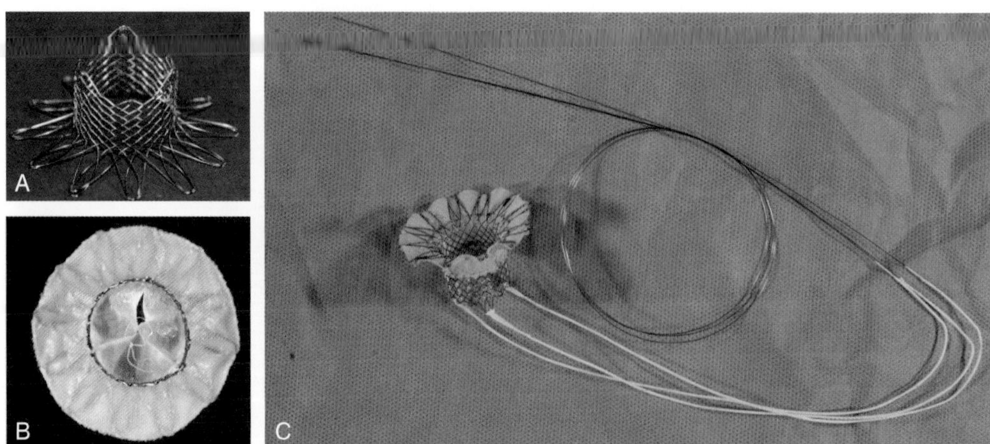

Figure 56.4 MitralSeal device for transcatheter mitral valve implantation. The device is constructed on a self-expanding Nitinol stent with a cuff, cylindrical body, and tether attachment points (A). The cuff portion of the device is covered with Dacron and the body houses bioprosthetic valve leaflets (B). Three tethers are attached to the ventral portion of the prosthesis for manipulation during deployment and anchoring after deployment (C).

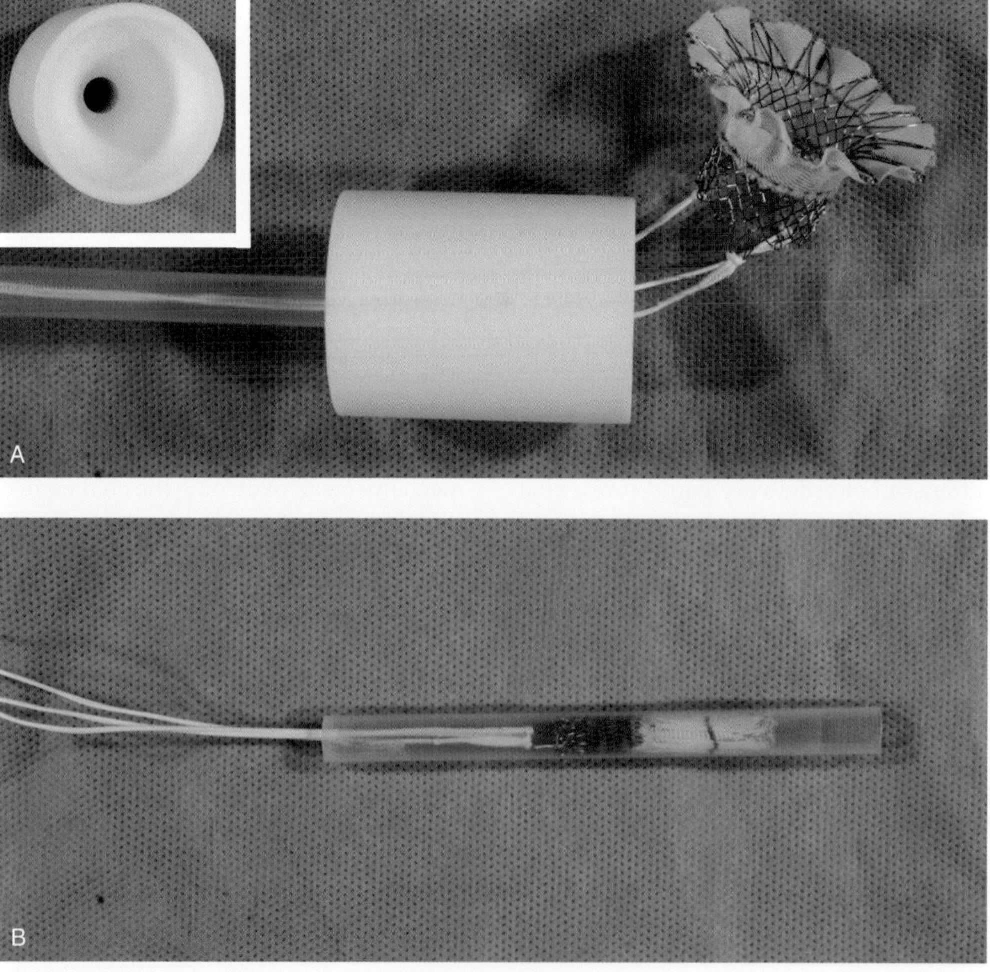

Figure 56.5 Loading of the MitralSeal device for transcatheter deployment. The MitralSeal prosthesis is compressed into the delivery loading tube using a cone device (inset) and traction on the tethers (A). Loading of the prosthesis is performed under water in cold saline to reduce entrapment of air bubbles. The compressed prosthesis and loading tube are then ready for "back-loading" onto the delivery catheter (B).

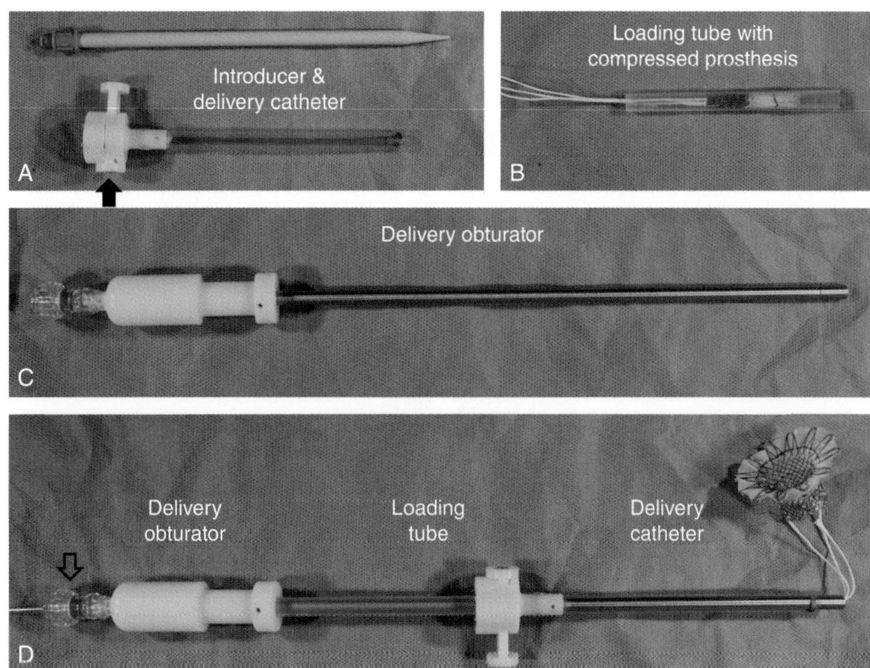

Figure 56.6 Delivery system for the MitralSeal prosthesis. The delivery system includes a delivery catheter with introducer and a hemostasis control device (solid arrow) on the proximal end (A). The introducer accepts a 0.032" guidewire. The system includes a loading tube for housing of the compressed prosthesis prior to deployment (B) and a delivery obturator (C). The delivery obturator is used to push the prosthesis through the loading tube and delivery catheter during deployment (D). The tethers are passed through the center of the delivery system to allow externalization of the tethers after the delivery system is removed. The delivery obturator has a hemostasis device to accommodate passage of the tethers (open arrow).

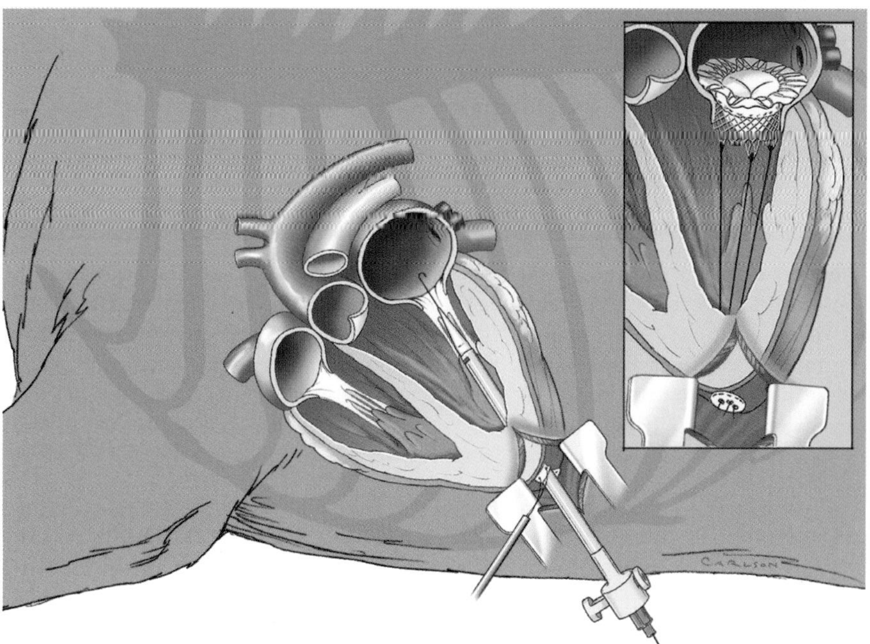

Figure 56.7 Hybrid surgical-transcatheter implantation of the MitralSeal valve prosthesis. A minimally-invasive left thoracotomy is performed over the cardiac apex (6th or 7th intercostal space). The pericardium is opened and two buttressed mattress sutures are placed in the cardiac apex and passed through tourniquets. A delivery catheter with introducer are introduced into the left ventricle and advanced into the left atrium over a guidewire. The prosthesis is deployed into the left atrium and positioned and fixed into the mitral annulus with the tethers (inset). The tethers are secured outside the cardiac apex using a pledget. The buttressed mattress sutures are then tied.

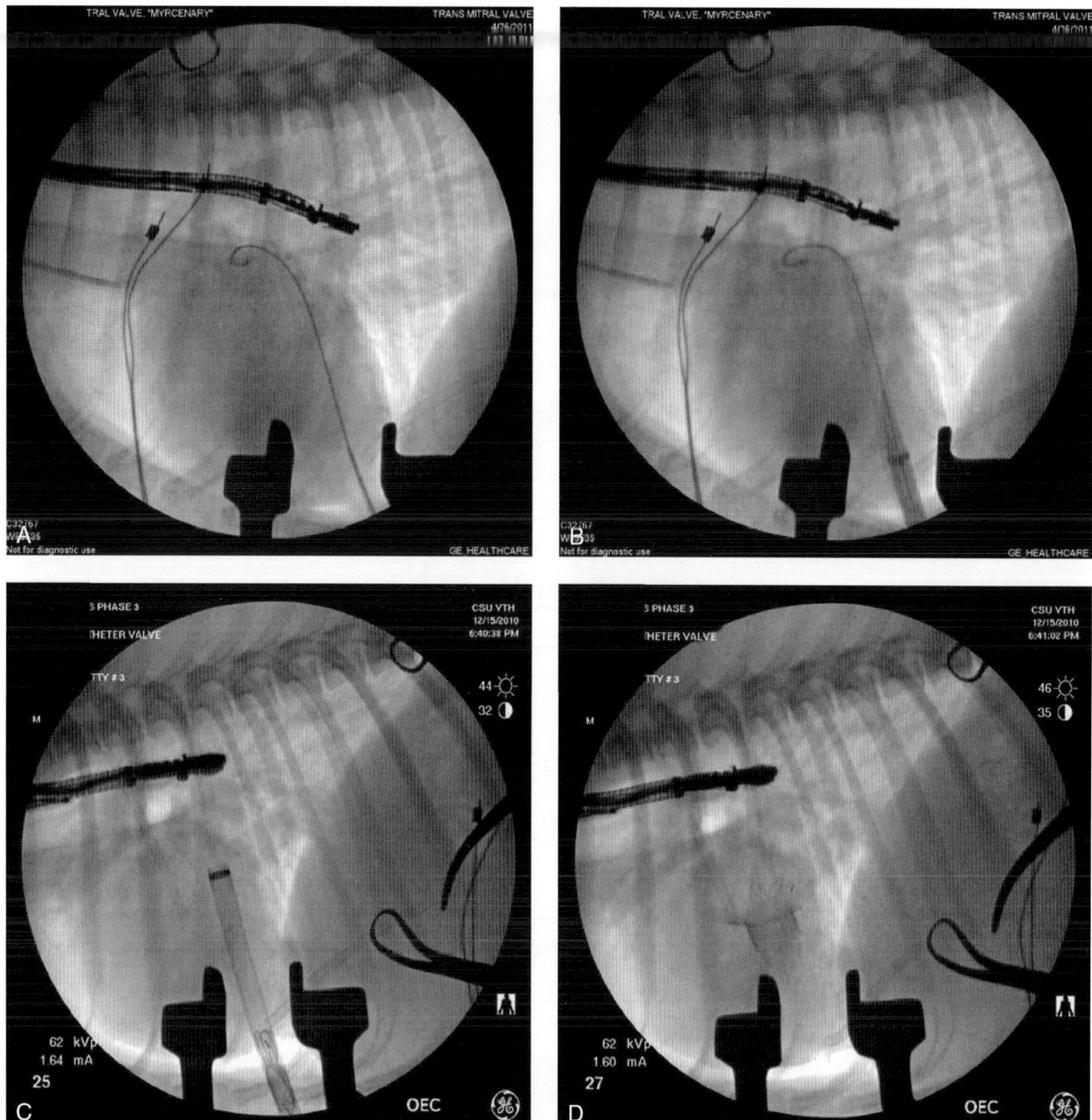

Figure 56.8 Deployment of MitralSeal prosthesis under fluoroscopic guidance. A 0.032″ guidewire is introduced through the left ventricular apex and passed through the mitral valve into the left atrium (A). The introducer and delivery catheter are introduced into the left ventricle via the cardiac apex and passed through the mitral valve into the left atrium along the guidewire (B). The guidewire and introducer are removed leaving the delivery catheter in the left atrium. The prosthesis is deployed into the left atrium using the delivery catheter (C). The delivery catheter is removed. The prosthesis is positioned into the mitral annulus using the externalized tethers (D).

(Figure 56.7). Access is gained to the left ventricular apex via a minimally invasive left thoracotomy. Two mattress sutures are placed in the left ventricular apex and passed through tourniquets to control bleeding during delivery. The device is deployed into the left atrium under fluoroscopic guidance (Figure 56.8). The anchoring tethers are passed through the delivery system so that the ends remain outside the heart when the delivery catheter is removed. The device is positioned into the mitral annulus by placing traction on the tethers. Tension is adjusted on the tethers to minimize paravalvular leak under transesophageal echocardiographic guidance (Figure 56.9). The tethers are fixed to the outside of the cardiac apex with an anchoring pledget.

The MitralSeal device has been successfully deployed into normal dogs and normal pigs out to 110 days (Figure 56.10). The device is scheduled for phase I clinical trial in dogs with severe degenerative MR at the time of writing.

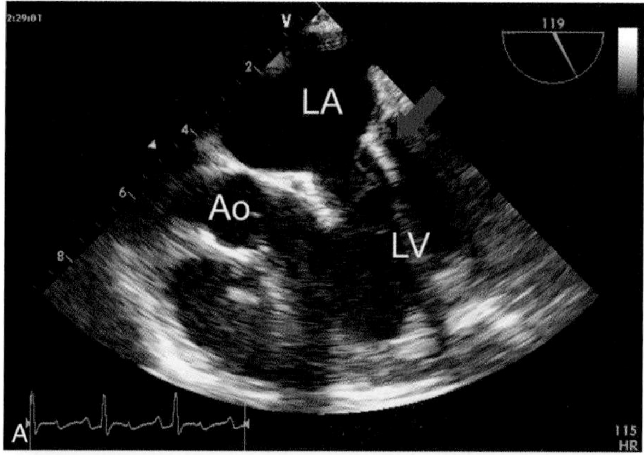

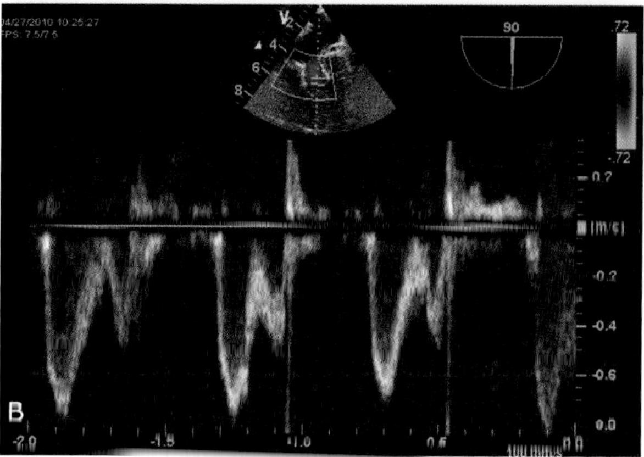

Figure 56.9 Transesophageal echocardiography (TEE) of the MitralSeal prosthesis. The position of the prosthesis (red arrow) is adjusted under TEE guidance to minimized paravalvular leak around the prosthesis (A). The prosthesis is interrogated with Doppler TEE to assess hemodynamic function (B).

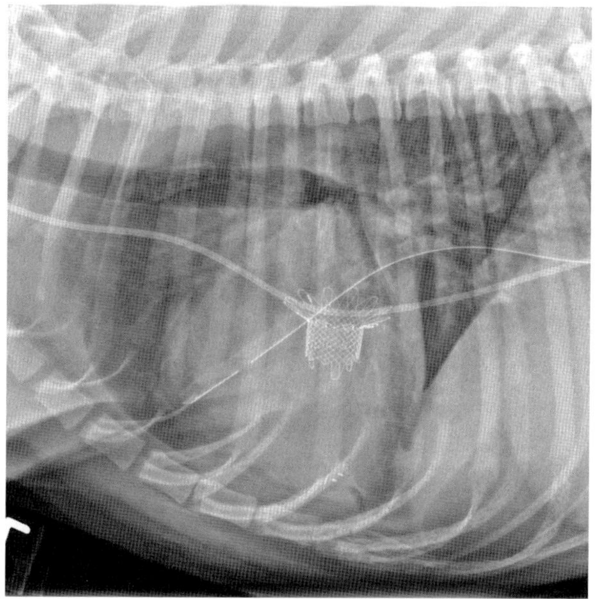

Figure 56.10 Thoracic radiograph of a dog after implantation of the MitralSeal prosthesis.

References

Alfieri O, De Bonis M, Lapenna E, et al (2004) "Edge-to-edge" repair for anterior mitral leaflet prolapse. *Semin Thorac Cardiovasc Surg* 16, 182–7.

Atkins C, Bonagura J, Ettinger S, et al (2009) Guidelines for the diagnosis and treatment of canine chronic valvular heart disease. *J Vet Intern Med* 23, 1142–50.

Bonow RO, Carabello BA, Chatterjee K, et al (2008) 2008 Focused update incorporated into the ACC/AHA 2006 guidelines for the management of patients with valvular heart disease: a report of the American College of Cardiology/American Heart Association Task Force on Practice Guidelines. *Circulation* 118:e523–661.

de Marchena E, Badiye A, Robalino G, et al (2011) Respective prevalence of the different carpentier classes of mitral regurgitation: a stepping stone for future therapeutic research and development. *J Card Surg* 26, 385–92.

Feldman T, Foster E, Glower DD, et al (2011) Percutaneous repair or surgery for mitral regurgitation. *N Engl J Med* 364, 1395–406.

Feldman T, Kar S, Rinaldi M, et al (2009) Percutaneous mitral repair with the MitraClip system: safety and midterm durability in the initial EVEREST (Endovascular Valve Edge-to-Edge REpair Study) cohort. *J Am Coll Cardiol* 54, 686–94.

Griffiths LG, Orton EC, and Boon JA (2004) Evaluation of techniques and outcomes of mitral valve repair in dogs. *J Am Vet Med Assoc* 224, 1941–5.

Harnek J, Webb JG, Kuck KH, et al (2011) Transcatheter implantation of the MONARC coronary sinus device for mitral regurgitation: 1-year results from the EVOLUTION phase I study (Clinical Evaluation of the Edwards Lifesciences Percutaneous Mitral Annuloplasty System for the Treatment of Mitral Regurgitation). *J Am Coll Cardiol: Cardiovasc Interv* 4, 115–22.

Uechi M, Mizukoshi T, Mizuno T, et al (2012) Mitral valve repair under cardiopulmonary bypass in small-breed dogs: 48 cases (2006–2009). *J Am Vet Med Assoc* 240, 1194–201.

CHAPTER FIFTY-SEVEN

Cardiac Tumor Palliation

Chick Weisse[1] and Brian A. Scansen[2]
[1]The Animal Medical Center, New York , NY
[2]Department of Veterinary Clinical Sciences, The Ohio State University, Columbus, OH

Background/Indications

Central venous obstruction can have profound systemic effects, particularly when venous return is affected. Interventional radiology techniques have been used to palliate both malignant and non-malignant causes of vascular obstruction for both intrinsic and extrinsic lesions. The authors' have been presented with dramatic cases of naturally occurring large cardiac masses resulting in right atrial compression or obstruction preventing adequate venous return to the heart with subsequent clinical signs associated with congestion (head swelling, pleural effusion, ascites, etc.). The authors have recently reported on the placement of transatrial stents for long-term decompression of cardiac tumor venous obstruction in three cases (Weisse et al, 2012).

This chapter will discuss the technical considerations for identifying and treating cases that might benefit from similar cardiac tumor obstruction interventions. While tumor embolization, chemoembolization, or ablation procedures have been considered for intracardiac tumors, these have not been performed clinically at this time in veterinary patients to the authors' knowledge. Intervention for pericardial effusion secondary to intracardiac tumors is discussed in Chapter 52.

Patient Preparation

All patients should receive a full physical examination and medical work-up prior to performing cardiac interventions. In addition, consultation with a cardiologist, oncologist, and surgeon should be performed to ensure current standard-of-care therapies have been discussed and a long-term plan has been formulated. Particularly close attention should be made during physical examination for signs associated with venous obstruction of the cranial (CrVC) or caudal (CdVC) vena cava, including jugular distension, head and neck swelling/edema, dull lung sounds consistent with pleural effusion, abdominal distension consistent with ascites, weakness, shortness of breath, arrhythmias, etc. Full bloodwork as well as blood pressure, coagulation panels, blood type, thoracic radiographs, ECG, and echocardiography should be performed. Cross-sectional imaging such as computed tomography angiography (CTA) and gated magnetic resonance angiography (MRA) (Figure 57.1A) can further elucidate the nature and anatomy of these obstructions as well as provide pre-operative measurements to make certain appropriate stent sizes and other related equipment are readily available. The contrast used during CTA may preclude performing an intervention under the same anesthetic episode due to iodinated contrast limitations. MRA may not have the same limitations but these imaging procedures can take much longer to perform.

These patients should be managed by a cardiologist prior to, during, and following any intervention when possible. Aggressive medical management should be instituted prior to general anesthesia or interventional management to best control any underlying cardiac disease or clinical signs associated with pleural or chylous effusions, massive ascites, head/neck swelling interfering with respiration, etc. Diuretics are often used (Table 57.1) in these cases but only provide partial relief when clinical signs are severe. Abdominocentesis can provide temporary relief to the patient and perhaps improve suitability for anesthesia. This procedure is best performed under ultrasound guidance as these dogs have elevated portal venous pressures (and therefore ascites) which can worsen potential hemorrhage should a vessel be punctured. In addition, the abdominal fluid will prevent the blood coagulation process,

Veterinary Image-Guided Interventions, First Edition. Edited by Chick Weisse and Allyson Berent.

Companion website: www.wiley.com/go/weisse/vet-image-guided-interventions

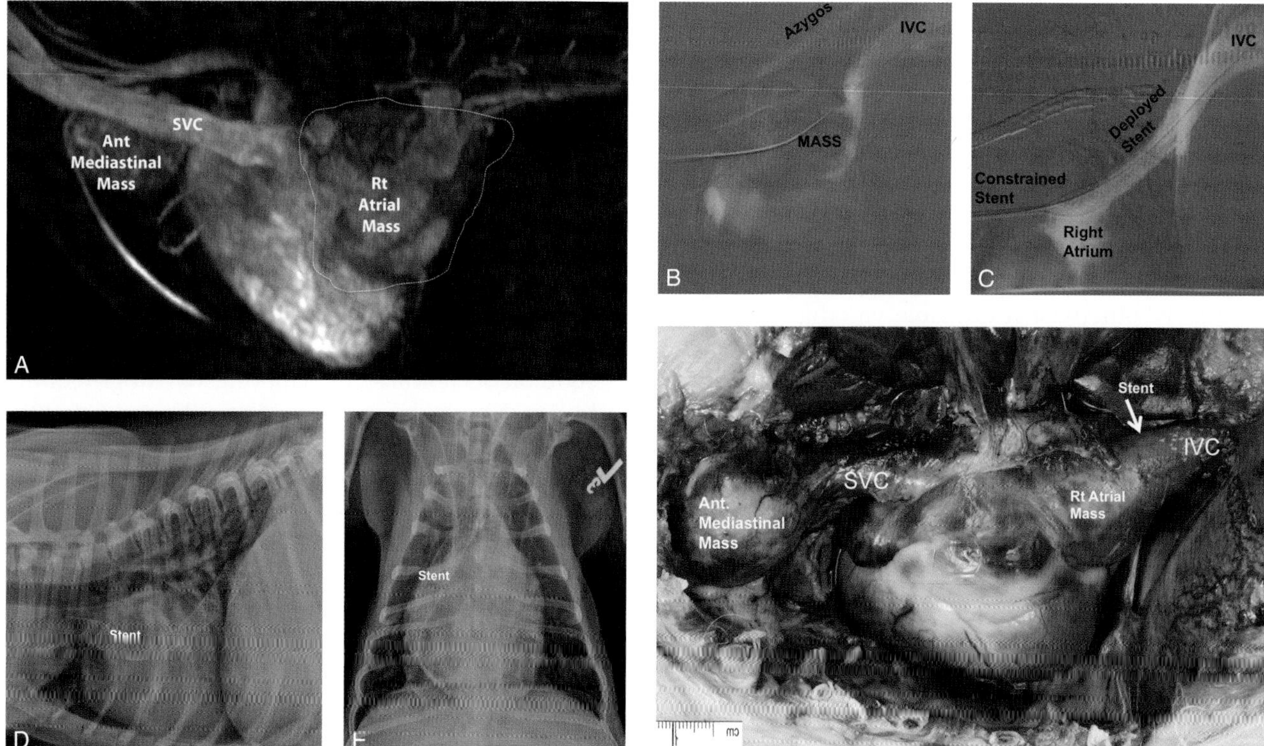

Figure 57.1 Multiple images of a dog with a right atrial mass, cranial mediastinal mass, and caudal vena cava (CdVC) obstruction. (A) Magnetic resonance angiography demonstrating large right atrial mass (white dotted line), patent cranial vena cava (SVC) but absent contrast enhancement of CdVC due to obstruction. (B) Digital subtraction angiogram (DSA) of caudal vena cava (IVC) showing obstructive mass preventing caudal venous return. Note decompression of venous system through the azygos vein entering the right atrium cranial to the mass. (C) Repeat DSA cavagram with partially deployed transatrial stent showing patent CdVC with contrast returning to right atrium and no azygos vein filling. Lateral (D) and ventrodorsal (E) radiographs postoperatively with transatrial stent in place. (F) Postmortem examination 21 months following initial stent placement following euthanasia due to progressive lethargy and metastatic chemodectoma.

TABLE 57.1
Pre- and post-procedural medical management

- Antibiotics:
  - Intraoperative: cefoxitin (30 mg/kg IV once, then 20 mg/kg IV q2 hr)
  - Postoperative: clavamox (13.75 mg/kg PO q12 hr × 10 days) or similar broad-spectrum antibiotic
- Diuretics:
  - Pre- and postoperative: furosemide (1.0–5.0 mg/kg PO q12–24 hr)
  - Pre- and postoperative: spironolactone (1.0–2.0 mg/kg PO q12 hr)
- Alpha blockers:
  - Pre- and postoperative: phenoxybenzamine (0.25–0.5 mg/kg q12–24 hr)
- Vasodilator:
  - Intraoperative: sodium nitroprusside (start at 1–2 μg/kg/min if systolic BP >200 mmHg)
- Beta-blockers:
  - Intra- and postoperative: esmolol (250–500 μg/kg slow bolus followed by 75–200 μg/kg/min CRI)
  - Postoperative: atenolol (0.25–1.0 mg/kg PO q12 hr)
- Anticoagulation: (see Chapter 47)
  - Pre-, intra-, or postoperatively: not routinely performed
- Analgesics (not standardly necessary):
  - Postoperative: tramadol (2–4 mg/kg PO q8–12 hr × 3 days)

further complicating the paracentesis procedure should bleeding occur.

These obstructions may also be associated with hormonally active neuroendocrine tumors so tachyarrhythmias and hypertension should be anticipated and prior discussion with the anesthesia team is mandatory. A plan should include potential use of both vasodilatory agents (ideally provided a few weeks prior to the procedure if systemic hypertension is documented preoperatively, otherwise a titratable vasodilator such as nitroprusside should be prepared preoperatively) and beta blockade intraoperatively if necessary (typically a beta-1 specific agent such as esmolol) (Table 57.1).

When performing anesthesia, intravenous catheter placement should take into consideration the location of the obstruction. If ascites is present due to the substantial caudal vena cava post-sinusoidal obstruction, hindlimb catheters will not deliver anesthetics to the patient appropriately. In the same respect, forelimb catheters placed in those patients with swollen heads and possible pleural effusions (cranial vena cava syndrome) will likely be ineffective as drugs pool in the venous system.

Potential Risks/Complications/Expected Outcomes

In the authors' limited experience with such cases, transatrial stent placement has been successful and resolution of ascites or head swelling/pleural effusion was achieved. Two of three dogs required additional stent placement for subsequent partial stent occlusion likely due to tumor ingrowth. In both cases, restenting resulted in ascites resolution or substantial reduction suggesting overlapping of open stents did not prevent bloodflow through the stent interstices.

Thrombosis or tumor embolism does not appear to be a substantial problem in the few cases performed to date; none of which received anticoagulant therapy. Cardiac venous return across the stent interstices appeared to be adequate in these dogs but cardiac output was not challenged. Neointimal formation across the stents interstices did not appear to be a major complication aside from those regions of the stent directly abutting vascular or cardiac endothelium. Substantial contact with the CrVC (and possibly CdVC) should be the goal to prevent migration into the atrium as stent expansion is difficult to anticipate during stent deployment (Figure 57.2). Ascites recurrence suggests progressive mass ingrowth through the interstices of the stent. For tumors in which survival is expected to be longer than 3–6 months, potential restenting should be anticipated.

Transatrial stenting from the inferior vena cava to the superior vena cava has been described for short-term management of ascites in two humans for intracardiac HCC extension (Wallace, 2003). The authors' of this chapter presented the first report of long-term palliative transatrial stenting for non-HCC tumors affecting venous return to the heart (cardiac tumors) in three dogs. In all cases, stent placement was successful and resolution of clinical signs achieved. Two dogs required additional stent placement in 14 months and 6 months, respectively, for stent occlusion. In both cases, restenting resulted in ascites resolution or substantial reduction. One dog was euthanized 21 months following initial stent placement for general systemic decline and return of moderate ascites. The second dog was euthanized 35 months following initial stent placement due to anorexia and general malaise. Severe ascites had recurred at the time of euthanasia though the stent remained patent on post-mortem examination (Figure 57.3). The third died of undetermined causes 5.5 months later; the stent was patent on post-mortem.

The stents were well tolerated in these dogs for whom surgical options were not possible and it appears that longer-term palliation (>3 months) is possible using this technique, as some dogs lived for years without clinical signs. Stent free ends within the atrium can theoretically result in cardiac perforation or migration into the ventricle (Prahlow et al, 1997), but this was not appreciated in any of the authors' cases.

Transatrial stenting may be considered in the future for similar patients in which traditional options are declined, not indicated, or may be associated with excessive morbidity or mortality, however potential stent shortening may be anticipated (so stent length should be longer than necessary) and careful monitoring is necessary to evaluate for stent occlusion.

Equipment

Recommended equipment is shown in Figure 57.4. Digital subtraction angiography is not required but highly recommended when performing the stenting procedure. Pressure transducers are generally easier to use and more reliable than water manometers in the authors' experience. Trans-esophageal echocardiography is not required but can be very helpful during stent deployment. A variety of different diameter and length self-expanding metallic stents (SEMS) should be available for these fairly long lesions.

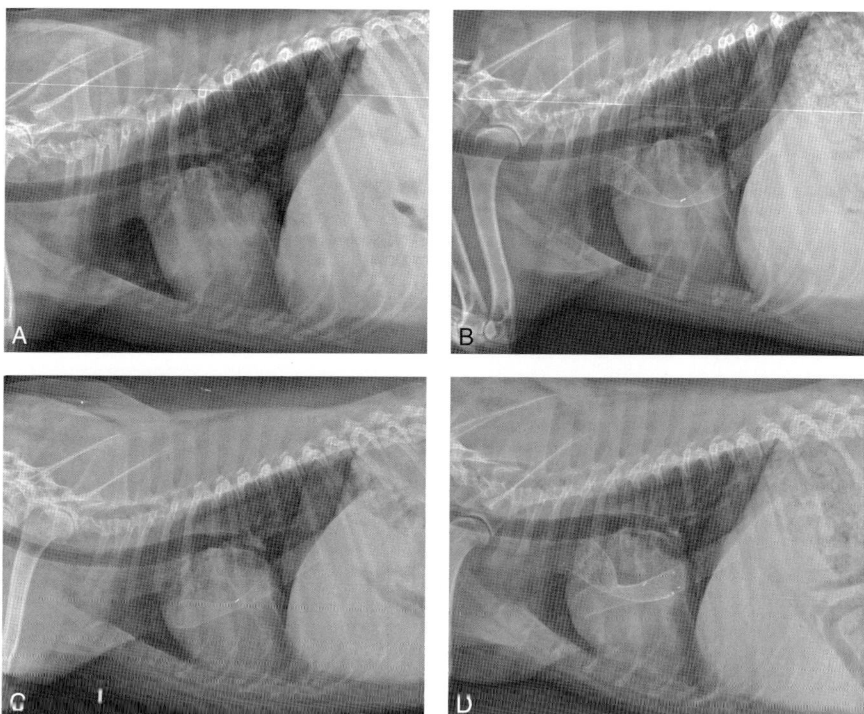

Figure 57.2 Serial lateral radiographs of a dog with a cardiac tumor and subsequent caudal vena cava obstruction. (A) Pre-stent radiograph. (B) Immediately following transatrial stent placement. (C) Follow up radiograph 4 months later demonstrating cranial aspect of the transatrial stent shortened and migrated into the right auricular appendage. The venous obstruction was still relieved. (D) Radiograph taken 7 months after first transatrial stent, following second transatrial stent delivered through the interstices of the initial stent and performed to prevent migration of the first stent as well as to improve caudal vena caval return.

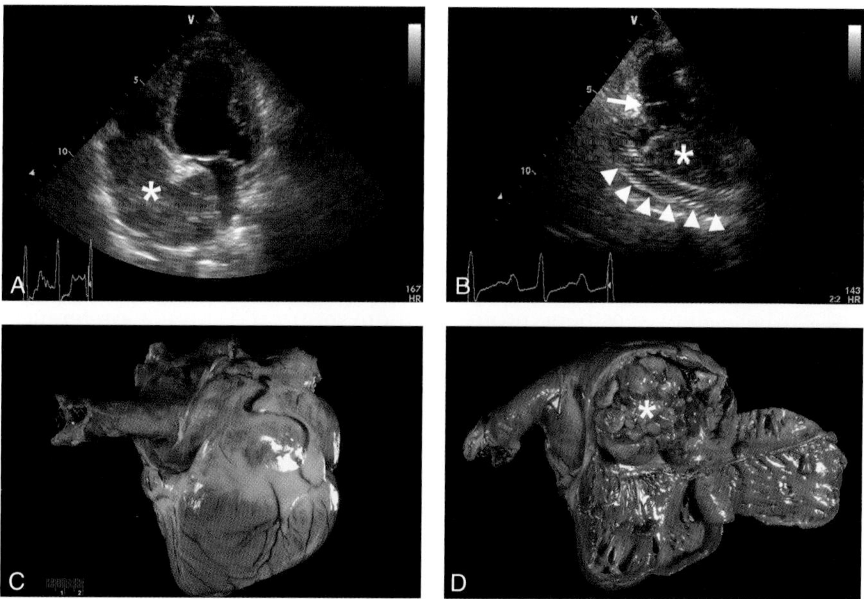

Figure 57.3 Echocardiographic and post-mortem images of the dog from Figure 57.2. The echocardiographic image in (A) was recorded at presentation and prior to transatrial stent placement, showing a large hyperechoic mass (*) filling the right atrial lumen. The echocardiographic image in (B) shows the stent (arrowheads) in position in the caudal vena cava and within the right atrial lumen, pushing the mass away from the tricuspid valve (arrow) and providing a path for caudal venous return. The dog lived for 35 months after first stent placement and post mortem images in (C) and (D) show the expansile mass (*) nearly obliterating the entire right atrial lumen.

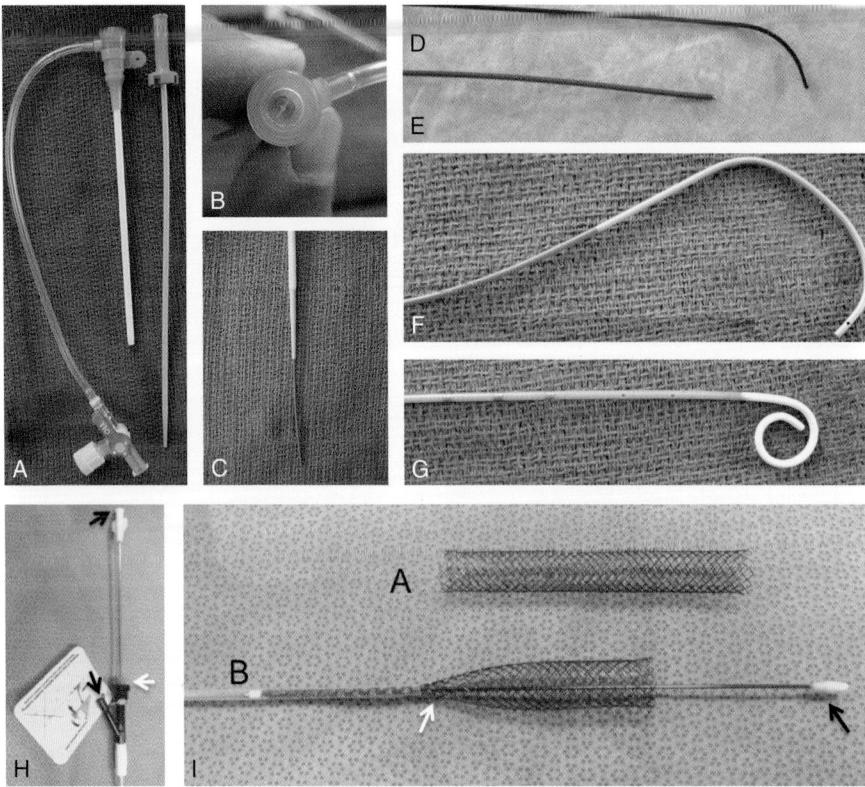

Figure 57.4 Equipment used for transatrial stenting procedure. 10 Fr or 12 Fr vascular introducer sheath and dilator (A) with hemostasis valve (B) and smooth transition from sheath to dilator to 0.035″ guide wire (C). (D) 0.035″ angled hydrophilic guide wire, typically 150 or 180 cm in length but may need 260 cm. (E) Floppy tip PTFE guide wire, typically 260 cm long. (F) 4 Fr Cobra catheter (alternatively can use Berenstein catheter). (G) Pigtail (shown here) or straight tip marker catheter. The radio-opaque marks are 10 mm from the beginning of one mark to the beginning of the next. (H) Close-up view of the mesh self-expanding metallic stent delivery system. Prior to use, sterile saline is injected in the proximal port and side port (black arrows) to remove air and moisten stent. The diaphragm is then unlocked by twisting the dial on the Y-piece (white arrow). I(A). Close-up view of deployed mesh SEMS. I(B). Partially constrained mesh SEMS. Prior to placement within the patient the stent is only slightly deployed to make certain everything is working. Note the partially constrained stent and partially deployed stent (white arrow). As the stent is deployed, it retracts away from the nose cone (black arrow).

Fluoroscopic Procedure

All procedures are performed under general anesthesia using standard cardiac-safety anesthetic protocols. Perioperative cefoxitin (or similar broad-spectrum antibiotic) is administered at 30 mg/kg once, followed by 20 mg/kg q2 hr during the procedure.

Patients are placed in dorsal recumbency, neck extended, with the hindlimbs extended and abducted to provide access to both groins. The ventral cervical region is clipped, scrubbed, and draped exposing the right jugular vein (preferred over the left jugular vein because of the straight path into the vena cava). If both jugular and femoral vein access is necessary, the contralateral femoral vein should be accessed; this facilitates access when the patient is turned into lateral recumbency. For instance, with right jugular vein access, if the patient is turned into left lateral recumbency (to keep jugular sheath up) access will be easiest with the groin sheath on the left side. The opposite is true for left jugular access; this decision is made based upon the room set-up and surgeon preference. See Chapter 44 for more information.

A 3–5 mm skin incision facilitates percutaneous placement of an 18-gauge over-the-needle catheter into the jugular vein. A 0.035″ angled, hydrophilic guide wire[1] is advanced through the catheter and into the cranial vena cava. The catheter is removed over-the-wire and replaced with either a 10 Fr or 12 Fr vascular introducer sheath[2] depending upon the anticipated stent delivery system size. The sheath is secured in place with a single nylon suture and the dilator removed. Femoral vein access is made via surgical cut-down (see Chapter 44) and sheath placement is performed the same as above. For CrVC obstructions, groin access may be easier due to swelling in the head and neck. In addition, it may be prudent to avoid placing sheaths or catheters in the external jugular vein when drainage of the head is a necessity. Often, single site access is sufficient but access "above and below" may be necessary in some cases.

Following vascular access, the patient is rotated in lateral recumbency. The authors finds it easier to view relevant anatomy in this position. In addition, rotating the patient typically provides improved visualization versus rotating the C-arm due to the wide table and anesthetic equipment typically running along the patient.

A combination hydrophilic guide wire and Berenstein catheter[3] or Cobra catheter[4] are used to gain access across the tumor obstruction (Figure 57.1, Figure 57.5, and Figure 57.6). Sometimes this process is more easily achieved after a contrast[5] study has been performed. Once access has been achieved, the Berenstein catheter is exchanged for a marker catheter[6]. Digital subtraction angiography is preferred when possible, and it is best to inject both above and below the lesion simultaneously to fully characterize the extent of the lesion. When access "above and below" is achieved, it may be prudent to snare the exchange length guide wire in order to pull it through the opposite sheath. This allows bilateral access across the obstruction and through the stent in case any problems occur.

Following angiography, pressure measurements are made to determine the gradient across the tumor obstruction; a patient with no pressure gradient will unlikely benefit from stent placement. It is prudent to measure pressures through the marker catheter (across the obstruction) and the introducer sheath rather than losing access across the tumor obstruction once it has been achieved. The marker catheter often has multiple side-holes distally so be certain all holes are beyond the obstruction when obtaining measurements.

At this time, fluoroscopic biopsy may be performed at the operator's discretion. Considering this is a palliative procedure without curative intent, the risk and benefits must be weighed in each individual case. The authors have performed a number of intravascular biopsies, all of them safe; however, diagnostic samples are often not obtained – rather blood clot is identified, likely on the outside of the tumor. In addition, it is not always clear if the tumor is within the vessel/heart (intrinsic), or invading the vessel/heart, or compressing it (extrinsic). This raises concern about biopsy of the (potentially compromised) vessel wall and risk for hemorrhage. Transesophageal echo or prior cross-sectional imaging may help identify preferred areas for biopsy. Following biopsy, repeat angiography should be performed to make sure there has been no contrast extravasation or hemorrhage.

The marker catheter bands are used to calculate radiographic magnification, the SEMS are chosen to be 10–20% larger in diameter than the normal vena cava and to extend well beyond the lesion and into both the CrVC and CdVC. Mesh SEMS[7,8] are often reconstrainable (laser-cut" SEMS typically are not) so may be preferred in this location; however, the associated fore shortening can make ultimate stent positioning more difficult to predict. Sometimes available stent diameters are insufficient to fill the entire vena cava lumen but the tumor tissue or tumor compression of the vessel will help hold the undersized stents in place;

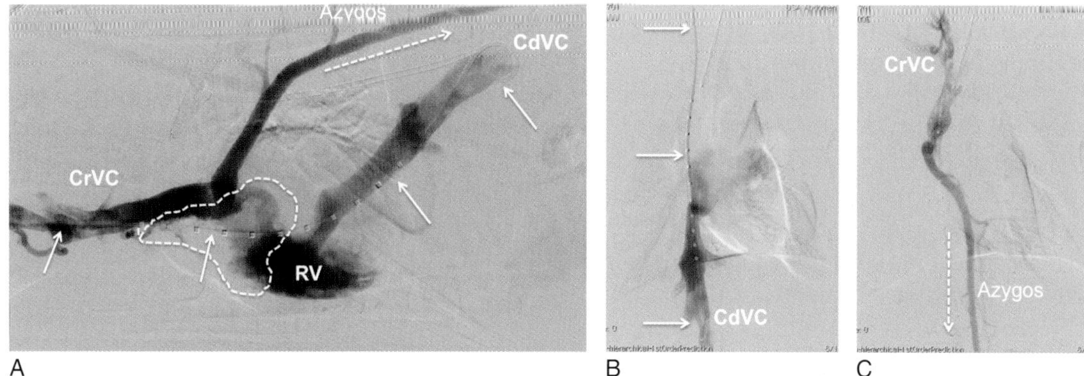

Figure 57.5 Serial pre-stent digital subtraction angiograms (DSA) in a dog with a cardiac tumor causing right atrial obstruction at the level of the cranial vena cava causing cranial vena caval syndrome and pleural effusion. (A) Dual lateral DSA angiogram in the caudal vena cava (CdVC) through a marker catheter (white arrows) and cranial vena cava (CrVC) through the introducer sheath showing the tumor filling defect (white dotted line), a patent CdVC filling the right ventricle (RV), and reverse bloodflow down the azygos vein to decompress the CrVC. (B) Ventrodorsal DSA CdVC venogram through the marker catheter showing a patent CdVC. (C) Ventrodorsal DSA CrVC venogram showing obstruction at the level of the right atrium with reverse blood flow decompressing through the azygos vein.

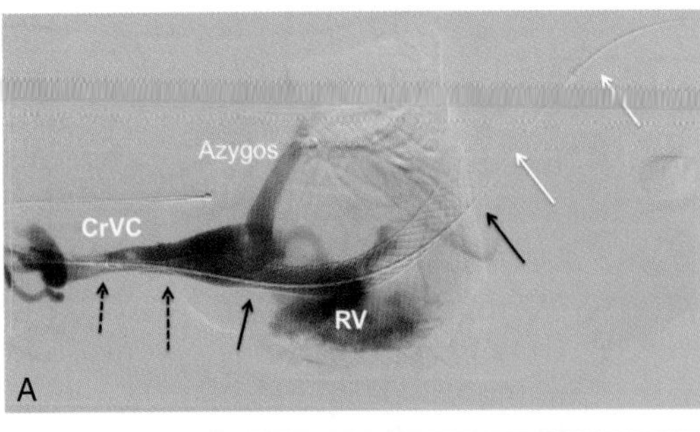

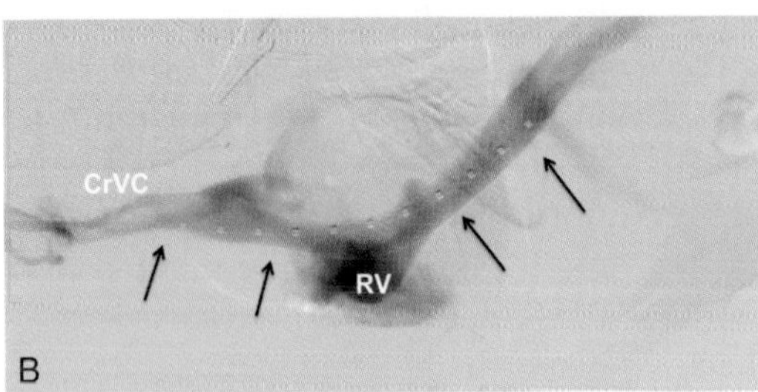

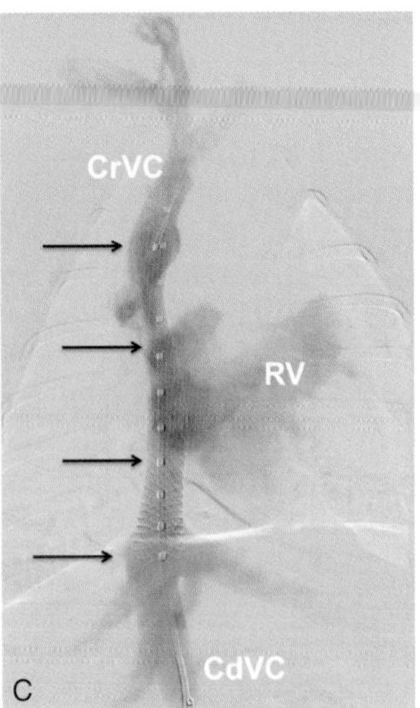

Figure 57.6 Serial post-stent digital subtraction angiograms (DSA) in the same dog as Figure 57.5. (A) Lateral DSA CrVC venogram before complete stent deployment. Note the guide wire (white arrows), the partially deployed transatrial stent (black arrows), and the partially constrained stent (black dotted arrows). Contrast can be seen passing through the stent interstices, across the previous obstruction, and into the right ventricle (RV). There is a small amount of reflux into the azygos vein but normal blood flow direction has resumed. (B) Dual lateral DSA angiogram in the caudal vena cava through a marker catheter and cranial vena cava (CrVC) through the introducer sheath showing the deployed stent (black arrows), re-established CrVC patency, and RV filling without azygos vein filling. (C) Dual ventrodorsal DSA CrVC venogram and CdVC venogram showing patent CrVC, transatrial stent (black arrows), lack of azygos vein filling, and contrast filled right ventricle (RV).

larger stents are preferred as they will permit more venous return. If stent lengths are insufficient, multiple overlapping stents can be placed to cross the entire lesion. If this is necessary, stents with wide interstices are preferred. The stents may cross the azygos vein or the hepatic vein ostia. Transatrial placement helps to avoid stent migration across the tricuspid valve by securing its position in both vessels. It also may prevent excessively large tumor thrombi from launching into the pulmonary circulation. Stent grafts (covered stents) should never be placed transatrially.

Following stent deployment, repeat angiography and pressure gradients should be performed. A superficial absorbable purse-string suture is typically placed at the entry site prior to removal of the sheath. If a large sheath was placed in the neck, it can be exchanged for a smaller multi-lumen catheter overnight to maintain access in case of emergency and to allow the stoma to close down. The multi-lumen catheter is typically removed the following day. The femoral vein is often ligated at completion of the procedure and the surgical site closed routinely.

Animals recover in the intensive care unit on intravenous fluid therapy (3–4 ml/kg/hr until awake and eating or longer if excessive contrast volumes administered) and antibiotics (Table 57.1). Analgesics are not routinely necessary.

Follow-Up

Patients can be discharged one or two days postoperatively and owners are instructed to continue all previous medications (as well as 10–14 days of an additional broad-spectrum antibiotic). Weights are obtained daily and accumulated fluid should be reabsorbed and excreted over the following 1–2 weeks at which time recheck and suture removal can be performed. This examination would be a good opportunity for the oncologist to meet again with the client to consider adjuvant therapies if indicated as any biopsy results will be available. Follow-up examination and testing should be considered on a case-by-case basis. In general, recheck examinations should take place no less frequently than every 3 months.

Special Considerations/ Alternative Uses/ Complication Examples

Heart base tumors such as chemodectomas can cause pulmonary artery compression leading to increased vascular resistance; a pulmonary artery stent has been placed in such situations resulting in reduced gradients (Figure 57.7).

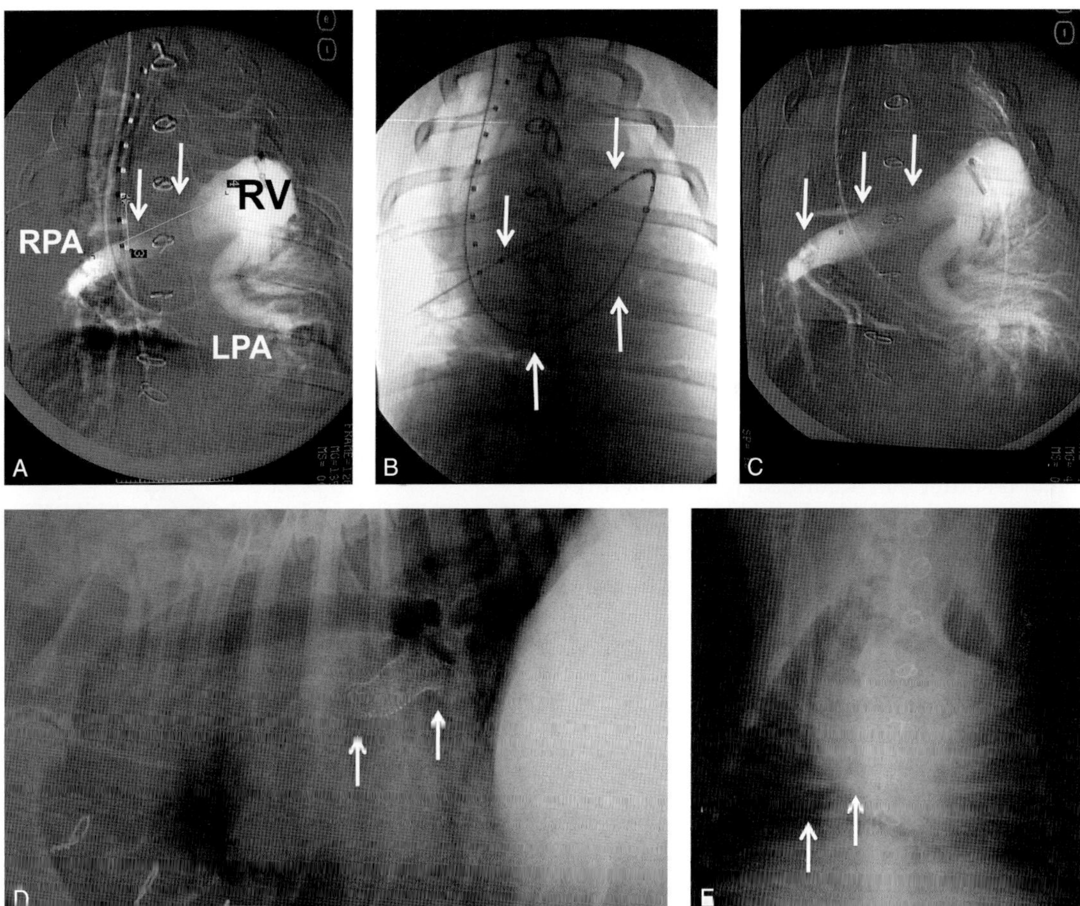

Figure 57.7 Serial images in a dog with a chemodectoma following previous surgical pericardiectomy and subsequent tumor growth and right pulmonary artery compression and obstruction. (A, B) Ventrodorsal images with the head to the top in each image. (A) DSA of the right ventricular (RV) outflow tract demonstrating a narrowed right pulmonary artery (white arrows) and little contrast filling of the right lung. The left pulmonary artery (LPA) can be seen as well. (B) A marker catheter (white arrows) is passed beyond the obstruction for pressure gradients and stent measurements. (C) Following stent placement, the RPA demonstrated better contrast filling (white arrows) with some improved contrast filling of the right pulmonary bed. The pressure gradient was reduced as well. (D, E) Lateral (D) and ventrodorsal (E) radiographs following right pulmonary artery stent (white arrows) placement.

Notes

(Samples; Multiple vendors available)

1. Weasel wire, Infiniti Medical, Menlo Park, CA.
2. 10 Fr or 12 Fr Vascular introducer sheath, Infiniti Medical, Menlo Park, CA.
3. Berenstein catheter, Infiniti Medical, Menlo Park, CA.
4. Cobra head catheter, Infiniti Medical, Menlo Park, CA.
5. Omnipaque (iohexol) injection, Amersham Health Inc., Princeton, NJ.
6. Measuring catheter, Infiniti Medical, Menlo Park, CA.
7. Vet Stent-Trachea, Infiniti Medical, Menlo Park, CA.
8. Wallstent, Boston Scientific, Natick, MA.
9. Vet Stent-Cava, Infiniti Medical, Menlo Park, CA.

References

Prahlow JA, O'Bryant TJ, and Barnard JJ (1997) Cardiac perforation due to Wallstent embolization: a fatal complication of the transjugular intrahepatic portosystemic shunt procedure. *Radiology* 205, 170–2.

Wallace MJ (2003) Transatrial stent placement for treatment of inferior vena cava obstruction secondary to extension of intracardiac tumor thrombus from hepatocellular carcinoma. *J Vasc Interv Radiol* 14, 1339–43.

Weisse C, Berent A, Scansen B, et al. (2012) Transatrial stenting for long-term management of tumor obstruction of the right atrium in 3 dogs. ECVIM Forum 2012, Maastricht, The Netherlands.

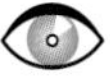

Video clips to accompany this chapter can be found in the online material at **www.wiley.com/go/weisse/vet-image-guided-interventions**

CHAPTER FIFTY-EIGHT

Patent Ductus Arteriosus

Christopher D. Stauthammer
Veterinary Medical Center, College of Veterinary Medicine, University of Minnesota, Saint Paul, MN

Background/Indication

Patent ductus arteriosus (PDA) is a common congenital cardiovascular disorder that occurs as a result of failure of vascular smooth muscle development within the fetal ductus arteriosus (Buchanan and Patterson, 2003). The hypoplastic ductal smooth muscle is largely replaced by non-contractile elastic tissue, thereby preventing postpartum constriction and fibrosis of the vessel. Its patency results in a volume overload and subsequent eccentric hypertrophy of the left heart (Kittleson, 1998, Oyama et al, 2005). Complications include systolic dysfunction, congestive heart failure, and arrhythmias. The majority of untreated dogs succumb to cardiac-related death within 1 year of diagnosis. Those that survive are likely to develop clinical signs and complications from their heart disease by a relatively young age.

Treatment Options

Surgical ligation has traditionally been a successful method of PDA occlusion. However, ligation has been associated with patient mortality, complications, and residual flow (Tobias and Stauthammer, 2010). Interventional methods of PDA occlusion have largely evolved to avoid thoracotomy, while lowering perioperative mortality and complication rates. A variety of devices have been evaluated with variable success. The reader is directed to the reference list at the end of this chapter for a detailed overview of the results obtained with the various occlusion devices.

The Amplatz Canine Duct Occluder (ACDO; AGA Medical Corporation) is the only commercially available device specifically developed for the canine ductus arteriosus (Tobias and Stauthammer, 2010). The device's casted shape includes a flat distal disc separated from a cupped proximal disc by a short waist (Figure 58.1). The distal disc resides in the pulmonary artery, while the cupped proximal disc resides in the ductal ampulla with the device waist traversing the ductal ostium (Figure 58.2). The ACDO consists of a multilayered nitinol mesh that is self-expanding yet highly compressible (Figure 58.3). The device is attached to a

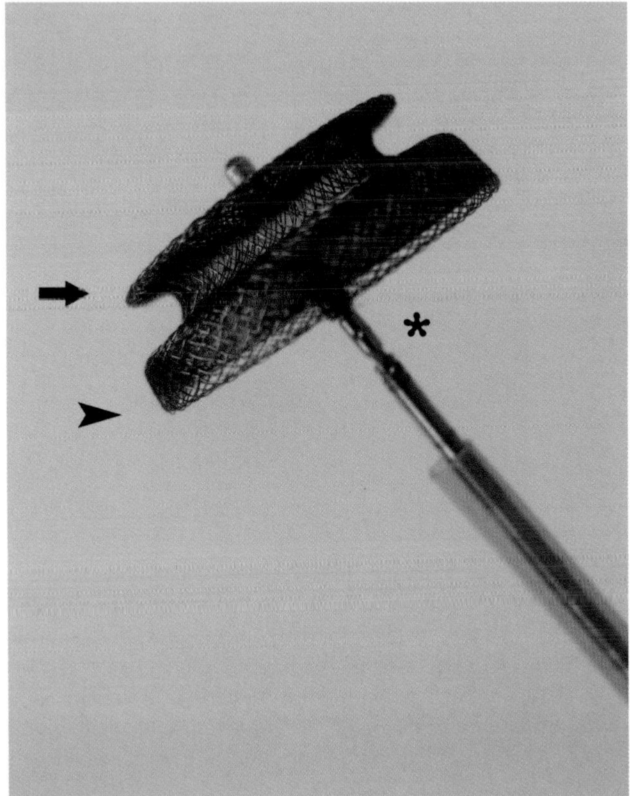

Figure 58.1 The Amplatz Canine Ductal Occluder (ACDO) is a multilayer nitinol wire mesh device consisting of a flat distal disc (arrow) and a cupped proximal disc (arrow head) separated by a short waist. A microscrew (*) within the proximal disc attaches the device to the delivery cable.

Veterinary Image-Guided Interventions, First Edition. Edited by Chick Weisse and Allyson Berent.

Companion website: www.wiley.com/go/weisse/vet-image-guided-interventions

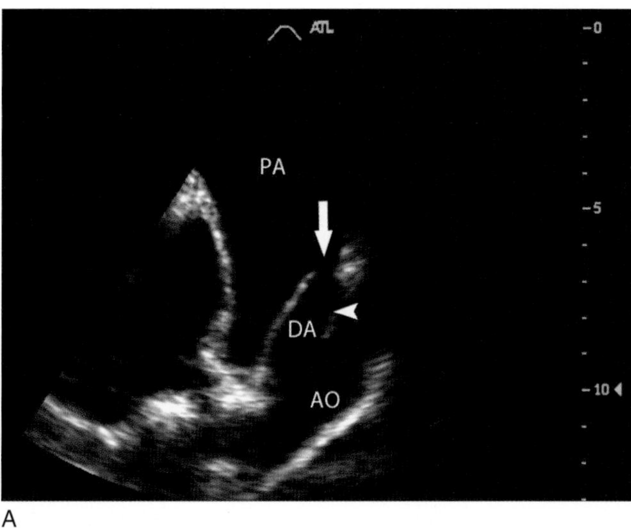

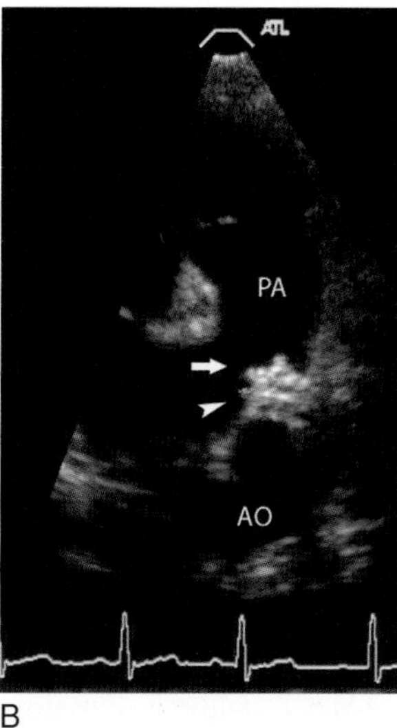

Figure 58.2 (A) An echocardiographic image taken from the left cranial parasternal view demonstrating the anatomy of the ductus arteriosus. The pulmonary artery (PA), descending aorta (AO) and ductus arteriosus (DA) are as labeled. The ampulla (arrow head) is the relatively wide region of the ductus located on the aortic side of the vessel. The pulmonary ostium (arrow) is the narrowed region of the ductus that directly communicates with the pulmonary artery. (B) An echocardiographic image taken from the same imaging plane as (A) demonstrating ductal occlusion with an ACDO device. The flat distal disc (arrow) is located within the pulmonary artery, and the cupped proximal disc (arrow head) resides within the ampulla. The narrowed device waist is located within the ostium.

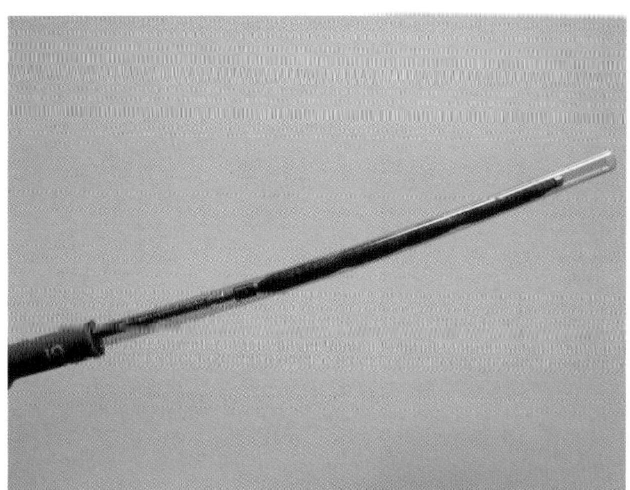

Figure 58.3 An ACDO device constrained within the manufacturer-supplied loader.

manufacturer-supplied delivery cable via a micro-screw within the proximal disc. The attached delivery cable allows for controlled delivery and the ability to recapture the device into a catheter or sheath.

The ACDO is a popular method for PDA occlusion and has recently been found to be superior to coils and the vascular plug for ease of use, complication rate, and degree of occlusion (Singh et al, 2012). Large studies evaluating ductal occlusion with the ACDO are unavailable. However, numerous small studies have demonstrated promising results with an overall 0% mortality rate, ≤6% residual flow and a low incidence of procedural abandonment (Nguyenba et al, 2008, Gordon et al 2010, Singh et al, 2012). The author has performed more than 60 PDA occlusion procedures with the ACDO with an overall 0% perioperative mortality rate, <2% residual flow, 3% embolization rate, and 1 case of procedural abandonment.

Potential Risks/ Complications/ Expected Outcomes

The primary procedural related concerns with PDA occlusion by ACDO include device infection, device embolization, and femoral arterial hemorrhage. Device embolization is exceptionally rare and is reported to be well tolerated if embolized into the pulmonary vasculature (Nguyenba et al, 2008, Gordon et al, 2010). The author's experience is in agreement with these reports in that an embolized device does not appear to complicate pulmonary function and can be left out in the pulmonary vasculature without compromising the patient. A snare could be passed through a sheath for device retrieval if deemed necessary. Device infection should be considered catastrophic as the infection will unlikely resolve with antibiotics and lead to septic emboli (Fine and Tobias, 2007). Infection is preventable by following aseptic technique within a clean catheterization environment. Patients should optimally be screened for evidence of an infection before the procedure with blood work and a urine culture. Although controversial, the author also administers perioperative antibiotics for an extended period of 1–2 weeks following the procedure. The patient is not allowed to undergo any elective surgical or dental procedure for 3 months. Following the 3-month window, the device is covered by vascular endothelium and no longer in contact with potential bacteremia (personal communication with AGA Medical). Tearing of the femoral artery is predominately a risk in small patients and is discussed under the Special Considerations section.

Successful PDA occlusion is considered a curative procedure with normalization of cardiac chamber dimensions within one year in uncomplicated patients (Corti et al, 2000, Bureau et al, 2005, Blossom et al, 2010, Stauthammer et al, 2013). The normalization in chamber dimensions is independent of patient age at time of procedure. Systolic dysfunction may persist post-occlusion, but is clinically unimportant as it does not influence survival times (median >11.5 years post-procedure) or result in congestive heart failure. There is a paucity of research evaluating the prognosis in complicated cases; although some studies have suggested that the presence of congestive heart failure, atrial fibrillation, or ventricular arrhythmias worsen the long-term prognosis (Oliveria, 2009). The author has also witnessed cases with heart failure and/or ventricular arrhythmias that demonstrated cardiac-related death within a short time period following the procedure. However, limited experience indicates that dogs in congestive heart failure have an excellent outcome if PDA occlusion is performed before one year of age.

Procedure

Patient Preparation

The presence of a PDA is often suspected when the characteristic continuous heart murmur is heard over the left heart base. However, echocardiography is required for a definitive diagnosis as other cardiac defects may result in a similar continuous murmur including aortopulmonary window and systemic to pulmonary arterial fistulae. Concurrent cardiac abnormalities may also be identified with echocardiography. The PDA is visualized from the left cranial parasternal view for assessment of ductal morphology and measurement of the ductal ostium diameter. Ductal morphology is described using the classification scheme reported by Miller et al (2006) (Figure 58.4).

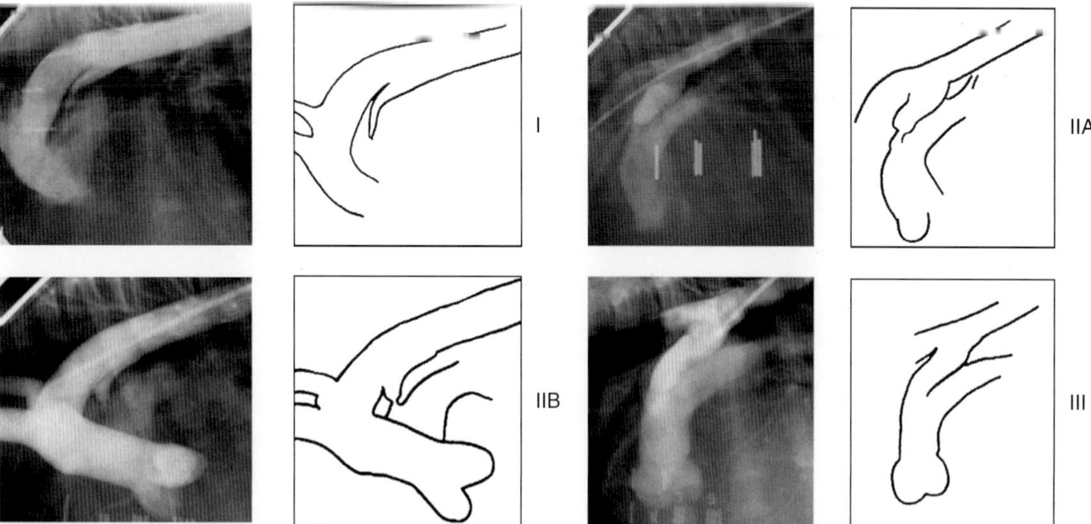

Figure 58.4 Representative aortic angiograms from dogs with left-to-right shunting PDA highlighting characteristic ductal morphology. To the right of each angiogram is the corresponding line drawing illustrating relevant morphologic features. All angiograms were obtained in the right lateral projection. (I) Type I PDA. Notice that the diameter of the ductus gradually decreases in size from the aorta to the pulmonary arterial location. (IIA) Type IIA PDA. Notice that the walls of the ductus are essentially parallel to one another, and that the ductal diameter abruptly decreases (>50%) at the point of insertion into the pulmonary artery. (IIB) Type IIB PDA. Notice that the diameter of the ductus decreases markedly from the aortic to the pulmonic side with the most narrow aspect being at the pulmonic insertion. (III) Type III PDA. Notice that the diameter of the ductus does not change substantially throughout its length, producing a tubular appearance. (From Miller MW, Gordon SG, Saunders AG, et al. Angiographic classification of patent ductus arteriosus morphology in the dog. J Vet Cardiol 2006; 8, 109–14; with permission.)

The ductal diameter measurements are useful in estimating a range of potential device sizes necessary for the procedure, though precise measurements of minimal ductal diameter by transthoracic echocardiography can be challenging in some dogs.

Equipment

Recommended equipment is shown in Figure 58.5. PDA occlusion may be performed under fluoroscopy, transesophageal echocardiography, or transthoracic echocardiography (Caivano et al, 2012). The author prefers fluoroscopy as it enables visualization of the entire occlusive device during the procedure ensuring proper device deployment and reducing the risk of embolization, valvular damage, and residual ductal flow. Fluoroscopy also allows the interventionalist to monitor the position of catheters, sheaths and exchange wires along their entire length during the procedure, facilitating the passage of equipment to the appropriate location and minimizing vascular and valvular damage as well as potential looping of equipment. The authors also rely on the angiographic measurement of the PDA for device size selection. This measurement cannot be substituted by transthoracic echocardiography as the limits of agreement between the imaging modalities are unacceptably large (Nguyenba and Tobias, 2007). Many interventionalists will utilize fluoroscopy and transesophageal echocardiography (TEE) during the procedure. The addition of TEE facilitates device positioning and assessment of residual flow. The authors also recommend the use of an angiographic power injector as discussed under angiography.

The ACDO may be delivered through a guiding catheter or a long sheath. The original procedural description recommended use of a guiding catheter due to enhanced tactile feedback (Nguyenba and Tobias, 2007). However, the author commonly utilizes a vascular sheath for ACDO delivery due to expense and limited availability of guiding catheters. Different sizing conventions are utilized for guiding catheters and sheaths with the French (Fr) size referring to the inner diameter of sheaths and the outer diameter of guiding catheters. The required guiding catheter is generally two Fr sizes larger than the required sheath.

Vascular Access

Access to the right femoral artery is obtained as described in Chapter 44. The selected size of the vascular access sheath (4–10 Fr) is dependent on vessel size and the required size of the delivery sheath for ACDO placement (Table 58.1). Ideally, the vascular access sheath should be 2 Fr greater in diameter than the required delivery sheath in order to accommodate passage of the delivery sheath. If guiding catheters are used in place of sheaths, then the required vascular access sheath should be selected to be of equal size as the guiding catheter. This is generally feasible for dogs weighing greater than 5 kg. Within smaller dogs, the femoral artery is too small to safely pass a 6 Fr access sheath, which is the smallest access sheath that will accommodate passage of the ACDO delivery system. Consequently, a 4 Fr access sheath is initially placed and exchanged with a 4 or 5 Fr delivery sheath during the later stages of the procedure.

Ductal Angiography

Ductal angiography is a critical step in transcatheter PDA occlusion as the information obtained will determine device size and success of the procedure. The patient should be positioned in right lateral recumbency without rotation. Excessive patient rotation often prevents adequate visualization of the ductal ostium. A pigtail angiographic catheter is advanced into the aorta immediately cranial or caudal to the ductal ampulla. Moving the catheter too cranial to the ductus may prevent adequate visualization of the ductal ostium due to summation with the ascending aorta and arch. Angiography is performed with a rapid rate of administration (20 ml/s; dependent on catheter flow limitations) of non-ionic contrast medium at a volume of 1 ml per kg bodyweight. The authors utilize an angiographic power injector to ensure an optimal rate of injection for angiography. Manual injections of contrast are feasible in smaller dogs. Image magnification is taken into account with use of a sizing angiographic catheter or a calibrated guide wire passed through the lumen of the pigtail. While the outer diameter of the angiographic catheter can be used as a reference point with 1 Fr = 0.33 mm, this practice is not encouraged as it is less precise and carries a greater risk of inaccurate ductal measurements. The angiogram is reviewed for identification of the narrowed contrast jet as it enters the pulmonary artery from the ductus (Figure 58.6, Video 58.1). This jet represents the minimal ductal diameter (MDD) or the pulmonary ostium of the ductus. The selected ACDO device should have a waist diameter ranging from 1.5 to 2.0 times the angiographic MDD. This oversize factor is necessary to prevent device embolization. However, selection of too large of a device will also likely result in embolization, as the ductal ampulla would be too small to accommodate the

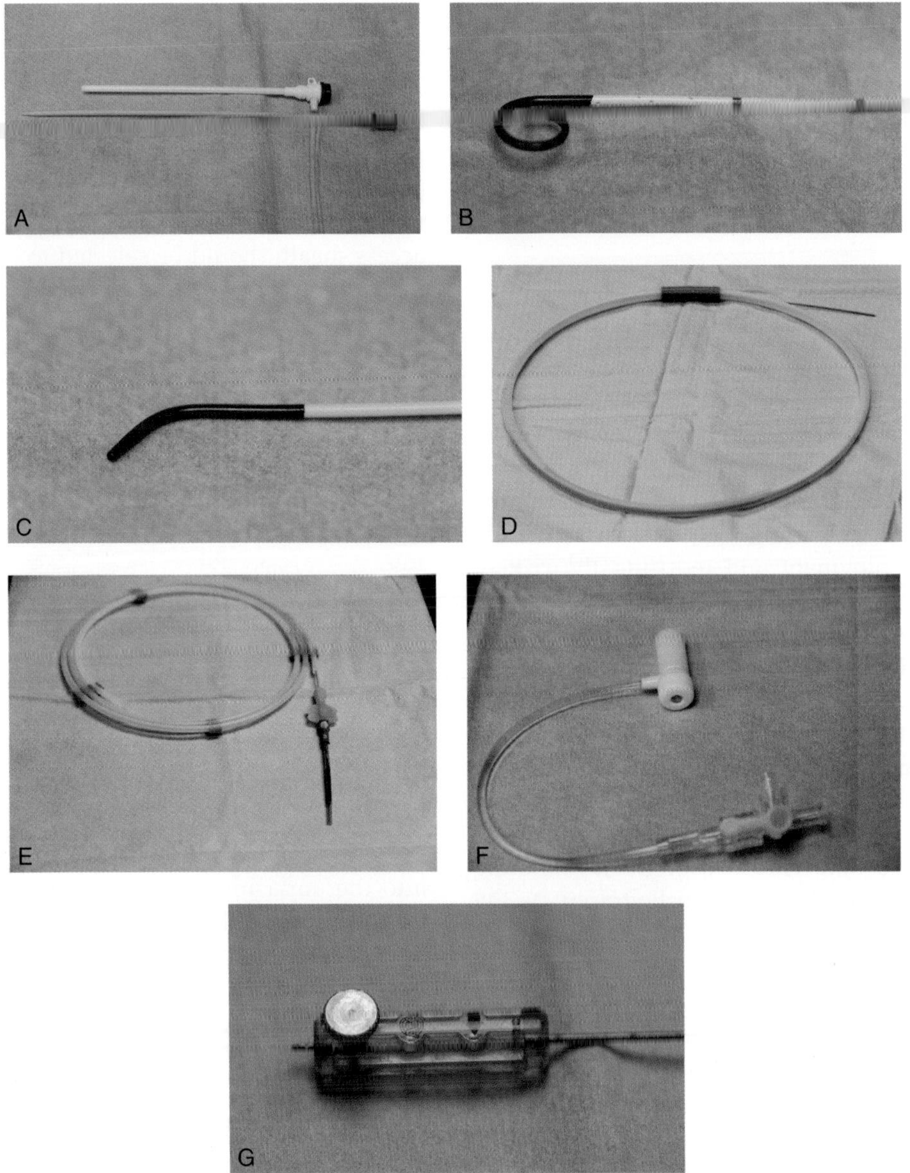

Figure 58.5 (A) Vascular access sheath and introducer. The vascular access sheath is required for most vascular interventional procedures. An access sheath is a relatively short sheath with an attached one way valve on the end. The sheath allows for access and passage of catheters and delivery sheaths into the vessel lumen while minimizing hemorrhage. The dilator reduces endothelial damage during passage of the access sheath. A side port allows for flushing of the sheath. (B) Pigtail angiographic catheter with calibration markers. A pigtail angiographic catheter is recommended for arterial contrast studies performed with a power injector. The shape of the catheter tip and numerous side holes prevent the forceful injection of contrast into the myocardium (i.e., myocardial staining), which can lead to ventricular arrhythmias and death. The catheter also allows for rapid dispersion of contrast providing for a more uniform angiogram. Calibration markers allow for image magnification to be accounted for during measurement of the ductal ostium. A calibrated guide wire could also be passed through the catheter lumen if markers are not present. (C) Angled end-hole catheter. An angled end-hole catheter is used to facilitate passage of an exchange wire across the ductus into the main pulmonary artery. The catheter directs the wire into the ductus from the descending aorta. A variety of angles could be used provided the internal catheter diameter accommodates the exchange wire. (D) Exchange wire. An exchange wire is necessary to direct the delivery sheath across the ductus into the main pulmonary artery. The wire length needs to be at least twice as long as the length of the angled end-hole catheter and delivery sheath. Generally, an 0.035″ flexible, straight tip, polytetrafluoroethylene (PTFE) wire 260 cm in length with a stainless steel core is selected for the exchange as demonstrated here. Hydrophilic, nitinol wires are not recommended due to the weight of the delivery sheath. (E) Loaded ACDO and delivery cable. The ACDO is packaged within the loader and attached to the delivery cable. The loader is necessary for passing the device into the delivery sheath. (F) Hemostasis valve. The hemostasis valve attaches to the catheter end and allows for passage of wire or device without hemorrhage. The hemostasis valve generally is similar to that included on a vascular access sheath. (G) Vice. The manufacturer-supplied vice grips the delivery cable facilitating the release of the device from the delivery cable.

TABLE 58.1
The recommended delivery system and vascular access sheath per selected ACDO device size

Device waist size (mm)	Delivery sheath (Fr)	Guiding catheter (Fr)	Vascular access sheath (Fr)
3	4	6	6
4	4	6	6
5	4	6	6
6	4	6	6
7	5	7	7
8	5	7	7
9	6	8	8
10	7	9	9
12	7	9	9
14	7	9	9

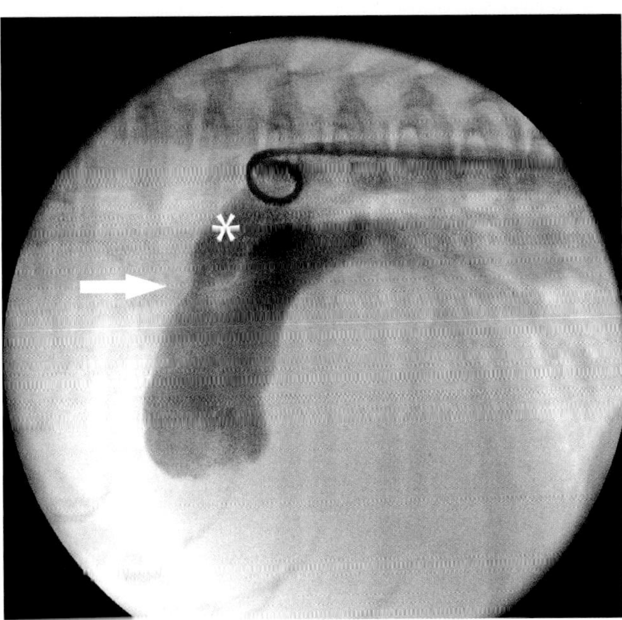

Figure 58.6 Ductal angiogram. The angiogram is performed with the pigtail catheter in the aorta. The ampulla of the ductus arteriosus (*) is ventral to the aorta. The narrowed jet of contrast (arrow) or minimal ductal diameter represents the ductal ostium. The selected ACDO device size is determined by the width of the contrast jet. The diameter of the ductal ampulla may be utilized to estimate maximal device size.

proximal cupped disc, preventing the device from resuming its original casted shape. As such, the angiographic diameter of the ductal ampulla should also be evaluated to aid in determination of maximal device size. Caution is urged in deploying a device with a proximal disc diameter exceeding three times the ampulla diameter.

ACDO Deployment

Following angiographic analysis, a size 4 or 5 Fr angled end-hole catheter is directed into the aorta and advanced to the level of the ductus. A variety of angled end-hole catheters may be utilized. The author prefers a catheter tip with an approximate 45 degree angle. A hemostasis valve is placed on the catheter end to prevent hemorrhage and allow passage of a wire. A 0.035″ straight, floppy tip exchange wire is then directed through this catheter lumen and advanced across the PDA into the pulmonary artery (Figure 58.7, Video 58.2). The length of the wire needs to be at least twice the length of the catheter to facilitate exchange of the catheter. The floppy end of the exchange wire is maintained within the main pulmonary artery (MPA), while the end-hole catheter is withdrawn.

Following removal of the catheter, the portion of the wire outside of the patient must be cleaned by a dampened gauze square to remove any blood droplets, which if clotted may prevent passage of the delivery sheath over the wire. The delivery sheath size (4 to 8 Fr) is determined by the selected ACDO size as outlined on the product label (Table 58.1). The sheath with its dilator in place is directed over the exchange wire and advanced across the ductus into the MPA. A hemostasis valve is generally not required on the end of the dilator as the wire fully occludes the dilator lumen. Use of the dilator is recommended to facilitate passage across the ductus and minimize the risk of ductal laceration and vascular endothelial damage. The location of the exchange wire must be controlled during passage of the sheath to prevent looping of the wire within the MPA or damage to the pulmonary valve. The dilator should also be carefully withdrawn into the sheath as the sheath tip crosses the ductus to minimize dilator contact and potential damage to the pulmonary valve (Video 58.3). Once the sheath tip is positioned within the MPA, the dilator and exchange wire are completely removed and a hemostasis valve applied if not already present on the sheath end.

Inspection of the ACDO device and its attachment to the delivery cable is recommended before implantation by exteriorizing the device from the loader. The degree of attachment is assessed by loosening, removing, and then re-tightening the device until resistance is felt; a good rule of thumb is to tighten the device completely and then rotate back a ½ turn. Do not over tighten. The device should then be reloaded under sterile saline to prevent air emboli during deployment. The distal tip of the device should be flush with the loader tip to facilitate passage into the delivery sheath. The

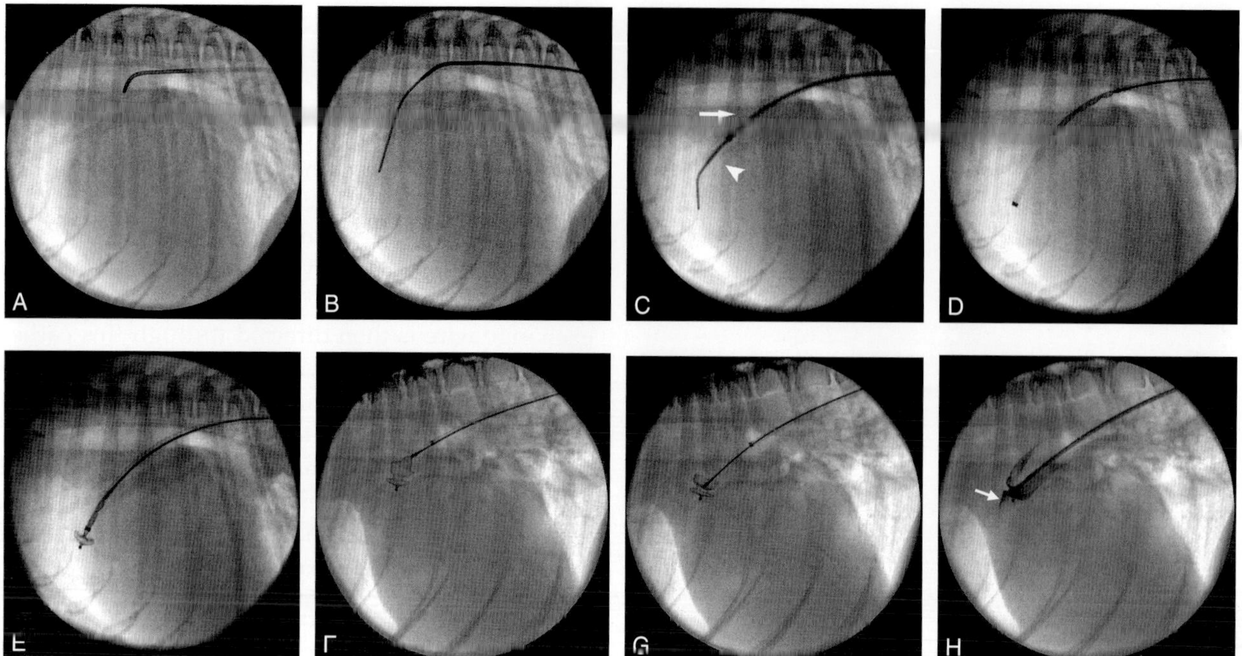

Figure 58.7 (A) The angled end-hole catheter is advanced in the aorta to the level of the ductus. The catheter tip is directed towards the ductal ampulla by rotating the catheter end. (B) The exchange wire is advance across the ductus into the main pulmonary artery. The wire is directed into the appropriate location by the end-hole catheter. Following placement of the exchange wire, the catheter is removed over the wire. (C) The delivery sheath (arrow) and dilator (arrow head) are advanced over the exchange wire into the main pulmonary artery. The dilator minimizes potential damage to the vascular endothelium and the ductal wall. The dilator should be slightly retracted into the sheath lumen to minimize contact with the pulmonary valve. The wire and dilator are subsequently removed, while the sheath tip is positioned within the pulmonary artery away from the valve. (D) The ACDO device is then loaded into the delivery sheath and advanced to the sheath tip. (E) The distal disc is exteriorized into the pulmonary artery away from the valve. The waist of the device should also be partially exteriorized. The distal disc is moved into apposition with the ductal ostium by simultaneously retracting the sheath and delivery cable. Tactile feedback and subtle changes in device motion signal proper device positioning. Additional retraction may result in exteriorization of the proximal disc. (F, G) The proximal disc is exteriorized by maintaining tension on the delivery cable via a gentle pulling motion on the delivery cable while retracting the sheath over the cable. Release of the tension on the delivery cable following exteriorization will allow for the proximal disc to reform its native shape. (H) Prior to device release, a small volume of contrast is administered through the sheath lumen to confirm proper device placement. Contrast is evident within the ductal ampulla and residual flow through the device (arrow) is common due to slight device displacement from the attached delivery cable.

loader tip will need to be fully inserted across the hemostasis valve on the sheath before advancing the device into the lumen. To prevent hemorrhage, the loader is withdrawn from the valve once the device is within the sheath. The device is then advanced through the sheath lumen with a gentle pushing motion on the delivery cable, while simultaneously maintaining the sheath tip within the MPA. The sheath tip should be withdrawn away from the pulmonary valve before exteriorizing the distal disc of the ACDO to prevent valvular damage from device entanglement. After the distal disc and a portion of the device waist have been exteriorized within the pulmonary artery, the sheath and device are withdrawn together until the distal disc engages with the pulmonary ostium, at which point resistance may be felt (Video 58.4). Often the device will exhibit a subtle change in direction of movement along with straightening of the delivery cable when the distal disc encounters the pulmonary ostium. Continuing to withdraw the sheath tip will initiate deployment of the proximal disc. The proximal disc should be deployed by maintaining tension with a steady, gentle traction on the delivery cable to keep the distal disc in contact with the pulmonic ostium (Video 58.5). The sheath is then slowly withdrawn over the cable while maintaining tension on the delivery cable until the proximal disc is fully exteriorized. Afterwards, a gentle pushing motion on the delivery cable may be necessary for the proximal disk to resume its cupped shape. Once the device has been exteriorized from the sheath, a small volume (3–5 ml) of contrast is administered by hand injection to document device position (Video 58.6). Marked resistance to the injection is often noted with smaller sheath sizes due to partial luminal occlusion from the delivery cable. Residual flow is common as the device is slightly distorted by the attachment of the delivery cable. Following the contrast injection, device stability is assessed with a moderate level of pushing and pulling on the delivery cable (Videos 58.7 and 58.8). The proximal disc shape should slightly distort while pulling on the cable. The delivery cable should bend dorsally with pushing on the cable. Excessive force on the delivery cable is not recommended as a properly sized device can be pushed or pulled through the ductus if sufficient strain is applied, with potential to result in ductal tearing.

If the device is dislodged with cable manipulation, it should be recaptured into the sheath with a gentle, steady pulling motion on the delivery cable while advancing the sheath over the cable. Following recapture, the angiogram and all measurements and calculations should be reviewed. The angiogram should be repeated if there is inadequate visualization of the MDD. If the original selected device size appears appropriate following the review, a new device should be selected with a waist diameter that is 2 to 3 mm larger than the first. The device may be released if it remains stable following the cable manipulation, and it has resumed its casted shape. The manufacturer-supplied vice pin or a hemostat is attached to the delivery cable and rotated in a counterclockwise direction until release of the device. Do not pull on the cable during the rotation of the vice pin as this could partially dislodge the device. Once the device has been released, the cable is withdrawn into the sheath lumen and the sheath and cable are then withdrawn together. If the vascular access sheath was removed as part of an exchange in a small dog, then the delivery sheath should remain within the descending aorta. An aortic angiogram is then performed as previously described to assess degree of ductal occlusion (Figure 58.8, Video 58.9). In small dogs where an exchange occurred, a 4 Fr angiographic catheter will fit through the lumen of a 4 Fr delivery sheath. The tip of the angiographic catheter should be advanced out of the sheath prior to injection. Alternatively, a manual injection may be performed through the delivery sheath. Occasionally, trivial to mild residual flow through the device will be noted immediately following device release. Such flow typically resolves within another 5 to 10 minutes.

The final step of PDA occlusion is removal of the vascular access sheath or delivery sheath. The author prefers to repair the entry site within the femoral artery with 6–0 non-absorbable suture material in a simple continuous pattern. Alternatively, the femoral artery may be ligated with non-absorbable suture material. The incision site is closed in a routine manner.

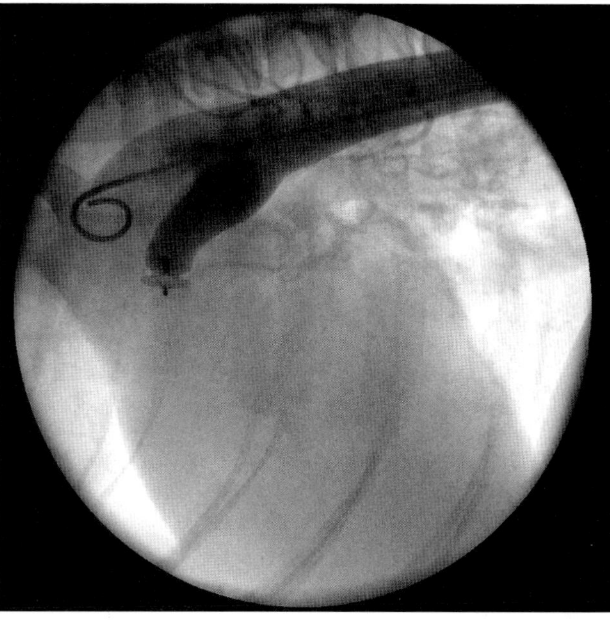

Figure 58.8 Post deployment angiogram demonstrating complete ductal occlusion secondary to proper positioning of the ACDO device across the ductus.

The patient is kept moderately sedated overnight and discharged the following morning. Moderate exercise restriction is recommended for the following two weeks.

Follow-Up

Follow-up recommendations are dependent on each individual case. An echocardiogram is performed the following morning before patient discharge. Device placement and residual flow are evaluated as well as left ventricular chamber dimensions and function. Residual flow is not an expected finding as closure is typically 100% complete at this time. Patients are rechecked 3 months and 1 year post procedure with an echocardiogram performed during these visits. The one year follow-up examination is not necessary if the 3-month echocardiogram reveals complete occlusion with normalization of left ventricular chamber dimensions.

Special Considerations

The ACDO is the recommended treatment for PDA. However, the device has limitations in regards to patient size and ductal morphology. Due to the required delivery catheter/sheath size, the ACDO is not feasible in patients less than 2.5 kg in body weight or in slightly larger chondrodystrophic breeds. The femoral artery in these smaller dogs is unable to accommodate a 4 Fr sheath and is at risk of tearing. These

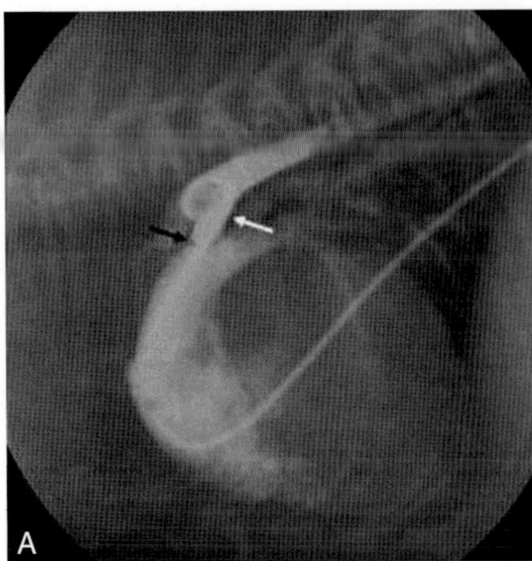

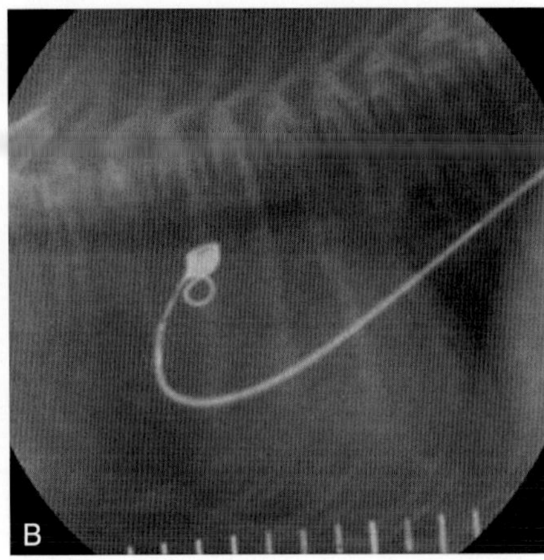

Figure 58.9 (A) Lateral angiogram of a small dog undergoing transvenous coil occlusion of the PDA. A pigtail catheter was advanced retrograde through the ductus into the aorta. Contrast is evident within the descending aorta, ductus, main pulmonary artery and right ventricle. The ductal ampulla (white arrow) and minimal ductal diameter (black arrow) are measured for coil selection. The coil loop diameter should be greater than twice the minimal ductal diameter. (B) Fluoroscopic image acquired before coil deployment. A detachable 0.038″ coil has been positioned within the ductal ampulla, leaving 1 loop in the pulmonary artery. (Images used with permission, from Henrich E, Hildebrandt N, Schneider C, Hassdenteufel E, Schneider M. Transvenous Coil Embolization of Patent Ductus Arteriosus in Small (≤3 kg) dogs. JVIM 2011; 25, 65–70.)

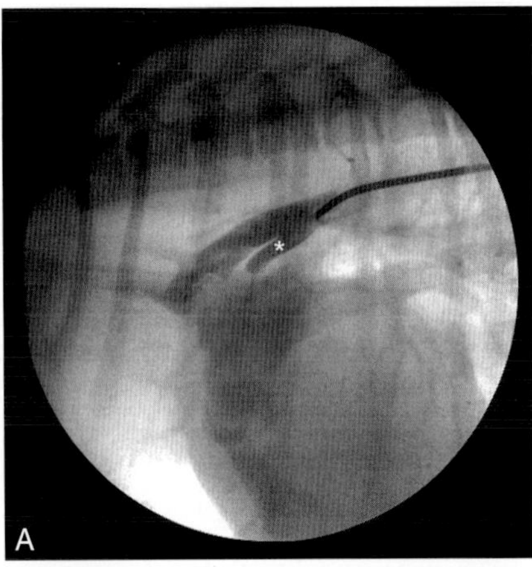

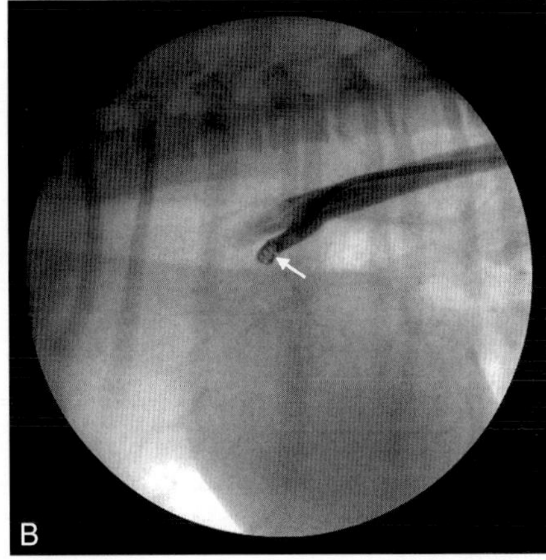

Figure 58.10 (A) Lateral angiogram of a small dog undergoing transarterial coil occlusion of a PDA. A 4 Fr KMP catheter has been advanced from the femoral artery to the descending aorta and contrast injection highlights the ductus arteriosus (*). The ductal ostium (minimal ductal diameter) in this dog is less than 1 mm and a small coil (0.035″, 2 mm × 3 cm) is chosen. (B) After advancement of the coil (arrow) by a standard 0.035″ guidewire into the ductal ampulla, repeat contrast injection shows complete occlusion of ductal flow. (Images courtesy of Brian A Scansen.)

patients should either undergo surgical ligation or occlusion with a different device. Coil embolization was the first reported means of transcatheter PDA occlusion in dogs and can be performed from either a venous or arterial approach (Gordon and Miller, 2005, Henrich et al, 2011). Excellent outcomes have been reported with coil embolization through a transvenous approach, whereby a 4 Fr catheter is inserted into the femoral vein and advanced from the pulmonary artery, across the ductus and into the aorta (Gordon and Miller, 2005) (Figure 58.9). An 0.052″ or 0.038″ detachable coil with a loop diameter of twice the diameter of the MDD is placed across the ductus with the majority of the coil loops extruded within the ductal ampulla and the remaining 0.5 to 1 loop extruded on the pulmonary side. The practice of leaving a small loop of coil on the pulmonary artery side of the ductus is commonplace in human interventional cardiology, but is now less commonly performed in animals due to a perceived greater risk of coil embolization.

The delivery of coils from a transarterial approach allows direct monitoring of post-coil angiography to verify the degree of occlusion and facilitates the addition of more coils if necessary (Figure 58.10). One

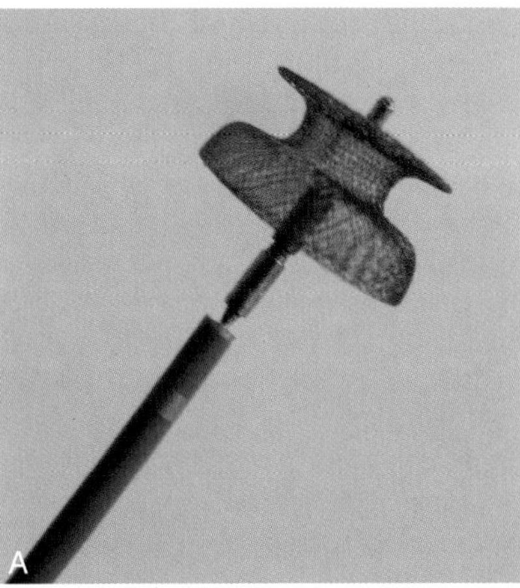

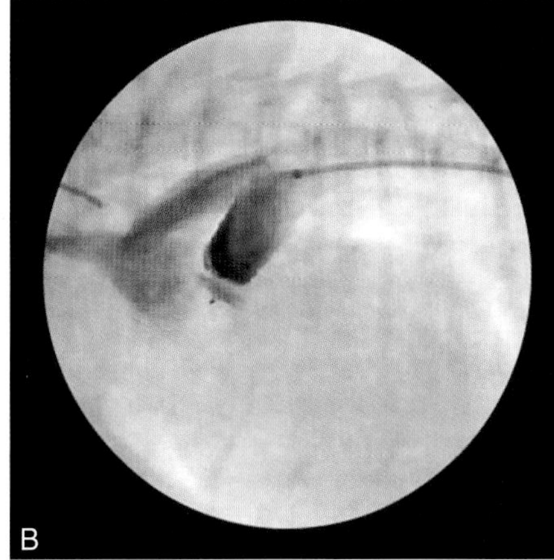

Figure 58.11 (A) Modified ACDO device designed to pass through a 4 Fr catheter. The device shape remains similar to the standard ACDO device. Reduced layers of the nitinol mesh confer greater device compressibility, allowing for passage through the smaller catheter. (B) Angiogram post deployment demonstrating complete ductal occlusion. Contrast is administered through the 4 Fr delivery catheter by hand injection.

drawback of coil embolization for PDA is the lack of controlled delivery as the coil is pushed out the delivery catheter via advancement of a guide wire and cannot be reconstrained or repositioned. The use of bioptome forceps or commercially-available detachable coils have been described for improved control during coil delivery and may be considered (Gordon and Miller, 2005, Olson et al, 2010, Singh et al, 2012). An additional disadvantage of coil embolization is the relatively higher proportion of dogs that have persistent flow across the ductus following the procedure as compared to the ACDO (Singh et al, 2012). The benefit of coil embolization for PDA is the reduced cost of the coils as compared to the ACDO. It should be noted that stainless steel coils, which were the traditional coil of choice for PDA embolization in dogs, are no longer available from the human market due to concerns for magnetic resonance imaging (MRI) compatibility. As such, platinum coils have been the only commercially-available option for PDA coil embolization and carry a higher cost than stainless steel, albeit less than the cost of an ACDO. Recently, inconel coils have been introduced, which are MRI compatible, but have the rigid characteristics of the older generation, discontinued stainless steel coils.

The author currently uses an investigational modified ACDO device designed to fit through a 4 Fr catheter (Olson et al, 2010) (Figure 58.11). The device is similar in design to the ACDO, with the exception of reduced layers of material, increasing compressibility. The device is deployed through an arterial approach in the same manner as described above for the ACDO.

The ACDO has been shown to successfully occlude PDAs of all morphology types (Nguyenba et al, 2008, Gordon et al, 2010, Singh et al, 2012). However, rare instances of procedural abandonment occur due to the ductal ostium being too large for the largest commercially available device (14 mm). Generally, these rare instances involve PDAs of type 3 morphology in which the ostium is of similar diameter as the ampulla. Most reported instances of procedural abandonment have involved German shepherd dogs with type 3 morphology (Nguyenba and Tobias, 2007). The author prefers to have a surgeon on back up when catheterizing such cases. An ACDO may be placed through a second procedure if the patient has significant residual flow on follow up evaluations.

References

Buchanan J and Patterson D (2003) Etiology of the patent ductus arteriosus in dogs. *J Vet Intern Med* 17, 167–71.

Blossom J, Bright J, and Griffiths L (2010) Transvenous occlusion of patent ductus arteriosus in 56 consecutive dogs. *J Vet Cardiol* 12, 75–84.

Bureau S, Monnet E, and Orton E (2005) Evaluation of survival rate and prognostic indicators for surgical treatment of left-to-right patent ductus arteriosus in dogs: 52 cases (1995–2003). *J Am Vet Med Assoc* 227, 1794–9.

Caivano D, Birettoni F, Fruganti A, et al. (2012) Transthoracic echocardiographically – guided interventional cardiac procedures in the dog. *J Vet Cardiol* 14, 431–44.

Corti L, Merkley D, Nelson O, et al (2000) Retrospective evaluation of occlusion of patent ductus arteriosus with hemoclips in 20 dogs. *J Am Anim Hosp Assoc* 36, 548–55.

Fine DM and Tobias AH (2007) Cardiovascular device infections in dogs: report of 8 cases and review of the literature. *J Vet Intern Med* 21, 1265–71.

Gordon S, Saunders A, Achen S, et al (2010) Transarterial ductal occlusion using the Amplatz canine duct occluder in 40 dogs. *J Vet Cardiol* 12, 85–92.

Gordon SG and Miller MW (2005) Transarterial coil embolization for canine patent ductus arteriosus occlusion. *Clin Techn Small Anim Pract* 20(3), 196–202.

Henrich E, Hildebrandt N, Schneider C, et al. (2011) Transvenous coil embolization of patent ductus arteriosus in small (≤3 kg) dogs. *J Vet Intern Med* 25, 65–70.

Kittleson MD (1998) Patent ductus arteriosus. In *Small Animal Cardiovascular Medicine*. (Kittleson MD and Kienle RD, editors). Mosby, St. Louis, pp. 218–30.

Miller MW, Gordon SG, Saunders AG, et al. (2006) Angiographic classification of patent ductus arteriosus morphology in the dog. *J Vet Cardiol* 8, 109–14.

Nguyenba T and Tobias AH (2007) The Amplatz canine duct occluder: A novel device for patent ductus arteriosus occlusion. *J Vet Cardiol* 9, 109–17.

Nguyenba TP and Tobias AH (2008) Minimally invasive per-catheter patent ductus arteriosus occlusion in dogs using a prototype duct occluder. *J Vet Intern Med* 22, 129–34.

Oliveira P (2009) Percutaneous closure of patent ductus arteriosus with Amplatz canine duct occluder in 46 dogs: outcome and prognostic survival factors. ECVIM – 19th Congress Porto, Portugal [Abstract].

Olson JLC, Tobias AH, Stauthammer C, et al (2010) Minimally invasive per catheter patent ductus arteriosus occlusion in small dogs (≤3 kg): preliminary results. ACVIM. Research Forum, Anaheim, CA. *J Vet Intern Med* 24, 694 [abstract].

Oyama M, Sisson D, Thomas W, et al (2005) Congenital heart disease. In *Textbook of Veterinary Internal Medicine*, 6th edn (Ettinger SJ and Feldman E, eds). Elsevier Saunders, St. Louis, pp. 972–87.

Singh MK, Kittleson MD, Kass PH, and Griffiths LG (2012) Occlusive devices and approaches in canine patent ductus arteriosus: comparison of outcomes. *J Vet Intern Med* 26, 85–92.

Stauthammer C, Tobias AH, Leeeder D, et al (2013) Structural and functional cardiovascular changes and their consequences following interventional patent ductus arteriosus occlusion in dogs. *J Am Vet Med Assoc* 242, 1722–6.

Tobias AH and Stauthammer C (2010) Minimally invasive per-catheter occlusion and dilation procedures for congenital cardiovascular abnormalities in dogs. *Vet Clin N Am Small Anim* 40, 581–603.

Video 58.1 Ductal angiogram. The angiogram is performed with the pigtail catheter in the aorta. The narrowed jet of contrast (minimal ductal diameter) is measured for selection of ACDO device size.

Video 58.2 The exchange wire is advanced across the ductus into the main pulmonary artery. The wire is directed into the appropriate location by the angled end-hole catheter.

Video 58.3 The delivery sheath and dilator are advanced over the exchange wire into the main pulmonary artery. The dilator extends beyond the sheath tip and should be slightly retracted into the sheath lumen to minimize contact with the pulmonary valve.

Video 58.4 The distal disc and portion of the waist are exteriorized into the pulmonary artery and moved into apposition with the ductal ostium. Additional retraction results in exteriorization of the proximal disc.

Video 58.5 The proximal disc is exteriorized while maintaining the distal disc in apposition with the pulmonic ostium. The ACDO resumes its casted shape following release of the tension applied to the delivery cable.

Video 58.6 After exteriorization, a small volume of contrast is administered through the sheath lumen to confirm proper device placement. The ductal ampulla is seen filling with contrast.

Video 58.7, 58.8 Prior to deployment, device stability is assessed with a moderate level of pushing and pulling on the delivery cable. The proximal disc shape slightly distorts while pulling on the cable (58.7). The delivery cable bows dorsally with pushing on the cable (58.8).

Video 58.9 Post deployment angiogram. Contrast fills the ductal ampulla but is prevented from shunting into the pulmonary circulation. The contrast swirls within the ampulla and eventually flows into the descending aorta.

These video clips can be found in the online material at **www.wiley.com/go/weisse/vet-image-guided-interventions**

CHAPTER FIFTY-NINE

Pulmonary Valve Stenosis

Brian A. Scansen

Department of Veterinary Clinical Sciences, The Ohio State University, Columbus, OH

Background/Indications

Congenital pulmonary valve stenosis (PS) has been reported as the third most commonly diagnosed congenital heart defect of dogs in North America (Buchanan, 1992). As in humans, valvular PS in dogs encompasses three principal forms: (1) a dome-shaped valve with commissural fusion; (2) a dysplastic and markedly thickened valve with or without hypoplasia of one or more leaflets; and (3) hypoplasia of the pulmonary annulus (Patterson et al, 1981). Variable degrees of all three forms may be present in a given animal, with purely fused valves (e.g., with normal valve anatomy and thickness) being less common in dogs as compared to humans. Without therapy, dogs with valvular PS are at risk for symptoms including exercise intolerance, syncope, sudden cardiac death, congestive heart failure, and cyanosis from a right-to-left shunt (Johnson et al, 2004; Francis et al, 2011).

Balloon pulmonary valvuloplasty (BPV) was first performed in a dog in 1980 and reported in a child in 1982. There is evidence that BPV improves the clinical outcome of human and canine patients with valvular PS, both with a reduction in clinical symptomatology and an improvement in survival. The procedure is now routinely performed in clinical canine practice with low morbidity and mortality for those patients with a severe gradient or the presence of clinical signs referable to their disease.

Although effective for many patients, human and canine studies suggest that patients with valvular dysplasia and a hypoplastic annulus show less reduction in pressure gradient following BPV than those with purely valvular fusion. This is understandable, as the principal benefit of BPV is tearing of commissural fusion; it is unable to alleviate obstruction secondary to annular hypoplasia or thick, redundant valve tissue. In a study of 30 dogs with valvular PS, 94% of the 18 dogs with a normal pulmonary annular diameter and minimal valve thickening had resolution of their clinical signs and survived more than 1 year after the procedure; however, for the 12 dogs with marked leaflet thickening and a hypoplastic pulmonary annulus, only 66.6% had a favorable outcome and only 50% showed a resolution in their clinical signs (Bussadori et al, 2001).

Patient Preparation

Preoperative Imaging

Prior to intervention, an attempt should be made to characterize the valve morphology and to estimate the balloon size required. Transthoracic echocardiography with Doppler is the current standard of care in veterinary cardiology for evaluation of pulmonary valve morphology, annular size, and severity of stenosis (Figure 59.1). The degree of valve fusion (leaflet doming in systole, tethering of the leaflet tips), valve thickening (redundant valve tissue), annular hypoplasia, subvalvular obstruction, tricuspid valve competence, and right ventricular (RV) hypertrophy should be assessed and recorded. The pulmonary annulus is considered hypoplastic when the ratio of the aortic annular diameter to pulmonary annular diameter is greater than 1.2 (Bussadori et al, 2001). Valves with severe dysplasia (redundant tissue, annular hypoplasia, or a subvalvular fibrous ring) are less likely to respond to BPV and clients should be so advised. The author still recommends BPV in such cases as it is difficult to quantify the degree of valvular fusion by echocardiography alone, and such fusion may still have a partial response to BPV. Additionally, the author has attempted stent implantation into the RV outflow tract and across the annulus of such dogs with fair improvement in clinical symptoms and a

Veterinary Image-Guided Interventions, First Edition. Edited by Chick Weisse and Allyson Berent.

Companion website: www.wiley.com/go/weisse/vet-image-guided-interventions

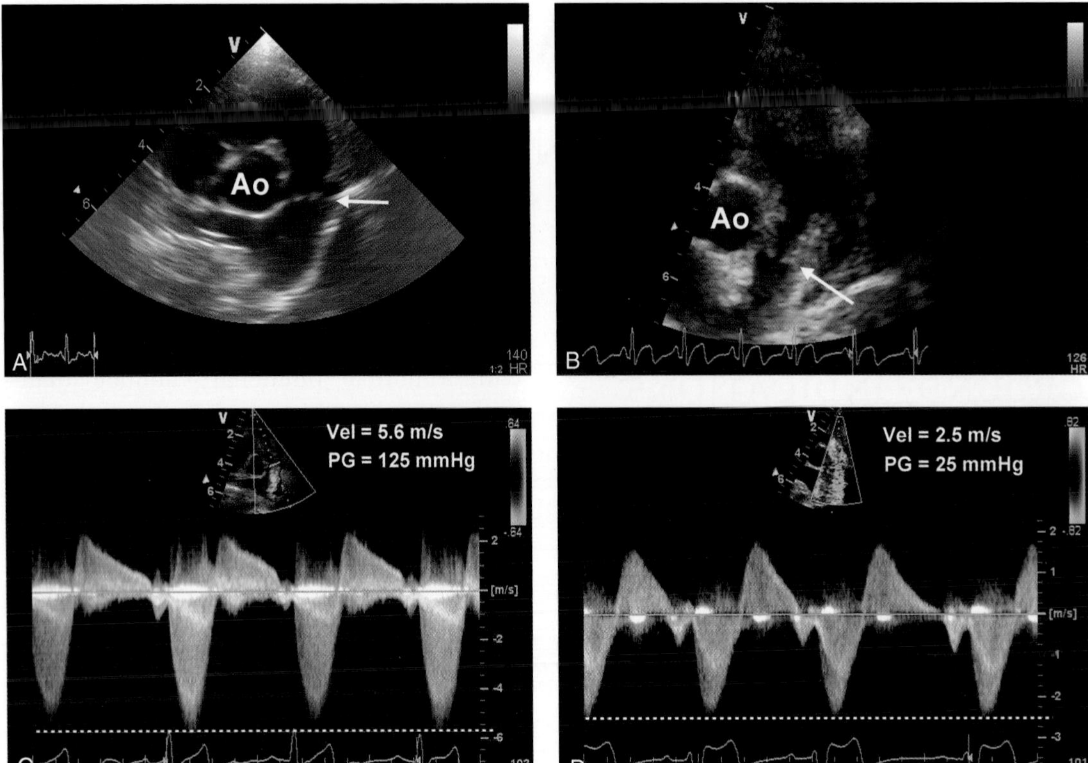

Figure 59.1 Transthoracic echocardiography with Doppler for the evaluation of pulmonary valve morphology, annular diameter, and stenosis severity in dogs with pulmonary valve stenosis. (A) A right parasternal short axis view of a dog with fused and doming valve leaflets, minimal valve thickening, and a pulmonary valve annulus (arrow) of comparable diameter to the aortic root (Ao); such morphology is optimal for balloon intervention. In contrast (B) shows a right parasternal short axis view of a dog with pulmonary valve hypoplasia characterized by a severely narrowed pulmonary valve annulus (arrow) as compared to the aortic root (Ao) and severe infundibular hypertrophy; such morphology is expected to have a less favorable outcome after balloon intervention. (C & D) Doppler interrogation of a dog before (C) and after (D) balloon pulmonary valvuloplasty, indicating a marked drop in the systolic velocity across the valve and consistent with a reduction of ~100 mmHg in the severity of the stenosis.

reduction in pressure gradient. Surgical reconstruction of the RV outflow tract of such dogs can also be considered if access to cardiopulmonary bypass is available.

An estimation of the pressure gradient across the stenotic valve is obtained by continuous wave spectral Doppler, guided by color Doppler imaging to optimize alignment parallel to the direction of the turbulent jet (Figure 59.1C). The modified Bernoulli equation is used to translate the peak systolic velocity as determined by Doppler into an estimated pressure gradient across the valve. Most cardiologists consider the stenosis mild at a gradient of 10 to 49 mmHg, moderate at 50 to 79 mmHg, and severe when the gradient is over 80 mmHg. The decision to pursue BPV should be made with the pressure gradient in mind, with greater benefit from the procedure likely in dogs with severe stenosis. Dogs with mild stenosis seldom develop clinical signs related to their disease and BPV is not recommended, while those with moderate stenosis are typically ballooned only if they display overt symptoms of the disease such as exercise intolerance, syncope, or cyanosis. As with all Doppler estimates, the velocity measured is dependent not only on the orifice of the valve, but also on the flow across the valve at the time of measurement and the systolic function of the RV. As such, changes in the dog's sympathetic tone, intravascular volume status, or intrinsic RV function can alter the velocity measured. While there are advanced echocardiographic ways to correct for some of these variables, the peak velocity and derived pressure gradient remains the sole, albeit imperfect, method of assessing disease severity and monitoring response to therapy by most veterinary cardiologists.

It has been estimated that 8% to 40% of dogs with PS have a patent foramen ovale, which can allow the shunting of poorly oxygenated systemic venous blood from the right to the left atrium in dogs with PS due to high right-sided pressure (Fugii et al, 2012). As such, the author typically performs an echocardiographic

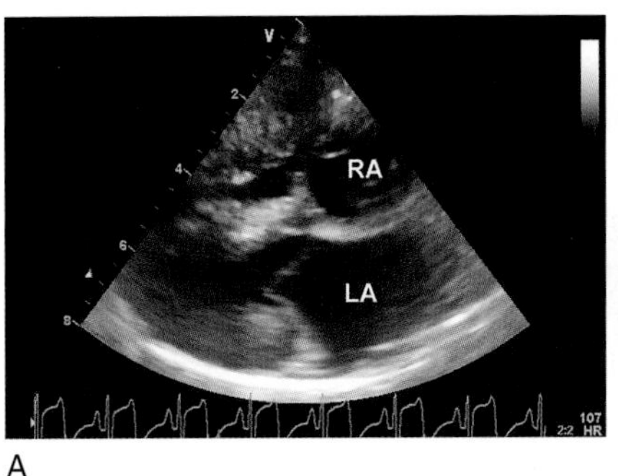

A

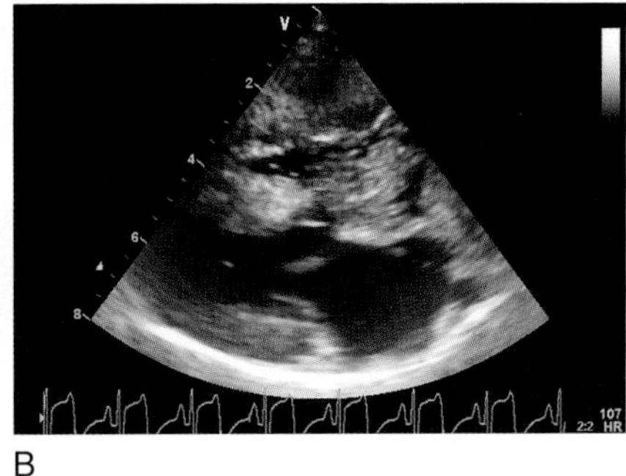

B

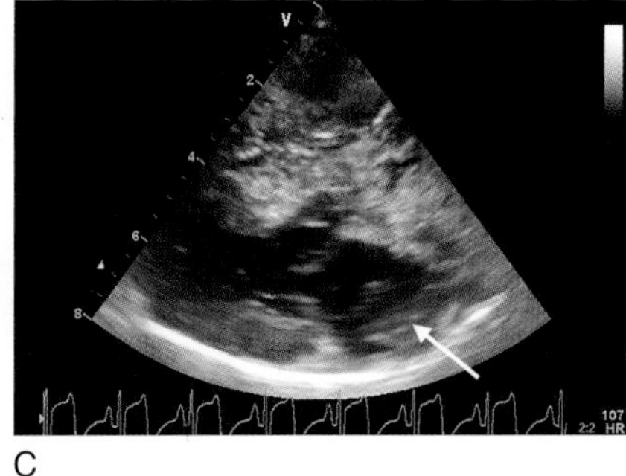

C

Figure 59.2 Contrast echocardiographic study using agitated saline to evaluate patency of the atrial septum in a dog with pulmonary valve stenosis. A right parasternal long-axis image is acquired (A) showing the right atrium (RA) and left atrium (LA), followed by injection of agitated saline into a peripheral vein that results in microcavitations seen first in the right atrium (B) and then in the left atrium (C; arrow).

contrast study in dogs with PS prior to BPV to inform the client of potential cyanotic risk and to be aware of the risk for paradoxical embolization of air or thrombi during the BPV procedure. In brief, two 12 ml Luer-lock syringes are connected to a three-way stopcock and filled with 5–10 ml of saline each. Air is *not* introduced into the syringes, but microcavitations are created by rapid mixing between the two syringes. The open end of the three-way stopcock is connected a peripheral IV placed in the dog (typically the cephalic vein) and the assistant rapidly agitates both syringes back and forth and then injects the agitated saline into the vein while an image of the atrial septum is recorded (Figure 59.2; Video 59.1). The microcavitations can be visualized as hyperechoic contrast on the echocardiogram. A digital loop is recorded of the injection and carefully analyzed to evaluate for the presence of microcavitations passing across the atrial septum and entering the left atrium. If microcavitations are noted in the left atrium only after three or more cardiac cycles following injection, they may represent physiologic intrapulmonary shunting and not true patency of the atrial septum. Last, it has been suggested the injection into a caudal vein (e.g. lateral saphenous vein) may increase the sensitivity of detecting PFO due to the preferential direction of caudal vena caval flow toward the atrial septum, though this has not been shown conclusively in animals.

Medical Therapy

The decision to medicate a dog with beta-blockers prior to BPV is made on a case-by-case basis. The author believes that most dogs with severe stenosis will benefit from starting atenolol for 2 to 4 weeks prior to the BPV procedure. Beta-blockade decreases the force of RV contraction, slows heart rate, and reduces myocardial oxygen consumption. These effects may reduce arrhythmic risk, improve anesthetic stability, reduce the dynamic component of stenosis that develops due to severe infundibular hypertrophy, and provide a slower heart rate during the procedure, which facilitates balloon inflation. A dose of 0.5 mg/kg PO q12 hr is typically started, increasing to 1 to 1.5 mg/kg PO q12 hr over the following 1–2 weeks. Those dogs with severe dynamic obstruction below the valve as a result of muscular hypertrophy may benefit from even higher doses of atenolol. Finally, waiting for a few weeks prior to BPV can be particularly beneficial in very young dogs as it allows for somatic growth that will reduce anesthetic risk and increase the likelihood of successful BPV. While dogs less than 1 kg can undergo BPV, their small vasculature and reduced RV lumen greatly complicate the passage of wires and catheters necessary for a successful procedure. As such, waiting until the animal is over 2 kg is preferred, particularly if they are asymptomatic.

Expected Outcomes

A successful procedure is defined as a reduction of more than 50% of the pre-BPV pressure gradient or a final gradient of less than 30 to 40 mmHg. Restenosis of the valve over time is uncommon, but is seen in some cases. In such cases, repeat BPV can be performed and may be associated with a further reduction in measured gradient. Pulmonary insufficiency is almost universally made worse by BPV, though is seldom of clinical significance. Progressive right heart dilation has been observed by the author in dogs with marked pulmonary insufficiency post-BPV, but cavitary effusions appear unlikely unless moderate to severe tricuspid regurgitation is also present. Long-term, dogs with residual mild to moderate stenosis have a favorable prognosis.

Those dogs with severe residual stenosis appear to have a greater risk for cardiac complications (right heart failure, syncope, exercise intolerance, cyanosis, sudden death), though individualized prognostication remains a challenge as a wide spectrum of outcome is encountered from dogs with comparable gradients.

Equipment

Balloon Selection

Correct balloon sizing is critical for successful BPV. The most important dimension for the balloon catheter is the diameter of the balloon, which is determined from measurements of the pulmonary valve annulus. A balloon-to-annulus ratio (BAR) of 1.2 to 1.4 is typically selected, with values below 1.2 not providing sufficient force to open the fused valve and ratios exceeding 1.5 being more likely to damage the valve and/or pulmonary artery. The pulmonary annulus diameter can be measured from echocardiography or angiography and at various phases of the cardiac cycle (Figure 59.3). In general, the author prefers to measure the pulmonary annulus diameter at the onset of systole from a right-parasternal short axis echocardiographic image optimized to be directly sagittal to the valve. However, if translational motion prevents an accurate measurement at the onset of systole, the end-diastolic or end systolic frames may also be used. The measurement is repeated during angiography (see below) to confirm the echocardiographic measurement; the author advances a calibrated marker catheter into the dog's esophagus so that an accurate calibration can be made at the same radiographic magnification as the heart.

If the measured pulmonary annulus diameter exceeds 20 mm, a double balloon technique should be considered (Estrada et al, 2005). The technique for double balloon will be described later, but the method for sizing a double balloon procedure is given here. Briefly, the effective diameter of two balloons during inflation is not merely the addition of each balloon's respective diameter. Rather, a correction factor must be considered where the effective diameter is calculated to be $[0.82 \times (D1 + D2)]$ where D1 and D2 are the diameters of the two selected balloon catheters. As an example, if the measured pulmonary annulus diameter is 21 mm, an effective balloon diameter of ~27 mm is desired (1.3 × the pulmonary valve annulus diameter). A 27 mm balloon takes considerable time to inflate and has a comparably low burst pressure; as such, a double

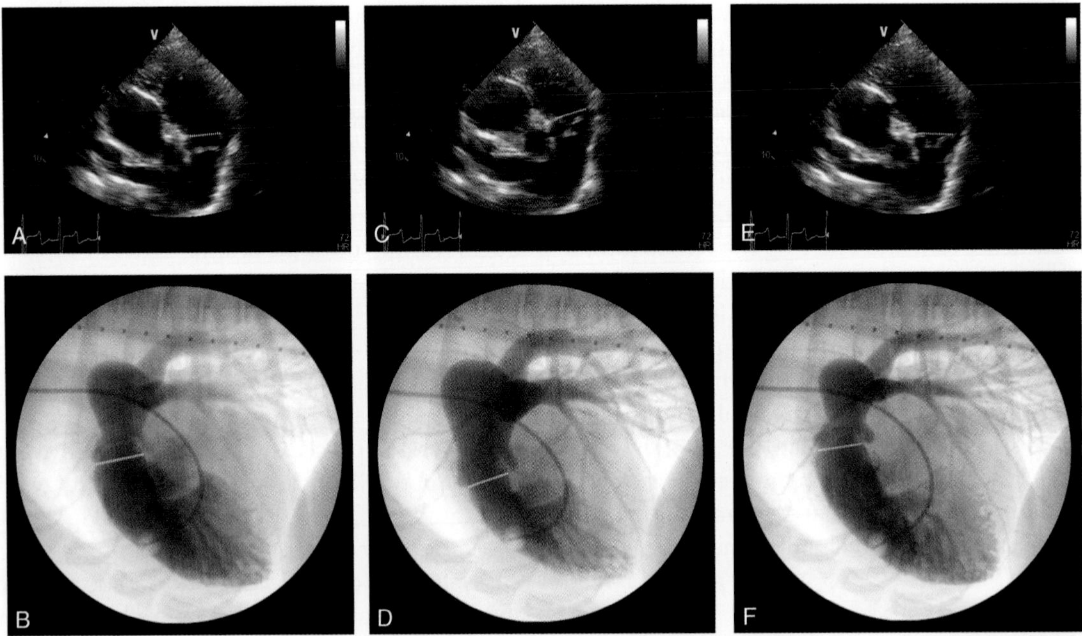

Figure 59.3 Measurements of the pulmonary valve annulus by echocardiography and angiography from the same dog with pulmonary valve stenosis. Both echocardiography (A, C, E) and angiography (B, D, F) can be used to determine the pulmonary annulus diameter for balloon sizing. The pulmonary valve diameter may be measured at the hinge point of the valve at the onset of systole (A & B), at the end of systole (C & D), or at the end of diastole (E & F) by both imaging techniques. The measurements are typically comparable by the two methods; the final determination should be the measurement where the operator can most clearly visualize the valve structures to obtain a reliable value. In the author's opinion, the onset of systole when the valve first opens is preferred (A & B). In the angiographic images, a marker catheter is present in the esophagus to calibrate the radiographic magnification of the image for measurement.

balloon technique is advised. The balloons selected for this example case might include a 15 mm balloon and an 18 mm balloon as the effective diameter would be ~27 mm [0.82 × (15 + 18)].

Calculation of the preferred balloon length is less important than the diameter, but remains a necessary consideration. The author measures 2, 3, and 4 cm distances on the echocardiographic images of the patient's RV outflow tract to assess the relative size of the balloon to the animal's cardiac anatomy. In general, a longer balloon provides for a smoother dilation as the valve annulus can be positioned in the middle of the balloon with greater ease; when the balloon is excessively short in length, the ejection of the RV pushes the balloon into the pulmonary artery and makes "landing" the center of the balloon at the valve annulus more challenging. However, an excessively long balloon may damage the tricuspid valve chordae or the distal pulmonary artery during inflation. In general, 2 to 3 cm length balloons are used for small dogs (less than 6 kg) and 3 to 4 cm length balloons are used for medium and larger size dogs.

There are many balloon dilation catheters available on the market, with varying profiles, materials, sizes, and maximal pressure. While a full categorization of all commercially available balloons is beyond the scope of this chapter, a few comments are pertinent. The cost of balloons typically precludes the veterinarian from maintaining a full inventory of all options. As such, most veterinarians that perform BPV carry a range of commonly used sizes of one or two different lines of balloon dilation catheters. If this is not feasible, the animal's pulmonary annulus diameter can be measured echocardiographically and two to three balloons around the estimated size can be purchased to have on hand; preoperative beta-blockade for 2–4 weeks before the procedure can provide sufficient time for the ordering and arrival of necessary equipment. Some veterinarians resterilize and reuse balloon dilation catheters; however, the author does not recommend this practice as it may alter the nominal and burst pressure of the balloon, it is challenging to reconstrain the balloon catheter to the same low profile as when it is new, and there is a theoretical risk of pyrogen reaction to proteins that remain on the resterilized balloon. Today's balloon dilation catheters are made for one-time use only and their cost is typically affordable for most clients. As such, new equipment is preferred for each animal, though a selection of resterilized balloons may be kept on hand for charitable cases.

The ideal balloon for BPV is made of a non-compliant material so that it will only expand to its stated size, is of a low profile meaning that it folds tightly over the shaft to form a small diameter for introduction into the vasculature, and exists on a flexible shaft that will accommodate an appropriately sized guide wire and offer good tracking and pushability when advanced into the heart (Mullins, 2006a). As some of the above characteristics are contradictory to one another, the balloon dilation catheter chosen is always a trade-off of characteristics and all should be considered with a given patient's size and valve anatomy in mind. Importantly, the selection of a balloon dilation catheter should consider the size of the introducer needed to access the animal's vasculature as very small dogs will have a limit on the maximal introducer that can be placed; the size and angulation of the RV lumen as small, thick hearts will not be able to tolerate stiff guide wires or inflexible catheter shafts; and the valve anatomy which will impact the diameter and length as well as the desired nominal and burst pressures of the balloon. A higher maximal pressure increases the radial force that the balloon can apply to a stenotic valve, however, higher pressure balloons are typically stiffer and have a larger profile necessitating a larger introducer. Within the same line of balloon dilation catheters, the larger the diameter a balloon is, the lower its maximal burst pressure. As such, very large balloons typically have a very low maximal pressure, further supporting the recommendation to utilize a double balloon technique in dogs with pulmonary valve diameters exceeding 20 mm.

The most commonly used balloon dilation catheters in veterinary medicine are made by a human pediatric device company[1] and include the TYSHAK™ and Z-MED™ lines of balloon dilation catheters. Importantly, a vendor[2] specific to the veterinary market is now the sole supplier for these two lines of balloon dilation catheters to veterinarians. While this veterinary vendor has only a limited selection of the full line of balloons available in stock, it is possible to order any desired balloon type and/or size; however, at the time of this writing delivery times may exceed 6 weeks for non-stock balloon catheters. The TYSHAK™ line of balloon dilation catheters are made of a thin, minimally compliant thermoplastic elastomer and have a relatively low maximal burst pressure. They are, however, low profile and most sizes can accommodate a 0.035" guide wire making them a commonly selected catheter for BPV in dogs. The Z-MED™ line of balloon dilation catheters are made from a thicker thermoplastic elastomer which provides a greater maximal burst pressure, though requiring a larger introducer size. Both the TYSHAK™ and Z-MED™ lines come in three generations of balloons – named I, II, and X. In general, the second-generation balloons (TYSHAK II™ and Z-MED II™) provide higher burst pressures than the first-generation and occasionally require a larger introducer. They also have a coaxial shaft to improve pushability. The X generation of these balloons (TYSHAK X™ or Z-MED X™) are mounted on a braided catheter shaft which accommodates a larger guide wire without requiring a larger introducer, improving the tracking and pushability of the catheter. The author uses the Z-MED™ line of balloon dilation catheters for BPV in dogs with dysplastic valves (thick, redundant tissue or a subvalvular fibrous ridge) and the TYSHAK™ line of balloons for those with pure valve fusion or small dogs whose vasculature is too small for the required Z-MED™ introducer size. There are additional balloon dilation catheters available, some of very high burst pressure, which can be used for BPV though experience in veterinary medicine with these catheters is fairly limited.

Procedure

Anesthesia of the PS Patient

A skilled anesthesia staff is critical for success during catheterization of the animal with PS. Anesthetic concerns for the dog with PS include arrhythmias, particularly during passage of catheters and wires within the heart. Lidocaine should be available and the author commonly instructs the anesthetist to bolus 2 mg/kg of IV lidocaine when the right heart is first catheterized and maintains the dog with a continuous infusion at 50 μg/kg/min during the BPV. Additional boluses of lidocaine may be necessary if rapid ventricular tachycardia is observed during the catheterization. It is common for dogs with PS to develop systemic hypotension during anesthesia; typically, this is preload responsive and a colloid or crystalloid bolus is often effective at normalizing blood pressure. Although the PS patient has heart disease, fluid administration during anesthesia should not be restricted in these dogs unless congestive heart failure (e.g., pleural effusion, ascites) is present prior to catheterization. Heart rate is an important consideration during BPV and these dogs are nearly always on chronic beta-blockade with atenolol. Atenolol is typically given the morning of the procedure, with some cardiologists preferring to give ½ the maintenance dose on the day of BPV. A slower heart rate during BPV will improve visualization of cardiovascular structures during angiography and make it easier to position the balloon during inflation. Last, the anesthetist should be aware of the potential for luminal collapse of the RV after BPV due to an acute drop in RV afterload, a condition that has been termed the "suicidal RV". In this condition, systemic hypotension develops rapidly after valvuloplasty due to hyper-contraction of the RV infundibulum that obstructs blood flow out of the right heart. Therapy includes fluid administration as well as esmolol, a fast-acting beta-blocker given as a 250 to 500 μg/kg IV bolus and continuous infusion at 75 to 150 μg/kg/min. Although suicidal RV should always be planned for prior to BPV, particularly in those dogs with severe RV hypertrophy and a small RV lumen, it remains a rare complication of BPV. Because of the risk of systemic hypotension both before and after BPV in dogs with PS, the author recommends continuous invasive arterial monitoring throughout the procedure. Non-invasive blood pressure monitoring can be used when arterial access cannot be obtained, but may fail to detect abrupt changes in systemic blood pressure as hemodynamic changes in these dogs can be sudden.

Pressure Recording and Angiography

BPV is performed from a transvenous approach, either via the external jugular vein or the femoral vein. In general, the jugular vein is preferred for small dogs as it affords a larger size vessel and therefore a larger introducer sheath than the femoral vein. The femoral vein is typically used when an arterial study is desired concurrently given the close relationship of the femoral artery and vein. In the author's experience, a femoral venous approach can also increase ease of catheter advancement across the pulmonary valve in dogs with a very small RV lumen, as the angle of approach is less severe than from the jugular approach. Percutaneous access with an appropriately sized introducer is achieved with the animal in lateral (for jugular vein access) or ventrodorsal (femoral vein) recumbency (see Chapter 44). Typically a vascular sheath is selected that is at least one French size larger than what is required by the anticipated balloon dilation catheter. A balloon wedge pressure catheter[3] (BWP) is prepped, flushed, and advanced under fluoroscopic guidance into the right atrium. The balloon is carefully inflated and the catheter is then advanced across the tricuspid valve and into the RV. *Note*: It is always preferable to cross cardiac valves antegrade with a flow-directed (balloon-tipped) catheter or one with a J-tip or pigtail. Theoretically, advancing an end-hold catheter across the valve can perforate a valve leaflet, ensnare chordae tendineae, or otherwise damage the valve apparatus. A balloon-tipped or pigtail catheter, however, will preferentially enter the true valve orifice and minimize trauma to the valve. The BWP catheter is then advanced

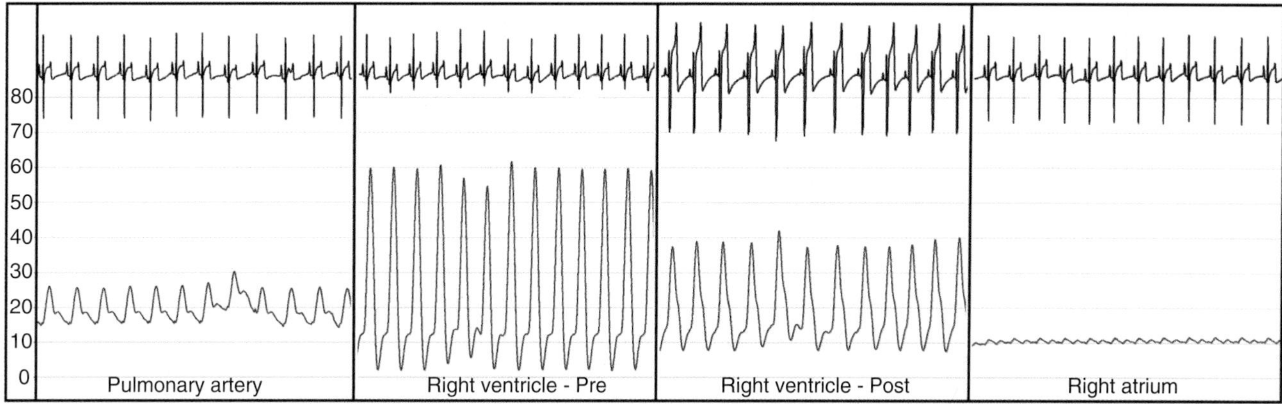

Figure 59.4 These pressure recordings were taken from a dog with pulmonary valve stenosis before and after balloon pulmonary valvuloplasty (BPV). The pulmonary arterial pressure is normal as seen on the far left and there is a step-up in pressure from the pulmonary artery to the right ventricle consistent with stenosis as shown in the second panel from the left. Following BPV, the peak right ventricular systolic pressure has fallen though there remains a mild gradient from pulmonary artery to right ventricle as seen in the third panel from the left. Note also the appearance of a right bundle branch block pattern in the lead II ECG following BPV; this is a common finding and is usually transient as the right bundle branch is easily damaged during passage and inflation of the balloon catheter. The final panel on the right shows the right atrial pressure, which is mildly elevated at 10 mmHg.

out the main pulmonary artery and pressures are recorded (Figure 59.4). The catheter is pulled back across the pulmonary valve and the step-up in pressure is documented as well as the pre-balloon RV pressure. It is preferable to measure all pressures prior to angiography as the contrast agent may affect cardiovascular function.

A catheter appropriate for right ventriculography (see Chapter 51 on Radiographic Cardiac Anatomy) is then prepped, flushed, and advanced into the RV for the angiographic study. In small dogs (less than 6 kg), a hand injection is usually sufficient to opacify the RV and delineate pulmonary valve anatomy. For medium-size and larger dogs, a power injector is preferred (see Chapter 51). The right ventriculogram is digitally recorded and saved for measurement of the pulmonary valve annulus and determination of cardiovascular anatomy. Particular attention is given to noting the level of obstruction (subvalvular, valvular, supravalvular), the presence of tricuspid regurgitation, the severity of dynamic muscular obstruction in the RV outflow tract, the morphology of the main pulmonary artery and branches, and the levophase for assessment of left heart structures and coronary arterial anatomy (Figure 59.5; Video 59.2). The coronary arterial anatomy is of particular importance in brachycephalic dogs; anomalous coronary arterial anatomy has been described in Bulldogs, Boxer dogs, and related breeds that can course cranial to the pulmonary annulus and lead to fatal coronary arterial damage during balloon inflation (Figure 59.5; Video 59.3). BPV may still be considered in dogs with anomalous coronary arterial circulations, but special measures should be taken as will be discussed below. Once the angiogram has been recorded, the pulmonary valve annulus is again measured using a calibrated image to correct for radiographic magnification (Figure 59.3). The author advances a marker catheter into the esophagus of the dog prior to BPV to provide a calibrated standard within the image during angiography. The angiographic measurement is compared to the echocardiographic measurement of pulmonary annulus diameter and a balloon is chosen with a diameter ~1.3 times the annulus diameter.

Balloon Dilation

Once a balloon dilation catheter has been selected, the BWP catheter is again floated across the pulmonary valve and out a distal branch pulmonary artery (Figure 59.6B). The left pulmonary artery (the dorsal branch pulmonary artery when viewed from a lateral image) is preferred as it provides a smoother and more secure path for advancement of the balloon dilation catheter as compared to the right pulmonary artery. Next, a J-tipped exchange length guide wire (typically greater than 180 cm length) is selected and advanced into the BWP catheter and placed within the distal branch pulmonary artery (Figure 59.6C). The J-tip is preferred as it will be less traumatic to the distal pulmonary artery. The diameter and stiffness of the guide wire chosen will depend on the size of the dog

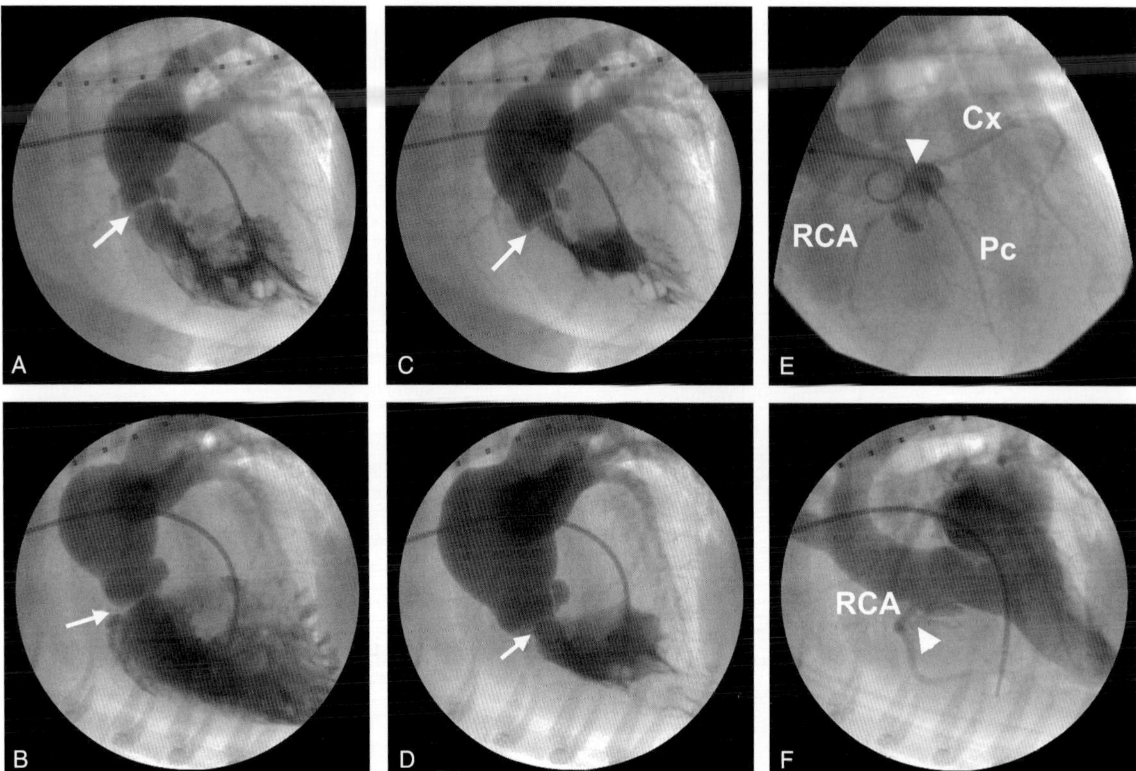

Figure 59.5 Angiography during balloon pulmonary valvuloplasty. Panels A through D are right ventriculograms from a Boxer (A & C) and an English Bulldog (B & D) with pulmonary valve stenosis. Panels A & B are taken at end-diastole and show right ventricular hypertrophy, post-stenotic dilation of the main and branch pulmonary arteries, and either thickened fused pulmonary valve leaflets (A) or a subvalvular ridge of tissue with a cranial filling defect (B). The systolic frames from each dog show similar findings though the dynamic subvalvular obstruction secondary to right ventricular hypertrophy is severe in (C) and the subvalvular ridge in (D) is more clearly visualized. (E) A still image taken from an aortic root injection from a Chesapeake Bay Retriever to show normal coronary arterial anatomy. In (E) the right coronary artery (RCA) can be seen arising from the cranioventral sinus of Valsalva, while the ostium of the left coronary artery (arrowhead) is seen arising at the caudodorsal sinus and divides into the paraconal coronary artery (Pc) that descends along the interventricular groove and the circumflex artery (Cx) that traverses around the atrioventricular groove. In comparison (F) is a levophase image from the same Bulldog in (B) and (D) showing a single right coronary artery (RCA) with the left coronary arterial circulation (arrowhead) arising from the right coronary artery. Note that the position of the single right coronary artery in F corresponds to the cranial indentation and subvalvular narrowing seen in the right ventricular outflow tract in panels (B) and (D).

and the stiffness of the balloon dilation catheter to be used. In general, 0.035″ guide wires in a standard stiffness[4] or super-stiff[5] are preferred for BPV. In small dogs or those with severe RV hypertrophy, the super-stiff guide wires place too much pressure on the tricuspid valve and the RV endocardium, particularly when they are advanced from a jugular venous approach. For larger dogs, the standard stiffness guide wires are typically too flexible and do not maintain the balloon in proper position during inflation; as such, super-stiff guide wires are preferred for large dogs or inflexible balloon dilation catheters. For very small dogs, the chosen balloon dilation catheter may not accept a 0.035″ guide wire. In such instances, a 0.018″ or 0.025″ guide wire[6] can be used, but such wires provide even less stability during advancement and inflation of the balloon dilation catheter and stiffer varieties should be selected. Once the guide wire is positioned in the distal pulmonary artery, the BWP catheter is removed under fluoroscopic guidance to maintain guide wire position. In some dogs, particularly small dogs with severe RV hypertrophy, it is not possible to advance a BWP catheter out the RV outflow tract or across the valve. In such cases, standard end-hole catheters with a reverse curve can be employed to direct the guide wire toward the outflow tract, although these are less desirable as they cross the tricuspid valve with a stiffer tip and increase the risk

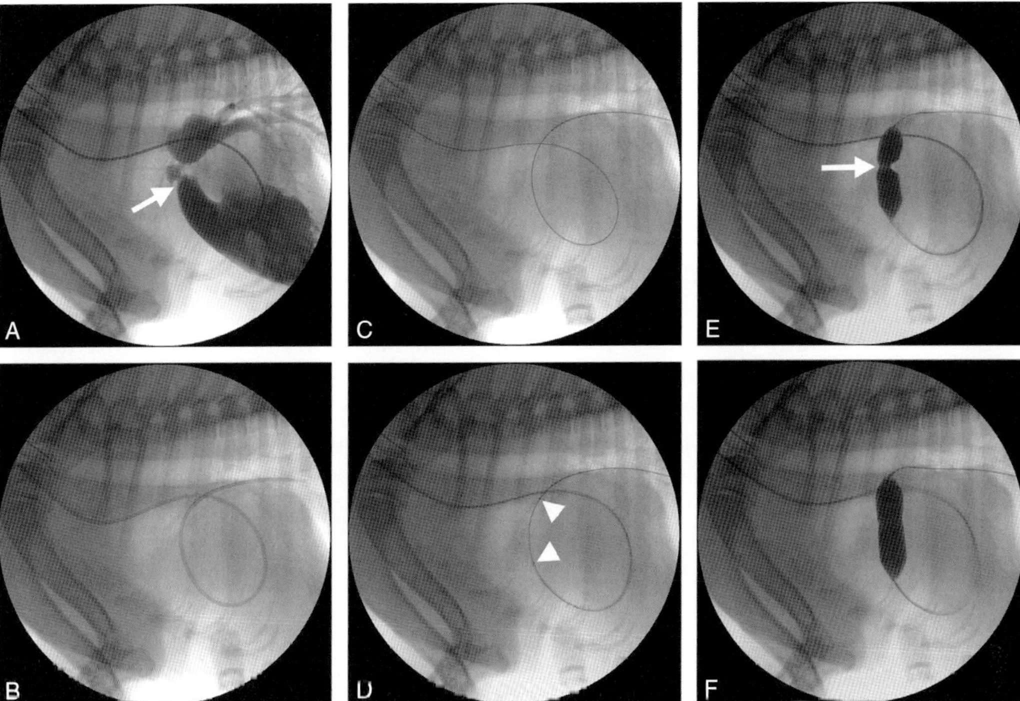

Figure 59.6 Balloon pulmonary valvuloplasty. A right ventricular angiogram is obtained to evaluate valve morphology and locate the site of stenosis (A); in this dog, valvular and supravalvular stenosis is apparent. A balloon wedge pressure catheter is then floated out the pulmonary artery and into a branch pulmonary artery (B); in this case the catheter was positioned in the right pulmonary artery as it provided sufficient stability, though the left is preferred. An appropriate guide wire is then advanced through the wedge pressure catheter and placed in the distal pulmonary artery (C); in contrast to this image, the distal end of the wire should always be visualized to avoid excessive advancement. The selected balloon dilation catheter is then advanced over the guide wire and the balloon markers (arrowheads) are used to position the balloon across the pulmonary valve annulus (D). With rapid inflation of the balloon, a central waist (arrow) is observed as the balloon engages the stenosis (E). With greater pressure, the waist resolves and the balloon takes its proper inflated shape as the valve fusion is torn (F).

of ensnaring tricuspid valve chordae tendineae. The author has had success with the Judkins left catheter shape, CHGB catheters, Cobra catheters, and even pigtail catheters (as the curl will slowly release and direct the guidewire toward the outflow tract if it is advanced with the pigtail positioned in the RV apex). In very tight valves with severe infundibular narrowing, an end-hole catheter with a straight or angled-tip (not a J-tip) hydrophilic guide wire may be the only means to successfully cross the valve. In these cases, extreme care should be taken to advance the guide wire with minimal force and allow it to find the true valve orifice; damage to the tricuspid valve, RV endocardium, or pulmonary valve is more likely with such a technique.

Once the guide wire is positioned out the branch pulmonary artery, the balloon dilation catheter is prepared. The protective plastic sheath around the balloon is first removed. A three-way stopcock is attached to the balloon catheter port and a pressure inflation device is connected to one port with a 12 ml Luer-lock syringe attached to the other port. Within the inflation device, a mixture of iodinated contrast and saline (from 1:1 to 1:3, contrast to saline) is drawn up and 3–4 ml of a similar mixture is drawn into the syringe. For larger balloons, a lesser proportion of contrast to saline should be used as the rate of balloon deflation is partially dependent on the viscosity of the fluid used for inflation; contrast is necessary to visualize inflation, but results in a slower deflation rate. The process of purging the balloon is then performed; briefly, negative pressure is applied to the balloon using the syringe and the three-way stopcock, which is released by turning the stopcock open to the inflation device and closed to the syringe. The air that was drawn into the syringe is then removed. This is repeated several times, with the balloon positioned vertically and tip-down, so that all air within the balloon is removed and a small amount of the contrast/saline mixture is within the shaft and lining of the balloon. The purpose of this procedure is to remove all air from the balloon, catheter, and inflation device so that rupture of the balloon will not result in an air embolus within the patient. The other catheter port through which the guide wire will be advanced is then similarly flushed with saline and the balloon dilation catheter mounted on the guide wire that has been placed in the patient's branch pulmonary artery. The balloon dilation catheter is then slowly advanced over the guide wire and positioned across the pulmonary valve annulus; an assistant makes this aspect of the procedure much easier as one can monitor and adjust the guide wire position while the balloon dilation catheter is advanced. Having a reference image projected of the RV angiogram can aid in proper positioning of the balloon; platinum marker bands on the balloon dilation catheter allow the operator to adequately center the annulus, or site of stenosis, to the balloon (Figure 59.6D). Rapid inflation of the balloon is then performed under live fluoroscopy to visualize the development of a waist at the site of stenosis (Figure 59.6E; Video 59.4) or to provide traction/ advancement of the catheter if the position changes. The pressure generated by the inflation device should be monitored and increased to the nominal pressure of the balloon. Exceeding this nominal pressure (the pressure at which the balloon reaches its advertised diameter) can be done if the stenotic waist persists, but the burst pressure of the balloon should not be exceeded. Once the desired pressure is reached, or if the balloon migrates from the site of stenosis, rapid deflation of the balloon is performed. The time of inflation should not exceed 5–6 seconds. The author prefers to have an assistant continuously call out the dog's systemic blood pressure during balloon inflation to monitor the duration and hemodynamic changes during BPV. A precipitous drop in systemic pressure is expected, with recovery rapid within the following 5–10 seconds. Deflation can be assisted with the Luer-lock syringe and three-way stopcock on the port of the balloon catheter. The desired outcome with BPV is resolution of the stenotic waist (Figure 59.6F) and the lack of waist on subsequent reinflations. Typically, two to four inflations are performed to confirm the waist was engaged and has resolved. If a waist persists, the measurements of the pulmonary annulus are verified and a larger balloon considered only if it will not exceed a BAR of 1.5. Following successful dilation, the wire is left in the distal pulmonary and the balloon dilation catheter removed over the wire. The BWP catheter is reintroduced over the wire and a final pullback pressure tracing is recorded from pulmonary artery to RV to evaluate the degree of change in RV pressure. While a substantial drop in RV pressure is ideal, the effect of anesthesia and dynamic muscular obstruction can complicate interpretation of the invasive pressure data. As such, the final decision to stop or attempt a larger balloon is made on the basis of how successful the initial inflation and waist resolution was felt to be, on how stable the dog is under anesthesia, and on the initial morphology of the valve. The vascular sheath is removed and hemostasis achieved with a purse-string suture around the access site as well as 5 minutes of pressure. A neck bandage is placed if the jugular vein was accessed to keep the site clean as the animal is recovered. Analgesia is given postoperatively and ECG-monitoring overnight performed if ventricular arrhythmias were frequent during the procedure. Echocardiography is performed the following morning in the awake animal to compare the gradient to pre-BPV values (Figure 59.1D) and to assess for the presence of any complications from the procedure (e.g., worsening tricuspid valve regurgitation, endothelial tears of the pulmonary artery, etc.).

Follow-Up

Dogs are typically discharged the day following BPV. Beta-blockade is continued at the same dose and a recheck is scheduled in one month to evaluate the Doppler gradient across the valve. Further reduction from the immediate 24-hour post-BPV gradient is occasionally seen, related both to a resolution of valve swelling and edema that was present at the 24-hour post-BPV echocardiogram as well as to regression of RV hypertrophy and dynamic obstruction.

Special Considerations/ Alternative Uses/ Complication Examples

Anomalous Coronary Arterial Circulations

As seen in Figure 59.5, dogs of brachycephalic stature are reported to be at risk for anomalous coronary arterial circulations characterized by either a single right coronary ostium or single left coronary ostium. In such cases, the coronary artery that lacks a patent ostium arises from the other coronary artery and passes adjacent and cranial to the pulmonary valve annulus (Figure 59.7). In these dogs, concurrent PS is frequently seen and BPV with a standard size balloon (BAR of 1.2 to 1.5) may result in coronary artery avulsion, damage, and/or death. BPV using a more conservative BAR of 0.9 to 1.0 in such dogs has been reported with some reduction in stenosis severity observed. The long-term benefit of this conservative ballooning in these dogs remains uncertain, but may be considered artery.

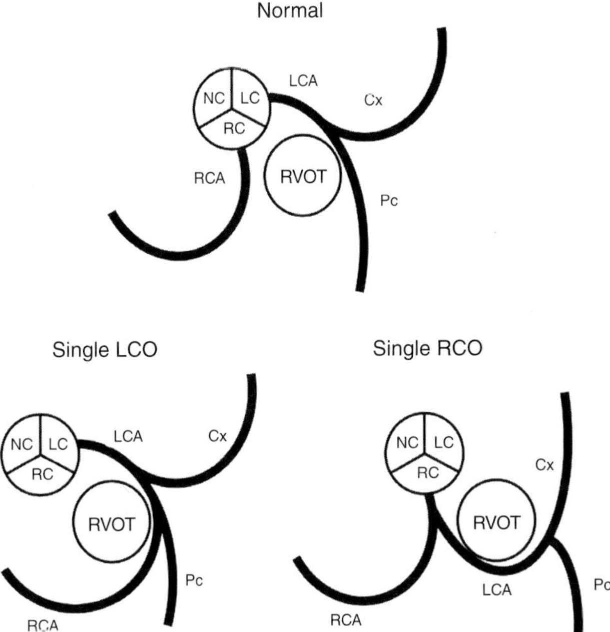

Figure 59.7 Schematic of the normal canine coronary artery anatomy (top) as compared to the anatomy of a single left coronary ostium (LCO) with an anomalous prepulmonic right coronary artery (bottom left) and a single right coronary ostium (RCO) with an anomalous prepulmonic left coronary artery (bottom right). Orientation is the animal's head to the bottom of the page and the left side of the animal to the right of the page. RCA = right coronary artery; LCA = left coronary artery; Cx = circumflex branch coronary artery; Pc = paraconal interventricular branch coronary artery; RVOT = right ventricular outflow tract; NC = non-coronary aortic cusp; RC = right coronary aortic cusp; LC = left coronary aortic cusp. (Reprinted from Journal of Veterinary Cardiology, 15, Visser LC, Scansen BA, Schober KE, Single left coronary ostium and an anomalous prepulmonic right coronary artery in 2 dogs with congenital pulmonary valve stenosis, pp. 161–169, 2013, with permission of Elsevier.)

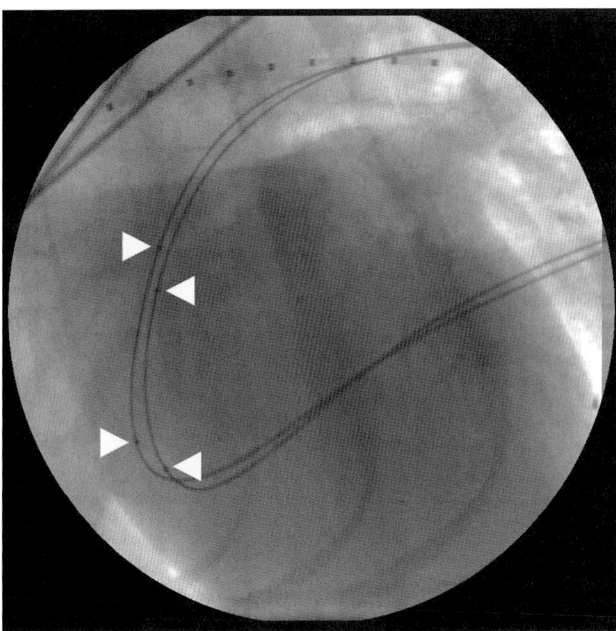

Figure 59.8 Positioning of guide wires and balloons for a double balloon pulmonary valvuloplasty. Both femoral veins have been accessed and two guide wires have been advanced across the pulmonary valve and placed in a branch pulmonary artery. Two balloon dilation catheters were then advanced and positioned across the stenotic pulmonary valve, the location of each balloon can be seen by the platinum marker bands (arrowheads). Simultaneous inflation of the two balloons takes less time and provides a greater radial force than inflation of a single balloon of comparable diameter.

Double Balloon Technique

In dogs with a pulmonary valve annulus exceeding 20 mm in diameter, a double balloon technique is preferred. Determination of the appropriate size for each balloon was discussed previously. Vascular access for this procedure is obtained from both femoral veins simultaneously. It is comparable to the technique described above for a single balloon, though two guide wires are advanced into the same branch pulmonary artery and two balloons are delivered to the same position and inflated simultaneously (Figure 59.8). At least two and preferably three operators are preferred when performing the double balloon technique as adjustment of catheter position and simultaneous inflation of both catheters is not possible with only one operator.

Double Chamber Right Ventricle

While the majority of dogs with PS have obstruction at the level of the valve annulus (or immediately sub- or supra-valvular), cases of stenosis in the mid-RV are also occasionally encountered. The nomenclature for such lesions is variable; the presence of anomalous muscle bundles in the mid-RV causing obstruction has been termed double chamber right ventricle (DCRV), while more localized fibrosis in the proximal RV outflow tract has been termed pulmonic infundibular stenosis. DCRV dogs present similarly to dogs with PS, though echocardiography shows the obstruction is in the mid-RV with a hypertrophied proximal chamber and a distal chamber of normal wall thickness (Figure 59.9). The pulmonary valve is typically normal. A high proportion of dogs with DCRV have concurrent ventricular septal defects. The author has ballooned dogs with DCRV and a reduction in gradient and improvement in clinical signs can be achieved (Figure 59.9). Typically, a very high pressure (Kevlar) balloon[7] or pre-dilation with a cutting balloon[8] is

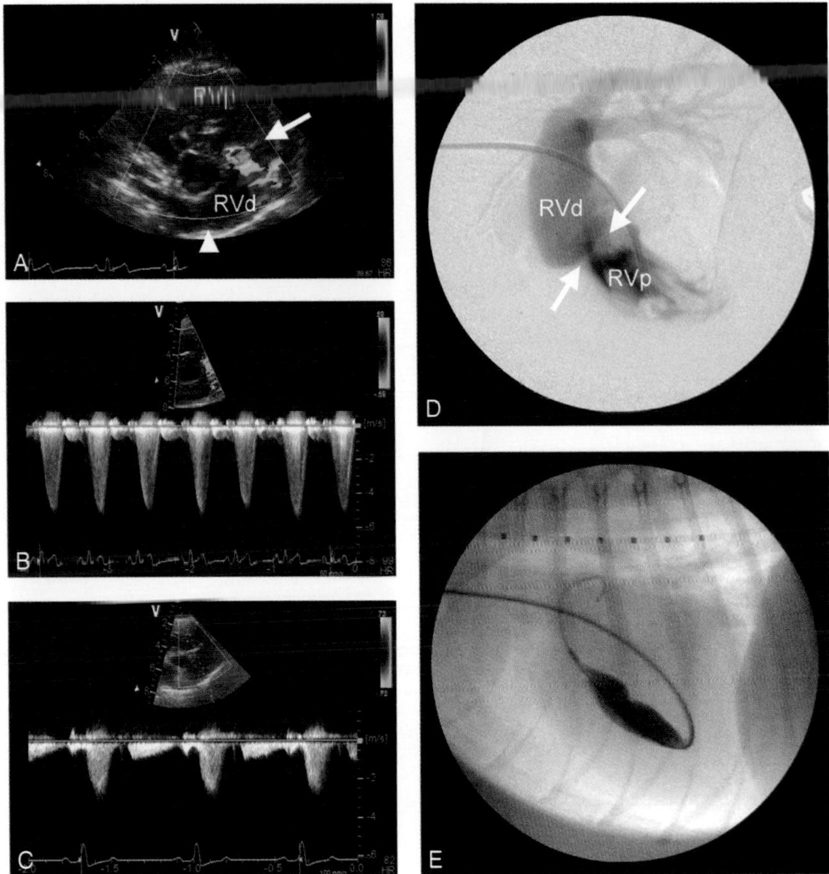

Figure 59.9 Balloon dilation of double chamber right ventricle in a dog. The echocardiographic image in A shows a proximal right ventricular chamber with severe muscular hypertrophy (RVp), a mid-ventricular fibromuscular band resulting in severe obstruction (arrow), and a distal RV chamber of normal wall thickness (RVd). The pulmonary valve is normal (arrowhead). Doppler gradients before (B) and after (C) balloon dilation of the obstructing membrane demonstrate a marked reduction in stenosis severity. Angiography under digital subtraction (D) confirms the mid-RV stenosis (arrows) and proximal RV hypertrophy. Balloon dilation with a high pressure balloon (E) highlights the stenotic waist in the mid-RV.

chosen as the obstruction in these dogs is often fibrous or fibromuscular. Reports of successful balloon dilation of infundibular stenosis in cats are also available in the literature (Schrope, 2008).

Notes

1. NuMED, Inc., Hopkington, New York, NY.
2. Infiniti Medical, LLC, Menlo Park, CA.
3. Balloon wedge pressure catheter; Teleflex Medical, Research Triangle Park, NC.
4. GuideRight Guidewire, St. Jude Medical Inc., St. Paul, MN.
5. Amplatz Extra-Stiff Wire Guide, Cook Medical Inc., Bloomington, IN.
6. V-18 ControlWire, Boston Scientific, Natick, MA.
7. Atlas PTA dilatation catheter, Bard Peripheral Vascular Inc., Tempe, AZ.
8. Flextome cutting balloon device, Boston Scientific, Natick, MA.

References

Buchanan JW (1992) Causes and prevalence of cardiovascular diseases. In: *Current Veterinary Therapy XI: Small Animal Practice* (Kirk RW and Bonagura JD, eds). WB Saunders Co., Philadelphia, pp. 647–54.

Bussadori C, deMadron E, Santilli RA, et al (2001) Balloon valvuloplasty in 30 dogs with pulmonic stenosis: effect of valve morphology and annular size on initial and 1-year outcome. *J Vet Intern Med* 15, 553–8.

Estrada A, Moise NS, and Renaud-Farrell S (2005) When, how and why to perform a double ballooning technique for dogs with valvular pulmonic stenosis. *J Vet Cardiol* 7, 41–51.

Francis AJ, Johnson MS, Culshaw GC, et al (2011) Outcome in 55 dogs with pulmonic stenosis that did not undergo balloon valvuloplasty or surgery. *J Small Anim Pract* 52, 282–8.

Fujii Y, Nishimoto Y, Sunahara H, et al (2012) Prevalence of patent foramen ovale with right-to-left shunting in dogs with pulmonic stenosis. *J Vet Intern Med* 26, 183–5.

Johnson MS, Martin M, Edwards D, et al (2004) Pulmonic stenosis in dogs: balloon dilation improves clinical outcome. *J Vet Intern Med* 18, 656–62.

Mullins CE (2006a) Balloon dilation procedures – general. In: *Cardiac Catheterization in Congenital Heart Disease: Pediatric and Adult*, 1st edn. Blackwell Publishing, Inc., Malden, MA, pp. 410–29.

Patterson DF, Haskins ME, and Schnarr WR (1981) Hereditary dysplasia of the pulmonary valve in beagle dogs. Pathologic and genetic studies. *Am J Cardiol* 47, 591–641.

Schrope DP (2008) Primary pulmonic infundibular stenosis in 12 cats: natural history and the effects of balloon valvuloplasty. *J Vet Cardiol* 10, 33–43.

Suggested Reading

Estrada A, Moise NS, Erb HN, et al (2006) Prospective evaluation of the balloon-to-annulus ratio for valvuloplasty in the treatment of pulmonic stenosis in the dog. *J Vet Intern Med* 20, 862–72.

Fonfara S, Martinez Pereira Y, Swift S, et al (2010) Balloon valvuloplasty for treatment of pulmonic stenosis in English Bulldogs with an aberrant coronary artery. *J Vet Intern Med* 24, 354–9.

Mullins CE (2006b) Pulmonary valve balloon dilation. In: *Cardiac Catheterization in Congenital Heart Disease: Pediatric and Adult*, 1st edn. Blackwell Publishing, Inc., Malden, MA, pp. 430–440.

Video 59.1 Contrast echocardiographic study using agitated saline to evaluate patency of the atrial septum in a dog with pulmonary valve stenosis. A right parasternal long-axis image is acquired and injection of agitated saline into a peripheral vein results in microcavitations that can be seen first in the right atrium and then pass into the left atrium and ventricle. Severe right ventricular hypertrophy is also apparent.

Video 59.2 Right ventricular angiogram with levophase in a dog with congenital pulmonary valve stenosis. An injection is made into the right ventricle showing a thickened, fused, and doming pulmonary valve, right ventricular hypertrophy, post-stenotic dilation of the main pulmonary artery and branch pulmonary arteries, and normal left-sided structures with normal coronary artery anatomy. A marker catheter is present in the esophagus to calibrate the radiographic magnification of the image for measurement.

Video 59.3 Right ventricular angiogram with levophase in an English bulldog with congenital pulmonary valve stenosis and an anomalous coronary arterial circulation. An injection is made into the right ventricle showing a narrowed pulmonary annulus with a discrete subvalvular ring and prominent cranial filling defect. Severe post-stenotic dilation of the main and branch pulmonary arteries is apparent. Severe right ventricular hypertrophy is also seen. On the levophase, only a single coronary ostium is visualized originating in the area of a suspected right coronary ostium (e.g., from the cranioventral aortic sinus). This coronary artery is enlarged and gives rise to both the left and right coronary arterial circulations. In addition, the left coronary arterial circulation is noted to have a prepulmonic course and passes cranial to the pulmonary annulus in the same position as the cranial filling defect noted in the right ventricular study. These findings are consistent with a single right coronary ostium and anomalous prepulmonic left coronary artery (so-called R2A anatomy) and is a relative contraindication to balloon pulmonary valvuloplasty. A conservative balloon may be considered with informed client consent. A marker catheter is present in the esophagus to calibrate the radiographic magnification of the image for measurement

Video 59.4 Balloon pulmonary valvuloplasty. Balloon inflation of the same dog shown in Figure 59.6. Rapid inflation of the balloon dilation catheter shows an initial stenotic waist at the level of the pulmonary valve, which resolves with increasing inflation pressure.

These video clips can be found in the online material at **www.wiley.com/go/weisse/vet-image-guided-interventions**

CHAPTER SIXTY

Aortic Valve Stenosis

Mandi E. Kleman

Background/Indications

Subaortic stenosis (SAS) is one of the most common congenital cardiac diseases in dogs. Severe SAS is a discouraging condition with a poor long-term prognosis and management of severe SAS in dogs remains a challenge, as treatment options are limited. Many dogs are asymptomatic; however, patients may present with exercise intolerance, rear limb weakness, syncope, left-sided congestive heart failure, or systemic illness secondary to valvular endocarditis. Ventricular arrhythmias and sudden death, with or without clinical signs, are common. Treatment modalities in veterinary medicine have included the use of β-adrenoceptor blocking drugs (i.e., atenolol) in combination with exercise restriction, balloon dilation/valvuloplasty of the stenotic region, and open heart resection of the fibrotic ridge or ring. Valvular aortic stenosis is uncommon in the dog and cat, although similar treatment options may be considered. Supravalvular aortic stenosis is rare.

Patient Selection, Echocardiography, and Preparation

The author currently offers balloon aortic valvuloplasty (BAV) for dogs with severe subaortic or aortic stenosis (peak left ventricular outflow tract pressure gradient greater than 80 mmHg as assessed by Doppler echocardiography). In addition to BAV intervention, treatment involves oral beta-blocker therapy (atenolol 0.5–1.0 mg/kg PO BID) and exercise restriction. Ideally this form of intervention should be performed early in life, prior to irreversible pathologic changes of the myocardium and the coronary arteries. Prior to performing BAV for severe SAS in canine patients, a thorough physical exam and diagnostic work-up including screening bloodwork, thoracic radiographs, electrocardiogram, and echocardiogram is recommended. A 24-hour ambulatory electrocardiogram (Holter monitor) may also be considered to screen for arrhythmic risk.

Dogs are evaluated with transthoracic echocardiography using all standard views and measurements (including color flow, pulsed wave, and continuous wave Doppler) in order to classify the severity of stenosis and assess myocardial function. A thorough echocardiographic examination is also necessary to rule out concurrent congenital heart defects. The subaortic region is interrogated from the right parasternal, left apical, and subcostal views to best appreciate the annulus diameter, subaortic lesion width, and peak left ventricular outflow tract velocity. The presence and magnitude of aortic regurgitation is assessed as mild, moderate, or severe utilizing color flow imaging of the proximal jet width and the rate of deceleration of the diastolic regurgitant jet to derive the pressure half-time. The aortic valve annulus and width of the subaortic lesion is measured from the right parasternal long-axis view. The diameter of the aortic valve annulus is determined at the hinge points. Care should be taken to avoid measuring the dilated sinuses of Valsalva typical of this condition. The ideal view is the image that most clearly shows the valve and supporting structures in any given patient. At least three measurements should be obtained so that a range and average of dimensions can be used to compare to angiographic measurements for the final selection of the balloon prior to BAV. If available, transesophageal echocardiography under general anesthesia may be used to further visualize and measure the diameter of the hingepoints of the aortic valve annulus and of the subvalvular stenotic region.

Veterinary Image-Guided Interventions, First Edition. Edited by Chick Weisse and Allyson Berent.

Companion website: www.wiley.com/go/weisse/vet-image-guided-interventions

Potential Risks/ Complications/ Expected Outcomes

Complications associated with BAV in dogs with severe subaortic stenosis include local arterial trauma, ventricular or atrial arrhythmias, bundle branch or atrioventricular block, worsening aortic regurgitation, acute mitral valve damage and regurgitation, ventricular perforation, systemic embolism, or cardiac arrest. These complications emphasize the importance of technique and are presumably related to factors inherent to the procedure and to the patient's underlying disease. The author has found that ventricular arrhythmias are common during the procedure, however aggressive anti-arrhythmic control during BAV prevents hemodynamically significant ventricular tachycardia in the majority of patients. Aortic regurgitation is a potential immediate and progressive complication; however, it is not a common clinical concern with appropriate balloon selection. A reduction in severity of ≥25–50% without a notable increase in aortic regurgitation is considered a successful outcome. However, it is unknown how a reduction of this magnitude affects long-term survival and quality of life in patients with severe SAS.

Interim analysis of 28 dogs that underwent cutting and high pressure BAV for SAS suggested that a significant decrease in the peak transvalvular pressure gradient can be expected, from a mean of 143 mmHg to 78 mmHg at day 1 post-BAV. Additionally, this reduction persisted at 1 to 24 months of follow-up in this study. However, an increase in transvalvular pressure gradient was noted in a minority of dogs over time and three dogs went on to develop progressive myocardial failure and left-sided congestive heart failure, two dogs died suddenly after the procedure, and one dog was euthanized for recurrent syncopal events (Kleman et al, 2013).

Equipment

In addition to fluoroscopy, recommended equipment can be found in Table 60.1. When ballooning SAS, the author recommends a high pressure and non-elastic dilatation balloon be chosen to apply a high radial force to the subaortic tissue. The fibromuscular ridge or ring in SAS is believed to require greater radial force to sufficiently tear and achieve an increase in effective orifice area as compared to the force required to tear fused valve leaflets as is the goal in balloon pulmonary valvuloplasty for dogs congenital pulmonary valve stenosis. A long balloon, extra stiff exchange wire, and low heart rate are essential to improve balloon stability for successful BAV in severe SAS. Due to severe obstruction, ventricular hypertrophy, and consequent suprasystemic left ventricular pressure, the balloon tends to be expelled from the ventricle after inflation. The high pressure balloon recommended here has very long tapered shoulders, which almost double the working length of the balloon. The long shoulders of this balloon prevent its use in smaller-breed dogs with small left ventricular chamber dimensions. However, in medium and large-breed dogs this balloon provides a stability advantage compared to standard balloons. Additionally, utilizing extra stiff guide wires is very important to stabilize balloon position. A less stiff wire of the same gauge will not prevent the balloon from being expelled into the post-stenotic dilation of the aortic arch during systole.

TABLE 60.1

Summary of catheterization supplies needed for cutting balloon and high pressure balloon valvuloplasty for subaortic stenosis

Supply	Size	Manufacturer
Vascular sheath introducer	9–12 Fr	Cordis Corporation, various
Pigtail catheter	7 Fr	Cook Medical, various
Exchange guide wire for cutting balloon	0.018″ diameter × 260 cm length	Cook Medical, various
Cutting balloon peripheral microsurgical dilatation device	8.0 mm × 2.0 cm × 135 cm	Boston Scientific
Inflation device	N/A	B. Braun, various
Extra stiff exchange guide wire for high pressure balloon	0.035″ diameter × 260 cm length, 3 mm J-tip	Cook Medical
ATLAS PTA balloon dilatation catheter (recommended for medium and large breed dogs)	12.0–26.0 mm × 2.0–4.0 cm balloon length 75 or 120 cm catheter length	Bard Peripheral Vascular
Z-MED II balloon dilatation catheter (recommended for small breed dogs)	5.0–25.0 mm × 2.0–5.0 cm balloon length 100 cm catheter length	B. Braun, various

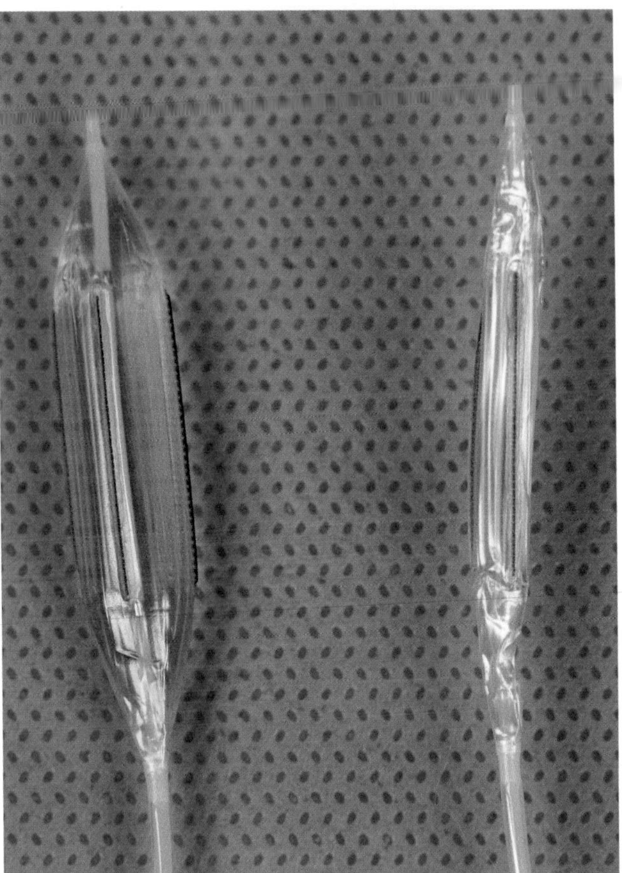

Figure 60.1 Two peripheral 8 mm cutting balloon dilation catheters. The catheter on the left demonstrates inflation. The atherotomes are fixed longitudinally on the outer surface of a balloon and expand radially during inflation. These atherotomes deliver longitudinal scores in the vessel or lesion to more effectively stretch and dilate the vessel during subsequent high pressure balloon valvuloplasty. The catheter on the right demonstrates the balloon following deflation. The unique design of the cutting balloon allows for the edges of the atherotomes to no longer be in contact with tissue when the balloon is deflated.

The use of a more aggressive cutting balloon valvuloplasty (CBV) technique combined with high pressure balloon valvuloplasty provides an alternative treatment to dogs with severe subaortic stenosis. The advantage of the cutting balloon, as compared to standard BAV, is the ability to increase vessel stretch while reducing vessel injury by scoring the vessel longitudinally. The artherotomes are fixed longitudinally on the outer surface of a balloon and expand radially to deliver longitudinal scores in the vessel or lesion. These scores create controlled tears that allow the second, high-pressure balloon to more effectively stretch and dilate the narrowed target. The unique design of the cutting balloon is engineered to protect the tissues from the edges of the artherotomes when it is deflated (Figure 60.1).

A pressure-monitored inflation device capable of generating and holding specific atmospheres of pressure is required for cutting balloon valvuloplasty and high pressure balloon valvuloplasty.

Procedure

Anesthesia

Patients should receive at least 0.5 mg/kg of oral atenolol twice daily for optimally 2 or more weeks prior to the BAV and should receive atenolol the morning of the procedure. On the day of the procedure, dogs may be premedicated with a combination of hydromorphone (0.1 mg/kg IM) and midazolam (0.2 mg/kg IM). Standard prophylactic intravenous antibiotics can be administered prior to carotid artery access and BAV. The author recommends administration of procainamide (10 mg/kg IM) and a bolus of lidocaine (2mg/kg IV) followed by a continuous infusion of lidocaine (50–75 μg/kg/min) prior to the interventional procedure. Dogs additionally may receive a continuous infusion of fentanyl (1–5 μg/kg/min IV) in order to maintain bradycardia during BAV. Maintaining an approximate heart rate of 50–70 beats per minute is helpful to improve balloon stability during BAV.

Carotid Artery Access

Following anesthetic induction and instrumentation, the patient is placed in left lateral recumbency and the lateral region of the right neck is clipped, prepped, and draped. Carotid artery access is obtained with a 4 to 5 cm vascular cut-down of the right carotid artery. The right carotid artery is isolated via blunt dissection and stabilized with stay sutures. The right carotid artery pulse can be palpated to assist with dissection; however, a blunted carotid pulse is expected in dogs with severe aortic obstruction. A 16-gauge short, over the needle catheter is advanced into the right carotid artery and through this catheter a 0.038″ guide wire is advanced into the lumen of the right carotid artery. Once the guide wire is in place the catheter is removed and an appropriately sized introducer and dilator (9 to 12 Fr) are then advanced over the guide wire. Once the introducer is positioned, the dilator and guide wire are removed, and the introducer is sutured in place to the skin or underlying muscle. The author recommends sizing 1 to 2 French sizes above the manufacturer's recommended introducer size, due to difficulty in removing the high-pressure balloon out of the introducer following inflation. The large size of introducer

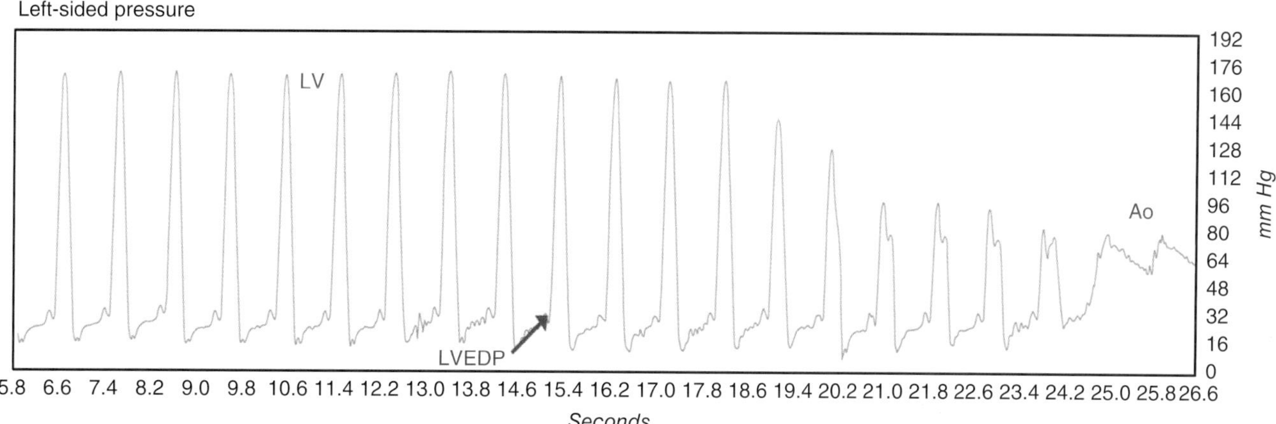

Figure 60.2 This pressure tracing demonstrates the withdrawal of a catheter from the left ventricle (LV) to the aorta (Ao) in a dog with severe subaortic stenosis. The peak-to-peak systolic pressure gradient in this dog is approximately 90 mmHg and consistent with a severe obstruction, especially considering the depressant effects of general anesthesia on LV function and pressure development. The four pressure waveforms with reduced systolic pressure and a low (ventricular) diastolic pressure prior to the Ao pressure waves are diagnostic for subaortic stenosis. The LV end-diastolic pressure (LVEDP) is elevated at approximately 25 mmHg, consistent with pressure overload, concentric hypertrophy, and decreased compliance.

required for high pressure BAV generally precludes using the femoral artery for retrograde left ventricular catheterization in most dogs.

Intracardiac Pressures and Angiography

A 6 or 7 Fr pigtail angiographic catheter should be carefully flushed to remove any air bubbles prior to being placed through the carotid artery introducer and advanced into the left ventricle to obtain left ventricular and aortic root pressures via a pull-back procedure. Special attention must be made to remove air bubbles. Frequent flushing of all catheters and valves is important to prevent potential air embolism during cardiac catheterization. A standard pigtail catheter with end- and multiple side-holes is effective as the initial left heart catheter in most cases as it can be advanced down the aorta and across the aortic valve with a low degree of difficulty and a low incidence of vascular or valvular trauma. The multiple side holes improve contrast opacification during angiography while minimizing myocardial staining and the end hole allows for guide wire placement. The pressure pullback from the left ventricle to the aorta should be recorded in order to calculate the peak-to-peak pressure gradient across the stenosis prior to BAV (Figure 60.2). After initial pressure measurements are obtained, left ventricular and aortic root angiography is performed by injecting 0.5 ml/kg of iodinated contrast medium though the pigtail catheter with a rapid pressure injector or via hand injection. (Videos 60.1 and 60.2). The diameter of the subvalvular obstruction and of the aortic annulus at the hingepoints of the semilunar cusps are again measured from a high quality angiographic image and a calibrated ruler or catheter (Figure 60.3). Care should be taken to avoid measuring the dilated sinuses of Valsalva typical of this condition.

Cutting Balloon Valvuloplasty

CBV should not be performed in dogs with purely valvular aortic stenosis, but has theoretical benefit in dogs with SAS. The cutting balloon diameter is sized approximately 1:1 to the diameter of the subaortic narrowing or stenotic waist. The width of the largest cutting balloon currently available, 8 mm in diameter, generally approximates the stenotic waist in most large breed dogs with severe SAS as measured by echocardiography and angiography. Immediately prior to CBV, a test inflation of the cutting balloon catheter may be performed with a mixture of 2:1 saline and contrast to remove as many air bubbles within the balloon as possible. Current cutting balloons utilize a 0.018″ × 260 cm guide wire for placement. This guide wire has a small diameter and is easily bent. Care is required to advance the 0.018″ guide wire into the left ventricle through a pigtail catheter. The pigtail catheter is then removed while maintaining a large loop of guide wire within the apex of the left ventricle. The deflated cutting balloon catheter is then advanced over the guide wire and passed to just below the center of the subaortic obstruction. The cutting balloon is inflated rapidly using an inflation device to consistently achieve the nominal pressure of 6 atm. Inflating the balloon initially below

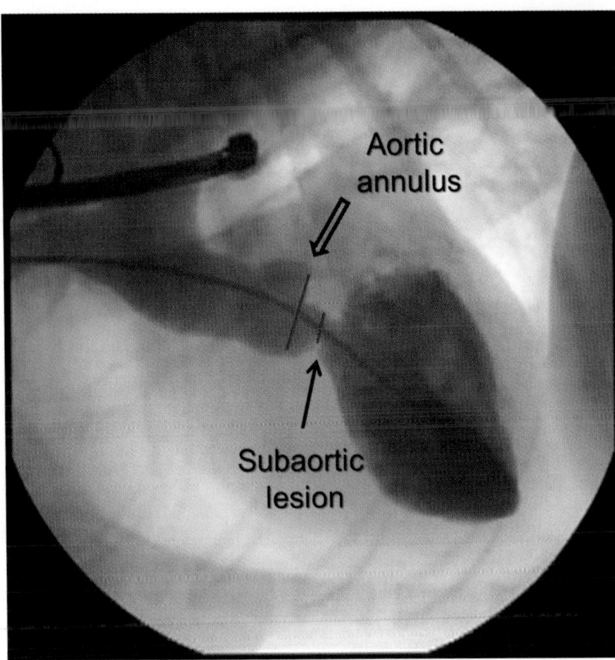

Figure 60.3 Still frame of a selective left ventricular angiogram in a dog with subaortic stenosis. Contrast is seen within the left ventricle and highlights the narrowing of the left ventricular outflow tract. There is also trace mitral regurgitation and post-stenotic dilation of the aortic arch and brachiocephalic trunk. Note the measurement of the diameter of width of the subaortic stenosis (arrow) and the measurement of the diameter of the width of the aortic annulus at the hingepoints (open arrow). Additionally, a transesophageal echocardiography probe is seen within the esophagus. This image complements Video 60.1.

the left ventricular outflow tract and then allowing contraction to push the partially inflated balloon into the subaortic stenotic lesion is helpful to engage the cutting balloon within the lesion. During initial inflation, gentle advancement pressure is applied to the cutting balloon catheter in order to prevent the balloon from being expelled into the aortic arch. The cutting balloon is typically inflated 2 to 3 times and can be effectively positioned within the stenotic lesion during the majority of inflations (Video 60.3). Following inflation, the cutting balloon is completely deflated to ensure protection of the vasculature from the blades. The cutting balloon and 0.018″ guide wire are then removed.

High-Pressure Balloon Valvuloplasty

The pigtail catheter is again flushed and placed within the introducer, across the aortic valve, and into the left ventricle. A high pressure balloon dilation catheter is selected to be approximately 90 to 100% the diameter of the aortic valve annulus primarily based on angiographic measurements from a left ventricular angiogram or aortic root angiogram. The author also utilizes transthoracic and transesophageal echocardiographic measurements of the aortic annulus to develop a tentative interventional plan, and the final balloon selection is based on all three measurements. The recommendation for balloon selection is based on human reports describing the use of a balloon:annulus ratio <0.9 as a risk factor for a suboptimal gradient reduction and the use of a balloon:annulus ratio >1.0 as a risk factor for severe aortic regurgitation.

Immediately prior to BAV, a test inflation of the high-pressure balloon is performed with a mixture of 2:1 saline to contrast to remove as many air bubbles as possible. The inflation device should be primed and the test inflation performed prior to advancement of the guide wire into the left ventricle in order to reduce morbidity secondary to ventricular arrhythmias. An extra stiff 0.035″ × 260 cm guide wire is then placed into the left ventricle through the pigtail catheter. A large curve in the extremity of the guide wire is cautiously maintained within the apex of the left ventricle. Molding a soft curve to the extremity of the guide wire prior to placement within the left ventricular apex may be helpful to decrease myocardial damage and clinically significant arrhythmogenesis. The pigtail catheter is then removed slowly while the guide wire is simultaneously manipulated to prevent any movement from the ideal curved position within the left ventricular apex. The high-pressure balloon dilation catheter is then advanced over the guide wire and across the center of the subaortic obstruction, while again simultaneously manipulating the guide wire to avoid excessive wire accumulation within the left ventricle. The high pressure balloon can then be inflated to approximately 10 atm using an inflation device. During inflation it is necessary to have two or three people performing the inflation. One person is needed to maintain the balloon position across the subaortic lesion via gentle traction or advancement and one or two people are required to inflate the balloon. In order to compensate for systolic contraction pushing the balloon forward, it is helpful to initially begin inflation with only one-third of the balloon above the lesion. Balloons sized at 20 mm or greater require more volume than can be delivered via the standard inflation device. Therefore, a three-way stopcock and a luer-lock syringe in combination with the inflation device are used to deliver an increased volume quickly while maintaining pressure within the inflation device. One person initially delivers 20 ml of sterile 2:1 saline and contrast mixture into the balloon

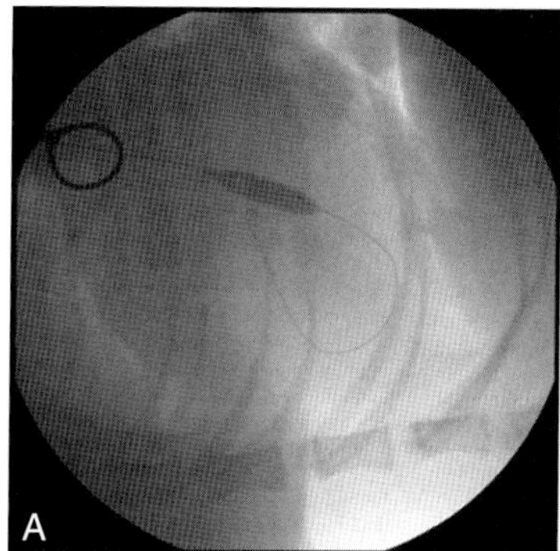

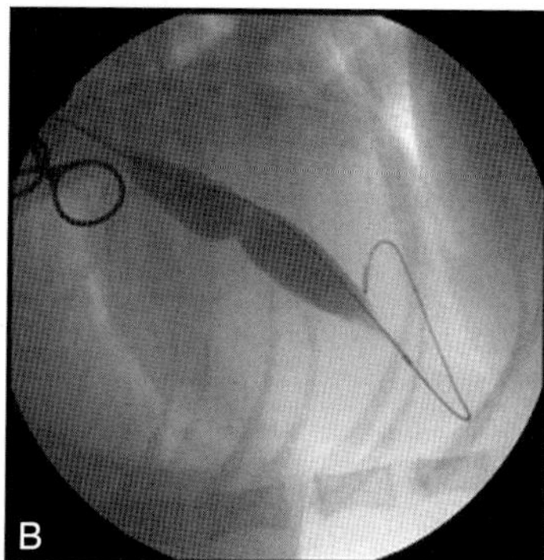

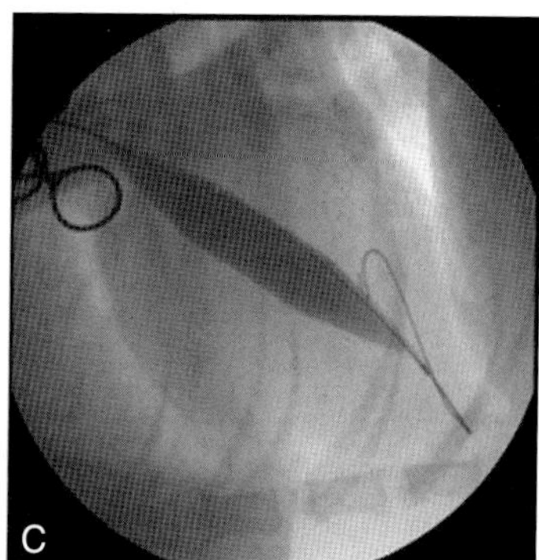

Figure 60.4 Still frame lateral fluoroscopic images of combined cutting balloon valvuloplasty and high pressure balloon valvuloplasty in a dog with subaortic stenosis. (A) An 8 mm cutting balloon inflated and engaged in the left ventricular outflow tract. (B, C) High-pressure balloon aortic valvulolplasty. (B) The typical hourglass shape prior to complete inflation of the high pressure balloon. (C) Complete inflation of the balloon with successful reduction of the previously noted waist. Note the longer tapered length of the high pressure balloon extending into the left ventricular apex as compared to conventional balloons. Note also the loop of wire seen within the left ventricle in both techniques. Ideally, the wire could have been withdrawn to decrease the length of the tip of the wire pointing dorsally towards the mitral valve. These images complement Videos 60.3 and 60.4.

followed by a second person delivering approximately 5 to 15 ml of sterile saline via the inflation device in order to achieve a working pressure of 10 to 12 atm. Visualization of the typical hourglass shape and successful reduction of the waist is routinely achievable in dogs with severe SAS (Figure 60.4; Video 60.4). Following one to three balloon inflations, the high pressure balloon dilation catheter and guide wire are then removed. Following completion of balloon valvuloplasty the pressure pull-back procedure should be repeated to assess the residual pressure gradient across the subaortic stenosis. Additionally, left ventricular and aortic root angiography may also be repeated to evaluate for the presence of worsened aortic regurgitation. Finally, the introducer is removed as the artery is ligated twice proximally and once distally with 2–0 silk suture. Alternatively, repair of the carotid artery may be performed. The incision is then closed routinely with three layers. The patient's neck is wrapped with bandage material to maintain light compression of the surgical site.

Follow-Up

The patient should be recovered and monitored in the intensive care unit overnight. Prophylactic antibiotic therapy following recovery from anesthesia is not routinely administered. β-adrenoceptor blocking therapy (atenolol 0.5–1.0 mg/kg PO BID) should be continued and pain control medications can be administered as necessary. It is not uncommon for patients to develop ventricular arrhythmias during the first 24 hours after BAV and continuous electrocardiography is recommended until discharge 24–48 hr after BAV. Sotalol (1–2 mg/kg PO BID) should be instituted, as alternative to atenolol therapy, if frequent and/or multiform ventricular arrhythmias or fast ventricular tachycardia is observed. Recheck transthoracic echocardiography is performed prior to discharge to evaluate response to BAV. A recheck examination is scheduled for 1 month, 3–6 months, and 1 year; examinations are then scheduled every 6 months to 1 year thereafter. Owners are instructed to monitor for weakness, changes in appetite, syncope, or difficulty breathing as these signs warrant immediate re-evaluation.

Reference

Kleman ME, Estrada AH, Tschosik ML, et al (2013) An update on combined cutting balloon and high pressure balloon valvuloplasty for dogs with severe subaortic stenosis. [Abstract] *J Vet Intern Med* 27(3), 632–3.

Suggested Reading

DeLellis L, Thomas W, and Pion P (1993) Balloon dilation of congenital subaortic stenosis in the dog. *J Vet Intern Medi* 7(3), 153–62.

Kienle RD (1998) Aortic stenosis. In Kittleson MD, Kienle RD: *Small Animal Cardiovascular Medicine*. Mosby, St. Louis, pp. 260–72.

Kleman M, Estrada A, Maisenbacher H, et al (2012) How to perform combined cutting balloon and high pressure balloon valvuloplasty for dogs with subaortic stenosis. *J Vet Cardiol* 14(2), 351–61.

Meurs K, Lehmkuhl L, and Bonagura J (2005) Survival times in dogs with severe subvalvular aortic stenosis treated with balloon valvuloplasty or atenolol. *J Am Vet Med Assoc* 227(3), 420–4.

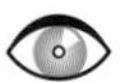
Video 60.1 A pigtail catheter is used to obtain left ventricular angiography in a dog with severe subaortic stenosis.

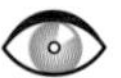
Video 60.2 A pigtail catheter is used to obtain aortic root angiography in a dog with severe subaortic stenosis.

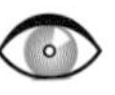
Video 60.3 An 8 mm cutting balloon is inflated and engaged within the subaortic region in a dog with severe subaortic stenosis.

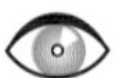
Video 60.4 A high pressure balloon is inflated and engaged within the subaortic region in a dog with severe subaortic stenosis.

These video clips can be found in the online material at **www.wiley.com/go/weisse/vet-image-guided-interventions**

CHAPTER SIXTY-ONE

Atrioventricular Valve Stenosis

Aaron C. Wey
Upstate Veterinary Specialties, PLLC, Latham, NY

Background/Indications

Atrioventricular (A-V) valvular dysplasias are uncommon cardiac conditions in veterinary patients but may cause significant clinical symptoms in severely affected animals. Genetic predispositions have been reported for both mitral and tricuspid dysplasia in the dog. Symptoms are most commonly attributable to valvular insufficiency resulting in volume overload and symptoms of either right or left-sided congestive heart failure. If options for medical management of these causes have been exhausted, few interventional options currently exist for management of severe valvular insufficiency other than valve replacement or repair, neither of which is routinely available at the time of this writing. Stenosis is a less common complication of A-V valvular dysplasia but can result in significant clinical signs if the transvalvular gradient causes marked elevations of atrial pressure (>10 mmHg in right atrium, >20 mmHg in left atrium) or reductions in forward cardiac output. Stenosis secondary to A-V valvular dysplasia may be amenable to minimally invasive balloon dilation depending on the anatomy of the dysplastic valve, but has been reported only rarely in the veterinary literature. All current case reports of tricuspid balloon dilation were dogs of retriever breeds (primarily Labrador retrievers), but too few mitral balloon valvuloplasty cases exist to identify breed predilection. While both mitral and tricuspid dysplasia/stenosis has been reported in the cat, no minimally invasive dilation procedures have been reported in the veterinary literature to date so intervention in feline patients will not be discussed. Case selection is important for these procedures, and associated comorbid conditions should be considered carefully before attempting balloon dilation. Patients most often considered for intervention in veterinary medicine have typically failed medical management and have refractory symptoms of congestive heart failure, syncope, severe exercise restriction, or have unacceptable side effects of medical therapy. With appropriate case selection, clinical outcome for palliative balloon dilation of a stenotic valve can be successful and can reduce the need for long-term medical therapy.

In addition to A-V valve stenosis secondary to valvular dysplasia, palliative balloon dilation may have applications for a variety of acquired forms of valvular stenosis. In human patients, these include rheumatic valve disease, stenosis of valvular prostheses, and stenosis secondary to endocardial lead wires. While only the latter pacing complication has been reported in the veterinary literature, anecdotal reports of the other conditions exist and palliative balloon dilation for selected cases may be clinically useful in the future.

Patient Preparation

Patients with congenital A-V valvular dysplasia in which significant stenosis is a component of the clinical presentation constitute the cases that may be amenable to balloon valvuloplasty. These cases may present with signs attributable to low cardiac output (i.e., exertional fatigue or syncope) or of congestive heart failure; either ascites or pleural effusion (in the case of tricuspid dysplasia/stenosis) or pulmonary edema (in the case of mitral dysplasia/stenosis). Patients with congenital mitral stenosis may also have post-capillary pulmonary hypertension resulting in concurrent symptoms of dyspnea, cyanosis, collapse, or right heart failure. Clinical evaluation of these patients should include thoracic radiography,

Veterinary Image-Guided Interventions, First Edition. Edited by Chick Weisse and Allyson Berent.

Companion website: www.wiley.com/go/weisse/vet-image-guided-interventions

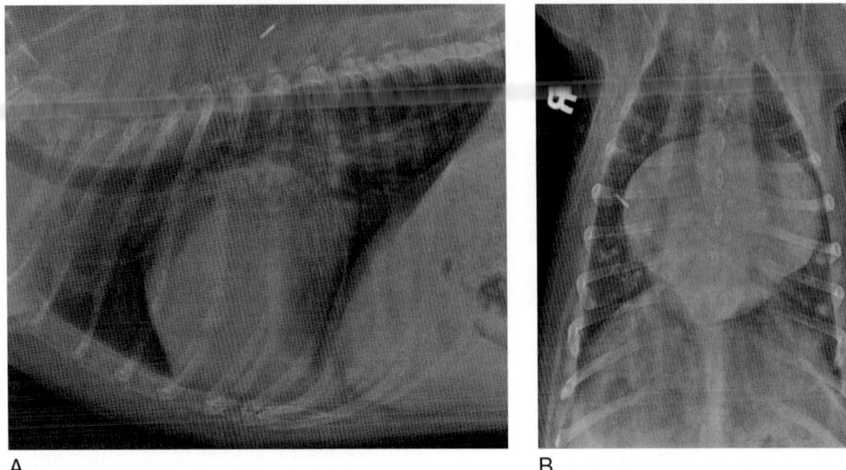

Figure 61.1 Right lateral (A) and DV (B) radiographic projections of a canine patient with severe mitral stenosis. The radiographs demonstrate severe left heart enlargement, particularly the left atrium, with enlarged pulmonary veins and a caudodorsal pulmonary interstitial pattern consistent with cardiogenic pulmonary edema. Image used with permission from Arndt, J.W., Oyama, M.A. (2013) Balloon valvuloplasty of congenital mitral stenosis. Journal of Veterinary Cardiology, 15(2), 147–151, Elsevier.

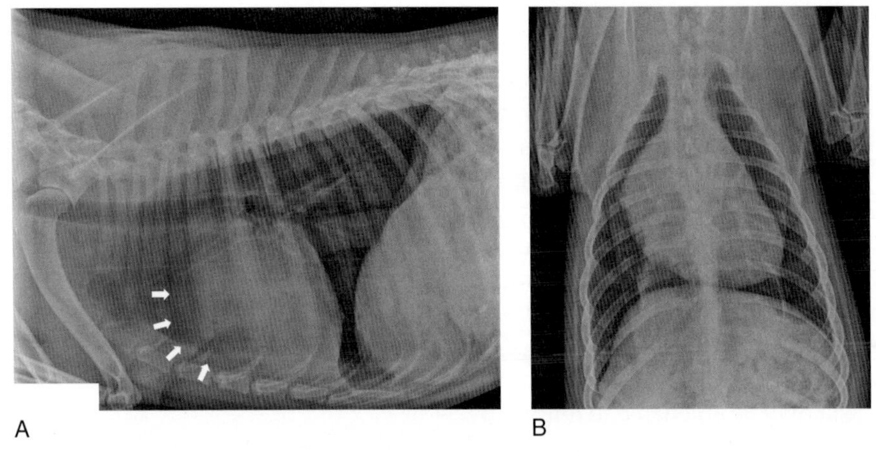

Figure 61.2 Right lateral (A) and DV (B) radiographic projections of a canine patient with severe tricuspid stenosis and minimal tricuspid regurgitation. The radiographs demonstrate right heart enlargement evident as increased sternal contact and loss of the cranial cardiac waist on the lateral projection (arrows), and increased volume of the cardiac silhouette in the right hemithorax on the DV view. The patient also has a distended caudal vena cava on both views, and the pulmonary vessels are subjectively attenuated, particularly on the lateral projection.

electrocardiography, echocardiography, and routine laboratory evaluation including complete blood count, biochemical profile, and urinalysis. Supraventricular arrhythmias (atrial fibrillation, atrial tachycardia) are common due to the atrial dilation that accompanies severe valvular stenosis. Although the atrial dilatation in these patients may be dramatic (Figure 61.1), radiographic cardiomegaly may be moderate in pure valvular stenosis due to the lack of any significant ventricular dilation (Figure 61.2).

Echocardiography with a complete spectral and color Doppler analysis by an experienced echocardiographer is critical to identify patients that have appropriate intracardiac hemodynamics, valvular anatomy, and a lack of concurrent cardiac pathology that might benefit from balloon dilation. Typical echocardiographic changes include thickened and tethered valve leaflets that have restricted diastolic motion ("doming") with variable degrees of valvular insufficiency. Acceptable candidates for intervention should be distinguished

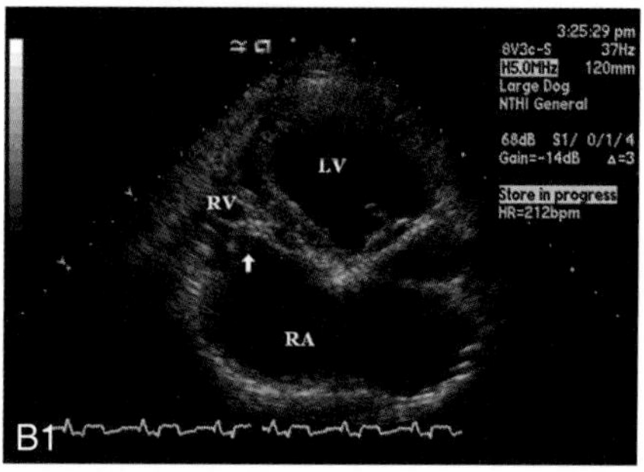

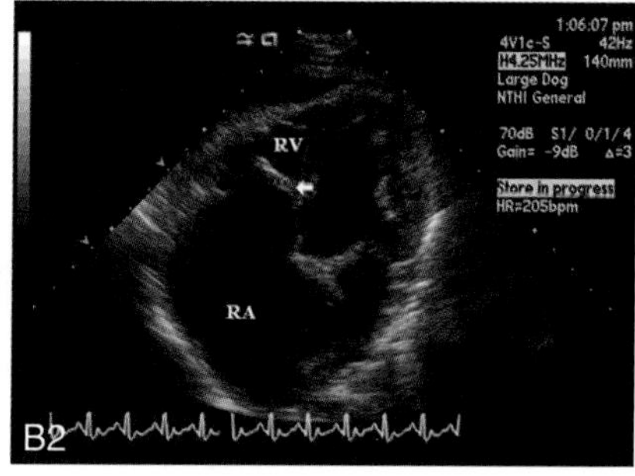

Figure 61.3 Two-dimensional echocardiograms from two canine patients with tricuspid stenosis and differing valvular anatomy. (A) A dog with valvular anatomy conducive to balloon dilation, including elongated and mobile valve leaflets with tethering only at the leaflet margins and doming of the leaflets in diastole (arrow), moderate length chordae tendineae, and minimal subvalvular attachment or tethering. This patient also had only mild tricuspid regurgitation. (B) A different dog with anatomy not considered optimal for balloon dilation, including markedly thickened and immobile valve leaflets (B1, arrow) and marked subvalvular tethering and leaflet immobility (B2, arrow). This dog also had subjectively moderate to severe tricuspid regurgitation. RV – right ventricle, RA – right atrium, LV – left ventricle.

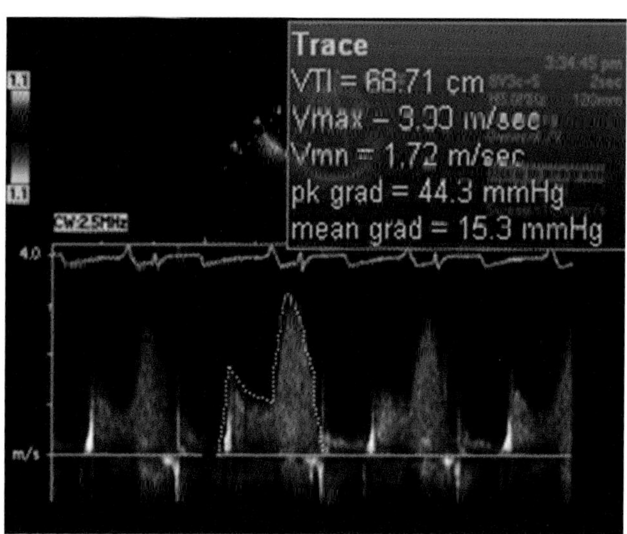

Figure 61.4 Spectral Doppler echocardiogram of a canine patient with tricuspid valve stenosis demonstrating markedly increased mean pressure gradients consistent with severe stenosis (mean gradient >15 mmHg).

from patients with valvular anatomy that is not amenable to balloon dilation (Figure 61.3; Videos 61.1 and 61.2). Stenotic orifice area may be calculated by a variety of methods (pressure half-time, Gorlin equation, or flow-convergence method) to help assess the severity of the stenosis. In humans, mean diastolic trans-valvular Doppler gradients >5 mmHg in the tricuspid position and >10 mmHg in the mitral position are considered severe (Figure 61.4), and stenotic orifice areas <1 cm^2 in either the mitral or tricuspid position are considered severe. However, patients with only moderate stenoses may still be symptomatic in the presence of significant tachyarrhythmias. Specific echocardiographic criteria have not been established to guide decisions regarding intervention in the veterinary literature. Consequently, the decision to perform balloon valvuloplasty has historically been based on valvular anatomy and the presence of clinical signs refractory to medical intervention. The Suggested Reading list should be consulted for a more complete description of the echocardiographic evaluation and determination of lesion severity in patients with valvular dysplasia/stenosis.

Medical management for symptomatic mitral or tricuspid stenosis often includes a variety of medications tailored to the individual patient. Therapy for congestive heart failure should include diuretics and angiotensin-converting enzyme (ACE)-inhibitors, but aggressive preload reduction should be avoided to minimize the risk of large reductions in atrial pressure that might reduce ventricular filling and cardiac output. The benefit of positive inotropic agents or inodilators (i.e. pimobendan) typically used in other forms of congestive heart failure may be negligible in patients with pure valvular stenosis due to the absence of ventricular systolic dysfunction or dilation, but these agents would be useful in the setting of concurrent severe A-V valvular insufficiency causing ventricular dilation and myocardial failure. Negative chronotropic therapy is important to maximize diastolic filling time and to address atrial tachycardia and/or atrial fibrillation, if present. Pulmonary vasodilators may also be indicated in the presence of severe pulmonary hypertension secondary to chronic mitral stenosis. Table 61.1 summarizes some common drugs and doses used in the management of complications of valvular dysplasia/stenosis in dogs and cats but should not be considered all inclusive. Patients that remain symptomatic after appropriate medical management with these or other therapies, or those that have unacceptable side effects

TABLE 61.1
Common oral medications for management of symptomatic tricuspid/mitral stenosis

Diuretics
- Furosemide: 1–4 mg/kg BID-TID
- Hydrochlorothiazide: 2–4 mg/kg BID
- Spironolactone: 1–2 mg/kg BID

ACE-inhibitors
- Enalapril: 0.25–0.5 mg/kg BID
- Benazepril: 0.25–0.5 mg/kg BID

Negative chronotropic agents
- Atenolol: 0.5–1.5 mg/kg BID
- Metoprolol: 0.5–1.5 mg/kg BID
- Diltiazem: 0.5–3 mg/kg TID
- Digoxin: 0.005–0.01 mg/kg BID

Pulmonary vasodilators (mitral stenosis)
- Sildenafil: 1–2 mg/kg TID
- Pimobendan: 0.25 mg/kg BID

from therapy should be considered candidates for balloon valvuloplasty.

Potential Risks/Complications

Due to the relatively small number of case reports in the veterinary literature for transvenous balloon tricuspid/mitral valvuloplasty (seven tricuspid stenosis, two mitral stenosis) the list of complications is largely anecdotal and/or extrapolated from the human literature. The most substantial risk associated with balloon dilation of an atrioventricular valve is chordae/valvular rupture that results in severe valvular insufficiency. This complication may counteract or overwhelm any potential benefit achieved through relief of the stenosis resulting in persistent or worsening clinical symptoms. It has been suggested in both the human and veterinary literature that iatrogenic valvular insufficiency may occur more frequently with selection of larger balloon sizes. Other life threatening complications common to any intracardiac intervention include new or life-threatening arrhythmia formation or cardiac perforation with hemopericardium, hemothorax, or cardiac arrest. Inadequate dilation and recurrent stenosis appear to be the most common pitfalls of the procedure. Prior to any intervention, the owners of a patient with severe mitral/tricuspid stenosis should be advised of these complications and the potential for a suboptimal outcome. As with most interventional procedures, the risk of complications decreases proportionately with the experience of the interventionalist, and can be largely avoided with knowledge of intracardiac anatomy, careful adherence to cardiac catheterization technique and protocol, and attention to detail.

Equipment

Interventional cardiology requires the availability of fluoroscopy with an adjustable angle of radiation, a procedure table compatible with fluoroscopy, appropriate radiation safety equipment, a defibrillator, and monitoring equipment with invasive pressure monitoring/recording capabilities. A "crash cart" with appropriate medications and equipment for cardiopulmonary resuscitation is also a necessity in the catheterization laboratory. Ideally, these catheterization procedures would be performed in a facility with surgical assistance for complications such as cardiac perforation and great vessel rupture. Radiation safety guidelines should be followed to minimize radiation exposure times for all individuals in the room, including appropriate collimation, magnification and use of lower radiation "scanning" modes when possible. Selected equipment necessary for general balloon valvuloplasty is shown in Figure 61.5. The balloons utilized for valvuloplasty are double-lumen configuration and are often specifically manufactured for this purpose (bougienage catheters and other dilators should not be used). Larger balloon sizes have less radial strength than smaller balloons, and a manometer attached to the inflation syringe is ideal to minimize the risk of balloon rupture during inflation. The size of the balloon chosen for balloon valvuloplasty in humans is recommended to be between 70 and 110% of the size of the valve annulus calculated via echocardiography. Dilation using these sizing criteria has been described in humans using a single balloon technique, double balloon technique, or Inoue balloon (hourglass shape). If using a double-balloon technique, the effective balloon diameter, defined as 80% of the combined diameters of both balloons, should be used in choosing two appropriately sized balloons for dilation. While balloon dilation in veterinary patients can be adequately performed using a single balloon, a double balloon technique may be preferable for larger breeds, in which larger catheter and/or balloon sizes are not available, to approximate 70–110% of the calculated annular size. The guide wire size necessary for a balloon catheter is often specified by the manufacturer, but in general should be stiff to minimize flexion of the balloon during dilation and should always have a flexible J-tip configuration to avoid cardiac or great vessel trauma/perforation.

Procedure

Tricuspid Stenosis

The anesthesia staff for A-V valve intervention should be knowledgeable about and experienced with

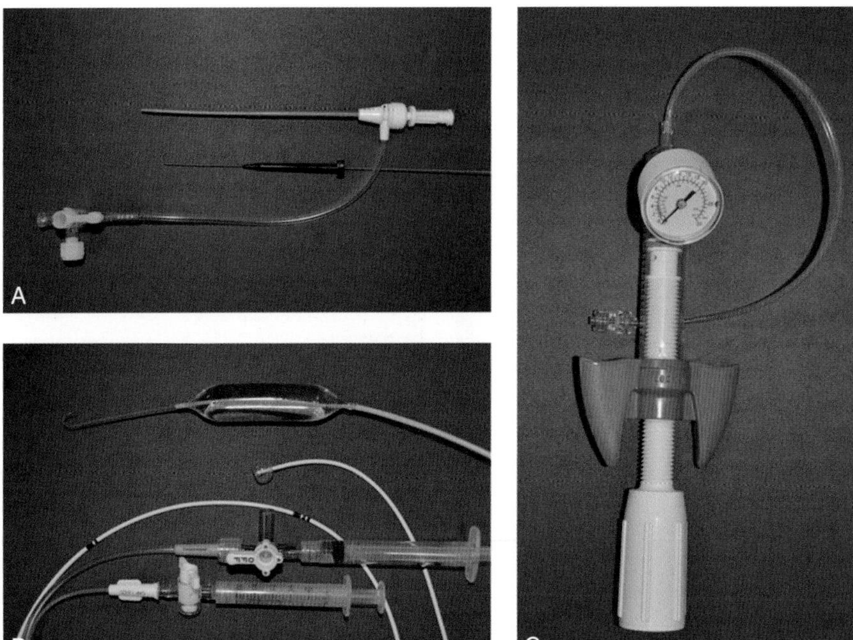

Figure 61.5 Equipment necessary for general balloon dilation procedures. (A) An introducing sheath with a hemostasis valve and dilator, supplied with a wire guide to secure intravenous access after percutaneous needle puncture. (B) A balloon dilation catheter is shown (top) with a wire guide inserted through the central channel of the catheter, leading with a flexible J-tip. A balloon wedge pressure (BWP) catheter is also displayed (bottom) with the distal balloon inflated. (C) An injection manometer may be helpful to monitor inflation pressure during balloon dilation.

cardiovascular hemodynamics and the management of patients with advanced cardiovascular disease; open communication between the interventionalist and the anesthesia staff regarding each individual patient's cardiovascular status and potential complications of the procedure is critical. The use of prophylactic antibiotics in the setting of balloon valvuloplasty is controversial, but due to the risk of endocarditis with congenital valvular anomalies and cardiac catheterization, the author prefers the use of a cephalosporin (cefazolin, 22 mg/kg IV) at the time of anesthetic induction and every two hours thereafter during anesthesia. Additional considerations should include a lidocaine CRI (20–50 µg/kg/min) to minimize the risk of life-threatening ventricular ectopy, and other antiarrhythmics should be on hand (20% lidocaine, 10% esmolol, 5% diltiazem). For cardiac catheterization that involves catheter and guide wire exchanges such as balloon valvuloplasty, it is easier, but not essential, to perform the procedure with two individuals. For a double-balloon technique, two interventionalists are required for simultaneous balloon inflations. Patient positioning for this procedure is often dictated by the preference of the individual performing the intervention based on their dominant hand for feeding catheters and guide wires, but lateral recumbency is preferred to allow the best visualization of the tricuspid and mitral valve. However, the annular plane of the canine tricuspid valve may not be perpendicular to a fluoroscopic beam, particularly in patients with severe right atrial dilation. Consequently, an adjustable fluoroscope is preferable to optimize visualization of the dilation balloon during inflation.

Venous access for the procedure (see Chapter 44) can be from either the jugular or femoral vein and is largely dictated by user preference as the procedure has been performed successfully from both approaches (Figure 61.6; Videos 61.3 and 61.4). Although there are some theoretical advantages to femoral vein access with respect to the angle of incidence of the catheter approaching the plane of the tricuspid annulus, these are often counterbalanced by the benefit of larger vessel size, ease of patient positioning and postoperative monitoring, and familiarity of many cardiologists with the jugular approach. A modified Seldinger (percutaneous) technique can be utilized to gain venous access for placement of an introducer sheath. Alternatively a cut-down procedure can be performed to directly isolate the preferred vein for venotomy. The latter protocol is preferred by some as it allows direct visualization of the vein and eliminates the need for placing an introducer sheath, potentially reducing anesthetic time and cost to the owner. This benefit may be overstated if an individual is adept at percutaneous introducer placement, or alternatively if an individual *not* accustomed to vascular surgical techniques attempts

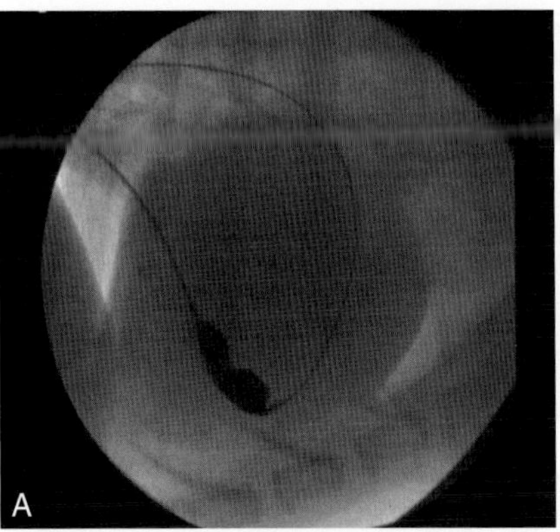

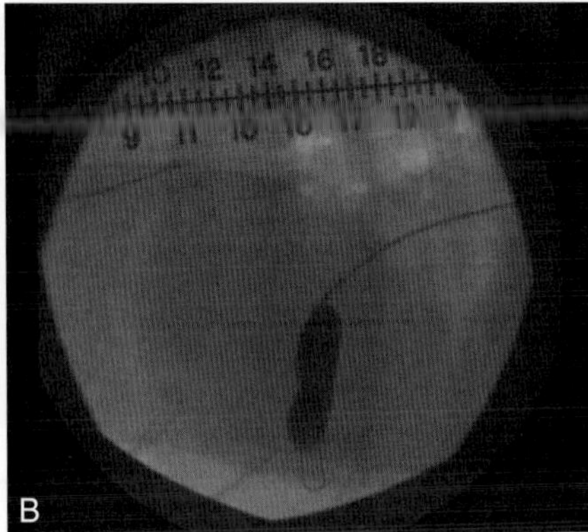

Figure 61.6 Still fluoroscopic images of two canine patients undergoing balloon valvuloplasty for severe tricuspid stenosis. (A) Femoral venous approach with partial balloon inflation across the stenotic orifice and appropriate positioning of the distal guide wire tip in the peripheral pulmonary arteries. (B) Jugular venous approach with partial balloon inflation across the stenotic orifice with inadequate extension of the guide wire tip (only into the right ventricle). In this example, antegrade migration of the balloon through the stenotic orifice under high pressure could result in right ventricular freewall trauma or cardiac perforation. Images used with permission of Dr. Geri Lake-Bakaar.

to salvage the vein after a cut-down procedure. If a percutaneous approach is preferred, an introducer should be chosen that is of appropriate size to accommodate the balloon dilation catheter. For smaller patients, this may require one or more introducer exchanges ("upsizing") to arrive at the appropriately sized introducer.

All catheters and associated connectors, three-way stopcocks, manifolds, and syringes should be flushed with heparinized saline (10 000 U/liter) and be free of any air prior to placement into a vein. Once venous access is achieved, a balloon wedge pressure catheter (BWP) is advised for passage through the great vessels and cardiac chambers in most patients. The balloon at the tip of the catheter should be inflated/deflated with the manufacturer's recommended volume of air prior to insertion to verify functionality. Catheter passage will be through the cranial vena cava (for jugular approach) or caudal vena cava (femoral approach), right atrium (RA), tricuspid valve, right ventricle (RV), pulmonary valve, and pulmonary artery (PA). Inflation of the balloon of the BWP catheter is advised to minimize the risk of endocardial or vascular trauma and to utilize venous flow to help with catheter advancement. A 45° angle pre-placed by the interventionalist is often helpful to direct the catheter tip ventrally toward the tricuspid orifice upon entering the right atrium. The catheter should then be connected to a pressure transducer for monitoring and recording intracardiac pressures. A right-heart pressure pullback is recommended after BWP placement with documentation of PA, RV, and RA pressures, and calculation of any transvalvular gradients prior to balloon dilation. Pressure recordings are advised prior to angiography so that hemodynamic reactions to contrast agents do not skew measurements. The catheter tip is then placed into the right atrium for angiography, typically utilizing 0.5–1 ml/kg of iodinated contrast agent delivered by hand-injection. Pressure injection is not typically needed due to impaired right ventricular filling/atrial emptying secondary to the stenosis. The angiogram documents the position of the stenotic orifice and rules out the presence of an atrial-level shunt (Figure 61.7, Video 61.5). A RV angiogram may also be performed to semiquantitatively assess the degree of tricuspid regurgitation and rule out a ventricular-level shunt, although this is not considered a necessity if there has been a complete preoperative echocardiographic evaluation. All angiograms should be recorded to allow playback and generation of a roadmap to aid in positioning of the balloon catheter(s).

After an adequate pressure pullback and angiogram have been performed, the BWP is again placed in the PA and the flexible J-tip of an appropriately sized guide wire is advanced through the catheter and into a distal pulmonary artery branch. If the catheter utilized for initial access was limited in size by a small patient, one or more catheter and guide wire exchanges may be necessary to allow placement of a guide wire with a diameter sufficient for the chosen balloon catheter (typically 0.035″ guide wire, 6 Fr BWP). If utilizing a double balloon technique, the second BWP and wire are placed at this time, either from the same vein (if the patient is large enough) or from a second venous access point (Figure 61.8). Once an appropriately sized guide wire(s) is (are) in place, the chosen balloon dilation catheter(s) is (are) advanced over the wire and positioned with fluoroscopic guidance across the tricuspid annulus. The fluoroscopy beam may need to be adjusted at this time to achieve optimal (perpendicular) alignment with the long axis of the balloon(s). Using an

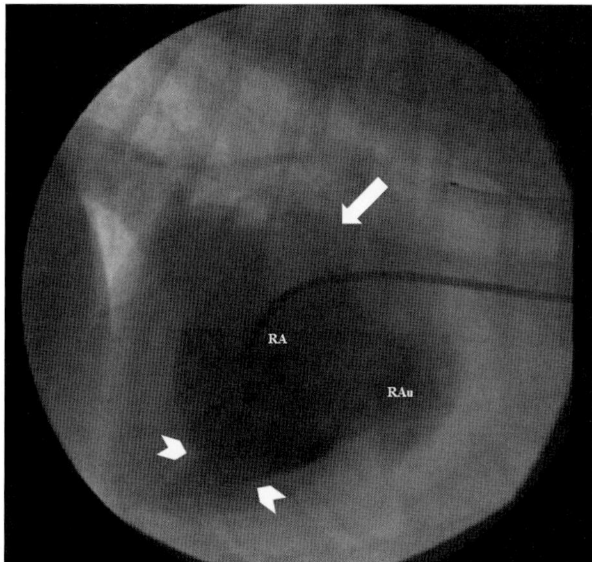

Figure 61.7 Still angiographic image obtained following injection of iodinated contrast with the catheter tip in the right atrium demonstrating a markedly dilated right atrium and right auricular appendage, retrograde filling of a distended caudal vena cava, a markedly stenotic tricuspid valve orifice (arrowheads) and faint blushing of a pulmonary artery (arrow). RA – right atrium, Rau – right auricular appendage. Image used with permission of Dr. Geri Lake Bakaar.

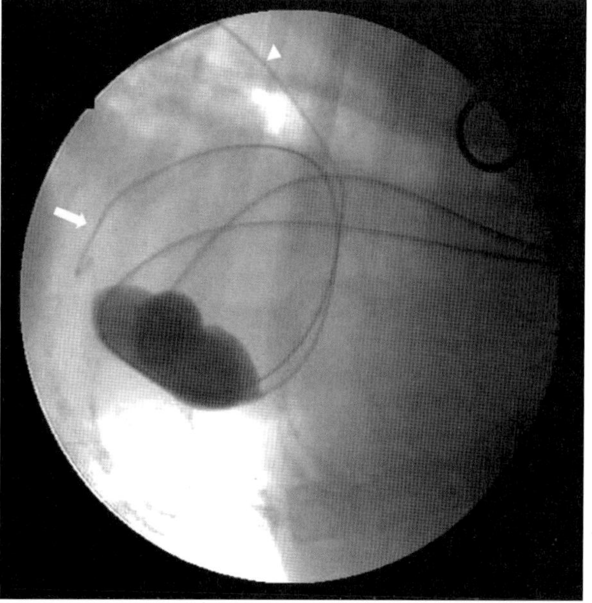

Figure 61.8 Still fluoroscopic image demonstrating a double technique using the jugular approach for both balloons in a canine patient with severe tricuspid stenosis and residual symptoms one year after balloon dilation with a single balloon. A jugular cut-down was utilized to facilitate passage of both balloons through a venotomy. Severe right atrial enlargement has resulted in displacement of the tricuspid annulus so that it is not perpendicular to the fluoroscopy beam. Ideally the fluoroscope would be adjusted to allow for better visualization of the long axis of the balloons during inflation. The guide wire tips are positioned in caudal (arrowhead) and accessory (arrow) pulmonary artery branches.

empty syringe, repeated aspiration is often performed to remove any air from the inflation balloon(s) and catheter(s) before balloon inflation. Once aspiration is negative for air, a syringe of adequate volume pre-filled with a 1:1 or 1:2 mixture of iodinated contrast and saline is used for balloon inflation(s). Inflation is recommended to the manufacturer's nominal pressure as rapidly as possible to attempt to engage the stenotic orifice. This often requires several attempts, with the most common pitfalls including improper balloon positioning, asynchronous inflation (double-balloon technique) or movement of an incompletely filled balloon antegrade or retrograde into the right ventricle or right atrium, respectively. As with other balloon dilation procedures, visualization of a "waist" in the balloon(s) at the level of the stenotic orifice is necessary to ensure that the affected valve has been engaged appropriately and that the chosen balloon is of sufficient diameter to effectively dilate the valve. Once subjectively adequate balloon dilation has occurred (ideally with a sudden disappearance of the balloon waist), the balloon(s) is (are) deflated as rapidly as possible to minimize reductions in cardiac output that occur with obstruction of the valvular orifice, and the balloons are removed while leaving the guide wires in place.

Post-dilation assessment involves replacing the BWP catheter over a guide wire and performing a post-dilation right heart pressure pullback. Although guidelines for successful balloon dilation have not been described in the veterinary literature, a reduction in the mean trans-valvular gradient to ≤5 mmHg has been adequate in the author's experience to result in resolution of right heart failure symptoms. If initial dilation attempts do not achieve an adequate reduction in RA pressure or transvalvular gradient, repeated balloon dilation with a larger balloon diameter, or converting to a double balloon technique, should be considered. Right atrial/ventricular angiography should also be repeated as described previously, with subjective evaluation of the stenotic orifice, severity of tricuspid regurgitation, and time of clearance of contrast from the RA after RA injection. Once adequate dilation of the stenotic orifice has been achieved and all catheters and introducers have been removed, a venotomy can be salvaged using a purse-string suture of 3–0 or 4–0 silk around the venotomy site. Closure of an open cut-down should follow standard surgical protocol to minimize dead space and provide an adequate number of closure layers. When percutaneous venous access has been utilized, an introducer can be

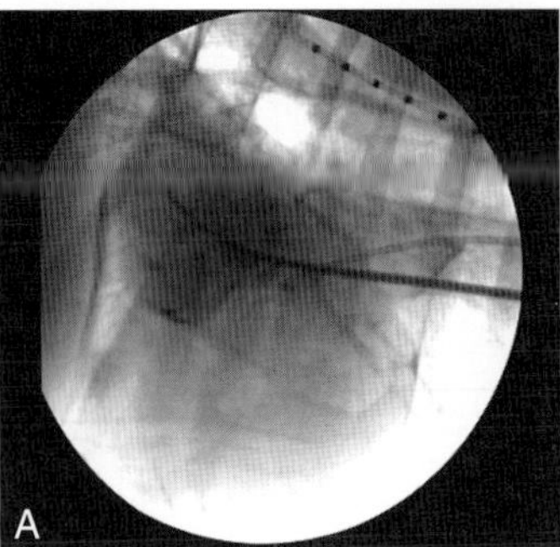

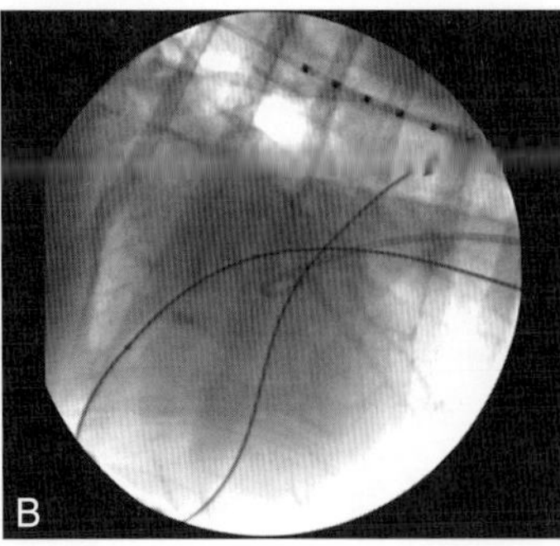

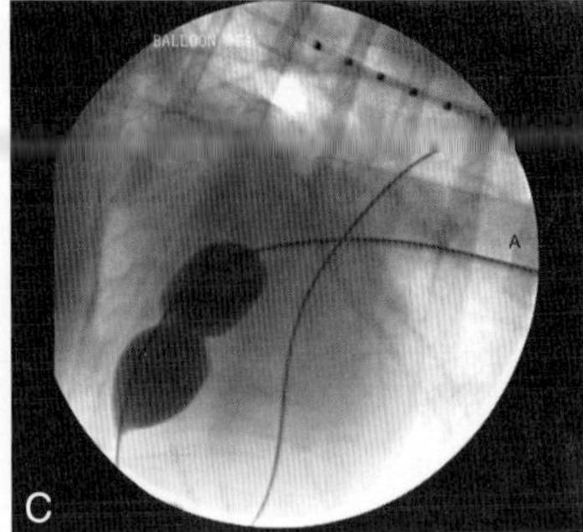

Figure 61.9 Still fluoroscopic images of a canine patient with severe mitral stenosis undergoing balloon dilation via a transseptal approach. (A) Left atrial angiogram recorded after the introducer has passed from the cranial vena cava and right atrium through an atrial septostomy created by a transseptal (Brockenbrough) needle. A pigtail catheter is visible in the ascending aorta. (B) Guide wire positioning for placement of a balloon dilation catheter. The wire course is as follows: cranial cava, right atrium, atrial septostomy, left atrium, mitral orifice, left ventricle, and aorta. (C) Partial balloon inflation has resulted in a waist at the level of the stenosis. Image used with permission from Arndt, J.W., Oyama, M.A. (2013) Balloon valvuloplasty of congenital mitral stenosis. Journal of Veterinary Cardiology, 15(2), 147–151, Elsevier.

left in place at the clinician's preference to provide central venous access postoperatively.

Mitral Stenosis

Until recently, minimally invasive balloon dilation of mitral stenosis had not been described in the veterinary literature and all case reports were anecdotal. The only current case reports utilize the standard human approach of atrial transseptal puncture or a hybrid surgical technique, introducing balloon dilation catheters directly through the left atrial wall via a thoracotomy. The Suggested Reading list should be consulted for detailed description of these procedures. In brief, venous access is similar to the tricuspid valve although only the jugular vein approach has been described in dogs. Transseptal catheterization is accomplished with use of an introducer through which a Brockenbrough needle is used to cross the interatrial septum. Transesophageal echocardiography may be beneficial in guiding needle placement and helping to avoid perforation of the atrial wall or the aorta. After traversing the atrial septum, the introducer is advanced through the septostomy and the Brockenbrough needle is retracted. A guide wire of appropriate size is passed through the introducer and then the mitral orifice. As with right heart procedures, the flexible J-tip should be passed first, and excess wire should extend into the left ventricle and proximal aorta to minimize the risk of damage from antegrade balloon movement during inflation. In smaller patients, wire manipulation and advancement may be difficult in the left ventricular apex, requiring passage of a snare or other intravascular retrieval device retrograde through the aortic valve via a carotid approach to grasp the distal end of the guide wire in the left ventricle. After an appropriate pressure pullback (aorta, left ventricle, left atrium), documentation of any transvalvular gradients, and left atrial/ventricular angiography as described for tricuspid stenosis, a balloon catheter is advanced over the guide wire and across the stenotic orifice for valvular dilation. With the exception of the modified surgical approach and transseptal puncture, the technique and protocol for catheter manipulation and balloon dilation is similar to balloon tricuspid valvuloplasty once access to the mitral valve is obtained. Figure 61.9 illustrates several steps in balloon mitral valvuloplasty including appropriate positioning of the wire guide and dilation balloon.

Follow-Up

As with other cardiac catheterization procedures, recovery should be in an intensive care unit where invasive pressure and continuous ECG monitoring are available. Because minimally invasive procedures are not particularly painful, post-operative analgesia is minimal and often provided by agents used for sedation. Patients should continue to receive IV fluid therapy until they are able to eat/drink voluntarily, as this will facilitate delivery of medication via continuous rate infusion if necessary (lidocaine, dobutamine, etc.). Continued antibiotic therapy is used at the discretion of the attending veterinarian. An echocardiogram should be performed the following day to evaluate the stenotic orifice area, transvalvular gradient, and degree of A-V valve insufficiency. The patient should be seen at the time of suture removal, and if receiving medical therapy prior to the procedure, weaning of individual medications can be considered at that time. Diuretic therapy may be weaned first, assuming adequate dilation of the affected valve and relief of the clinical signs of congestion. The decision whether to wean or discontinue other cardiac medications should be individualized to the patient's specific condition, residual symptoms, and comorbidities (persistent arrhythmias, pulmonary hypertension, additional congenital anomalies, etc.). Additional follow-up evaluations should be individualized as well, although once yearly recheck echocardiography should be considered at a minimum to monitor for evidence of restenosis or other complications.

Suggested Reading

Arndt JW and Oyama MA (2013) Balloon valvuloplasty of congenital mitral stenosis. *J Vet Cardiol* 15(2), 147–51.

Ashraf T, Pathan A, and Kundi A (2008) Percutaneous balloon valvuloplasty of coexisting mitral and rricuspid stenosis: Single-wire, double balloon technique. *J Invas Cardiol* 20(4), 1–5.

Boon JA (2011) Stenotic lesions. In: *Veterinary Echocardiography*, 2nd edn Wiley-Blackwell, Chichester, UK. pp. 477–525.

Boccuzzi G, Gigli N, Cian D, et al (2009) Percutaneous transcatheter balloon valvuloplasty for severe tricuspid valve stenosis in Ebstein's anomaly. *J Cardiovasc Med* 10, 510–15.

Brown WA and Thomas WP (1995) Balloon valvuloplasty of tricuspid stenosis in a Labrador retriever. *J Vet Intern Med* 1(6), 419–25.

Egred M, Albouaini K, Morrison WL, et al (2006) Balloon valvuloplasty of a stenosed bioprosthetic tricuspid valve. *Circulation* 113, e745–e747.

Harle T, Kronberg K, Motz R, et al (2010) Balloon valvuloplasty of a tricuspid valve stenosis in a double balloon technique. *Clini Res Cardiol* 99, 203–5.

Hussain T, Knight WB, and McLeod K (2009) Lead-induced tricuspid stenosis – successful management by balloon angioplasty. *Pace* 32, 140–2.

Kunze CP, Abbott JA, Hamilton SM, et al (2002) Balloon valvuloplasty for palliative treatment of tricuspid stenosis with right-to-left atrial-level shunting in a dog. *J Am Vet Med Assoc* 220(4), 491–6.

Lake-Bakaar G, Griffiths LG, and Kittleson MD (2013) Balloon valvuloplasty of tricuspid valve stenosis: a retrospective study of 5 labrador retrievers. *J Vet Intern Med* 27, 641–2, Abstract C-46.

Oyama MA, Weidman JA, and Cole SG (2008) Calculation of pressure half-time. *J Vet Cardiol* 10(1), 57–60.

Patel TM, Dani SI, Shah SC, et al (1996) Tricuspid balloon valvuloplasty: A more simplified approach using Inuoe balloon. *Catheteriz Cardiovasc Diagn* 37, 86–8.

Ribiero PA, al Zaibag M, and Idris MT (1990) Percutanous double balloon tricuspid valvotomy for severe tricuspid stenosis: 3 year follow-up study. *Eur Heart J* 11, 1109–12.

Sancaktar O, Kumbasar SD, Semiz E, et al (1998) Late results of combined percutaneous balloon valvuloplasty of mitral and tricuspid valves. *Catheteriz Cardiovascr Diagn* 45, 246–50.

Sharma S, Loya YS, Desai DM, et al (1997) Percutaneous double valve balloon valvotomy for multivalve stenosis: Immediate results and intermediate term follow-up. *Am Heart J* 133, 64–70.

Trehiou-Sechi E, Behr L, Chetboul V, et al (2011) Echo-guided closed commissurotomy for mitral valve stenosis in a dog. *J Vet Cardiol* 13(3), 219–25.

Video 61.1 Left apical four-chamber echocardiogram from a canine patient with severe tricuspid stenosis and valvular anatomy that may be amenable to balloon dilation. Echocardiography reveals elongated, relatively mobile tricuspid valve leaflets that are tethered at their margins resulting in doming of the valves in diastole and minimal subvalvular pathology or tethering. This patient also had mild tricuspid regurgitation.

Video 61.2 Left apical four-chamber echocardiogram from a canine patient with severe tricuspid stenosis and valvular anatomy that is not conducive to balloon dilation. The valve leaflets are tethered and relatively immobile, with significant subvalvular pathology and marked apical displacement that would make manipulation of catheters/balloons difficult.

Video 61.3 Fluoroscopic video of a canine patient undergoing balloon valvuloplasty for severe tricuspid stenosis utilizing a femoral venous approach. The video demonstrates appropriate positioning of the distal guide wire tip in the peripheral pulmonary arteries. Video used with permission of Dr. Geri Lake-Bakaar.

Video 61.4 Fluoroscopic video of a canine patient undergoing balloon valvuloplasty for severe tricuspid stenosis utilizing a jugular venous approach. The guide wire tip is only into the right ventricle. In this example, antegrade migration of the balloon through the stenotic orifice under high pressure could result in right ventricular freewall trauma or cardiac perforation. Video used with permission of Dr. Geri Lake-Bakaar.

Video 61.5 Angiogram obtained from injection of iodinated contrast with the catheter tip in the right atrium demonstrating a markedly dilated right atrium and right auricular appendage, retrograde filling of a distended caudal vena cava, a markedly stenotic valve orifice, and opacification of the right ventricle and pulmonary artery in the late stages of the angiogram. Video used with permission of Dr. Geri Lake-Bakaar.

These video clips can be found in the online material at **www.wiley.com/go/weisse/vet-image-guided-interventions**

CHAPTER SIXTY-TWO

Cor Triatriatum

Bruce W. Keene and Sandra P. Tou
North Carolina State University, College of Veterinary Medicine, Raleigh, NC

Introduction

Cor triatriatum is the Latin term for a triatrial heart – literally, a heart with three atria. First reported in humans in 1868, cor triatriatum is a congenital heart defect in which either the right (cor triatriatum dexter) or left atrium (cor triatriatum sinister) is divided into two compartments by a membrane, a fold of tissue, or a fibromuscular band. Because the clinical presentation of cor triatriatum depends entirely on which atrium is affected, the right- and left-sided forms of cor triatriatum are outlined separately below.

Cor Triatriatum Dexter

Background/Indications

Cor triatriatum dexter (CTd) is a rare congenital cardiac defect in human and veterinary medicine, resulting from persistence of the right valve of the sinus venosus. CTd is thought to account for only 0.1% of human congenital heart disease, and only 0.3% of canine congenital heart disease. While CTd has been well described in the dog, the condition remains unreported in cats.

During embryogenesis, the right horn of the sinus venosus is incorporated into the developing right atrium to form the smooth posterior portion of the right atrium. The true embryologic right atrium forms the remaining anterior (trabeculated) portion of the right atrium. The larger right valve of the sinus venosus, which guards the right horn, partially divides the right atrium and functions during early fetal life to direct oxygenated blood from the caudal vena cava across the foramen ovale. Failure of the right sinus valve to regress causes CTd, and the resulting intra-atrial membrane separates the smooth from the trabeculated portions of the right atrium, dividing the right atrium into a cranial and caudal chamber. Most commonly, the cranial chamber communicates with the cranial vena cava, tricuspid annulus and right auricular appendage, while the caudal chamber (termed the sinus venarum) receives the caudal vena cava and coronary sinus. The fossa ovalis is typically present in the caudal chamber, and may result in a right-to-left shunt if patent. Although a single perforation in the abnormal membrane dividing the right atrium appears to be the most common manifestation of the defect, the abnormal membrane can take a variety of forms, ranging from a partial reticulum to a complete, imperforate sheet of tissue. The obstruction to blood flow between the caudal and cranial portions of the right atrium created by the abnormal membrane causes high intravascular pressures within the caudal right atrial chamber. This pressure gradient drives continuous, usually turbulent, blood flow across whatever fenestration is present in the abnormal membrane.

The severity of the clinical signs caused by CTd depends on the severity of obstruction to intra-atrial blood flow. High intravascular pressures in the caudal chamber cause elevated caudal caval and hepatic venous pressures that may result in hepatomegaly and ascites. In cases in which the abnormal membrane is extensively fenestrated, CTd may go undetected. Severely affected animals often present with symptoms commonly associated with right heart failure, including abdominal distension (ascites), lethargy, inappetence, weight loss and diarrhea. As the cranial vena cava typically enters the low-pressure cranial right atrial chamber, jugular venous distension is absent. In humans, other symptoms may relate to concurrent cardiac defects. In dogs, CTd has generally been reported as an isolated defect.

Veterinary Image-Guided Interventions, First Edition. Edited by Chick Weisse and Allyson Berent.

Companion website: www.wiley.com/go/weisse/vet-image-guided-interventions

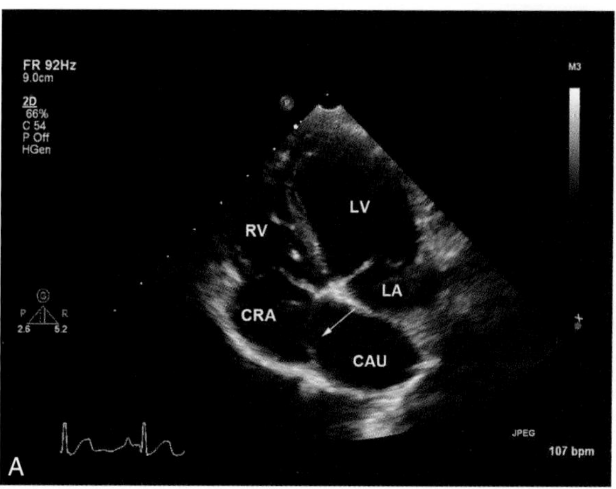

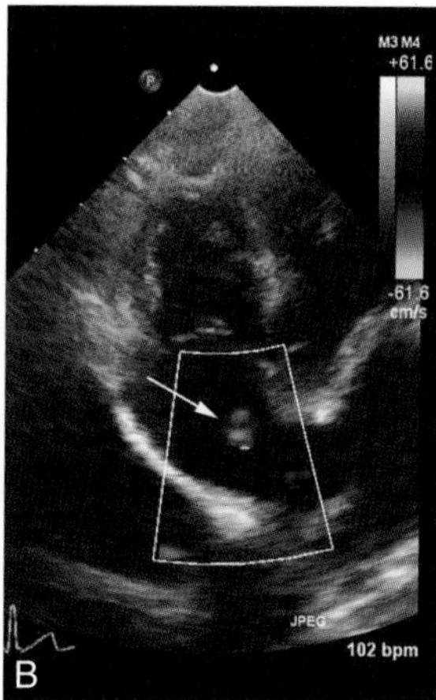

Figure 62.1 Echocardiographic left apical views of the heart of a dog with cor triatriatum dexter. (A) A membrane divides the right atrium into cranial (CRA) and caudal (CAU) portions; the arrow denotes the anomalous membrane. Also visualized are right ventricle (RV), left ventricle (LV), and left atrium (LA). (B) Color flow Doppler shows blood flow disturbance across a perforated intra-atrial membrane. The arrow indicates abnormal color flow across the membrane. From LeBlanc et al. Cutting balloon catheterization for interventional treatment of cor triatriatum dexter: 2 cases. J Vet Cardiol 2012;14:525–530. Used with permission from Elsevier.

Patient Preparation

Animals are typically placed on medical therapy consisting of furosemide 2–4 mg/kg PO, q8–12 hr and enalapril 0.5 mg/kg PO, q12 hr if ascites is present. However, resolution of the obstruction to caudal venous return is the only way to adequately control abdominal effusion in these patients. Complete preoperative echocardiography with color and spectral Doppler imaging is required and a definitive diagnosis of CTd can usually be obtained with two-dimensional (2-D) echocardiography. Right- and left-sided views reveal the abnormal membrane, which divides the right atrium into discrete subchambers (Figure 62.1A). Color and spectral Doppler interrogation of the resulting blood flow demonstrates continuous, relatively low-velocity flow across the membrane if a fenestration is present (Figure 62.1B). Applying the modified Bernoulli equation, flow velocity can be used to estimate caudal chamber pressure. Bowing of the membrane towards the cranial chamber may occur during ventricular systole. An agitated saline contrast (i.e., microbubble) study can aid in the diagnosis of CTd, as microbubbles from a cephalic vein injection opacify the cranial right atrial chamber, while a saphenous vein injection opacifies the caudal chamber and best demonstrates the stenosis (Arndt and Oyama, 2008). In cases with an imperforate or severely restrictive membrane, anomalous venous drainage (e.g., via a dilated azygous vein) around the complete obstruction and/or retrograde flow into the coronary sinus and great cardiac vein can typically be identified.

Potential Risks/Complications/Expected Outcomes

The prognosis for dogs undergoing successful catheter-based dilation of the CTd membrane is considered good to excellent. Ascites typically reduces and resolves within days. While no survival data exists for dogs treated medically, reports from dogs treated by balloon dilation imply routine long-term survival. Complications associated with catheter-based dilation of CTd are not well described, but anecdotal reports of right atrial or vena caval rupture, hemorrhage, and death exist.

Procedure

The traditional treatment for symptomatic patients was surgical excision of the dividing membrane. The option of open heart surgery in veterinary patients remains limited to few institutions equipped and experienced with cardiopulmonary bypass (Tanaka et al, 2003). Other invasive surgical techniques have been reported with variable success, including septectomy under inflow occlusion, modified patch-graft technique and use of a valve dilator. Over the past 10 years, transvenous catheter-based balloon dilation has been performed in dogs with CTd and is now widely considered an accepted and effective alternative to invasive surgery (Adin and Thomas, 1999, Johnson et al, 2005, LeBlanc et al, 2012).

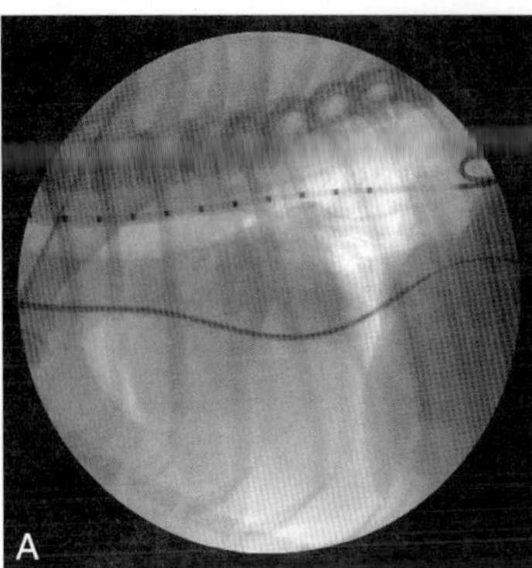

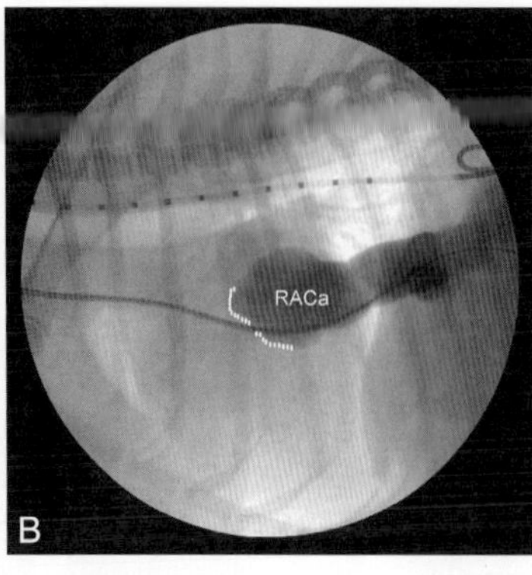

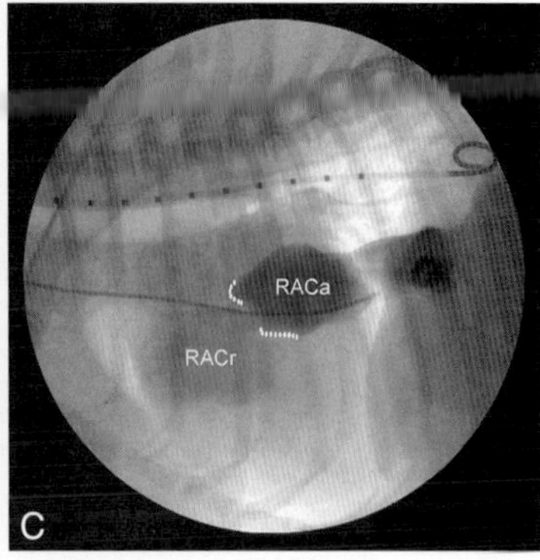

Figure 62.2 Angiographic images from a dog with cor triatriatum dexter. (A) A guidewire has been advanced from the jugular vein antegrade across the restrictive membrane and down the caudal vena cava. A double lumen catheter (to allow maintenance of wire position) was then advanced over the guide wire with the tip positioned in the caudal vena cava. (B) Iodinated contrast is infused through the second port of the double lumen catheter to highlight the caudal vena cava, caudal right atrium (RACa) and obstructive membrane (dashed line). Note that contrast does not opacify the cranial right atrium. (C) Following balloon dilation, contrast can be seen streaming into the cranial right atrium through a larger fenestration in the anomalous membrane (dashed line) and the cranial right atrium (RACr) can now be visualized. Image courtesy of Brian A. Scansen.

The use of a cutting balloon catheter followed by traditional balloon dilation is the treatment of choice at the authors' institution for dogs with CTd (LeBlanc et al, 2012). In contrast to conventional balloon inflation that causes stretching and irregular tearing of the abnormal membrane, cutting balloons contain 3–4 embedded blades (microtomes), designed to create regular, radially-oriented cuts when inflated (Coe et al, 1996). Although successful traditional balloon dilation of CTd has been described in dogs, unsuccessful (Miller et al, 1989) and anecdotal reports of fatal balloon dilation attempts associated with atrial wall fracture also exist. Because some membranes may be more fibrotic, the use of a cutting balloon prior to balloon dilation may improve both the efficacy of the subsequent dilatation as well as the safety of the procedure. In a presumably analogous situation, using a cutting balloon followed by a traditional atrial septostomy balloon has been demonstrated to create cleaner and more consistent tearing of the interatrial septum in humans (Coe et al, 1996).

Under general anesthesia, an introducer sheath is placed into the femoral vein either percutaneously or directly by surgical cutdown using the modified Seldinger technique (see Chapter 44). If the femoral vein is deemed inadequate in size to accommodate the appropriate size introducer, venous access can be obtained percutaneously through a right jugular approach, and the guide wire advanced antegrade through the ostium (Figure 62.2). An end-hole multipurpose catheter is advanced into the caudal vena cava under fluoroscopic guidance. Selective angiography is performed using a nonionic, iodinated contrast material (e.g., iohexol) for confirmation and location of the membrane (Figure 62.2). Contrast injection into the caudal chamber reveals a dilated subchamber with varying amounts of contrast flow across the abnormal membrane's fenestration(s).

The diameter of the membrane ostium can be determined by angiography or transesophageal echocardiography. The catheter is then advanced to obtain pressure readings within the caudal and cranial atrial subchambers. An 0.014 or 0.018″ diameter × 260 cm long exchange wire (sized as recommended by the cutting balloon manufacturer), is placed across the membrane orifice and a cutting balloon is advanced over the wire and centered across the membrane. The cutting balloon is sized according to the diameter of the ostium, with optimal diameter being not more than 2 mm larger than the diameter of the opening. The balloon is then inflated three times to a maximal inflation pressure. When deflating a cutting balloon, slow and steady withdrawal of fluid is key to allow proper refolding of the cutting blades into the balloon. The cutting balloon is then removed, and a conventional balloon catheter is advanced over the wire, centered in the defect and inflated in a similar manner (Figure 62.3). The size of balloon is determined as the approximate diameter of the membrane or caudal vena cava. Pressure measurements are repeated following balloon withdrawal prior to completion of the procedure.

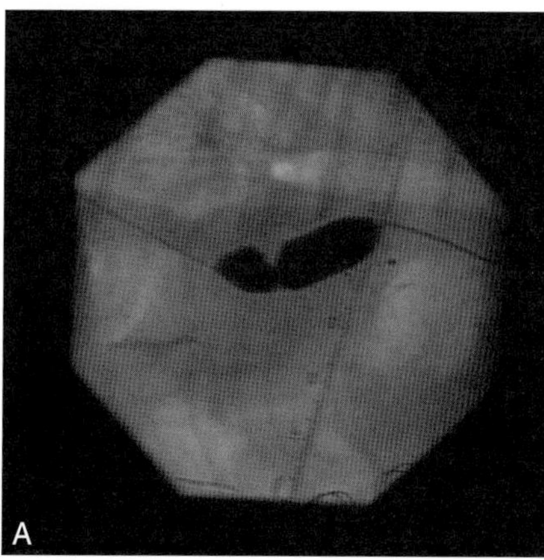

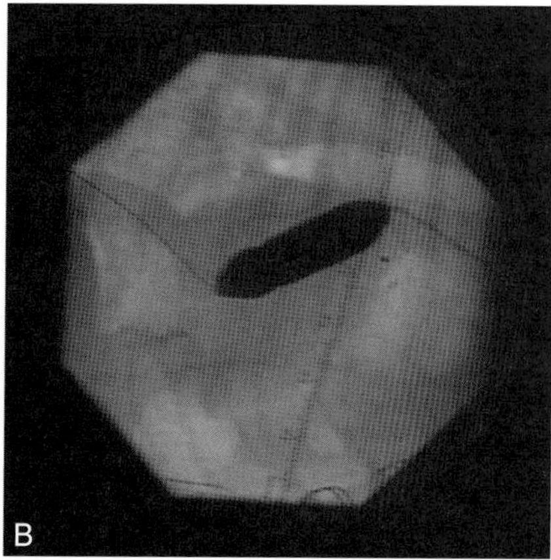

Figure 62.3 Fluoroscopic views of conventional balloon dilation after cutting balloon dilation in a dog with cor triatriatum dexter. (A) The catheter waist is formed by the scored anomalous septum dividing right atrium into cranial and caudal chambers. (B) With further balloon inflation and increased pressure, the waist is relieved consistent with tearing and opening of the restrictive membrane. From LeBlanc et al. Cutting balloon catheterization for interventional treatment of cor triatriatum dexter: 2 cases. J Vet Cardiol 2012;14:525–530. Used with permission from Elsevier.

Follow-up

Diuretic therapy may be weaned over the subsequent 12 weeks pending response to the intervention. Repeat echocardiography is advised in 1 month and again in 1 year. If no change in the transmembrane gradient is detected at that time, further follow-up is likely unnecessary unless clinical signs recur.

Cor Triatriatum Sinister

Background/Indications

Cor triatriatum sinister (CTs) is a rare congenital cardiac defect characterized by the presence of an abnormal membrane subdividing the left atrium into two segments. Because CTs is far more common that CTd in humans, many authors mean CTs when they refer to cor triatriatum. In animals, CTd appears more common in the dog while CTs is seen most frequently in the cat.

The most widely accepted cause of CTs is failure of incorporation of the common pulmonary vein into the left atrium during embryogenesis. The result is an abnormal fibromuscular diaphragm that divides the left atrium into a posterosuperior (proximal or caudal) accessory chamber and an anteroinferior (distal or cranial) true left atrial chamber. In most cases, the proximal chamber receives all the pulmonary veins, while the distal chamber connects with the left atrial appendage, the fossa ovalis and the mitral valve orifice. Less commonly, partial or total anomalous pulmonary venous connections are present. The partitioning membrane of CTs typically contains a single fenestration or ostium, but the membrane morphology can vary from multiple fenestrations to imperforate. The degree of communication between chambers produces varying degrees of obstruction of pulmonary venous return and that obstruction determines the severity of clinical signs. Patients with initially non-obstructed flow may experience a delayed onset of symptoms, or may remain asymptomatic throughout their lifetime.

Pathophysiologically, the fibromuscular membrane obstructs/impedes pulmonary venous flow into the left atrium and creates an intra-atrial pressure gradient. The associated elevation in pulmonary venous pressure may cause pulmonary edema in the lung lobes drained by the obstructed veins, and may result in reactive pulmonary arterial hypertension.

The clinical presentation of affected patients is dependent on the degree of pulmonary venous obstruction. Humans with CTs are typically symptomatic at birth, and affected animals generally show symptoms of congestive heart failure within a few years of life. Affected cats may present with symptoms such as respiratory distress, lethargy, anorexia and coughing (Wander et al, 1998, Heaney and Bulmer, 2004, Stern et al, 2013).

Patient Preparation

Most cases of CTs can be diagnosed accurately with 2-D transthoracic echocardiography, the diagnostic modality of choice for classic CTs in humans. The partitioning membrane is seen proximal to (i.e. above) the mitral valve, creating a double-chamber left atrium

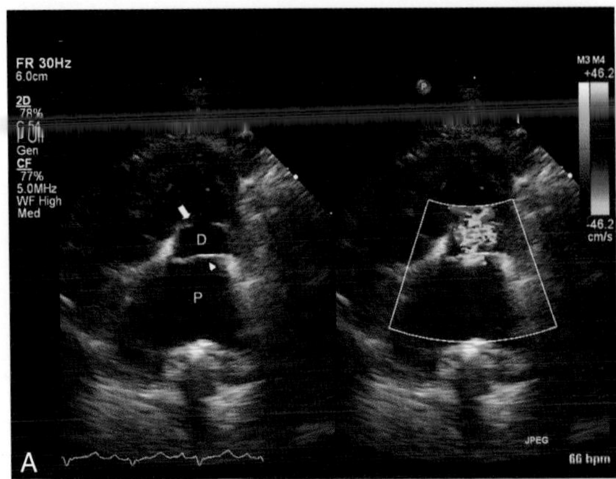
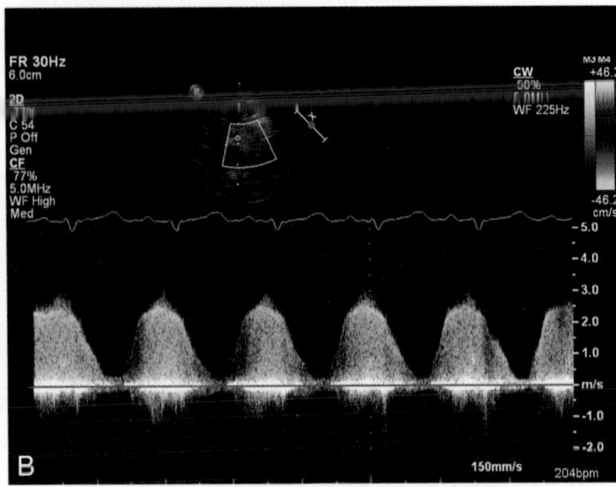

Figure 62.4 Two-dimensional left apical views of the heart of a cat with cor triatriatum sinister. (A) An anomalous membrane divides the left atrium into proximal and distal subchambers. A small communication is visible within the membrane. (B) Spectral Doppler shows high velocity diastolic flow across the membrane. From Stern JA et al. Hybrid cutting balloon dilatation for treatment of cor triatriatum sinister in a cat. J Vet Cardiol 2013; 15:205–210. Used with permission from Elsevier.

(Figure 62.4A). Color-flow Doppler shows relatively high-velocity, turbulent flow across the membrane orifice, allowing for calculation of the intra-atrial pressure gradient, using the modified Bernoulli equation (Figure 62.4B). Bowing of the membrane towards the mitral orifice may occur during diastole. Identification of the left atrial appendage and its relationship to the membrane distinguishes cor triatriatum from the primary differential diagnosis of supravalvular mitral valve stenosis (Fine et al, 2002). Transesophageal echocardiography may offer improved assessment of atrial morphology, and may be particularly useful intraoperatively to evaluate repair success. Other diagnostic modalities, including three-dimensional echocardiography, computerized tomography and magnetic resonance imaging, may aid in the diagnosis of CTs, particularly in patients with concurrent cardiac defects.

The cat should be stabilized with medical therapy prior to intervention. For cats in congestive heart failure, this includes furosemide (1 to 3 mg/kg PO, q12 hr), enalapril (0.5 mg/kg PO, q12–24 hr), and clopidogrel (18.75 mg/cat PO, q24 hr). Immediately prior to the procedure, thoracic radiographs, complete blood count, biochemical profile, blood type, and repeat echocardiography should be evaluated.

Potential Risks/Complications/ Expected Outcomes

Long-term prognosis is considered excellent in humans undergoing complete surgical excision of the diaphragm. An excellent prognosis also appears to be a reasonable expectation for cats undergoing surgical correction using a valve dilator (Wander et al, 1998) or balloon dilation through a hybrid approach (Stern et al, 2013). Complications of balloon dilation of CTs in animals are not reported, but risk of hemorrhage, fracture of the atrial wall, or an inability to dilate the stenotic membrane are theoretical risks of the procedure.

Procedure

Definitive treatment of CTs is complete surgical excision of the membrane, and surgery is recommended in all symptomatic human patients. Successful surgical membrane excision in small animals is limited by the need for cardiopulmonary bypass. Successful surgical correction of CTs without cardiopulmonary bypass using a valve dilator introduced through a left atriotomy has been reported in the cat (Wander et al, 1998). Other anecdotal reports utilizing this technique show mixed long-term results, with at least one patient experiencing "restenosis" of the membrane months after the initial dilatation (E. Hardie, personal communication, 2013). Percutaneous balloon dilation has been successfully reported as an alternative nonsurgical treatment option in humans (Huang et al, 2002). In such cases, access to the accessory left atrial chamber is typically obtained through a transseptal approach from the femoral vein, followed by inflation of a balloon angioplasty catheter or Inoue balloon catheter across the membrane orifice. A similar method in veterinary medicine is complicated by the small size of the feline atrium and limited sheath size that can be accommodated by the jugular or femoral vein of a small cat. At the authors' institution, a hybrid surgical approach is used involving surgical exposure of the heart and interventional balloon dilation of the CTs membrane (Stern et al, 2013). A left lateral thoracotomy is performed to access the left atrium and a purse string suture is placed in the apex of the left auricular appendage prior to left auricular access via an 18-gauge needle. An 0.014 or 0.018″, 180 cm, J-tip guide wire, sized as specified by the cutting balloon manufacturer, is advanced into the left auricle and true left atrium. The wire is then directed across the membrane ostium into the accessory left atrial chamber under transesophageal echocardiographic control. A sheath introducer (5 Fr, 4 cm) is then passed over the guide wire across the membrane ostium and into the caudal, high pressure chamber. A cutting balloon catheter is then prepped, purged, and flushed and advanced into the sheath, and centered across the ostium, followed by inflation of the cutting balloon to score and dilate the membrane. The cutting balloon is sized as for CTd, ideally 1 mm (and not more than 2 mm) larger than the ostial diameter. The procedure is then repeated using a standard valvuloplasty balloon (e.g., sized to approximate the membrane diameter) to dilate the scored membrane. Transesophageal or epicardial echocardiography is used to verify improved ostial opening and a reduction/elimination of the estimated intra-atrial pressure gradient. The sheath and wire are then removed and the purse-string suture tied to close the auricular access. The thorax is closed routinely after placement of a chest tube for evacuation of air and fluid from the thorax. Recovery should take place in an intensive care unit with standard monitoring and analgesia. This method has been reported in a cat, with excellent results and no evidence of restenosis at 12 month follow-up (Stern et al, 2013).

Follow-Up

The membrane's patency should be assessed by echocardiography the day following the procedure, and again at the time of suture removal. Diuretic therapy may be discontinued in the week following intervention pending respiratory status and thoracic radiographic resolution of pulmonary edema. Benazepril and clopidogrel are typically continued for an additional 3 months prior to discontinuation. Standard echocardiographic rechecks are advised in 3 months and at 1 year, if the cat is stable.

References

Adin DB and Thomas WP (1999) Balloon dilation of cor triatriatum dexter in a dog. *J Vet Intern Med* 13, 6176–19.

Arndt JW and Oyama MA (2008) Agitated saline contrast echocardiography to diagnose a congenital heart defect in a dog. *J Vet Cardiol* 10, 1291–32.

Coe JY, Chen RPC, Timinsky J, et al (1996) A novel method to create atrial septal defect using a cutting balloon in piglets. *Am J Cardiol* 78, 13231–326.

Fine DM, Tobias AH, and Jacob KA. (2002) Supravalvular mitral stenosis in a cat. *J Am Anim Hosp Assoc* 38, 4034–6.

Heaney AH and Bulmer BJ (2004) Cor triatriatum sinister and persistent left cranial vena cava in a kitten. *J Vet Intern Med* 18, 8958–98.

Huang TC, Lee CL, Lin CC, et al (2002) Use of Inoue balloon dilation method for treatment of cor triatriatum stenosis in a child. *Catheteriz Cardiovasc Intervent* 57, 2522–56.

Johnson MS, Martin M, DeGiovanni MM, et al (2004) Management of cor triatriatum dexter by balloon dilatation in three dogs. *J Small Anim Pract* 45, 162–70.

LeBlanc N, DeFrancesco TC, Adams AK, et al (2012) Cutting balloon catheterization for the treatment of cor triatriatum dexter: 2 cases. *J Vet Cardiol* 14, 5255–30.

Miller MW, Bonagura JD, DiBartola SP, et al (1989) Budd-chiari-like syndrome in two dogs. *J Am Anim Hosp Assoc* 25, 2772–83.

Stern JA, Tou SP, Barker PC, et al (2013) Hybrid cutting balloon dilatation for treatment of cor triatriatum sinister in a cat. *J Vet Cardiol*, 15, 205–10.

Tanaka R, Hoshi K, Shimizu M, et al (2003) Surgical correction of cor triatriatum dexter in a dog under extracorporeal circulation. *J Small Anim Pract* 44, 3703–73.

Wander KW, Monnet E, and Orton EC. (1998) Surgical correction of cor triatriatum sinister in a kitten. *J Am Anim Hosp Assoc* 34, 383–6.

Suggested Reading

Atkins C and DeFrancesco T (2000) Balloon dilation of cor triatriatum dexter in a dog. *J Vet Intern Med* 14, 471.

Kittleson MD (1998) Other congenital cardiovascular abnormalities. In: *Small Animal Cardiovascular Medicine* (Kittleson MD and Kienle RD, eds). Mosby, Inc., St. Louis, MO, pp. 2822–96.

CHAPTER SIXTY-THREE

Septal Defects

Sonya G. Gordon
Department of Small Animal Clinical Science, College of Veterinary Medicine and Biomedical Science, Texas A&M University, College Station, TX

Background and Indications

Hemodynamically significant atrial and ventricular septal defects (ASD, VSD) occur relatively infrequently as solitary congenital defects in the dog and cat. Some breeds are reportedly predisposed. Depending on the size and position of the defect, both ASD and VSD may be amendable to catheter based occlusion either via a percutaneous or a hybrid procedure that utilizes a thoracotomy. There are reports of both ASD and VSD occlusion with a variety of Amplatzer™ heart occluders (AHO) in individual dogs via both methods and one case series report on transcatheter atrial septal defect closure with the Amplatzer™ atrial septal occluder[1] (ASO) in 13 dogs. The author is unaware of any reports of catheter-based ASD or VSD occlusion in the cat. Publications in the veterinary literature to date, although scarce, have provided valuable information for those who wish to consider the use of these devices in clinical cases and this chapter will attempt to summarize this information. Since the majority of the available information pertains to ASD repair this chapter will emphasize this technique and highlight any relevant differences between ASD and VSD repair where warranted. Much of the information is summarized in Table 63.1.

Patient Preparation

In general, the most important criteria to consider for transcatheter (percutaneous or hybrid) ASD or VSD closure is the identification of a hemodynamically significant left-to-right shunt. The shunt fraction (Qp/Qs), typically determined by a comprehensive echocardiographic assessment, should be greater than 1.6 with accompanying evidence of secondary volume overload (ASD – right atrial and ventricular dilatation; VSD – left atrial and left ventricular dilatation) and pulmonary overcirculation.

Hemodynamically significant ASD and VSD can lead to congestive heart failure (CHF) that can manifest as pulmonary edema, with or without ascites and the commensurate clinical signs. Regardless of whether definitive repair is being considered, the initial treatment for CHF from a shunt is comparable to other causes: abdominocentesis as required, furosemide (2 to 4 mg/kg PO, q8–12 hr), angiotensin-converting enzyme inhibitor such as enalapril (0.5 mg/kg PO, q12 hr), pimobendan (0.25 mg/kg PO, q12 hr), and spironolactone (1 to 2 mg/kg PO, q12–24 hr). Sildenafil (2 mg/kg PO, q8–12 hr) and L-arginine (250 mg PO, q12 hr) may also be useful if pulmonary hypertension (PH) is documented.

Large left-to-right septal shunts (ASD or VSD) can lead to the development of PH. If and when pulmonary vascular resistance exceeds systemic vascular resistance, shunting can become right-to-left (Eisenmenger's physiology), which is a contraindication for definitive repair of the defect. Likewise, severe pulmonary valve stenosis (PS), in conjunction with ASD or VSD, represents a contraindication for repair unless the PS can also be palliated with balloon pulmonary valvuloplasty. Definitive repair can be considered in patients with ASD or VSD that have mild to moderate PH or PS. For example, if echocardiography shows that the direction of shunt flow is of low velocity but predominantly left-to-right, closure may still be considered. In fact, PH may decrease in severity and/or resolve following definitive repair, as may signs of CHF. Decisions regarding the feasibility of definitive repair in these types of cases need to be made on a case-by-case basis with careful consultation from a veterinary cardiologist.

Veterinary Image-Guided Interventions, First Edition. Edited by Chick Weisse and Allyson Berent.

Companion website: www.wiley.com/go/weisse/vet-image-guided-interventions

TABLE 63.1

Case selection, equipment, and potential approaches for transcatheter closure of septal defects in small animals

			Atrial septal defects	Ventricular septal defects
Septal defect case selection for closure with an Amplatzer™ heart occluders			• hemodynamically significant with or without clinical signs • left to right shunting • dogs • hybrid procedures should be considered for small dogs (puppies) and possibly cats whose size may limit percutaneous approaches, limited vascular access, e.g., persistent left cranial vena cava with absent right cranial vena cava	
Amenable defects			• secundum type defects • patent foramen ovale (PC) • 4<38 mm in size • adequate rim tissue (rim tissue 75% of circumference	• muscular, muscular perimembranous defects (>3–5.5 mm from aortic or AV valves) • 3<5.5 mm • 4<17.5 mm
Approach	Percutaneous	Arterial	NA	Femoral artery
		Venous	Jugular vein (preferred by author) Femoral vein	Jugular vein
	Hybrid		Transatrial through a right thoracotomy: Palpation of the ASD and TEE facilitated the placement of an introducer placed via a modified Seldinger technique through the right atrial wall adjacent to the ASD through which the ASO was deployed under TEE guidance Open transatrial approach through a right thoracotomy: transatrial deployment of ASO as described above followed by active ASO fixation through right atriotomy under temporary inflow occlusion.	Transventricular through a sternal thoracotomy: ventral midline pericardial incision over the right ventricular outflow tract. Palpation of the VSD through the RV wall in combination with epicardial echocardiography and TEE allowed placement of an introducer via a modified Seldinger technique, through which an ADOII was deployed under TEE guidance (PC)
Defect measurement and occluder selection (Note; TTE can be used to estimate device size prior to the procedure to facilitate acquisition of appropriate device inventory)			TEE, stop-flow balloon inflation under TEE and fluoroscopy, ICE	TEE, angiography, ICE, epicardial echocardiography (hybrid)
Occluder selection			None to minimal (0.5–2 mm) upsizing once largest diameter is measured. In general the device selected should be as close to the maximum measured diameter as possible. If there is no device in that size then select the next one up. Note: with the exception of the MFSO most devices increase in size by 1–2 mm increments and the device size pertains to the diameter of the deployed waist Other considerations for device selection include the size and proximity of the retention disks to adjacent cardiac structures (adequate margins to prevent erosion), volume of the chambers where the retention disks are deployed must be sufficient to accommodate the disk and the length of the waist (for VSD devices) must be sufficient to bridge the IVS.	
Amplatzer™ heart occluders used for septal defect closure			ASO [for ASD] sizes 4 to 38 mm PFO [for PFO] (PC) sizes 18 to 35 mm	mVSDO sizes 4 to 18 mm ADOII sizes 3 to 6 mm

(*continued*)

TABLE 63.1
(continued)

	Atrial septal defects	Ventricular septal defects
Delivery systems	Amplatzer™ TorqVue™ delivery systems include: delivery cable, delivery sheath & dilator, hemostasis port, loader, plastic vice. Sheath French sizes; 6, 7, 8, 9, 10, 12. All sheath sizes are available with a 45° tip angle and some can be ordered with 180°. Most are available in 60 cm length and some in 80 cm length. The Amplatzer™ TorqVue™ LP (low profile) delivery systems include the same supplies but come in a 4 and 5 French size through which the ADOII can be deployed Note: neither of the available tip angles are optimum for percutaneous deployment in the dog but the 45° is preferred by the author.	
Other equipment	0.35″ J-tipped exchange guide wire, and other basic supplies required for diagnostic catheterization Amplatzer™ sizing balloon II (20, 27,40 mm diameter)	
Intraoperative concerns	Heparinization during the procedure has been reported by some authors, but may not be necessary as long as the saline used to flush the device, sheath and catheters is heparinized Device embolization (this risk is minimized by gentle manipulation of the device prior to release, but due to the awkward angle we are forced to work with (re the sheath) it is sometimes difficult to assess because the proximal retention disk frequently does not take its native shape until it is released; likewise residual flow is sometimes not resolved until after the device is released.	
Perioperative concerns	An antithrombotic plan is recommended for 6 months beginning as soon as the dog wakes up (clopidogrel ± aspirin) Device embolization	

ASO, Amplatzer™ septal occluder; mVSDO, Amplatzer™ muscular VSD occluder; ADOII, Amplatzer™ duct occlude II; PFO, Amplatzer™ patent foramen ovale occlude; PC, personal communication; TTE, transthoracic echocardiography; TEE, transesophageal echocardiography; ICE, intracardiac echocardiography.

Criteria for Device Selection

Patients considered for ASD or VSD closure require careful evaluation of the morphology of the defect to confirm the patient is a reasonable candidate for transcatheter closure and to determine the size of the closure device needed. Such evaluations are made by a combination of transthoracic (TTE; Figure 63.1) and transesophageal echocardiographic (TEE; Figure 63.2) and/or intracardiac echocardiographic (ICE) imaging. Three-dimensional echocardiographic (3D) evaluation may also be useful if available. Direct epicardial imaging may also be useful during hybrid procedures. For ASD closure, sizing with a balloon catheter[2] (Amplatzer™ sizing balloon II) under fluoroscopic guidance at the time of the procedure is also recommended. Although actual device selection is typically made during the procedure, TTE or even preliminary TEE or ICE can be used to estimate device size prior to the procedure so appropriate inventory can be ordered and on hand.

The caliber of venous access must be sufficient to accommodate a delivery system of appropriate size for the selected Amplatzer™ occluder. In cases where this is not possible, a hybrid procedure should be considered.

ASD criteria

The atrial septal defects amenable to transcatheter closure are those of the secundum type with adequate rim tissue (Figure 63.1 and Figure 63.2). Adequate rim tissue is defined as the presence of atrial septal tissue around a minimum of 75% of the ASD circumference, which is necessary for secure deployment of the ASO. The atrial volumes must be sufficient to accommodate the retention disks once the device is deployed. Emphasis should be made on attempting to confirm that there are adequate margins between the retentions disks and adjacent cardiac structures (e.g., mitral and tricuspid valves). The ASD should not have a size estimate in excess of 38 mm as this is the largest available ASO. *Note*: Determination of the adequacy of ASD rim tissue is very

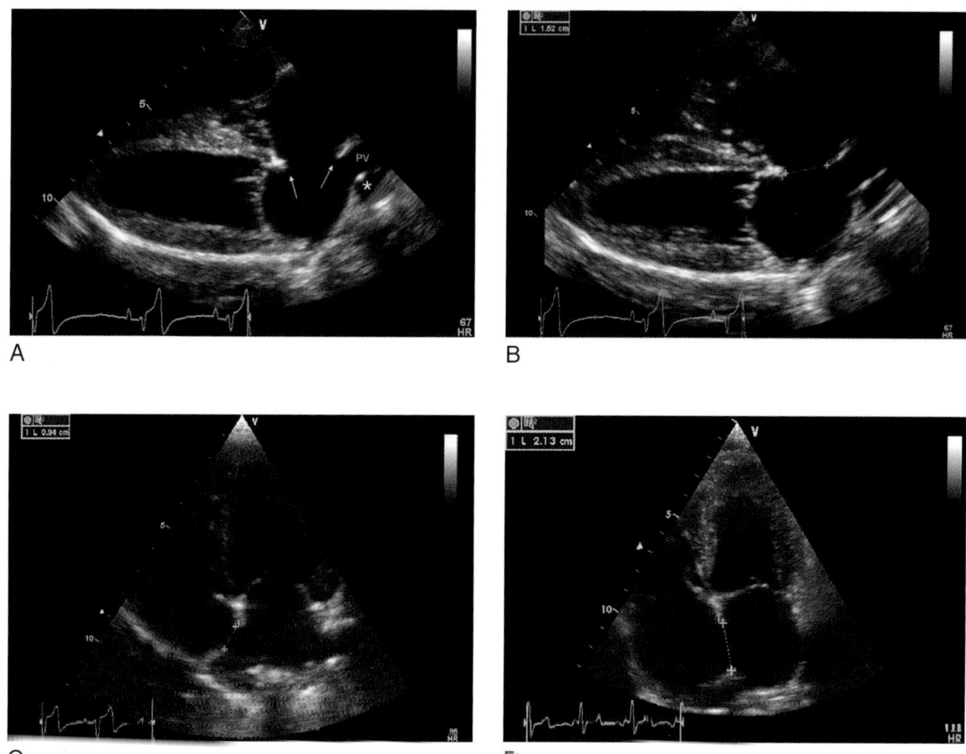

Figure 63.1 (A) Right parasternal 4-chamber long axis transthoracic echocardiographic (TTE) image demonstrating a large secundum type ASD. This image plane optimizes visualization of the defect – with the pulmonary vein in long axis (PV) and the right pulmonary artery (*) in short axis. This is typically the best TTE image plane to measure the ASD and correlates best with transesophageal echocardiography (TEE) and stop-flow balloon sizing of the defect. The arrows point at the edges of the defect in this plane and suggest the presence of sufficient rim tissue in this plane. (B) This is the same image plane as in A and demonstrates measurement of the ASD. Rim tissue in this image also appears adequate. (C) This image demonstrates measurement of an ASD from the left apical four-chamber TTE plane. This is a relatively small ASD and rim tissue in this plane appears adequate. (D) This image demonstrates measurement of a different ASD from the left apical four-chamber TTE plane. This ASD is larger than the one in C and the adequacy of the rim tissue along the ventral aspect of the defect in this plane is difficult to assess but appears inadequate. Other imaging planes and/or TEE would be necessary to better assess the adequacy of rim tissue in this large defect.

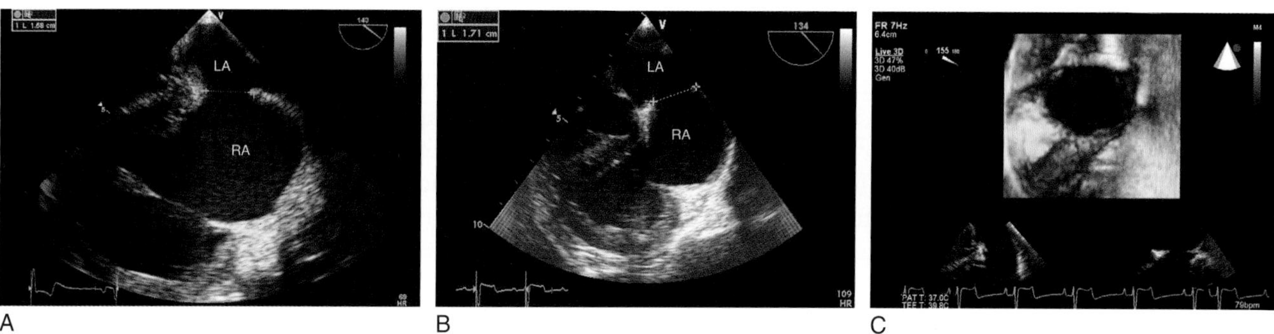

Figure 63.2 (A) This is a transesophageal echocardiographic (TEE) image that was optimized for measurement of the ASD. The rim tissue on the left hand side of the defect in this plane appears inadequate. Other planes would be necessary to better assess the adequacy of rim tissue in this large defect. (B) This is a TEE image from a different ASD for measurement determination. In this plane, the rim tissue on the right hand side of the defect appears inadequate. Other planes would be necessary to better assess the adequacy of rim tissue in this large defect. (C) This is a real time three-dimensional (4D) TEE image from a dog with a large secundum ASD. Along the bottom the orthogonal 2D views can be seen and the 3D rendering is above. The 3D rendering (particularly in real time) facilitates visualization of rim tissue and assessment of its adequacy as well as measurement. LA = left atrium; RA = right atrium.

difficult with large defects. The most promising imaging modalities to accomplish this are 3D-TEE and -ICE. In the author's experience, even if there is uncertainty about the presence of sufficient rim tissue to ensure secure deployment of the ASO, the best way to tell may be to deploy the device and see if it seats securely. In defects with inadequate rim tissue it is typically impossible to deploy the ASO securely. In addition, most ASDs are not perfectly round, and thus some apparent diskrepancies in defect measurements may reflect the fact that the defect is not round but rather oval/ellipsoid in shape. Care must be taken not to oversize the defect in cases like this. The stop flow balloon sizing, as discussed below, should be relied on in these cases.

VSD criteria

The VSDs most amenable to transcatheter closure are those surrounded on all sides by muscular septum (muscular VSDs). Perimembranous defects that are at least 3–5.5mm from the aortic and atrioventricular valves may also be amenable to device closure and specific devices with asymmetric disks for perimembranous VSD closure are available on the human market. The defect should also be between 3 to17.5mm in size as the largest Amplatzer™ muscular ventricular septal defect occluder[3] (mVSDO) is 18mm. Single case reports of transcatheter closure of both muscular (Margiocco et al, 2008) and perimembranous VSDs (Bussadori et al, 2007, Saunders et al, 2013) exist in the veterinary literature. Transcatheter closure of doubly-committed juxtaarterial (also called subarterial or supracristal) VSDs as well as perimembranous VSDs within 3mm of the aortic valve is not recommended.

Potential Risks/ Complications/Expected Outcomes

Potentially life-threatening complications appear to be more common with this catheterization procedure, as compared to other transcatheter procedures commonly carried out in veterinary medicine. In particular, inadvertent ASO release or unexpected ASO embolization/dislodgement requiring emergency device retrieval could be fatal if appropriate surgical support is not immediately available. Percutaneous retrieval is very difficult/impossible once the device is released from the cable and leaving the embolized device in place is not an option. If inadvertent release or dislodgement following release occurs during the procedure or when the dog is still anesthetized, then a thoracotomy should be done over the chamber or vessel where the device is lodged and it should be retrieved through an atriotomy (if in right atrium or left atrium) or arteriotomy (if in main pulmonary artery). The author has had two ASO devices dislodge after release: one was intraoperative (within in 2–3min of release) and the device was embolized into the right atrium and the second was discovered the day after surgery during a planned TTE evaluation and was lodged in the main pulmonary artery, the dog was asymptomatic. The first dog had the device removed while still under anesthesia and ultimately (a few days later) had its ASD definitively repaired with an open-heart hybrid procedure using an ASO. The second dog had the device removed as soon as it was discovered via thoracotomy and pulmonary arteriotomy. In this dog, a second repair procedure was not attempted as it was felt embolization of the device was evidence that the dog had inadequate ASD rim tissue. Both dogs that underwent ASO retrieval procedures recovered uneventfully. The author is unaware of any late (after discharge) ASO embolizations.

The other two complications the author has experienced are thrombosis of the ASO and supraventricular tachyarrhythmias. Thrombosis was detected in two dogs perioperatively. Since that time clopidogrel and not aspirin has been used for 6 months after the procedure. In humans, aspirin is recommended for 6 months following implantation. Both dogs with thrombosis of the ASO resolved the majority of the thrombus over time while on clopidogrel and aspirin. Clinically significant supraventricular arrhythmias developed late, more than 6 months after implantation, in two dogs. Supraventricular arrhythmias have been reported in human patients as well. It is possible/probable that other complications may arise in larger cohorts or with long-term follow-up.

The clinical outcome in the dogs undergoing ASD occlusion has been very good. These dogs have long duration of event free survival. Mild residual shunting detectable by TTE may be present in as many 50% of dogs the day after the procedure. Typically, any residual shunting is reduced or resolved over the following 6 to 12 months. In addition, pre-procedural PH and cardiomegaly tend to resolve as well. Lastly, any dogs that required treatment for CHF prior to the procedure can likely have those medications reduced and ultimately discontinued.

Percutaneous and transcatheter hybrid ASD occlusion with Amplatzer™ ASO appears to be a reasonably safe and efficacious option in many dogs. Very large ASD may not be amenable to this technique without significantly increasing the risk of potentially life threatening complications due to lack of sufficient tissue rim to retain the device. Percutaneous and transcatheter hybrid occlusion of some VSDs with either the Amplatzer™ mVSDO or Amplatzer™ ADOII are

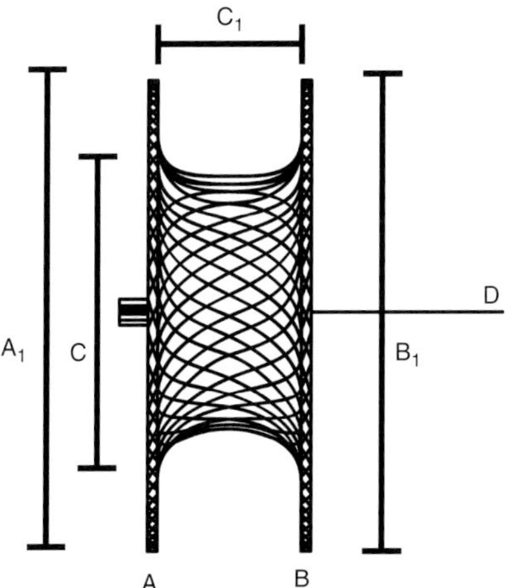

Figure 63.3 This is a diagram of a generic Amplatzer™ heart occluder that demonstrates the various components and measurements. There are two retention disks; a proximal disk (B) that is attached (screwed) to the delivery cable (D). There is a distal retention disk (A) and a waist that has both a diameter (C) and a length (C_1). A_1 = diameter of the distal retention disk; B_1 = diameter of the proximal retention disk. The retention disk diameters are larger than the waist and may or may not be equal in diameter; in addition, their contour and width may be variable. The device size selected (with the exception of the PFO occluder) is based on the diameter of the waist (C) when it is deployed. The length of the waist is also variable depending on the device (VSD > ASD). The device is made of nitinol and may or may not have polyester filler.

feasible in the dog and represent a good alternative to open-heart procedures.

Equipment

Amplatzer™ Heart Occluders (AHO)

In general, AHOs have two retention disks, a proximal disk (which is attached to a delivery cable and released once deployed) and a distal disk (Figure 63.3 and Figure 63.4). The contour of the retention disks is somewhat variable from device to device. The retention disks are equal in diameter, width and contour for some devices (mVSDO, Amplatzer™ duct occluder II[4] [ADOII]) and unequal with a larger distal disk in ASO and larger proximal disk in the Amplatzer™ patent foramen ovale occluder[5] (PFO). The waist is smaller than the retention disks and the deployed diameter of the waist is selected to fill the defect without oversizing (unlike the Amplatz Canine Duct Occluder for patent ductus arteriosus). The width of the waist is also device dependent (wider for VSD than ASD). The size in mm of the mVSDO, ADOII, and ASO are based on the size of the waist in the deployed state. The retention disks are 1–3 mm bigger than the waist. For the PFO the waist is very small and the size of the device is based on the retention disk size.

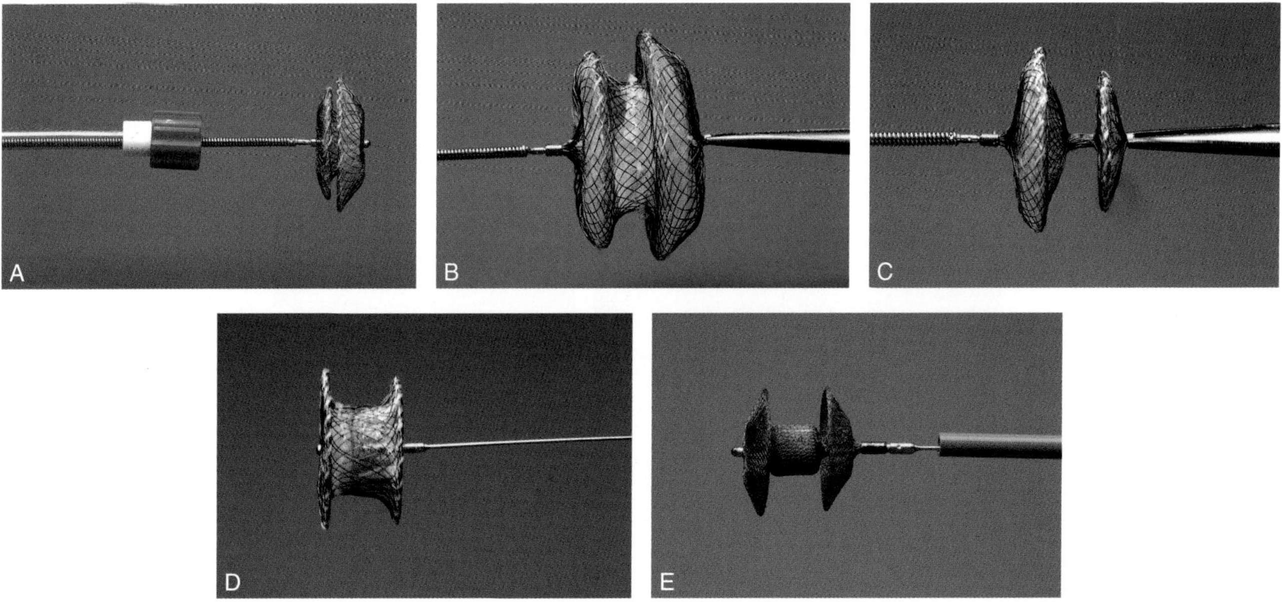

Figure 63.4 (A) An Amplatzer™ septal occluder (ASO) attached to a delivery cable. (B) An ASO attached to a delivery cable (left). Forceps have grasped the distal retention disk (right) to demonstrate the waist and the relative size of the proximal to distal retention disks (distal > proximal) and the polyester filler. (C) An Amplatzer™ patent foramen ovale occluder (PFO) attached to a delivery cable (left). Forceps have grasped the distal retention disk (right) to demonstrate the very small waist and the relative size of the proximal to distal retention disks (proximal > distal) and the polyester filler. (D) An Amplatzer™ muscular VSD occluder (mVSDO) attached to a delivery cable. Notice that, unlike the ASO and PFO, no retraction is necessary to visualize the waist in its deployed state. E. An Amplatzer™ duct occluder II (ADOII) attached to a delivery cable.

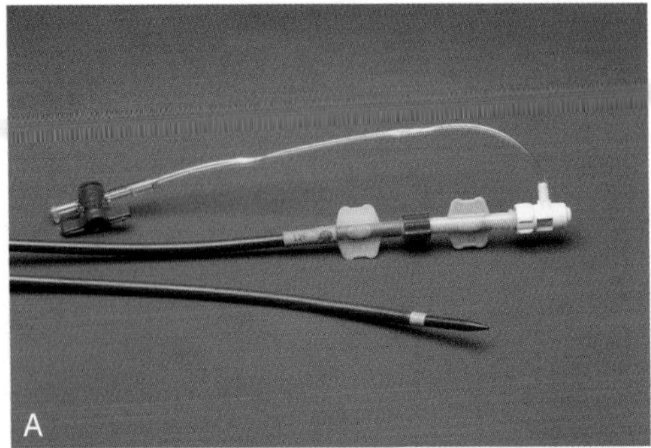

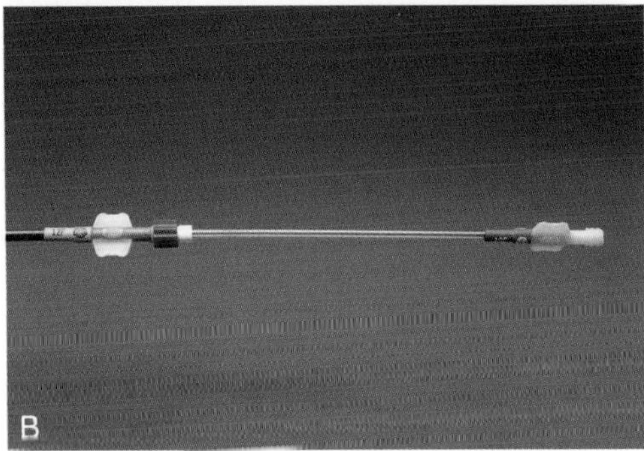

Figure 63.5 (A) The Amplatzer™ TorqVue™ delivery system sheath with dilator within and the hemostasis port. (B) The Amplatzer™ TorqVue™ delivery system device loader.

Delivery Systems

Appropriate delivery systems of different French sizes (6 through 12) that contain the majority of the supplies required to perform the procedure are supplied by AGA Medical (Amplatzer™ TorqVue ™ delivery systems[6], Figure 63.5). Delivery systems include: delivery cable, delivery sheath and dilator, hemostasis port, loader, and plastic vice. All sheath sizes are available with a 45° tip angle and some can be ordered with a 180° tip. Most are available in 60 cm length and some in 80 cm length. The Amplatzer™ TorqVue™ LP[7] (low profile) delivery systems include the same supplies but come in a 4 and 5 French size through which the ADOII can be deployed. It is worth noting that neither of the available sheath tip angles are optimum for percutaneous device deployment in the dog but the 45° is preferred over the 180° by the author for ASD occlusion.

Other Required Supplies

A 0.035″ J-tipped 150 to 180 cm hydrophilic guide wire is needed as well as a variety of end-hole catheters that can be used to cross the defect. For ASD, a Amplatzer™ sizing balloon II is also recommended (Figure 63.6A).

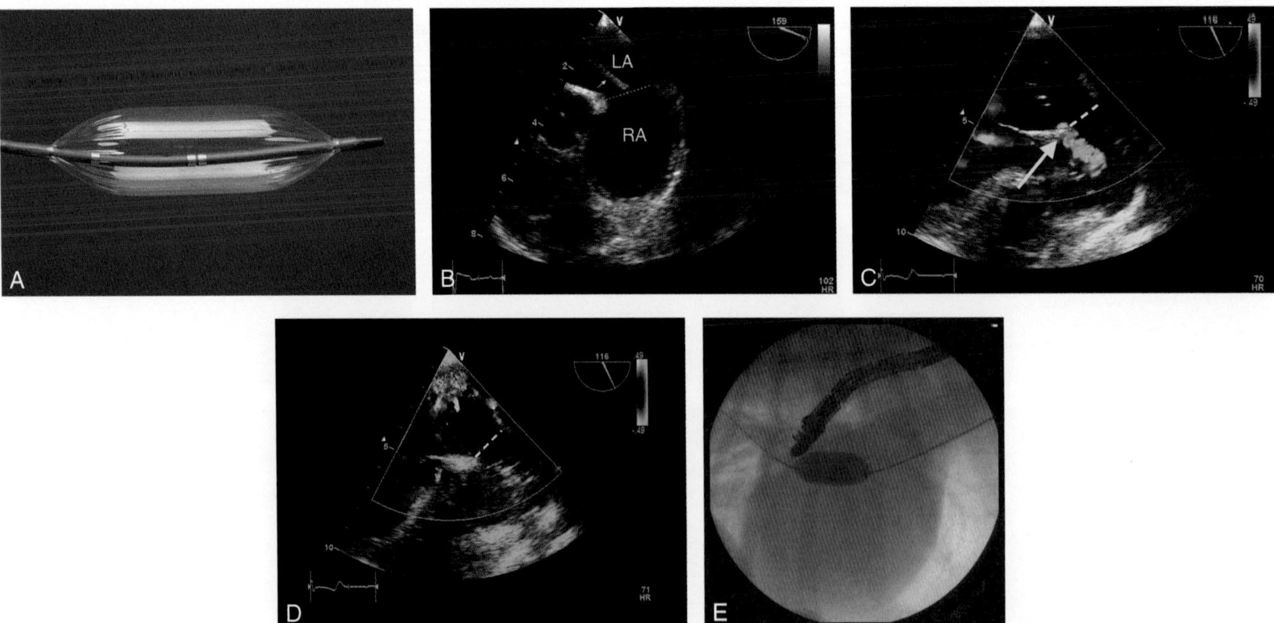

Figure 63.6 (A) The Amplatzer™ sizing balloon II inflated with air. Note the calibrated marker bands on the catheter shaft. (B) This is a transesophageal echocardiographic (TEE) image that was optimized for visualization of the ASD and the deflated balloon sizing catheter (arrow) can be seen across the defect within the left atrium (LA). RA = right atrium. (C) This is the same TEE image plane from B. The balloon has been inflated partially but there is still flow (arrow) across the defect around the balloon. (D) This is the same TEE image plane from B and C. The balloon has been inflated more and there is now no flow apparent, the stop-flow balloon volume has been reached. The diameter of the balloon in short axis can now be measured by both TEE (dashed line) and fluoroscopy. (E) This is the accompanying fluoroscopic image taken once the stop-flow volume of the balloon was reached. Notice there is no waist seen in the balloon, which is a common finding.

Other basic catheterization supplies may also be needed e.g. introducer, contrast agent, etc.

Imaging Requirements

A high quality C-arm fluoroscope with rotational capabilities is recommended. Intraoperative cardiac ultrasound (TEE or ICE) is also necessary for optimal defect measurement and device positioning.

Procedure

Anesthetic Concerns

As for other catheterization procedures in patients with structural heart disease, animals with ASD or VSD are at risk for the development of pulmonary edema and significant ventricular and supraventricular arrhythmias. An experienced anesthesia staff and frequent, open communication between interventionalist and anesthesia staff is critical to procedural success.

Percutaneous Procedures

The animal is placed in left lateral recumbency and the skin over the right external jugular vein is clipped and surgically prepped. The procedure begins with percutaneous placement of an introducer of an appropriate size to allow passing of the desired delivery sheath into the animal's right external jugular vein; a jugular venous cut-down may alternatively be performed. At this time, another unsterile operator should be performing TEE for visualization and measurement of the defect.

A relatively small diameter (4 or 5 French) end hole catheter and an 0.035″ J-tipped hydrophilic guide wire are advanced under fluoroscopic guidance to gain access to the left atrium (or left ventricle for VSD) across the ASD. The guide wire should be passed deep into the right caudal pulmonary vein (Figure 63.7A). For VSD the wire should be advanced into to the LV. TEE can be very helpful with this aspect of the procedure to direct wire positioning.

The end-hole catheter should then be exchanged for the ASD sizing balloon of appropriate size based on TTE and TEE estimate of ASD size. The ASD size is then determined by the recommended stop flow balloon inflation technique. This is not done for VSD. To determine ASD size, the balloon should be positioned across the ASD over the preplaced guide wire and inflated with a mixture of sterile saline and nonionic contrast while simultaneously imaging with TEE and fluoroscopy. ASD size can then be determined by measuring the maximal diameter of the balloon after no further shunting can be seen around the edges of the balloon on TEE (Figure 63.6). *Note*: the balloon will not always have an indentable waist, and waisting is not always consistent with the stop flow balloon inflation size. Once the stop flow balloon size is reached, the defect is measured from TEE and/or a fluoroscopic image. Once the diameter of the ASD is determined, an ASO equal to or slightly larger than the defect (if the identical size is not available) is selected. *Note*: oversizing is to be avoided.

The device is then prepared prior to introduction into the patient. The delivery cable is passed through the loader and securely attached to the ASO. The ASO is immersed in sterile saline and retracted into the loader while still immersed in saline. This should be done several times to ensure that all air bubbles trapped within the device are removed. The loader should then be flushed through the side port with the ASO inside the loader to further ensure that no air bubbles are present. *Note*: precautions to limit the introduction of any air bubbles is critical in these procedures because of the potential to introduce them into the systemic arterial circulation.

The dilator should then be loaded into the Amplatzer™ Delivery Sheath and secured with the locking mechanism. The sheath and dilator should be passed over the preplaced guide wire and advanced across the ASD into the left atrium. Once the sheath reaches the right atrium, the dilator should be removed to allow back bleeding which ensures all air bubbles are purged from the system. Next, and before advancing the sheath into the left atrium, the hemostasis valve supplied in the delivery system package should be affixed to the sheath and the system flushed. The sheath should then be advanced over the guide wire and into the right caudal pulmonary vein, at which time the guide wire is removed.

The sheath position can be verified with TEE and/or a hand injection of contrast under fluoroscopic imaging. The previously prepared loader and ASO should then be inserted into the hemostasis port on the sheath. The ASO should be advanced by pushing it into sheath with the attached cable. *Note*: It is very important not to accidently rotate the cable while advancing, positioning, and repositioning the ASO as this can lead to inadvertent release and percutaneous retrieval is very difficult if not impossible and can lead to devastating consequences.

Under fluoroscopic and TEE guidance, the first/proximal retention disk and part of the waist should deployed in the left atrium (Figure 63.7B). The ASO and sheath should then be retracted gently against

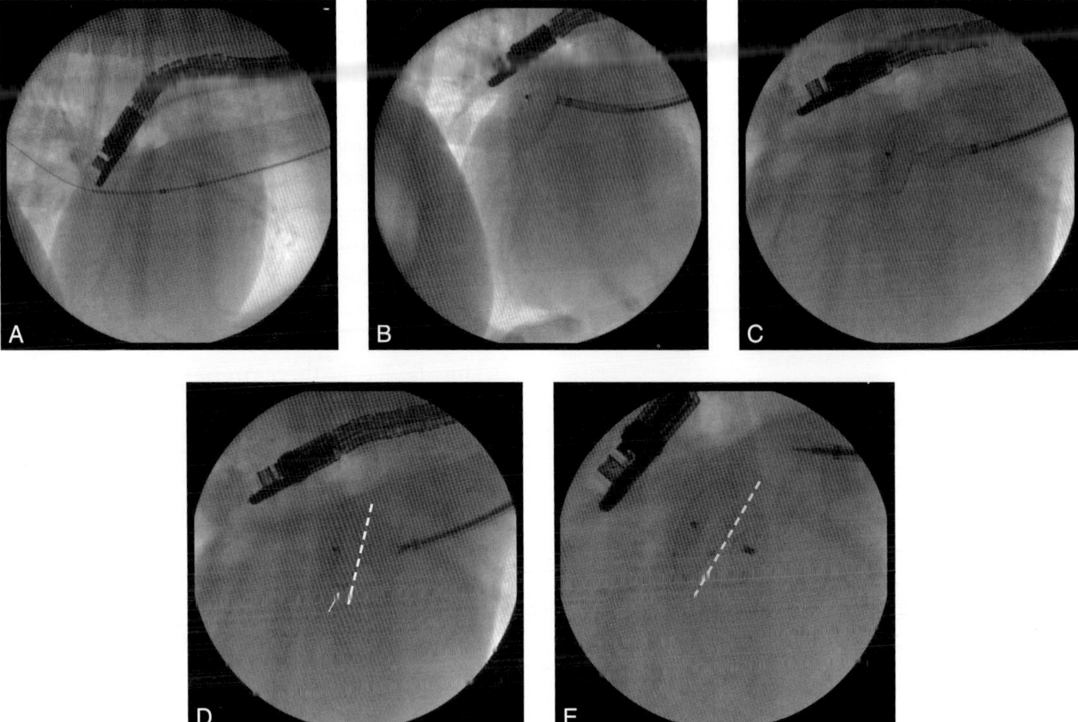

Figure 63.7 (A) Lateral fluoroscopic image during deployment of an Amplatzer™ septal occluder (ASO); cranial is to right of the image and caudal is to the left. There is a transesophageal echocardiography probe in the esophagus dorsal to the heart. There is a hydrophilic guide wire placed deep in a pulmonary vein and a catheter is present over the wire. The catheter and wire were advanced down the right jugular into the right atrium and then through the ASD into the left atrium and pulmonary vein. (B) The same image view as in A. The distal retention disk of the ASO has been deployed in the left atrium. (C) The same image view as in A. The distal retention disk and part of the waist of the ASO have been deployed and gentle traction on the delivery cable has been used to bring the distal retention disk up against the intra-atrial septum. The distal disk is in the left atrium and the partially deployed waist is across the defect. (D) The same image view as in A. The distal retention disk of the ASO has been deployed in the left atrium and the proximal retention disk has been deployed in the right atrium. The device is still affixed to the delivery cable and the resultant unavoidable back tension on the proximal disk (due to the angle of approach) has not allowed the proximal retention disk to take its true shape. The dashed line demonstrates the orientation of the intra-atrial septum. The arrow is pointing to the ventral lip of the distal retention disk that is putting a lot of tension on the ASD rim tissue in that region. This often leads to dislodgement of the distal disk into the right atrium during deployment of the proximal disk and may require multiple attempts to gain a secure deployment. This problem can be overcome by a hybrid procedure. (E) The same image view as in A. The distal retention disk has been deployed in the left atrium and the proximal retention disk has been deployed in the right atrium. The device has been released from the cable and the relative shape of the device (in particular the proximal retention disk) is appropriate and the orientation of the device now, in comparison to when it was still affixed to the delivery cable in D, shows the degree of unavoidable back tension on the device until it is released. This makes it difficult to assess positioning of the retention disks and security of the device prior to release and also makes deployment of the proximal disk without dislodgment of the distal retention disk more challenging.

the atrial septum, which can typically be felt by the operators and observed on TEE and fluoroscopy (Figure 63.7C). Gentle back tension should be maintained on the delivery cable and the sheath should be retracted, such that the second/distal retention disk is unsheathed within the right atrium (Figure 63.7D). The tension on the delivery cable should then be gradually released and the sheath retracted an additional 5 to 10 cm. *Note*: Recommendations in humans are to then exert gentle to-and-fro motion on the cable to confirm secure ASO positioning prior to deployment. However, due to the angle of approach to the atrial septum in the dog when using transjugular access, this degree of manipulation and resultant tension may dislodge even a securely positioned ASO (Figure 63.7D, E, Figure 63.8, and Figure 63.9). The author typically depends on visualization of secure ASO positioning by TEE and TTE. Secure positioning can be assumed if the ASO takes its original shape and one retention disk is visible in both atria with uniform separation of the retention disks (Figure 63.10).

The ASO almost always requires repeated attempts at repositioning to achieve a secure position, particularly in

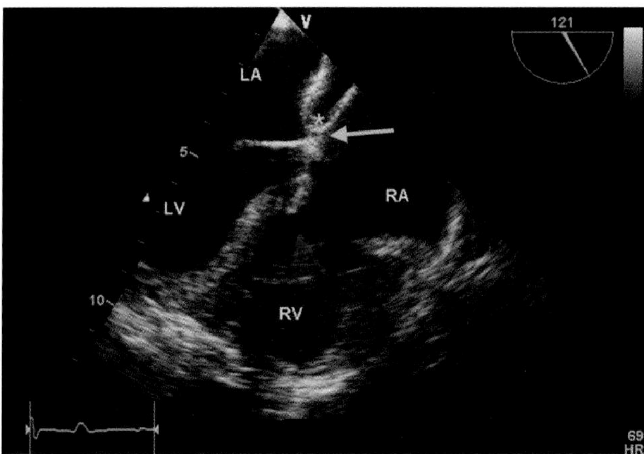

Figure 63.8 This is a transesophageal echocardiographic image. The distal disk of the ASO has been deployed in the left atrium and the * identifies the ventral portion of distal retention disk. The arrow is pointing at the rim of the ASD in this position and the angle of back-tension on the ASO as the proximal retention disk is deployed.

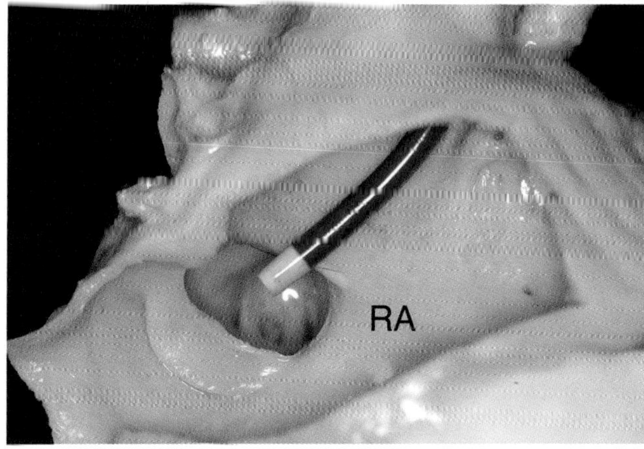

Figure 63.9 This is a gross image of the heart of a dog with a secundum type ASD. The right atrial wall has been removed and the ASD is visible. The guiding sheath used to deliver an ASO is being advanced into the right atrium from the cranial vena cava. The acute angle of incidence from cranial vena cava to the defect is apparent.

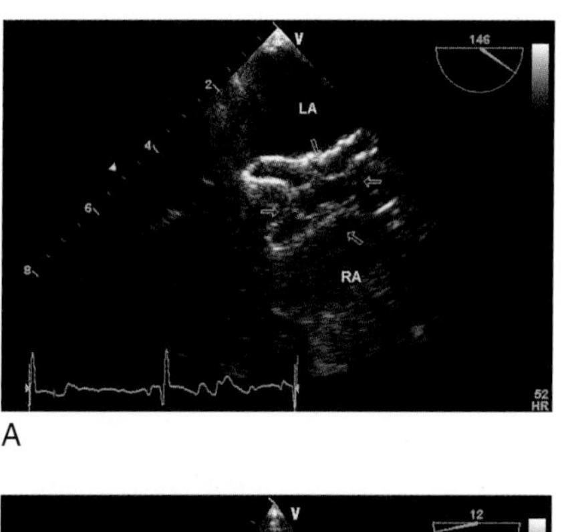

A

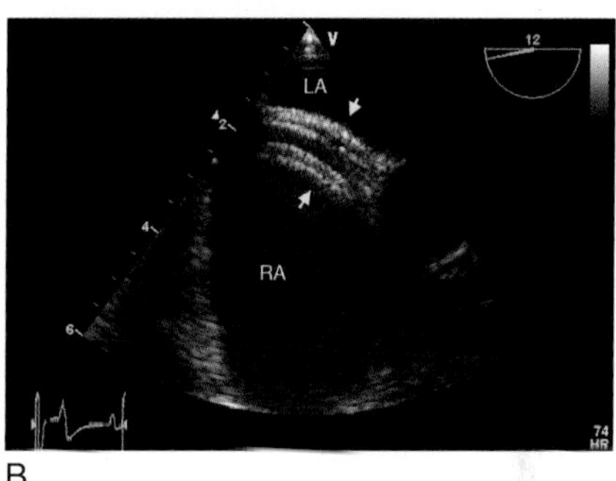

B

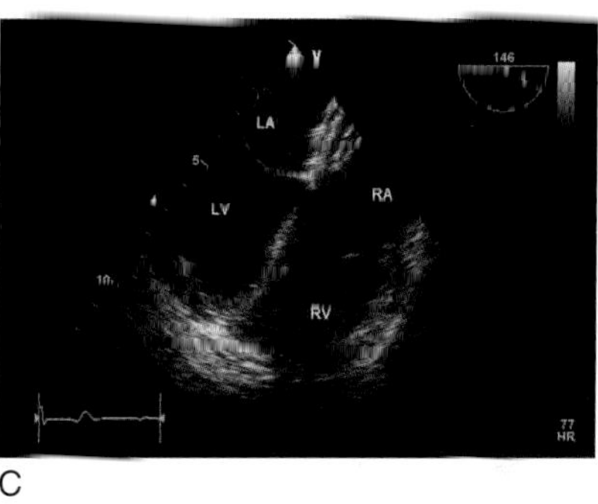

C

Figure 63.10 (A) This is a transesophageal echocardiographic (TEE) image of an Amplatzer™ septal occluder (ASO) that has been completely deployed and released from the delivery cable. The ASO is securely positioned. (B) This is a TEE image of an ASO that has been completely deployed and released from the delivery cable. The ASO is securely positioned. This image is a different plane than that shown in A. (C) This is a TEE image of an ASO that has been completely deployed and released from the delivery cable. The ASO is securely positioned. This image is a different plane than that shown in A and B. Multiple TEE planes are typically used to assess ASO position.

larger defects. Following confirmation of secure positioning, the ASO can be released from the cable by attaching the provided plastic vise (delivery system) to the cable and rotating counter clockwise while under observation with fluoroscopy and TEE until the cable is free of the device (Figure 63.7E). The cable and sheath and introducer can then be withdrawn.

Hybrid Procedures

These are procedures that utilize surgical exposure to the heart, combined with transcatheter tools to occlude defects. Hybrid procedures offer the advantage of allowing access to small animals (maybe even cats) or animals whose defect would require a device and accompanying delivery system that is larger than the available venous access. They also provide an optimal angle for deployment that cannot be achieved with percutaneous approaches and the currently available delivery systems (45°, 180°). Last, hybrid procedures typically do not require fluoroscopy as all guidance is by TEE or epicardial echocardiography. As the delivery system and other catheterization supplies are not required in hybrid procedures, consumable equipment costs may be reduced.

Hybrid procedures allow the positioning of an introducer of appropriate size to facilitate device deployment directly into the right atrial or right ventricular wall adjacent to the ASD or VSD, respectively. Purse string sutures are secured with Rumel tourniquets and, in the case of the right ventricular approach, pledgets may be necessary to obtain and maintain a secure hemostatic entry and facilitate closure at the end of the procedure. Simultaneous catheterization is often not necessary eliminating the need for fluoroscopy. These procedures are typically done with TEE guidance, although ICE and or direct epicardial imaging could be considered.

For hybrid ASD closure, a right thoracotomy is performed. Palpation of the ASD and TEE facilitate the placement of an introducer placed via a modified Seldinger technique through the right atrial wall adjacent to the ASD through which the ASO can be deployed under TEE guidance. An open trans-atrial approach has also been employed through a right thoracotomy whereby the ASO is deployed as described above, followed by active ASO fixation through right atriotomy under temporary inflow occlusion.

The author's team has achieved hybrid VSD closure via a median sternotomy with a ventral midline pericardial incision over the right ventricular outflow tract. Palpation of the VSD through the right ventricular wall in combination with epicardial echocardiography and TEE allowed placement of an introducer via a modified Seldinger technique through which an ADOII was deployed under TEE guidance.

Follow-Up/Prognosis

The patient should be recovered routinely in an intensive care unit with respiratory and cardiac rhythm monitoring. Transthoracic echocardiography should be performed the day after the procedure to confirm ASO position and determine the presence and severity of any residual flow. Chamber size and function should also be re-assessed. Dogs are typically discharged the day after the procedure. Severe exercise restriction is advised for 4 weeks and then limited activity for 6 months. Clopidogrel (1–3 mg/kg PO, q24 hr) is prescribed for 6 months. Follow-up echocardiography is also performed in 6 months or sooner if any change in clinical condition is observed.

Long-term follow-up should be determined on a case-by-case basis. If the defect is completely closed at the 6 month recheck and the heart is normal in size and function, then additional follow-up may only be necessary if new clinical signs develop that could be consistent with heart failure, embolization or arrhythmias. Additional indications my include the detection of a new murmur or arrhythmia or if the dog develops signs of sepsis or another disease condition that is associated with procoagulability.

Notes

1. Amplatzer™ septal occluder, AGA Medical Corporation, Goldenvalley, MN.
2. Amplatzer™ sizing balloon II, AGA Medical Corporation, Goldenvalley, MN.
3. Amplatzer™ muscular VSD occluder, AGA Medical Corporation, Goldenvalley, MN.
4. Amplatzer™ Duct Occluder II, AGA Medical Corporation, Goldenvalley, MN.
5. Amplatzer™ patent foramen ovale occluder, AGA Medical Corporation, Goldenvalley, MN.
6. Amplatzer™ TorqVue ™ delivery systems, AGA Medical Corporation, Goldenvalley, MN.
7. Amplatzer™ TorqVue™ LP (low profile) delivery systems, AGA Medical Corporation, Goldenvalley, MN.

References

Bussadori C, Carminati M, and Domenech O (2007) Transcatheter closure of a perimembranous ventricular septal defect in a dog. *J Vet Intern Med* 21, 1396–400.

Margiocco ML, Bulmer BJ, and Sisson DD (2008) Percutaneous occlusion of a muscular ventricular septal defect with an Amplatzer® muscular VSD occluder. *J Vet Cardiol* 10, 61–6.

Saunders AB, Carlson JA, Nelson DA, Gordon SG, and Miller MW (2013) Hybrid technique for ventricular septal defect closure in a dog using an Amplatzer® Duct Occluder II. *J Vet Cardiol* 2013 Sep;15(3):217–24. doi: 10.1016/j.jvc.2013.06.003. Epub 2013 Aug 17.

Suggested Reading

Gordon SG, Miller MW, Roland RM, et al (2009) Transcatheter atrial septal defect closure with the Amplatzer® atrial septal occluder in 13 dogs: short- and mid term outcome. *J Vet Intern Med* 23, 995–1002.

Gordon SG, Nelson DA, Achen SE, et al (2010) Open heart closure of an atrial septal defect by use of an atrial septal occluder in a dog. *J Am Vet Med Assoc* 236, 434–9.

Sanders RA, Hogan DF, Green HW, et al (2005) Trans catheter closure of an atrial septal defect in a dog. *J Am Vet Med Assoc* 227(3), 430–4.

Saunders AB, Carlson JA, Nelson DA, et al (2013) Hybrid technique for ventricular septal defect closure in a dog using an Amplatzer® Duct Occluder II. *J Vet Cardiol*, 15, 217–24.

SECTION EIGHT

Musculoskeletal/ Neurological Systems

Edited by William T.N. Culp

CHAPTER SIXTY-FOUR

Tumor Ablations – Soft Tissue and Skeletal

William T.N. Culp
School of Veterinary Medicine, University of California – Davis, Davis, CA

Background/Indications

In veterinary medicine, surgical treatment of solid tumors is generally recommended whenever possible. In those cases where surgery is either not elected or not recommended, other techniques should be considered. Chemotherapy and radiation therapy may demonstrate efficacy against certain tumor types, but the tumor response from these modalities is often limited for bulky disease. Procedures performed via image-guidance such as intravascular delivery of chemotherapy and/or embolic agents and loco-ablative treatments can be considered in these cases as a primary therapy or in the neoadjuvant setting. As many tumors are diagnosed at a stage when resection is not possible, tumor ablation offers an alternative option for treatment that may benefit our veterinary patients.

Tumor ablations are procedures resulting in cellular destruction via the administration of either chemical or thermal ablative techniques; in addition, newer technologies such as cementoplasty and irreversible electroporation are also being utilized. Chemical ablation techniques involve the intratumoral injection of liquid agents, most commonly ethanol. Thermal ablation is based on the delivery of heat or freezing agents directly to a tumor to cause death of the cells that are targeted. Most of the human literature concerning thermal ablation procedures has focused on radiofrequency ablation and cryoablation (Nazario and Tam, 2011), and these techniques will be discussed in detail in subsequent sections. Other techniques that are more regularly being utilized in humans include microwave ablation, laser ablation, high-intensity focused ultrasound, cementoplasty, and irreversible electroporation, and brief descriptions of these procedures will also be included.

Patient Preparation

As part of a preanesthetic assessment and the general evaluation of a patient with cancer, bloodwork (complete blood count and biochemistry profile), urinalysis and chest radiographs should be performed. An ultrasound exam is a useful diagnostic tool to assess tumor size and location. For tumors in the cervical region, thorax or abdomen, ultrasonography can be utilized both as a pre- and post-treatment assessment tool as well as a tool to facilitate the performance of an ablation procedure. Computerized tomography (CT) and magnetic resonance imaging (MRI) are excellent modalities for precisely assessing tumor location and monitoring alterations in tumor volume. A fine-needle aspirate or biopsy should be obtained prior to therapy for definitive diagnosis.

Potential Risks/Complications/Expected Outcomes

When performing tumor ablation techniques, a comprehensive knowledge of regional anatomy is essential. Many tumors being treated by ablation are adjacent to essential organs and trauma to these organs can result in significant morbidity. Additionally, there is often a goal of treating a region of normal tissue ("margin") around the tumor to increase the level of confidence that the entire tumor has been treated. In regions such as the liver, where there is often abundant tissue surrounding the tumor, this may be easily accomplished; however, when treating tumors in more difficult locations (e.g., prostate), concern for adjacent organs (e.g., urethra, colon, nerves, blood vessels) is paramount.

Veterinary Image-Guided Interventions, First Edition. Edited by Chick Weisse and Allyson Berent.

Companion website: www.wiley.com/go/weisse/vet-image-guided-interventions

Pain control is essential, and this is often the most commonly reported complication that occurs in human patients undergoing ablative therapies (Ong et al, 2009, Zavaglia et al, 2008). Pyrexia has been reported regularly after ablative therapies in humans as well (Ong et al, 2009). Other complications may arise pending the location of the tumor that has been treated. Normal organs that are located adjacent to tumors should be monitored for signs of side effects. For cryoablation of bone lesions, fracture of the treated site and surrounding bone can occur (Nazario and Tam, 2011). While uncommon, trauma to the gallbladder can be noted during ablation of hepatic tumors (Akahane et al, 2005, Bhardwaj et al, 2010, Ding et al, 2013, Kudo, 2010). In reported cases of lung tumor ablation, pneumothorax can occur with varying levels of frequency and may require treatment (Carrafiello et al, 2012, Vogl et al, 2011, Zhu et al, 2008). Treated tumor sites in parenchymal organs can develop abscessation post-treatment leading to signs such as nausea, vomiting and diarrhea (Akahane et al, 2005, Bhardwaj et al, 2010, Ding et al, 2013, Kudo, 2010). While these represent a few specific examples of complications that can arise, it is important to consider each individual organ that is undergoing ablation and the potential risks that can occur both in that organ and adjacent organs.

Inappropriate placement of grounding pads can lead to severe burns, which may result in significant morbidity and can require surgical treatment (Akahane et al, 2005, Sutherland et al, 2006, Vogl et al, 2011). Seeding of tumors is also possible, as the probes are placed percutaneously when performing these techniques with image-guidance (Akahane et al, 2005, Vogl et al, 2011, Zavaglia et al, 2008). Clinicians considering ablative therapies should be well trained prior to pursuing these techniques, as experience and appropriate technique will likely decrease the development of many complications.

Due to the paucity of veterinary literature describing these techniques, there is still much that remains unknown. Ablative therapies hold promise for veterinary patients both as a primary treatment for soft tissue and bone tumors as well as a means of pain control. These differing goals have been extensively evaluated in human patients, and the results are encouraging. Further investigation into the role of ablative therapies for different tumor types in companion animals will hopefully elucidate the efficacy of these procedures and add another option to our currently commonly employed treatments.

Ablation Therapies

Equipment and General Principles

Veterinary patients undergoing tumor ablation need to be placed under general anesthesia. When an ablation procedure is being performed via image-guidance (as opposed to laparoscopy/thoracoscopy or an open surgery), the patient is positioned in a manner that allows for simplified use of the chosen image-modality (fluoroscopy, ultrasonography, CT and/or MRI). With certain modalities, a grounding pad is necessary, and it is essential that this pad be placed with close adherence to the skin to prevent burns; clipping of the fur in the region of the pad is mandatory.

Most thermal ablation techniques require specialized equipment and some examples include: Covidien Cool-tip™ RF Ablation System[1], Galil Medical Cryoablation System[2], Evident™ Microwave Ablation system[3] and ExAblate® 2000 high-intensity focused ultrasound system[4]. A thorough understanding of each specific device is essential to performing the procedure safely and effectively, and training is always recommended.

Radiofrequency ablation

Radiofrequency ablation (RFA) works by causing coagulative necrosis of cells (Bhardwaj et al, 2010). RF waves are produced in a generator and then transferred to a probe that is positioned directly into the desired tissue. The mechanism of action of the tissue destruction is based on the effect that the waves cause within the tissue; as RF waves are delivered, the ions in the tissue tend to follow the current which results in heat and subsequent coagulative necrosis within a certain distance of the probe (Bhardwaj et al, 2010, Carrafiello et al, 2008a, Ni et al, 2005).

General anesthesia, conscious sedation, and regional anesthesia have all been used in humans to eliminate motion and provide pain control (Callstrom and Charboneau, 2007, Decadt and Siriwardena, 2004); in companion animals, general anesthesia is a necessity. Monopolar RFA works by passing electricity from an active or positive electrode (placed in the tissue) to a negative electrode (pad placed on the skin); for bipolar systems an active probe containing both a positive and negative electrode is placed within the tumor tissue (Carrafiello et al, 2008b, Mahnken et al, 2009, Ni et al, 2005). Probes can be inserted into tissue percutaneously with ultrasound, fluoroscopic, CT, or MRI guidance. Probes can also be positioned into tissue during both laparoscopic/thoracoscopic or open surgical procedures (Bhardwaj et al, 2010). For lesions less than 3 cm, only one ablation field is generally needed, and the time of ablation generally ranges from 5–10 minutes to reach the target temperature (100 °C). For larger lesions, overlapping fields can be established through the placement of multiple probes (Callstrom and Charboneau, 2007, Nazario and Tam, 2011).

RFA is commonly utilized in human patients in the treatment of hepatic malignancies (Brown, 2005, Kurup and Callstrom, 2010, Ni et al, 2005). Other tumors that are regularly treated include renal, adrenal, breast and lung tumors. Additionally, primary and metastatic bone tumors are often treated with RFA (Brown, 2005, Kurup and Callstrom, 2010). RFA has been used to treat canine primary hyperparathyroidism (Pollard et al, 2001, Rasor et al, 2007) and feline hyperthyroidism (Mallery et al, 2003), but data regarding the clinical use of RFA to treat malignant neoplasia in companion animals is lacking.

Cryoablation

The mechanism of action of cryoablation is complex and mulitifactorial. Freezing causes the production of intracellular ice crystals that cause cellular damage (Bhardwaj et al, 2010). Additionally, gradual cooling that occurs away from the probe causes osmosis across the cell membrane with secondary cellular dehydration (Carrafiello et al, 2008b). The vascularity in the treated zone can also become altered which results in subsequent cellular hypoxia leading to further cell death (Bhardwaj et al, 2010). Both liquid nitrogen and argon gas have been investigated as coolants during the performance of cryoablation, and these substances have tremendous ability to significantly decrease local temperatures (Bhardwaj et al, 2010, Nazario and Tam, 2011).

As with RFA, cryoablation can be performed percutaneously, via endoscopic-guidance or in an open surgical setting. To perform cryoablation, a cryoprobe is inserted into the tissue where destruction is desired and cell destruction is controlled via alternating periods of freezing and thawing. After the probe has been inserted and the location confirmed via imaging techniques, a period of freezing is initiated. An ice ball is created when the coolant is delivered to the tissue containing the probe (freeze). The size of the ice ball is affected by the length of the insulated tip of the probe, the volume of gas delivered, and the length of time that freezing was performed (Callstrom and Charboneau, 2007, Callstrom and Kurup, 2009). Cell death occurs to a point that is within millimeters of the outer rim of the ice ball, and a single probe generates an ice ball that ranges in size and up to about 3.5 cm diameter (Callstrom and Charboneau, 2007, Callstrom et al, 2006, Callstrom and Kurup, 2009, Carrafiello et al, 2008b). When multiple probes are placed, these are generally arranged in a parallel formation, and an attempt is made to create a 1 cm outer margin (Callstrom and Kurup, 2009).

Most reports discuss a freeze–thaw cycle of a 10 minute freeze with a 5 minute thaw; after this, an additional 10 minute freeze is performed (two freeze–thaw cycles in general) (Callstrom and Charboneau, 2007, Callstrom and Kurup, 2009, Nazario et al, 2011). Most newer systems utilize the infusion of argon gas for freezing purposes, and the infusion of helium for thawing (Callstrom and Kurup, 2009). The most effective means of monitoring the area affected by the ice ball is with CT; however, ultrasonography can be used as well (Callstrom and Charboneau, 2007). Cryoprobes should be warmed by the infusion of helium gas prior to removal.

Cryoablation has been utilized in the treatment of many different organ systems in humans and has been documented in the treatment of prostate, kidney, liver, uterine, and bone tumors, specifically in patients that are not surgical candidates (Callstrom and Kurup, 2009, Carrafiello et al, 2008b, Kurup and Callstrom, 2010, Nazario and Tam, 2011). Two reported cases of cryoablation in the treatment of nasal and maxillary tumors exist in the veterinary literature (Murphy et al, 2011, Weisse et al, 2011). In one dog with a nasal adenocarcinoma, serial CT scans demonstrated primary tumor resolution secondary to a cryoablation procedure (Murphy et al, 2011). Combination therapy with transarterial embolization, systemic cyclophosphamide and cryoablation was used to treat a dog with a maxillary fibrosarcoma; partial tumor remission was noted at a 4-week recheck examination (Weisse et al, 2011).

Microwave ablation

Microwave ablation has a similar mechanism of action to RFA in that tissue destruction is a result of cellular coagulative necrosis (Bhardwaj et al, 2010, Carrafiello et al, 2008a). This necrosis occurs when current is applied to tissue resulting in the realignment of molecules and the subsequent generation of heat (Ong et al, 2009). As with RFA, a generator produces the current and this is delivered to the tissue via a probe (Bhardwaj et al, 2010). Microwave ablation has the advantage of being able to achieve higher temperatures than RFA, a faster ablation time, and no loss of heat to a vessel in close proximity to the probe (heat sink effect) (Carrafiello et al, 2008b, Kurup and Callstrom, 2010, Padma et al, 2009). Microwave ablation does not require grounding pads, providing an additional advantage over RFA (Kurup and Callstrom, 2010, Simon et al, 2005).

Microwave ablation has tremendous potential; however, there are still limited studies assessing the effectiveness and outcomes in human patients (Carrafiello et al, 2008a). Some of the human tumors that have been treated with microwave ablation include liver, renal, adrenal, pulmonary, pancreas, and bone (Carrafiello et al, 2008a, Ong et al, 2009, Simon et al, 2005).

Laser ablation

To perform laser ablation, absorbed light is converted into heat to cause cell death (Gough-Palmer and Gedroyc, 2008, Kurup and Callstrom, 2010) Rapid cell death secondary to coagulative necrosis tends to occur at temperatures above 60° C, and temperatures above 100° C cause vaporization. (Gough-Palmer and Gedroyc, 2008, Kurup and Callstrom, 2010). The neodymium: yttrium-aluminum-garnet, or Nd-YAG, is the most commonly utilized device for laser ablation (Gough-Palmer and Gedroyc, 2008). The extent of necrosis is proportional to the amount of deposited energy; as an example, when 1200 J is applied, a necrotic region of up to 15 mm diameter can be generated (Sabharwal et al, 2009). The use of ultrasound and MRI guidance have both been described, and these modalities assist in the percutaneous performance of this procedure (Gough-Palmer and Gedroyc, 2008).

High-intensity focused ultrasound

High-intensity focused ultrasound (HIFU) has been utilized in humans to treat bone, kidney, liver, prostate, and pancreas (Ji et al, 2009, Padma et al, 2009, Rebillard et al, 2008). When performing HIFU, the ultrasound beams are targeted directly into the tissue, and tissue necrosis occurs secondary to increased temperatures (above 60°C) (Ji et al, 2009). This procedure is directed with the use of either ultrasonography or MRI and has been shown to be safe and effective (Kurup and Callstrom, 2010, Zhang and Wang, 2010). While evidence is still limited, early results are promising especially in the treatment of human bone cancer (Kurup and Callstrom, 2010, Zhang and Wang, 2010). MRI-guided HIFU has been reported in one dog with a hepatocellular adenoma (Kopelman et al, 2006). The treatment was able to cause ablation of significant volumes of the tumor, and tumor necrosis was noted to correlate with the planned treatment region (Kopelman et al, 2006).

Ethanol ablation

The local delivery of ethanol has been utilized for many years in humans to provide pain relief and tumor destruction. The mechanism of action of ethanol is to cause cellular dehydration, vascular thrombosis, and subsequent ischemia and cellular necrosis (Kurup and Callstrom, 2010). To perform this procedure, a needle (20–25 gauge) is directed into the area of interest via image-guidance (ultrasonography and computed tomography), and 95% ethanol is injected directly into the lesion (Carrafiello et al, 2008b, Kurup and Callstrom, 2010, Padma et al, 2009). A needle with a closed, conical tip is often preferred as this allows for a more uniform administration of ethanol (Mahnken et al, 2009). Prior to the instillation of alcohol a test injection utilizing a mixture of iodinated contrast (25%) and lidocaine 1% (75%) can be performed to determine the extent of diffusion that will occur when the ethanol is injected; this also provides local anesthesia as this procedure is painful (Sabharwal et al, 2009).

Percutaneous ethanol injection is generally only recommended for tumors with a size of 3 cm or less (Saldanha et al, 2010). Ethanol has been investigated in the treatment of hepatocellular carcinoma in several human studies (Lencioni and Crocetti, 2013, Mahnken et al, 2009, Padma et al, 2009, Shiina et al, 2012, Yin et al, 2012). Additionally, ethanol injected percutaneously has been utilized in the treatment of other tumor types such as bone cancer (Callstrom et al, 2006). A study evaluating canine cases of hyperparathyroidism, compared the performance of parathyroidectomy, heat ablation, and ethanol ablation. In that study, 18 cases underwent ethanol ablation, and of those, 72% experienced control of hypercalcemia (Rasor et al, 2007).

Other ablation techniques

Cementoplasty, the intralesional injection of polymethylmethacrylate, has several useful properties. This procedure can be used for percutaneous stabilization of bone lesions and stabilization of bone that has undergone another ablative procedure (Castaneda Rodriguez and Callstrom, 2011, Lane et al, 2011, Sabharwal et al, 2009, Saldanha et al, 2010). Additionally, the cement can have direct thermal and cytotoxic effects on tumor cells (Kurup and Callstrom, 2010). Cementoplasty is performed by placing a 10–15 gauge cementoplasty trocar into the bone lesion (Gangi and Buy, 2010, Katsanos et al, 2010).

Irreversible electroporation (IRE) alters cell membrane permeability by the administration of electrical pulses (Guo et al, 2010, Sabharwal et al, 2009, Saldanha et al, 2010). IRE has the advantage of avoiding the heat-sink effect that is seen with RFA as well as avoiding strictures of nearby structures such as the biliary system or ureter. Ultrasonography is a useful method to monitor the ablative effect (Saldanha et al, 2010). Early preclinical studies with IRE provide evidence that this treatment may be useful in the treatment of liver tumors (Guo et al, 2010).

Follow-Up

Patients undergoing tumor ablation should be monitored closely post-treatment for pain control as well as for trauma to the treated and adjacent organs. Hospitalization is often required for patients to receive intravenous opioid medications in the immediate post-treatment time period. Generally, several days of post-treatment oral pain medication is required due to discomfort associated with the procedure.

Ultrasonography is useful for the assessment of the development of abscesses but long-term evaluation of tumor response is more effectively performed with CT or MRI. Additionally, recurrence of neoplasia in the treated site or metastatic progression can also be monitored with these imaging modalities. Pending the results of these studies, further treatments may be considered or planned.

Notes

(Examples: Multiple vendors available)

1. Cool-tip RF™ Ablation System, Covidien, Mansfield, MA.
2. SeedNet™ Cryoablation System, Galil Medical Inc., Arden Hills, MN
3. Evident™ MWA System, Covidien, Mansfield, MA
4. ExAblate® 2000, InSightec Ltd., Tirat Hacarmel, Israel

References

Akahane M, Koga H, Kato N, et al (2005) Complications of percutaneous radiofrequency ablation for hepato-cellular carcinoma: imaging spectrum and management. *Radiographics* 25(Suppl 1), S57–68.

Bhardwaj N, Strickland AD, Ahmad F, Dennison AR, and Lloyd DM (2010) Liver ablation techniques: a review. *Surg Endosc* 24, 254–65.

Brown DB (2005) Concepts, considerations, and concerns on the cutting edge of radiofrequency ablation. *J Vasc Interv Radiol* 16, 597–613.

Callstrom MR and Charboneau JW (2007) Image-guided palliation of painful metastases using percutaneous ablation. *Tech Vasc Interv Radiol*, 10, 120–31.

Callstrom MR and Kurup AN (2009) Percutaneous ablation for bone and soft tissue metastases--why cryoablation? *Skeletal Radiol*, 38, 835–9.

Callstrom MR, Charboneau JW, Goetz MP, et al (2006) Image-guided ablation of painful metastatic bone tumors: a new and effective approach to a difficult problem. *Skeletal Radiol*, 35, 1–15.

Carrafiello G, Lagana D, Mangini M, et al (2008a) Microwave tumors ablation: principles, clinical applications and review of preliminary experiences. *Int J Surg*, 6(Suppl 1), S65–9.

Carrafiello G, Lagana D, Pellegrino C, et al (2008b) Ablation of painful metastatic bone tumors: a systematic review. *Int J Surg* 6(Suppl 1), S47–52.

Carrafiello G, Mangini M, Fontana F, et al (2012) Complications of microwave and radiofrequency lung ablation: personal experience and review of the literature. *Radiol Med* 117, 201–13.

Castaneda Rodriguez WR and Callstrom MR (2011) Effective pain palliation and prevention of fracture for axial-loading skeletal metastases using combined cryoablation and cementoplasty. *Tech Vasc Interv Radiol* 14, 160–9.

Decadt B and Siriwardena AK (2004) Radiofrequency ablation of liver tumours: systematic review. *Lancet Oncol* 5, 550–60.

Ding J, Jing X, Liu J, et al (2013) Complications of thermal ablation of hepatic tumours: Comparison of radiofrequency and microwave ablative techniques. *Clin Radiol* 68, 608–15.

Gangi A and Buy X (2010) Percutaneous bone tumor management. *Semin Intervent Radiol* 27, 124–36.

Gough-Palmer AL and Gedroyc WM (2008) Laser ablation of hepatocellular carcinoma--a review. *World J Gastroenterol* 14, 7170–4.

Guo Y, Zhang Y, Klein R, et al (2010) Irreversible electroporation therapy in the liver: longitudinal efficacy studies in a rat model of hepatocellular carcinoma. *Cancer Res* 70, 1555–63.

Ji X, Bai JF, Shen GF, and Chen YZ (2009) High-intensity focused ultrasound with large scale spherical phased array for the ablation of deep tumors. *J Zhejiang Univ Sci B* 10, 639–47.

Katsanos K, Sabharwal T, and Adam A (2010) Percutaneous cementoplasty. *Semin Intervent Radiol* 27, 137–47.

Kopelman D, Inbar Y, Hanannel A, et al (2006) Magnetic resonance-guided focused ultrasound surgery (MRgFUS). Four ablation treatments of a single canine hepatocellular adenoma. *HPB (Oxford)* 8, 292–8.

Kudo M (2010) Radiofrequency ablation for hepatocellular carcinoma: updated review in 2010. *Oncology* 78(Suppl 1), 113–24.

Kurup AN and Callstrom MR (2010) Ablation of skeletal metastases: current status. *J Vasc Interv Radiol* 21, S242–50.

Lane MD, Le HB, Lee S, et al (2011) Combination radiofrequency ablation and cementoplasty for palliative treatment of painful neoplastic bone metastasis: experience with 53 treated lesions in 36 patients. *Skeletal Radiol* 40, 25–32.

Lencioni R and Crocetti L (2013) Image-guided ablation for hepatocellular carcinoma. *Recent Results Cancer Res* 190, 181–94.

Mahnken AH, Bruners P, and Gunther RW (2009) Local ablative therapies in HCC: percutaneous ethanol injection and radiofrequency ablation. *Dig Dis* 27, 148–56.

Mallery KF, Pollard RE, Nelson RW, Hornof WJ, and Feldman EC (2003) Percutaneous ultrasound-guided radiofrequency heat ablation for treatment of hyperthyroidism in cats. *J Am Vet Med Assoc* 223, 1602–7.

Murphy SM, Lawrence JA, Schmiedt CW, et al (2011) Image-guided transnasal cryoablation of a recurrent nasal adenocarcinoma in a dog. *J Small Anim Pract* 52, 329–33.

Nazario J and Tam AL (2011) Ablation of bone metastases. *Surg Oncol Clin N Am* 20, 355–68, ix.

Nazario J, Hernandez J, and Tam AL (2011) Thermal ablation of painful bone metastases. *Tech Vasc Interv Radiol* 14, 150–9.

Ni Y, Mulier S, Miao Y, Michel L, and Marchal G (2005) A review of the general aspects of radiofrequency ablation. *Abdom Imaging* 30, 381–400.

Ong SL, Gravante G, Metcalfe MS, Strickland AD, Dennison AR, and Lloyd DM (2009) Efficacy and safety of microwave ablation for primary and secondary liver malignancies: a systematic review. *Eur J Gastroenterol Hepatol* 21, 599–605.

Padma S, Martinie JB, and Iannitti DA (2009) Liver tumor ablation: percutaneous and open approaches. *J Surg Oncol* 100, 619–34.

Pollard RE, Long CD, Nelson RW, Hornof WJ, and Feldman EC (2001) Percutaneous ultrasonographically guided radiofrequency heat ablation for treatment of primary hyperparathyroidism in dogs. *J Am Vet Med Assoc* 218, 1106–10.

Rasor L, Pollard R, and Feldman EC (2007) Retrospective evaluation of three treatment methods for primary hyperparathyroidism in dogs. *J Am Anim Hosp Assoc* 43, 70–7.

Rebillard X, Soulie M, Chartier-Kastler E, et al (2008) High-intensity focused ultrasound in prostate cancer; a systematic literature review of the French Association of Urology. *BJU Int* 101, 1205–13.

Sabharwal T, Katsanos K, Buy X, and Gangi A (2009) Image-guided ablation therapy of bone tumors. *Semin Ultrasound CT MR* 30, 78–90.

Saldanha DF, Khiatani VL, Carrillo TC, et al (2010) Current tumor ablation technologies: basic science and device review. *Semin Intervent Radiol* 27, 247–54.

Shiina S, Tateishi R, Imamura M, et al (2012) Percutaneous ethanol injection for hepatocellular carcinoma: 20-year outcome and prognostic factors. *Liver Int* 32, 1434–42.

Simon CJ, Dupuy DE, and Mayo-Smith WW (2005) Microwave ablation: principles and applications. *Radiographics* 25 Suppl 1, S69–83.

Sutherland LM, Williams JA, Padbury RT, Gotley DC, Stokes B, and Maddern GJ (2006) Radiofrequency ablation of liver tumors: a systematic review. *Arch Surg* 141, 181–90.

Vogl TJ, Naguib NN, Lehnert T, and Nour-Eldin NE (2011) Radiofrequency, microwave and laser ablation of pulmonary neoplasms: clinical studies and technical considerations–review article. *Eur J Radiol* 77, 346–57.

Weisse C, Berent A, and Solomon S (2011) Combined transarterial embolization, systemic cyclophosphamide, and cryotherapy ablation for "Hi-Lo" maxillary fibrosarcoma in a dog. *Proceedings 8th Annual Meeting Veterinary Endoscopy Society*, 22.

Yin XY, Xie XY, Lu MD, et al (2012) Percutaneous ablative therapies of recurrent hepatocellular carcinoma after hepatectomy: proposal of a prognostic model. *Ann Surg Oncol* 19, 4300–6.

Zavaglia C, Corso R, Rampoldi A, et al (2008) Is percutaneous radiofrequency thermal ablation of hepatocellular carcinoma a safe procedure? *Eur J Gastroenterol Hepatol* 20, 196–201.

Zhang L and Wang ZB (2010) High-intensity focused ultrasound tumor ablation: review of ten years of clinical experience. *Front Med China* 4, 294–302.

Zhu JC, Yan TD, and Morris DL (2008) A systematic review of radiofrequency ablation for lung tumors. *Ann Surg Oncol* 15, 1765–74.

CHAPTER SIXTY-FIVE

Transarterial Embolization and Chemoembolization

Sarah Boston
Small Animal Clinical Sciences, University of Florida, Gainesville, FL

Background/Indications

Transarterial embolization (TAE), or bland arterial embolization, is the catheter-directed delivery of an embolic agent to particular arteries. In the context of oncology, the goal of TAE is embolization of the tumor arterial bed (Weisse et al, 2002). Transarterial chemoembolization (TACE) is the intra-arterial (IA) administration of chemotherapeutic agents to the tumor bed in addition to embolization (Weisse et al, 2002). IA chemotherapy followed by embolization works in concert because it allows for a much higher local concentration of the drug (Avritscher and Javadi, 2011, Weisse et al, 2002) prior to metabolism, and embolization increases the retention time in the tumor through the slowing of blood flow, ischemia, and damage to tumor cells (Chu et al, 2007, Weisse et al, 2002).

The two main indications for TAE/TACE in human orthopedic oncology are preoperative down staging prior to resection, and as adjunctive therapy for palliation of bone lesions for metastatic cancers (Barton et al, 1996, Chu et al, 2007, Gupta and Gamanagatti, 2012, Radeleff et al, 2006, Munk and Legiehn, 2007). TACE has been shown to decrease intraoperative blood loss and facilitate dissection through tumor consolidation (Barton et al, 1996, Chu et al, 2007, Gupta and Gamanagatti, 2012). TAE can also be performed immediately prior to surgical resection with the sole goal of decreasing blood loss (Radeleff et al, 2006). The goal of the procedure is the embolization of the entire tumor capillary bed and not just the main arterial feeder as this can lead to the opening of collateral circulation and revascularization (Gupta and Gamanagatti, 2012, Radeleff et al, 2006).

Patient Preparation

The patient preparation should be consistent with the tumor type. Minimum testing should include three-view thoracic radiographs to assess for metastasis and high quality radiographs of any affected limbs. A large amount of iodinated contrast material may be used during TAE and TACE, as well as potentially a chemotherapeutic agent, therefore assessment of renal and hepatic function is critical. Pretreatment with intravenous fluids is recommended. Because some embolic agents require an intact clotting cascade, assessment of clotting function is also recommended (Owen, 2010). Prior to TAE/TACE in humans, bone scan, magnetic resonance imaging (MRI) and/or computerized tomography (CT) are performed to assess the arterial blood supply and proximity of vital structures that share the arterial supply (Owen, 2010, Munk and Legiehn, 2007, Avritscher and Javadi, 2011). A CT angiographic scan is recommended prior to TAE and TACE in veterinary patients to assess tumor vascularity and proximity to adjacent structures and it is imperative an arterial phase is performed.

Selection criteria for patients has not been well-established in veterinary medicine as this is a developing field. Two potential applications of this technique for primary bone tumors in dogs are palliation of bone pain and down staging of disease prior to a limb spare procedure. For palliative cases, severe bone lysis is a contraindication for this procedure due to the potential for pathological fracture, unless additional stabilization is part of the treatment. When used for down staging, the most common site would be the distal radius, where TAE or TACE could be used for preoperative tumor consolidation. These treatments

Veterinary Image-Guided Interventions, First Edition. Edited by Chick Weisse and Allyson Berent.

Companion website: www.wiley.com/go/weisse/vet-image-guided-interventions

may also be considered for down staging prior to stereotactic radiosurgery.

Potential Risks/ Complications/ Expected Outcomes

Potential risks that should be discussed with the owners include nontarget embolization that may lead to necrosis or paresis, ischemic pain, tumoral hemorrhage, post-embolization syndrome, and the risk of pathological fracture (Marciel et al, 2011).

The most serious potential complications are due to nontarget embolization, which can lead to ischemic neuropraxia and tissue necrosis (Munk and Legiehn, 2007, Chu et al, 2007). There have been no reports of human death or limb loss with this procedure (Avritscher and Javadi, 2011). Non-target embolization can be avoided by being as selective as possible with the microcatheter and by using a dilute solution of embolic beads and embolizing slowly. It is important to monitor the embolization carefully as soon as the contrast flow begins to slow through the target vessels. Retrograde flow of the embolic material due to decreased forward flow can lead to nontarget embolization.

Postembolization syndrome is the most common complication reported in humans and results in local skin redness, swelling, pain, fever and a burning sensation (Zhang et al, 2009, Munk and Legiehn, 2007, Avritscher and Javadi, 2011). This generally resolves within 1–5 days, but may require hospitalization and pain relief medication. Pain relief after TACE of human appendicular osteosarcoma has been reported within 7 days (Chu et al, 2007).

There are three reports of TAE in the veterinary literature for palliation of musculoskeletal tumors in dogs. Two were for the management of large limb soft tissue sarcomas (Sun et al, 2002, de La Villeon et al, 2011), and one was for the management of a metastatic osteosarcoma to the proximal humerus (Weisse et al, 2002). These reports have shown that TAE is a technically feasible procedure for the palliation of musculoskeletal tumors in dogs. Sun et al and de La Villeon et al reported similar case reports in two dogs with large (>15 cm) soft tissue sarcomas of the pelvic limb that were deemed non-resectable without limb amputation. In both cases, the goal was palliation. Bland embolization was carried out using glue embolization (de La Villeon et al, 2011) and gelatin sponge (Sun et al, 2002). In both cases there was a measurable decrease in tumor size; this was a durable response in one dog (de La Villeon et al, 2011).

Bland embolization using 350 µm polyvinyl alcohol particles was reported by Weisse for the management of a metastatic osteosarcoma of the proximal humerus. The dog had been previously treated for a tibial osteosarcoma with amputation and chemotherapy. TAE resulted in palliation of the bone tumor pain over a period of two weeks post-procedure. Unfortunately, the dog developed a pathological fracture at this site and a lumbar spine metastatic site and was subsequently euthanized (Weisse et al, 2002). Postembolization edema can weaken the treated bone but it can go on to heal; The weakened bone and increased weight-bearing following pain palliation likely contributed to the pathological fracture in this case. In humans, weight-bearing bones are embolized with caution for this reason.

If this technique is used for palliation, a multimodal approach to bone pain palliation should be employed. The technique is new and consistent expectations to prepare the clients are not available. Drawing from the human literature, the goals of TAE or TACE when used to palliate painful neoplastic bone lesions are decreased pain and a decreased need for analgesics (Marciel et al, 2011).

Equipment

A commercially-available interventional radiology pack[1] is recommended for this procedure. For vascular access, a hypodermic needle or IV catheter (18 g), 0.035″ 180 cm hydrophilic guide wire with angled tip[2] and vascular introducer sheath (4–6 Fr)[3] is required and an adapter to allow for continuous flow of saline to flush the catheter. Iohexol (350 mgI/ml)[4] and sterile saline are required throughout the procedure, bearing in mind that the maximum recommended dose is ~5 ml/kg, based on package insert recommendations for angiography in pediatrics. The risk of side effects is increased with an increased dosage and a goal of 2 ml/kg is recommended. The catheters used for selective catheterization will depend on the limb affected. For forelimb lesions, a 100 cm Berenstein catheter[6] is recommended. For hind limb lesions, either a 65 cm Berenstein catheter[5] or a Cobra catheter[6] are recommended (100 cm lengths may be necessary for larger patients). For superselective catheterization, a 1.9–3 Fr 180 cm microcatheter[7] and 0.010–0.018″ 180 cm microwires[8] are required (different microcatheters have different internal diameters so make certain the microwire is of compatible size). Some consideration must be given to the size of the dog and the site of the lesion. The author has used a 180 cm mosquito wire and microcatheter with femoral artery access in a large St. Bernard for embolization of a distal radial lesion with success.

A variety of embolic agents have been reported. Liquid agents are often alcohol or glue based. These agents can be more difficult to use with an increased risk of nontarget embolization (Owen, 2010). If multiple feeder vessels are present, liquid glue agents will increase costs because a separate microcatheter may be required for each superselective catheterization (Radeleff et al, 2006). Particulate embolization materials include gelatin and acrylic copolymer microspheres, polyvinyl alcohol particles, and Gelfoam (Chu et al, 2007, Owen, 2010). Gelfoam is considered a temporary occlusive agent and could be considered if the procedure is performed immediately prior to resection, with the goal of decreased intraoperative hemorrhage. Microspheres are used most commonly, with the advantages of ease of delivery and a lower potential for recanalization (Marciel et al, 2011). Microspheres are available in a range of sizes (45–1000 μm) with 300–500 μm being the most commonly reported sizes for TAE/TACE in dogs and humans (Marciel et al, 2011, Radeleff et al, 2006, Weisse et al, 2002). Undersized particles carry an increased risk of non-target embolization, while oversized particles carry a risk of proximal vessel thrombosis that can lead to recanalization (Weisse et al, 2002). Microspheres are recommended for ease of use and to minimize potential complications in veterinary patients. The microspheres[9] (or another embolic agent) are delivered using a three-way stopcock and 1 ml polycarbonate high-pressure syringe[10] to enable delivery through the microcatheter.

The chemotherapeutic agent of choice and associated protective equipment for chemotherapy administration and radiation exposure are also required. Ideally, the fluoroscopy unit has the ability to do real-time fluoroscopy, rapid-sequence filming, digital subtraction angiography, road mapping, and magnification. A wide variety of chemotherapeutic agents have been reported in the human literature for TACE. Generally the systemic dose and protocol for chemotherapy are administered. In dogs, carboplatin at the standard systemic dose is most commonly used. See Chapter 3 for additional information.

TAE and TACE Procedure

Patients should be under general anesthesia and on intravenous fluids throughout the procedure. Prophylactic antibiotics have been reported in veterinary patients (Weisse et al, 2002) and are used routinely by the author. Patients are placed in dorsal recumbency. For hind limb lesions, the contralateral femoral artery is used for access; alternatively, the carotid artery can be used as an access location. For forelimb lesions, either femoral artery can be used. The inguinal area is clipped and prepared in a sterile fashion. A large commercial drape is used to cover the patient and prevent contamination. Strict asepsis is maintained throughout the procedure.

The method for arterial vascular access can be found in Chapter 44 (Figure 65.1, Figure 65.2, Figure 65.3, and Figure 65.4). After placement of the introducer sheath, the guide wire is advanced into the aorta. A 4–5 Fr Berenstein or Cobra catheter is advanced over the guide wire. Using an angiographic map created with 50:50 iodinated contrast material and sterile saline, the guide wire and catheter are advanced under fluoroscopic guidance to the axillary artery (forelimb) or femoral artery (hind limb). A non-selective angiogram is performed to visualize the arterial supply to the limb and tumor and to create a road map. Ideally, orthogonal images of the limb can be viewed without moving the patient. However, with some fluoroscopy units this is not possible and patient repositioning may be necessary to facilitate superselective catheterization of the vessels supplying the tumor. This must be done before the introduction of the microcatheter and microwire or both may be damaged during repositioning. Once the patient is in the correct position and the catheter has been advanced to the main feeding artery of the tumor, a repeat angiogram is performed to serve as the road map for superselective catheterization (Figure 65.5 and Figure 65.6). If more than one feeding vessel is identified, superselective catheterization is repeated for each vessel to allow for extensive embolization of the tumor.

A microcatheter and mosquito wire are then introduced coaxially into the 4–5 Fr catheter to allow for superselective catheterization and repeat angiography. Whether TAE or TACE is performed will depend on the goals of therapy. If the goal is to decrease intraprocedural blood loss, TAE is performed. It is likely that the goals in veterinary patients will be to administer a high dose of chemotherapy to the tumor and to follow with embolization. The exact technique for administration varies, but the author has used a combination of microspheres and carboplatin at the standard systemic dose in clinical cases. The chemotherapeutic agent is administered via the microcatheter prior to embolization. It is possible to give a small amount of the embolic agent first, to allow for slowing of the chemotherapeutic agent in

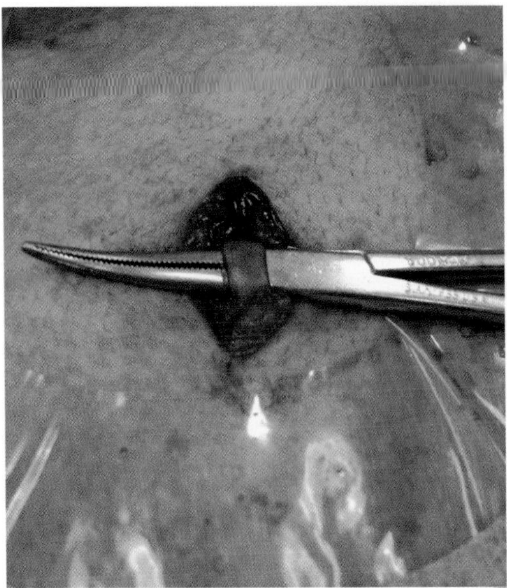

Figure 65.1 Minimal surgical approach to isolate femoral artery.

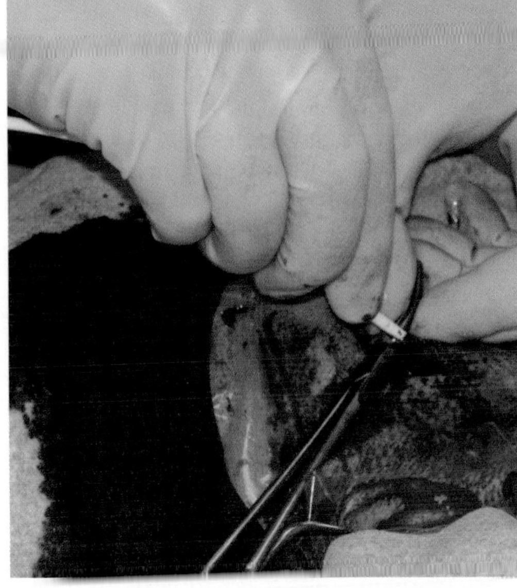

Figure 65.3 Vessel dilator passed over the 0.035″ guide wire.

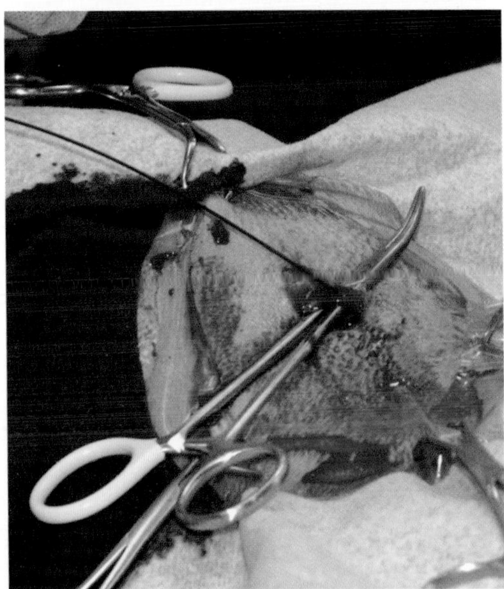

Figure 65.2 Seldinger technique to obtain vascular access via an 18 g hypodermic needle passed into femoral artery, followed by a 0.035″ guide wire through the needle.

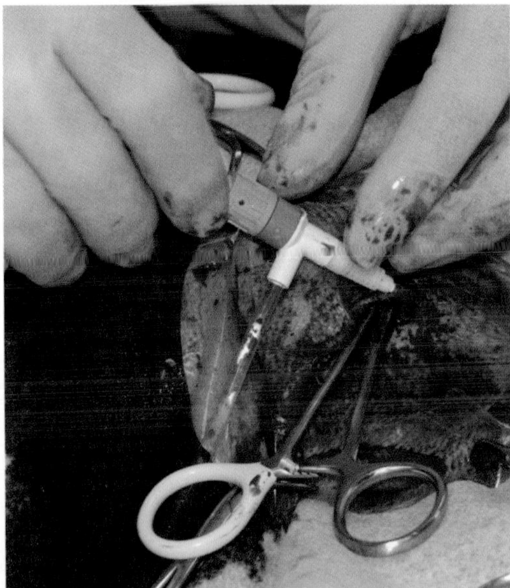

Figure 65.4 Vascular access sheath placed.

the target. Drug-eluting beads have been developed for chemoembolization and will likely become more available in veterinary medicine in the future. The microspheres are suspended in dilute contrast material and attached to the microcatheter via a three-way stopcock. A 1ml high-pressure syringe is attached to the three-way stopcock to allow for vigorous mixing of the microspheres and contrast material. The embolic material is gradually injected using the 1 ml syringe under fluoroscopic guidance. If a small amount of embolic agent is administered prior to chemotherapy, this administration is performed slowly until the contrast media dose not immediately dissipate after injection. Embolization is then performed. The end-goal is loss of the tumor blush (>75%) and avoidance of efflux of embolic material out of the feeding artery, as this can lead to non-target embolization (Figure 65.7). A final angiogram is obtained.

The vascular sheath is then removed and the femoral artery is either ligated, repaired, or manual pressure is applied after removal of the sheath. Manual pressure or vascular closure devices are the techniques most often reported in humans as these allow for repeat

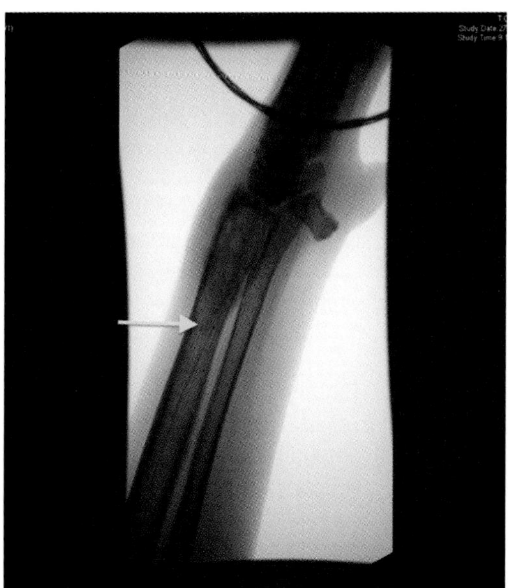

Figure 65.5 Superselective catheterization via a microcatheter in the tumor feeding vessel (arrow) for a distal radial osteosarcoma.

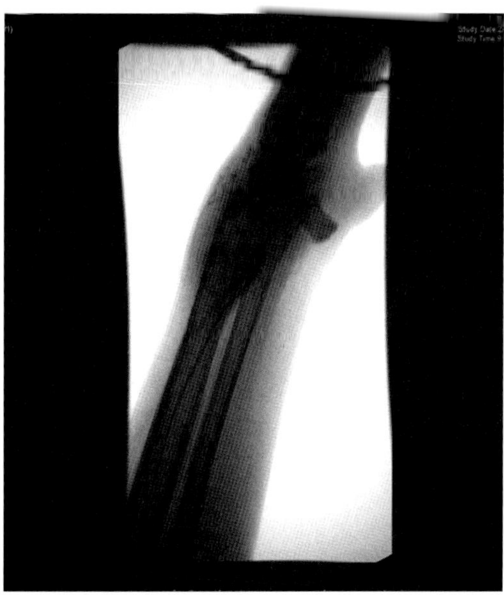

Figure 65.6 Angiogram via microcatheter.

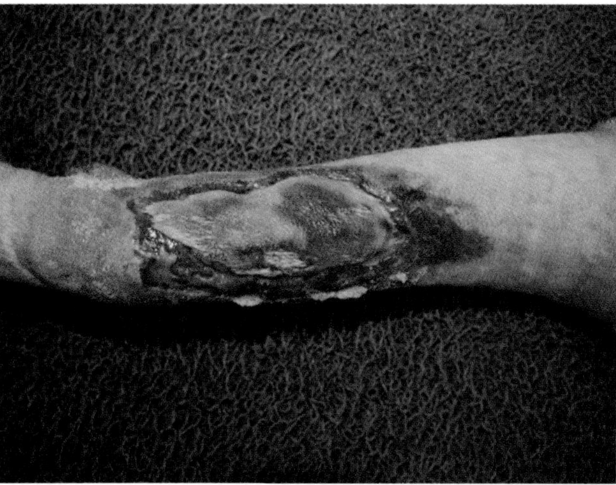

Figure 65.7 Post amputation image of a dog with distal radial osteosarcoma that developed an area of skin necrosis due to non-target embolization. (Image courtesy of Dr. Heindrich Snyman.)

TAE/TACE procedures and patency of the blood vessel. These techniques require percutaneous vascular access via ultrasonography and strict bedrest post-procedure to prevent hemorrhage from the artery.

Follow-Up

Hospitalization overnight for monitoring, pain management, and intravenous fluid diuresis is recommended. Patients may experience pain secondary to postembolization syndrome or postembolization edema, and analgesia with opioids and non-steroidal anti inflammatory drugs (if not contraindicated) are recommended. The follow-up will be dependent on the goals of therapy. Re evaluation in 2 and 4 weeks post-procedure and radiographs in 4 and 8 weeks post procedure are recommended. Repeat procedures are possible, but each case much be evaluated on an individual basis to determine if this is advisable. The progression of lysis of a bone tumor would be a factor to consider prior to repeat embolization. For palliative procedures, both monitoring of clinical response and sequential radiographs are recommended. If the goal of the procedure is down staging for limb spare, CT scan of the limb in 4 weeks is recommended to assess tumor response and for surgical planning.

Special Considerations/ Alternative Uses/ Complication Examples

Bland embolization (TAE) is most appropriate when this technique is used immediately prior to resection, when the goal is to decrease blood loss at the time of surgical limb spare. TAE may also be considered in cases where systemic cytotoxic chemotherapy is not desirable due to patient comorbidities or owner concerns. TACE will allow for the administration of a high concentration of chemotherapy to the tumor, as well as the ability to embolize the feeding vessels.

Notes

(Examples) Multiple vendors available)

1. IR pack, Infiniti Medical, Menlo Park, CA.
2. Weasel wire, Infiniti Medical, Menlo Park, CA.
3. Check-Flo Performer Introducer Sheath, Cook Medical, Bloomington, IN.
4. Omnipaque 300 mgI/ml, GE Healthcare, Princeton, NJ.
5. Berenstein catheter, Infiniti Medical, Menlo Park, CA.
6. Cobra Catheter, Infiniti Medical, Menlo Park, CA.
7. Microcatheter, Infiniti Medical, Menlo Park, CA.
8. Mosquito Wire, Infiniti Medical, Menlo Park, CA.
9. Embosphere, Biosphere Medical, Rockland, MA.
10. 1 ml Polycarbonate syringe, Infiniti Medical, Menlo Park, CA.

References

Avritscher R and Javadi S (2011) Transcatheter intra-arterial limb infusion for extremity osteosarcoma: technical considerations and outcomes. *Techn Vasc Intervent Radiol* 14(3), 124–8.

Barton PP, Waneck RE, Karnel FJ, et al (1996) Embolization of bone metastases. *J Vasc Intervent Radiol* 7(1), 81–88.

Chu J, Chen W, Li J, et al (2007) Clinicopathologic features and results of transcatheter arterial chemoembolization for osteosarcoma. *Cardiovasc Intervent Radiol* 30(2), 201–6.

de La Villeon G, Louvet A, Behr L, et al (2011) Transcatheter glue arterial embolization of a mass in the hind limb of a dog. *Can Vet J* 52(3), 289–94.

Gupta P and Gamanagatti S (2012) Preoperative transarterial embolisation in bone tumors. *World J Radiol* 4(5), 186–92.

Marciel A, Van Zandt BL, and Baxter AJ (2011) Transcatheter arterial embolization for the palliation of painful bone lesions. *Techn Vasc Intervent Radiol* 14(3), 141–9.

Munk PL and Legiehn GM (2007) Musculoskeletal interventional radiology: applications to oncology. *Semin Roentgenol* 42(3), 164–74.

Owen RJT (2010) Embolization of musculoskeletal bone tumors. *Semin Intervent Radiol* 27(2), 111–23.

Radeleff B, Eiers M, Lopez-Benitez R, et al (2006) Transarterial embolization of primary and secondary tumors of the skeletal system. *Eur J Radiol* 58(1), 68–75.

Sun F, Hernández J, Ezquerra J, et al (2002) Angiographic study and therapeutic embolization of soft-tissue fibrosarcoma in a dog: case report and literature. *J Am Anim Hosp Assoc* 38(5), 452–7

Weisse C, Clifford C, Holt D, et al (2002) Percutaneous arterial embolization and chemoembolization for treatment of benign and malignant tumors in three dogs and a goat. *J Am Vet Med Assoc* 221(10), 1430–6.

Zhang H, Yang J, Lu J, et al (2009) Use of intra-arterial chemotherapy and embolization before limb salvage surgery for osteosarcoma of the lower extremity. *Cardiovasc Intervent Radiol* 32(4), 672–8.

CHAPTER SIXTY-SIX

Analgesic Nerve, Neuraxial, Articular and Soft Tissue Interventions

Andrea L. Looney
InTown Veterinary Group (IVG) Hospitals, Woburn, MA

Background/Indications

The role of interventional radiology in veterinary practice varies widely from institution to institution and from practice to practice. Pain management in animals is yet another application of image-guided procedures to benefit veterinary patients.

Interventional analgesic techniques refer to a group of minor or major non-surgical procedures that can be used to control painful conditions. These include, but are not limited to, trigger point injections, peripheral nerve and nerve root branch blocks, sympathetic plexus blocks, intravenous infusions, radiofrequency lesioning, botulinum toxin injections, intraarticular and peritendonous injections, and spinal or epidural administration of analgesics. These procedures are indicated for a variety of acute, chronic, oncologic, degenerative, and post-traumatic painful conditions. Although some patients respond to interventional procedures as unimodal therapy, most chronic pain patients respond best when such interventions are part of a multidisciplinary approach (usually coupled with physical rehabilitation as well as medications).

Patient Preparation

Informed consent is essential before any procedure is undertaken. Sterile technique should be used for all procedures. Clipping of fur, sterile preparation and gloving, as well as draping of sites is required for most cases, particularly acute or perisurgical interventions.

In veterinary patients, conscious sedation is a minimal necessity for interventional techniques in order to provide immobilization, positioning of imaging equipment, proper intervention placement, and analgesia for the disease and level of pain, let alone the intervention. The author commonly employs a combination of butorphanol, hydromorphone, oxymorphone, or methadone, with dexmedetomidine and midazolam administered intravenously or intramuscularly for small animal patients, and detomidine or xylazine with butorphanol for large animal patients to provide sedation. This can easily be supplemented with low-dose ketamine, propofol, or inhalant anesthetic. Resuscitative and reversal drugs, oxygen, and airway management equipment should be readily available and maintained.

Clinical sedation protocols for interventional techniques in small animal patients are as follows:

- Healthy feline: butorphanol 0.2 mg/kg, dexmedetomidine 5–10 μg/kg, midazolam 0.2 mg/kg combined and administered IM or alternatively in 1/3 boluses to effect IV
- Healthy canine: butorphanol 0.2 mg/kg, dexmedetomidine 1–5 μg/kg, midazolam 0.2 mg/kg combined and administered IM or alternatively in 1/3 boluses to effect IV
- Higher-risk (worsened physical status) feline and canine patients: fentanyl 5 μg/kg, ketamine 1 mg/kg, midazolam 0.4 mg/kg combined and administered IV.

The use of a "test dose" of local anesthetic is normally employed in humans prior to more permanent interventions, especially when dealing with the complaint of "back pain", for which the list of differential diagnoses is vast. Whereas large animal practitioners commonly utilize diagnostic blockade when dealing

Veterinary Image-Guided Interventions, First Edition. Edited by Chick Weisse and Allyson Berent.

Companion website: www.wiley.com/go/weisse/vet-image-guided-interventions

with equine lameness, small animal practitioners are not as proficient with these techniques. Regardless, this author advocates the use of such in canine and feline patients. The use of mepivacaine and lidocaine can prove help in identifying areas, distributions, or dermatomes of issue even with the multiproblematic painful veterinary patient.

Potential Risks/Complications/Expected Outcomes

Potential complications of locoregional techniques in veterinary patients include, but are not limited to, sedation or anesthesia complications, intravascular injections, inappropriate placement of intervention due to lack of communicating the pain location, anaphylactoid or other drug reactions, enhanced pain from intraneural administration, motor nerve or sympathetic impairment, infection and sepsis, catheter or substance migration, and mechanical injury to already damaged structures and surrounding tissue. Risk of any of these complications has been minimized with the use of imaging modalities in both veterinary and human patients.

There are difficulties and disadvantages of interventional procedures but the strongest potential benefit is to provide superior pain relief without the side effects of more potent and stronger analgesics, or without the use of heavy inhalant anesthesia for acute pain treatment. Both opioid dependence and inhalational anesthesia have been associated with morbidity, mortality, longer hospital stays, postoperative cognitive and sympathetic dysfunction, and disability in human medicine. In the veterinary acute or perioperative arena it is fully understood that these techniques have several benefits for surgical patients. First, local blockade permits reduction of inhalant requirements that is inherently safer for patients. Second, local anesthesia permits comfortable and quick arousal from anesthesia with little potential for unwanted systemic effects such as sedation or respiratory depression. Third, recovery to mobility, appetite return, and cognitive function are vastly better when local techniques are employed in the perioperative plan. Lastly, local anesthetics are recognized to have many beneficial effects beyond blocking nerve conduction including broad anti-inflammatory effects (reduced production of eicosanoids, thromboxane, leukotriene, histamine, and inflammatory cytokines; and scavenging of oxygen free radicals) and even antimicrobial, antifungal and antiviral effects (Cassuto et al, 2006). Benefits of interventional techniques in chronic veterinary pain management appear to be more confined to epidural, intraarticular, peritendonous, or trigger point indications and are historically more popular in large animal arenas than small animal practice.

Overview of Imaging Modalities, Instrumentation and Techniques

Radiography is useful as a baseline screening tool for articular and skeletal interventions. The injection of contrast while obtaining radiographs has allowed confirmation of spinal and epidural injections and catheters (Figure 66.1). However, newer modalities such as computerized tomography (CT) allow even better resolution of boney structure and disruption with spatial resolution. Fluoroscopy has proved very fruitful for larger joint or facet injections, epidural and spinal injections, but requires ionizing radiation as well. Magnetic resonance imaging (MRI) and functional MRI has been ultimately linked to incredible advances in pain management, specifically concerning human neurologic disease/neuropathic pain and soft tissue disease (such as fascial, tendon, ligament and intra-articular/periarticular structures) but both require general anesthesia and cost is considerable for veterinary patients.

In recent years ultrasonography has been recognized as a noninvasive, practical method for localizing peripheral nerves, plexi, difficult joints (facets), tendons, and even epidural spaces that may improve

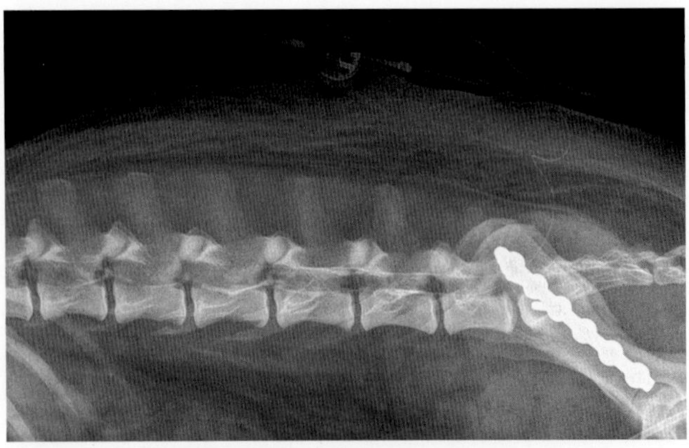

Figure 66.1 Radiograph of epidural catheter being confirmed by contrast injection through catheter. Courtesy of Dr. Peter Scrivani, Cornell University.

block success and safety. It is this author's choice of diagnostic modality for analgesic interventions[1,2]. Ultrasonography has many advantages in that it is low in cost, less cumbersome, and faster than fluoroscopy and CT. There is also greater anatomic detail, and the window or viewing angle can be changed at will. The entire procedure can be performed by a single trained clinician and contrast material is not necessary. Benefits of ultrasound-guided interventions include no need for anesthesia, shortened procedure time, quicker block onset, improvement in block quality, prolonged block duration, and decrease in block related complications such as vascular puncture.

Neurolocation of structures is often combined with ultrasonography and is a technique whereby electric current is directed onto nerve fibers suspected of supplying a painful or potentially painful (upcoming surgery) area. Neurostimulation techniques have been identified for major nerves, nerve roots, and plexi in both human and veterinary patients (Chambers, 2008, Mahler and Adogwa, 2008). These techniques have guided major perioperative and acute intensive pain control with local anesthetics for the past decade in veterinary medicine. Neurostimulation location requires a nerve stimulator, specialized sheathed needles, and catheters designed to deliver a low enough current to assure proximity to nerves, nerve roots, plexi, or ganglia[3–6].

Neuraxial (epidural and spinal) interventions performed blindly, by neurolocation or echolocation, require appropriate spinal and epidural needles, catheters, pumps, stimulation or infusion devices.[7–11] Larger surgical areas may require "soaker" catheters or wound infusion catheters and medication reservoirs.[12,13] A variety of materials used in interventional analgesic techniques is shown in Figure 66.2, Figure 66.3, Figure 66.4, and Figure 66.5, and the

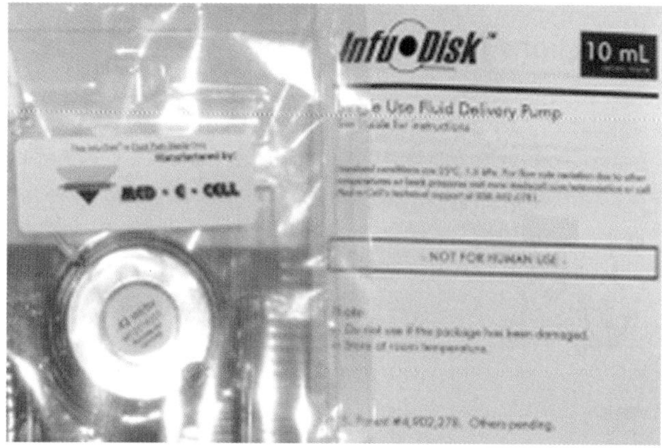

Figure 66.3 Med-E-Cell lightweight elastomeric fluid delivery pump.

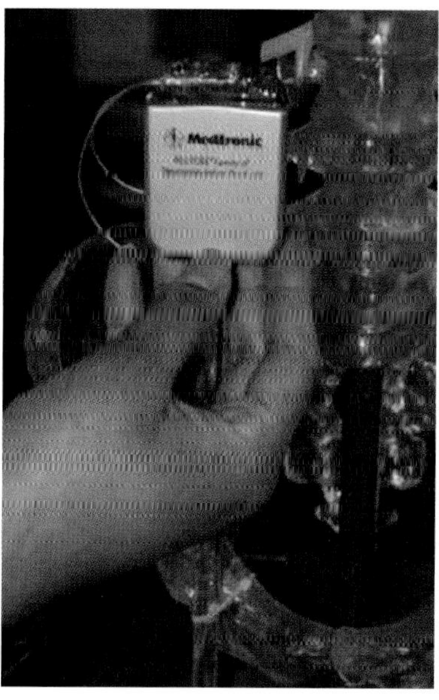

Figure 66.4 Medtronic spinal cord stimulator.

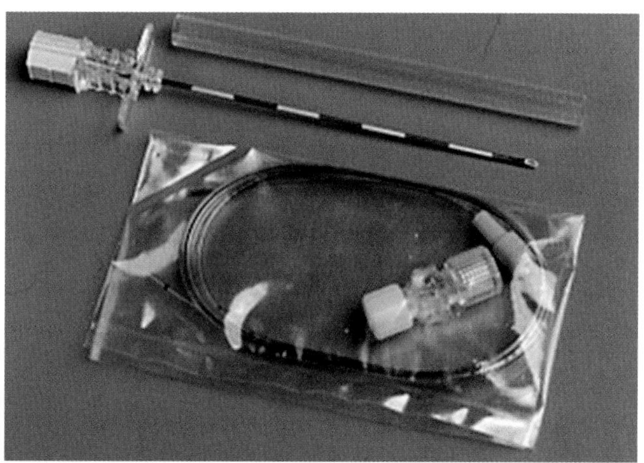
Figure 66.2 Epidural catheter set.

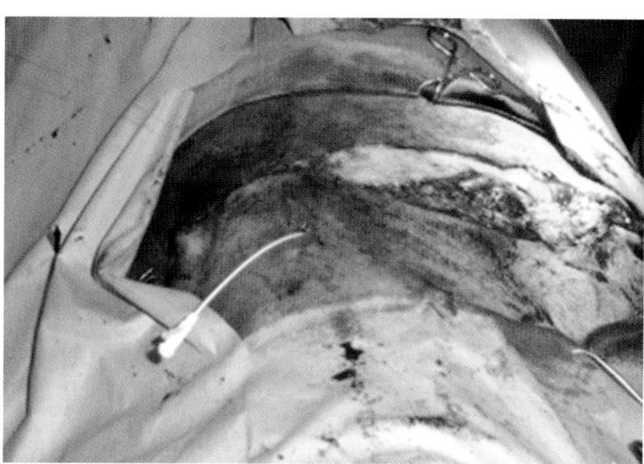
Figure 66.5 Mila soaker catheter in a forelimb amputation surgical site.

author's major equipment preferences are listed in the chapter footnotes.

A plethora of injectable substances are used in interventional pain management techniques. Choice of agents and dilution are often unique to each blockade, and dependent on the target tissue (nerve, plexus, fascia, tendon, or ligament); these are discussed at length below. There can be neuraxial (epidural or spinal), perineural (near to major nerves and plexi), intra-articular, tendon or trigger application, and there may be a single shot (one time) or continuous application (usually through a catheter). Substances can be used for immediate (surgical), long-term (repository or encapsulated), or even (semi-) permanent neurolytic effect.

Ultrasound-Guided Analgesic Procedures

Before beginning it is prudent to clip the fur and clean the surface of the skin. Also important is the need to interrogate the proposed area using both grayscale and Doppler imaging, vessels should be noted and avoided. A general site of approach is then approximated and bony landmarks/skin may be marked if desired. Needle and syringe selection is joint-, tendon-, and nerve-specific and should be prepared prior to injection.

A sterile ultrasound probe cover can be used. It is necessary to place a small amount of acoustic coupling gel inside the transducer cover; otherwise air trapped between the face of the transducer and the latex cover will seriously degrade the ultrasound image. The ultrasound probe should then be positioned with the long axis of the beam in line with the needle entry site. The beam should be directed obliquely at the needle and advancement is directly visualized (Figure 66.6). The needle (stylet in place) is oriented parallel to the ultrasound beam keeping in mind that the ultrasound beam is only millimeters thick. The tip of the needle is directed underneath the ultrasound transducer and advanced through skin and subcutaneous structures into the given area where sampling may occur prior to injection. During the injection, circumferential spread of drug around a nerve or tendon, ligament, or other pathologic structure confirms appropriate placement. A special ultrasound visible needle (echogenic) may be used to improve visualization, although scoring the shaft of the distal needle with a scalpel blade has a similar effect.

In ultrasound longitudinal view, muscles appear as relatively hypoechoic structures with fine, oblique echogenic striations representing fascia. Likewise, tendons are hyperechoic and composed of multiple organized parallel lines surrounded by a minimal amount of anechoic fluid. The tendon sheath appears thin and hyperechoic at the peritendon-superficial soft tissue interface. It is imperative that the transducer remain parallel to the linear fiber pattern of the tendon to prevent artifact.

Ultrasound location of facets has been well described in horses (Mattoon et al, 2004). Articular processes have a characteristic hyperechoic appearance created by the strong reflection of the ultrasound beam by the bone. Some cranial and caudal articular processes form a characteristic "S-shaped" curvilinear echogenic interface. This is referred to as the "chair" sign; the cranial articular process forming the seat and the cranial margin of the caudal process forming the chair back (Figure 66.7). The joint space is located at the junction of the cranial and caudal processes, identified as an anechoic gap between the two articular processes.

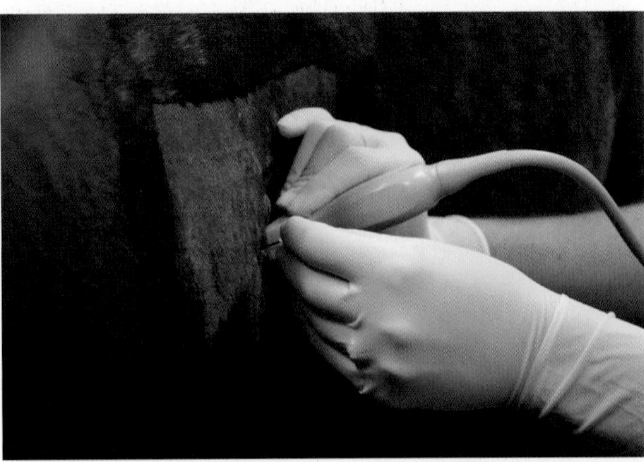

Figure 66.6 Ultrasound beam directed obliquely at needle as it enters a facet joint left side cervical in an equine patient. Courtesy of Dr. Sally Ness, Cornell University.

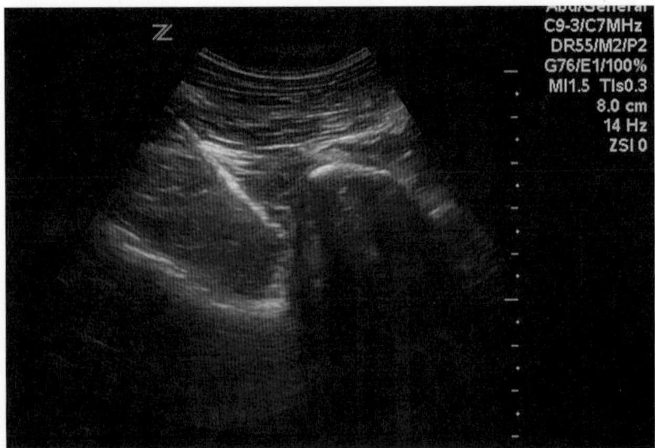

Figure 66.7 Cranial and caudal articular processes form a characteristic "S-shaped" curvilinear echogenic interface in an ultrasound guided facet block of an equine patient. Courtesy of Dr. Sally Ness, Cornell University.

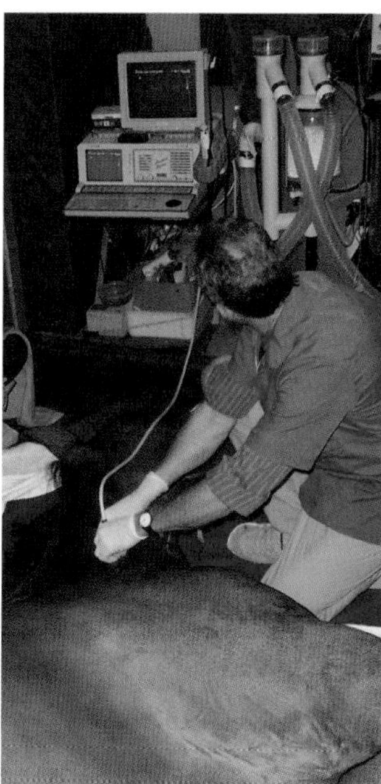

Figure 66.8 Clinician performs an ultrasound guided facet block in an anesthetized equine patient; ultrasound identifies the joint.

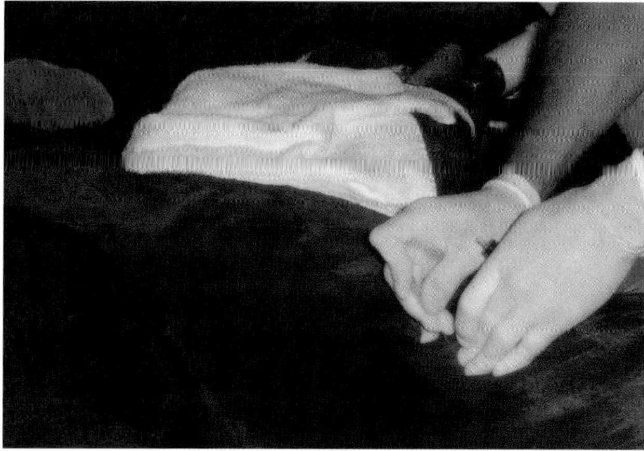

Figure 66.9 Same patient as in Figure 66.8. Syringe is ready to obtain synovial fluid to confirm entry.

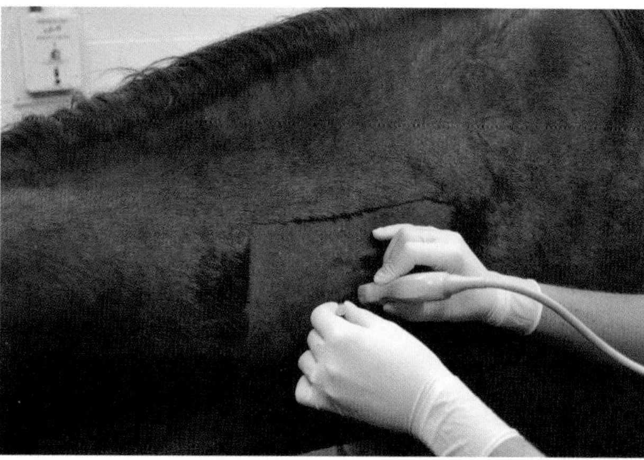

Figure 66.10 Ultrasound guides a facet block between C3 and C4 left in an awake equine patient. As sedation drops the head, resting the horses chin via padded halter and cross ties often "opens" the joint for easier access. Courtesy of Dr. Sally Ness, Cornell University.

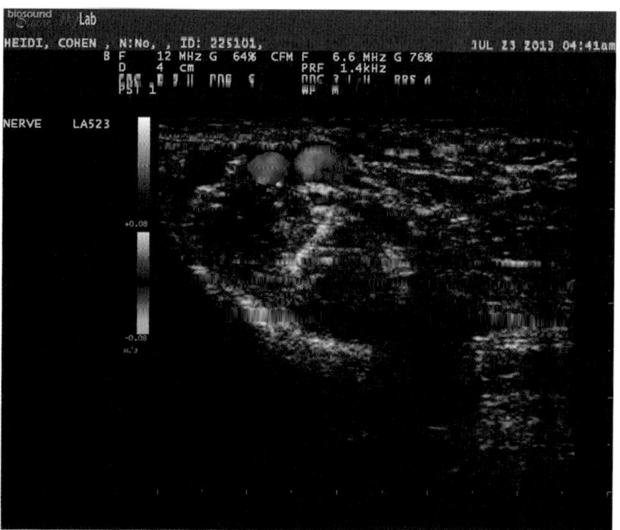

Figure 66.11 Ultrasound pictures of a femoral nerve block in a canine patient. Actual photo of blockade. Courtesy of Dr. Luis Campoy, Cornell University.

Figure 66.8, Figure 66.9, and Figure 66.10 illustrate ultrasound-guided facet block in a horse.

Ultrasound identification of nerves in cross section can be challenging. They often appear round to ovoid and demonstrate different echogenicity. They are hypoechoic or dark showing the neural component or hyperechoic /bright showing the connective tissue component. Needle imaging during advancement provides real-time visual guidance to minimize random needle movement as the block needle is advanced toward the target nerve. Visualization of nerves, termed echolocation, is often combined with neurostimulation location to best identify major landmarks of fascia and vessels and then avoid intraneural injection through fine tuning current used to obtain motor response. Figure 66.11 and Figure 66.12 illustrate an ultrasound guided femoral nerve block in the dog.

Neurostimulation-Guided Perineural or Neuraxial Techniques

Nerve blockade is an extremely effective intervention in acute and chronic pain management. The goal of any local or regional anesthetic technique should be to use the lowest appropriate volume of local anesthetic agent as close to the nerve of question as possible in

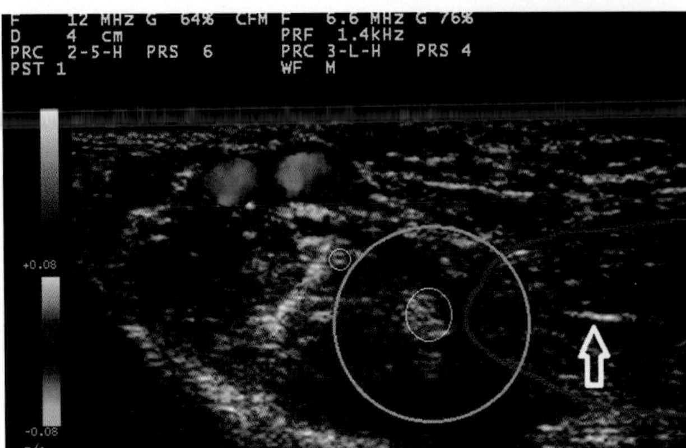

Figure 66.12 The local anatomy. Femoral artery and vein are seen via characteristic blue/red color flow Doppler signals. Large white circle outlines the femoral nerve. Small white circle outlines the lateral cutaneous saphenous nerve. Red outlines the vastus medialis muscle. Large arrow points toward echogenic needle. Blue circle shows approximate deposition of nerve block substance just deposited by needle. Courtesy of Dr. Luis Campoy, Cornell University.

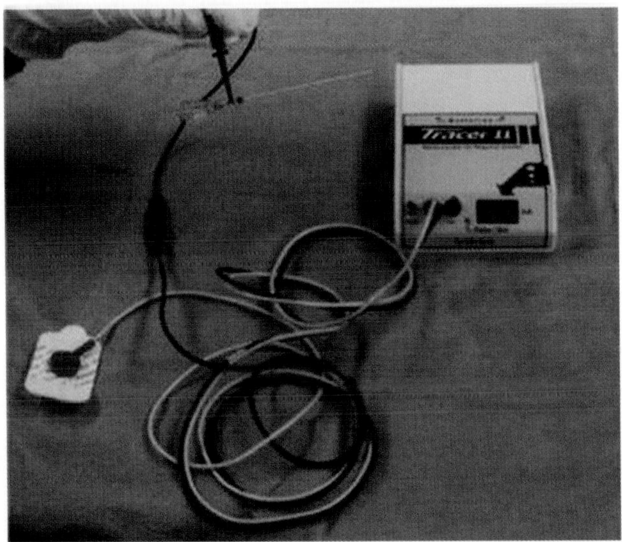

Figure 66.13 Life tech Tracer II nerve stimulator with black lead attached to nerve block needle and red lead attached to grounding electrode pad which can be placed anywhere on the patient's body.

order to treat the intended issue. One way to assist the operator with finding or identifying the nerve root or nerves involved in painful transmission is to electrically stimulate the nerve.

This technique has many names (amongst them, neuro-electrostimulation, electrostimulation location, or neuro-location), and it requires a small current to be directed onto the tip of the needle that approximates the nerve, plexus, or ganglia. The current is produced by a stimulator such as the one seen in Figure 66.13. Peripheral nerve stimulators used for nerve location should have short pulse durations such that motor responses can be elicited without causing discomfort or pain to the patient (i.e., in human pain management these are used in awake patients without causing discomfort). Veterinary patients are normally under conscious sedation and/or general anesthesia pre-nerve blockade. A general knowledge of local anatomy and technique is essential to initiate the nerve block and several good synopses are available to guide the clinician or technician in the process (Lemke and Dawson, 2000, Campoy, 2008).

Using a nerve stimulator, electric current is directed onto nerve fibers suspected of supplying a painful or potentially painful (upcoming surgery) area. If the nerve contains motor fibers, the nerve will depolarize and contractions of the innervated muscle bodies will occur. The 'searching' (black) electrode of the nerve stimulator should be attached to the needle and the surface electrode should be placed near the site of needle insertion; recent research has shown that the specific anatomic location of the surface electrode is not important and that it can be attached anywhere on the body that is convenient. This is followed by adjustment of the initial current stimulator for 1 to 2 mA and the duration of the stimulus for 100 μs, with a frequency of 2 Hz. The needle is inserted until a contraction or muscle spasm is identified visually. After identification of the contraction, current amplitude is decreased until the contraction disappears. Further insertion of the needle continues until a new contraction appears. This procedure is repeated until the applied current is 0.3 mA and a muscle contraction is visible. At this point, the needle tip is from 1 to 2 mm distance from the motor nerve and the injection of local anesthetic solution should provide a satisfactory blockade. Appropriate nerve blockade is assured by increasing current and observing lack of motor response post injection. Figure 66.14 illustrates a neurolocation of the brachial plexus for blockade in a canine patient. Figure 66.15 shows a peripheral nerve stimulating catheter that can be placed near a major nerve, plexus, or root using neurolocation for continuous administration of analgesic agents.

Image-Guided Interventions

Intraarticular Interventions

Analgesic intra-articular interventions in veterinary medicine are required for multiple reasons, including, most commonly, ligamentous injury, immune-mediated

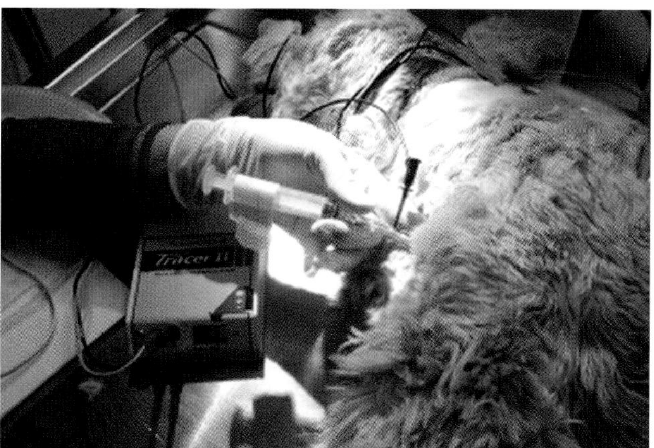

Figure 66.14 Nerve stimulator used to perform a left brachial plexus blockade on a canine patient.

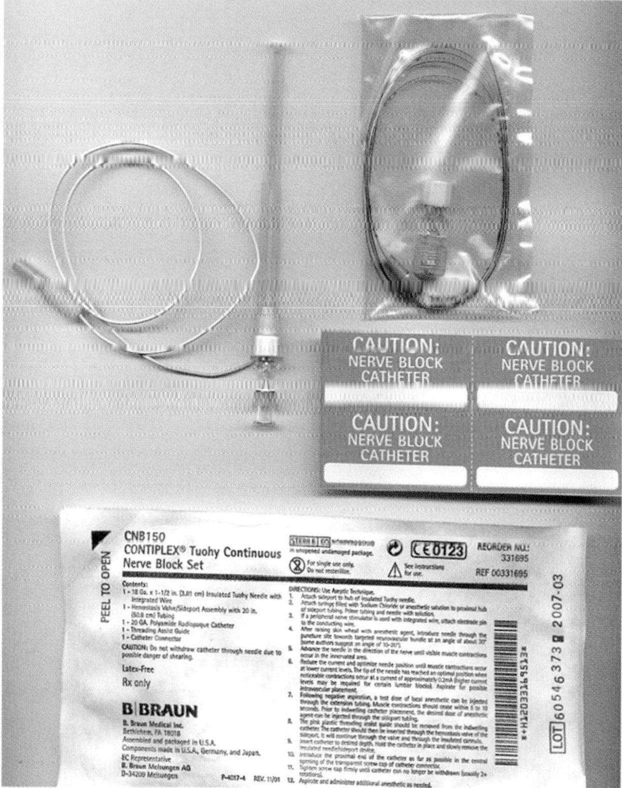

Figure 66.15 Peripheral nerve stimulator catheter set used to provide continuous (days to weeks) perineural blockade.

or degenerative arthopathy (e.g., osteoarthritis in dogs, facet disease in horses), perioperative analgesia, traumatic arthopathy, infectious arthopathy, and developmental disease (e.g., osteochondritis dissecans in horses and dogs, elbow and hip dysplasia in dogs) (Black et al, 2007). Most reports and summaries on intra-articular interventions concern blinded (non-image guided) elbow and stifle interventions such as the one illustrated in Figure 66.16. Evidence exists on

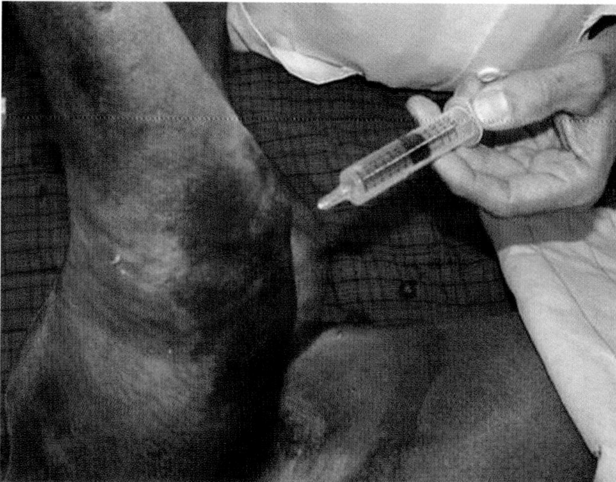

Figure 66.16 Intra-articular block in medial compartment of left hind limb stifle in a canine patient.

ultrasound-guided equine intra-articular interventions to include treatment for chronic pain or disability (wobbler) treatment in both axial (facet) joints as well as appendicular joints. Veterinarians have historically used "blind" injections, given that veterinary education historically lacked image guidance for joint therapies, and relied on bony landmarks.

Some individuals identify correct placement of intra-articular substances with procurement of synovial fluid; however, fluid may not be readily evident in chronic degenerative disease and inflammation may result in periarticular fluid accumulation resulting in inappropriate placement. Suggestions have been made at the very least, to allow image guidance in patients who do not respond to blindly injected therapy. Ultrasonography seems to be clearly improving a majority of equine facet intra- and periarticular interventions.

A review of pharmacologic agents for both diagnostic and therapeutic use in canine and equine patients is available (Van Vynckt et al, 2010), as well as reports of use for surgical pain, septic arthritis, post-surgical healing, and chronic degenerative disease; most recent reports involve cell-based regenerative therapies, hyaluronate, triamcinolone, local anesthetics, and opioids. Local anesthetics can be employed in almost all interventional techniques, although their use in intra-articular administration has recently been questioned due to chondrotoxicity potential. Antibiotics, particularly aminoglycosides (gentamicin, amikacin), whether in parenteral or encapsulated form, can be added to intra-articular or tendon injections to avoid infection.

Viscosupplementation refers to the use of substances such as hyaluronate delivered intra-articularly; this

BOX 66.1

Intra-articular pain management intervention: clinical case example

Indications: 8-year-old MC Great Dane with left-sided neck pain and complaints of stumbling in the forelimbs non-responsive to non-steroidal anti-inflammatories and tramadol.

Physical exam findings: occasional left forelimb CP deficits, pain on extreme lateral deviation/flexion of neck to the left.

Pertinent diagnostic imaging: MRI rules out spinal cord compression significant enough to warrant surgical intervention with T2 weighted sagittal acquisition confirming mild central canal diameter reduction over the C4–C5 disc space; radiographs show increased C4–C5 facet periarticular increased radio-opacity, indicative of spondylarthritis.

Intervention: Ultrasound guidance allows sampling of joint fluid (subsequently found to be degenerative and inflammatory) and injection of C4–C5 facet joint with 1 ml mepivacaine, utilized because of its spared chondrotoxicity. Upon waking, the dog was significantly less painful in next 24 hours but still has mild stumbling in the front limbs, and altered proprioception in the left forelimb. Owners were given options of systemic prednisone, gabapentin, and methocarbamol therapy, chiropractic treatment, or injection of joint. Later that week the dog, was resedated and an intra-articular facet injection of 5 mg sodium hyaluronate, 1.25 mg bupivacaine, and 2 mg triamcinolone was given into the left C5–C6 facet under ultrasound guidance. The dog's improved ambulation and pain free status were sustained for 3.5 months following this injection, during which time physical rehabilitation techniques (exercise therapy, distraction, therapeutic ultrasound) were employed to allow sustained pain relief, improved coordination, and diminished muscle spasm/atrophy.

intervention for equine performance preceded use in humans. Although the actual indwelling time of injected hyaluronate is days, the beneficial effects are variable, lasting from days, to months, even up to a year. Some argue that the use of autologous biologic therapies such as cell-based (embryonic and mesenchymal stem cells, fibroblasts, and tenocytes), or factor-based (platelet-rich plasma (PRP), and interleukin-1 receptor antagonist protein (IRAP)), has driven clinical usage to the point that it has outpaced, or perhaps even bypassed, scientific investigation into their use (Textor 2011). A case example is presented in Box 66.1.

Tendon Analgesic Interventions

Tendon injuries occur commonly in both horses and dogs, and analgesic interventions are required commonly for conditions such as trauma and injury, overuse and strain, and occasionally, systemically displaced infection. Flexor tendinitis and desmitis are common injuries in the sport and racehorse. In dogs, shoulder (biceps, supra- or infraspinatus) tendonitis, calcaneal tendonitis and tendon rupture, patellar tendonitis secondary to cruciate damage and repair, or patellar luxation, sesamoiditis, and carpal/tarsal injuries in the working dog frequently require interventions. Iliopsoas muscle and musculotendinous injury should also be included in this group. Tendon injuries most likely to occur in horses involve the palmar and plantar distal limbs and have been well described diagnostically in veterinary imaging. In canine medicine, ultrasound diagnostic imaging has proven useful historically for tendon and muscle injury as well as joint disease. Contrast radiology has also been helpful in evaluating the biceps area in the canine patient. MRI has been used in small animal musculoskeletal disease to identify shoulder, elbow, carpus, and stifle problems.

Modern interventional treatments are confined to substance injection, neurectomy, regenerative therapies (Fortier and Smith 2008), infusion therapies as well as standard therapeutic ultrasound and topical and extracorporeal shockwave therapies. Interventional intra- or peritendinous injections are commonly performed via ultrasound guidance (just as in intra-articular interventions) due to ease of handling/positioning the imaging modality, and performing the injection simultaneously See Box 66.2 for a case example. In contrast to equine desmopathies (which currently rely heavily on regenerative therapies), canine interventions often involve steroids, homeopathic preparations (Arnica, Traumeel), sterile water, dextrose, or even local anesthetics.

Steroids are commonly employed neuraxially, perineurally/periplexus, intraarticularly and within or around tendons. Triamcinolone is postulated to have more pronounced repository effect than methylprednisone due to larger particle size. Regenerative and cell-based therapies seem most utilized when considering intra-articular or tendon based interventions in veterinary medicine. Scientific evidence indicates that PRP can provide a scaffold and growth factor concentrate to enhance the cellular repair of musculoskeletal lesions in both soft and orthopedic tissues (Textor 2011). PRP is an attractive product because of its autologous nature, non-invasive

BOX 66.2

Peritendinous pain management intervention: clinical case example

Indications: 2-year-old FS German Shorthaired Pointer with sudden LH lameness after rough play.

Physical exam findings: Grade 4/5 non-weight bearing LH lameness with painful swelling 3 cm proximal to tuber calcanei and mild evidence of increased hock flexion angle with stifle extension. Subtle plantigrade stance is noted compared to opposite limb when dog does bear weight and toes are not hyperflexed.

Pertinent diagnostic imaging: Ultrasound using linear high frequency probe shows hypoechoic areas interspersed among hyperechoic strands at the gastrocnemius musculotendinous junction, as well as 30% loss of linear areas of normal tendon seen more distally. Insertion of tendon on calcaneus shows irregular hyperechoic areas. Radiographs show terminal insertional dystrophic mineralization indicative of enthesitis of the calcaneal tendon.

Intervention: To determine which area (tendon insertion or musculotendinous intersection) is more responsible for acute signs, 10 mg of lidocaine is first injected blindly closest to tuber calcanei and dog is allowed to walk. No change in lameness was seen, so 10 mg of lidocaine was then injected blindly at disrupted mid-tendon and dog became weightbearing. A Dyna splint was then applied over mid crus, extending to the metatarsals of LH limb to allow immobilization with support and gradual flexion over course of weeks. Ultrasound was used to guide 1.5 ml of PRP into LH common calcaneal tendon at the area of musculotendinous disruption and at insertion (tuber calcanei). Ultrasound also guides peritendinous injection of microdoses (0.1 ml) of homeopathic Arnica (Traumeel) along the length of the common calcaneal tendon. Three injections of PRP were administered 2 weeks apart. Ultrasound showed reduction in hypoechoic areas at 3 weeks and mild increase in hyperechoic areas (presumptive fibrosis) at 4 weeks, at which time, shockwave therapy was utilized as flexion of the Dyna splint commenced.

collection process, and rapid preparation (Zachos and Bertone, 2005) Periligamentous injections of steroids with or without Adequan (Luitpold Pharmaceuticals) or Sarapin (High Chemical Company, Levittown, PA) have been successfully used to treat desmitis in horses with acute onset of the condition without significant ultrasonographic changes.

Therapeutic Nerve Blockade (Plexus, Peripheral Nerve, and Sympathetic Blockades)

Locoregional or nerve blockades are used in both small and large animal arenas for treatment of acute and surgical pain. Using various combinations of agents (mostly local anesthetics with or without saline, ketamine, or opioids), they provide for reduced need for inhalant, improved pain relief, surgery without need for heavier agents, and quicker recovery. Blind or non-guided peripheral nerve blocks have been used diagnostically in the equine patient as well.

Therapeutic nerve blocks have been used in chronic pain management in humans through several venues, albeit medial branch blocks for chronic lower back pain, neurolytic blocks for cancer pain, and specific or selective nerve, nerve root or plexus blocks for chronic post-traumatic or neuropathic pain (Petersen et al, 2008). Short-term therapies include fluoroscopic- or ultrasound-guidance of catheters for infusions via intermittent injections or pumps, or stimulating catheters (Chambers, 2008). They are used in veterinary chronic pain patients with similar success, although usage is limited at this time to more palliative care for degenerative and oncologic disease.

When considering the use of therapeutic nerve blockade, it is important to recognize that the area in which the patient reports the pain may be distal to the site of the pathology causing it; the intervention has to be undertaken proximal to the site of pathology if it is to be completely effective. As such, knowledge of nerve distribution, dermatome localization, and referred pain phenomena is extremely important. Though chemical neurectomy has been used in horses for laminitis and navicular pain, neurolysis is a technique best reserved for discrete areas with refractory pain, especially in the context of cancer pain when quality of life is often more important than longitudinal functional status. Reports of neurolysis in veterinary patients are few, but reports using resiniferintoxin perineurally showed promising results in reducing inflammatory hyperalgesia. Risks of (semi-) permanent neurolysis include impermanence, neuritis, neuroma formation, motor deficits, and structural/functional damage to non-neural structures. Due to plasticity and the fact that cell bodies are usually spared, pain relief is rarely permanent and averages somewhere between 2–30 weeks in patients with stable disease. Imaging technology has improved success of peripheral neurolytic blocks in people via US, CT and fluoroscopic guidance. CT guidance has been particularly helpful in delivering visceral nerve blockade procedures in people. In veterinary patients both neurostimulation and echolocation, or both

BOX 66.3

Locoregional perineural pain management intervention: clinical case example

Indications: 13-year-old female spayed calico with left forelimb mass and progressive disuse of limb.

Physical exam findings: Atrophy of forelimb extensors, with painful bony mass occupying head of radius and barbering/self-excoriation noted distally along craniodorsal radius and medial carpus of entire left forelimb (presumptive sensory neuropathy).

Pertinent diagnostic imaging: Radiographs showed osteolytic and productive mass emanating from radial head. Ultrasound using 10–14 mHz linear head showed entrapment of radial nerve within growth.

Intervention: Under sedation, neurostimulation at 0.4 mA was used to guide a brachial plexus block of 2 mg bupivicaine and 4 mg methylprednisolone acetate via standard approach (cat in lateral recumbency) while patient received pamidronate infusion. Within 2 hours, less focusing/barbering of limb and weight bearing were noticed and sustained for 4 days. Under repeat sedation and ultrasound guidance, a neurolytic block injection of 0.3 ml of 0.75% sarapin, 2 mg bupivacaine were injected under ultrasound guidance via an axillary approach, which provided for 5 weeks of substantially lessened barbering/no self-mutilation and improved, but not full, weight bearing. This block was repeated once alternating with a repeat pamidronate infusion to provide palliative quality care totaling 3.5 months, when euthanasia was elected. Non-steroidal therapy (robenacoxib) was used starting at week 3.5 post initial block. Transmucosal buprenorphine was used 6 weeks post initial block.

used simultaneously, have guided successful neuroanalgesia.

Neurolytic blockade using alcohol, ammonium salts, phenol, glycerol, and hypertonic saline have all been utilized to produce Wallerian degeneration when administered neuraxially or perineurally in patients with limited life expectancy, usually those suffering from intractable pain and cancer pain (Burton et al, 2009, Petersen et al, 2008). Sarapin is a derivative of the pitcher plant and has been evaluated in equine models of soft tissue pain and in human lower back pain (Manchikanti et al, 2001). Alongside irritated nerves, local anesthetics are commonly placed and combined with opioids and corticosteroids in neuraxial administration where they exert an anti-inflammatory effect, as well as purportedly helping with steroid crystal dissolution for lengthier reduced inflammation (Hogan et al, 1991, Chambers, 2008).

In addition to all of the above substances, fluoroscopy, ultrasound, and CT have been utilized to guide placement of a wide variety of devices in including continuous infusion catheters, stimulating catheters, radiofrequency ablation probes, and cryoneurolysis probes into perineural areas for peripheral, central (spinal and epidural) and sympathetic neurolysis in people. These have been used for decades to alleviate suffering in degenerative disease, staged surgical disease, and in cancer patients with intractable pain (Burton et al, 2009). Recently, encapsulated local anesthetics and addition of other substances (steroids, opioids) to local anesthetics have added a new dimension to utilization of locoregional blockade in veterinary patients which has the potential to provide extended pain relief without neurolysis (Chahar and Cummings, 2012). In veterinary patients, this author has utilized ultrasound guidance and electrostimulation location to allow placement of combinations of encapsulated local anesthetics, butamben, alcohol, ammonium chloride, sarapin, bupivacaine, and triamcinolone or methylprednisolone acetate near nerves whose distribution encompasses painful tumors, surgical sites, self-mutilatory disorders, sensory neuropathies, and radiation-induced dermatologic injury. With these techniques, pain relief without motor or apparent sympathetic complications has been provided over periods of days to weeks and has allowed quality of life to veterinary patients with chronic, oncologic, and terminal pain. See Box 66.3 for a case example.

Epidural and Spinal Interventions

Epidural injections have been used to treat acute and perioperative pain in humans and in veterinary patients for decades. Although pain relief associated with epidural analgesia can be outstanding, clinicians expect more from this invasive, high-cost, labor-intensive technique. The number of indications for the use of epidural analgesia seems to be decreasing for a variety of reasons, most of these having to do with the advent of perineural or locoregional analgesia, even in veterinary patients. Though recent focus in veterinary medicine has been use of peripheral nerve blocks, specifically for surgical patients, epidurals still fare favorably in comparison. Spinal injections have been used for surgical MAC reduction and postoperative analgesia in dogs and for human chronic malignant,

BOX 66.4

Epidural pain management intervention: clinical case example

Indications: 1-year-old MC bulldog HBC.

Physical exam findings: Right-sided ilial wing and ischial fractures, abdominal wall/inguinal hernia, traumatic dermatitis ventral abdominal skin.

Pertinent diagnostic imaging: Radiographs confirmed fractures and FAST scan allowed identification of intact and patent urinary tract and rectum with no abdominal effusion present.

Intervention: Following cardiorespiratory stabilization and in provision of perisurgical analgesia, epidural catheterization was elected. Due to the nature of the pelvic fractures, landmarks for blind placement were not available, so under general anesthesia, fluoroscopy was utilized to allow placement of 22 gauge epidural catheter through lumbosacral space advanced to above L3–4 disk space. Bupivacaine infusion of 0.5 mg/hr began through elastomeric pump and catheter. Ilial wing and ischial repair were completed 14 hours later. Infusion continued at 0.2 mg/hr for an additional 48 hours, at which time ventral wall hernia was repaired.

Roughly 4.3 weeks post surgery, patient represented for sudden bouts of peracute non-weightbearing lameness, and right hind limb focusing, decreased hair growth over the right ilium and self-mutilation of the right cranial hock skin. On physical exam, pain was elicited over the L6–L7 disk space. Radiographs showed mild lucency around one screw utilized in ilial wing repair. Due to hardware fixation and financial constraints, MRI could not be utilized to examine whether disk protrusion and nerve root entrapment or soft tissue impingement/inflammation by screw was responsible for paroxysmal painful events. Owners elected to allow proximal screw removal at which time (under anesthesia), an epidural with 3 mg triamcinolone, 2.5 mg bupivicaine, and 1 ml saline was administered under similar fluoroscopy. Recovery was uneventful and allowed pain-free movement and cessation of foot chewing for remainder of recuperation and fracture healing.

ischemic, and degenerative pain (Kedlaya et al, 2002) While epidural and spinal local anesthetics have been the mainstay of acute pain management, steroids provide relief of chronic pain when administered epidurally and intrathecally via anti-inflammatory effects through inhibition of action of phospholipase (A2), as well as diminished transmission of impulses along the unmyelinated C-fibers.

Epidural steroid injections (ESIs) are the most widely utilized pain management procedure in the human medical world, their use supported by placebo-controlled studies and dozens of systematic reviews (Kedlaya et al, 2002). In veterinary patients, Janssens et al (2009) found resolution of signs in 53% of affected dogs for 5–66 months and improvement in signs in 79% of dogs with lumbosacral disease when methylprednisone was delivered epidurally. Epidural opioids penetrate the dura and gain entry into the cerebrospinal fluid as do spinally administered opioids. The theoretical advantage of neuraxial delivery in proximity to the spinal site of action is to allow a significant reduction in effective dose compared to systemic administration, potentially reducing the incidence of side effects.

Recent evidence has suggested a role for the spinal *N*-methyl-D-aspartate (NMDA) receptor subunit in cancer bone pain, and development of targeted therapies (e.g., ketamine, an NMDA blocker) injected perineurally or neuraxially may herald future analgesic opportunities. Ziconotide is a compound based on the neurotoxin produced by the cone snail. Combination of this agent with morphine has been used for chronic refractory pain when administered neuraxially. Resiniferatoxin is a potent capsaicin analog. Intrathecal administration leads to selective, prolonged opening of the transient receptor potential V1 ion channel, which is localized mainly to C-fiber primary afferent nociceptive sensory neurons. Although associated with transient hemodynamic effects, spinal administration in dogs with bone cancer produces a prolonged antinociceptive response (Brown et al, 2005).

Imaging to guide both epidural and spinal interventions in both human and veterinary patients is usually performed via fluoroscopy and injection of a small amount of contrast material confirms appropriate placement. The prolific availability of fluoroscopy has allowed the growth of a transforaminal/selective nerve root block technique in humans, although a common entry point is the lumbosacral interspace in veterinary patients because it is so often accessed blindly.

Epidural catheterization has been utilized and studied well in veterinary patients (Box 66.4) and placement through both anterior and caudal approaches. Ultrasonography has been described to identify spinal space, obtain cerebrospinal fluid, and inject contrast in selected animal models. Both fluoroscopy and ultrasonography are routinely used in human patients for epidural and spinal interventions. Advanced imaging, such as CT, is thought to better allow interventions in veterinary patients due to the variety of species, breed, and individual variations in spinal soft tissue and osseous anatomy. Fluoroscopy, ultrasonography, and CT have been used in human pain management to allow transforaminal approaches to both spinal and epidural drugs, as well as indwelling device (catheter) placement.

Follow-Up

Patients receiving interventional pain relieving techniques, whether for acute pain, intensive care, presurgical pain, or chronic pain, and especially those receiving a local anesthetic within their blockade, should be observed post sedation or general anesthesia for any evidence of hypotension, impaired motor function, respiratory status decline, or paraesthesia. Observation for 2–6 hours post intervention, as well as monitoring of respiratory rate and character, pulse rate and character, oxygenation status and blood pressure if needed, all assist in reducing periprocedural morbidity.

Intraarticular and peritendinous injections may be treated post procedure with cold therapy to reduce inflammation and pain. Perineural and neuraxial blockades should be monitored for motor and sympathetic impairment, the latter of which may appear as inability to regulate body temperature, vascular tone, and urinary or fecal control, especially when surgery or general anesthesia has been performed as well. Use of low volumes and concentrations of local agents, limited use of opioids, use of C fiber sensitive substances (sarapin) and guided placement (ultrasound, neurolocation, and fluoroscopy), have allowed most post-intervention complications to be avoided.

Outcomes assessment of therapies for chronic pain alleviation can be readily assessed in a clinical practice setting via pressure mat, gait analysis, or stance analysis for musculoskeletal therapies. Chronic pain scoring is best determined for companion animals via quality of life measures, several of which exist for osteoarthritis, cancer, spinal, or intervertebral disk disease, etc. These scoring systems provide framework for owner questionnaires and can guide not only response to therapy/lack thereof, but future interventions if needed. Ultrasonography is a fantastic therapeutic monitoring tool in terms of soft tissue (articular and tendon) recovery as well.

Special Considerations/Alternative Uses/Complication Examples

Despite the use of imaging to allow more accurate, focused and efficacious analgesic interventions, there are a few caveats still to the use of these techniques in veterinary patients. First and foremost, they are rarely relied upon as sole agents of pain relief in the chronic setting; they are often part of a multimodal scheme involving altered lifestyle, rehabilitation techniques, complementary (e.g., acupuncture and chiropractic) therapies, classic analgesics (e.g., non-steroidal anti-inflammatory drugs, tramadol, oxycodone, chondroprotectants) and non-classic analgesics (e.g., anti-epileptic drugs, selective serotonin receptor inhibitors). Second, in the acute care setting, depending on the agents used, these techniques may be potent and may potentiate anesthetic plane, cause cardiorespiratory depression and allow reduced usage of inhalant and supplemental (e.g., infusion) agents. Third, potential exists for inadvertent intravascular or intraneural injections, as well as cardiorespiratory decline secondary to agent uptake. Epidural and spinal agents, particularly those wherein local anesthetics are used, can cause sympathetic and motor paralysis. Patients must be stable in terms of cardiocerebrorespiratory status and agents must be chosen appropriately to not only improve success, but to avoid morbidity and mortality. Finally, none of these techniques are meant to supplant traditional medical or surgical diagnostics or therapeutics. They are meant to reduce pain and inflammation, enhance better healing, overall return to function, and quality of life in patients who have followed primary medical and surgical therapeutic routes. No joint injection (despite the thousands of stem cells, healing proteins, or neurochemicals it contains) is currently capable of re-attaching two ends of a torn cruciate ligament.

Pain is a multidimensional experience formed by an ever changing neuromatrix; this complex array of peripheral and central components can no longer be addressed with the simple principles of parenterally administered drugs, even when multimodal therapies are considered. As veterinary pain management becomes more like human pain management in offering patients a broader range of strategies to treat acute and chronic pain, interventional techniques described above will become more commonplace. Inherent in this trend is the need for more comprehensive training in imaging and subsequent use of imaging techniques to better identify pathology and to guide techniques alleviating pain. Although interventional approaches to analgesia have a more technical dimension than those generally used in practice and even academia, the specific skills and training for their quality performance depends on experience and research. The use of the above techniques still properly belong in the context of a multimodal approach to pain therapy. Our hope is to encourage use of image-guided interventions that complement rather than replace the standard use of analgesic drugs in veterinary pain management.

Notes

1. My Lab diagnostic ultrasound, Esaote Indianapolis, IN.
2. M-turbo diagnostic ultrasound, Sonosite, Bothell, WA.
3. Stimuplex® HNS12 Nerve Stimulator, BBraun, Bethlehem, PA.
4. Stimulplex and Ultraplex Single Shot Nerve Block needles, BBraun, Bethlehem, PA.
5. EZ Stim Nerve Stimulator, Life-Tech/Kimberly Clark, Roswell, GA.
6. ProBloc II insulated regional block needles, Life-Tech Inc/Kimberly Clark, Roswell, GA.
7. Spinal needles and Tuohy epidural needles, Mila International, Erlanger, KY.
8. Perifix epidural sets, BBraun, Bethlehem, PA.
9. Elastomeric Pump, Infu-Disk, and SpringPowered Syringe Pump, Mila International, Erlanger, KY.
10. Med E Cell Infu Disk, www.medecell.com
11. Restore Ultra Neurostimulator, Medtronic, Minneapolis, MN.
12. Diffusion Wound Catheter, Mila International, Erlanger, KY.
13. ON-Q pain buster pump, iFlo, Lake Forest, CA.
14. AmbIT pain control pump, Summit Medical Products, Sandy, UT.

References

Black LL, Gaynor J, Gahring D, et al (2007) Effect of adipose-derived mesenchymal stem and regenerative cells on lameness in dogs with chronic osteoarthritis of the coxofemoral joints: a randomized, double-blinded, multicenter, controlled trial. *Vet Ther* 8(4), 272–84.

Brown D, Iadorola MJ, Perkowski SZ, et al. (2005) Physiologic and antinociceptive effects of intrathecal resiniferatoxin in a canine bone cancer model. *Anesthesiology* 103(5), 1052–9.

Burton AW, Phan PC, Cousins MJ, et al. (2009) Treatment of cancer pain: role of neural blockade and neuromodulation. In: *Cousins and Bridenbaugh's Neural Blockade in Clinical Anesthesia and Pain Medicine*, 4th edn (Cousins MJ, Carr DB, Horlocker TT, and Bridenbaugh PO, eds). Lippincott Williams & Wilkins, Philadelphia, pp. 1117–33.

Campoy L (2008) Fundamentals of regional anesthesia using nerve stimulation in the dog. In: *Recent Advances in Veterinary Anesthesia and Analgesia: Companion Animals* (Gleed RD and Ludders JW, eds). International Veterinary Information Service, Ithaca, NY (www.ivis.org).

Cassuto J, Sinclair R, and Bondervocic M. (2006) Anti-inflammatory properties of local anesthetics and their present and potential clinical implications. *Acta Anaesthesiol Scand* 50(3), 265–82.

Chahar P and Cummings KC. (2012) Liposomal bupivacaine: a review of a new bupivacaine formulation. *J Pain Res* 5, 257–64.

Chambers WA (2008) Nerve blocks in palliative care. *Br J Anaesth* 101(1), 95–100.

Fortier LA and Smith RKW. (2008) regenerative medicine for tendinous and ligamentous injuries of sport horses. *Vet Clin North Am Equine Practice* 24(1), 191–201.

Hogan Q, Haddox JD, Abram S, et al (1991) Epidural opiates and local anesthetics for the management of cancer pain. *Pain* 46(3), 271–9.

Janssens L, Beosier Y, and Daems R. (2009) Lumbosacral degenerative stenosis in the dog. The results of epidural infiltration with methylprednisolone acetate: a retrospective study. *Vet Comp Orthop Traumatol* 22(6), 486–91.

Kedlaya D, Reynolds L, and Waldman S (2002) Epidural and intrathecal analgesia for cancer pain. *Best Pract Res Clin Anaesthesiol* 16(4), 651–65.

Lemke KA and Dawson SD (2000) Local and regional anesthesia. *Vet Clin North Am* 30, 839–57.

Mahler SP and Adogwa AO (2008) Anatomical and experimental studies of brachial plexus, sciatic, and femoral nerve-location using peripheral nerve stimulation in the dog. *Vet Anaesth Analg* 35(1), 80–9.

Manchikanti L, Pampati V, Rivera JJ, et al (2001) Caudal epidural injections with sarapin or steroids in chronic low back pain. *Pain Physician* 4(4), 322–35.

Mattoon JS, Drost WT, Grguric MR, et al. (2004) Technique for equine cervical articular process joint injection. *Vet Rad & Ultrasound* 45(3), 238–40.

Petersen BD, Davis KW, Choi J, et al (2008) Selective nerve root blocks. In: *Pain Management in Interventional Radiology* (Ray CE, ed.). Cambridge University Press, New York, pp. 112–17.

Textor J (2011) Autologous biologictreatment for equine musculoskeletal injuries: platelet-rich plasma and IL-1 receptor antagonist protein. *Vet Clin North Am Eq* 27, 275–98.

Van Vynckt D, Polis I, Vershooten F, et al (2010) A review of the human and veterinary literature on local anaesthetics and their intra-articular use. Relevant information for lameness diagnosis in the dog. *Vet Comp Orthop Traumatol* 23(4), 225–30.

Zachos TA and Bertone AL. (2005) Growth factors and their potential therapeutic applications for healing of musculoskeletal and other connective tissues. *Am J Vet Res* 66(4), 727–38.

Index

Indexer: Dr Laurence Errington

Illustrations are comprehensively referred to from the text. Therefore, significant items in illustrations (figures and tables) have only been given a page reference in the absence of their concomitant mention in the text referring to that illustration.

Veterinary Image-Guided Interventions, First Edition. Edited by Chick Weisse and Allyson Berent.

Companion website: www.wiley.com/go/weisse/vet-image-guided-interventions